Health promotion strategies through the lifespan

Health promotion strategies through the lifespan

Canadian Edition

RUTH BECKMANN MURRAY
St. Louis University

JUDITH PROCTOR ZENTNER
Director of Health Services, Hickory Hill Furniture Corporation

VERNA PANGMAN
University of Manitoba

CLARE PANGMAN
University of Manitoba

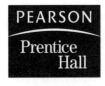

PEARSON

Prentice
Hall

Toronto

Library and Archives Canada Cataloguing in Publication

Health promotion strategies through the lifespan / Ruth Beckmann
Murray ... [et al.]. — Canadian ed.

Includes index.
ISBN 0-13-143365-2

1. Nursing assessment—Textbooks. 2. Health promotion—Textbooks.
3. Life cycle, Human—Textbooks. 4. Developmental psychology—Textbooks. I.
Murray, Ruth Beckmann

RT48.H44 2006   613   C2004-906491-6

Vice President, Editorial Director: Michael J. Young
Executive Editor: Sam Scully
Executive Marketing Manager: Cas Shields
Associate Editor: Stephen Broadbent
Production Editor: Kevin Leung
Proofreader: Susan Broadhurst
Production Coordinator: Andrea Falkenberg
Manufacturing Coordinator: Susan Johnson
Photo and Literary Permissions: Sandy Cooke
Page Layout: Laserwords
Art Director: Julia Hall
Interior and Cover Design: Gillian Tsintziras
Cover Image: Veer Inc.

Statistics Canada information is used with the permission of the Ministry of Industry, as Minister responsible for Statistics Canada. Information
on the availbility of the wide range of data from Statistics Canada can be from Statistics Canada's Regional Offices, its World Wide Web site at
http://www.statcan.ca, and its toll-free number 1-800-263-1136.

Printed and bound in the USA.

1 2 3 4 5 10 09 08 07 06
ISBN: 0-13-143365-2

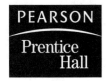

Contents

Acknowledgments

We wish to acknowledge and graciously thank all of those dedicated individuals who gave freely of their precious time to assist us in the completion of this Canadian adaptation.

In particular, we wish to acknowledge and to express our thanks to the following:

Administration and colleagues at the Faculty of Nursing, University of Manitoba, for their unending support and encouragement. We would not have been able to complete this work without their significant encouragement and contributions.

Research assistants for their enthusiasm and unending work in assisting us to collect data from various scholarly books and journals.

Library administration and staff, who many times pointed us in the right direction in our literature searches and provided us with many creative ideas and suggestions.

We are grateful to the following reviewers who provided valuable feedback on all or part of the manuscript:

- Charlene Beynon (University of Western Ontario)
- Doris Callaghan (Okanagan University College)
- Benita Cohen (University of Manitoba)
- Claudette Kelly (University College of the Cariboo)
- Melanie MacNeil (Brock University)
- Joanne Toornstra (University of Alberta)
- Linda McDevitt (Algonquin College)
- Susan Brajtman (University of Ottawa)
- Judy A. Hurst (Loyalist College)

The entire editorial and production staff at Pearson Education Canada, and in particular: Stephen Broadbent, Kevin Leung, Valerie Adams, and Samantha Scully for their talents and patience.

Dedication

This book is dedicated to
Students—for their inspiration
Friends—for their assistance
Our families—for their patience

Ruth Beckmann Murray

Judith Proctor Zentner

We dedicate this book to our loving parents,
Rose and William, and Essie and Harvey, whose spirits inspired us
in our journey to create and complete the first
Canadian edition with care and consideration.

Verna Pangman

Clare Pangman

Health Promotion in Canada

Health promotion is the continuous process of enabling people to increase control over and to improve their well-being and health. According to Maville and Huerta, Canada is recognized as having launched health promotion in the global community.[1] In fact, other countries have adopted several of the Canadian theoretical frameworks for health promotion in order to instigate their own health promotion programs.[2] The most significant challenge in implementing health promotion strategies is the ongoing paradigm shift from a medical model of treatment to a primary health care model.

Developmental Perspectives

In 1974, the federal government report entitled "A New Perspective on the Health of Canadians" outlined a framework for health comprised of four main elements: lifestyle, environment, human biology, and health care organization.[3] This report was received favourably by Canadians, and it continues to receive national and international acclaim. The report led to the development of successful health promotion programs associated with personal behaviours and lifestyles.[4]

One important global initiative related to health promotion was the World Health Organization (WHO) Conference in 1978. This conference identified primary health care as the route to achieve "Health for All" by the year 2000.[5] Member states of the WHO, including Canada, decided to act towards the principles of "Health for All."[6] Canada hosted the first International Conference on Health Promotion in 1986. Two key documents released at that time, *The Ottawa Charter on Health Promotion* and *Achieving Health for All: A Framework for Health Promotion*,[7] alerted Canadians to the underlying conditions within society that determine health.

The Ottawa Charter called for action in five areas: (1) to build healthy public policy to ensure that policies contribute to health promoting conditions; (2) to create supportive environments; (3) to strengthen community action so that communities have the capacity to set priorities and take action on issues affecting their health; (4) to develop personal skills, so that people have skills to meet life challenges, and (5) to reorient health services to focus on the needs of the entire person and invite a collaboration among providers and users of services.[8] *The Ottawa Charter* has been translated into over 40 languages, and it serves as a guide for health promotion around the world.

Achieving Health for All focused attention on three key health promotion challenges for Canadians: (1) reducing inequities in health, (2) increasing the emphasis on prevention of disease, and (3) increasing people's skills to cope with chronic disease and disability.[9] The framework put forward three mechanisms to meet these challenges: self-care, mutual aid, and health environments. It also suggested three strategies: community participation, strengthening community health services, and health public policy.[10]

To continue the journey of Canada's involvement in health promotion, it is important to state that, in 1989, the members of the Population Health Program at the Canadian Institutes for Advanced Research (CIAR) began to increase the understanding of multiple and interactive factors that influence health status and function, including social, economic, genetic, and health care, as well as the complex interrelationships among them.[11] Taking into account the work of CIAR, in 1994 the federal and provincial health ministers released their report—*Strategies for Population Health: Investing in the Health of Canadians*.[12] The contents of this report included timely and relevant information on the determinants of health. Most importantly, it proposed a population health conceptual framework based on five categories of determinants which underpin the health of a population: (1) personal health practices, (2) individual capacity and coping skills, (3) the social and economic environment, (4) the physical environment, and (5) health services.[13]

The Canadian government established the National Forum on Health in October 1994.[14] Its purpose was to inform and involve Canadians, and to advise the federal government on creative ways to improve health. Further, the mandate of the National Forum on Health was to ensure that Canada's health care system was equipped for the challenges of the future.[15] The National Forum recommended transforming knowledge about health into action, mainly through a broader awareness of the determinants of health.[16] In 1997, the National Forum on Health delivered its report and made recommendations that support the following four principles of primary health care: (1) public participation, (2) accessibility, (3) health promotion and disease prevention, and (4) intersectorial collaboration. The one principle not supported by the National Forum is the principle of appropriate technology.[17,18] The National Forum on Health officially ended its operations in June 1997.[19]

Since the late 1980s, the term "population health" has been used to explain an approach that focuses on the range of individual and collective elements and conditions, and the interactions among them, that determine the health and well-being of Canadians.[20] The goals of a population approach are intended not only to maintain, but to improve, the health and well-being of an entire population, and to decrease inequities in health status among various population groups.[21] Further deliberations at Health Canada have led to the following list of determinants for future population health policy and research directions: income and social status; social support networks; education, employment, and working conditions, social and physical environments; biology and genetic endowment; personal health practices and coping skills; healthy child development; and health services.[22] As a result of recent discussions within Health Canada, gender and culture have been added to this list of determinants.[23]

In the mid-1990s, Hamilton and Bhatti of the Health Promotion Development Division of Health Canada constructed a population health promotion model, which explains the relationship between population health and health promotion.[24] Hamilton and Bhatti's model emphasizes that to improve people's health, we must take action on the full range of health determinants.[25] That is, the model illustrates how a population health approach can be implemented through comprehensive health promotion strategies to influence the factors and conditions that determine health. This model also stresses the need for evidence-based decision-making procedures to ensure the development of population health promotion activities.[26]

Reforming primary health care has been a constant message since the early 1980s.[27] Now that we've reached the new millennium, what is the status of health promotion in the lives of Canadians? According to the Canadian Institute for Health Information, health and health care continue to be top priorities for Canadians.[28] As part of the Action Plan for Health System Renewal in September 2000, federal, provincial and territorial first ministers agreed that improvements to primary health care are critical to the renewal of health services that touch Canadians in all facets of their lives.[29] The federal government established an $800 million primary health care transition fund in September 2000 by to support the efforts of provinces and territories to develop and implement transitional primary health care reform initiatives.[30] The suggested changes to the structure of primary health care were intended to help achieve the following: (1) better health for citizens by placing the focus on preventing illness and promoting health, (2) better access to, and integration of, primary health care services, and (3) greater job satisfaction for health care providers by encouraging them to use their skills to full potential, and by improving working conditions.[31]

Recently, the combined results of the Romanow Commission on the Future of Health Care in Canada, the Kirby Senate Committee Final Report on the State of the Health Care System in Canada, and several provincial reports (including those of Clair, Fyke, and Mazankowski) indicated specifically that Canadians not only want, but expect, improved access to quality services from the health care system.[32] Specifically, Roy Romanow recommended the creation of a Health Council of Canada, which would help foster collaboration and cooperation among provinces, territories, and the federal government. The council would play a key role in establishing common indicators to measure the performance of the health care system and reporting the results to Canadians on a regular basis.

It is interesting to note that some concerns are reported in the literature regarding meaningful health promotion, or disease prevention aspects, within the health care system. It has been stated, for example, that in order for health promotion to flourish in Canada, a great deal of community involvement is necessary.[33] Certain difficulties appear to be inherent in federally driven programs that emphasize the community participation of disadvantaged groups.[34] Other difficulties in implementing health promotion projects stem from limited funding and understaffing.[35] Given these issues, to what extent can we, as Canadians, expect answers from the health ministers as they meet to deliberate and make decisions regarding the state of our health?

The Role of Health Practitioners

For the past two decades, the Canadian Nurses Association (CNA) has been promoting primary health care as a helpful strategy to guide the reform of the health care system.[36] The influence of the CNA has been clear because it was the only national health association to advocate primary health care. In 2000, the Nursing Strategy for Canada was made public by the federal, provincial, and territorial health ministers, after significant consultation with nurses and other health care stakeholders.[37] The goal of the strategy was to put mechanisms in place and to maintain an adequate supply of nursing personnel who are well educated, well distributed, and deployed to meet the health needs of Canadians.[38] The final report of the Nursing Strategy for Canada, released in September 2003, indicated that the collaborative approach has resulted in significant progress towards the objective that nurses play a vital and effective role in the delivery of health care in Canada.[39] However, you might ask, where does the concept of primary health care stand among nurses? Exerting influence on the implementation of primary health care will require concerted action on the part of nurses throughout the country.[40] Nurses can take many measures to ensure that the changes taking place in the health care system reflect the primary health care model. Notably, nurses can lobby their local politicians to ensure that health care plans reflect the realities of their communities.[41] Nurses need to play a broader role in today's society by being visible and making certain that the nursing voice is heard at the decision-making table as the health system moves towards primary health care.

As you read and reflect upon how the Canadian concepts of health promotion interact with and connect with the material retained from earlier editions of this work, you will note that the theme of health promotion is indeed directed toward individuals and families throughout the life span. Think carefully about the health promotion strategies presented in the text. At the same time, consider alternate strategies that you, as an individual, might devise and implement under various circumstances you encounter as a health care professional. We hope you will seek to help clients and their families to deal with day-to-day health issues as they strive to lead healthy lives.

ENDNOTES

1. Maville, J.A., and C.G. Huerta, *Health Promotion in Nursing.* Albany, NY: Delmar Thompson Learning, Inc., 2002.
2. *Ibid.*
3. Lalonde, M., *A New Perspective on the Health of Canadians: A Working Paper.* Ottawa: Government of Canada. Quoted in M.J. Stewart, *Community Nursing: Promoting Canadians' Health* (2nd ed.). Toronto: W.B. Saunders, 2000.

4. Health Canada, *Population Health Approach*, Appendix A: The Evolution of the Population Health Paradigm, Website: www.hc-sc.gc.ca/hppb/phdd/docs/common/appendix_a.html, August 2004.

5. World Health Organization, *Primary Health Care: Report on the International Conference on Primary Health Care,* Alma Alta, USSR, 6–12 September 1978. Quoted in M.J. Stewart, *Community Nursing: Promoting Canadians' Health* (2nd ed., p. 34). Toronto: W.B. Saunders, 2000.

6. Lemire Rodger, G., and S.M. Gallagher, The Move Toward Primary Health Care in Canada: Community Health Nursing from 1985 to 2000, in M.J. Stewart, ed., *Community Nursing: Promoting Canadians' Health* (2nd ed., pp. 37–38). Toronto: W.B. Saunders, 2000.

7. Health Canada, *Population Health Approach—Population Health Promotion: An Integrated Model of Population Health and Health Promotion*, Website: www.hc-sc.gc.ca/hppb/phdd/php/php2.htm, August 2004.

8. *Ibid.*

9. *Ibid.*

10. West, L., *Trends and Issues in Health Care*. Toronto: McGraw-Hill Ryerson Ltd., 2003.

11. Health Canada, *Population Health Approach*, Appendix A: The Evolution of the Population Health Paradigm.

12. *Ibid.*

13. Health Canada, *Population Health, Population Health Approach—* Appendix B: Population Health Framework, Website: www.hc-sc.gc.ca/hppb/pfdd/docs/common/appendix_b.html, August 2004.

14. Noseworthy, T.W., Continuing to Build on our Legacy: National Forum on Health, 1994–1997, in M.J. Stewart, ed., *Community Nursing: Promoting Canadians' Health* (2nd ed., pp. 33–37). Toronto: W.B. Saunders, 2000.

15. *Ibid.*

16. *Ibid.*

17. Lemire Rodger and Gallagher, *op. cit.*

18. Stewart, M.J., Framework Based on Primary Health Care Principles, in M.J. Stewart, ed., *Community Nursing: Promoting Canadians' Health* (2nd ed., pp. 58–59). Toronto: W.B. Saunders, 2000.

19. Health Canada, *Health Care—National Forum on Health*, Website: www.hc-sc.gc.ca/english/care/health_forum/forum_e.htm, August 2004.

20. Health Canada, *Population Health Approach—Towards a Common Understanding: Clarifying the Core Concepts of Population Health:* Introduction, Website: www.hc-sc.gc.ca/hppb/phdd/docs/common/intro.html, August 2004.

21. Health Canada, *Population Health Approach—The Statistical Report on the Health of Canadians 1999: An Overview*, Website: www.hc-sc.gc.ca/hppb/phb/phdd/report/stat/over.html, August 2004.

22. Health Canada, *Population Health Approach—Towards a Common Understanding: Clarifying the Core Concepts of Population Health: Core Concepts of the Population Health Approach*, Website: www.hc-sc.gc.ca/hppb/phdd/docs/common/chap2.html, August 2004.

23. *Ibid.*

24. Health Canada, Population Health—*Population Health Promotion: An Integrated Model of Population Health and Health Promotion*, Website: www.hc-sc.gc.ca/hppb/hppb/phdd/php/php4.htm, August 2004.

25. *Ibid.*

26. Health Canada, *Population Health Approach—Population Health Promotion: An Integrated Model of Population Health and Health Promotion*, Website: www.hc-sc.gc.ca/hppb/hppb/phdd/php/php4.htm, August 2003.

27. Statistics Canada, *2002 Health Care in Canada*, Ottawa: Canadian Institute for Health Information, 2002.

28. *Ibid.*

29. Health Canada, *Primary Health Care in Canada*, Website: www.hc-sc.gc.ca/english/media/releases/2002/2002_50bk1.htm, June 2003.

30. Health Canada, *$13.6 Million to Strengthen Primary Health Care in New Brunswick*, News Release, Website: www.hc-sc.gc.ca/english/media/releases/2003/2003_68.htm, September 2003.

31. Health Canada, *Primary Health Care in Canada*.

32. West, *op. cit.*

33. Segall, A., and N.L. Chappell, *Health and Health Care in Canada*. Toronto: Pearson Education Canada Inc., 2000.

34. Boyce, W.F., Influence of Health Promotion Bureaucracy on Community Participation: A Canadian Case Study. *Health Promotion International,* 17 no. 1 (2002), 61–68.

35. *Ibid.*

36. Lemire Rodger, G., Canadian Nurses Association, in M. McIntyre and E. Thomlinson, eds., *Realities of Canadian Nursing: Professional, Practice, and Power Issues* (pp. 124–137). Philadelphia: Lippincott, 2003.

37. Health Canada, *A Report on the Nursing Strategy for Canada*, Website: www.hc-sc.gc.ca/english/media/releases/2003/2003_67bk1.htm, November 2003.

38. *Ibid.*

39. Health Canada, *Nursing Strategy for Canada*, Website: www.hc-sc.gc.ca/english/for_you/nursing/index.htm, November 2003.

40. Canadian Nurses Association, Primary Health Care—The Time Has Come, *Nursing Now: Issues and Trends in Canadian Nursing,* 16 (September 2003), 1–4.

41. *Ibid.*

Part 1

INFLUENCES ON THE DEVELOPING PERSON AND FAMILY UNIT

CHAPTER 1

SOCIOCULTURAL INFLUENCES ON THE PERSON AND FAMILY

CHAPTER 2

ENVIRONMENTAL INFLUENCES ON THE PERSON AND FAMILY

CHAPTER 3

SPIRITUAL AND RELIGIOUS INFLUENCES ON THE PERSON AND FAMILY

Chapter 1

SOCIOCULTURAL INFLUENCES ON THE PERSON AND FAMILY

The culture and subcultures into which we are born encompass us and direct us for life. We learn an identity, values, beliefs, norms and habits of life, language, relationships, time, space, work, play, right, wrong, and physical and mental health practices.

Ruth Beckmann Murray

Caring relationships based on respect are central to a multicultural environment.

P. Moffitt and J. Wuest, *Spirit of the Drum: The Development of Cultural Nursing Praxis,* Canadian Journal of Nursing Research, 34, No. 4 (2002), 115.

OBJECTIVES

STUDY OF THIS CHAPTER WILL ENABLE YOU TO:

1. Identify population groups in Canada and the United States.

2. Define *culture* and *subculture* and describe various types of subcultures.

3. Examine the general characteristics of any culture and determine how they affect those under your care.

4. Identify the dominant cultural values in Canada and the United States and discuss how they influence you as a health care worker as well as the client and family.

5. Compare and contrast dominant traditional and emerging values with values of other racial or ethnic groups in Canada and the United States.

6. Describe the beliefs and values of Middle Eastern, Greek, Latino, and Japanese cultures in relation to the family unit, male–female relationships, childrearing patterns, the group versus privacy, time orientation, work and use of leisure, education, and change.

7. Contrast attitudes toward health and illness of persons of North American and other cultures.

8. Analyze the influences of socioeconomic levels on the health status of the person and group.

9. Determine how knowledge of cultural and socioeconomic level values and attitudes toward daily living

practices, health, and illness can contribute to the effectiveness of your health care.

10. Evaluate ways to meet the needs of a person with cultural values and a socioeconomic level different from your own.

11. Apply knowledge about the teaching–learning process to a health promotion education program for a person or family from a particular culture or socioeconomic level.

12. Design a plan of care for a person or family from another culture and socioeconomic level.

13. Identify your own ethnocentric tendencies regarding the health care system.

SOCIOCULTURAL INFLUENCES

When people talk or act differently from you, consider that to them you may also seem to talk or act differently. Many such differences are cultural and should be understood rather than laughed at or ignored.

J. Zentner

CRITICAL THINKING

In what ways has your particular culture influenced the manner in which you speak to and behave with others?

Humans are unique because we have culture. Culture includes using language, art forms, and games to communicate with others; cooperating in problem solving; deliberately training children; developing unique interpretations; forming organizations; and making, saving, using, and changing tools. Humans are heir to the accumulation of the wisdom and folly of preceding generations, and, in turn, they teach others their beliefs, feelings, and practices. The client, family, and you are deeply affected by the culture learned during the early years, often more so than by cultural knowledge acquired later.

CULTURAL POPULATIONS IN CANADA AND THE UNITED STATES

An understanding of cultural and socioeconomic class systems and their influence on the development of behaviour is essential to understanding yourself and the person under your care.

Did you know that Canada was the first nation in the world to declare multiculturalism as an official policy? Consequently, the *Canadian Multiculturalism Act* was passed in 1988.[1] One of the objectives of the Act is to recognize the need to assist people to overcome barriers in order to participate effectively in society. According to Census Canada 2001, Canada has close to 30 million inhabitants.[2] This population reflects a cultural, ethnic, and linguistic profile that has become a permanent aspect of Canadian society. With the *Canadian Multiculturalism Act*, racial and cultural equalities are protected by law.

Over the past 100 years, immigration has shaped Canada, adding not only to the nation's ethnic composition, but to its cultural makeup as well. Since the 1980s, Canada has had a proportionately higher annual intake of immigrants than either the United States or Australia.[3] Today, the primary source of immigrants is most likely to be Asian countries. In fact, of the 1.8 million immigrants who arrived between 1991 and 2001, 58 percent came from Asia, including the Middle East.

The growth of the visible minority population during the last several decades is the result of immigration patterns. That is, while earlier immigrants were mainly of European descent, new arrivals were more likely to have been born in non-European countries. However, some visible minority groups, such as Japanese and blacks, are more likely to be Canadian-born. It is important to note that the visible minority (those other than the Aboriginal peoples who are non-Caucasian in race or non-white in colour, as defined by the *Employment Equity Act*) is growing faster than the total population.[4]

According to the Report of the Royal Commission on Aboriginal Peoples, "the term Aboriginal obscures the distinctiveness of the First Peoples of Canada, namely Inuit, Métis and First Nations".[5] Among the First Nations alone, there are more than 50 distinct groupings, and among Inuit, several dialects exist within Inuktitut. The Métis people speak a variety of First Nations languages, such as Cree, Objibwa, or Chipewyan, as well as Michif, a language which evolved from their varied ancestry. The cultural and linguistic variations among these particular groups are greater than the variations among the European nations.[6] It is interesting that in the Canada 2001 census, the population reporting Aboriginal identity had reached nearly one million in 2001.[7]

Meanwhile, to consider the American situation for comparison purposes, the Asian, Asian-American, and Pacific Islander populations are the fastest growing in the United States. They include the Japanese, Chinese, Filipinos, Koreans, Vietnamese, Asian Indians, Thais, Hmong, Malaysians, Indonesians, Pakistanis, Cambodians, Laotians, and those from Singapore, Taiwan, and Hong Kong. Pacific Islanders include Polynesians (Hawaiian, and Samoans), Micronesians (such as Chamorros, the indigenous people of Guam), and Melanesians (such as Fijians). Twelve million new arrivals to the United States in the 1990s is a rate that exceeds the largest previous wave of 10 million immigrants from 1905 to 1914.[8]

The Latino (Spanish-speaking, or Hispanic) population is the second fastest growing population in the United States, many of whom are young. About 30 percent have incomes below the poverty level; 28 percent of these families are headed by women with children under age 18. However, there is a growing middle class.[9]

Despite the growth patterns, non-whites continue to be separate from the white population and mainstream culture. Even if they are not segregated physically, they may be separated by lack of mutual understanding.

DEFINITIONS

A number of definitions are presented to assist you in the correct use of words for all the cultures. These words also relate to assessment. However, before you begin to read and to study this section, take a moment to reflect on your own meaning of "culture."

Culture *is the sum total of the learned ways of doing, feeling, and thinking, past and present, of a social group within a given period.* These ways are transmitted from one generation to the next or to immigrants who become members of the society. Culture is a group's design for living, a shared set of socially transmitted assumptions about the nature of the physical and social worlds, goals in life, attitudes, roles, and values. Culture is a complex integrated system that includes knowledge, beliefs, skills, art, morals, law, customs, and any other acquired habits and capabilities of the human being. All provide a pattern for living together.

Manifest culture *reveals what people are actually saying and doing daily.* **Ideal culture** *refers to beliefs, practices, and feelings which people believe in or hold as desirable but do not always practise.*[10]

A **subculture** *is a group of persons within a larger culture of the same age, socioeconomic level, ethnic origin, education, or occupation, or with the same goals, who have an identity of their own but are related to the total culture in certain ways.*

Ethnic, regional, socioeconomic, religious, and family subcultures also exist. A description of each follows.

The term **ethnic** pertains to *a group of people, distinguished from other people by race or nationality, that possesses common physical and mental traits as a result of heredity, cultural traditions, language or speech, customs, and common history.* **Ethnicity** refers to *a national group.* In Canada, there are many European ethnic subcultures, for example, Slovakian (German, Italian, Polish, or Slavic), Scandinavian (Danish, Norwegian, Icelandic, Finnish, or Swedish), Swiss, French, Dutch, and Russian. There are also ethnic subcultures from the United Kingdom: English, Irish, Welsh, and Scottish. The markers of racial or ethnic identity are every conceivable hue of colour and sometimes as much a matter of socialization, ideology, and attitude as pigmentation. Courtney[11] describes the challenges and hurts that he has encountered because he is biracial. He states that being biracial has frequently meant denying half of his identity, depending on whether he was with white or black people. Tiger Woods, a professional golfer, is an example of a new generation of multiracial individuals who believe ethnic diversity and ambiguity confer both individuality and a sense of shared values.[12]

According to Census Canada 2001, ethnic origin refers to the ethnic or cultural group(s) to which an individual's ancestors belonged.[13] In that census, more than 200 different ethnic origins were reported. The reported list includes cultural groups associated with Canada's first peoples, North American Indian, Métis, and Inuit. (Note: For statistical and other purposes, the Federal Government of Canada usually divides the Aboriginal population into four categories: (1) North American Indians registered under the *Indian Act*, (2) North American Indians not registered under the *Indian Act*, (3) Métis, and (4) Inuit.[14] Other cultural groups included were associated with the founding of Canada, such as the French, the English, the Scottish, and the Irish. The list also reflects the history of immigration to Canada in the past 100 years, with such groups as German, Italian, Chinese, Ukrainian, Dutch, Polish, and others. A host of new ethnic origins has emerged as a result of changing sources of immigrants to Canada and includes: Kosovars from Yugoslavia, Azerbaijani and Georgians from Central Asia; Pashtun from Afghanistan, Yemeni and Saudi Arabians from the Middle East; Khmer from Southeast Asia; Nepali and Kashmiri from South Asia; Congolese, Yoruba, and Ashanti from Africa; and Bolivians, Maya, and Caribbean Indians from Central and South America.[15] How far back can you trace your own ethnic or cultural group in Canada?

In both the 1996 and 2001 censuses, an increased number of people have reported being either Canadian, or Canadien, as part of their ethnic heritage. It is important to note that those people had English or French as a mother tongue, were born in Canada, and had both parents born inside Canada.[16] English and French are Canada's official languages as well as being the two languages most likely to be spoken in the country.[17] The *Official Language Act*, adopted in 1969, gave these languages equal status, rights, and privileges in federal institutions. The other languages are recognized as non-official or heritage languages. In parts of Canada, where Aboriginal groups are prevalent, a small portion of the population speaks neither English nor French. Furthermore, in large ethnic communities, this same phenomenon also occurs because many immigrants have never learned either official language.

Canadian health professionals are observing an increase in non-official languages being spoken. In society generally, however, English and French predominate; but more than 100 other languages are being spoken.[18] The effects of a rapid cultural shift have caused an impact on health care, especially in the area of medical communication. Many Canadians who have a relatively low level of literacy in either official language cannot use the printed health information available to them. Census Canada 2001 reports, the largest visible minority group surpassing one million for the first time was Chinese. With this figure in mind, it appears that a growing need exists for cross-cultural services in various health care settings.

CRITICAL THINKING

What types of cross-cultural service do you see being implemented in an urban hospital?

Regional culture refers to *the local or regional manifestations of the larger culture.* Thus, the child learns the sectional variant of the national culture, for example, rural or urban. Regional culture is influenced by geography, climate, natural resources, trade, and economics; variations may be shown in values, beliefs, housing, food, occupational skills, and language. One type of regional culture is **urban**, which is defined as *a city of 50 000 or more people or an area of at least 50 000 persons that is part of a region with a population of at least 100 000.*[19] One particular type of population to consider is **rural**. The term *rural* is difficult to define, in part because it prompts different images for different people.

Most of Canada's vast land area is sparsely populated. In addition, with each passing decade, a greater proportion of the total population is found in urban areas. On the basis of defined rules with respect to the total population and population density, all land in Canada is defined by Statistics Canada as either urban or rural. An urban area has a minimum population concentration of 1000 persons and a population density of at least 400 persons per square kilometre. By default, all territory outside urban areas is classified as rural.[20]

Rural dwellers use the same adaptive strategies and products as urban dwellers, and value systems may be similar. Differences may depend more on the geography, climate, and history of the area than on socioeconomic status, race, ethnicity, or religion. Yet several characteristics are common in rural areas:

1. Isolation from or scarcity of at least some necessary resources to promote health and, sometimes, geographic isolation from people
2. Assumption that what is done locally is the norm, for example, "we've always done it this way," in spite of rules and regulations on a provincial, state, or national level
3. Lack of anonymity, because everyone knows, directly or indirectly, everyone else for miles around, and sometimes, the family history for generations
4. A sense of independence or autonomy, for example, a desire to be one's own boss and to be left alone

These characteristics may have a negative impact on the health care provided to those in rural areas, even though isolation, independence, and lack of anonymity are seen as positive attributes by them.

Population density, population size, and distance from health care facilities are criteria frequently used in defining rural areas. *Ruralness* is a matter of perspective; to some people, it means "smaller than here." Differences within rural populations and among rural areas are substantial. Age, income, race, ethnicity, and occupation all contribute to different values and customs and definitions of health among rural people. To consider health resources in rural communities, a study was conducted within a Canadian provincial regional health authority to explore and analyze mental health services and other resources used by rural consumers, and it produced some interesting findings.[21] One such finding revealed that access to mental health services was challenging for residents of many rural communities. Another finding was that a number of programs and services available for the rural people in some communities were not available in others.

Socioeconomic level is *a cultural grouping of persons who, through group consensus and similarity of financial position or wealth, occupation, and education, have come to have similar status, lifestyle, interests, feelings, attitudes, language, and overt behaviour.* The more the economic level of a group becomes fixed, the more predictable are its patterns of attitudes and behaviour. Children learn the patterns of their own group and the group's attitude toward a group at another level. The attitude patterns make up a culture's **value system**, *its concept of how people should behave in various situations as well as which goals they should pursue and how.* The value systems of the general culture and those of the subculture or socioeconomic level may conflict at times. Further, in Canada or other Western countries, people may, at times, move up or down from their economic or prosperity levels, but the original values may be maintained.

All cultures, subcultures, and ethnic groups possess certain values, customs, and practices common to every culture; share certain values, customs, and practices with some other cultures; and have certain values, customs, and practices unique only to that group of people. **Religious culture** *also influences the person, for a religion constitutes a way of living, behaving, and thinking and therefore is a kind of culture.* Religious influences on values, attitudes, and behaviour are discussed in Chapter 3.

Family culture *refers to family life, which is part of the cultural system.* The family is the medium through which the large cultural heritage is transmitted to the child; family culture consists of ways of living and thinking that constitute the familial and sexual aspects of group life. These include courtship and marriage patterns, sexual mores, husband–wife relationships, status and relationships of men and women, parent–child relationships, childrearing, responsibilities to parents, and attitudes toward unmarried women, children, divorce, homosexuality, and various health problems.

The family name gives the child a social position as well as an identity; the child is assigned the status of the family and the reputation that goes with it. Family status has a great deal to do with health and behaviour throughout life because of its effect on self-concept.

Family rituals are the collective way of working out household routines and using time within the family culture and are indicators of family values. **Ritual** is *a system of definitely prescribed behaviours and procedures.* It provides exactness in daily tasks of living and has a sense of rightness about it. The more often the behaviour is repeated, the more it comes to be approved and therefore habitual. Thus, rituals inevitably develop in family life as a result of the intimacy of relationships and the repetition or continuity of certain interactions. Rituals change from one life cycle to another, for example, at marriage, after childbirth, when children go to school, and when children leave home. Rituals are important in child development for several reasons:

■ They are group habits that communicate ways of doing things and attitudes related to events, including family etiquette, affectionate responses between family members, organization of leisure time, and education for group adjustment.

■ They promote solidarity and continuity by promoting habitual behaviour, unconsciously performed, that brings harmony to family life. Many rituals continue to the next generation, increasing the person's sense of worth, security, and family continuity or identity.

■ They aid in maintaining self-control through disciplinary measures.

■ They promote feelings of euphoria, sentimentality, or well-being, for example, through celebrations on special occasions.

■ They dictate reactions to threat, such as at times of loss, illness, or death.[22, 23]

CRITICAL THINKING

In what ways have the rituals that you grew up with come to affect you in your adult life?

Family influences are dealt with more extensively in Chapter 4.

CHARACTERISTICS OF CULTURE

Understanding the characteristics of culture will help you understand and work with people from various cultures. Take a moment to reflect on the cultural differences that you recall seeing in your childhood friends and in your neighbourhood. What stands out for you?

Culture Is Learned

The first of the three basic characteristics of culture is that it is learned. People function physiologically in much the same way throughout the world, but their behaviour is learned and therefore relatively diverse. Because of culture, a child is ascribed or acquires a certain **status** or *position of prestige.* The child also learns or assumes certain **roles**, *patterns or related behaviours expected by others, and later by oneself, that define behaviour and adjustment to a given group.* The behaviour, values, attitudes, and beliefs learned within the culture become a matter of tradition, even though the culture allows choices within limits. What the person learns during development is of great significance. Culture determines the kinds of experiences the person encounters and the extent to which responses to life situations are unhealthy, maladaptive, and self-defeating or healthy, adaptive, constructive, and creative.[24, 25] What the person has learned from the culture determines, first, how and what you as the health care provider will be able to teach him or her, and, secondly, what approach you might take during care.

Culture Is Stable but Changing

The second characteristic of culture is that it is subject to and capable of change in order to remain viable and adaptive, although it is basically a stable entity. The culture of a society, like a human body, is dynamic but maintained at a steady state by self-regulating devices. In advanced countries throughout the world, there is often much overt change occurring. Yet, underneath the manifested lifestyle changes, certain basic values of most people within a group are unlikely to be changed because behaviour is defined by the culture. The stabilizing features are traditions, group pressure, and the ready-made solutions to life's problems that are provided for the group, enabling individuals to anticipate the behaviour of others, predict future events, and regulate their lives within the culture. Everyone within the same culture does not behave in exactly the same way. Norms and customs that persist may have a negative influence on the group.[26] Food taboos during illness and pregnancy, pica, a diet high in animal fat, and crowding of people into a common dwelling that becomes an incubator for the spread of contagious diseases are some examples.

A culture makes change, stability, or adaptation possible through its ideas, inventions, and customs. Together with physiological adaptive processes, culture is a powerful force. Humans, for example, are able to live in a wide variety of climates because the human body has adjusted gradually to permit survival. We have constructed a variety of lifestyles and patterns of social relationships to guarantee our survival and free ourselves from the limits of physical environments. Prescribed cultural norms are the most effective adaptive mechanisms that humans use. They affect physical, social, and mental well-being; aid adaptation to diverse situations, environments, and recurring problems; and teach about other environments to which we may have to adapt. In addition, some adaptive modifications are achieved through genetic, physiological, and constitutional capacities that have been transmitted for generations through natural selection or cultural conditioning.

Another stabilizing aspect of culture is the use of language, even though the meanings of words change over time.[27] Although language forms vary from culture to culture, the terms for *mother* and *father* sound very much alike across cultural lines, perhaps because certain vocalizations are easy for a child to articulate and learn.[28] Language is also a means by which culture is transmitted from one generation to the next. Canadians are aware of the importance of language to culture. Even though Canada is officially bilingual, French-speaking majorities exist mainly in Quebec and northern New Brunswick, and English is spoken elsewhere in Canada.[29] The Aboriginal culture, being oral in nature, is transmitted through speech, rather than through the written word. The Aboriginal languages, which are symbols of Aboriginal culture and group identity, are many and diverse. Language not only serves as a means of interacting but also connects people with their past and grounds their emotional, social, and spiritual self. Despite the efforts of the Canadian Aboriginal peoples to preserve their languages, these languages are endangered; if they are lost, the consequences will have a profound effect on the cultural survival of the Aboriginal peoples.[30]

CRITICAL THINKING

What may be the factors contributing to the potential loss of Aboriginal languages?

The meeting ground between cultures is in language and **dialect**, a variety of a language spoken by a distinct group of people in a definite place. Dialects are related to racial and ethnic backgrounds, geographic regions, and neighbourhoods. If the words are not understood in relation to the culture, there is breakdown of communication and relationships. Choice of words, syntax, intonation, and level of emotion in speech all convey meanings.[31,32,33] As Chinese Canadians have made gains in education and employment, they have also made conscious efforts to develop a sense of community and to increase the awareness of Chinese culture.[34] Although Chinese people read and write with the same characters, they employ any of the several dozen dialects. The "official" dialect taught in schools in China is Mandarin, which is the dialect of Beijing, the capital of China.[35]

Because of the increasing variety of languages which we now encounter in Canada, it is important for health professionals to listen carefully to the language spoken, be accepting of the dialect, and validate meanings of words when necessary during that assessment and intervention phase of health care delivery.

Immigrants and refugees vary in their ability to speak and understand English, depending upon the extent to which English was taught in the country of origin and the age of the person. Usually, the children of these families learn English quickly enough and become interpreters for the family. Use of nonverbal language also varies by cultural background.

CONTROVERSY DEBATE

Elizabeth is a fourth-year student in a Baccalaureate Nursing degree program. She is a lone parent with three school age children and has maintained a 3.8 grade point average since year 1. After graduation, she wants to work in a Toronto hospital's paediatric unit. In her Transcultural Nursing course, she has learned that in Toronto, after English, Chinese, with its various dialects, is the most predominantly spoken language and that Chinese is the first language of more than 355 000 Toronto residents.[36] In order to prepare herself maximally for the position, she is wondering whether or not she should register for a Chinese language course for Anglophones one evening per week January through April. Elizabeth seeks your advice on the matter.

1. What relevant issues should Elizabeth consider in arriving at her decision?

2. Would the completion of the course help significantly to prepare her for the position?

Language emphasizes the particular values of a culture. For example, neither the language of the Nootka Indians on Vancouver Island nor that of the Hopi in the American southwest has separate subject and predicate or parts of speech, as does English. These languages describe an event as a whole with a single term. However, North Americans are complex, abstract, and fragmentary in their descriptions of the world around them.

The Indo-European languages, including English, emphasize *time*. Cultures using these languages keep records, use mathematics, do accounting, use clocks and calendars, and study archeology to study their historical past. In contrast, past, present, and future tenses do not exist in the Hopi language; the validity of a statement is not based on time or history but on "fact," memory, expectations, or customs. The Navaho language has hardly any mention of clock time and instead emphasizes type of activity, duration, or aspects of movement.

Moreover, Indo-European languages, such as English, describe *nonspatial relationships* with *spatial* metaphors, for example, *long* and *short* for duration; *heavy* and *light* or *long* and *short* for intensity; or *rise* and *fall* for tendency. The natives in Alaska have numerous concepts about the varieties of *space*, whereas Americans have more words for the concept of *time*. Inuktitut, the language of the Inuit, is widely used throughout the North, and thus the Inuit from across the Arctic can understand one another. Even though dialects and accents vary from region to region, Inuktitut is considered a single language.[37] One thing a person new to the language might notice is that a single word may be spelled in many different ways.

CRITICAL THINKING

Do you think that the Inuit may experience their world differently because of their language, which has its own distinct symbols?

Conceptualizations and language influence the values, behaviour, stability, strength, connectedness, and progress of a culture. Assessment of the person's intellectual ability must consider culture as well as age. People from non-Western cultures may learn differently and at a different rate because of different language and perceptual skills and value orientations.[38] Most cultures are less technical and less verbal than the North American culture.

Analyses of the habits and practices of various peoples show that traditional language and behaviour patterns practised by parents and children within a culture are related to the interactions between employer and employee, among peers, and between caregiver and patient, making for predictability and stability. Stability of culture promotes adaptability and economy of energy.[39,40]

Cultures also change, sometimes imperceptibly, so that norms—the usual rules for living—are modified to meet the group's needs as new life challenges arise. What have been some of the cultural changes you have experienced?

Cultures change for various reasons:

- Technological changes or innovations
- Competition among groups for geographical regions to meet members' sustenance and safety needs
- Use of another culture's inventions, art forms, or life ways
- Education of the group
- Use of deferred gains for members to induce them to work for the good of the culture, as in Communist countries
- Change in political leadership, as in China, Russia, Iran, and Central America
- Increased scientific and industrial complexity

- Increased or decreased population growth
- Change in economic practices and standards, such as the change from feudalism to industrialism seen in some African and Asian countries
- Use of behaviour modification techniques by groups in power
- Promotion of values, lifestyles, and products through mass media programming and advertisements[41]

Culture is continually shaped by forces and people outside our awareness. Many industrial societies, including Canada and the United States, are moving into a **postindustrial** or **postmodern society**. Daniel Bell, a sociologist in 1973, coined the term *post-industrialism* to refer to technology that supports an information-based economy.[42] Production, in postindustrial societies focuses on computers and other electronic devices that not only create but also process as well as store and apply information. Individuals in postindustrial societies concentrate on learning skills for jobs in high-tech communication. The following are some of the problem areas of postmodern society:

- Need for more professional knowledge
- Greater expectations by the public
- More goods considered to be public goods
- Lack of measurements to show what is actually needed and thus where money and resources should be directed
- A changing demography with more urban concentration
- Increased life expectancy
- Changing values, with little understanding of historical roots of the culture
- Power struggles between groups.[43,44]

CRITICAL THINKING

In what ways does the postindustrial era affect the practice of health care professionals?

Adaptation failure and illness are likely to occur unless people come to grips with rapid social changes, such as frequent shifting of families from one place to another; alterations in bureaucratic structures that may overwhelm the worker in change; diversity of options; continuing novelty in many life situations; and loss of faith in basic truths, realities, and societal foundations. A disposable, transient culture makes it difficult for people to establish roots or pass on culture as a guideline to future generations. Not all people can cope with continual rapid change.[45] Risk of illness can be predicted from the amount of change. If a person is in the equivalent of the alarm stage of the stress syndrome continually, body defences weaken (see Chapter 5). Extreme examples of persons caught in rapidly changing environments are the combat soldier, the disaster victim, the culturally dislocated traveller, the homeless person, and the migrant worker. Other examples include elderly persons who are uprooted and the person who moves from a rural environment to an urban environment.

Significant numbers of people may begin to respond differently to one or more facets of a culture, and this factor may cause others in the society to realize that a particular custom or norm is no longer useful. Such customs might pertain to marriage, burial, childrearing, or moral codes. If a group of people (or isolated persons) can consistently adapt and at the same time imperfectly follow a particular norm, they may establish a new norm, which may be gradually adopted by others until that becomes the generally established pattern. Thus, the culture and the people in it can be changed in spite of initial resistance. Such changes can have a positive or negative influence on health.[46]

Each culture is a whole, but not every culture is integrated in the same way and to the same extent. Some cultures are so tightly integrated that any change threatens the whole. Other cultures are characterized by traditional patterns that are easy to manipulate and change.

Culture Has Components and Patterns

The third characteristic of culture is that every culture has certain components or patterns, regardless of how "primitive" or "advanced" the culture may be.[47] Understanding these components and patterns can help you understand yourself, your client, and the health care system in which you work.

Table 1-1 describes the various components of cultures, with examples.[48,49,50,51,52]

All the foregoing components and patterns influence and are influenced by adaptation to climate, use of natural resources, geography, sanitation facilities, diet, group biological and genetic factors, and disease conditions and health practices.

COMPARISON OF CULTURES

Knowledge of cultural values is essential for providing culturally sensitive care as you interact with, assess, teach, and intervene with people from various cultures.

Cultural Values in Canada

Multiculturalism

In 1971, the focus of the multicultural policy was on the fact that Canada had no official culture but recognized those of all ethnic backgrounds. The *Canadian Multiculturalism Act* passed in 1988 to preserve Canada's multicultural heritage. Both racial and cultural equalities are now protected by law due to the passage of this Act.[53]

TABLE 1-1 Components of All Cultures		
Component of the Culture	Purpose or Meaning	Examples
Provision of physical welfare; feeding, clothing, and shelter patterns	Survival and maintenance of population. Health promotion.	Production and processing of food, shelter, clothing. Personal and health care patterns. Production and use of tools. Manufacturing, industrialization. Change of land terrain for home building, farming, industry. Health care services.
Communication systems	Basis for interaction and cohesion. Vehicle for transmission and preservation of the culture. Distinguishes groups from each other.	Language and dialects. Vocabulary and word taboos. Nonverbal behaviour. Voice tone, rhythm, speed, pronunciation. Facial expressions, gestures, symbols. Mass media. Computers. Music. Art. Satellites.
Exchange of goods and services	Production and distribution of goods and services. Work roles. Payment. Obtain at least necessities or luxury, depending on culture.	Barter. Trade. Commerce. Financial institutions. Economic policies. Regulatory mechanisms. Health care institutions and services.
Travel and transportation	Provision for obtaining goods and services. Mobility within and across cultures, societies, nations.	Walk. Use of animals, such as dog, llama, horse, oxen. System of car, truck, railway, air travel transport.
Social controls; institutions of government	Maintenance of order. Organization of people, society, government. Regulation of time and activity. Power systems.	Mores, *morally binding attitudes.* **Customs,** *long-established practices having force of unwritten laws.* Value systems. Laws. Policies. Regulations. Public or group opinion. Political offices; kingships; dictators.

(continued)

TABLE 1-1 *(continued)*
Components of All Cultures

Component of the Culture	Purpose or Meaning	Examples
Forms of property	Necessities to maintain survival. May contribute to person's worth, status, social position.	Personal belongings. Personal property. Real estate. Financial institutions and systems.
Human response patterns	Family relationships structure other relationships and "taken-for-granted" activities to maintain the group. Values, beliefs, attitudes taught for socialization of person into culture. Ready-made solutions to life problems and goal achievements. Relationships structured by age, sex, status, wealth, power, number of kin, wisdom.	Rules for all social interaction, handling competition, conflict, cooperation, and games. Intimate habits of daily living personally and in groups. Manner in which one's body, home, property perceived. Daily "taken-for-granted" activities and interactions. Use of time and space. Health care roles and practices.
Family and sexual patterns	Maintain structure for care and support of others. Regulate relationships for survival, harmony, generational longevity.	Wedding ceremonies. Birth, childbearing practices. Family division of labour. Roles assigned to men, women, children. Inheritance rights. Care of elderly. Guardianship. Forms of kinship. Divorce proceedings, or removal of undesired member, such as infanticide, burial of woman with husband, or elders leaving tribe to die. Use of time and space.
Knowledge	Survival and expansion of group and desired practices. Contributes to improved living standards through inventions, products, practices, services. Technologic innovation, mobility to higher social status.	Reasoning process. Education system, informal and local, formal and national. Skills. Values. **Science,** *systematized knowledge based on observation, study, experimentation.* Traditions. Folklore. Folk and scientific medical, nursing, and health care practices.
Belief system	Guides behaviour of individuals and group during daily life, at special events, occasions, celebrations. Provides meaning to life and death. Indicates priorities. Guides health and illness behaviour.	Religion. Ethical codes. Magical ideas and practices. Taboos. Rituals. Methodology. Philosophy. Organized institution of the church. Values and norms.
Artistic and aesthetic expression	Expression of meaning in life and death, feelings ranging from joy to sorrow, depending on situation. Spiritual expression. Expression of individual talents. Health promotion. Therapy and rehabilitation in illness.	Painting. Music. Dance. Architecture. Sculpture. Literature. Aesthetic expressions also in body adornment. Use and decoration of space and surrounding environment, such as floral gardens.
Recreation and leisure activities	Socialization. Use of leisure time. Travel to other cultures.	Play activities and tools. Games. Organized sports. Leisure activities depend on climate, terrain, available time, resources.

CRITICAL THINKING

What may be some of the criticisms of multiculturalism in Canada?

Canada stands as a nation, both diverse and cohesive, tied together by a set of shared values that includes respect of the individual's dignity and rule of law, freedom, equality, compassion, and fairness. In addition, Canada's framework for diversity recognizes that respect for cultural distinctiveness is intrinsic to an individual's sense of self-worth, which, in turn, encourages participation, achievement, and eventually attachment to the nation.[54] The Government of Canada is working with the provincial and territorial governments, as well as with different community groups, nonprofit organizations, the corporate sector, and the private sector, to help strengthen the nation's institutions and build safer communities in order to reinforce shared values.

Immigration

Immigration continues to influence the cultural composition of the population of Canada. One prediction is that by the year 2016, 1 out of every 5 Canadians and 1 out of every 4 children will be a member of a visible minority group. These figures bear directly on our understanding of the implications for health care delivery in the nation.

Social Value Groups

A sociologist and pollster, Michael Adams, examined Canadian social values in his book *Sex in the Snow,* published in January 1997.[55] According to Adams, when Canadians are divided according to their social values, 12 distinct psychographic "tribes," or social value groups emerge. These can be organized under three categories: (1) the elders category (over age 50) comprises three subgroups; (2) the baby-boomers category (age 30–49) comprises four subgroups; and (3) the Generation-X category (age 15–29) has five subgroups. The fact that the greatest number of social value groups exists among the Generation-Xers reflects a trend toward increasingly diverse Canadian values. Adams has attributed this trend to the effects of technological advances, such as the Internet, which allow Canadians to cross cultural boundaries and in doing so to explore a host of diverse values.[56] Canada's own techno-evangelist Don Tapscott believes that the Net Generation, also called Generation-Y, has grown up with computers and is wired for cyberspace.[57] They are as young as five years and as old as 20 and are more racially diverse than ever before. For example, in this group, one in three is non-Caucasian.[58]

Adams states that in the years 1997–1999, some untoward reactions occurred following how Canadians perceive their own lives on the one hand and the changing context of the Canadian society on the other. The overwhelming economic and technological forces appear to be going beyond the control of Canadians, leaving them with a growing sense of insecurity.[59]

Canadian National Values

However, Canada remains a nation strongly embedded in distinctive national values. According to Kirton, who is the Director of the G8 Research Group at the University of Toronto, there appear to be seven core enduring values embedded in Canada's constitution that unify Canadians at home and set them apart from the citizens of other countries.[60] See Table 1-2.

TABLE 1-2 Canada's Distinctive National Values	
Core Value	Focus Points
1. Globalism	a. Canadians believe they are an integral part of a completely connected global community.
	b. Canadians have a powerful incentive to look outward to the global community.
	c. They seek support for their accomplishments at home, and
	d. They give expression to those accomplishments abroad.
2. Multiculturalism	a. Within multiculturalism lies a tolerance for diversity and respect for the rights of minorities
	b. British subjects who arrived to settle Canada sought political accommodation with French settlers who were already well established there.
	c. Both French and English settlers depended for survival upon the many First Nations who had lived there for centuries before
	d. Initially was the need to make a virtue of necessity, then accept, and later celebrate multiculturalism.
	e. The same sequence has been reinforced by successive waves of immigration from ever more diverse places around the world.
	f. Most immigrants have been quickly accepted as full citizens of Canada regardless of their bloodlines or place of birth.
	g. Consequently Canada has become a country of multicultural minorities, which reinforces its sense of global connection and community to this day.

(continued)

TABLE 1-2 *(continued)*
Canada's Distinctive National Values

Core Value	Focus Points
3. Openness	a. Beyond Canada's openness to the outside world regarding her multicultural people, Canada is also open in regard to common and civil law legal systems. b. Canada is open to ideas, education, goods, services, investments, finance and ecological flows. c. Most goods and services produced in the private sector are destined for export, mostly to USA.
4. Anti-militarism	a. An aversion to military force in general, and to nuclear weapons in particular, has been an important source of influence in the world. b. Generally, Canada has acquired, or kept, her vast territory, from Atlantic to Pacific and through the Arctic Ocean to the North Pole, **without** the use of military force. c. Canada was among the first countries, in the late 1940s, capable of having her own nuclear weapon but chose not to—then and ever since.
5. Environmentalism	a. Virtually every Canadian carries an enduring conviction that global environmental protection should be the first priority in Canadian foreign policy. b. Canada is one of the world leaders in ecological and energy resources, but it has a strong conservationist instinct, reflected, for example in its instinctive aversion to exporting water in bulk.
6. Egalitarianism	a. Egalitarianism for Canadians includes the belief that a strong state must act to provide all of its citizens with the high minimum standards of living and social services they require for a civilized life. b. This value is reflected in Canada's constitutionally entrenched equalization payments, in which monies are transferred by the federal government from the affluent provinces of oil-rich Alberta and high-tech Ontario, to the eight less wealthy provinces and the three northern territories.
7. International Institutionalism	a. Generally Canada seeks to join most new international institutions to be able to connect Canada with others. b. The Commonwealth connects Canada to more than 50 countries, almost all historically attached to Britain, and who Canada has never considered as foreign.

Source: John Kirton, "Canada and its values: Policy priorities and practices" Lecture 10, G8 Online 2002, <http://www. library.utoronto.ca/ g7/g8online/english/2002/10.html>. Used with permission.

CRITICAL THINKING

What is your understanding of a global community?

It is important to note that the *Canadian Multiculturalism Act* challenges nurses and other health care professionals to work with culturally diverse groups at the individual, family, community, and societal levels. Stewart claims that this will be a continuing role for health care professionals as Canada becomes even more of a diverse nation.

CRITICAL THINKING

What have you learned about multiculturalism that you can apply to your daily interactions with your fellow students, friends, and family?

Blacks in Canada

One ethnic group that bears attention is the black families in Canada. Blacks have been in Canada for more than 300 years and have always occupied a subordinate position in economic, political, and ideological relations.[61] The survival of black families against extreme hardship and oppression indicates their endurance and resilience. In order for their families to survive, black women have needed to be strong; and many have had to work outside the home. This outside work has led them to become relatively independent. Many black families in Canada develop racial socialization strategies in order to create positive self-concepts and a pride in racial identity, which together assist their children to deal more effectively with racism. Many black parents emphasize the value of education to their children and, in the face of racism, motivate their children to believe that they need to be better than the whites. Many Olympic champions have succeeded by following such guidelines.

Television and Internet

In Canadian homes, television is a common feature and a major recreational activity. In fact, 49.7 percent of homes have two or more colour television sets.[62] Television has increased not only our knowledge of the diverse cultures in Canada but has provoked discussion of current issues relating to diversity. Some of the concerns are that some television programming may reinforce harmful social, cultural, and gender stereotypes and cause an increase in violence and aggressive behaviours in children. To counter these negative aspects of television on children's development, a number of educational programs, such as *Sesame Street*, have been designed to promote prosocial interactions and greater academic competence, especially in children from families of low socioeconomic status. One of the fastest-growing media,[63] the Internet is highly beneficial, especially in providing knowledge about people and countries around the world. However, on a note of caution, children who spend a lot of time surfing the Internet may be vulnerable to certain dangers and thus may be in need of parental supervision.

National Identity

There is now a growing recognition of the importance of culture to Canada's national identity at home and abroad. In addition, culture is viewed as a stimulus to job creation and economic growth. For example, many tourists are drawn to Canada by its festivals, museums, art galleries, performing arts, historic and archeological sites, or its open spaces and natural landscape. All levels of government play a vital role in supporting Canadian culture, for example, by providing government funding and employing new technologies to disseminate Canada's heritage.[64] (See Table 1-2.)

Cultural Values in the United States

The United States has been described as a **melting pot**, in that many cultural groups make up the population and have contributed to the value system. Over the years, many ethnic minorities have resettled in the United States and obtained citizenship. More recently there has been a large influx of refugees and immigrants from other European countries. Both *traditional* (middle-class, or mainstream) and *emerging* (changing) *values* are increasingly seen in the United States among ethnic populations as well as among Caucasians. Table 1-3 lists both the traditional and emerging values found in the United States. Some values show conflict between ideal and manifested values and behaviours that have been based on those held by different earlier generations, and the erosion of some basic values over the years.[65,66,67,68,69,70,71,72,73]

TABLE 1-3
Values of Dominant Culture in the United States

Traditional Values	Emerging Values
1. Marriage and children. Romantic love basis for marriage. Family stability; try to resolve or live with issues.	1. Variety of alternate lifestyles. Marriage not considered permanent or only way of life. Divorce expected, a way out of issues or if lack of self-satisfaction.
2. Sexual activity in relationships if there is affection and commitment. Heterogeneous relationships acceptable.	2. Sexual relationships for self-satisfaction. Same-sex and bisexual relationships acceptable.
3. Willingness to sacrifice for good of family members, children. Role of parents/family to discipline and guide children, help children find answers.	3. Less investment in having children; less sacrifice for children. Children given less discipline and guidance, expected to care for self, solve problems.
4. Work ethic. Commitment to cause. Goal of work is provisions for life, status, success. Loyalty to employer. Follow routine. Quality workmanship.	4. Decreasing work ethic, increasing emphasis on leisure and recreation. Freedom to indulge self. Routine work seen as dull, to be avoided. Work should be fun. Loyalty to self and technology.
5. Rules of conduct, etiquette. Socially acceptable behaviour. Formal responses. Sensitive to effect of behaviour on others.	5. Decreased emphasis on etiquette. Informal approach; disregard rules of behaviour. Lack of respect for others. Don't care about effect of behaviour on others. Less gentleness.
6. Puritanical. Preferred way to behave. Concern about effect on others. Cleanliness.	6. Sensual. Societal obsession with sex, alternate lifestyles, experimentation, violence. Less concern with cleanliness in environment or life.
7. Materialistic. Thrift. Economic security for present and future.	7. Materialistic consumerism for present excitement, enjoyment, prestige. Money taken for granted.

(continued)

TABLE 1-3 *(continued)*
Values of Dominant Culture in the United States

Traditional Values	Emerging Values
8. Equality of people an ideal. Recognize differences. Inequality accepted based on personal abilities or background.	8. Equal opportunity for people. Differences accepted and diversity expected. More freedom for personal choices. Respect for ability to perform. Desire to reduce inequality.
9. Rugged individualism but also cooperation with group on larger projects. Superordinate–subordinate relationships.	9. Do your own thing. Group conformity during school and teen years, while seeking individuality. Peer relationships.
10. Competition; emphasis on individual. Achievement. Success. Status consciousness.	10. Competition, with emphasis on team. Aggressive behaviour. Manipulate others to be successful. Disrespect for social status of others.
11. Authoritarian outlook. Accept institutional and political leadership. Patriotism. Democracy. Freedom.	11. Democratic outlook. Question all leadership and institutions. Apathy to or disrespect for leaders and country. Freedom means self-gratification.
12. Self-reliance. Responsible behaviour.	12. Increasing dependency. Lack of planning. Use others in system. Irresponsible behaviour.
13. Youth; beauty; health; strength.	13. Youth; beauty. Health is a right.
14. Future orientation. Interest in long-term goals. Willing to defer immediate satisfaction.	14. Present outcome emphasized. Immediate answers and satisfaction expected.
15. Education for social, geographic, economic, occupational mobility. Basic subjects. Science. Advanced degrees.	15. Education for immediate goals. Experiment with methods. Mass media as an education tool, used to manipulate ideas and values, create desire for products, change practices.
16. Problem-oriented; systematic; specific. Thoughtfulness valued; time for thinking.	16. Process-oriented; concerned about process even if no solutions. Focus on external and immediate experience. Inner experience or contemplation not valued. Power oriented.
17. Use of practical or functional goods or products. Keep objects considered valuable or sentimental. Maintain basic knowledge and skills.	17. New products. Technology. Automation. Use of disposable goods; recycle items for environment or for book fairs. Constant updating of knowledge and skills.
18. Speed. Change. Progress. Efficiency. Time important, scheduled.	18. Increasing demand for immediate output. Change even more rapid. Sense of hurry and no control over time or schedules.
19. Exert will over environment. Use of environmental resources for societal and own needs.	19. Environment represents a course; effort to save environment and resources in conflict with demand for products, waste.
20. Sense of humanitarianism, concern for others in trouble or disaster. Continued caretaking.	20. Depersonalization. Robot or machinelike performance by people is expected. Concern about effects on self from helping others (legal or co-dependency).
21. Books, media used to develop social conscience.	21. Mass media, information systems, electronic games used for personal enhancement and to influence masses. Education potential.

Although research indicates that value differences exist among different racial and ethnic groups and economic levels, similarities also exist among most families in the same geographical area.

Several trends are important to health care: the emphasis on an information society; high-technology, high-touch care; the long-term perspective; decentralization of services; use of self-help practices; use of networking; seeking of multiple options; the rise of more women in leadership positions; and decline of the welfare state. The concepts of aggression and violence vary from culture to culture. In American culture, aggression is regarded as an innate force that has survival value and that requires appropriate channels for its expression; it is considered an integral part of social success.

People react differently to constant exposure to violence: they may tolerate it, develop disease symptoms, project their own aggression onto others, develop a neurotic preoccupation with it, or act violently themselves to discharge rage. We see examples of each reaction in society in the form of physical, emotional, and social illness.

Americans teach their children to be independent and emphasize the importance of the adolescent or young adult leaving home. Psychiatric therapy in the United States is often directed toward these goals. In Asian and many Asian-American cultures, however, indirect communication, modesty, and cooperation with and conformity to the group are valued, rather than assertiveness of the individual. Touch or physical contact between business colleagues is avoided. Young adults may be castigated for abruptly leaving home or striving for independence. Consideration for family elders is more important than one's desires to pursue personal goals. In the American culture, a well-developed ego is considered necessary for maturity. In Asian cultures, personal preoccupation with the ego is considered absurd.

Use of time varies with the culture and historical era. For example:

- Before the Industrial Revolution, the smallest unit of time was the day.
- After the Industrial Revolution, money and minutes became important.
- In the Western world, time is seen as a progression of events, of new beginnings. Timetables are important. Appointments are to be kept. Mass transportation and mass media have timetables.
- In both present-day Canada and the United States, people are often hasty and impatient; they want things quickly, immediately, and easily. Canadians and Americans often seem to have lost the ability to sit still. Is it because we live in a hurried culture?
- Measurement of time is now in milliseconds; the societal clock tyrannizes and may be counter to the person's internal clock.

Health may be compromised by how the person uses time, or lets time use him or her. Nurses and health care providers must be attuned to the effects of use of time on themselves and the clients and families they care for.

Comparison of Cultures: Greek, Latino, Japanese, and Middle Eastern

Tables 1-4 through 1-10 (pages 15–21) contrast Greek culture, Latino culture, and Japanese culture. Discussion centres on the family unit, male–female relationships, childrearing, the group versus privacy, time orientation, work and use of leisure time, education, and attitudes toward change. Although many nationality groups fit under the Spanish-speaking category, and each has its unique values and customs, the values, norms, customs, and behaviours described in the tables are applicable to people who have a Spanish or Latino background, whether they are from Spain, Mexico, Puerto Rico, the Caribbean Islands, Central America, or South America. There are variations in these values as individuals or families get integrated into mainstream North American culture. Furthermore, values may be lived differently, outwardly, if the person resides in

Greece, Mexico, or Japan, rather than in North America. Yet, much of the behaviour of a third- or fourth-generation family or person from any of these countries reflects the original cultural and ethnic values. That fact explains differences among groups of people and should not be considered abnormal. Middle Eastern culture is described in the section that follows this one.

The discussion then compares the attitudes of North American residents toward health and illness with the corresponding attitudes in each of these cultures.

Table 1-11 (page 22) summarizes Kluckhorn's presentation of five basic value questions, the range of beliefs derived from these questions, and examples of some subcultural groups adhering to these beliefs. You may wish to assess your clients and their families according to these values and the characteristics presented in Tables 1-4 through 1-10. Although they present neither a comprehensive study nor stereotypes of those in these cultures, these comparisons indicate that subtle as well as obvious differences, along with some similarities, exist among different groups' values and behaviour. Understand that these cultural patterns will be followed by persons in each culture in varying degrees, ignored by some, and not identified yet taken for granted by others. Chapter 4 discusses some of these values in relation to the family culture of the United States and that of Canada.

Focus: Middle Eastern Culture

Many people from the Middle East are migrating to North America because of political unrest in the region and somewhat easier travel possibilities.[†] Many first-generation immigrants come here to study and then become permanent residents in North America. These people strongly maintain their cultural and religious values and practices, which makes them a unique set of clients to provide care for. Even though many of these clients identify with their countries of origin, many also identify with particular families, such as the Seyeds of Iran; with a city or a village they lived in; or with a religion.

Roles. In many Middle Eastern countries, Islam is a dominant religion, and roles in families are dictated by the religion, as well as by the culture of the country. The older generation generally reveres ancestors and authority of family and state, and to a lesser extent, the younger generation also follows these traditions. Men tend to have earning positions in the household, and thus they either cannot or will not help with most or all of the household duties. Women, on the other hand, tend to be in control of household affairs. These roles are clearly divided but complementary. There are some women in these Islamic countries who have professional jobs outside their homes. But in a traditional society and environment, roles tend to be held in a status quo: The woman stays at home, and the man is the wage earner. Children are taught to respect gender role differences.

[†]This section is was written by Caroline Samiezadé-Yazd, RN, PNP, MSN.

TABLE 1–4
A Comparison of Cultures: The Family Unit

Component	Greek	Spanish-speaking	Japanese
Basis for marriage	Social and family welfare. All of society patterned on family.	Family welfare centre.	Value family and household lineage. Family gives sense of purpose.
Type of family system	Paternalistic. Extended. Monogamy. Marriage bond strong.	Paternalistic. Extended. Monogamy. Marriage bond strong. Family cares for ill, needy. Closely knit.	Traditional value on authority of father and elders. Family strongly identified with father. Subordinate position of women and arranged marriage still accepted by older generation.
Family size	Want many children.	Children validate marriage. Large, so parents not alone in old age.	Home, family, children are focus of women. Family planning, including use of abortion to control size in modern family.
Pattern of interaction	Authoritarian; man dominant in conversation and decision making. Man head of house and disciplinarian. Sex roles traditional male and female. Mother powerful in own way; credited with sustaining child with moral strength. Children subordinate. Oldest son responsible for family if husband not present. Child not focus of family activity. No special activities for child; even birthday a time to wish family long happiness with child rather than focus on child. Family together most of time with child learning to enjoy adult behaviour and anticipate adulthood. Peer contacts through family.	Authoritarian. Man head of house. Woman subordinate socially, carries out family decisions. Sex roles traditional male and female. Child not sole focus of attention. Avoid admiration of child for fear of "evil eye." Child proud of home responsibilities. Familism reinforces attachment. Needs of family more important than needs of individual. Age, authority figures, and traditions highly respected. Family loyalty strong. Obedience emphasized. Emphasize affiliation over confrontation; cooperation over competition. Interdependence over independence. Family ties may extend beyond biological relatives, including godparents (compadres), the boss. Warm, demonstrative behaviour. Stand close, touch used. Child may avoid direct eye contact. Modesty about body care and functions and sexuality. Person's dignity important.	Family revered as an institution. Close family relationship although may not express spontaneous companionship and warmth. Major decisions made by family. Subordination of individual to family interest. Traditional autocratic family system stronger in rural areas, with eldest son inheriting family property and hesitant to rebel against father. Young generation choosing own marriage partner, establishing own household, and daughter-in-law gaining freedom from mother-in-law's dominance. Increasing premarital and extramarital sexual affairs.

TABLE 1-5
A Comparison of Cultures: Childrearing Patterns

Component	Greek	Spanish-speaking	Japanese
Process of childbirth	Considered normal process, not to be feared.	Considered normal process. Husband little involved. Prefer woman's presence. Special practices surrounding process.	Considered normal process.
Philosophy of childrearing	Effectiveness sought as parent, not as pal. Child raised to be strong, hard, firm, straight, for that is ideal personality. Wishes of elders put before child's wishes.	Effectiveness sought as parent, not as pal. Child taught to do as parents do, to listen to parents' advice, learn from their experience, and not advance further than their parents.	Traditionally child to be dutiful, disciplined, responsible, respectful to elders. Young urban generations not bound as firmly by traditions.
Practices of childrearing	Mother firm, not over-protective. Baby kept in straight position when carried or in bed. Follow rigid schedule, consistent.	Consistent, traditional, faith in own judgment. Tradition of breastfeeding needs reinforcement if in Anglo health care setting.	Mother enveloping child in warmth during early years, but when child older, relationship more distant. Oldest son reared differently from other brothers, and brothers from sisters, so every child aware of his or her place.
Responsibility for child care	Primarily mother, but older children involved in daily activities, including care of younger siblings. Attitude of love and responsibility among siblings; new baby not seen as competition.	Husband ultimately responsible as head of household. Any family member, including siblings and cousins, responsible at times.	Mother primarily, but all of family involved.
Discipline	Consistent. Obedience very important and taught to child at early age. Child praised when good and told when bad; taught that it is important to be good and not shame family. Use group pressure to set limits on behaviour.	Consistently correct child when behaviour is bothersome and warned not to act in a way to provoke father. Instil fear of consequences Instil pride in self-control and fear of being shamed. Seldom told he or she is "good" or "bad."	Firm, consistent, lack strong emotional expression. Emphasis on responsibility, duty, loyalty, patience, orderliness, cleanliness. Promote feeling of insecurity when doing wrong.

(continued)

TABLE 1-5 *(continued)*
A Comparison of Cultures: Childrearing Patterns

Component	Greek	Spanish-speaking	Japanese
Training of child	Taught to value interdependence, cooperation. Sibling rivalry when new baby arrives but does not last long. Mother delighted with new baby but shares self equally with older child, including offer of free breast during feeding. Older child invited to share excitement about baby. Parents never clown for child's amusement or give many material things.	Taught to value interdependence, companionship Little sibling jealousy. Freely show affection and attention. May use child as translator for family if they are not bilingual.	Taught to value interdependence but responsible for own behaviour. Taught to carry out obligation regardless of personal cost and to control behaviour to avoid personal shame and disgrace of group. Develop strong sense of responsibility, loyalty to family or work group. Poor communication between generations because of differences in experiences, education, language comprehension, and values, fostering problems in modern society. Women's etiquette differs from that for men. Women taught to be passive, modest.

TABLE 1-6
A Comparison of Cultures: Interaction with Others versus Privacy

Component	Greek	Spanish-speaking	Japanese
Basic values of person and behaviour	Strong sense of self-esteem. Inner core of personality not to be exposed or shamed. Value equality, individuality. Aloneness not sought, but borne with fortitude. Pride in glorious past of Greece.	Anxiety about being alone and concern for people who are alone. Not considered proper to compete, push self forward in group through achievements. Better to submit than provoke anger in another. Self-restraint emphasized. Violence atypical.	Strong sense of self-respect and important to be treated respectfully by others. Privacy defined differently than in Canada; seen as loneliness. Group relationships sought and valued.
Personal possessions	Value in shared living and sharing possessions, especially with family and friends.	Sharing of possessions. One's own house nebulous; frequent unannounced visiting among family and friends.	Possessions not highly valued. Shared living space and possessions in family.
Status of person	Valued for what he or she is rather than position or achievement. Family unit valued, not individual.	Valued for what he or she is, depends on family. Child has mother and father's surname, respectively; hyphenated name common.	Belonging to right clique or faction important to status and future success. Try to join influential group at early age.

(continued)

Component	Greek	Spanish-speaking	Japanese
Interaction among persons	Resentment when treated impersonally, mechanically, or like a number on a chart.	Much neighbourhood socializing, especially among women, to borrow, help, consult, discuss, or exchange gifts.	Suppression of emotion and pain in many situations.
	No word for "group," but born into group of family and friends.	Interchange of gifts and services frequent.	Most docile with strong urge to conform.
	Extended family working together for benefit of each other.	Accepting as gracious as giving, and person not satisfied until he or she has returned a gift to show appreciation; return gift not necessarily same kind or form.	Pleasant, polite, correct but aloof behaviour to others in all classes.
	Units of cooperation retained from past, not created.		Use of polite, honorific, correct language to avoid being rude, to show respect and modesty.
	Work to achieve common goal with those to whom individual feels loyalty.	Strangers not completely accepted unless related to established family by marriage.	Concern about language use.
	Speech important because it establishes interactions; expressive of feelings.	Interdependence between family and close friends does not extend to broader community.	Avoids handshake or body contact.
			Restrained, formal, hierarchal relationships in family, company, and political party rather than horizontal, comradely behaviour.
			Ceremonious, at ease, and apologetic to acquaintances and friends but less so with strangers.
			Man unappreciative of domineering woman.
			Wish to avoid confrontation; strive to save face in conflictual situation.
Social activities	Family basic social group.	Few formalized social groups.	Fondness for crowds and physical proximity of people.
	Circle of friends important.	Suspicious of outsiders.	
	Enjoy social affiliations, great loyalty to all groups to which one belongs.	Dependency on others accepted.	Participation and spectator roles in social activities and sports enjoyed.
	Food important with social activities.	Family basic social group.	
		Women thought of as one social group, men another.	
		Remain close to own social group for job or marriage partner.	
		Use of diplomacy, tact, concern, respect for other's feelings.	
		May appear to agree when does not.	
		Child may avoid eye contact or not verbalize feelings, out of deference to elder.	

TABLE 1-7
A Comparison of Cultures: Time Orientation

Component	Greek	Spanish-speaking	Japanese
Concept of time	Present important but prepare for something in future that is sure part of the life. No automatic faith in future. Distasteful to organize activities according to clock. Life regulated by body needs and rhythms, daily pattern of light and dark, and seasons.	Present important but validated by past. Expect future to be like present. Perform with distinction in present rather than emphasize efficiency, quantity. Life not regulated by clock but by body needs and rhythms, light and dark, seasons, religious holidays.	Time neither an absolute nor objective category but a process—the changing of nature with the person as part of it. Planning for future valued. Present considered important, and past priceless. Time is eternal, subjective.
Use of time	Time used spontaneously; not time conscious. Elastic attitude toward time; governed by cycles of nature. "Tomorrow" thought of as tomorrow, next week, or never. Activities and appointments usually not starting on time, person not hurried.	Time used spontaneously; not time conscious. Little emphasis on long-range planning. "Right now" means now or later. May arrive after scheduled appointment time.	Appreciation and effective use of time. Calmness and time for daily ceremony highly valued. Ceremony carried out in spite of rush of work. Emphasize long-range planning.

TABLE 1-8
A Comparison of Cultures: Work and Use of Leisure Time

Component	Greek	Spanish-speaking	Japanese
Concept of work	Work thought of as life, a joy and dignity, not drudgery. Work interrupted primarily for religious reasons, not as claim to idleness or leisure. Women work as hard as men. Tenacious and resourceful at making the best of what they have and coping with difficulty. Person not to be hurried but works efficiently at own pace.	Work considered inevitable part of daily life. Not done just to keep busy or earn more money if present needs met. No moral corruption in being idle. Work at own pace and no specially defined working hours if possible. Everyone expected to cooperate and do his or her part. Work shared to decrease loneliness. Work roles of sexes and age groups distinct but each aware of tasks performed by others. Able to take over work roles of other family members. Child a part of work, of home and family, and feels important. No special rewards.	Enjoyment of work more important than money earned. Industriousness and hard work emphasized. Strong ties between person, the job, and the company. Work hard for success. Job mobility frowned on; loyalty to company valued. Independence in work traditionally valued but younger workers adjusting to Western concept of employment. Seek perfection on job. High sense of responsibility for job; quiet achievement. Consensus management emphasized.

(continued)

TABLE 1-8 *(continued)*
A Comparison of Cultures: Work and Use of Leisure Time

Component	Greek	Spanish-speaking	Japanese
Concept of leisure	Leisure an attitude, a dimension of all life and work. Not confined to certain time but a continual expression of internal freedom, at work or rest.	Leisure synonymous with free time. No emphasis on leisure for own sake. Intersperse work with rest, socialize during work. Free time spent visiting.	Some leisure time used in solitude. Much leisure time spent in travelling with peers and family. Freer expression of emotion in recreational pursuits. Leisure should be useful or educational activity. Little leisure time for children; school studies and work emphasized.

TABLE 1-9
A Comparison of Cultures: Education

Component	Greek	Spanish-speaking	Japanese
Value on education	Highly prized, especially professional education. Curiosity and creativity valued. Educated person accorded much respect. Use of creative intellect and being a cultured citizen valued, but can be achieved through life's experiences and work as well as by education.	Learns that which interests him or her. Absent from school if learning little or if something more interesting going on elsewhere. Not seen as only way to achieve.	Respect for school and teacher. Education highly valued, with emphasis on scientific information. Parents involved in education. Eager to learn. Memorization emphasized. Believe in value of practical experience as well. Choice of college influences status in life. Much competition in education.
Educational methods	Emphasize quickness, curiosity, cleverness, realism, reason. Education applied to matters of life.	No emphasis on excelling or competing against other family members for high grades or honours. Use of native language may interfere with success in school. Competition in learning is avoided if possible.	Educational reforms brought about by American occupation after World War II are counter to traditional methods, which emphasized learning by rote, moral training, unquestioning acceptance of authority, strict discipline, competition for grades, and work rather than leisure activities.

TABLE 1-10
A Comparison of Cultures: Attitudes Regarding Change

Component	Greek	Spanish-speaking	Japanese˙
Value of change	Not valued for itself. Progress hoped for but not taken for granted. Change does not necessarily bring progress or improvement.	Change condemned if simply because it is change. Patience and postponing personal desires emphasized. Appreciate gentle approach. Little faith in progress or control over own destiny.	Physical world considered transient. Person appreciative of but does not cling to things; thus change accepted. Traditional activities, religion, family, and ancestors valued.
Pace of change	Deliberate.	Deliberate. Slow. Fearful or suspicious of change.	Able to adjust lifestyle to rapid economic, industrial, and urban changes.
Effect of change	No value on unlimited progress. Wants what is better than present but what is known and can be achieved. A plan to a Canadian is synonymous with a dream to a Greek. Use material goods. Do not discard useful articles. Repair objects to maintain usefulness. Traditional Greek culture changing, becoming westernized, affecting behaviour of young.	Value system seen as constant. Feel many individuals not amenable to change by human endeavour. Adjust to environment. Use material goods to capacity. Generally remain near traditional home, maintain stable relationships with people. Change in main culture affecting behaviour of young, causing insecurity in elders.	Urgency of Western-like activity a new phenomenon. Breaking traditional patterns and solidarity; increased individualism, competition, and individual insecurity. Youth seeking new values to replace old dogmas.

Muslim society tends to be paternalistic. Children carry the last name of their father as their legal name through their entire life. Even after marriage, women continue to maintain their fathers' family names. Men have a great need to feel in control of situations relating to self and the family, and this may be viewed in Western culture as excessive control of women or family members. The controlling male brings great compliance into the family system through his role of a leader.

Therefore, in the health care setting, it is best to ask the man's permission or opinion with regard to anything that relates to his family members. If this aspect is neglected, the man may feel insulted, and mistrust may develop. In Western culture, this practice is viewed as a type of ownership by the man over his family. However, the Muslim man perceives this as protecting the family for which he is responsible. This

protection can be seen especially with a new mother and baby. In the absence of the husband, the health care provider can communicate through the woman's father or father-in-law, a designated brother or uncle of the husband, or the husband's mother.

In the Middle East, a large portion of a traditional village's female population is illiterate. Therefore, the woman's ability to bear and raise children is the major source of self-esteem and identity. This affords one of the greatest opportunities for a woman to realize her potential as a person. Because women are highly respected for their role as mother, children, even into adulthood, place their mother's needs as paramount. Often, this is done before considering even the wife's or family's needs, which can create an internal strain within the family structure.

TABLE 1–11
Basic Values of Cultures with Selected Cultural Examples

Example of Cultural or Subcultural Value	Range of Beliefs	Group Adhering to Value
Human Nature (What is innate nature of man?)	The person is basically *evil but capable of achieving goodness* with self-control and effort.	Puritan ancestors. Protestants of Pentecostal or Fundamentalist background. Appalachian subculture.
	The person is a *combination of good and evil*, with self-control necessary but lapses in behaviour understood.	Most people in Canada.
	The person is basically *good.*	Some religious groups, such as Society of Friends. Some philosophical groups, such as humanistic psychologists and members of ethical society.
Person–nature (What is relation of person to nature or supernatural?)	The person is *subjugated* to *nature* and cannot change whatever is destined to happen.	Spanish-speaking cultures. Appalachian subculture. Japanese and other Asian cultures.
	The person is to gain *mastery* over *nature;* all natural forces can be overcome.	Middle- and upper-class and highly educated people in Canada.
Time (What is temporal focus of human life?)	*Past time* is given preference; most important events to guide life have happened in the past.	Historic China.
	Present time is the main focus; people pay little attention to the past and regard the future as vague.	Spanish-speaking cultures. Appalachian subculture.
	Future is the main emphasis, seen as bigger and better; people are not content with the present.	Educated, professional, and middle-class people in Canada.
Activity (What is the main purpose in life?)	*Being orientation.* The person is important just because he or she is and may spontaneously express impulses and desires.	Appalachian subculture. Although no culture allows complete expression of impulses and all cultures must have some work done, the Mexican fiesta and Mardi Gras in New Orleans are manifestations of this value.
	Becoming-in-being orientation. The person is important for what he or she is, but must continue to develop.	Most religious cultures. American Indian subcultures. Greek culture.
	Doing orientation. The person is important when active or accomplishing something.	Most people in the United States.
Relational (What is one's relation to other people?)	*Individualistic relations.* These emphasize autonomy; the person does not have to fully submit to authority. Individual goals have primacy over group goal.	Most *Gemeinschaft* societies, such as folk or rural cultures. Yankee and Appalachian subcultures. Middle-class America, with emphasis on nuclear family.
	Collateral relations. These emphasize that the person is part of a social and family order and does not live just for the self. Group or family goals have primacy.	Most European-American ethnic groups, especially Italian-American, Spanish-speaking cultures. American Indian tribal subcultures. Most cultures adhere somewhat through sibling relations in family.
	Lineal relations. These emphasize the extended family and biological and cultural relationships through time. Group goals have primacy.	Cultures that emphasize hereditary lines. Upper-class America. Oriental cultures. Middle East cultures. British culture.
	Relations are impersonal, focused on role behaviour.	Business interactions, upper middle class, and those moving up the social ladder.

Adapted from References 74 and 75

Sexuality and Parenthood. Women do not practise contraception in the Middle East as much as in the West because the traditional role of the female is to bear children. There are, however, many misconceptions about conception, for instance, that conception will not occur during lactation. Such misconceptions are held even by the most educated people. By Islamic law, when contraception is used, it must be a form that will not destroy an already united egg and sperm, such as birth control pills or a condom, because Muslims hold to the belief that life begins at conception. Arabs and Iranians may use

abortion as a form of birth control, although it is not openly recommended or talked about and is clearly prohibited by Islamic law. Selective abortions are resorted to in the case of an illegitimate pregnancy, to maintain the society's integrity, because having illegitimate children and engaging in unsanctioned sexual practices carry grave consequences.[76]

Many Middle Eastern persons possess a feeling of fatalism; they do not plan excessively for future events but rather resign themselves to the will of God. Thus, many women do not seek prenatal care; only when delivery is imminent do they go to the hospital or call a midwife to come to the home for the birthing. Often, women do not plan the layette or select a name until after the baby is born. Traditional as well as modern Middle Eastern women tend to breastfeed for extended periods; the Koran spells out a requirement to breastfeed for two years.[77]

Children in the Middle East are viewed not only as a commodity but also as a blessing to the family. They are something to be cherished; therefore, families invest a great deal emotionally in their children and tend to be lenient in disciplinary matters. Children are usually not physically or verbally abused. Rather, they are distracted away from whatever they are doing that is bad and encouraged to do good things.

Many Middle Eastern parents tend to base the success of their parenthood not on the cognitive skills of their children, but rather on their weight gain, health, and normality. They do not accept any deviations from the normal health status. This author knew a woman from Kuwait who had a younger sister with Down syndrome. While introducing her family, she said, "This is my mother, and this is my abnormal sister." She did not feel her sister was worthy enough to be introduced by her name.

Need for Affiliation. An important aspect of caring for Middle Eastern clients is to recognize their need for affiliation and belonging, which, to them, is central and critical to survival. The strength and importance of the individual are directly related to family members and friends, who are an integral part of their life. Although men and women may be socially segregated, there is considerable and extensive socialization. Middle Eastern people are known for their hospitality, and they emphasize family relations. Visiting among members of the extended family and their friends is a social obligation on all occasions, and children of all ages are included in the visits.

Cleanliness. Although Middle Eastern families may live in crowded situations within their homes, they employ basic measures to ensure cleanliness. They not only maintain strict personal hygiene, they keep their homes in a continuously clean state. The expression "You can eat off the floor" is literally true here because the family does eat off the floor, as well as sit, lie down, and sleep on it. These homes generally have no furniture or are sparsely or very selectively furnished. When you walk into such a home, you are required to remove your shoes to keep the carpet and the floors clean so that everything is done in clean areas. For the Middle Easterner, there exists a definite feeling of separation between the external world and the internal world of their home.

Health Care Practices. Muslims and other Middle Eastern people often have home cures for common health problems. They may believe that cures can be obtained through the use of such remedies as herbs, concentrated sugar preparations, and hot or cold foods. Although they accept the superiority of Western medicine, they do not always trust it; therefore, they use home-remedy medicine alongside modern Western medical practices. If these home or cultural remedies do not harm the client, you should allow the person to apply them. This will serve to build trust in the relationship and show respect for the client.

In the case of medical treatments or drug prescriptions, these clients believe that intrusive measures are of more value than nonintrusive measures. For example, they may believe

that medication given intravenously will be more effective than that given intramuscularly, injections are better than pills, and coloured pills are better than white ones.

Another example of a cultural practice is that when a baby is delivered, parents want to say a prayer in the newborn's ears. Muslims believe that the first thing a child hears should be words from the Koran in praise of and supplication to God. This practice does not hurt the baby, but allowing it will go a long way toward building trust into the relationship with the parents and family.

In the health care setting, the long and crowded visits by family and friends can pose difficulties for the institution that will have specific visiting hour rules and regulations. But for the Middle Eastern client, these visits play an extremely important role in how the person perceives his or her condition and adapts to it. Lack of visitors may make the client think that he or she is gravely ill and close to death when this is not the case at all but only the result of the hospital policy about visitors. Visiting for such clients should be allowed on a more lenient basis. These visits from family members can serve other useful purposes. Middle Eastern clients do not expect personal care from health care providers; family members are expected, and are willing, to provide physical care for the person in the hospital.

Communication. Islam dictates that family affairs remain in the family; they are not the business of the rest of the world. This can be seen in many situations, for example, in the matter of modesty in dress. Women dress differently when they go outside the home from how they do inside the home. The body is completely covered, and only parts of the face and the hands and feet can be seen. For Muslim women residing in the West, this manner of dress is usually modified but still retains the quality of conservative fashion. Thus, respecting the client's modesty during health care or medical procedures is essential. For reasons of modesty, there is a difference in how information is given to various people. Very personal information is shared only with intimate contacts; nonintimate or general information can be shared with almost anyone. Thus, assessment has to be done in gradual steps and with respect. You may never be able to obtain certain information from the client or family.

Communication in the Middle East is an elaborate system. It can be either very intimate in terms of content and word usage, or it can be very stilted, using only proper nouns and formal forms of verbs. The choice depends on whom you are talking to and the subject of discussion. A person may knowingly say the opposite of what he or she is thinking to avoid being rude. There are communication methods to avoid, especially in nonintimate conversations, because they are perceived as offensive and rude. First, showing anger and speaking words that might seem insulting are considered bad manners. Emotion can be shown only with intimate persons but not with nonintimate contacts. Second, being abrupt or interrupting when someone is speaking, especially with elders, is unacceptable. Third, in preliminary casual conversation that is part of business or professional association, a man must not ask another man about the female members of his family, including his wife, sisters, or daughters after they reach age of puberty. A woman asking about female members is considered acceptable. It is important to use the person's title (Mr., Mrs., Dr., and so on) until permission is given by the client to do otherwise.

As in all populations, communication and teaching become critical issues related to health outcome. Individuality should never be viewed as noncompliance. There are generally reasons for a Muslim's behaviour or choice of action. Not carrying out a health care professional's instructions does not mean that the Muslim patient is being uncooperative. You should reassess the situation in terms of its cultural totality.

Language Barriers. Interpreters or family members can be used to assist with teaching when the client's language is not known by the health care worker; however, family members may withhold information that they feel may be too upsetting for the client to hear or inappropriate to disclose about the client. If interpreters are used, they should be of the same language, religion, and country of origin. A mistake was made in one agency when a Muslim woman from Iraq was asked to interpret in Arabic instructions to a new Muslim mother from Saudi Arabia, without first having obtained her husband's consent. When the father of the baby discovered this arrangement for his wife to learn newborn care through an Iraqi woman, he became angry and would not allow it. Involve family members when doing client teaching, and always attempt to involve both the husband and the wife in discussions. In the event that the health care provider needs to talk to a woman about her husband, extreme tact should be used at all times during the discussion.

Language barriers can cause a great amount of misunderstanding. It can take many years for a foreign person to learn a language, and usually building a vocabulary is the most difficult part of any language mastery. However, with many foreigners, even though their English vocabulary may not be strong, their grammar and word usage are correct. It would, therefore, be useful to listen to the themes of whatever is being discussed, rather than to the exact words being used.

When giving educational instructions to an individual or a family, remember that some people, to avoid embarrassment and to save face, may pretend to understand your communication, when in reality they do not understand enough to take responsibility for their own or their family's health needs or care. It is best in these situations, if an interpreter cannot be procured, to use short simple sentences containing easy-to-understand words and to speak slowly and clearly (but not loudly!). It is also best to communicate with the client using the same sentence each time. Saying, "How are you today?" one day and then, "How are you feeling?" the next time may be confusing to someone who is struggling with the language. It is also best to avoid slang and unconventional English because, like many other non-English-speaking people, most Middle Easterners, when learning English, learn and cling to the security of proper English.

Sometimes you may have to rely on nonverbal means of teaching. Although there may be cultural differences in body language, some nonverbal communication methods to express certain emotions, such as fear, pain, and sadness, may be similar in any culture. Teaching can also be accomplished by physically demonstrating on yourself or on the patient himself or herself. Pictures can be drawn to illustrate something, or bilingual flash cards can be used to aid teaching. Bilingual cards can be particularly useful because the teacher and the learner will both know what the cards are saying and therefore have some

basis for communication. These cards can be used at other times when interpreters and family are not available, for example, during the night when the client wants to use the bathroom, to communicate basic instructions to the client. Although this appears to be a simplistic means of communication, it can be very effective and serve to decrease frustration and anxiety in both the client and the health care professional.

Differences in Values. Middle Eastern clients do not give too much importance to time schedules; this Western value and practice is usually an imposition on Middle Eastern people. Time factors for these people tend to be in terms of what is important at that moment, rather than rigid projections into the future as to what is important. This can cause conflicts in a health care setting, where tests and other health care appointments are scheduled at particular times and the client may not feel that these appointments have to be kept. The client may view taking a bath and being clean as more of a priority and assume that the test can wait or be rescheduled for later.

Middle Eastern clients expect health care practitioners to find effective cures without asking many questions or using numerous diagnostic tests, which are often needed for a correct diagnosis. They believe that if a doctor or nurse asks too many questions or orders too many tests, the practitioner lacks confidence and experience and has a narrow perspective and poor understanding and therefore should not be trusted. These clients prefer older male doctors, preferably heads of departments in their specialty area, rather than younger or female doctors. The exception is that a female obstetrician or gynecologist is usually required for a woman who is pregnant or has a gynecological disorder. Generally, many Middle Eastern clients do not trust doctors completely because they feel doctors are too expensive, ask too many questions, and often lack experience.

Islamic laws strictly prohibit deviant sexual practices, premarital sex, adultery, and use of illegal drugs or alcohol. Thus, the associated diseases (e.g., AIDS, other sexually transmitted diseases, alcoholism, fetal alcohol syndrome, and so on) are virtually nonexistent in this population.

These clients prefer dealing with the same caregiver each day; this increases trust and acceptance in the relationship and decreases suspicion of the health care provider in the client and the family. Having the same caregiver also helps decrease mistrust of Western medicine, which these clients really do not understand thoroughly. A nurse can achieve positive relationship outcomes by being the consistent caregiver.

The Middle Eastern and Latino client believes that if somebody compliments a person about something that is good or of value, such as jewellery or a new baby, or even looks at it in admiration, this behaviour will bring about the "evil eye." The **evil eye** is a form of superstitious jealousy and mistrust of the admirer by the owner of the object being complimented.

In the health care setting, avoid being suspected of having the evil eye by directing compliments to the owner or to God (Allah), rather than to the object itself. This is considered to convert the possibility of the evil eye and misfortune into a blessing instead.

Legal Documents. An important area of client concern is legal documents. It is recommended that birth certificates and other legal documents be signed by both the father and the mother of the baby. In the United States, statistical agencies of state governments feel that only the mother is the verifiable parent of a child. This consideration can be very insulting to a patrilineal father. By having both parents sign the birth certificate or legal documents, the possibility of the father feeling insulted can be avoided and both the state and family will have their needs met.

Consent forms are generally not used in the Middle East. First, the client does not feel he or she has the knowledge to assume responsibility for health decisions and therefore would prefer to leave this responsibility to the health care professional who has been trained to make these decisions. Second, in Islam, a man's word and agreement, especially in front of witnesses, are considered binding, and written documentation is therefore deemed not necessary. When a consent form needs to be signed after an agreement has been made, the client and his or her family can interpret such a request with mistrust and suspicion toward the health care provider. To avoid this, one physician found that if the consent form was just presented in an institutionally oriented, matter-of-fact way, mistrust was minimized, and clients carried through with the required procedures.

Religious Beliefs. Not all Middle Eastern clients are Muslims; some may be followers of other religions, and their lifestyle and health care practices may be influenced by their religious beliefs. Chapter 3 discusses additional practices to be considered in a person's care based on different religious beliefs.

Without a proper understanding of Middle Eastern culture, caring for these patients can be a very frustrating experience, but when you understand that the values of this culture have meaning for these Middle Eastern clients, it becomes an enjoyable and rewarding experience. When you have established trust with the person and his or her family, you will see other aspects of their lives opening up to you. This new perspective will enrich your relationship with your client and the quality of the care you provide to him or her.

Attitudes toward Health and Illness

How health is identified, physically and emotionally, varies from culture to culture, as do ideas about the factors related to health and disease.

Canadian Culture. In the Canadian culture literature, new definitions of health have evolved from a medical (physiological) to a behavioural (lifestyle) approach. These definitions have not only enlarged the scope of social objectives but have improved Canadians' understanding of what makes them healthy and well. This shift to a behavioural approach has led to a focus on developing interventions linked to disease prevention and health promotion.[78] Primary Health Care (PHC), which has been adopted by the World Health Organization (WHO) and Canada, is essential health care that focuses on preventing illness and promoting health.[79]

The recent health care trend indicates that many Canadians are making impressive efforts to improve their health. One of the key determinants that influences population health is personal health practices and coping skills. Almost half of the Canadian population age 12 and older reported changing some behaviour to improve their health prior to the 1997–1998 National Population Health Survey. Behaviour changes toward improved health were reported most often in Ontario (50%) and least often in Saskatchewan (39%). However, there remains considerable room for improvement in personal health practices. The proportion of overweight men and women in Canada has increased steadily between 1985 and 1996–1997: from 22 to 34 percent among men, and from 14 to 23 percent among women. Body weights above the healthy weight range (i.e., Body Mass Index over 27) are linked to a variety of health problems, including cardiovascular disease, diabetes, and some forms of cancer.[80] A Canadian study estimated the direct costs related to the treatment of, and research into, obesity in Canada in 1997. The result indicated that the total direct cost was estimated to be over 1.8 billion dollars.[81] In addition, Martin states that the Health Canada Report, "Economics: Burden of Illness in Canada 1998," estimates that the direct and indirect costs associated with illness, injury, and premature death in Canada reached $159.4 billion in 1998, or roughly $5,310 for every Canadian. Males accounted for 52.4 percent of the total.[82]

CRITICAL THINKING

In what ways can costs associated with illness, injury, and premature death be reduced for the male population?

For Canadians, health care has become the top national priority as observed in the recent federal election.[83] In the past decade, a review of polls, surveys, and reports indicates that Canadians cherish a number of values related to health care. In fact, the most in-depth examination of Canadians' values related to health and health care was completed by the National Forum on Health during the mid-1990s.[84] The National Forum established four working groups. One group was the values working group, which identified eight values that are supported widely by the Canadian public. These values are: (1) equality of access, (2) compassion, (3) dignity and respect, (4) efficiency/effectiveness, (5) collective responsibility, (6) personal responsibility, (7) quality, and (8) thriftiness/responsible stewardship/accountability.[85] Canadians identified equality of access and quality of care as the critical values in relation to the health care system. Equality of access refers to everyone having equal access to care based on need and not the ability to pay. This value was viewed as the key feature of Canada's health care system and illustrated the difference in values between Canada and the United States.[86] Measurements of support for the principles of the 1984 *Canada Health Act* are undertaken frequently in order to determine whether or not Canadians support the fundamental values of their health care system. Results have indicated that out of the five principles (universality, accessibility, portability, comprehensiveness, and public administration), the highest supported principle has been universality, while the lowest support measured was public administration,[87] which has indicated clearly that Canadians still believe in universality and that Medicare is highly valued. At a symbolic level, Canadians believe that Medicare is part of Canada's identity; and Canadians resist changes that might destroy or weaken that symbol.[88] The result of a 1999 Ekos survey indicated that 72 percent of Canadians agreed with the statement "Universal publicly funded health care is part of what it means to be Canadian and reflects our core values: we would be a poorer society if we shifted to a two-tier system".[89]

In the past two decades, Canadians' values have gradually shifted toward greater personal autonomy, empowerment, and the desire to make choices on their own in a wide range of areas. They are collaborating with their health care providers about their treatments, accessing health information online, and discussing the information that they have obtained with their family physician. Mendelsohn states that one must be cautious not to overstate the extent to which Canadians are prepared to use the Internet for health related matters. Few Canadians buy health products online, and many are still wary of the Internet. Many older Canadians, who are more economically vulnerable, will probably never be comfortable with computers.[90]

CRITICAL THINKING

What is your personal view regarding the value of Medicare?

American Culture. Attitudes in the United States toward health are influenced considerably by society's emphasis on mastery of the environment as opposed to adjustment to it. Illness is seen as a challenge to be met by mobilizing resources: research, science, funds, institutions, and people. Because independence is highly valued, even the weak are expected to help themselves as much as possible, and self-care is emphasized. A person is evaluated on productivity or "doing well." Because the ability to be productive depends, in part, on health, individual health is highly valued. Health, in the broadest sense, is considered necessary for successful interaction with others, educational accomplishment, ability to work, leadership, childrearing, and capacity to use opportunities. Medical, nursing, and other health sciences and technology are considered important. The physical causes of illnesses are generally accepted. Recently, however, the psychological and sociocultural causes of diseases have come to the forefront.

The United States is proud of the scope of its medical research, technologically advanced medical care, and highly qualified health care professionals. It devotes a large share of national income to medical care. Yet, it is more economical, more effective, and easier to keep people healthy than it is to cure disease. Doctors, researchers, and medical care facilities have little effect on general health if the population lacks basic disease prevention and health promotion measures.

Common trends that continue to affect health and health care in the United States and the United Kingdom include the following:[91,92,93]

- Increasing numbers of elderly people, both well and ill
- High mortality from cancer, stroke, and heart disease
- Use of advanced technology in medicine and nursing

- New emphasis on family practice
- Greater acuity of illness in hospitalized patients
- Reduced length of stay in hospitals
- Greater need for aftercare in the community
- Expansion of hospital-based practice into the community
- Continuing inequities in health care

In the United States, and to some extent in other countries, there is continuing health care crisis, in the form of (1) escalating costs, (2) a shifting of burden of payment from the federal to state and local governments and the individual, (3) less regulation of health care planning, (4) expanding corporate enterprise in health care services, (5) greater competition among health care facilities and higher enrolment in prepaid group medical practices or health maintenance organizations, and (6) a rising level of consumer activism in individual and community health matters. People are increasingly concerned about and involved in caring for themselves and others as the health care system faces decreasing economic resources.[94,95,96]

There is increasing focus on:

- Interdisciplinary care, coordination, and integration of services
- Health care practitioners being responsible for changes in the health care system, and health care based on societal changes
- Wellness and prevention programs
- Care of populations and communities
- Awareness and reduction of risk factors
- Intensive use of information
- Consumer or client evaluation of services
- Outcomes of intervention, rather than process of intervention
- Providing same or better care, with fewer resources, as a result of Medicare, Medicaid, and welfare reform

Greek Culture. In Greece, health is important and desired, but it is not a preoccupation. The attitude is that one should not pamper the self. Straight living gives a healthy body; thus, fortitude, hardiness, and simple living are pursued. Excesses in living—in eating, drinking, or smoking—are avoided, and, in general, the level of public health is high. Because children are prized, their health needs take precedence over adults' needs.

Staying in bed is considered a sign of weakness, except for certain recognized disease. People do not go to a physician unless there is something seriously wrong; but then they expect the physician, who is a father figure, to have the answers to all their health problems. Home remedies and the services of an herbalist are tried first as treatment. Prayers are said, and vows are made. Illness is thought to arise from evil or supernatural sources that can be counteracted through the practice of magic. The hospital is seen as the last resort. The whole family becomes involved when one member is sick; each person has a specific role to play, and a role gap exists in the family during illness.

The organs of highest significance are the eyes, for they are believed to reflect the real person. Next in importance are the lips because of the words that come out of them. A girl's hair and a man's moustache are important symbols of sexual identity and attractiveness. The genital organs are not openly discussed but are respected for their reproductive functions. The body is meant to be kept covered, and exposed only when necessary. Dress and ornamentation are essential to complete one's body image.

Childlessness is unfortunate and the woman may be held responsible. Women generally dislike any examination or treatment of the reproductive organs and are resigned to gynecological problems; they would not seek medical care for fear that the treatments may affect their fertility. Special care is given to women during pregnancy, when special regulations about hygiene, rest, activity, and a happy environment are followed.

Handicapped persons are not easily accepted because of the emphasis on a whole, strong, firm body. To be crippled, blind, or lame means that one is not a whole person, is dependent, and is unable to do anything for oneself.

Greek-Americans adhere to some or many of the aforementioned values and practices, depending on how close their cultural ties are.

Latino Culture. Attitudes among Latinos in the American southwest (or other Spanish-speaking people) are very unlike attitudes in mainstream America. Spanish-American people consider the self to be a whole person; thus, "better health" has no meaning. Good health is associated with the ability to work and fulfill normal roles; for one can gain and maintain respect by meeting one's responsibilities. Criteria of health are a sturdy body, ability to maintain normal physical activity, and absence of pain.

Acculturation, *the process of change occurring as a result of contact between cultural groups*, is demonstrated by a minority group's adoption of the larger group's cultural mores. It is assumed that the Latinos who retain Spanish as their first language and who do not follow American norms and values are much less likely than their more assimilated counterparts to use health services. Access to and availability of services, attitudes toward screening processes, values about privacy, and sociodemographic factors are strong determinants of Latino health practices.[97,98]

The role of the family is important in time of illness. The head of the house, the man, determines whether illness exists and what treatment is to be given. The affected person goes to bed when too ill to work or move. Treatment from a lay healer is sought if family care does not help. A physician is called only when the person becomes gravely ill. There is a a lot of visiting, and so the sick person does not get the rest and isolation advised by health care professionals in the majority culture. The sick person does not withdraw from the group; doing so would only make him or her feel worse. Acceptance of fate amounts to saying, "If the Lord intends for me to die, I'll die." The discomfort of the present is considered, but not in terms of future complications. Being ill brings no secondary advantage of care or coddling. Communicable diseases are hard to control, for resistance to isolation is based on the idea that family members, relatives, and familiar objects cannot contaminate or cause illness. Taking home remedies, wearing special objects, and performing special ceremonies are accepted ways to achieve getting and staying well. The person feels he or she will keep well by observing the ritual calendar, being brotherly, and being a good Catholic and member of the community. If the health care provider uses any procedure, such as a diagnostic x-ray, it is considered to be the treatment that should cure the person.[99,100]

Accidents are feared because they disrupt the wholeness of the person. In addition, Latinos fear surgery, the impersonality of the hospital and nurses, and any infringement on their sense of modesty. The hospital represents death and isolation from family and friends. The "professional" (Anglo) approach of the majority culture is regarded as showing indifference to their needs and as causing anxiety and discomfort.

Several authors have described the specific health care practices of Spanish-speaking people and families and the nursing implications, including those for childbirth, childbearing, and prevention of communicable diseases. They also discuss customs related to the use of folk medicine, use of surnames, and customs of interaction.[101]

Japanese Culture. Attitudes in Japan toward health strongly reflect the belief in a body–mind–spirit interrelationship. Spiritual and temporal affairs in life are closely integrated; thus, health practices and religion are closely intertwined, influenced considerably by the magico-religious practices of Shinto, Japan's ancient religion. Bathing customs stem from Shinto purification rites, for example, and baths are taken in the evening before eating, not only for cleanliness but for ceremony and relaxation as well.

There is strong emphasis on a healthy diet (low in fat and sugar), physical fitness, an intact body, physical strength, determination, family and group relationships, and long life. Self-discipline in daily habits is highly valued, as are the mental, spiritual, and aesthetic aspects of the person. All of these values and traits not only promote health but also remain equally important to the sick person to promote recovery.

As a child, the individual is taught to minimize reactions to injury and illness. Hence, to the Westerner, a sick person

1-1 BONUS SECTION IN CD-ROM
Attitudes toward Health and Illness—Latino

Did you ever hear an older person speak of someone giving an "evil eye"? This section provides some insight into where the expression might have originated. You will learn as well about some of the attitudes that Latino people have about health and illness.

may appear unnecessarily stoic. Part of the reserve in express-ing emotion and pain is due to the influence of childrearing and interaction practices, which emphasize correct behaviour and suppression of emotion. Yet the sick person, as much as one who is well, expects to be treated with respect and resents being addressed abruptly or informally by first name. Japanese also resent people entering the hospital room with-out knocking. The Japanese man resents being dominated by a woman, and he may feel uncomfortable with an American female health care professional because he may misinterpret her demeanour as overbearing. Japanese are eager to cooper-ate with the medical care program and wish to be included in planning and decisions regarding care. The normal profes-sional approach of the average North American health care provider is likely to offend the average Japanese person, although he or she may be too polite to say so.

Culture and Nursing Care

By studying life patterns of people in various cultures (espe-cially those of patients to whom you provide nursing care) and by taking into account the factors discussed in the follow-ing chapters on religion and family, you can better under-stand and handle varying levels of health, health problems, and care of different groups of patients. Vargus and Koss-Chioino, in their edited book, present strategies for caring for children and adolescents of a number of ethnic and racial cultures, including foster-care children and middle-class African-American adolescents, American Indian youth, Asian-American youth and first-generation American families, Hispanic children and Latino gang members, and Southeast Asian families.

SOCIOECONOMIC LEVEL SUBCULTURE

Research on social stratification indicates that a person's class position is influenced by economic and social status

and political power of the family and affects the formation of values, attitudes, and lifestyles. Each class in any country tends to have a more or less specified set of values and role expectations regarding practically every area of human activity: sex, marriage, male–female and parent–child responsibilities and behaviour, birth, death, education, dress, housing, home furnishings, leisure, reading habits, occupational status, politics, religion, and status sym-bols.[102] In turn, health status in Canada and the United States is closely linked to income level. What seems natural and logical in determining status to some people may be rejected by others.

Vulnerable populations *are social groups, often poor, but they may be in the middle or even upper economic levels. They are people who are often subordinated or discriminated against, mar-ginalized, or disenfranchised.* They have low social status and lack power in social and political relationships and experience relatively more illness, premature death, and lower quality of life overall than comparable groups; these misfortunes are related to lack of resources and increased exposure to risk.

Some of these populations, especially ethnic people of colour, are viewed as a threat to job security of others, and any one of the vulnerable population groups are frequently threat-ened with or are targets of violence.[103]

As you gain general knowledge about values and lifestyles of people in various economic levels, realize that no one person encompasses all that the literature describes. Knowledge about lifestyles is generally useful to your prac-tice, but you should avoid stereotyping people based upon this knowledge.

Profile of Socioeconomic Levels in Canada

Defining socioeconomic classes in Canada is difficult because one's social class standing on one dimension contradicts, or is inconsistent with, that individual's position on another dimen-sion.[104] For example, counsellors may enjoy high prestige but

NARRATIVE VIGNETTE

Note: Prior to addressing the issues raised in this Narrative Vignette you will need to obtain a blank Nursing Assessment Form.

You are the coordinator of a Nurse-Managed Clinic recently opened in a culturally diverse segment of the city. You have a staff of four nurses working with you. Two members of your staff are recent graduates, and the others have considerable experience working in hospitals in the same district. While unpacking materials for the new unit, you notice a box of standard nursing assessment forms. You read the instrument with special attention to how it will

apply to the diverse cultural array of clients who appear at your clinic.

1. What information, beyond that addressed on the stan-dard form, should be included on a form used in a cul-turally diverse setting?
2. Are the questions on the standard form culturally acceptable? Consider, for example, questions concern-ing allergies, family support, and discharge plans.
3. What changes, if any, will you make for the Nursing Assessment Form to be used in your clinic?

yet receive low pay. Social mobility, which occurs during one's life, may blur the boundaries of social class. Consider the implications when someone wins a lotto and immediately begins to climb the social class ladder. However, despite such problems of categorizing people, four general social classes are considered in Canada: the upper class, the middle class, the working class, and the lower class.[105]

The Upper Class
In Canada, some 3 to 5 percent of the population's income is inherited or acquired from such investments as stocks and bonds or real estate. Income, however, is only one aspect of wealth, and for the upper class, wealth often comes from inheritance.[106] One significant feature of this upper class is that its members attain the highest level of education. The upper class may be divided into two levels. The upper-upper class comprises the 1 percent of the Canadian population referred to as "society." Children from such families attend private schools and well-known universities. The lower-upper class comprises the remaining 2 to 4 percent of the upper class. These people are seen as the "working rich"; and they usually depend upon their earnings as their primary source of income, rather than their inherited wealth.

The Middle Class
The Canadian middle class comprises around 40 to 50 percent of the population. This segment of the population encompasses a much wider ethnic and racial diversity than does the upper class; consequently, it exerts great influence on the patterns of North American culture. This broad middle class also includes two levels. The upper-middle class reflects incomes ranging from $50 000 to $100 000 per year. They tend to have a nice home and accumulate property, such as recreational property. Most people in this class have a university education and prestigious occupations, such as lawyer, engineer, or professor. The other middle class is known as the average-middle class. These people usually work in white collar positions, such as bank teller, or are middle managers. Most of them are high-school graduates, own a comfortable home, and send their children to a local college or university.

The Working Class
The working class contains about one-third of the population and is sometimes referred to as the lower-middle class. They occupy blue-collar jobs and their salaries tend to be below the national average. Their homes are likely to be in lower-cost neighbourhoods, and their children are less likely to attend universities.

The Lower Class
In Canada, the lower class makes up about 20 percent of the population and has the lowest family income. This section of the population is known as the "working poor" because their income is unable to meet all of the basic necessities, such as food, shelter, and clothing. Some of this population survive on social welfare. Those who are employed often have jobs that provide a minimal income and little inner satisfaction. Many in this class are functionally illiterate.

Canada is, thus, a stratified society in which certain groups are more vulnerable to poverty than others due to the unequal distribution of both income and wealth. Most of these disadvantaged people are women, children, persons with disabilities, or Aboriginal people.[107,108] In fact, family poverty is deep and widespread in Canada today.[109]

What then can be said about Canada's socioeconomic classes and the health of Canadians? Roos and Mustard claim that health varies with socioeconomic status.[110] One example is that those who are better educated and have higher incomes can expect to have better health. According to these researchers, the general health status of the lower and middle socioeconomic groups will depend primarily on changes in social policy, such as improvement of educational opportunities. One study, conducted by Kosteniuk and Dickinson (Department of Sociology, University of Saskatchewan) found that higher household income, being retired, and growing older are significantly associated with lower stress levels.[111] Higher-income Canadians experience greater levels of control and social support, while older Canadians experience lower rates of social support but higher rates of social involvement. When the effects of low income on infant health were studied, the researchers concluded that less than sufficient household incomes were associated with poorer health and higher hospital admissions in the first five months of life. This occurred even after adjusting for factors known to affect infant health, including the mother's level of education.[112] Similar results were found by another group of Canadian researchers who concluded that children from poor families have more health problems than do children from better-off families. Furthermore, children of single mothers have more health problems than do children from two-parent families.[113] Another Canadian study of 6748 women age 20–64 years found that women in the lowest income group are about five times more likely to report poor or marginal health. Not surprisingly, those with higher incomes are more likely to report better health.[114]

CRITICAL THINKING

What is your perception of the socioeconomic class system in Canada? As a health professional, how can you effectively deal with social inequality as you endeavour to promote health for all?

Profile of Socioeconomic Levels in the United States

The Upper-Upper, Affluent, or Corporate Level
This level consists of a relatively small number of people who own a disproportionate share of personal wealth and whose income is largely derived from ownership of investments, business, and property. One percent of the population

in the United States owns about one-third of the nation's wealth.

For these privileged few, destiny is abundance and limitless possibility. They are confident that life will be rewarding. Even crisis, such as illness or surgery, can be made into something basically pleasant, for the best of specialized health care professionals and comprehensive facilities can be obtained, and convalescence frequently involves a trip to and rest at a secluded place.[115,116,117]

The Lower-Upper Level

This group consists of people whose wealth is more recently acquired and who have become well-known and influential. These 9 percent own about one-third of the nation's wealth. These people are well-known entertainers; chairpersons of technology, data information, and banking systems; famous doctors or lawyers; and athletes. Or they may be less famous, such as stock and insurance investors and brokers, manufacturers, international businessmen, or employees who have benefited from their company's stock options. They have large incomes, homes, and opulent lifestyles that show off their money. These individuals who are billionaires and millionaires have accumulated wealth through the stock market and also technology rather than by traditional methods, such as manufacturing. They have social position and prestige because of what they *do*.

The Over Class

The United States now has a new social class, the **over class**, *professionals and managers who are upwardly mobile, know wealth and intelligence are not the same, and have earned this lifestyle through hard work*. Although people in this group have interests and a culture in common, they are the new American elite, a part of businesses or fields of work that bright and ambitious people want to enter (not political leadership). Members of this group are likely to be urban singles and couples without children. If the couple has children, they are likely to employ a nanny instead of using daycare.

The Upper-Middle Level

This group, the top third of the middle class, is described as those who are well off and are considered to be the backbone of the community. Income is high but varies, depending on occupation and geographic area, and accumulating property and investments is important. Each spouse is college-educated and at least one is a professional—doctor, dentist, engineer, business manager, or lawyer. The main work of these people is intellectual instead of manual, requires professional training, and offers upward mobility. The workplace is as important to the spouse as to the employed member.

This group has a relatively carefree lifestyle because money is not a major issue. Movement, gaiety, creativity, leisure activities, fun in indoor or outdoor sports, dancing, theatre, museums, travel or educational experiences, acquiring a deeper self-knowledge and self-control, and remaining

youthful are major foci. One image is that of the serious-minded sportsman.[118,119,120,121]

The Middle Level

The middle economic level sometimes is divided in two categories: those who reached the American dream and those who have a comfortable existence. Members of the American dream group have education above the high-school level in a professional or specialized school and include business people with small or medium-sized enterprises, self-employed business people, artists, skilled workers, office and sales workers, and public or private school teachers, and clergy. Nurses and other health care professionals typically are in this level. Members of the *comfortable existence* group tend to have less education and fewer material goods than the first group, but they live comfortably. They have more than the necessities and are somewhat active in the community.[122,123,124,125,126,127,128,129,130]

The people in this group use the internist, family-practice physician, paediatrician, and nurse practitioner for routine health care, but the services of specialists are used when indicated. They see themselves as knowledgeable about health and appreciate and try to use additional information. The group's values correspond closely to those of the dominant society previously described (Table 1-3).

The Lower-Middle or Working Level

This group is often perceived as those who are just getting by. Generally both spouses have graduated from high school and may attend community college. They both have jobs as industrial or blue-collar workers, clerical or service workers, agricultural wage earners, technicians, skilled or semiskilled workers, telephone operators, or waitpersons.[131,132,133] Chances for advancement are minimal unless the person pursues further education. Job security is threatened by the effects of automation in the workplace. Many workers who are a part of this economic level are proud of their work, do it very well, and know that they make an important contribution to society. They value traditional values listed in Table 1-3.

Health care is sought when a person is too sick to work—the group's definition of illness. Prevention is emphasized less than in the foregoing economic levels. People may try home or folk remedies first and then seek medical care. The neighbourhood health centre will be used if one exists. Dental care is more likely to be neglected than other medical care. Individuals and families in this level respond well to an approach that is respectful, personable, prompt, and thorough. They do not understand why health care should be so costly, and they may omit very expensive treatments or drugs whenever possible.[134]

The Upper-Lower Level

This group is perceived as those who are having a really hard time. The family is often only one step away from poverty and welfare. An individual has fewer chances of acquiring education. Thus, people work at menial tasks, usually in non-union jobs, but are proud to be working. Wages and job benefits are a concern.[135] Individuals may work as domestics, gardeners, hospital or school maintenance or cafeteria workers, junk collectors, garbage collectors, or street cleaners. Often neither husband nor wife has completed high school.

Values of individuals in this level are similar to the traditional values of the lower-middle level, with greater emphasis on thrift and conformity to external authority (see Table 1-3).

The Underclass

Poor people, the underclass, include those who are in acute poverty and those in chronic poverty. These comprise children, adults, elderly people, the homeless, migrant workers and their families, refugees, and new immigrants. Chronically ill and divorced women with low incomes are also included in this category. According to Free,[136] one-fourth of American families is, or will be, poor at some time. It is estimated that 45 percent of poor persons in the United States are children. Children reared by single mothers, especially if African-American or Hispanic, are more likely to be living in poverty. The mothers frequently have jobs, but the pay is too low to lift the family out of poverty.[137] *Elderly people* continue to be at risk for poverty because of legislative and economic trends in the United States. Elderly people in rural areas are more likely to be poor than are urban elderly persons, and the poverty increases with age. People over age 85 are especially vulnerable. Migrant workers and their families also suffer poverty and its effects. The **migrant family** *is one with children under age of compulsory school attendance that moves from one geographic region to another for the purpose of working in agricultural production and harvest of tree and field crops and that receives 50 percent of its income from this activity.* Refugees and newly arrived immigrants face harsh economic and social conditions, which places them in acute and chronic poverty.

Poverty in North America

Poverty has two definitions. **Poverty** is *having inadequate pretax money or source of income to purchase a minimum amount of goods and services.* Poverty is also a power issue. It is the relative lack of an individual's access to and control over environmental resources. Poverty reflects class and racial stratification and hopelessness and is seen in increasing homelessness and health problems that result from the conditions of poverty. The person or family in **acute poverty** *has reduced economic means for a limited time because of given circumstances but anticipates being able to return to work and a better lifestyle.* The person or family in **chronic poverty** *has a long family history of being unemployed and without adequate economic means and is unlikely to see much opportunity for improvement,*[138] which is compounded by lack of access to affordable housing or health benefits. **Near poverty** *is defined as families with incomes between 100 and 185 percent of the federal poverty line.* **Extreme poverty** *is defined as families with income of less than half of the poverty line.*[139]

Who Is Poor?

Children, adults, elderly people, homeless people, migrant workers and their families, refugees, and new immigrants are poor. Further, chronically ill and unemployed persons and divorced women all may become poor. Poor people may be of any race or ethnic group.

Children are poor. Too many children born and reared in poverty never grow up to be economically productive members of society. They are more likely to drop out of school, have children out of wedlock, and be unemployed.

Elderly people continue to be at risk for poverty, especially in the United States because of legislative and economic trends. *Elderly people in rural areas* are more likely to be poor than are urban elderly persons, and the poverty increases with age. *People over age 85* are especially vulnerable. Poverty rates are higher for all rural demographic subgroups, including ethnic minorities, than for all urban demographic subgroups because of past employment experiences, education, and living arrangements. Often elderly people have had less pension or insurance coverage and less lifetime earnings, and thereby, they have less accumulated economic resources and lower Social Security benefits. Older women are particularly dependent on the marital union for economic well-being. To prevent poverty in future elderly people, employment prospects and strategies for retirement planning for today's young adults and middle-agers are highly important. Policies related to death and divorce benefits are also critical.[140]

Homeless people are also poor, sometimes acutely or newly poor. The duration of homelessness varies from a short time to many years, depending on the cause and the type of social services and assistance available to the person. People of all ages and all walks of life are among the homeless. Becoming a single parent or working at low-paying jobs adds to the risk of living on the street, especially if living with family members is not an alternative. The homeless population is younger and better educated; there are an increasing number of women with children and even entire family units. The homeless are represented by all racial groups and geographic areas. About one-third are chronically mentally ill, and about one-third are chemically dependent; however, being homeless for some period also brings stressors that contribute to a decline in both physical and mental health.

Refugees are poor. According to the U.S. *Refugee Act* of 1980, a *refugee* is a person who is involuntarily living outside the habitual residence or country of nationality, who is persecuted or fears persecution on return because of race, religion, nationality, social group membership, or political opinion. Refugees have a physical health screening before they leave their home country to come to Canada or the United States. However, immunizations are given on arrival. Because of their life experiences as refugees, a variety of physical health problems may arise after arrival. Mental health problems may arise because of losses suffered in the country of origin, living in refugee camps, torture, as well as culture shock and scapegoating on arrival in Canada and the United States and thereafter.[141]

Refugees who are suddenly displaced because of war, such as we have seen in Southeast Asia, Europe, and the Middle East, may be forced to a country that is not their choice with only the meagre goods they can carry. Physical and mental health is taxed, often to the point of death. These scars, physical and mental, have to be considered when they arrive in Canada or the United States. Posttraumatic stress disorder is to be expected. Other diseases may also be present

Immigrants *from other lands choose to come to a specific location, with the intention of taking up permanent residence, reunification with family, and employment.* Various events in the country of origin may cause the shift:

1. Political upheavals
2. Religious strife
3. Failure of national economic policies
4. Ethnic conflict, humanitarian crises
5. Wars, warlords vying for power, and separatist movements
6. Warring criminal factions, such as drug cartel conflicts in some South American and Caribbean nations
7. Multiple natural disasters, famines

Some immigrants are children being adopted and brought to a new home.

Whatever the reason for immigrating, many immigrants may have economic problems but are less likely to be in poverty than refugees. Health status among immigrants varies because they do not have systematic health screenings before leaving their country or on arrival in Canada or the United States. Health care providers should screen for parasites; tuberculosis; infectious diseases, such as hepatitis; female genital mutilation; HIV infection and untreated sexually transmitted diseases; cancer; trauma; malnutrition; dental problems; and posttraumatic stress disorder. The local health department is a useful resource for newly arrived immigrants.[142,143]

Both refugee and immigrant families may keep their children home from school because of fear, scapegoating, and language difficulties or to act as interpreters.

Where Are the Poor People?

Poor people live anywhere: in the better areas of a city as well as in inner city areas, in rural areas, and in all geographic areas of Canada and the United States. Poverty is found among *all* racial and ethnic groups—wherever they live—city, town, farm, reservation, mountain areas.[144]

Rural poverty is on the rise. Poverty is more prevalent among rural females than males, especially among female-headed households. Children in rural areas are more likely to live in poverty. Because of the economic losses of farmers during the past decade, an increasing number now also work off the farm at least part-time.[145]

Images of crime, drugs, gangs, out-of-wedlock births, AIDS, and unemployed men are as much a part of the white underclass as they are a part of any group that is poor in the inner city, including the black underclass. Children born to single mothers, many of whom have below-average IQs, are not likely to be successful. Pregnant elementary and high-school students insist that having a baby gives them someone to love and someone who loves them. The father of the baby disappears after the child's arrival—many times before the arrival. Often, the girl is fleeing an abusive family, only to find abuse in the new relationships with men. The cycle can be repeated in the next generation.[146]

Patterns of childrearing and family relationships of the long-term or very poor affect the children, who are the next generation of parents. These characteristics may include the following:

- Misbehaviour is regarded in terms of overt outcome; reasons for behaviour are infrequently considered.
- Lack of goal commitment, impulsive gratification, fatalism, and lack of belief in long-range goals or success result from effects of chronic poverty on a person's motivations and lifestyle. Immediate needs must be met first.
- Communication between family members is more physical than verbal; explanations may not be given to the child, affecting curiosity and learning.
- Families are frequently large; each member acts to get whatever gratification he or she can. Previously unmet needs in the parent cause the parent to be poorly equipped to meet the dependency needs of children. The child, as an adult, continues the cycle of previously unmet needs and inability to nurture.
- Mother is the chief childcare agent. The milieu of the home is authoritarian, whether or not the father is in the home.
- Discipline is harsh, inconsistent, and physical, often makes use of ridicule, and is based on whether or not the child's behaviour annoys the parent.
- Aggressive behaviour is alternately encouraged and restrained, depending primarily on the consequences to the parent of the child's behaviour. Such inconsistency causes the child to learn how to get away with certain behaviour and does not teach impulse control.[147,148,149,150]

Parental low self-esteem provokes feelings of shame, guilt, defensiveness, and decreased self-worth in children. Such childhood experiences can be the cause of low self-esteem in children; and these feelings continue into adulthood. Consequently, as parents, these individuals inflict the same feelings they suffered as a child.[151]

Authoritarian or harsh childrearing practices have as their explicit objective the development of toughness and self-sufficiency for survival; however, parents are warm and expressive. A loving attachment exists between parent and child. In their own home, children are likely to be expressive, although they may seem restrained with strangers. Children are often given adult responsibilities early; they are not the focus of the family in the way that middle-class children are. They must fend more for themselves.[152]

Most minority and ethnic cultures value kinship ties and the emotional, social, and economic support that the extended family provides, in contrast to the middle-class, which values individualism and independence. Much visiting goes on between relatives in the lower and working levels; assistance is sought and appreciated. All get along better by sharing meagre resources or by working together to gain resources. The grandmother (and grandfather, if living) is valued as carrier of the culture and as caregiver for the child if the mother works. Ability to delay gratification appears related to the situation. Frequently, poor people learn early that they are at the mercy of the system, whether the system is legal-political, economic, educational, or health care.

Children learn to delay gratification if they can trust that what is needed will be there when needed. Poor children may seldom have this opportunity. If meagre resources are used to meet today's needs, it is difficult or impossible to plan ahead, save, or anticipate that planning and saving have merit.

Impaired verbal communication and problem-solving ability may be present, not because the poor person is cognitively deficient but for other reasons. Many ethnic or minority groups speak a dialect in the home; the child then has difficulty understanding Standard English or being understood. Essentially, the child must become bilingual to be successful in school.[153] Parents often wish to help children learn more; in fact, most poor parents repeatedly emphasize that their children must get an education so that they can achieve more than their parents did. Poor parents often lack the education, energy, time, or resources to help their children advance educationally or even keep up minimally. Yet, most poor parents are receptive to suggestions on how to make the best possible use of their limited resources or what specific measures to follow to enhance child development.[154]

Poverty and ill health are related. Long-term ill health may contribute to poverty. Poverty predisposes to certain illnesses or causes a person to suffer adverse consequences of illness. As income level drops, health status declines. The ill child who is poor is less likely to attend school. Poor people have higher infant and maternal mortality rates and a higher number of deaths from accidents. Preventive measures, such as immunization of children, are less likely to be carried out in the family.

A poor person defines illness in terms of being unable to work for days or weeks, and first uses folk or home remedies when ill or may go to a traditional healer. Reluctantly, and only when absolutely necessary, he or she might enter the modern health care system. A person in chronic poverty may not seek professional, scientific care at all because of lack of knowledge, money, transportation, or an inadequate sense of self-worth. Many a poor person is suspicious of health care professionals or feels that there is a distance between him or her and the practitioner. These feelings can be overcome only by a gentle, respectful, courteous, prompt approach and straightforward speech. Moreover, poor people are unfamiliar with or unlikely to use community agencies without assistance. Because they often do not have the resources to practise preventive physical or dental care, they

may be very ill—even irreversibly—on entry into the health care system.[155] Living in poverty takes its toll physically, emotionally, and mentally. Consequent behaviour and health patterns, therefore, should not be viewed judgmentally.

INFLUENCES OF CULTURE ON HEALTH

Culture creates a milieu that influences the health beliefs and practices of an individual and his or her family living in a community. Because every culture is complex, it can be difficult to determine whether health and illness are the result of cultural or other elements, such as physiological or psychological factors. Yet, there are numerous accounts of the presence or absence of certain diseases in certain cultural groups and reactions to illness that are culturally determined. **Culture-bound illness or syndrome** *refers to the features of an illness that vary from culture to culture.*

Culture and climate influence food availability, dietary taboos, and methods of hygiene. The influence of cultural folkways on health has been studied. Race, social class, ethnic group, and religion influence the distribution rates of disease and death. Differences exist among cultural populations and people from different races and socioeconomic levels with respect to risk for disease and distribution of disease and death. These broad factors influence education, occupation and lifestyle, as well as decisions about health care. These differences are important in planning health promotion programs for a community and a nation.[156,157]

Canada's population is diverse in nature, and, largely due to the *Canadian Multiculturalism Act* (1988), each cultural group has been able to retain its identity.[158] Most Canadians enjoy a relatively high level of health.[159] However, the overall high standard of health is not shared equally by all Canadians. For example, life expectancy, which is an important indicator of population health, varies from region to region. Life expectancy is generally higher in southern urban areas in, or west of, Ontario. Meanwhile life expectancy is generally lower in remote regions or in the northern parts of certain provinces. Many of these regions have significant proportions of Aboriginal people. Interestingly, life expectancies that are somewhat lower than those in other regions are not linked with any one specific cause; the mortality rates in these regions are higher for most causes of death.[160]

The Aboriginal population is not a single homogeneous group but comprises three groups, the North American Indian, the Inuit, and the Métis, each of which is linguistically and culturally distinct.[161,162] The Aboriginal People's Survey 2001 presents a statistical portrait of the well-being of the Aboriginal population living in non-reserve areas across Canada. Also included are those who did not identify themselves as Aboriginal but were registered under the *Indian Act* and/or were members of a Band or First Nation. The results indicate that, overall, the Aboriginal non-reserve population rated its health status as lower than that of the total Canadian population.[163]

According to Kue Young, health research may be the answer to why such disparities exist and to solutions for eliminating them.[164] The rate of Type 2 diabetes has become a more serious health problem among the non-reserve Aboriginal population than among the total Canadian population.[165] However, according to Health Canada, evidence exists that the prevalence of diabetes is even higher among the Aboriginal population living on reserves.[166] Five other chronic conditions known to be more prevalent in the off-reserve Aboriginal population are high blood pressure, arthritis or rheumatism, asthma, stomach problems or intestinal ulcers, and heart problems. It is interesting to note, however, that about 69 percent of Aboriginal people aged 15–24 in non-reserve areas rated their health as very good or excellent compared with 71 percent of the total population in the same age group (see Table 1-12). While Aboriginal young people report levels of health status similar to those reported by the general Canadian youth population, the perceived health status of Aboriginal people, with each successive age group, declines more rapidly than it does in the total Canadian population (see Table 1-12).[167]

One exceptional point regarding Aboriginal youth has been made by Tester and McNicoll.[168] Their claim is that the Government of Nunavut in the Canadian Eastern Arctic faces a severe problem of high suicide rate, particularly among young Inuit males, which is among the highest in the world.[169]

Jenkins and his colleagues at the Department of Epidemiology and Biostatistics, McGill University, examined the health status of Inuit infants and focused on Canadian Inuit communities with reference to other circumpolar regions.[170] Their results indicated that a wide range of interrelated factors affect the health of Inuit infants. Some of these factors are their demographic, social, economic, and physical environments as well as personal health practices and the availability of quality, culturally appropriate health services. In addition, throughout the Arctic, Inuit infants experience higher mortality and poorer health than their non-Inuit counterparts. They also suffer disproportionately from bacterial and viral infections.[171]

To address the growing health concerns, in September 1999, a proposal was made for creating a research institute solely for Aboriginal health.[172] A group of leading Aboriginal and non-Aboriginal Canadian health researchers urged the federal government to consider funding dedicated to Aboriginal health research. This group strongly believed that such an approach would contribute significantly to the overall health and well-being of Aboriginal people. The Canadian Institute of Health Research (CIHR) was presented with the group's recommendations and launched the Institute of Aboriginal Peoples' Health (IAPH) in early 2000.[173] One of the goals of the CIHR-IAPH is to present the results of health research to the

TABLE 1-12
Self-Rated Health Status by Age Group for the Aboriginal Identity Non-Reserve Population 15 Years and Over for Canada, Aboriginal Peoples Survey 2001[1,2,3]

	Total self-rated health status[4]		Excellent or very good		Good		Fair or poor		Invalid or not stated	
	Number	%	Number	%	Number	%	Number	%	Number	%
Total Aboriginal identity non-reserve population aged 15+	547,870	100.0	308,530	56.3	144,830	26.4	94,220	17.1	300E	0.0E
15–24	136,750	100.0	94,640	69.2	33,640	24.5	8,400	6.1	80E	0.0E
25–34	120,060	100.0	77,500	64.5	30,800	25.6	11,660	9.7	100E	0.0E
35–44	131,440	100.0	72,970	55.5	36,440	27.7	21,990	16.7	x	x
45–54	86,670	100.0	39,880	46.0	23,990	27.6	22,780	26.2	x	x
55 and over	72,940	100.0	23,540	32.2	19,960	27.3	29,390	40.2	x	x

[1] Excludes the population that did not answer the Health Section of the APS questionnaire and those with invalid or unstated ages.

[2] Aboriginal Identity population includes those people who reported on the APS at least one of the following: 1) Identification as North American Indian, Métis and/or Inuit; 2) Registered Indian status and/or; 3) Band membership.

[3] Non-reserve population includes Aboriginal people that do not live on Indian reserves, with the exception of the Northwest Territories, in which case the total (on and non-reserve) Aboriginal population is included.

[4] The sum of the values of each category may differ from the total due to rounding.

Source: Statistics Canada, Catalogue No. 89–589 of Aboriginal Peoples Survey 2001—Initial Findings: Well-Being of the Non-Reserve Aboriginal Population. Chart1: Excellent or Very Good Self-Rated Health Status, Page 12. Used with permission.

Aboriginal people in a way that is accessible, appropriate, and easily understood.[174]

According to the Martin Spigelman Research Associates, HIV/AIDS may be the most devastating infectious disease in the world since the bubonic plague that decimated Europe in the 14th century.[175] At the end of 2002, an estimated 56 000 people in Canada were living with HIV (including those who also had AIDS); this number is a significant increase from the estimated 49 800 HIV infections in 1999.[176] The largest group of people living with HIV/AIDS are gay men, although the number of women is gradually increasing in the HIV-positive population.[177] The frequency of reports of HIV/AIDS has been in large numbers in the Aboriginal community, particularly amongst Aboriginal women.[178] It has been noted that the Canadian Government, 2004–2008, will have a single goal, namely, to organize, align, and direct Canadian efforts and resources to prevent effectively an AIDS epidemic among the Aboriginal people.[179] In May 2001, the National Aboriginal Council on HIV/AIDS (NACHA) was formed to create a single council to inform and to advise Health Canada on HIV/AIDS issues that affect all of Canada's Aboriginal peoples.[180]

One concern that arises in examining the issue of cultural minorities and health is that of various conflicting explanations. In Canada, as well as in the United States, many members of cultural minorities are economically deprived.[181] This fact makes it not only complicated but difficult to determine how much cultural uniqueness, or economic disadvantage, or some combination of both, is responsible for health status. These Canadians who experience inadequate income, dependency on welfare, stresses, substandard living conditions, physical violence, sexual abuse, and substance abuse understandably suffer worse health than other Canadians.[182] For example, infant mortality is almost twice as high among the disadvantaged children from these groups compared with the general population.[183]

CRITICAL THINKING

In what ways does being an unemployed Canadian affect one's mental health? Think deeply about this question, putting yourself in the place of an unemployed person.

In both Canada and the United States, the most dramatic change in the health of the population in the last decade has been the sharp decline in the health of blacks. The most disadvantaged person is the black male, whose life expectancy is steadily decreasing. The exact causes of the worsening health of blacks have not been conclusively identified, but strong evidence suggests that they are at greater risk because of smoking, high blood pressure, high cholesterol levels, alcohol and other drug intake, excess weight, and diabetes—health problems often associated with lower income and stressful life circumstances.[184]

Both the extent of education and income level exert an influence upon a person's decision to seek health care. Poor, less educated black as well as white women seek diagnostic and treatment services for breast cancer later than did their counterparts who had higher incomes and education. Cancer screening programs are therefore needed in these populations; however, women of the lower socioeconomic level also have less access to preventive and medical care, and asymptomatic women may not make use of preventive health services unless they are created specifically for them.[185] Nurses are in a good position to institute screening procedures, teach about warning signs, and explain mammography and other cancer-screening tests to such women. In British Columbia, one research study, conducted to examine women-centred care in the context of cervical cancer screening in ethno-cultural groups, concluded that women found Pap test clinics more approachable because they expected to be able to discuss health care concerns with a female health provider.[186]

1-2 BONUS SECTION IN CD-ROM

Culture-Bound Illness and Behaviours

Many culture-bound illnesses and behaviours are unfamiliar to us. This section identifies and explains briefly 16 such interesting types. Some might be familiar to you, but several will be new to you.

There is a growing awareness that variations in dietary practices among ethnic groups may explain some interethnic differences in morbidity and mortality. For example, research suggests that dietary practices and nutrient intake of Mexican-American women may protect them against lung and breast cancer. Dietary practices may also explain their low rates of low birth weight babies, despite low income and education.

Immigration is a complex experience that exacts a great toll from immigrants in terms of mental and physical health, occupational and socioeconomic status, and total life ways. The *crisis of immigration* appears to be manifested as follows:

- During the first year, the immigrants/refugees experience relief, euphoria, and relatively high levels of happiness and life satisfaction.
- During the second year, exile shock occurs, with high levels of depression and unhappiness.
- During the third year, emotional improvement and increased adaptability are manifested.[187,188]

Canada's immigrants, who come from diverse backgrounds, comprise about 16 percent of the population.[189] Although they are a diverse group, such factors as length of residence in Canada, country of origin or ethnicity, as well as gender, age, level of education, and economic position may all be factors contributing to variations in health status.[190,191,192] Ali and Perez studied the Canadian immigrant's health status

---

EVIDENCE-BASED PRACTICE

Health Promotion among Immigrant Women from India Living in Canada

A small convenience sample of 20 first-generation immigrant women, ages 40–70 years, were interviewed individually, in their homes, and in their own language by a middle-aged female researcher who had immigrated to Canada from India over 30 years earlier. Questions asked during the 1- to 3-hour interview included the following:

- What is the meaning of health and well-being?
- What value does the woman place on health?
- What cultural norms and values influence health and health practice?
- What did the woman do to keep healthy before living in Canada?
- What does she do now to remain healthy?

The results showed that:

1. Women place great value on health. The health status of the family and others is spoken about more than that of self.
2. Health includes being happy, free of worry and stress, not being a burden on anyone, and being independent.
3. A healthy life style includes:
   (a) Eating home-cooked, simple foods (lentils, bread, fruits, vegetables, milk, and yogurt) at the right times of the day.
   (b) Being active, with work in the home, taking regular walks, and controlling weight.
   (c) Taking a daily nap and keeping a private time.
   (d) Worshipping, praying, and listening to religious music.
   (e) Having a close relationship with family, and visiting friends.
   (f) Using traditional herbal and home remedies to manage health and illness.

Practice Implications

A considerable number of Indian women, not being highly proficient in the Canadian official languages, are more likely to learn about health care through interaction than from printed material. Indian women have been taught to suppress their needs and to focus on children and family. They have also learned to preserve gender roles, family heritage, and tradition.

In Canada, distance, the lack of a transportation vehicle, and cold weather can cause feelings of isolation. Both mental and physical well-being can be adversely affected. Indian women should be encouraged to maintain a network with family, friends, and the broader community.

The goals of health care should be congruent with cultural ways.

Women should be helped to adapt to and use available health care practices.

Source: Choudhry, U. K., Health Promotion among Immigrant Women from India Living in Canada, Image: Journal of Nursing Scholarship, 30, no. 3 (1998), 269-274. Blackwell Publishing Ltd. Used with permission.

(mental and physical health) by utilizing data from Statistics Canada Cross-sectional 2000/2001 Canadian Community Health Survey.[193,194] After analysis of the data, Ali found that immigrants who arrived in Canada in recent years had the lowest rates of depression and alcohol dependence compared with those immigrants who were in Canada 30 years or longer.[195] Rates of alcoholism and depression among immigrants from Asia, Africa, South and Central America, and the Caribbean were significantly lower than the Canadian-born average. Perez found that the results for chronic disorders generally indicate a gradient, wherein the health of immigrants becomes progressively worse with increasing length of stay in Canada.[196] These results for chronic conditions in general corroborate well with other previous Canadian findings.[197] This indicates that the health status of immigrants who have resided in Canada for decades deteriorates over time and tends, eventually, to match the health status of the Canadian-born population.

CRITICAL THINKING

In what ways might dietary habits influence health status differences between the new immigrants and the general Canadian population?

HEALTH CARE AND NURSING APPLICATIONS

Importance of Cultural Concepts

Because of the increasing predominance of scientific medical practices and specializations, many consumers of health care in Canada and the United States are voicing a preference for caring behaviours and cultural practices. Especially the poor, middle-to-lower socioeconomic groups and rural and ethnic or racial populations find the cosmopolitan approach to medical care too complex, too questionable, too difficult to understand and attain, and too expensive.

In the mid-1960s, Leininger, the founder and pioneering leader of transcultural nursing, came into Canada to begin to promote ideas, definitions, and functional concepts of transcultural nursing.[198] She assisted health care providers to recognize the important and growing need to establish a body of research-based knowledge and skills to provide informed cultural care to Aboriginal people and immigrants. **Transcultural nursing** *is the humanistic and scientific study and comparative analysis of different cultures and subcultures throughout the world in relation to differences* *and similarities in caring, health, illness, beliefs, values, life ways, and practices so that this knowledge can be used to provide culture-specific and cultural-universal nursing care to people.* The goal is to develop a body of knowledge so that transcultural nursing concepts, theories, and practices are an integral part of nursing education, service, and research. Leininger has developed *general principles* to guide transcultural practice, education, and research. She has emphasized the importance of knowing and respecting the cultural background, values, and practices of people to provide appropriate, meaningful, and satisfying care to people. These principles emphasize human rights and ethical considerations related to cultural care. Leininger describes the importance of the nurse being prepared for worldwide nursing and that transcultural nursing education should be worldwide.[199] Other authors have also written about educational and practice models that build on cultural concepts.[200,201,202,203]

A slow and uneven development of transcultural nursing in Canada has transpired over the past several decades. In the early 1990s, a nursing research study of Greek Canadians by Rosenbaum was the first major step, as well as an excellent example, to show the value of Culture Care Theory and to discover new knowledge.[204] Lately, several mainstream organizations in Canadian society have developed specific multicultural initiatives, or outreach activities, to encourage the people in the community to use the available services.[205] Even though the Canadian nursing profession recognizes cultural diversity, a critical need still exists for transcultural education, research, and practice to care for the many ethnic groups and the increasing number of immigrants and refugees who come into Canada.

What is essential to practice is awareness of cultural values, sensitivity to different beliefs and practices, and the concept of **cultural relativity** *(behaviour that is appropriate or right in one culture may not be so defined in another culture)* versus **ethnocentrism** *(behaviour based on the belief that one's own group is superior).*[206] In an article on exploring perinatal health in Indo-Canadian women, the authors cite that an important strategy to improve pregnancy outcomes in Indo-Canadian women is the importance of providing resources within the health care system as well as in the community.[207] In reflecting on what you have learned about culture, how would you approach the following critical thinking question?

CRITICAL THINKING

You are asked to do an assessment on an older lady who has just been admitted to your unit in the hospital. Her cultural background is very different from your own. How would you find out about her cultural beliefs and practices in order to begin a nursing care plan?

Attitudes Related to Culture

If you live or work in a culture different from your own, initially you may suffer **culture shock**, *feelings of bewilderment,*

confusion, disorganization, frustration, and stupidity, and the inability to adapt to differences and word meanings, activities, use of time, and customs that are part of culture.[208]

Brink and Saunders describe *four phases of culture shock:*[209]

1. **Honeymoon phase:** This stage is characterized by excitement, exploration, and pleasure. This phase may be experienced by a short-term visitor.

2. **Disenchanted phase:** The person feels stuck, depressed, and irritated, and realizes that the environment is unpredictable and no longer exotic. The normal cues for social intercourse are absent, and the person is cut adrift. The person may become physically ill.

3. **Beginning resolution phase:** New cultural behaviour patterns are adopted. Friends are found. Life becomes easier and more predictable.

4. **Effective function phase:** The person has become almost bicultural and may experience reverse culture shock on return to the home country.

An antidote for culture shock is to look for similarities between the native culture and the new culture. To adapt to a new culture, the person has to be interested in the new culture and be prepared to ask questions tactfully and to give up some of the old habits. It is important to learn the language, customs, beliefs, and values to the greatest extent possible. A support system will provide an environment where the new immigrant can be himself or herself, validate ideas, and help adapt.[210,211] Leininger[212] and Weiss[213] give a number of specific suggestions for adapting to another culture. Other authors in the reference list also discuss techniques that assist individuals in making the transition from one culture to another. Recognizing that one's own patterns of life and language are peculiar to one's culture will help avoid making inaccurate judgments of another culture.

Multiculturalism, a fundamental feature of Canadian society, focuses on the equal participation of individuals and communities of all origins and the preservation of multicultural heritage.[214] As you probably know, Canada's ethno-cultural diversity is increasing. The Canadian Nurses Association (CNA) has been examining ways to incorporate cultural practices into health promotion activities.[215] The four key responsibilities set out by the CNA for nurses who wish to provide culturally appropriate care are as follows:

- **Self-assessment**—nurses need to spend time to explore their own personal attitudes and values about health in order to appreciate not only their own experiences but others' understanding of health as well.

- **Cultural knowledge**—involves the true understanding of others' health beliefs and values that can affect their responses to such personal events as birth practices, death and dying, spirituality, and alternative or traditional therapies.

- **Verbal and non-verbal communication**—are both essential for clients and families to access the services they require. Facilitative techniques, such as listening, respecting, empathizing, and, particularly, being open are helpful.

- **Partnerships among clients, providers, and funding agencies**—are essential for quality care. It frequently becomes necessary to develop ways that incorporate culturally diverse practices into health care services to optimize health outcomes for the client. The development of partnership (intersectoral collaboration) is an important principle of health promotion.

All health professionals, not only nurses, can contribute to achieving the goal of health promotion to clients and their families in different communities. As part of this effort, cross-cultural services are becoming a growing need in the health care system in both urban and rural communities.

During the course of delivering health care, some Caucasian health care professionals may sometimes feel that Asian parents are noncompliant, for example, because they are not as forceful as Caucasian parents in having the chronically ill child carry out prescribed exercises when the exercises cause pain. This may, in turn, cause Asian parents to be less responsive to the health care professionals. Health care professionals are often unaware of the complex factors that influence client responses to treatment and care. Some clients may not follow the treatment because they have different priorities.

The Aboriginal Nurses Association of Canada embraces a common vision of wellness for Aboriginal people. Members of that Association have reinforced the practice of drawing on traditional healing practices for Aboriginal health issues.[216]

CRITICAL THINKING

What do you know about traditional healing practices?

All people have some **prejudice**, which is *unfavourable, intolerant, injurious preconceived ideas formed before facts are known.*

Do not make value judgments that interfere with your relationship with the patient and with objective care. There are too many unknown factors in people's lives, and therefore it is wrong to set up stereotyped categories. Try to accept people as they are, regardless of culture or social class. Picture the world through the eyes of those you care for. In this way, you can maintain your own personal standards without being shocked by those of others. The box entitled "Self-Assessment of Cultural Attitudes" is a questionnaire that can help you assess your own cultural attitudes and perceptions.

Assessment

Holistic nursing *is nursing practice that has as its goal the healing of the whole person.* **Holism** *involves understanding the relationships among the biological, psychological, social, and spiritual dimensions of the person, that the whole is greater than the sum of the parts, and that the person is an integrated being interacting with internal and external environments.*[217,218,219,220]

CASE SITUATION

You are a Nurse Unit Manager (NUM) in the Health Services Unit in a rural hospital in Northern Alberta. Over the past year, you have noticed that the rate of admission for First Nations people with diabetes, from all of the neighbouring communities (some 4000 residents), has increased by 15 percent overall, with a range of 11 to 18 percent, with the highest increase found in the remotest community. When you reported the results of your survey at an interdisciplinary health team meeting, the members decided to form a specific task force group including yourself. The mandate of the task force, referred to as the "Down with Diabetes Operation—Task Force Group" (DDO-TFG) was to develop, within a month's time, a set of health promoting strategies. The health team unit agreed to implement the strategies as soon as they were developed. It was agreed that the strategies should be developed in cooperation with the communities—and, where possible, on site within the communities to promote as much joint commitment as possible.

1. What guidelines will you suggest at the first meeting (tomorrow) that should be followed by the DDO-TFG as it begins to build a valuable community health program with the First Nations People?
2. Fortunately, at the first meeting of the DDO-TFG, after you were resoundingly commended for the excellent set of guidelines you presented, you were urged, by the members, to now provide the preliminary design of an initial assessment/evaluation tool to be used in the communities when the full operation, the Down with Diabetes Operation (DDO), becomes active.
   a. What will be your first steps in creating such an instrument? What help will you need? Who, or what agencies, might provide assistance for you?
   b. What procedural steps will you propose to the DDO-TFG to test and refine the instrument in time for the expected opening of the DDO a few weeks from now?

Health promotion assessment includes the following:[221,222,223]

1. Health history and physical assessment.
2. Health-promoting behaviours, including nutritional practices, physical activity, and stress management.
3. Health-protecting behaviours, including avoiding abuse of tobacco, alcohol, and chemical substances, and exposure to environmental hazards and injuries.

Be aware that when you assess a client, your questions may seem intrusive. For example, among some Indian tribes,

Self-Assessment of Cultural Attitudes

To become more aware of your own attitudes toward and feelings about people of other racial and ethnic backgrounds, ask yourself the following questions:

1. What is your cultural or subculture background?
2. What is your earliest memory of racial or ethnic differences?
3. What are the messages you have received in your life about black, Asian, Aboriginal, and Slavic people?
4. What messages have you received in your life about Caucasians of various nationality backgrounds?
5. How much experience did you have with any person from a racial or ethnic minority group different from your own while you were growing up?
6. In what way have these experiences affected your behaviour toward people from the group(s)?
7. Describe people from other racial or ethnic minority groups with whom you have felt comfortable or uncomfortable.
8. What features or characteristics are dominant in people from other racial or ethnic minority groups with whom you have had contact?
9. What have you observed about the racial or ethnic composition of your community?
10. What have you observed about the interaction of people from diverse cultural backgrounds at your school, church, or workplace or in organizations to which you belong?
11. Do you consider yourself to be nonracist or racist? (A member of any race can be a racist against a different racial group.)
12. What do you plan to do to increase your understanding of a person different from you?

a question carries with it assumptions and obligations. If the person is asked a question, it implies that he or she must have the answer and that the answer is needed by you. Otherwise, there is no reason for you to have asked the question. If the person does not know the answer, the person starts to talk about something else which is probably the customary practice in the culture to save face and dignity. You may be able to obtain information by more indirect means, without putting the person on the spot. You may also need to use an interpreter (Table 1-13). Interpreters may be trained or untrained. One important aspect is that all interpreters must keep confidentiality and accuracy of information as the first and foremost considerations while relating to the client and family.

Learning about another's cultural background can promote feelings of respect and humility. It can enhance one's understanding of the person and the family—their needs, likes and dislikes, their behaviour, attitudes, care and treatment approaches and whether or not they might be influenced by sociocultural causes of disease.

Leininger described nine major domains to consider while doing a cultural assessment: (1) patterns of lifestyle, (2) specific cultural norms and values, (3) cultural taboos and myths, (4) worldview and ethnocentric tendencies, (5) general features that the client perceives as different or similar to other cultures, (6) health and life care rituals and rites of passage to maintain health, (7) folk and professional health-illness systems that are used, (8) degree of cultural change and acculturation needed, and (9) methods of caring for self and others in regaining health.[224,225]

According to Tripp-Reimer, Brink, and Saunders, a thorough cultural assessment guide would include the following components:[226]

- *Values* about health, human nature, relationships between the person and nature, time, activity, relations, and others
- *Beliefs* about health (health maintenance, causes and treatment of illness), religion, other practices
- *Customs* about communication (verbal and nonverbal), decision making, food, diet, grief, dying, religion, family roles, and role of the patient
- *Social structure,* including family lines of authority, education, ethnic affiliation, physical environment, religion, use of economic resources, health care facilities, use of art and history, and cultural change
- *Preferences* about their health care situation

The Transcultural Assessment Model by Giger and Davidhizar focuses on (1) the person as a unique cultural individual; (2) communication patterns, including language use, use of silence, and nonverbal communication; (3) preference for touch; (4) preferred space or distance between person and others; (5) family relationships; (6) belief system; (7) other social characteristics, such as work; (8) time orientation; (9) sense of control over environmental events; (10) use of home remedies; and (11) biological variations resulting from race or ethnicity. During the assessment, the model encourages discussion to determine how well the person is assimilated into the mainstream culture and specific cultural practices related to health, food, religious belief, and general lifestyle.[227] The assessment model is applicable to children. (See Davidhizar, R., Havens, R., and Bechtel, G., "Assessing Culturally Diverse Paediatric Clients," *Pediatric Nursing,* 25, no. 4, 1999, pp 371–375.)

The assessment must consider the complexity and coherence among (1) the individual life span; (2) development and aging; (3) biological and physiological factors; (4) contextual and interaction models of intellectual functioning; (5) personality development and expression; (6) social interaction; and (7) family and social support systems in relation to racial, ethnic, and cultural status as well as spiritual, religious, and philosophical beliefs and values. Racial or ethnic minority groups may experience a very different process of development and aging and manifest illness differently from Caucasians. Variability within racial or ethnic groups and between men and women is also apparent. There is lack of research data on normative development and mental health characteristics over the life course and on manifestation of psychiatric symptoms among various racial and ethnic groups.[228]

TABLE 1-13
Guidelines for Using a Language Interpreter

1. Hospital translators, in contrast to family members, may not be as familiar with a particular dialect, but may be more neutral and better at interpreting technical aspects of health care.

2. Patients and family members may be embarrassed to answer some questions or reveal some information in the presence of each other but would be willing to talk with an interpreter. Clients may request a specific translator or bring their own.

3. Family members, in contrast to an interpreter, have knowledge of the patient and may be able to insert additional information in context, but may be guarded with personal information.

4. Family members, in contrast to an interpreter, may have issues about what is meant, how much is translated, and how much is condensed or omitted.

5. Plan what you want to say ahead of time. Avoid confusing the interpreter by backing up, inserting a proviso, rephrasing, or hesitating. Be patient.

6. Address the person or family directly. Avoid directing all comments to and through the interpreter.

7. Assure the person or family and interpreter of confidentiality.

8. Use short questions and comments. Technical terminology and professional jargon (e.g., "psychotropic medication") should be reduced to plain English.

9. When lengthy explanations are necessary, break them up and have them interpreted piece by piece in straightforward, concrete terms in the foreign language by the interpreter.

10. Use language and explanations the interpreter can handle.

11. Make allowances for terms that do not exist in the target language.

12. Try to avoid ambiguous statements and questions.

13. Avoid abstractions, idiomatic expressions, similes, and metaphors. It is useful to learn about the use of these grammatical elements in the target language.

14. Avoid indefinite phrases using "would," "could," "if," and "maybe." These can be mistaken for actual agreements or firm approval of a course of action.

15. Ask the interpreter to comment on the client's word content and emotions.

16. Invite correction and induce the discussion of alternatives: "Correct me if I'm wrong, I understand it this way... Do you see it some other way?"

17. Pursue seemingly unconnected issues raised by the client. These issues may lead to crucial information or may uncover difficulties with the interpretation.

18. Return to an issue if you suspect a problem and get a negative response. Be certain the interpreter knows what you want. Use related questions, change the wording, and come at the issue indirectly.

19. Provide instructions in list format. Ask clients to outline their understanding of the plans. If alternatives exist, spell each one out. Check the quality of translated health-related materials by having them back translated.

20. Clarify your nursing limitations. The willingness to talk about an issue may be viewed as evidence of "understanding" it or the ability to "fix" it.

Adapted from Murray, R., and M. Huelskoetter, Psychiatric/Mental Health Nursing: Giving Emotional Care *(3rd Ed.). Stamford, CT: Appleton & Lange, 1991, p. 109.*

Cultural differences should be anticipated not only in refugees, immigrants, and first-generation immigrants but also in persons even further removed in time from their country of origin and in persons from other regions within your country. A person's behaviour during illness is influenced by *cultural definitions* of how he or she should act and the meaning of illness. Understanding this situation and seeking reasons for behaviour help avoid stereotyping and labelling a person as uncooperative and resistant just because the behaviour is different. As you consider alternative reasons for behaviour, care can be based on understanding of individual differences. People from different cultural backgrounds classify health problems differently and have certain expectations about how they should be helped. If cultural differences are ignored, your ability to assess and help the clients and their ability to progress toward a personally and culturally defined health status may be hampered. You should be able to translate your knowledge of the health care system into terms that match the concepts of your clients.

Knowledge about socioeconomic levels and cultural groups may help explain such behaviours as late or broken appointments, which may have resulted from fear, or feelings of inferiority, lack of transportation, or not having someone to babysit the children, rather than from lack of interest in health. An Aboriginal person, a black person from the low-income group, or a recent immigrant, for instance, may not be accustomed to keeping a strict time schedule or appointments, because a strict clock-time orientation is not valued as highly as in the North American society. Take time to talk with the person, and you will learn of fears, problems, aspirations, and concerns for health and family. You will begin to feel human warmth.

Assessment involves observing, listening, and talking with the client and, frequently, the family. Some people communicate best in their first (or native) language when they are ill. Further, an elderly person may speak only his or her own language at home, having never learned English. There is currently an emphasis on any group maintaining its language because language provides the strength and connectedness of a community.

Because of the diversity of cultures found in Canada and the United States, there are a number of people for whom English is not the first language. Hence, you may need to use an interpreter to assist you with assessment, care planning, and intervention. Become acquainted with people in the community who speak other languages fluently and can be interpreters or translators for health care professionals. Table 1-13 gives guidelines for an interpreter. Learn key words of languages. Use language dictionaries or a card file of key words. Try your best to overcome language barriers so that your assessment is more accurate and care measures are understood by the patient.

As you assess clients, particularly during a physical assessment, remember that people differ not only culturally but also biologically (Table 1-14). Studies on biological baselines for growth and development or normal characteristics have usually been done on Caucasian populations. These norms may not be applicable to non-Caucasians. Biological features, such as skin colour, body size and shape, and presence of enzymes are the result of genetically transmitted biological adjustments to the environment in earlier times.[229,230] Yet, people of different races from different geographical areas are also similar in many ways. Study of the 24-hour hormone profiles of Caucasians in temperate climates and Africans living at the Equator showed a similar cycle of cortisol and thyroid-stimulating hormone (TSH) concentrations. In both groups, concentrations of TSH and cortisol increased with awakening and decreased during slow-wave sleep. Fluctuation

TABLE 1-14
Clinical Assessment of Skin Colour

Characteristic	White or Light-skinned Person	Dark-skinned Person
Pallor Vasoconstriction present	Skin takes on white hue, which is colour of collagen fibres in subcutaneous connective tissue.	Skin loses underlying red tones. Brown-skinned person appears yellow-brown. Black-skinned person appears ashen grey. Mucous membranes, lips, and nail beds are pale or grey.
Erythema, Inflammation Cutaneous vasodilation	Skin is red.	Palpate for increased warmth of skin, oedema, tightness, or indurations of skin. Streaking and redness are difficult to assess.
Cyanosis Hypoxia of tissues	Skin, especially in earlobes, as well as in lips, oral mucosa, and nail beds, has bluish tinge.	Lips, tongue, conjunctiva, palms, soles of feet are pale or ashen grey. Apply light pressure to create pallor; in cyanosis, tissue colour returns slowly by spreading from periphery to the centre.
Ecchymosis Deoxygenated blood seeps from broken blood vessel into subcutaneous tissue	Skin changes from purple-blue to yellow-green to yellow.	Oral mucous membrane or conjunctiva show colour changes from purple-blue to yellow-green to yellow. Obtain history of trauma and discomfort. Note swelling and indurations.
Petechiae Intradermal or submucosal bleeding	Round, pinpoint purplish-red spots are present on skin.	Oral mucosa or conjunctiva show purplish-red spots if person has black skin.
Jaundice Accumulated bilirubin in tissues	Skin, mucous membranes, and sclera of eyes are yellow. Light-colour stools and dark urine often occur.	Sclera of eyes, oral mucous membranes, palms of hand, and soles of feet have yellow discoloration.

of plasma renin activity (PRA) during nighttime sleep was also similar for both groups.[231]

Pain assessment must consider cultural factors: different population groups have about the same physical thresholds of pain, although there is individual variation within each group; however, how people express pain varies according to whether or not the individuals were taught in their culture to speak about or give evidence of their pain (physical and emotional). It is necessary to look for subtle cues of pain among Northern European, Asian, and Aboriginal people and to avoid overmedicating others who tend to be more expressive, such as the Italian or Jewish people. Family members may also react in different ways when they see the patient in pain. Families of Eastern European patients tend to be proactive and assertive on behalf of the patient. Patients also respond differently when family members are present. In some cultures, the patient is not expected to talk about the pain with the family.[232]

Among the various physical differences that are known to exist are **Mongolian spots**, *the hyperpigmented, bluish discoloration only occasionally seen in Caucasian neonates but normal in many Asians, Aboriginal people, and blacks.* The shape of the female pelvis, the shapes of the teeth and tongue, fingerprint pattern, blood type, keloid formation, and presence of the enzyme lactase all vary among different ethnic groups. Adults who have **lactose intolerance** *are deficient in lactase, the enzyme required for digestion and metabolism of lactose in milk and milk products.* They become ill on ingestion of these foods and have such symptoms as flatulence, distension, abdominal cramping, diarrhea, and colitis. Only people of Northern European Caucasian extraction and members of two African tribes tolerate lactose indefinitely; even some elderly Caucasians have lactose deficiency.

Other biological variations exist. It is commonly known that persons with certain blood types are more prone to certain illnesses. Rh-negative blood type is common in Caucasians and rarer in other groups. Myopia is more common in Chinese people; colour blindness is more common in Europeans and East Indians. Nose sizes and shapes correlate with ancestral homelands. Small noses (seen in Asians) evolved in cold regions, high-bridged noses (e.g., in Arabs and some American Indian tribes) were common in dry areas; and the flat, broad noses of some black persons were the result of adaption to moist, warm climates.[234]

Susceptibility to illness also varies among racial groups. For example, sickle cell anemia is considered the most common genetic disorder in the United States and occurs mostly among African-Americans. Hypertension, both primary and malignant, is more common in African-Americans of all age groups than in other racial groups. G6PD, a hematological disease, occurs in 35 percent of African-Americans. A fluorescent spot test that screens for the deficiency that causes G6PD should be part of the blood transfusion procedures for African-Americans, including infants.[235] In Canada, until recently, Aboriginal people had lower-than-average rates of heart disease. However, the figures from the Regional Health Surveys indicate higher rates. The results of these surveys are somewhat questionable, and future surveys are needed to verify the results. Type 2 diabetes is extremely common in the Aboriginal and Inuit populations. Further, suicide rates are high, and cancer rates are increasing among this population.[236]

CRITICAL THINKING

What do you think may be some causes of Type 2 diabetes among the Aboriginal and Inuit people? What health promotion strategies could be planned for these people who live in northern communities?

To aid assessment, learn about significant religious customs and the everyday practices of hygiene, eating, types of foods eaten, sleeping, elimination, use of space, and various rituals that are a part of a person's culture. Because the client and the practitioner may have different perspectives of health and illness, answers to the following questions can enhance understanding about the client's viewpoint:

- What do you think caused your problem?
- Why do you think it started when it did?
- What do you think this illness does to you? What problems has it caused you?
- What do you fear most about your illness?
- How severe is your illness?
- What kind of treatment have you already tried? What else would help?
- What would you like health care providers to do for you? What results do you expect from treatment?

For persons from another country, a thorough physical examination should include the components listed in the box entitled "Physical Examination of Foreign-born Immigrants".[237]

Nursing Diagnoses

The nursing diagnoses in the box entitled "Selected Nursing Diagnoses Related to Transcultural Nursing" may be applicable to working with people from various cultural backgrounds. Leininger discusses the importance of including non-anglicized cultural concepts in the North American Nursing Diagnosis Association (NANDA) taxonomy, rather than focusing solely on Anglo-American, Western cultural values. Further, the diagnostic categories should include positive health descriptors and assets of cultures in dealing with human conditions.[238]

It is important to use wellness nursing diagnoses to help clients focus on health, progress, and strengths, and not focus only on problems. Wellness diagnoses could include (1) gaining new information, (2) learning new skills, (3) acquiring new roles, and (4) achieving developmental tasks.[239] Throughout the remainder of this text, the wellness diagnoses are included to promote health, prevent illness, and capitalize on the strengths of clients and their families; these steps are imperative to provide comprehensive, meaningful nursing care.

Physical Examination of Foreign-Born Immigrants

Screening Tests

- PPD for tuberculosis, even if there is a history of Bacillus Calmette-Guerin (BCG) vaccination
- Chest x-ray if the tuberculosis skin test is positive or if there are symptoms of pulmonary disease
- Hepatitis B serology, surface antigen, and core antibody tests, to determine if the person is infectious
- Hemoglobin and hematocrit (anemia may be caused by parasites, malaria, and malnutrition)
- Stool tests for ova and parasites (giardiasis, ascariasis, amebiasis, pinworms, hookworms, tapeworms, whipworms, and fluke are common)

Complete History and Physical Examination

- Include gross nutritional status, vision and hearing, dental examination, and identification of high-risk pregnancy. Question bowel habits; and inquire about abdominal pain to detect salmonella, shigella, and parasites.

Immunization Update

- Persons age 18 and older are often overlooked for history of vaccination for measles, mumps, rubella, tetanus, diphtheria, hepatitis B, and polio.

Selected Nursing Diagnoses Related to Transcultural Nursing

Pattern 3: Relating

Impaired Social Interaction
Social Isolation
Risk for Loneliness

Pattern 5: Choosing

Ineffective Individual Coping
Potential for Enhanced Community Coping
Ineffective Community Coping
Decisional Conflict
Health-Seeking Behaviours

Pattern 6: Moving

Altered Health Maintenance

Pattern 7: Perceiving

Powerlessness

Pattern 8: Knowing

Knowledge Deficit
Many of the NANDA nursing diagnoses are applicable to an individual in any culture who is ill.

Source: North American Nursing Diagnosis Association, *NANDA Nursing Diagnoses Definitions & Classification 1999–2000.* Philadelphia: North American Nursing Diagnosis Association, 1999.

Chen, Ng, and Wilkins argue that when immigrants arrive in Canada, they are, generally speaking, a healthy group of individuals.[240] One obvious reason is that individuals in good health are more inclined and better able to emigrate than those in poor health. Another reason is that employability, which is a factor in granting permission to immigrate to Canada, includes a certain health status. Finally, potential immigrants, before they are admitted, undergo medical screening to ensure that that they do not suffer from serious medical conditions (see *Immigration Act*, Section 11 and Section 91).[241]

It is imperative to note that in 2001, the anthrax cases reported in the United States heightened public awareness of bio-terrorism. While the probability of such attacks in Canada is low, should one occur, the consequences would be severe. It is, therefore, important to have emergency plans in place. These plans are critical for the health care system to respond effectively. Note that in 2003, the outbreak of severe acute respiratory syndrome (SARS) in several Canadian cities brought home the importance of coordinated efforts of all levels of governments as well as international agencies.[242]

Wellness-oriented nursing diagnoses serve several purposes. The nurse and the client, as well as the family, are encouraged to examine the positive, adaptive, or previously successful behaviours that contribute to identified healthy functioning.[243]

CRITICAL THINKING

Develop a list of wellness diagnoses related to Transcultural Nursing.

Concepts of Culturally Based Intervention

Caring *is understood to be assistive, supportive, or facilitative actions directed toward another person or group with evident or anticipated needs to ameliorate or improve a human condition or life way.*[244] Nurses in different cultures tend to know and emphasize different care constructs, such as support, comfort, and touch. In several non-Western cultures, nurses and clients perceive care as protective with a sociocultural emphasis. Depending on the culture, Leininger states, the concept of care can mean any of these different things:

Comfort	Stress alleviation
Support	Restoration
Attention	Direct assistance
Compassion	Helping the dependent

Touch	Tenderness
Love	Trust
Stimulation	Instruction
Presence	Succorance
Protection	Empathy
Surveillance	Medical or technical assistance
Personalized help	Assistance
Nurturance	Maintenance of well-being

Care and caring are basic to health, health promotion, and illness prevention. For more information, see the box "Key Definitions Related to Health and Health Promotion." Health is desired universally, and in most societies, health is linked with goals of human development, satisfaction of basic needs, work, quality of life, and social well-being. Yet, in the war-torn or very poor countries of the world, health may scarcely be a memory, let alone a perceived state in the current reality.

Economic, political, and environmental factors that contribute to poor health must be addressed in health planning and policy formation. Community participation increases access to health care; provides for greater efficiency, effectiveness, and coordination of services; and leads to equity in and self-reliance of a population. It requires time, energy, cultural knowledge, trust and respect, common goals, and constant dialogues. Nurses are in a key position to foster this model of health and the consequent empowerment.[249,250,251]

In Canada, the need for effective nursing and health care leadership has been recognized as being critical for client and family care in all settings, including the development of policies and health promotion strategies. Nursing leadership encompasses a wide range of challenges and competencies to ensure quality client outcomes. What are such competencies? They include caring, modelling, and mentoring, as well as envisioning and decision making. At the Conference on Leadership in Ottawa 2003, the three areas of focus for nursing leaders were identified: (1) building practice environments; (2) developing primary health care; and (3) promoting evidence-based practice.[252] It is clear, then, that the effective nurse of today must not only plan nursing care for the client and families but must collaborate, in a cooperative manner, with members of the health care team to reach the common goal of quality care for all.

Leininger, in her Theory of Cultural Care Diversity and Universality, proposes that client therapy goals should be congruent with cultural values, beliefs, and life ways. The Anglo-American and Western European cultural values of individualism, autonomy, independence, self-reliance, self-control, self-regulation, self-management, and self-care may be in conflict with non-Western cultural values. In non-Western cultures throughout the world and among some people in some groups in Canada and the United States (those of Mexican, African, Asian, or American Indian origin), *other-care,* rather than *self-care,* is the value and norm. People promote and retain the role of

others to care for their people, reflecting caring values, such as interdependence, interconnectedness, understanding, presence, and being responsible for others. *Other-care* values are essential for the survival of extended families, sub-clans, clans, and tribes.[253,254]

Cultural care congruence will explain and predict outcomes. Three principles for client therapy goals are: (1) cultural

Key Definitions Related to Health and Health Promotion

- **Health:** State of well-being in which the person is able to use purposeful, adaptive responses and processes physically, mentally, emotionally, spiritually, and socially, in response to internal and external stimuli (stressors) to maintain relative stability and comfort and to strive for personal objectives and cultural goals.
- **Wellness:** Ability to adapt, to relate effectively, and to function at near-maximum capacity; includes self-responsibility, nutritional awareness, physical fitness, stress management, environmental sensitivity, productivity, expression of emotions, self-expression in a variety of ways, creativity, personal care, and home and automobile safety.[245]
- **Bio-psychosocial or holistic health:** High level and total view of health; unity of body, mind (feelings, beliefs, attitudes), and spirit, and person's interrelatedness with others and the environment.[246]
- **Health promotion:** Activities that increase the levels of health and well-being and actualize or maximize the health potential of individuals, families, groups, communities, and society.[247]
- **Health-protective behaviour:** Any behaviour performed by a person, regardless of the perceived or actual health status, to protect, promote, or maintain health, whether or not that behaviour is actually effective.[248]
- **Primary prevention:** Activities that decrease the probability of occurrence of specific illness of dysfunction in an individual, family, group, or community and reduce incidence of new cases of disorder in the population by combating harmful forces that operate in the community and by strengthening the capacity of people to withstand these forces.
- **Secondary prevention:** Early diagnosis and treatment of the pathological process, thereby shortening disease duration and severity and enabling the person to return to normal function as quickly as possible.
- **Tertiary prevention:** Restoring the person to optimum function through rehabilitation and within the constraints of the problem when a defect or disability is fixed, stable, or irreversible.
- **Risk:** Exposure to possible loss, injury, or danger; the *probability* of occurrence of a particular event.
- **Risk factor:** Factors or characteristics *associated* with an increased probability of experiencing a particular event. Association means the risk factor and the condition often occur together, but the risk factor may or may not be a cause.

care preservation or maintenance, (2) cultural care negotiation or accommodation, and (3) cultural care repatterning or restructuring. These principles are defined as follows:

- **Cultural care preservation** refers to assistive, facilitative, or enabling acts that preserve cultural values and life ways viewed as beneficial to the client.
- **Cultural care accommodation** refers to assistive, facilitative, or enabling acts that reflect ways to adapt or adjust health care services to fit clients' needs, values, beliefs, and practices.
- **Cultural care repatterning** refers to altered designs to help clients change health or life patterns that are meaningful; the cognitive way that one recognizes different attributes and features of a culture for new patterns of care to become evident and for retention or preservation of selected values, beliefs, or practices of the culture.[255,256,257,258]

Cultural competence is the ability of a health care provider, agency, or system to respond to the unique trends of the populations whose cultures are different from that of the mainstream or dominant society. The importance of culture on all levels—client, provider, administration, and policy—is acknowledged and incorporated into health care. Basic beliefs about the nature of health and disease vary widely among cultures; it is not necessary to know everything about the person's culture to treat or give care competently. Cultural competence is an educational process that includes self-awareness, cultural knowledge, and the ability to develop working relationships across lines of difference, to be flexible, and to use intercultural communication skills. It is also acknowledging that the patient or client and family may not want a health care worker from the same country of origin to provide care, in case that person is familiar with the patient or family.

Nontraditional, Complementary, and Alternative Methods to Health Care

The use of Complementary Therapies and Alternative Health Care (CAHC) is becoming increasingly widespread in Canada with significant implications for health delivery.[259] In 1997, the results of a survey conducted by Angus Reid indicated that 42 percent of the respondents had used some type of complementary or alternative therapy.[260] What may be an issue is that many people are venturing forth and utilizing complementary therapies and alternative health practices—with or without the involvement of mainstream practitioners.[261] This issue, which may involve a degree of complexity, may bring a variety of questions to the minds of many health care professionals. For example, what may be the processes used to integrate complementary and alternative health practices with mainstream health care? Reflect on the following critical thinking question for a few minutes before responding.

CRITICAL THINKING

What are some ethical issues that accompany the use of CAHC?

Alternative Therapies

To be able to comprehend the meaning of alternative therapies, one may be drawn to the definition provided by Montbriand for her research project. She notes that alternative therapies entail a wide scope of health-related products or healing practices initiated or prescribed by self, family, network of friends, or an alternative health care practitioner who does not have the recognized authority to prescribe given by the provincial Colleges of Physicians and Surgeons or the Canadian Medical Association.[262] Montbriand's results are most informative for health professionals. For example, one of her findings indicates that all three groups of professionals (doctor, nurse, and pharmacist) saw the need for evidence-based information about alternative therapies.

To conclude, Health Canada indicated in a 1998 Report on Natural Health Products that it was imperative to have a balance between access and safety. Today, many nurses are involved in the debate on complementary and alternative therapies. Mulkins, Morse, and Best state that complementary therapy is congruent with health promotion and disease prevention.[263] Thorne and a group of researchers studied a geographically diverse Canadian population with inflammatory bowel disease (IBD) and found that the use of complementary/alternative medicine (CAM) is common among them and is generally perceived by the users to be beneficial and safe.[264] In a study by a Harvard University team, the folk remedy of drinking cranberry juice for urinary tract infections has been found to be effective in preventing recurring infection.

CRITICAL THINKING

What do you know about herbal remedies?

While some controversy may remain about CAM therapies, it is imperative that nurses know the position of their provincial/territorial regulatory body on the provision of alternative therapies.

Some insurance plans are now paying for nontraditional and alternative methods because they are less costly. These methods avoid hospitalization and focus on nontechnological methods. The possible danger in this is that some people will not get the needed life-saving medication or surgery—at least not soon enough.

Specific Culturally Based Interventions

Your approach to and way of speaking *to* the client will set the tone for how the client reacts to you and everyone else on the team. Call the person by title and last name until the person gives you permission to use the first name. Calling someone by his or her first name without leave may suggest that he or she is in a subservient position to you.

Be sensitive also to how you speak *about* the person. Often, in this context, people have experienced racial discrimination to the extent that it has affected their lifestyle and health outcomes.

As you intervene, teach, or counsel, adjust your communication approach with and behaviour toward clients from another cultural background accordingly because people from most ethnic or racial groups feel uncomfortable initially when interacting with someone who is different. Although you may be communicating in a way that is natural to you, someone from another culture may perceive that behaviour as too forward or aggressive, too passive, or not empathetic enough. While you cannot put on a different mask for each person you interact with, be aware that the client may misinterpret your well-intentioned behaviour. Use general knowledge about a culture, and simultaneously see the individual, unique differences of people. Unfortunately, not many nurses are bilingual. This poses difficulties when the client for whom English is a second language does not speak or understand English adequately for you to effectively assess, teach, or intervene in other ways.

Learn what the client considers a priority in care. Include the person's ideas in planning and giving care. Often, you may have to negotiate with the individual or family to carry out the essential medical treatments and nursing care, as well as include the cultural practices or spiritual healing rituals they hold most dear.

In male-dominated households (Asian, Middle Eastern), the male head of house must be included in all decisions and health teaching if you expect to obtain cooperation. In many such families, an older female relative, such as an aunt, mother-in-law, or grandmother, is often the designated health care provider for that family. She must also be included in decision making and health teaching. Speaking to the important family elder with respect will gain you a staunch ally; the desired behaviour change is almost certain to be achieved.[265] Relations between the client and the family may at times seem offensive or disharmonious to you. Differentiate carefully between patterns of behaviour that are culturally induced and expected and those that are harmful to the health of the persons involved.

Respecting the person's need for privacy or need to have others continually around is essential. Understand that some clients or families will not be expressive emotionally or verbally. Respect this pattern, recognizing that nonverbal behaviour also is significant. The meaning of a gesture differs from country to country. A wave of the hand may be friendly or an insult, depending on hand position. Be aware, too, that word meanings may vary considerably from culture to culture so that the person may have difficulty understanding you, and vice versa. Be sure the gesture or touch you use conveys the message you intend to convey. If you are unsure, avoid nonverbal behaviour to the extent that you can.

Interference with normal living patterns or practices adds to the stress of being ill. You will encounter and need to adapt care to the following customs; what is drunk with meals, when the main meal of the day is eaten, undressing in front of a strange person, special hair care, avoiding use of the bedpan because someone else must handle it, maintaining special religious or ethnic customs, refusing to bathe daily, refusing a pelvic exam by a male doctor, moaning loudly when in pain, and showing unreserved demonstrations of grief when a loved one dies.

A client with a strict time orientation feels it is important to take medicines and receive treatments on time—or feels neglected. You are expected to give prompt and efficient, but compassionate, service to this patient and family. Time orientation determines one's correctness in making appointments for the clinic, planning for medication routines, or returning to work after discharge. Time orientation even influences a person's ideas about how quickly he or she should get well. Clients with little future-time orientation have difficulty planning a future clinic appointment or a long-term medication schedule. They cannot predict now how they will feel at a later date and may think that clinic visits or medicines for a future time are unnecessary if they feel all right at the moment.

For some clients, the hurrying behaviour of the nurse or other health care providers is distressing; it conveys a lack of concern and lack of time to give adequate care. In turn, the person expresses guilt feelings when it is necessary to ask for help. Although you may look very efficient when scurrying about, you are likely to miss many observations, cues, and hidden meanings in what the person or family says. Examine your own attitude toward activity and inactivity to help others consider leisure as part of life. The disabled person for whom inability to work carries a stigma must develop a positive attitude about inactivity and may need your help. Think for a moment about how you may help this disabled person.

Your knowledge of cultures will enable you to practise **holistic care** that includes cultural values and norms as part of the nursing process. Holistic healing practices combine the best of two worlds: the wisdom and sensitivity of the older cultures and the technology and precision of the modern world. Although holistic practitioners use conventional therapies in many cases, the emphasis on the whole person—his or her physical, emotional, intellectual, spiritual, and sociocultural dimensions—remains. The focus is on disease prevention and health promotion as the individual takes responsibility for his or her own health and well-being. Multiple techniques are used to restore and maintain the balance of body energy. These techniques include exercise, acupuncture, massage, herbal medicine, nutritional changes, manipulation of joints and spine, medications, stress management, and counselling. The nurse–client relationship is the key to holistic nursing care, for the person has come to expect a caring interaction from the healer.

An important part of transcultural care is providing health services for refugee and immigrant populations. Be aware that newcomers to this country may be suspicious of screening processes; extra time must be spent in explaining why each component is necessary. You may need to use an interpreter (see Table 1-13).

Many immigrants find jobs in the food industry. When they first come to Canada or the United States, it is essential to ensure that they are in good health and not carrying any diseases. Foreign exchange students, visitors, and tourists may not be required to undergo medical clearance; however, their possible exposure to diseases may, in turn, endanger others around them.[266]

Some recent immigrants may continue to adhere closely to traditional practices. Others may not. Your care cannot be based on assumption or stereotyping. Immigrants may combine traditional cultural practices and Western practices. What is pertinent is the assessment of individual factors and cultural backgrounds that can help health care professionals anticipate and deal with difficulties experienced by immigrants and refugees with regards to seeking health care.[267]

Many Chinese throughout North America practise Western-oriented activities of exercise, religious practices, lifestyle, and illness behaviour activities. Four influencing variables are significant in their described health beliefs, dietary practices, and sick behaviour measures:[268,269,270] (1) the familiarity of the participant with Western health care systems, (2) language, (3) occupation, and (4) religion. Yep shares information on how nurses can better care for clients from an Asian culture:[271]

- Talk to the person in a way that shows respect. Call the person by title and last name. Do not talk down to the person or family.
- Older people may not be fluent in English, even if they have lived in Canada or the United States for many years. Speak slowly, but not loudly, to the client; invite the family to help interpret to the client and communicate feelings or questions to the health professional. The client is unlikely to admit that he or she does not understand.
- Generally, clients value care that reflects silence, patience, smooth relationships, and protecting self-esteem.
- Asian clients probably will not want to bother the practitioners with their complaints and problems. Most Asians believe suffering is part of life and must be quietly accepted; however, the client is likely to complain to family members. Include family in your assessment, and question the client repeatedly and in several different ways to assess pain.
- Illness may be viewed as the result of an imbalance between *yin* and *yang,* an evil spirit, improper food, or something bad in the family.
- Having the family bring familiar foods makes the hospital stay more comfortable for the Asian client. Some are accustomed to having rice at every meal.
- Most Asians highly respect and even fear authority; doctors and nurses represent authority. Thus, the client expects a formal relationship and may become confused by an informal approach.
- Explanations should be given slowly and repeatedly in simple language; the client is likely to be too intimidated by the authority figure to ask questions. The family should also be given the explanations so that they can clarify for the client, if necessary.
- Older Asian people may associate hospitals with death; it is the last place to go. On the other hand, hospitals also represent power and dominion. Hospital routines may not be understood. For example, an Asian person views his or her blood as finite in supply, as vital energy, and a life source; thus, taking frequent blood samples may cause much fear.
- Asian adults do not touch much and are not usually demonstrative. A smile conveys caring much better than a touch, as does performing little extras for the client without being asked, such as refilling the water pitcher.
- Use the family as an important resource. Let them know that they can visit frequently and for long hours, if they desire. They can assist in care; in fact, the client may expect them to. Cooperation with treatment and care routines will be fostered through communication with and involvement of the family.[272]

In some cultures, such as in the traditional Philippine, it is believed that illness is the result of evil forces and that treatment involves protection from or removal of these evil forces. For example, the body is viewed as a container that collects debris, so cleansing it involves stimulating perspiration, vomiting, flatus, or menstrual bleeding to remove evil forces from the body. Use of heat and control of cold through herbs, teas, water, and fire is believed to help maintain a balanced internal temperature. Mental illness may be thought to be the result of a spell; carrying an oval stone, or wearing a cross if the person is a Christian, is meant to serve as an antidote or protection.

In Canada, the Aboriginal cultural revival is beginning to have an effect on the mainstream society.[273] It is important, while caring for Aboriginal people and their families that the health care professionals be aware of the Aboriginal people's nationalism and cultural pride. Culturally appropriate health care takes into account the health beliefs, practices, and traditional healing systems that the clients and their families prefer. In fact, within the Canadian health care delivery system, it is nurses who provide the majority of health services to the Aboriginal people in various settings.[274]

As you care for clients from different cultures, be aware of barriers to accessibility or receptivity to health care services. For example, barriers to health care in a rural community may include the following:

- Heavy work schedule
- Economic difficulties
- Lack of health insurance coverage, high deductibles
- Lack of accessible health care services, long distances to services
- Negative attitudes toward health care services
- Lack of information about prevention or health maintenance, ignorance of warning signs of disease
- Inadequate prenatal care
- Less attention to or care for chronic illnesses
- Value of self-reliance and risk-taking behaviours

Gwyther and Jenkins describe barriers and services for a specific rural group in their article "Migrant Farm Worker Children: Health Status, Barriers to Care and Nursing Innovations in Health Care Delivery." (See *The Journal of Pediatric Health Care,* 12, no. 12 (1998), pp. 60–66.)

The changes in society may cause a variety of problems to families. Be a supportive listener, validate realistic ideas, and prepare the family to adapt to a new or changing environment, and be aware of community agencies or resources that can provide additional help. See Table 1-15 for guidelines on making referrals. When a client has no family nearby and seems alone and friendless, you may be able to provide them with significant support. Develop a better awareness of your own personal philosophy that promotes a feeling of stability in your life so that you, in turn, can assist the client and family to explore feelings and formulate a philosophy for coping with change.

Health teaching is one way to have a lasting effect on the health practices of a different cultural group. Health education specifically transmits information, mobilizes the inner resources of the person, and helps people adopt and maintain healthful practices and lifestyles. Others cannot make decisions for a person, but the person should be provided with sufficient information concerning alternative behaviours so that they can make intelligent choices themselves. Table 1-16 lists teaching principles and methods.

Various pressures interfere with attempts at health teaching. Behind poor health habits lies more than ignorance, economic pressure, or selfish desires. Motivation plays a great part in continuing certain practices, in spite of your efforts at education. Motivation, moreover, is influenced by a person's culture, and his or her status and role in that culture and by social pressures for conformity. Starting programs of health promotion can be difficult when people place a low value on health, cannot recognize cause-and-effect relationships in disease, lack future-time orientation, or are confused about the existence of preventive measures in their culture. Thus, preventive programs or innovations in health promotion must be shaped to fit the cultural and health profiles of the population. Long-range health promotion and disease prevention goals stand a better chance of implementation if they are combined with measures to meet immediate needs. A mother is more likely to heed your advice on how to prevent her sick child's condition getting worse if you give the child immediate care and attention.

IMPROVING HEALTH CARE PRACTICE AND ADVOCACY

With your knowledge about cultures and ways to care for people from different cultures, you can be an advocate for a client from a different culture to ensure accessibility and appropriateness of services. Moreover, you can help the health care system be more culturally sensitive in the care of clients, or you can work together with several agencies toward that goal.

What does good health mean to you and your family? According to Health Canada, good health is a major resource for personal, social, and economic development and an important aspect of quality of life. Health promotion strategies aim at making these conditions favourable through advocacy.[275] Health professionals should be visible and accessible, and they

---

TABLE 1-15
Guidelines for Making a Referral

1. Know the available community resources and the services offered.
2. Recognize when you are unable to further assist or work with the client; be honest about your own limits and your perceived need for a referral. Avoid implying rejection of the client.
3. Explore client readiness for referral. The client may also have ideas about referrals and sources of help or may be unwilling to use community agencies.
4. Determine which other professionals had contact with the client and confer with them about the possibility of referral. Various ethnic and racial groups prefer using the extended family or church.
5. Discuss the possibility of referral with a specific person at the selected agency before referral.
6. Inform parents of your recommendations and obtain their consent and cooperation if the client is a minor.

7. Be honest in explaining services of the referral agency. Do not make false promises about another agency's services or roles.
8. Describe specifics about location, how to get to the referral place or person, where to park and enter, and what to expect on arrival.
9. Have the client (or parent) make the initial appointment for the new service if he or she is willing to do so; some people may prefer you to make the initial contact. Tell the person that you have called the agency and that he or she is expected.
10. Do not release information to the referral agency or person without written permission from the client (or parent).
11. Ask the client to give you feedback about the referral agency or person to help you evaluate your decision and to help you make a satisfactory referral selection if needed for future needy individuals or families.

TABLE 1-16
Principles and Methods of Teaching

General Approach

1. Convey respect; be genuine.
2. Reduce social distance between self and others as much as possible.
3. Promote sense of trust and an open interaction; a trusting relationship fosters self-understanding and motivation to follow a teaching plan.
4. Elicit description of feelings from the client about the subject matter or situation to relieve tension and meet the learner's needs.
5. Be organized in presentation.
6. Use a comfortable setting and audiovisual aids as indicated.
7. Encourage questions, disagreement, and comments to ensure that your presentation stays focused on client needs and meets teaching goals.
8. Encourage, support, and reinforce as you present content.

Teaching Specific Content

1. Begin at knowledge level of client; consider readiness to learn.
2. Determine what client wants to know and already knows.
3. Answer the client's questions first; the client will then be more receptive to the information presented.
4. Build on what the client knows. Gently refute myths or misunderstandings.

5. Relate information to behaviour patterns, lifestyle, and sociocultural background to increase likelihood of their being followed by the client.
6. Assist client in reworking your ideas to fit cultural, religious, or family values and customs to ensure that the material to be learned will be practised.
7. Be logical in sequence of content.
8. Present more basic or simpler content before more advanced or complex information.
9. Present one idea or a group of related ideas, at a time, rather than many diverse ideas together.
10. Demonstrate as you describe directions, suggestions, or ideas, if possible.
11. Break content into units and a series of sessions, if necessary. Do not present too many ideas at one time.
12. Teach the family as thoroughly as the client to ensure that suggestions on interpersonal relationships and other concerns will be followed.
13. Present the same information to friends, employer, occupational health nurse, schoolteacher, clergyman, or significant community leader, if possible and relevant.
14. Provide written instructions in addition to oral presentations.
15. Provide feedback and reinforcement to the client as you provide opportunity for practice and review.

need to speak for health in its broadest sense. It is the essence of caring.

Group Teaching

Client groups provide a channel through which feelings and needs can be expressed and met, especially if the clients have similar concerns, such as colostomy or diabetes. Thus, you can use the group process to enhance health teaching or for therapy to aid coping with problems (Figure 1-1). You may work with a group that has formed to accomplish some specific goal, such as losing weight, promoting research to find a cure for cancer, or providing guidance to parents with mentally retarded children. In some cases information is not enough. Social support is also necessary, especially when engaging in a lesser-valued activity—such as avoiding excessive consumption of sweet foods.

Individual Teaching

Programmed Learning

Material is presented in carefully planned sequential steps through program instruction books or a computer program. One frame of information is presented at a time. The learner then tests his or her grasp of the information in the frame

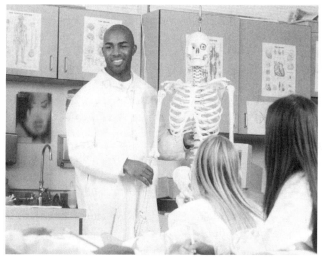

FIGURE 1-1

Group teaching provides an opportunity to provide health teaching to individuals with similar health concerns and problems.

Source: Berger, K. J., and M. B. Williams, Fundamentals of Nursing: Collaborating for Optimal Health. *Stamford, CT: Appleton & Lange, 1992, p. 181.*

by writing, or, in the case of a computer, keying in, a response to a question, usually a multiple-choice type. The book or computer then gives the correct response. If the learner's response was incorrect, the program presents a repetition of the information, or it might provide a more detailed explanation.

Literature

Pamphlets and brochures describe preventive measures, signs and symptoms of disease, and major steps of intervention. These are published by many health care organizations and agencies, often for specific diseases or groups.

Autobiographies of persons with certain disease processes and "how-to" books by persons who have experienced certain health problems directly or indirectly pass along suggestions to others.

Audiovisual Material

A player and cassettes explaining preventive measures, disease processes, or specific instructions can be loaned to the client. He or she can stop the cassette at any point and replay necessary portions until satisfied with the learning. "Talking Books" is a program that records information for the visually impaired. Closed-circuit television or videotape setups allow the person to hear and view material.

Note that these methods of individual instruction are individual only to a certain point. Only when the client can check learning with a *resource person,* ask further questions as necessary, and have help in making personal applications will learning become more significant. That process involves you. The person does not learn from a machine alone.

Computer/Internet

Instructions for prevention and health care for any condition as well as other information related to growth and development and care of the child, adolescent, and adult of any age is available through computer-assisted instruction formats. Computer programs for client teaching are available to home care and health care agencies. For example, a diagram along with instructions can teach a patient about bypass surgery. A parent can be shown exactly how tubes will be placed in a child's ear.

Evaluation of Teaching

1. Check frequently to determine if content is of interest or being understood.
2. Have client repeat content or give examples of application of content.
3. Have client review previously covered content, and its application, at each teaching session.
4. Determine the amount of learning that has occurred.

Telehealth

Telehealth—*electronically transmitted clinician consultation*—has improved access to care for people in rural or underserved areas but is also increasingly used in health promotion

education, illness prevention, and prevention of unnecessary hospitalizations. Telehealth can also reduce the number of home care visits through computer monitoring that is possible through audiovisual transmission over phone lines, so that the client and care provider can see and hear each other. The client controls the video monitor, which prevents any intrusion into privacy. You can also use this modern technology to continue learning about cultural care and to contribute to improved care.

The Advisory Council of Health Infrastructure for Canada describes Telehealth as using information and communication technologies to provide and deliver health information, services, and professional expertise over short and long distances.[276] In Manitoba, the Telehealth Network has extensively increased rural access to health care. A satellite or ground link connects health care providers with clients, or with each other. Participants at each end can talk with, hear, and see each other. Additional specialized equipment, such as digital cameras, digital otoscopes, and document cameras improve assessment and information sharing. Manitoba's Provincial Health Minister stated that Manitoba's Telehealth Network was a significant move toward a greater prevention of disabling illness and the promotion of health.[277] In Halifax, the establishment of the Izaak Walton Killam (IWK) Telehealth Program, by Chris-Anne Ingram, has not only been challenging but rewarding in bringing health care to clients and their families. Furthermore, Telehealth is able to bring continuing education to clinicians regardless of the distance.[278]

The National Initiative for Telehealth Framework of Guidelines was developed over a 20-month period and involved many steps and activities. Its focus is related to the rendering of clinical services (e.g., teletriage, telecare, and teleconsultation). The Guidelines will serve as a useful point of reference; and they will undoubtedly contribute to the general development of the Telehealth field in Canada.[279]

The Canadian Nurses Association (CNA), on a statement on telepractice, acknowledges the growing importance of telehealth and roles nurses can play in this area. The organization's position underlines the importance for safe, competent, and ethical involvement in Telehealth. Further, CNA implies that nurses must provide nursing telepractice services consistent with the Codes of Ethics for Registered Nurses.[280]

CRITICAL THINKING

Arrange for an observational experience to meet with a Telehealth contact. What kinds of questions would you like to have answered to be more informed about Telehealth?

Community Health Protection

Community health protection involves risk reduction behaviours and changing harmful environmental and social conditions. Screening and immunizations continue to be important, but changing personal health behaviours of people before the clinical disease develops is essential. Frequency and specific facets of the periodic health examination should be tailored to the unique health risks, age, and sex of the individual patient or client. Counselling and education that help the person, family, or group assume greater responsibility for health may be of more value than screenings every year.

However, health promotion and protection must focus on the community as well. Strengths of a community-based approach compared with individual approaches include the following:[281,282]

1. The power of intervention is greater, owing to the opportunity for diffusion and change of social norms.
2. Public awareness of health-promoting behaviours and barriers to such behaviours is increased, providing a basis for informed social action.
3. Programs are geared to the "real world" in which people live.
4. Programs can be delivered to larger groups than services targeted to individuals in circumscribed clinical settings.
5. Costs are generally lower for community programs than for one-on-one clinical services.
6. An environment of social support can be developed for risk-lowering and health-enhancing behaviours.

Community health protection strategies must be carefully planned and well coordinated. The following guidelines are useful for community health programming:[283,284]

1. Involve as many small groups, organizations, interorganizational networks, community-wide structures, and respected community leaders as possible.
2. Obtain official endorsement of your program from governmental agencies, local school districts, and religious organizations in the community.
3. Focus on intensive community action with a trained and well-organized health service structure and the media as backup.
4. Plan so that adequate time is allowed for each program phase and the overall time frame is manageable.
5. Develop and maintain a sense of community ownership and control of the program; enlist community volunteers as change agents.
6. Incorporate strategies to promote both maintaining healthful lifestyles and acquiring new habits.
7. Attend to ethnic and sociocultural aspects of the community in designing the program and tailoring health-promotion strategies to subpopulations. Monitor and evaluate the success of the program and provide feedback to participating populations concerning progress in reaching program goals.

Sites for Health Promotion and Wellness Programs

Traditionally the main health concerns for employees in the workplace were safety and accident prevention. A yearly physical examination was also included in many industries. Today industries and some hospitals and other work settings are adding programs for their employees that generally include emphasis in four areas: stress reduction, exercise, smoking cessation, and nutritional and weight guidance, particularly with reference to obesity and sodium and cholesterol dietary reduction. Some industries have also established employee assistance programs to help any employee with substance abuse problems so that he or she is a safe, dependable worker. Some settings offer daycare services to workers with young children to reduce stress that is related to child care. Others have stress management programs for their employees and their clients. Some companies have nearly 24-hour facilities comprising fully equipped exercise rooms, gyms, handball courts, whirlpool baths, and so on.

Health promotion sites could also be established in retirement centres, on campuses, in daycare centres, stores, housing projects, neighbourhood community centres, schools, churches, laundry facilities, or senior nutrition centres. Such sites would be more acceptable for health screening, well-child checkups, immunizations, or counselling to many cultural populations than is the hospital or traditional outpatient setting. Innovative city and regional public health agencies have for years used nontraditional settings for health promotion and illness prevention. The graduate-prepared nurse practitioner and clinical nurse specialist frequently work in a nontraditional site or, like other graduate-prepared nurses in any specialty, engage in entrepreneurial opportunities or faculty practice, combining practice, research, and academic roles.

Health care services must be provided in nontraditional sites to reach the homeless, refugees, or immigrants. Consistency in services and personnel will help such individuals to develop a trusting relationship and seek and accept health care. The health clinic adjacent to the day treatment program or walk-in meal site must be open at flexible hours and employ staff who are accepting and provide a variety of services besides health screening, primary care, or referral to other care agencies. Of greater importance than health services are food, clothing, showers, and personal care supplies, a safe place to rest, shelter from the weather and especially at night, and laundry facilities. In addition, the site should provide telephone and either employment counselling or referral to employment services. Helpful information on housing and paralegal services must be made available. Paralegal services can assist with obtaining entitlements, such as Social Insurance, disability benefits, or pensions. Giving the person a personal identification card that includes name, address, and phone number of a treatment facility is beneficial. One author (R.M.) has worked for more than 15 years with a community service agency in a metropolitan area that provides the above services for the poor and homeless, including the severely and persistently mentally ill and chemically dependent.

Among the factors creating the need for nurse entrepreneurs are the change in public attitudes and values and the growing emphasis on prevention. The present trend of reducing hospital use and curtailing health care costs has called for more cost-effective health care providers. Nurses are the perfect professional group to participate in the expansion of such primary health care and prevention services.

Each state in the United States or each province in Canada differs in the legal authority, reimbursement practices, and the prescription authority given to nurses in advanced practice. These factors greatly influence how much of an entrepreneur a nurse can be. A 1998 survey in the United States found that in all the states, advanced practice nurses (clinical nurse specialists, nurse midwives, nurse anaesthetists, and nurse practitioners) who are certified can be reimbursed for client care.[285]

The Canadian Nurses Association position statement on the Clinical Nurse Specialist (CNS) indicates that the CNS contributes significantly to the health of Canadians within a primary health care framework. Did you know that, historically speaking, the role of the CNS was introduced into the Canadian health care system in the 1960s? As health care became more complex, the trend toward specialization intensified and the result was the development of advanced nursing practice roles.[286] The CNS, as a practitioner, provides expert client care based on in-depth knowledge of a wide scope of nursing and other relevant sciences. Most importantly, the regulation of CNS practice is within the current scope of nursing practice and existing regulatory approaches.[287]

Because of change and uncertainty, a whole new set of nursing career opportunities are available. The future belongs to those who are able to respond to new demands and who have the courage to follow their convictions. In turn, people with diverse backgrounds will have a choice in selecting the type of health care service that best meets their needs. Then, culturally based care can become a reality.

INTERESTING WEBSITES

STATISTICS CANADA

http://www.statcan.ca

This website links you to numerous sources of information on population statistics. *The Daily* is a feature which provides the day's news releases through an easy-to-use A to Z index. Check it out.

CANADIAN CULTURE

http://www.culturecanada.gc.ca

This is the Government of Canada's Web access to government Culture, Heritage and Recreation Services. The extensive index provides alphabetically listed links from Archaeology to Provincial and Territorial Information with numerous options between them.

CANADIAN CITIZENSHIP AND IMMIGRATION

http://www.cic.gc.ca

Canadian Citizenship and Immigration was established in 1994 to link immigration services with citizenship registration.

One purpose was to help build a stronger Canada. This site can link you with The Minister, What's New, and the Statistical Newsletter.

GOVERNMENT OF NUNAVUT

http://www.stats.gov.nu.ca

At the time of accessing, this developing website showed an evaluation report on building Nunavut and several statistical reports on 2001 Census population counts including community level population estimates.

CANADIAN MULTICULTURALISM

http://www.mta.ca/faculty/arts/canadian_studies/english/about/multi

Details are provided here on Early Immigration, Modern Immigration, and Multicultural Policy.

INDIAN AND NORTHERN AFFAIRS CANADA

http://www.ainc-inac.gc.ca

This informative site lists services available for First Nations people along with a branch Performance Report for 2002–2003.

SUMMARY

1. You will encounter diverse value systems and customs in your care of clients and families.
2. Understanding the cultural and subcultural backgrounds enhances your care of the client, family, group, and community.
3. People from the *same* culture are uniquely different from each other; but they also share similarities.
4. People from *different* cultural backgrounds share similarities as well as differences in various life patterns and values.
5. Cultural background has a major influence on development and health.
6. You will practise principles of cultural care, based on concepts in this chapter, in every health care setting.
7. Engage in lifelong learning about your own and others' cultures to interact with, relate to, assess, intervene with, and care for the client as effectively as possible.

ENDNOTES

1. Canadian Heritage, Multiculturalism: Strength Through Diversity, 2003 [database online] Ottawa [cited 13 Aug. 2003] available from World Wide Web @ http://www.pch.gc.ca/progs/multi/reports/ann98-99/multic_e.cfm?nav=2
2. Statistics Canada, Population and Dwelling Counts For Canada, Provinces and Territories, 2001 and 1996 Census—100% Data, 2002 [database online] Ottawa [cited 13 Aug. 2003] available

from World Wide Web @ http://www12.statcan.ca/english/census01/ products/standard/popdwell/Table_PR.cfi

3. Statistics Canada, Census: Ethnocultural Portrait: Canada, 2003. [database online] Ottawa [cited 14 Aug. 2003] available from World Wide Web @ http://www12.statcan.ca/english/census01/ products/analytic/companion/etoimm/canada

4. *Ibid.*

5. Canada, *Royal Commission on Aboriginal Peoples: Report of the Royal Commission on Aboriginal Peoples, Vol. 2 Looking Forward, Looking Back,* 1996. Minister of Supply and Services Canada, Ottawa.

6. Kirmayer, L. J., G. M. Brass, and C. L. Tait, In Review: The Mental Health of Aboriginal Peoples: Transformations of Identity and Community, *Canadian Journal of Psychiatry,* 45, no. 7 (2000), 607–616.

7. Statistics Canada, 2001 Census—Release 5, Jan. 21, 2003: Ethnocultural Portrait of Canada [database online] Ottawa [cited 14 Aug. 2003] available from World Wide Web @ http:// www12.statcan.ca/english/census01/release/release5.cfm

8. Lester, N., Cultural Competence: A Nursing Dialogue, Part I, *American Journal of Nursing,* 98, no. 8 (1998), 26–34.

9. United States Bureau of the Census, *Statistical Abstract of the United States,* 1996. Washington, D.C.: 1996.

10. Leininger, M., Transcultural Care Principles, Human Rights, and Ethical Considerations, *Journal of Transcultural Nursing,* 3, no. 1, (1991), 21–22.

11. Courtney, B., Freedom From Choice, *Newsweek,* February 13 (1995), 16.

12. Leland, J., and G. Beals, In Living Color, *Newsweek,* May 5, 1997, 58–60.

13. Statistics Canada, Census: Ethnocultural Portrait: Canada, 2003.

14. Canada, *Royal Commission on Aboriginal Peoples: Report of the Royal Commission on Aboriginal Peoples, Vol.2 Looking Forward, Looking Back,* 1996.

15. Statistics Canada, Census: Ethnocultural Portrait: Canada, 2003.

16. Statistics Canada, Census: Ethnocultural Portrait: Canada, 2003.

17. Canadian Heritage, Bilingualism in Canada, 1999. [database online] Ottawa [cited 18 Aug. 2003] available from World Wide Web @ http://www.pch.gc.ca/progs/lo-ol/publications/facts/ bilingualism.html

18. Mackay, B., News: Changing Face of Canada is Changing the Face of Medicine, *Canadian Medical Association Journal,* 168, no. 5 (2003), [database online] Toronto [cited 12 Aug. 2003] available from World Wide Web @ http://www.cmaj.ca/cgi/content/ full/168/5/599

19. United States Bureau of the Census, *Statistical Abstract of the United States,* 1996.

20. Statistics Canada, 2001 Census Handbook: Reference, Minister of Industry, 2003 Ottawa. ISBN 0-662-31156-6.

21. Ryan-Nicholls, K. D., F. E. Racher, and J. R. Robinson, Providers' Perceptions of How Rural Consumers Access and Use Mental Health Services, *Journal of Psychosocial Nursing,* (2003), 41, no. 6, 34–43.

22. Andrews, M., and J. Boyle, *Transcultural Concepts in Nursing Care* (2nd ed.). Philadelphia: J. B. Lippincott, 1999.

23. Seifert, K., R. Hoffnung, and M. Hoffnung, *Lifespan Development.* Boston: Houghton Mifflin, 1997.

24. Mead, M. (ed.). *Cultural Patterns and Technological Change.* New York: Greenwood Press, 1985.

25. Popenoe, D., *Sociology* (10th ed.). Englewood Cliffs, NJ: Prentice-Hall, 1995.

26. Popenoe, *op. cit.*

27. Elliott, M., Here to Stay: An Adopted Son Embraces the Land of 'More,' *Newsweek,* July 10 (1995), 36–37.

28. Popenoe, *op. cit.*

29. Macionis, J., and L. Gerber, *Sociology: Fourth Canadian Edition,* Toronto, Pearson Education Canada Inc. 2002.

30. Kendall, D., R. Linden, and J. Lothian Murray, *Sociology in Our Times: The Essentials* (Second Canadian Edition). Scarborough: Nelson Thomson Learning, 2001.

31. Andrews, *op. cit.*

32. Giger, J., and R. Davidhizar, *Transcultural Nursing: Assessment and Intervention* (2nd ed.). St. Louis: C. V. Mosby, 1995.

33. Graham, J., *Another Mother Tongue.* New York: Beacon Press, 1990.

34. Kendall, *op. cit.*

35. Macionis, *op. cit.*

36. Mackay, *op. cit.*

37. Meekitjuk Hanson, A. with contributions from J. Otokiak (nd), Language. [database online] Nunavit [cited 25 Aug. 2003] available from World Wide Web @ http://www.google.ca/ search?q=cache:2jwkXJkdnUAJ:www.arctictravel.com/chapters/ languagepage.html

38. Graham, *op. cit.*

39. Mead, *op. cit.*

40. Popenoe, *op. cit.*

41. Mead, *op. cit.*

42. Macionis, *op. cit.*

43. Naisbitt, J., and P. Aburdene, *Megatrends 2000: Ten New Directions for the 1990s.* New York: William Morrow, 1990.

44. Zbilut, J., Contradictions of Nursing in a Post-modern World, *IMAGE: Journal of Nursing Scholarship,* 28, no. 3 (1996), 188–189.

45. Popenoe, *op. cit.*

46. Mead, *op. cit.*

47. Hecker, M., and F. Heike, eds., *The Greeks in America, 1528–1977.* Dobbs Ferry, NY: Oceana, 1978.

48. DeMott, B., *The Imperial Middle.* New York: William Morrow, 1990.

49. Macionis, J., *Sociology* (7th ed.). Englewood Cliffs, NJ: Prentice-Hall, 1999.

50. Naisbitt, *op. cit.*

51. Popenoe, *op. cit.*

52. Zbilut, *op. cit.*

53. Stewart, M. J. *Community Nursing: Promoting Canadians' Health, Second Edition.* Toronto: W. B. Saunders, 2000.

54. Canadian Heritage, Multiculturalism: Strength Through Diversity, 2003, *op. cit.*

55. Adams, M. *Book Summary: Sex in the Snow—Canadian Social Values at the End of the Millennium.* Toronto: Viking, 1997. [database online] [cited 24 Aug. 2003] available from World Wide Web Business Summaries @ http://www.bizsum.com/ sexinsnow.htm

56. Kendall, *op. cit.*

57. Kostash, M. *The Next Canada: In Search of our Future Nation.* Toronto: McClelland and Stewart Inc., 2000.

58. Neuborne, Ellen, with Kathleen Kerwin. 1999. Generation Y. *Business Week,* February.

59. Adams, M. *Clouds Over Canada: The New Social Climate.* Toronto: Environomics Research Group Ltd., 1999.

60. G8 online, 2002 Course, 10 Canada and its Values: Policy Priorities and Practice, John Kirton, U of T G8 Information Centre. [database online] Toronto [cited 24 Aug. 2003] Available from World Wide Web @ http://www.library.utoronto.ca/g7/g8online/english/ 2002/10.html

61. Calliste, A., *Black Families in Canada: Exploring the Interconnections of Race, Class, and Gender,* In Voices: Essays on

Canadian Families, Second Edition. Chapter 9. (Scarborough: Nelson Thomson Learning), 2003.

62. Baker, M., *Families: Changing Trends in Canada* (Fourth Edition). Toronto: McGraw-Hill Ryerson, 2001.

63. Ward, M., *The Family Dynamic: A Canadian Perspective* (Third Edition). Scarborough: Nelson Thomson Learning, 2002.

64. Statistics Canada, Canadian Culture in Perspective: A Statistical Overview, 2000 Edition, Minister of Industry, 2000. Ottawa. ISSN: 1480-879X.

65. Adler, J., The Rise of the Over-class, *Newsweek,* July 31 (1990), 32–46.

66. Case, E., The Good News About Black America, *Newsweek,* June 7, 1999, 29–40.

67. Gailey, P., In Search of the Real Middle Class: Debunking Some of the Defining Myths, *St. Petersburg Times.* Internet accessed. http://www.texnews.com/1998/opinion/mid0322.html.

68. Giger, *op. cit.*

69. Gilbert, D. A., *Compendium of American Public Opinion.* New York: Facts on File, 1989.

70. Gingrich, N., *To Renew America.* New York: HarperCollins, 1995

71. Macionis, *op. cit.*

72. Naisbitt, *op. cit.*

73. Popenoe, *op. cit.*

74. Kluckhorn, F., Family Diagnosis: Variations in Basic Values of Family Systems, *Social Casework,* 32 (February–March 1958), 63–72.

75. Kluckhorn, F., and E. Strodtbeck, *Variations in Value Orientations.* New York: Row, Petersen, 1961.

76. Meleis, A., Arab American Women and Their Birth Experience, *MCN,* 6, no. 3 (1981), 171–176.

77. *Koran,* 2: 223. Translation and Commentary by A. Yusef Ali.

78. Health Canada, *Population Health, Towards a Canadian Understanding: Clarifying the Core Concepts of Population Health: Introduction,* (2002). [database online] Ottawa [cited 29 August, 2003] Available from the World Wide Web @ http://www.hc-sc.gc.ca/hppb/phdd/docs/common/intro.html

79. Canadian Nurses Association. Nursing Now: Issues and Trends in Canadian Nursing, No. 5, Nursing with Communities-Making the Transition, 1998 [database online]. Ottawa [cited 1 September, 2003] Available from the World Wide Web @ http://www.cna-aiic.ca/pages/issuestrends/nrgnow/nrg_with_common.htm

80. Health Canada, *Population Health, Towards a Healthy Future: Second Report on the Health of Canadians,* 1999, Minister of Public Works and Government Services Canada, Ottawa. ISBN 0-662-27625-6.

81. Birmingham, C. L., J. L. Muller, A. Palepu, J. J. Spinelli, and A. H. Anis, 1999. The Cost of Obesity in Canada. *Canadian Medical Association Journal,* 160, no. 4, 484–488.

82. Martin, S., 2003. The staggering Cost of Illness and Injury. *Canadian Medical Association Journal,* 168, no. 3 (February 4), http://80-www-cmaj-ca.proxy1.lib.umanitoba.ca/cgi/content/full/168/3/332-a (accessed 28 August 2003).

83. Frank, James G. Canadians' Values and Attitudes on Canada's Health Care System: A Synthesis of Survey Results. Presentation—The Conference Board of Canada, Toronto, October 17, 2000. www.conferenceboard.ca

84. Vail, Stephan. 2001. Canadians' Values and Attitudes on Canada's Health Care System: A Synthesis of Survey Results. *The Conference Board of Canada,* January 2001. http://secure.conferenceboard.ca/Health/documents/307-00df.pdf

85. National Forum on Health, Canada Health Action: Building on the Legacy, Vol. 11, Values Working Group Synthesis Report, page 3, 1997. Quoted in Stephan Vail 2001. Canadians' Values and Attitudes on Canada's Health Care System: A Synthesis of Survey Results. *The Conference Board of Canada,* January 2001. http://secure.conferenceboard.ca/Health/documents/307-00df.pdf

86. Martin, *op. cit.*

87. Vail, *op. cit.*

88. Mendelsohn, Matthew. 2001. Canadians' Thoughts on Their Health Care System: Preserving the Canadian Model Through Innovation. A paper submitted to the Royal Commission on the Future of Medicare in Canada, November 2001. http://www.arts.waterloo.ca/~gboychuk/psci491/mendelsohn.doc

89. Ekos Research Associates, Health Canada Benchmark Survey, Final Report, November 23, 1999. Quoted in Stephan Vail, 2001. Canadians' Values and Attitudes on Canada's Health Care System: A Synthesis of Survey Results. *The Conference Board of Canada,* January 2001. http://secure.conferenceboard.ca/Health/documents/307-00df.pdf

90. Mendelsohn, *op. cit.*

91. Barnes, D., et al, Primary Health Care and Primary Care: A Confusion of Philosophies, *Nursing Outlook,* 43, no. 1 (1995), 7–16.

92. Flynn, B., The Caring Community: Primary Health Care and Nursing in England and the United States, in Leininger, M., ed., *Care: Discovery and Uses in Clinical and Community Nursing.* Detroit: Wayne State University Press, 1988, pp. 29–38.

93. *Healthy People 2000 National Health Promotion and Disease Prevention Objectives: Healthy People 2000 Review 1998–1999.* Hyattsville, MD: U.S. Department of Health and Human Services, 1999.

94. Barnes, *op. cit.*

95. Flynn, *op. cit.*

96. *Healthy People 2000 National Health Promotion and Disease Prevention Objectives: Healthy People 2000 Review 1998–1999.*

97. Andrews, *op. cit.*

98. Giger, *op. cit.*

99. Andrews, *op. cit.*

100. Giger, *op. cit.*

101. Giger, *op. cit.*

102. Popenoe, *op. cit.*

103. Flaskerud, J., Preface: Emerging Care of Vulnerable Populations, *Nursing Clinics of North America,* 34, no. 2 (1999), XV–XVI.

104. Gilbert, D., and J. Kahl. *The American Class Structure: A New Synthesis,* 3rd Edition. Homewood IL: The Dorsey Press, 1987.

105. Macionis, *op. cit.*

106. Kendall, Diana, Rick Linden, and Jane Lothian Murray. *Sociology in Our Times: The Essentials,* Second Canadian Edition. Scarborough: Nelson Thomson Learning, 2001.

107. Kendall, *op. cit.*

108. Harman, Lesley D., *Family Poverty and Economic Struggles,* in Canadian Families: Diversity, Conflict, and Change, Second Edition. 188, 189 (Nancy Mandell and Ann Duffy, Harcourt Canada 2000).

109. Gilbert, *op. cit.*

110. Roos, N. P., and C. A. Mustard, 1997. Variation in Health and Health Care use by Socioeconomic Status in Winnipeg, Canada: Does the System Work Well? Yes and No. Abstract. *Milbank Quarterly,* 75, no. 1, 89–111.

111. Kosteniuk, Julie G. and Harley D. Dickinson. 2003. Tracing the social gradient in the health of Canadians: Primary and

secondary determinants. *Social Science & Medicine,* 57, no. 2, 263–276.

112. Seguin, Louise, Qian Xu, Louise Potvin, Maria-Victoria Zunzunegui, and Katherine L. Frohlick. 2003. Effects of low income on infant health. *Canadian Medical Association Journal,* 168, no. 12, 1533–1538.

113. Dooley, Martin D., Lori Curtis, Ellen L. Lipman, and David H. Feeny. 1998. Child health and family socioeconomic status. *Policy Options* (September): 13–18.

114. Ing, Joan D., and Linda Reutter. 2003. Socioeconomic status, sense of coherence, and health in Canadian women. *Canadian Journal of Public Health,* 94, no. 3, 224–228.

115. Coles, R., The Children of Affluence, *The Atlantic Monthly,* September 1977, 53–66.

116. Phipps, L. Confusion of a Young WASP, *New York,* 21, no. 34 (1991), 24–31.

117. Statistics Canada, 2001 Census Handbook: Reference, Minister of Industry, 2003.

118. Ing, *op. cit.*

119. Macionis, *op. cit.*

120. Popenoe, *op. cit.*

121. World Health Organization, *Global Strategy for Health by All by the Year 2000.* Geneva: World Health Organization, 1981.

122. No More Pity for the Poor, *Money,* May (1995), 122–127.

123. DeMott, *op. cit.*

124. Gailey, *op. cit.*

125. Giger, *op. cit.*

126. Lamont, M., *Money, Morals, and Manners.* Chicago: University of Chicago Press, 1992

127. Macionis, *op. cit.*

128. Popenoe, *op. cit.*

129. Topolnicki, D., Five Trends to Bank On, *Money,* May (1995), 102–103.

130. Crane, M., Queen of the Charity Ball, *St. Louis Magazine,* May (1991), 39–41.

131. Gilbert, *op. cit.*

132. Gingrich, *op. cit.*

133. Popenoe, *op. cit.*

134. Macionis, *op. cit.*

135. Popenoe, *op. cit.*

136. Free, K., Who's Poor in America and Why, *Missouri Nurse,* 67, no. 1 (1998), 4–5.

137. Seifert, *op. cit.*

138. Popenoe, *op. cit.*

139. Free, *op. cit.*

140. McLaughlin, D., and L. Jensen, Poverty Among Older Americans: The Plight of Nonmetropolitan Elders, *Journal of Gerontology,* 48, no. 2 (1993), S44–S54.

141. No More Pity for the Poor.

142. De Santis, L., Building Healthy Communities with Immigrants and Refugees, *Journal of Transcultural Nursing,* 9, no. 1 (1997), 20–31.

143. Fisher, L., Health Care Recommendations for Treating Immigrant Populations, *Health Line Ink,* Fall (1994), 1, 7.

144. Free, *op. cit.*

145. Face of Rural Poverty, *Farmweek,* December 5 (1994), 7.

146. Whitman, D., D. Friedman, A. Linn, C. Doremus, and K. Hetter, The White Underclass, *U.S. News and World Report,* October 12 (1994), 4ff.

147. Courtney, *op. cit.*

148. Graham, *op. cit.*

149. Macionis, *op. cit.*

150. Popenoe, *op. cit.*

151. Macionis, *op. cit.*

152. Seifert, *op. cit.*

153. Courtney, *op. cit.*

154. Graham, *op. cit.*

155. Giger, *op. cit.*

156. Sorlie, P., E. Backland, and J. Keller, U.S. Mortality by Economic, Demographic, and Social Characteristics: The National Longitudinal Mortality Study, *American Journal of Public Health,* 85, no. 7 (1995), 949–956.

157. Susser, M., Editorial: Social Determinants of Health-Socioeconomic Status, Social Class, and Ethnicity, *American Journal of Public Health,* 85, no. 7 (1995), 903–904.

158. Canadian Heritage, Multiculturalism: Strength Through Diversity, 2003.

159. Health Canada, *Population Health, Towards a Healthy Future: Second Report on the Health of Canadians.*

160. Gilmore, J. and B. Wannell. Life Expectancy. *Health Reports* (Statistics Canada, Catalogue 82-003) 1999, 11, no. 3, 9–24.

161. Statistics Canada, Aboriginal Peoples of Canada: A demographic profile, 2001 Census: analysis series. Minister responsible for Statistics Canada, 2003. Ottawa. Catalogue 96F0030XIE2001 007.

162. Tjepkema, Michael. 2002. The health of the off-reserve Aboriginal population. *Supplement to Health Reports.* (Statistics Canada, Catalogue 82-003) Volume 13, 73–88.

163. Statistics Canada, Aboriginal Peoples Survey 2001—Initial Findings: Well-being of the non-reserve Aboriginal population. Minister of Industry, 2003. Ottawa. Cat. No. 89-589-XIE, ISBN 0-662-34985-7.

164. Young, T. Kue. 2002. Review of research on Aboriginal populations in Canada: relevance to their health needs. *British Medical Journal,* 327, 23 August, 419–422.

165. Statistics Canada, Aboriginal Peoples Survey 2001—Initial Findings: Well-being of the non-reserve Aboriginal population.

166. Health Canada. 2000. Diabetes Among Aboriginal (First Nations, Inuit and Métis) People in Canada: The Evidence, Health Canada, Ottawa.

167. Statistics Canada, Aboriginal Peoples Survey 2001—Initial Findings: Well-being of the non-reserve Aboriginal population.

168. Tester, Frank J. and Paule McNicoll, "Isumagijaksaq: mindful of the state: social constructions of Inuit suicide," *Social Science & Medicine* (forthcoming).

169. Young, *op. cit.*

170. Jenkins, A. L., T. W. Gyrokos, K. N. Culman, B. J. Ward, G. S. Pekeles, and E. L. Mills. 2003. An overview of factors influencing the health of Canadian Inuit infants. *International Journal of Circumpolar Health,* 62, no. 1, 17–39.

171. Health Canada. 2000. Diabetes Among Aboriginal (First Nations, Inuit and Métis) Peoples in Canada: The Evidenca.

172. Reading, Jeff, and Earl Nowgesic. 2002. Improving the health of future generations: The Canadian Institutes of Health, Research Institute of Aboriginal Peoples' Health. *American Journal of Public Health,* 92, no. 9, 1396–1401.

173. Tester, *op. cit.*

174. Reading, *op. cit.*

175. Martin Spigelman Research Associates. 2003. *Getting Ahead of the Epidemic: The Federal Government Role in the Canadian Strategy on HIV/AIDS 1998–2008*. Prepared for Health Canada and the Five Year Advisory Committee. June. Executive Summary.

176. Health Canada, Canada's Report on HIV/AIDS. 2003. [database online] Ottawa [cited 6 December 2003] Available from World Wide Web @ http://www.hc-sc.gc.ca/hppb/hiv_aids/report03/index.htm

177. Reading, *op. cit.*

178. Ship, S., and L. Norton. 2001. HIV/AIDS and Aboriginal Women in Canada. *Canadian Woman Studies,* 21, no. 2, 25–31.

179. Jenkins, *op. cit.*

180. Health Canada, Canadian Strategy on HIV/AIDS, National Aboriginal Council on HIV/AIDS. 2002. [database online] Ottawa [cited 6 December 2003] Available from World Wide Web @ http://www.hc-sc.gc.ca/hppb/hiv_aids/can_strat/aboriginal/main.htm

181. Segall, Alexander, and Chappell, Neena. *Health and Health Care in Canada.* Toronto: Prentice Hall, 2000.

182. Ship, *op. cit.*

183. Macionis, *op. cit.*

184. Giger, *op. cit.*

185. Giger, *op. cit.*

186. Bottorff, J. L., L. G. Balneaves, L. Sent, S. Grewal, and A. J. Browne. 2001. An Explanation of Women-centred Care in the Context of Cervical Cancer Screening in Ethnocultural Groups. *Research Bulletin: Centres of Excellence for Women's Health,* 1, no. 2, 8–9.

187. American Psychiatric Association, Committee on Nomenclature and Statistics, *Diagnostic and Statistical Manual of Mental Disorders-IV.* Washington, D.C.: American Psychiatric Association, 1994.

188. McLaughlin, *op. cit.*

189. Statistics Canada, Mental health of Canada's immigrants, Jennifer Ali. Supplement to Health Reports, vol. 13, 2002. Statistics Canada Catalogue 82–003.

190. Bottorff, *op. cit.*

191. Statistics Canada, Health status and health behaviour among immigrants, Claudio E. Perez, Supplement to Health Reports, vol. 13, 2002. Statistics Canada Catalogue 82–003.

192. Dunn, James R., and Isabel Dyck, 2000. Social Determinants of Health in Canada's Immigrant Population: Results from the National Population Health Survey. *Social Science & Medicine,* 51, no. 11, 1573–1593.

193. Bottorff, *op. cit.*

194. American Psychiatric Association, Committee on Nomenclature and Statistics.

195. Bottorff, *op. cit.*

196. American Psychiatric Association, Committee on Nomenclature and Statistics.

197. Dunn, *op. cit.*

198. Leininger, M. and M. McFarland. *Transcultural Nursing: Concepts, Theories, Research, and Practice* (Third Edition). New York: McGraw-Hill, 2002.

199. Leninger, *op. cit.*

200. Morgan, L., *And the Land Provides: Alaskan Natives in a Year of Transition.* Garden City, NY: Anchor Press/Doubleday, 1974

201. Davis, L., et al., AAN Expert Panel Report: Culturally Competent Health Care, *Nursing Outlook,* 40, no. 6 (1992), 277–283.

202. Giger, *op. cit.*

203. Capers, C., Mental Health Issues and African-Americans, *Nursing Clinics of North America,* 29, no. 1 (1994), 57–64.

204. Rosenbaum, J., Culture Care of Older Greek Canadian Widows within Leininger's Theory of Culture Care, *Journal of Transcultural Nursing,* 1990, 2, no.1, 37–47.

205. Srivastava, Rani, and Madeleine Leininger. "Canadian Transcultural Nursing: Trends and Issues." Chapter 31 of *Transcultural Nursing: Concepts, Theories, Research and Practice* (Third Edition), by Madeleine Leininger and Marilyn McFarland, 493–502, New York: McGraw-Hill, 2002.

206. Cravener, P., Establishing Therapeutic Alliance Across Cultural Barriers, *Journal of Psychosocial Nursing,* 30, no. 12 (1992), 10–14.

207. Lynam, M. Judith, Baldir Gurm, and Ranjit Dhari, 2000. Exploring perinatal health in Indo-Canadian women. *The Canadian Nurse,* 96, no. 4, 18–24.

208. Lipson, J. G., and A. Meleis, Culturally Appropriate Care: The Case of Immigrants, *TCN,* 7, no. 3 (1985), 48–56.

209. Brink, P., and J. Saunders, Culture Shock: Theoretical and Applied. In Brink, P., ed. *Transcultural Nursing: A Book of Readings.* Englewood Cliffs, N.J.: Prentice-Hall, 1978, pp. 128–138.

210. Brink, *op. cit.*

211. Lipson, *op. cit.*

212. Leininger, M., *Nursing and Anthropology: Two Worlds to Blend.* New York: John Wiley & Sons, 1970.

213. Weiss, O., Cultural Shock, *Nursing Outlook,* 19, no. 1 (1971), 40–43.

214. Canadian Heritage, Multiculturalism: Strength Through Diversity, 2003.

215. Canadian Nurses Association, 2000. Cultural diversity—changes and challenges, *Nursing Now: Issues and Trends in Canadian Nursing,* no. 7, February.

216. Aboriginal Nurses Association of Canada, Strengthening the circle of wellness, 2003. [database online] Ottawa [cited 9 August 2003] Available from World Wide Web @ http://www.anac.on.ca/

217. Davis, *op. cit.*

218. Dienemann, J. (ed.), *Cultural Diversity in Nursing: Issues, Strategies, and Outcomes.* Waldorf, MD: American Nurses Association, 1997.

219. Dossey, B., and L. Dossey, Body-Mind-Spirit, Attending to Holistic Care, *American Journal of Nursing,* 98, no. 8 (1998), 35–38.

220. Haddon, R., An Economic Agenda for Health Care, *Nursing and Health Care,* 11, no. 1 (1990), 21–30.

221. Aboriginal Nurses Association of Canada, Strengthening the circle of wellness, 2003.

222. Edelman, C., and C. Mandel, *Health Promotion Throughout the Life Span* (4th ed.). St. Louis: C. V. Mosby, 1998.

223. Meleis, A., and C. LaFever, The Arab American and Psychiatric Care, *Perspectives in Psychiatric Care,* 22, no. 2 (1984), 72–86.

224. Leininger, M., *Transcultural Nursing: Concepts, Theories, and Practices.* New York: John Wiley & Sons, 1978.

225. Leininger, M., *Transcultural Nursing.* New York: Masson, 1979.

226. Tripp-Reimer, T., P. Brink, and J. Saunders, Cultural Assessment: Content and Process, *Nursing Outlook,* 32, no. 2 (1984), 78–82.

227. Giger, *op. cit.*

228. Leininger, *op. cit.*

229. Giger, *op. cit.*

230. Roach, L., Assessment: Color Changes in Dark Skin, *Nursing '77,* 7, no. 1 (1977), 48–51.

231. Goichot, B., A. Buguet, P. Bogui, et al. Twenty-Four Hour Profiles and Sleep-Related Variations of Cortisol, Thyrotropin, and Plasma Renin Activity in Healthy African Melanoids, *European Journal of Applied Physiology and Occupational Therapy,* 70, no. 3 (1995), 220–225.

232. Davitz, L., Y. Sameshima, and J. Davitz, Suffering as Viewed in Six Different Cultures, *American Journal of Nursing,* 76, no. 8 (1976), 1296–1297.

233. Zbilut, *op. cit.*

234. Giger, *op. cit.*

235. Snow, L., Traditional Health Beliefs and Practices Among Lower Class Black-Americans, *The Western Journal of Medicine,* 139 (1983), 830–838.

236. Assembly of First Nations National Indian Brotherhood, 2002. First Nations and Inuit Regional Health Survey Report, chronic diseases. [database online] Ottawa [cited 9 August 2003.] Available from World Wide Web @ http://www.afn.ca/Programs? Health%20Secretariat?chronic_conditions.htm

237. Fisher, *op. cit.*

238. Leininger, M., *Ethical and Moral Dimensions of Care.* Detroit: Wayne State University Press, 1990.

239. Edelman, *op. cit.*

240. Statistics Canada, Health Statistics Division, 1996. The health of Canada's immigrants in 1994–95. *Health Reports,* 7, no. 4, 33–45.

241. Morrocco, F. N., and H. M. Goslett (eds.). *The Annotated Immigration Act of Canada.* Toronto: Thomson Professional Publishing, 1993.

242. Shah, Chandrakant P. *Public Health and Preventative Medicine in Canada,* Fifth Edition. Toronto: Elsevier Canada, 2003.

243. Houldin, Arlene D., Susan W. Saltstein, and Kathleen M. Ganley. *Nursing Diagnoses for Wellness: Supporting Strengths,* Philadelphia: Lippincott, 1987.

244. Leininger, M., *Care: The Essence of Nursing and Health.* Detroit: Wayne State University, 1988

245. Edelman, *op. cit.*

246. Alternative Medicine, *Harvard Women's Health Watch,* 1, no. 10 (1994).

247. Pender, Nola J., Carolyn L. Murdaugh, and Mary Ann Parsons, *Health Promotion in Nursing Practice* (4th ed.). Upper Saddle River: Pearson Education; 2002.

248. Pender, *op. cit.*

249. Haddon, *op. cit.*

250. *Healthy People 2000 National Health Promotion and Disease Prevention Objectives: Healthy People 2000 Review 1998–1999.*

251. Stoto, M., and J. Durch, National Health Objectives for the Year 2000: The Demographic Impact of Health Promotion and Disease Prevention, *American Journal of Public Health,* 81, no. 11 (1991), 1456–1465.

252. Canadian Nurses Association, Nursing Leadership Development in Canada—A Descriptive Status Report and Analysis of Leadership Programs, Approaches and Strategies: Domains and Competencies; Knowledge Skills; Gaps and Opportunities. Prepared for CNA by Dr. Heather Lee Kilty, March, 2003.

253. Leininger, M., Self-Care Ideology and Cultural Incongruities: Some Critical Issues, *Journal of Transcultural Nursing,* 4, no. 1 (1992), 2–4.

254. Villarruel, A., and M. Denyes, Testing Orem's Theory With Mexican Americans, *IMAGE: Journal of Nursing Scholarship,* 29, no. 3 (1997), 283–288.

255. Leininger, M., *Care: Discovery and Uses in Clinical and Community Nursing.* Detroit: Wayne State University Press, 1988.

256. Leininger, *op. cit.*

257. Leininger, M., Southern Rural Black and White American Lifeways with Focus on Care and Health Phenomena, in Leininger, M., ed., *Care: The Essence of Nursing and Health.* Detroit: Wayne State University Press, 1988, pp. 133–159.

258. Leininger, M., *Culture Care Diversity and Universality: A Theory of Nursing.* New York: National League for Nursing, 1991.

259. Canadian Nurses Association, Complementary Therapies— finding the right balance, *Nursing Now: Issues and Trends in Canadian Nursing,* 1999, no. 6, July.

260. Angus Reid Group Inc., 1998b. *Use and danger of alternative medicines and practice: Parts I and II.* Consumer poll conducted by CTV/Angus Reid Group Poll in August 1997.

261. Health Canada, Health Care Network, Perspectives on Complementary and Alternative Health Care, 2003. [database online] Ottawa [cited 12 June 2003] Available from World Wide Web @ http://www.hc-sc.gc.ca/hppb/healthcare/pubs/ comp_alt/ intro.html

262. Montbriand, Muriel, 2000. Alternative Therapies: health professionals' attitudes. *The Canadian Nurse,* 96, no. 3, 22–26.

263. Mulkins, Andrea, Janice M. Morse, and Allen Best, 2002. Complementary Therapy Use in HIV/AIDS. *Canadian Journal of Public Health,* 93, no. 4, 308–312.

264. Thorne, Sally, Barbara Paterson, Cynthia Russell, and Annette Schultz, 2002. Complementary/alternative medicine in chronic illness as informed self-care decision making. *International Journal of Nursing Studies,* 39, no. 7, 671–683.

265. Giger, *op. cit.*

266. Fisher, *op. cit.*

267. Andrews, Margaret M., and Joyceen S. Boyle. *Transcultural Concepts in Nursing Care,* Fourth Edition. Philadelphia: Lippincott Williams & Wilkins, 2003.

268. Giger, *op. cit.*

269. Webster, R., Asian Patients in the CCU, *Nursing 4,* no. 31 (March 28–April 10, 1991), 16–19.

270. Yep, J., An Asian Patient. How Does Culture Affect Care? A Family Member Responds, *Journal of Christian Nursing,* 6, no. 5 (1991), 5–8.

271. Yep, *op. cit.*

272. Yep, *op. cit.*

273. Ponting, J. Rick. *First Nations in Canada: Perspectives on Opportunity, Empowerment, and Self-Determination.* Toronto: McGraw-Hill Ryerson Ltd., 1997.

274. Clarke, Heather F., Rhea Joseph, Michele Deschamps, T. Gregory Hislop, Pierre R. Band, and Richard Atleo, 1998. Reducing Cervical Cancer among First Nations Women. *The Canadian Nurse,* 94, no. 3, 36–41.

275. Health Canada, Population Health Approach, Ottawa Charter for Health Promotion, 2002. [database online] Ottawa [cited 20 June 2003] Available from World Wide Web @ http://www.hc-sc.gc.ca/hppb/phdd/docs/charter/

276. Telehealth, Medico-Legal Implications of Telehealth in Canada, 2003. [database online] Toronto [cited 20 February 2004] Google search: Telehealth Medico Legal Implications. Available from World Wide Web @ http://www.Ininnovationlaw.org/ Bell_Labs/pages/Medico-Legal%20Implications%20of%20 Telehealth%20-%20CST%202003%20-%20V2.0.pdf

277. Manitoba Telehealth, Manitoba Government, Telehealth network increases rural access to health care, 2002 [database online] Winnipeg [cited 20 February 2004] Available from World Wide Web @ http://www.gov.mb.ca/chc/press/top/ 2002/02/2002-02-25.

278. Sibbald, Barbara, 2003. A Telehealth Pioneer. *Canadian Nurse,* 99, no. 3, 52.

279. National Initiative for Telehealth Guidelines, 2003. National Initiative for Telehealth (NIFTE) Framework of Guidelines. Ottawa: NIFTE.

280. Ross-Kerr, Janet C., and Marilyn J. Wood. *Canadian Nursing: Issues and Perspectives,* Fourth Edition. Toronto: Elsevier Science Canada, 2003.

281. Alternative Medicine, *Harvard Women's Health Watch.*

282. Leininger, *op. cit.*

283. Meleis, *op. cit.*

284. Stanhope, M., & J. Lancaster, *Community Health Nursing: Promoting Health of Aggregates, Families, and Individuals* (4th ed.). St. Louis: C. V. Mosby, 1997.

285. Pearson, L., Annual Update on How Each State Stands on Legislative Issues Affecting Advanced Nursing Practice, *The Nurse Practitioner,* 24, no. 1 (1999), 16–83.

286. Canadian Nurses Association, Position Statement, Clinical Nurse Specialist [database online] Ottawa [cited 20 February 2004] Available from World Wide Web @ http://www.cna-nurses.ca/pages/policies/Clinical%20Nurse%20Specialist_March%202003.pdf.

287. Stanhope, *op. cit.*

Chapter 2

ENVIRONMENTAL INFLUENCES ON THE PERSON AND FAMILY

Earth does not belong to us;
we belong to the earth.

Chief Seattle

OBJECTIVES

STUDY OF THIS CHAPTER WILL ENABLE YOU TO:

1. Examine the scope of environmental pollution, both outdoors and indoors.

2. Identify sources of air pollution in your community and specify resulting hazards to human health.

3. List types of water pollution and describe resultant health problems.

4. Determine substances that cause soil pollution and specify their effects on health.

5. Examine types of food pollution and consider their effects on health.

6. Identify sources of noise pollution in various settings.

7. Contrast different types of surface pollution and resultant health problems.

8. Describe health hazards encountered in the home and on the job and the major effects of these contaminants.

9. Analyze ways that you can prevent or reduce environmental, food, and noise pollution.

10. Evaluate your professional responsibility, in the practice area, in assessing for illness caused by environmental pollutants.

Although ecology is a well-publicized subject, the physical environment in which we live is often taken for granted and overlooked as a direct influence on people and their health. You may wonder why a book discussing major influences on the developing person, family unit, and their health contains a chapter about humans and their environment. Yet where we live and the condition of that area—its air, water, and soil—determine to a great extent how we live, what we eat, the disease agents to which we are exposed, our state of health, and our ability to adapt. This chapter focuses primarily on noxious agents to which many people in Canada and the United States are exposed in the external environment. Because of the interdependence of people, only those living in isolated rural areas escape the unpleasant effects of our urban, technologically advanced society. Yet even the isolated few may encounter some kind of environmental pollution, whether through ground water contaminated from

afar, food shipped into the area, smog blown from a nearby city, or contaminated rain or snow. Further, the pollutants that are discussed are observed worldwide.

Nursing in the past was concerned primarily with the client's immediate environment in the hospital or home. Today nursing and health care are extended to include assessment of the family and community as well as the individual. Interventions are directed toward promoting a healthy environment for individuals and families, well or ill, and maintaining public health standards and federal regulations. Understanding some specific environmental health problems and their sources and effects will enable you to function both as a citizen and as a health care professional in working with clients and their families in the hospital or community.

HISTORICAL PERSPECTIVE

The entire environment has been and is a vital part of our existence. Human skill in manipulating the environment has produced tremendous benefits; but none has been without a price, the high price of pollution. Pollution of our environment not only is a health threat but also offends aesthetic, spiritual, social, and philosophic values. Environmental pollution is a complex, significant problem requiring multiple solutions (Figure 2–1).

The world appears to be shrinking in size mainly due to the rapid advances in technology, be it communication or transportation. Global attention has been given to effects of acid rain on forests, depletion of the ozone layer, and global warming. People appear to be more linked together due to the outbreak and expansions of diseases around the world, such as severe acute respiratory syndrome (SARS). The health of the earth and the health of its people are becoming more inseparable. Today, the public faces the challenge and the need to become highly aware of the connection between environmental hazards and human health.[1]

The official recognition of the status of the earth's environmental problems and the impact of these problems on human health was first stated by governments at the 1992 Rio Earth Summit.[2] At the Rio summit, it was acknowledged that a clearer understanding and a precise identification of these environmental health issues, which were global in nature, were required. It was also evident that a collective stance was needed among communities and countries to act on these issues.[3] Environmental health may be defined as the study of those aspects that influence both human health and the well-being of the population.[4] Such aspects may include exposure to environmental contamination, hazards, or pollutants that are detrimental to health. What is most imperative is the

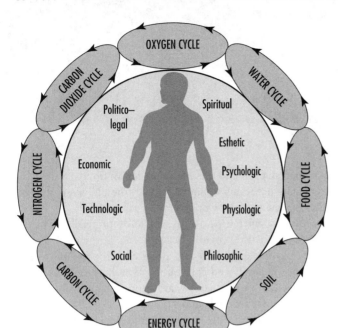

FIGURE 2-1

Human interrelationship with the environment.

attention that is needed now, to comprehend the effect that our environment exerts on human health. If we are to attain the goal of health for all, this attention must be continued to be addressed relentlessly. An overview of environmental health in Canada is available in several publications by Health Canada, including *Environment and Health: A Handbook for Health Professionals*.[5] It is most important for health professionals, such as nurses, to be knowledgeable regarding the ways of how environmental hazards impact upon human health. Similarly, health professionals must be alert to environmental health issues that surface in various settings and in various regions in the world.[6]

In October 2000, the Quebec City Consensus Conference on Environmental Health Indicators was held to examine the challenges facing environmental health monitoring and surveillance. It was held to discuss the possibility of developing consensus on many of these and related issues.[7] According to Shah, an indicator is a statistic that provides a meaningful indirect representation of the health of a community.[8] Examples include the infant mortality rate (IMR) as an indicator of the health status of a community, or the rise in ambient climatic temperatures as an indicator of climate change worldwide.[9] Hodge and Longo argue that, while selecting a particular indicator is important, an even more critical task is that of identifying and tracking the change, synthesizing meaning—often from contradictory indicators—and communicating the results to key players.[10]

CRITICAL THINKING

What other indicators can you think of that might effectively measure the health status of a community?

It is noteworthy to state that the *Canadian Environmental Protection Act* (CEPA) was enacted in 1988 to provide a means

of assessing, identifying, evaluating, and managing toxic chemicals. The act, administered jointly by Health Canada and Environment Canada, has many key elements; but it is designed mainly to protect human health and the environment by reducing or eliminating toxic substances and controlling the entry of new substances into Canada that may pose a threat to health and the environment.[11] In 1994, the House of Commons Standing Committee on Environment and Sustainable Development was given the task of conducting a five-year review of CEPA. The committee recommended a new approach whereby the emphasis in CEPA should shift from the *management* of pollution to the *prevention* of pollution.[12] The CEPA is designed to protect the environment and human health. It provides the federal government with the authority to confront pollution problems on land, in water, and through all layers of the atmosphere.[13] Thus the new CEPA is in harmony with the Canadian provinces and territories regarding environmental protection. Further, the New Substance Notification Regulations (NSNR) of CEPA (1999) specifies that all relevant information be provided to government offices if a substance, intended for import or manufacture, is considered new to Canada.[14] The cornerstone of CEPA (1999) is pollution prevention. Adequate prevention of pollution and harmful waste production helps to decrease risks to the environment and to human health.[15] Other methods of protecting the environment focus mainly on managing waste and pollution after they have been detected. Adhering to a preventive approach helps us manage risks to human health by protecting the quality of air, land, ecosystems, and nature (Figure 2–2).[16] The National Pollutant Release Inventory (NPRI) is a database of information on annual releases to air, water, and land. The same database maintains records of off-site transfers for disposal or recycling.[17] The NPRI is the only nationally legislated, publicly accessible, inventory of its kind in Canada. The inventory was established in 1992 and mandated under CEPA. It requires companies to report specific information on the release and transfer of pollutants to the federal government on an annual basis.[18] Other federal legislation on the protection of the environment includes the following:

- The *Arctic Waters Pollution Prevention Act*, which prohibits depositing waste of any type in the Arctic.
- The *Fisheries Act*, which prohibits the depositing of harmful substances in water that is frequented by fish.
- The *Canada Shipping Act*, which monitors the discharge of garbage and oil or oily substances from ships.
- The *Motor Vehicle Safety Act*, which establishes standards on emissions from gasoline- and diesel-powered motor vehicles.[19]

It is important to recognize that, in Canada, many federal and provincial environmental laws overlap. For example, the federal government and the province of Ontario have both enacted environmental statutes aimed at regulating similar matters. That is, both Canada and Ontario have an *Environmental Protection Act*.[20]

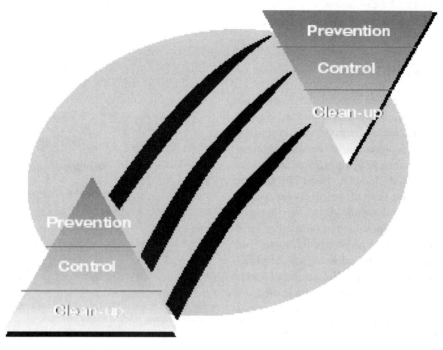

FIGURE 2–2

The pollution paradigm shift.

Source: Informing Canadians on Pollution, 2003, ISBN: 0-662-36412-0, Catalogue No. En40-7771 2003E, URL: www.ec.gc.ca/npri/communities, Figure 3–The Pollution Prevention Paradigm Shift. Year of Publications 2003.

CRITICAL THINKING

In what ways can municipal governments collaborate with the provincial and federal governments in dealing with environmental issues?

The recognition of the interdependence of human health and the health of the global ecosystems is growing.[21] A serious concern exists over the condition of the environment and the effects of chemical and biological contamination. Interestingly, this concern includes not only contamination effects on human health, but the viability of the ecosystems and numerous species. Public attention has been drawn to the many reports linking environmental exposure to unfavourable human health responses in our industrialized society.[22] For example, the literature, which examines the effects of chemicals on the hormone systems of humans and animals, is increasing. Due to the identification of a newly identified illness pattern—the sick building syndrome—indoor air quality in modern buildings has also been investigated.[23] Even though uncertainty may be associated with many environmental health problems, health care professionals remain the most credible source of information regarding health effects of environmental exposures.[24]

Before leaving this section, it is again important to note that a new way of managing the environment has emerged over the last few years. Environmental agencies are establishing mechanisms for ensuring that information is easily accessible and readily understood. These efforts have been aided by recent advances in information and communication technology. According to the Task Force on a Canadian Information System for the Environment to the Minister of the Environment, Canada is one of the most connected countries in the world. It is the world leader in the use of geographic information systems and satellite-based remote sensing technology for data collection on the environment.[25]

The following material is divided into discussions of air, water, soil, food, noise, and surface pollution, and occupational hazards. However, these categories overlap. To illustrate, when a person inhales harmful particles from the soil that have become airborne, soil pollution becomes air pollution; and soil or surface pollution becomes water or food pollution if the harmful particles are swept into the water, consumed first by fish and then by people. Further, in the workplace the person may encounter any of the pollutants described in this chapter.

AIR POLLUTION

*This most excellent canopy, the air, look you,
this brave o'erhanging firmament, this majestical
roof fretted with golden fire—why, it appears no
other thing to me than a foul and pestilent
congregation of vapors.*

Hamlet (II, ii, 314–315)

In various settings, you will care for clients and their families who have diseases caused by air pollution. It is critical to prevent these diseases by reducing all forms of pollution described in this section.

Problems of Air Pollution

Of course, air pollution is not a new problem; people have known for centuries that air can carry poisons. Natural processes, such as forest and prairie fires, volcanic eruptions, and wind erosion, have long contaminated the air. A dramatic example of natural air pollution in the United States was caused by the 1980 eruption of Mount St. Helens in the state of Washington. Gases and dust from the volcano were spewed into the atmosphere, and local communities were covered with volcanic ash. Human activities, such as burning of fossil fuels, surface mining of coal, incineration of solid wastes, and manufacturing processes, are recognized as sources of pollution. The current problem of toxic air pollution came sharply into focus in late 1984 when more than 2500 people died and as many as 100 000 were left with permanent disabilities as a result of a gas leak from a Union Carbide Corporation fertilizer plant in Bhopal, India.[26]

Air pollution and water pollution act interchangeably; together they present a world problem. All people on the earth share the oceans and the air. Significant local pollution of either can greatly affect distant areas, especially if the oceans cannot, by the processes of precipitation, oxidation, and absorption, cleanse the atmosphere before harmful effects occur. Given enough time, the oceans can cleanse the atmosphere; but if the amount of pollution exceeds the ocean's capacity to neutralize the waste, harmful materials are dispersed into the atmosphere, and we realize the effects by breathing contaminated air.[27]

For Canada, and for most countries in the world, the effects of air pollution and global warming are contributing highly to anxiety about the environment. The reason for this anxiety is that a potential exists for extensive adverse health effects and devastating climate change.[28] Air pollution levels tend to increase with higher temperatures. Such a relationship reflects the fact that the causes of global warming and air pollution are similar.[29] Edwards claims that almost two of every three Canadians claim that pollution has made their health worse (Figure 2–3).[30] Further, more than half of the population of Canada express their concern about air quality.[31]

An increasing prevalence of asthma is occurring in many industrialized countries, including Canada.[32] Asthma is a disease that causes breathing problems. The most common factors affecting the asthma client include allergens, respiratory irritants, and viral infections.[33] Examples of outdoor pollutants that can exacerbate asthma include ground-level ozone and sulphur dioxide. Meanwhile, the indoor irritant of tobacco smoke represents an even greater risk.[34] Manfreda and his coresearchers examined the variability of asthma-related manifestations and medication use in six sites across Canada (Vancouver, Winnipeg, Hamilton, Montreal, Halifax, and the province of Prince Edward Island). Their findings were then compared to those from sites that had participated in a recent

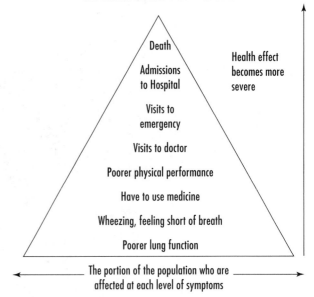

The Health Effects of Air Pollution

The health effects of air pollution may vary from subtle problems, to troubling symptoms, to hospital visits and early deaths.

FIGURE 2–3
The health effects of air pollution.

Source: Reproduced with permission of the Canadian Public Health Association. Originally published in *Canadian Journal of Public Health*, Vol. 92, no. 3, May/June 2001.

European survey. They concluded that the significant variation in the prevalence of asthma symptoms and attacks, and the use of asthma medication between Canadian sites and international sites, suggest environmental influences.[35] In the management of asthma, environmental control and education should be instituted for all asthma clients and their families.[36]

CASE SITUATION

Jean-Paul is a ten-year-old boy admitted to the Emergency Unit of the large urban hospital where you work. Jean-Paul's mother has informed you that he is highly allergic to cats and smoke and that anxiety appears to exacerbate his asthma attacks. The doctor has discussed Jean-Paul's asthmatic management with the mother and has discharged him with several prescriptions for asthma drugs. As Jean-Paul's nurse, you decide to conduct some discharge teaching.

QUESTIONS

1. What issues will you address in your discharge teaching episode with Jean-Paul and his mother?
2. List the relevant health promotion strategies in this case.
3. The mother's main question for you is: "How likely is Jean-Paul to have another asthmatic attack?" How do you answer her?

Sources of Air Pollution

The five most common pollutants found in the air are carbon monoxide, sulphur oxides, nitrogen oxides, suspended particles, and hydrocarbons (Table 2–1). The sources of these air pollutants vary, and the effects on humans differ according to length and degree of exposure to the pollutant. Air pollution is most harmful to the very young, the very old, and persons with respiratory and cardiac disease.[37–51]

A major cause of air contamination is imperfect or incomplete combustion. **Perfect or complete combustion** exists only in chemistry books and is the *result of hydrogen and carbon uniting completely with oxygen, thereby relinquishing heat, water vapour, light, and carbon dioxide to the air.* **Imperfect or incomplete combustion** refers to the *additional liberation of carbon monoxide, sulphur oxides, nitrogen oxides, and hydrocarbons into the air.*

Canada's National Ambient Air Quality Objectives (NAAQOs) are national goals for outdoor air quality. They protect not only public health but also the environment and certain aesthetic properties of the environment.[52] The establishment of NAAQOs is a dynamic and continuous process. Air quality objectives are developed to reflect the current state of understanding about an air pollutant, to establish a national indicator for assessing the quality of air in all parts of Canada, and to provide guidance to governments for implementing risk management decisions such as planning control strategies and setting local standards.[53] Air quality is monitored by both the federal and provincial governments. The Air Quality Index (AQI), also referred to as the Index of the Quality of Air (IQUA), is an indicator of overall air quality developed to inform the public about the general or prevailing air quality in their community.[54] For example, the lower the index on the AQI, the better the air quality is. The AQI values can be obtained from the Ontario Ministry of the Environment's website at http://www.airquality-ontario.com.[55] It is important to note that the NAAQOs do not provide a measure of overall air quality. They only provide a means of evaluating the levels of individual pollutants. In Ontario, an Air Quality Index network provides the public with air quality information across the province.[56]

Four additional air pollution problems should be mentioned: (1) depletion of the upper atmosphere ozone layer, (2) increasing levels of atmospheric carbon dioxide, (3) acid rain, and (4) radioactive substances. As noted, a thin layer of ozone surrounds the earth and blocks much of the sun's ultraviolet radiation from reaching the earth's surface. The ozone layer is in danger of being depleted by the continued use of fluorocarbons (Freon) and chlorofluoromethanes that release chlorine into the stratosphere to combine with ozone. The continued use of fluorocarbon-propelled aerosol products and supersonic transport planes adds to that danger.[57–59]

Large sport utility vehicles, with their low gas mileage, are exacerbating global warming because of the amount of carbon dioxide produced. For information about the amount of carbon dioxide produced by cars of all sizes and makes, visit http://www.toowarm.org. The pollution-free automotive vehicle is a fantasy at this point because of consumer indifference.[60]

In Canada, the federal government is developing an integrated strategy: (1) for clean air for vehicles and the fuels that power them, (2) for transboundary air pollution with the United States and other countries, (3) for industrial pollution, and (4) for encouraging Canadians to develop solutions to clean air issues.[61]

The *car driven daily to work,* in contrast to mass transit systems, can be considered an enemy to the environment and even society. Emissions from Canadian and U.S. cars are among the largest contributor to global-warming greenhouse-effect gases. The required paving covers fertile farmland and wetlands and encourages urban sprawl and its effect on traffic and longer commutes; community development; air, water, and noise pollution; habitat disruption; and wildlife loss. Limitless mobility has created an environmental nightmare in the Western world, and increasingly in developing countries. Some cities and groups such as Ottawa's "Communities Before Cars" are working to create communities that require less vehicle use; encourage walking, bicycling, or mass transit use; and have more open space and greenbelts.[62]

In Caucasians short-wavelength ultraviolet sunlight is thought to cause melanoma and nonmelanoma skin cancer that would increase in incidence if there were a reduction of the ozone layer. In addition, studies have shown that an increase in ultraviolet radiation damages the immune system of humans.[63,64]

Increasing Carbon Dioxide

The atmospheric content of carbon dioxide has increased significantly in the past century. Carbon dioxide is added to the atmosphere by burning fossil fuels. The increased level of atmospheric carbon dioxide alters the heat balance of the earth. Sunlight passes through the carbon dioxide, but the *radiation of heat away from the earth is slowed, producing what is known as the* **greenhouse effect.** Such changes might eventually result in melting of the polar ice caps, flooding of large coastal plain areas, and disruption of food production.[65–68] Some scientists fear the *opposite may occur*—the **refrigerator effect.** The carbon dioxide concentration would eventually prevent enough of the sun's rays from reaching earth that cooler temperatures would occur, again affecting food production and health factors.[69–71] Scientists find signs of a shift in distribution of invertebrate species that suggest a rapid warming of the Northern Hemisphere, which affects the food chain overall. According to the United Nations Development Report, Canada ranks second highest in the world in the amount of carbon dioxide emissions per individual. Canada's annual greenhouse gas emissions, for example, contribute about 2% of the global total of human-made emissions.[72]

CRITICAL THINKING

In addition to the burning of fossil fuels, what are other sources of carbon dioxide emissions?

TABLE 2–1
Common Air Pollutants

Pollutant	Characteristics	Source	Where Found	Effects
Carbon Monoxide (CO)	Colourless Odourless Tasteless Poisonous Contributes to photochemical smog	Motor vehicle, car exhaust Cigarette smoking Forest fires Faulty or unvented furnaces or kerosene or wood space heaters	Garages Tunnels Heavy traffic areas Basements and homes that are poorly ventilated CO detector monitors excess levels, prevents poisoning	**Hypoxia,** *decreased oxygen level in blood* Dizziness Hypotension Tachycardia Headaches Cherry-red lips and skin Fatigue Drowsiness Impaired perception and thinking; odd behaviour; brain damage Dangerous to people with heart or respiratory disease or anemia; pregnant women; children Fetal growth retardation and brain damage Death: exposure to 0.05% CO air concentration can be fatal in 30 minutes from respiratory or heart failure
Sulphur Oxides Sulphur dioxide (SO_2) Sulphuric acid (H_2SO_4)	 Heavy poisonous gas Heavy, corrosive colourless liquid	 Factories that burn coal or oil that contains sulphur Sulphur trioxide (SO_3) reacts with water vapour to form mist	 Coal that contains sulphur Industrial and urban areas	Irritation of mucous membranes: eyes, nose, throat, lungs Causes or aggravates respiratory disease Death Damage to plants Corrosion of metals

(continued)

TABLE 2–1 *(continued)*
Common Air Pollutants

Pollutant	Characteristics	Source	Where Found	Effects
Nitrogen Oxides Nitrogen dioxide	Gaseous end products Visible red-brown gas Toxic Foul-smelling	Burning fossil fuel Motor vehicles Other transportation modes Burning natural gas, oil, and coal in power plants	Coal Oil Natural gas Urban areas Rural areas if power or industrial plants present Nitrous oxide reacts in sunlight to produce smog and ozone	Irritation of mucous membranes of throat Altered night vision Respiratory disease Heart disease Cancer
Suspended Particles	Minute particles Dust Dirt Soot Aerosols Fly ash	Industrial processes Power and heating plants Wood or coal burner in homes Wind erosion Forest or building fires Incineration of solid wastes Surface mining	Urban industrial areas Rural mining areas Observable on surfaces in homes	Irritation to mucous membranes: eyes, nose, throat Respiratory disease Damage to surfaces
Asbestos particles	Asbestos material deteriorates, releases fibres in air	Factories Homes Public buildings Roadways Brake linings Clutch facings Now regulated or prohibited	Building insulation Shingles Sidings Floor and ceiling tiles Patching compounds Textured paints Appliances	Respiratory disease Rate of lung cancer 5 times greater in person with asbestosis than if no asbestos scarring; person with asbestosis who smokes 1 pack of cigarettes daily is 50 times more likely to develop lung cancer.
Tobacco smoke	Direct or passive smoke in environment	Tobacco cigarettes	Anywhere someone smokes tobacco products	Cardiac disease Respiratory disease Cancer Low birth weight in infants Parental smoking affects birth weight of baby

(continued)

TABLE 2–1 *(continued)*
Common Air Pollutants

Pollutant	Characteristics	Source	Where Found	Effects
Hydrocarbons	Volatile organic compounds of hydrogen and carbon	Natural sources: 85% Decomposition of organic matter Evaporation of gasoline from motor vehicles Vapours from chemical reactions Incomplete combustion	Atmosphere Forests Coal, gas, and petroleum fields Industrial and chemical manufacturing plants	React in presence of sunlight to produce smog or ozone
Ozone	Pungent Colourless Toxic gas	Lower atmosphere: formed in air by chemical reactions between nitrogen oxide and hydrocarbons	Upper atmosphere: a protective barrier against excess sunlight Lower atmosphere	Irritates eyes and mucous membranes of nose and throat Respiratory distress Cardiac distress Nausea Headaches Decreased tolerance to exercise Affects venous system Severely affects children, elderly, chronically ill Causes plants to turn yellow, reducing photosynthesis
Photochemical Smog	Chemical reaction between nitrogen oxides and hydrocarbons stimulated by sunlight			Eye irritation Cardiac distress Lung damage Decreased tolerance to physical activity

Acid Rain

Acid rain is the *end product of chemical reactions that begin when sulphur dioxide and nitrogen oxides enter the atmosphere from coal-, oil-, and gas-burning power plants, iron and copper smelters, and automobile exhaust.* These gases undergo changes and eventually react with moisture to form sulphuric acid and nitric acid. One-half to two-thirds of the pollution falls as acid rain or snow; some of the remainder is deposited as sulphate or nitrate particles that combine with dew and mist to form dilute acids.[73] Most of the northeastern United States; portions of the upper Midwest, Rocky Mountains, and West Coast; and parts of Ontario, Quebec, Nova Scotia, and Newfoundland now receive strongly acidic precipitation. It is somewhat gratifying, however, to know that Canada and the United States will increase their cooperation to reduce cross-border air pollution. Three major pilot projects designed to promote greater opportunities for coordinated air quality management between the two countries have been announced jointly by each government's environmental agency.[74]

Although acid rain's full effect on the environment is not understood as yet, increased acidity in soil, streams, and ponds can be documented. Certain freshwater ecosystems are particularly sensitive to acid; fish, frogs, and some aquatic plants die. Acid rain leaches compounds out of soil, damaging the root systems of plants, so forests die and crops are damaged. With continued episodes of acid rain, limestone and marble statues and buildings are dissolved, and homes and other structures weather more quickly.[75–77] At present, the only solution is to decrease the emissions of sulphur and nitrogen oxide into the atmosphere. Over the last two decades, Canada has reduced its sulphur dioxide emissions by more than half. In spite of this progress, however, the recovery of natural ecosystems has been much slower than anticipated. Beyond its injurious effects upon our lakes, forests, and wildlife, acid rain affects our health as well. For example, the sulphur dioxide contained in acid rain can react with other chemicals in the air to form sulphate particles, which can lodge in the lungs to cause respiratory problems.[78]

Radioactive Substances

Radioactive substances are *produced by mining and processing radioactive ore and by nuclear fission and radiation procedures* used in industry, medicine, and research. Pollution from radioactive materials poses a serious threat to our ability to reproduce and to our gene structure. It is also related to an increase in leukemia and other cancers, as demonstrated in persons working with radioactive materials over long periods without adequate safeguards and in survivors of the bombings in Hiroshima and Nagasaki, Japan. A small fraction (1% to 3%) of all cancers in the general population is attributable to natural radiation. Occupational irradiation produces an increase over the natural incidence.[79–82]

Indoor Air Pollution

Some significant indoor pollutants are carbon monoxide, asbestos particles, nitrogen oxides, formaldehyde, and radon. Office workers and others in North America and Europe who work in buildings with inadequate ventilation systems that create poor mechanical airflow regularly report a *variety of nonspecific but illness-producing symptoms.* The buildings have been referred to as "sick buildings," giving rise to the **"sick building syndrome."** Symptoms include the following:

- Irritation of the skin, eyes, nose, and throat
- Mental and physical fatigue
- Headache; difficulty concentrating
- Dizziness
- Eye, nose, throat irritation
- Frequent respiratory infections
- Hypersensitivity reactions

Exposure to other indoor pollutants, such as cigarette smoke and inhalants, increases the symptoms.[83–89]

It is somewhat disconcerting to note that only minimal attention has been placed on indoor pollutants issues in schools and on students. Poor indoor air quality affects the capacity to concentrate and learn. Further, it increases the likelihood for bacterial and viral infections, and mould growth to occur.[90] A multidisciplinary research team from Dalhousie University in Halifax, with sponsorship from Health Canada, has begun a three-year exploration of the issue of indoor air quality. The aim of the project is to develop standard guidelines and recommendations that will be pilot-tested in various schools across Canada.[91]

Formaldehyde, *a colourless gas characterized by a strong, pungent odour*, escapes into the air from foam insulation, particleboard, plywood, fibreboards, and carpets. Volatile organic compounds (benzene, chloroform, and formaldehyde) may be given off by paints, vinyl, printed documents, telephone cables, solvents, and some furniture. Tobacco smoke, which contains volatile organic compounds and other gases and particles, is dirtier than the usual air the smoker inhales. Carbon dioxide levels may be well above that considered healthy. Formaldehyde gas in newly insulated homes has reached concentrations high enough to cause dizziness, drowsiness, nausea, vomiting, rashes, nosebleeds, and diarrhea. It is extremely hazardous and probably is a carcinogen. Nitrogen oxides are released from unvented gas stoves and space heaters. As they accumulate in the home, these pollutants can affect sensory perception and produce eye irritation.[92,93]

Radon, a *natural radioactive gas produced by the decay of uranium 238,* is the most serious health threat of the common indoor pollutants, causing serious respiratory problems. It seeps into basements through cracked floors and diffuses out of brick and concrete building materials. Radon is responsible for thousands of deaths from lung cancer each year.[94–100] Homes in geographic areas with high levels of radon and high numbers of energy-efficient homes should be tested and home repairs made if needed.[101]

Particles such as dust, soot, ash, and cigarette smoke may be inhaled into the lungs. Tobacco smoke is linked to an increase in asthma and respiratory infections, especially in children.[102] In Canada, De Groh and Morrison state that the rates of home exposure to environmental tobacco smoke vary dramatically by province. Nevertheless, it appears that passive smoking produces elevated risks for coronary heart disease that are similar to low-level active smoking (about one cigarette per day).[103] Many household products such as cleansers, drain openers, and paint removers have toxic ingredients; fumes cause respiratory irritation, and eye or skin irritation occurs on contact. Some are carcinogenic when fumes or particles are inhaled over time. Chemicals from wall coverings and carpets; carbon dioxide and nitrous oxide from stoves; moulds; and pet dander also cause sickness.[104] Fungi, mould, dust mites, algae, pollen, and bacteria from humidifiers and air-conditioning systems can cause allergies or Legionnaires' disease and aggravate asthma.[105]

CRITICAL THINKING

What health program could you develop in your area of work to promote smoke-free homes?

Hospitals have a unique form of indoor air pollution. Fumes from disinfectants, such as glutaraldehyde, a sterilizing agent for instruments; surgical smoke or laser plume from tissue being cut, vaporized, or coagulated; and waste gases from anaesthetic agents affect health care workers and patients. A small amount of glutaraldehyde fumes can cause respiratory and dermatologic problems. Surgical smoke or laser plume can cause respiratory symptoms, burning and watery eyes, nausea, and viral contamination and regrowth. Nurses who work in the recovery room are likely to feel fatigue from breathing the patients' exhaled anaesthesia gases.[106]

Exposure to volatile organic compounds at home, such as those used in furniture stripping or home decorating, can cause local irritation and systemic effects—especially if used in a confined space. Chemical exposure can precipitate an asthma or angina attack, or even myocardial infarction.[107]

Indoor air pollution can be controlled by several measures: proper venting of gas stoves, heaters, and wood stoves; painting over materials that emit radon and formaldehyde; and daily airing of the house. Houseplants, especially spider plants, can be used to absorb air pollutants in the home.

Only in becoming aware of these factors as personal health threats will we seriously consider alternatives to using two or three cars, seek to know the serious hazards in our jobs, become concerned about houses downwind from an industrial site or the amount of ultraviolet light we receive, and use less dangerous products for many household tasks.

WATER POLLUTION

Pollution of the water from the natural processes of aquatic animal and plant life, combined with human-made waste, constitutes another hazard to the delicate state of human health. Human-made water pollution has two major origins—*point sources* and *nonpoint sources*. Point sources are those that discharge pollutants from a well-defined place (e.g., outlet pipes of sewage treatment plants and factories). Nonpoint sources consist of runoff from city streets, construction sites, farms, and mines.

Types of Water Pollution

The most common water pollutants are common sewage, pathogenic organisms, plant nutrients, synthetic chemicals, inorganic chemicals, sediment, radioactive substances, oil, and heat (Table 2–2).[108–115] Water pollution is a global problem, as is air pollution. As our environment changes, can we believe that all of our water sources will remain pristine? The fact is that preserving clean and safe drinking water sources is becoming a priority because of global pollution.[116] The link between human health and a fresh clean water supply is critical. McQuigge claims that human, industrial, and agricultural waste productions are escalating. Unfortunately, these wastes find their way into the groundwater, which increases the risk of pathogens such as bacteria and viruses. These same waste production sources are also largely responsible for the presence of chemicals in the water.[117] In Ontario, and elsewhere in Canada, the standards for potability of 30% to 40% of private wells are below standard.[118] In addition, the quality of surface water can change due to inputs of human wastes, nutrients, and chemicals, resulting in higher drinking water risks.[119]

Health Canada, in cooperation with the Federal-Provincial-Territorial Committee on Environmental and Occupational Health, published the April 2003 *Summary of Guidelines for Canadian Drinking Water Quality*, which supersedes all previous versions.[120] The summary provides guidelines for microbiological, chemical, physical, and radiological parameters for drinking water quality. For example, the microbiological parameter regarding public drinking water systems states that water samples should show no Escherichia coli (E. coli). E. coli denotes fecal contamination as well as the chance of enteric pathogens being present. Both may unfavourably affect human health. If E. coli is detected, municipal officials may issue a boil-water advisory, which advocates boiling water for one minute to ensure safety for drinking purposes.[121] Corrective actions directed toward a detected source of contaminated water supply should be taken. For all semi-public and private drinking water supply systems, water samples are expected to contain no E. coli, and no water sample should contain total coliform bacteria. In nondisinfected well water, the presence of total coliform bacteria, when E. coli is absent, implies that the well is prone to surface water infiltration and is at risk of fecal contamination.[122] It is important to note that in disinfected water systems, the presence of total coliform bacteria implies a failure in the disinfection process.[123] Currently, the microbiological parameters for bacteria, protozoa, and viruses are under review. To gain further insights into requirements for Canadian drinking water, see the *Summary of Guidelines for Canadian Drinking Water Quality* at http://www.hc-sc.gc.ca/hecssesc/water/pdf/summary.pdf.

CRITICAL THINKING

Of what importance is it for a health professional to know the difference between total coliform bacteria and fecal coliform bacteria?

TABLE 2–2
Common Water Pollutants

Pollutant	Characteristics	Source	Where Found	Effects
Common Sewage	Traditional waste from domestic or industrial sources	Sewage disposal system: septic tanks, cesspools, outdoor toilets	Sewage drains into water source, and water unable to deal with waste	Waste uses oxygen needed by aquatic plant and animal life Water rendered useless Death of aquatic life Human gastrointestinal diseases Infectious diseases
Pathogenic Organisms	Various disease-producing microorganisms	Sewage contamination	Rivers, lakes, streams Drinking water Farm areas Rural or urban areas where population is dense and public utilities are limited	Infectious gastroenteritis Hepatitis Typhoid fever Giardiasis, cholera
Plant Nutrients	Nutrients, especially phosphates and nitrates that nourish plant life	Sewage Livestock and human excrement Soil erosion Industrial wastes Chemical fertilizer	Rural ground water and drinking supplies Nutrients not easily removed by water treatment centres may inadvertently change substances into usable mineral form, causing more plant growth	Unpleasant odour and taste in water Disturbs normal food web in body of water Infant illness and death from nitrate-induced methemaglobinemia
Synthetic Chemicals	Synthetic chemical substances, such as detergents, cleaning agents, pesticides	Homes Industries	Widespread	Poisonous to aquatic life Unpleasant taste and colour in water Possible disease

(continued)

TABLE 2–2 *(continued)*
Common Water Pollutants

Pollutant	Characteristics	Source	Where Found	Effects
Inorganic chemicals	Mineral substances Toxic materials	Mining Manufacturing processes	Waste supplies Toxic waste materials may be dumped into water or land areas	Corrodes water treatment equipment Kills plant and animal life Disease in humans
Sediment	Particles of dirt or sand	Soil erosion		Reduced photosynthesis for aquatic plants in water where soil suspended; causes reduced food chain for animals Disrupts reproductive cycles of aquatic animals; clogs streams Prevents natural reservoirs from filling with rain Increased cost of water treatment
Radioactive material	Synthetic or natural	Waste from nuclear power plant		Contamination of water and food Cancer
Oil spills		Dumping of waste oil Flushing ship bilges Oil refinery discharge Accidental spills account for small percentage of spill		Death to birds and other aquatic life Presence in food web of humans, unknown effects
Heat	High temperature Reduces ability of water to absorb oxygen	Industrial processes		Ecologic balance of lakes and rivers permanently upset Interference with food chain for humans and animals

Let us move now, from the concerns of drinking water safety to consideration of our oceans. One of the most frightening results of water pollution is the threat to the oceans. The collective practice of the world's nations of ocean dumping of sewage may permanently pollute the oceans. An international conference on the dumping of wastes at sea was held in London, England, in 1972. This conference resulted in the *Ocean Dumping Act* of 1972. Amendments to the act followed; and in 1975, Canada joined over 50 other countries to ratify the Convention on the Prevention of Marine Pollution by Dumping Waste and Other Matter. This convention is a powerful weapon in the battle to protect the sea, including food resources, from lethal forms of pollution. In 1988, the *Ocean Dumping Control Act* was incorporated into the *Canadian Environmental Protection Act* (CEPA).[124]

Problems in Water Purification

The common denominator of all major water pollution is called **biologic oxygen demand (BOD)**, *the amount of free oxygen that extraneous substances absorb from water.*[125] The natural water purification process involves the action of bacteria, which use oxygen to decompose organic matter. If too much waste is dumped into a given body of water, this natural cleansing process cannot take place or at least does not take place fast enough. Further, once the water in the underground aquifer is contaminated, it is nearly impossible to guarantee a safe water supply.

When water contains pollutants in ever-increasing amounts, it becomes a threat to human health. At present, the quality of water service for countless people must be improved. Many inhabitants of rural areas and small towns obtain their drinking water from polluted sources.[126–130] The outbreak of E. coli in the water supply of Walkerton, Ontario, and Cryptosporidium species found in the water in North Battleford, Saskatchewan, were events that compromised public health.[131] Manure from cattle farms in the area, together with inadequate water treatment processes are the suspected causes of these outbreaks. The disease outbreaks which resulted from the public drinking water systems drew the attention of several levels of government and the public to the critical need of questioning and examining water safety and for having a supply of safe drinking water available in communities.[132]

Pollution of marshes and shorelines has severely impaired breeding habitats for many types of shellfish and deep-water species, thereby subsequently affecting the food supply. Polluted water cannot be used for recreational purposes; backpackers, campers, swimmers, windsurfers, and water skiers have all felt the impact of water pollution. In addition to the health risk, the odour of decay and the unsightliness of polluted water destroy the beauty of any natural setting.

Store-bought water may be safe, but the container that sits for weeks or months at room temperature is an ideal breeding ground for bacteria. Expiration dates are not required on the bottles. Further, traces of biphenyl A, an endocrine disrupter that can alter reproductive development in animals, has been found after 39 weeks in water held at room temperature in large polycarbonate containers (the office or home cooler). *The chemical is leached from the plastic water container.* Glass bottles of water are safer because they are not made from petrochemicals.[133]

Pip conducted a survey of bottled drinking water available in Manitoba. She claims that the bottled water samples studied indicated great variation in quality. Some exceeded the Canadian Water Quality Guidelines for drinking water for total dissolved solids (TDS), chloride, and lead.[134]

CRITICAL THINKING

What do you need to know to better understand the quality of drinking water?

CONTROVERSY DEBATE

Drinking Well Water: What Is the Risk?

While enjoying some well-earned time alone in a quiet restaurant you find yourself seated next to a family of four (two children under 12 years of age). This family is joined by an older couple who have obviously known the younger family from a common rural community some distance away. From their animated conversations you realize they have all been evacuated to your community from a region you heard about on the radio. This region had experienced a rapid spring thaw and heavy rains causing both small rivers in the area to overflow their banks and cause some flooding. Flooding, it seems, has never been experienced in this community in living memory. The two families have just received word that transportation is available the next day to return them to their homes after a two-week absence The women mention their anticipation to be home again doing their own cooking. Although home damage has been light in their neighbourhood, considerable ground flooding has occurred—especially near the hog-producing ranch and the beef cattle operation located in their community. Both operations, you learn, are close to where they live.

As a health care professional, you wonder about the water supply for the home community of these folks next to you.

1. What do you feel is your responsibility to these six people regarding your concerns about their water supply?

2. If you decide to introduce yourself to consider the matter with them, how do you start?

3. If you learn from them that no official contact person has been made available to them regarding their safety on returning home, what will you say to them?

4. What health-promoting options are open to you to assist these people?

5. Is it possible that there is no issue here and that you could be considered a "busybody" for interfering?

Some health problems associated with contaminated water could be eliminated by proper legislation, and needless sickness and death could be avoided. For the province of Manitoba, the *Water Protection Act* will set out water quality standards, objectives, and guidelines. This proposed act, designed to protect water at the source, is complementary to the *Drinking Water Safety Act* (2002), which was developed to protect water at the tap. The legislation will allow water management zones and watershed planning authorities to be established for the design of watershed management plans.[135]

The matter of joint Canada–United States responsibilities for dealing with trans-boundary pollution emergencies is covered at the national level by two contingency plans. One plan deals with marine spills and the other covers inland pollution.[136]

The health of future generations and their chance to enjoy the beauty, taste, and power of the water depend on those of us who are so carelessly polluting it. Water, like oxygen, is essential to life, development, and health.[137]

SOIL POLLUTION

Health problems from this source are increasingly being confronted. Knowledge is essential for recognition, treatment, and prevention. Soil contamination can cause long-term health problems because certain crops and vegetables can absorb soil contaminants.[138]

Canada has become one of the world's foremost agricultural nations due to its abundance of rich farmland. Canada's soils must be kept free from bacteria, fungal, and insect pests in order to produce high yields of quality crops. The federal government has developed the Pest Management Regulatory Agency (PMRA), which is responsible for the protection of human health and the environment by decreasing the risks associated with pest-control products.[139] All pesticides sold, used, or imported into Canada and which are intended to manage, attract, destroy, or repel pests, are regulated by the PMRA. These products include chemicals, devices, and

Effects of Pesticide Soil Pollutants

Source	Where Found	Effects
Pesticide manufacturing plants	Farms	May be undiagnosed
Exposure by inhalation of dust or spray, direct skin contact, ingestion of contaminated food and water, contact with contaminated equipment	Industry	Toxic effects vary, but most remain in soil long periods, causing water, soil, and food pollution, and disease
	Homes	Cholinesterase inhibition
	Gardens	Central nervous system depression or stimulation:
	Government agencies	Forgetfulness
	Storage bags	Attention impairment
	Spray equipment	Short attention span
	Surface water contamination by dust or spray	Anxiety
	Rain washes into streams and lakes, affecting food supply	Depression
		Nervousness
		Hyperirritability
		Insomnia
		Skin rashes and diseases
		Eye disease
		Respiratory disease
		Digestive disorders
		Reproductive problems
		Birth defects
		Cancer
		Leukemia
		Destruction of insects, bees, and birds reduces cross-pollination essential in food chain
		Water pollution from spray, dust, or rain affects food chain
		Destruction of earthworms and rodents interferes with food cycle for animals and people
		Farmers, workers in pesticide-manufacturing plants, agricultural workers, commercial pest-control operators are at high risk

organisms. The use of pesticides is regulated by the *Pest Control Products Act* as well as provincial/territorial legislation.[140] In fact, all pesticides which are sold in Canada must be registered under the *Pest Control Products Act* through Health Canada. It is a legal requirement to have labels on all registered pesticides, and it's very important to read and understand the contents and instructions on the label before purchasing and using a pesticide.[141] The *New Pest Control Product Act* (2002) has initiated somewhat more rigorous requirements for manufacturers by requiring them to provide safety data on their products and to conduct post-registration surveillance.[142]

In the United States, the *Federal Environmental Pesticide Control Act*, passed in 1972 and amended in 1975 and 1978, requires that all pesticide products sold or distributed in that country be registered with the U.S. Environmental Protection Agency.[143] See the box entitled "Effects of Pesticide Soil Pollutants" for a summary of sources, locations, and effects of pesticides, such as insecticides, herbicides, and fungicides.[144–154]

Dioxin is considered a toxic, synthetic, complex, organic chemical compound. It is insoluble in water but dissolves in organic solvents mixed with water. It is strongly attracted to lipids: fatty tissues in the body, oils, related lipid substances, and soil particles. The chemical remains in lipids or soil for many years and, during a flood or soil erosion, can move through water with solvents, soil particles, or colloids to which it is attached. Dioxin is also part of many other chemical compounds (e.g., chlorophenols, herbicides, and the antiseptic hexachlorophene). It can be generated by incineration of industrial, commercial, and municipal wastes that contain chlorinated aromatics, chlorophenols, or polychlorinated biphenyls (PCBs).[155–159]

Dioxin produces a wide range of harmful effects in animals and humans; some are chronic and long term:[160–163]

- Liver damage
- Birth defects
- Spontaneous abortions and sterility
- Some types of cancer
- Nerve and brain damage; decreased sensory perception
- Disturbed enzyme production
- Reduced immunity to infections
- Chloracne, a disfiguring and painful affliction of the skin that may last many years
- Damage to the gastrointestinal tract, with weight loss
- Damage to the immune system

Where additional sites of dioxin contamination may be found is not yet known, but dioxin is being found in many areas of the United States and Canada, including the Canadian Arctic.[164–168] In the Arctic, concern is being expressed as dioxins bio-accumulate in the marine food web and in animals that are hunted and eaten by Inuit.[169]

CRITICAL THINKING

How can you lobby industries for the reduction of dioxin?

FOOD POLLUTION

Canada's food supplies are regarded among the safest in the world. In fact, the Canadian food and safety system is recognized as a world-class system.[170] Yet, in spite of such recognition, contamination of food products continues to be a serious concern in Canada. The major sources of food contamination are microbial and environmental contamination, naturally occurring contaminants, pesticide residues and chemicals in meat and milk products, and food additives and preservatives.[171]

Food additives are natural and synthetic chemicals that assist in preserving, flavouring, and colouring food products. However, the addition of chemicals added to processed food has attracted much attention due to safety concerns.[172] Although many Canadians remain unconvinced about the safety of food additives, scientific consensus supports the notion that certain chemical additives do, in fact, contribute to the stability and appearance of Canada's food supply. Actually, the amount of additives used is relatively insignificant in the total diet of consumers.[173] Vitamins and minerals are added to many common foods such as milk, cereal, and flour. Such fortification and enrichment has helped to reduce malnutrition at home and abroad.

It should be noted that the question of toxicity of additives is an international concern. As a result, the Food and Agriculture Organization's Joint Expert Committee on Food Additives (part of the World Health Organization) meets regularly to evaluate the toxicity of food additives.

In Canada, food additives are subjected to review and safety testing before they are even considered for approval by the Health Protection Branch of Health Canada.[174] Only those food additives listed in the Food Additives Tables in the Food and Drug Regulations are permitted to be used in food. Foods containing additives are continuously monitored for adverse reactions and hazards. If, at any time, a food additive is considered harmful, the food containing that additive is removed from the market. Guinea green, diethyl pyrocarbonate, and saccharin are examples of additives that have been deleted from the Canadian market in recent years.[175] It is important to note that Aspartame (known as NutraSweet or Equal) does not cause cancer. However, it is advisable to use these artificial sweeteners in moderation.[176] The Food and Drug Administration in the United States regulates the use of food additives, using guidelines similar to those developed in Canada. The use of additives has made possible much of the variety in our food supply. Research and development on the use of food additives has become extremely important in Canada, especially as the population continues to increase, and food additive research is clearly of major importance when it comes to improving nutrition in undernourished areas in the world.[177]

Preservatives retard product spoilage caused by air, bacteria, mould, fungi, and yeast. Antioxidants are preservatives that prevent fats and oils in baked goods from becoming rancid. Sodium nitrate is extremely effective in inhibiting the growth of bacteria, which causes botulism.[178]

NARRATIVE VIGNETTE
Food Additives

You have been diagnosed recently with type 2 diabetes. Your doctor is quite insistent that you must reduce the sugar intake in your diet and develop a plan of exercise. You have always enjoyed your morning coffee (and, come to think of it, your desserts!) sweetened. Now, with diabetes on your mind, your thoughts turn to artificial sweeteners. However, you recall some media articles that claim that artificial sweeteners cause cancer. You live alone and do your own cooking and meal preparation. It now seems that you must readjust some of your living habits.

1. What is an artificial sweetener? Which one has been removed from the market? Why was it removed?

2. What other health-promoting strategies might you implement to decrease your sugar levels?

3. What do you plan to do now about your physical activity?

4. What measures will you implement to help yourself to maintain your plans?

The Canadian Nurses' position statement—"Food safety and security are determinants of health"—addresses several food-related health hazards. One such health hazard is obesity in Canadian adults and children. Another hazard is the public concern of food products developed through genetic engineering. The concern points to the transparency and scientific evaluation of environmental and human health outcomes.[179] The Royal Society of Canada, in 2000, reviewed the safety issues of new food products being developed through the use of genetic engineering. Their recommendations were driven mainly by concern for the protection of human health.[180] A working group led by the Canadian Standards Board is now considering the options for labelling food products that have been developed using genetic engineering.[181]

Another area of concern regarding food quality is the presence of persistent organochlorine residues in foods.[182] The Canadian Food Inspection Agency (CFIA), created in 1997, is responsible for testing foods to ensure that residues remain below the maximum allowable levels. The CFIA's main priority is food safety. That is, it strives to ensure that regulated procedures for safe food production and accurate labelling practices are carried out—all to ensure the health of Canadians.[183]

In January 2003, Health Canada proposed the Nutritional Labelling Regulations making nutrition labelling mandatory on most food labels. The new Nutrition Facts table usually appears in a standard format helping consumers to make informed choices about the foods they buy and eat.[184] The new labelling requirements apply only to prepackaged foods. The foods that are exempt, for example, include fresh fruits and vegetables.

Antibiotic and hormone residues from drugs, which are fed to animals for growth promotion and disease prevention, cause side effects. In people, these residues have resulted in (1) allergy and increased drug toxicity or resistance to pathogens when the *same* family of antibiotics is later administered therapeutically and (2) change of normal bacterial flora in a body area so that invasion by pathogens is more likely, causing infection or disease. Synthetic estrogen, diethylstilbestrol (DES), was used in cattle feed to promote rapid weight gain. Studies have linked DES to increases in a rare reproductive-tract tumours in women whose mothers were given DES

while pregnant. As a result of these studies, use of DES has been restricted. An attempt to ban the use of other sex hormones as feed supplements is also underway.[185–187]

In Canada, pesticides are strictly regulated by federal and provincial laws. Pesticides cannot be sold without approved testing and subsequent registration by Health Canada's Pest Management Regulatory Agency (PMRA).[188] The PMRA determines the amount of pesticide residue, if any, remaining on food without posing an unacceptable health risk to consumers.[189]

2-1 BONUS SECTION IN CD-ROM

Pesticides

Pesticides are ingested by eating fruits and vegetables grown in Mexico, the U.S., and even in Canada. Learn here about procedures for dealing with pesticides in food.

It is important to understand the vast interrelatedness of food preparation practices that result from federal, provincial, and territorial legislation. The resulting policies and regulations related to food supplies and health are extensive. For example, in all provinces, agriculture departments advise farmers regarding chemical applications and spraying programs. Health departments and environmental agencies regulate or assist in the control, distribution, and handling of pesticides.[190]

In Canada's north, the Inuit are discovering that food is slowly being contaminated by pollutants. On the average, Inuit women have levels of polychlorinated biphenyls (PCBs) in their breast milk five to ten times higher than women in southern Canada.[191] The Northern Contaminants Program (NCP) has provided an avenue in assisting the Inuit to eliminate pollutants harmful to their health and the health of their environment.[192]

CRITICAL THINKING

What may be some health-promoting strategies to address food supplies for the Inuit in the Arctic?

Biopesticides, or **biological pesticides**, are *pesticides derived from natural materials such as animals, plants, bacteria, and certain minerals.* For example, canola oil and baking soda are biopesticides.[193] There are three main types:[194]

1. *Microbial pesticides* contain a bacterium, fungus, virus, or protozoan that controls bugs, weeds, or plant diseases.

2. *Plant pesticides* are substances that plants produce from genetic material that has been added to the plant. Then the plant manufactures the substance that destroys the pest.

3. *Biochemical pesticides* are naturally occurring substances that control pests by nontoxic mechanisms, in contrast to conventional pesticides, which are synthetic and kill or inactivate the pest. For example, pheromones interfere with growth or mating of a pest.

Biopesticides have the following advantages:

1. They are less harmful than conventional pesticides.

2. They affect the target pest in contrast to a broad spectrum that affects many organisms.

3. They are effective in small quantities and decompose quickly, avoiding pollution problems.

4. They decrease use of conventional pesticides, even if not used alone.

Other food pollution hazards are *radioactive materials* such as strontium 90, which has been traced in milk; mercury, found in swordfish; worms; and mould, which may be present without noticeable change in the food's appearance, taste, or smell. Food handlers may introduce their infectious diseases into food by touching it or the equipment with soiled hands or by coughing onto it. Aluminium contained in cookware, utensils, and food wrappings can increase the presence of aluminium in foods. Studies have shown, however, that contamination from this source is generally negligible.[195] Copper and brass cookware sold in Canada are coated with a protective metal; but coated copper cookware can lose its protective coating if scoured. Therefore, badly scratched or uncoated copper cookware should not be used to cook, or even store, food.[196] Food sources may become contaminated by the chemicals and metals used in fertilizers and pesticides. In the future, diseases from food additives may assume as much significance in humans as do the **zoonoses**, *diseases transmitted between animals and humans,* such as trichinosis, brucellosis, tuberculosis, psittacosis, salmonellosis, typhus, roundworms, and rabies.[197]

For more information on how to reduce contamination from pesticides, herbicides, and insecticides on food, read the article "The Organic Revolution" by J. Bourne[198] in the March–April 1999 issue of *Audubon. Sierra* and other environmental organic gardening journals are also sources of information. Another related source is the *Health and Environment Handbook for Health Professionals*[199] compiled by Health Canada.

NOISE POLLUTION

You will care for people of all ages, in any setting, who have a hearing deficit—sometimes from noise pollution. The following information is useful for education and prevention activities. Sensory stimulation plays a major role in psychological and physiologic development and is therefore directly related to physical and mental health. Sound is but one form of sensory stimulation. **Sound overload**, *unwanted sound that produces unwanted effects,* and sound deprivation can be hazards to health.[200–202] One means of determining the potential hazard of any sound is to measure its loudness. The *measurement of sound loudness is stated in* **decibels.** Table 2–3 lists examples of common sound pollutants and their decibel readings.

In Canada, the federal, provincial, and municipal levels of government have different roles and responsibilities regarding noise-related issues (see http://www.cbc.ca/consumers/market/files/home/noise/noise_regulations.html).

Effects of Noise Pollution

Sound overload affects everyone at some time by intruding on privacy and shattering serenity. In addition to hearing loss, it can produce impaired communication and social relationships, irritability, chronic headache, tinnitus, insomnia, depression, fatigue, and tension. Although is not directly related to mental illness, it can induce latent mental disorders.[203] Noise has also been associated with elevated blood cholesterol levels, atherosclerosis, and accident proneness. In addition, research indicates that less obvious physiologic changes in the digestive, cardiovascular, endocrine, and nervous systems can occur. Humans do not adapt to excessive sound, as was once thought, but learn to tolerate it. Even when a person is asleep, noise cannot be shut out completely. He or she awakens exhausted by the efforts to sleep in the midst of excessive external stimuli. Awareness of environmental stress factors can aid an individual to reduce or to cope with them.[204–206] What, for you, are examples of excessive noise levels?

Although not every harmful form of sound can be avoided, certain measures can decrease the risk of hearing loss:

- Wear protective ear coverings.
- Shorten exposure time.
- Have regular hearing examinations.
- Seek immediate medical attention for any ear injury or infection.
- Wear ear plugs when exposed to loud noise for a long time or intense sound even for a short time.
- Use sound-absorbing materials to reduce noise at home and at work.
- Do not use several noisy machines at one time.
- Do not drown out unwanted noise with other noise.

You can educate the public about the hazards of excess noise and ways to reduce noise in the home environment:

- Hang heavy drapes over windows closest to outside noise sources.
- Use foam pads under mixers and blenders.
- Use carpeting in areas of heavy foot traffic.
- Use upholstered instead of hard-surfaced furniture.
- Install sound-absorbing ceiling tile in the kitchen.

TABLE 2–3
Common Sound Pollutants and Their Decibel Reading

Sound	Decibels	Sound	Decibels
Rustle of leaves	10	Air compressor	95
Library whisper	30	Power lawnmower	80–95
Normal conversation	60	Dirt bike	95
Electric shaver	60–86	Farm tractor	98
Car	60–90	Power drill	100
Office (busy)	70–85	Street sweeper	100
Vacuum cleaner	72–75	Chain saw	100–110
Dishwasher	76–96	Outboard motor	102
Minibike	76	Jet flying at 300 metres	103
Shop tools	80–95	Ambulance siren	105
Loud street noise	80–100	Stereo headset	110
Alarm clock	80	Riveting gun	110
Washing machine	80	Jackhammer	115–130
Video arcade	80–105	Motorcycle	115
Subway	80–114	Live rock music	120
Snowmobile	85–120	Gunshot	130–140
Heavy city traffic	90–95	Jet plane at takeoff	150
Food blender in home	93	Rocket engine	180
Pneumatic hammer	95		

The hospital, considered a place to recuperate and rest, may actually contribute to symptoms because of the noise levels in certain areas. Noise levels in infant incubators, the operating room, the recovery room, and acute care units are high enough to act as a stressor and stimulate the hypophyseal-adrenocortical axis.

SURFACE POLLUTION

The management of waste has become one of the most pressing issues throughout the world. Waste management is seen as the disposal, removal, or storage of solid waste and sewage (including industrial discharges and nuclear waste).[207] Canada is one of the world's prime producers of municipal solid waste, producing over 1000 kg of waste per capita each year (including commercial and construction waste).[208]

In Canada, three main approaches to solid waste disposal exist.[209] One is burial—in up-to-date sanitary landfills that satisfy guidelines related to aesthetics, health, and the monitoring and prevention of leaching. Leaching is the diffusion of materials into groundwater from the landfill site. The second approach to solid waste disposal is incineration, which is sometimes used to burn solid waste under controlled conditions. Incineration reduces the stress on landfills but produces other environmental problems, such as the emission of acid gases, carbon dioxide, and toxic chemicals that must be treated with expensive air-control equipment.[210] The third approach to waste management is transformation. An example of this process is the anaerobic digestion by microorganisms or pyrolysis (chemical decomposition caused by combustion in an oxygen deprived environment), which can reduce waste volume by 91%.[211]

Waste management is everyone's responsibility—not only in Canada but worldwide. In April 1989, the Canadian Council of Resource and Environment Ministers (now known as the Canadian Council of Ministers of the Environment) agreed that targets and schedules for waste minimization be established. One such target included a 50% reduction of waste generation by the year 2000.[212] For society, the best way to manage waste is to incorporate the 4Rs, which are listed in order of preference— reduce, reuse, recycle, and recovery.[213] Reducing the amount of waste is the most effective way to fight the flow of garbage into a landfill. Reusing material and products is the next best option. The process of recycling involves using material from old products to develop new products. Finally, recovery involves harvesting energy or worthwhile products from waste materials. The fourth R is difficult to place into practice by individuals, and is geared more toward industry.[214]

CRITICAL THINKING

What products could you reuse in your own home rather than disposing of them?

In Canada, Waste Reduction Week is organized by a coalition of nongovernmental, not-for-profit, environment groups from each of the 13 provincial and territorial jurisdictions in Canada. Waste Reduction Week informs and engages Canadians by providing them with "themed" specific facts and statistics on current wasteful practices. Individuals and families are then provided with practical strategies that encourage them to contribute to the solutions and successes of waste-free living.[215] (Visit http://www.wrwcanada.com/ for more information on this interesting topic.)

2-2 BONUS SECTION IN CD-ROM
Surface Pollution and Solid Waste Disposal Methods

Research shows that each person generates about 1.5 kg (3.5 pounds) of trash daily. Four basic ways of discarding solid waste are described: (1) open dumps, (2) in landfills, (3) by incineration, and (4) as salvage.

Hazardous Waste Disposal

The U.S. Environmental Protection Agency (EPA) has defined **hazardous waste** as *discarded material that may pose a threat or hazard to human health or the environment.* These wastes can be solids, liquids, sludge, or gases. They are toxic, ignitable, corrosive, infectious, reactive (react with air, water, or other substances, resulting in explosions and toxic fumes), or radioactive. It is estimated that 10% to 15% of all garbage produced in North America is considered hazardous.[216–220] Canadians produce more than 30 million tons of solid waste per year, of which 8 million tons are considered hazardous waste.[221]

Hazardous waste handling and disposal practices fall under the combined jurisdictions of federal, provincial and territorial agencies. Although provincial legislation is not in place at this time for biotechnology wastes, hazardous and biomedical waste management acts and regulations must be followed precisely for infectious or poisonous wastes.[222] Interestingly, prior to 1980 the transportation of hazardous wastes was partially regulated by more than 20 different statutes. In 1980, however, the federal *Transportation of Dangerous Goods Act* (TDGA) was established. This act and its pursuant regulations now present a blueprint of cooperation by all levels of government responding to public concerns on the need for the safe transportation of dangerous goods and hazardous wastes. For example, in the province of British Columbia, the *Waste Management Act* and Special Waste Regulation address the requirements for handling special waste, which includes dangerous goods that are no longer used for their original purpose, and waste pest control products (as defined by the *Pest Control Products Act*). British Columbia makes specific reference to biohazardous waste in the Occupational Health and Safety Regulation.[223]

Although most hazardous wastes are generated by the manufacturing industries, the military, with their obsolete explosives and herbicides, contribute significantly to the total volume. Hospitals, medical research laboratories, mining operations, service stations, retailers, and householders also contribute to the problem of hazardous-waste production. Only a small percentage of the hazardous waste currently generated is disposed of in an environmentally sound manner. The rest threatens our water and air quality and our water and land ecosystems.

Hazardous wastes can become a threat to human health in various ways: direct exposure of persons at or near the disposal site; direct exposure to persons as a result of accidents during transport of the wastes; exposure to polluted air during improperly controlled incineration; and contamination of groundwater and food.[224]

Nuclear Waste
One type of hazardous-waste product that has attracted considerable attention is radioactive waste. Some fission products that must be stored are cesium 137, strontium 90, iodine 131, and plutonium 239. Some decay rapidly in hours or days, whereas others require thousands or millions of years to lose their radioactive potency. No satisfactory method of permanent disposal has been developed; the cost and fear of leakage from the storage area have been stumbling blocks.[225]

The use of nuclear energy or power produced by fission reactors has caused much concern and debate among the people of both Canada and the United States. The concerns centre around two major issues: the long-term disposal of radioactive wastes and the safety of the reactors.

When a utility shuts down a reactor at the end of its period of usefulness, the utility is faced with the problem of what to do with intensely radioactive materials. At present, only three means of disposal exist: dismantlement of the reactor, with the debris shipped to a burial site; entombment of the reactor in a concrete structure; and protective storage that would prevent public access for 30 to 100 years. Even though nuclear power is about 30 years old, the problem of safe disposal of radioactive waste has not been solved.

The seriousness of problems associated with the safety of nuclear reactors for generating electricity is well illustrated by a highly publicized event in 1986. At a nuclear power plant at Chernobyl in the former Soviet Union, a fire in the plant's nuclear reactor sent a cloud of deadly radiation into the air. Some people in the plant died immediately, and hundreds of people in the vicinity developed radiation sickness. Contamination was so severe that the escaped radiation was detected around the world by monitoring devices.[226] The management of such life-threatening events of radiation exposure is both difficult and challenging.

The fear, anger, and confusion felt by the Chernobyl community is shared internationally, and many people now have serious concerns about the safety and reliability of nuclear power.[227] Diminishing planetary resources are leading to the need for alternative energy sources, such as solar and wind power. The problems in this area must be explored.

Hospital Waste

The amount of solid waste produced by hospitals should be a primary concern to health workers. Hospitals add tonnes of pathologic materials yearly to the waste load. This increase in hospital wastes can be attributed to the increase in disposable products: syringes, needles, surgical supplies, styrene dishes and utensils, various plastic products, linens, uniforms, and medication containers. Many hospitals use disposable products because they are considered cheaper, yet hospitals often fail to consider the cost or inconvenience of transporting or discarding large quantities of these contaminated objects. In the past, much of a hospital's solid waste, often contaminated by infectious organisms, was removed to open dumps or sanitary landfills without proper initial sterilization, thus spreading pathogens to land, water, and air.[228,229] Most hospital workers did not consider the implications of casually using disposable items;[230,231] however, laws have been tightened on the disposal of infectious and related waste.

One study conducted in an urban area with 16 participating hospitals revealed that the nurse influences decisions about the purchase of patient care items more than any other hospital worker. If these decisions are largely your responsibility, know how much trash your hospital creates, where the waste goes, the decontamination procedures used before disposal, the cost of disposal, why your agency uses disposable products, and how much your agency contributes to environmental pollution. Form an interdepartmental committee, perhaps of administrators, nurses, doctors, and patients. Report your findings to them, and together consider all the advantages and drawbacks of various products. Consider cost, convenience, infection control, and quality. Give each new product a careful clinical trial and adopt it for use only after careful consideration about contributions to patient care.

Encourage health workers in homes to demonstrate and teach proper disposal of such items as syringes and dressings, especially at this time of increasing incidence of infectious diseases, including AIDS. Work to reduce the huge volume of solid waste that is taking space and depleting natural resources,[232] and advocate disposal of infectious wastes in nonpolluting incinerators, which many cities and hospitals do not yet have.

In Canada, incineration has been the main disposal method of the broad range of combustible materials that constitute biomedical waste in hospitals. This method can significantly reduce the volume of waste material, and it can destroy unwanted organic matter. The Canadian Council of Ministers of the Environment has recently proposed new incinerator standards that will reduce current dioxin and mercury emissions by 80%.[233] However, driven by rising waste-disposal costs and public disfavour toward incineration, several Canadian hospitals have implemented programs recently to downsize the amount of misclassified biomedical waste entering the waste system. Over 18 months, a Toronto hospital reduced the volume of biomedical waste produced each month from 14 800 kg to 6300 kg. The resulting monthly saving amounted to $5599.[234]

CRITICAL THINKING

Through what methods did the Toronto hospital reduce the volume of biomedical waste?

Lead Poisoning

According to Sanborn, Abelsohn, Campbell, and Weir, lead levels in North American children and adults have decreased in the past three decades.[235] However, lead persists in the environment in lead paint, old plumbing, and contaminated soil.[236] Blood lead levels considered safe are now known to cause subtle but chronic health problems. Lead-based health problems include developmental neurotoxicity; reproductive dysfunction; and toxicity to the blood, kidneys, and endocrine system. Most lead exposures are preventable. Diagnosing lead poisoning is a fairly simple process compared to diagnosing health effects of exposures to other environmental toxins. The accurate assessment of lead poisoning, however, requires specific knowledge of its possible sources, such as lead smelters or battery recycling plants. In addition, the accurate assessment of lead poisoning is improved by knowing about possible high-risk groups, such as people who live in pre-1950s homes with lead paint. Finally, knowing about appropriate laboratory tests to detect lead poisoning is highly important.[237] One important high-risk group for lead poisoning is children. It is somewhat alarming to know that the population at risk from low-level lead exposure and toxicity has been expanded beyond the young child to include the fetus, adults, and the aged.[238]

The effect of a child's exposure to environmental hazards is likely to be greater than and/or different from the effects shown by adults. Children have immature immune and detoxification systems and are less able to cope with environmental exposures. Children absorb more lead and other substances through the gastrointestinal tract than adults do.[239] By implementing effective health-promoting strategies, case finding, and treatment interventions for lead exposure, the child or individual, the family, and the larger community reap the benefits of better health.

The National Pollutant Release Inventory (NPRI) provides Canadians with access to information on industrial and commercial pollution in their communities.[240] The NPRI is an important document that Environment Canada makes available to Canadians as an annual public report on pollutant releases. The NPRI may be accessed easily through an online database.

OCCUPATIONAL HAZARDS

Increasingly we learn of the health hazards that many workers face daily at their jobs, including indoor air pollution as well as other hazards discussed earlier. Monotony, paced work, and performance pressures are major sources of stress in many jobs and can contribute to disease pathology. The muscle strains, backaches, fractures, burns, eye injuries, effects of excess heat or cold and other accidental emergencies are taken for granted by the public. But workers may not suffer the consequences of the hidden environmental hazards—the chemicals or radiation they work with directly or indirectly—until years later. Often in the past the cause of the physical illness remained unsolved. Not only do miners and factory workers become ill because of their work environment, *hospital and other health care* workers also may suffer.

Health care workers provide services that expose them to serious short- and long-term health problems: Nonfatal occupational injuries and diseases are more common in hospital establishments and nursing care facilities than in private industry. There are five categories of hazard exposure:

1. *Biological or infectious:* Exposure to HIV and hepatitis viruses (causes chronic liver disease) is most common.
2. *Chemical:* Exposure to germicidal sterilizing agents, chemotherapy agents, and latex (Table 2–4).
3. *Environmental and mechanical:* Lifting, use of poorly designed equipment or work stations, lack of assistive devices, and inadequate staffing cause back and musculoskeletal injuries.
4. *Physical:* Shift work, causing biologic rhythm disturbance, sleep-wake cycle disruptions (cause gastrointestinal problems, chronic fatigue, accidents); physical injury from violent patients; exposure to heat, cold, vibration, radiation, natural rubber latex, laser non-ionizing radiation (Table 2–4), and noise (causes high blood pressure, headaches); computers (cause muscle and eye strain).
5. *Psychosocial:* Shift work causing biologic rhythm disturbance and sleep-wake cycle disruptions (cause depression, interpersonal conflicts); noise (causes irritability, lowered concentration); job stress from work overload, shift-work, inadequate staffing and resources, organizational politics, dealing with dying and death, and various illnesses, injuries, and accidents.[241]

In Canada, the enforcement of health and safety legislation in the workplace lies primarily with the provinces and territories. Although variations in legislation and regulations governing occupational health may exist, both the employer and employee have obligations to maintain high quality standards under the health and safety legislation.[242] For example, in Alberta employers must comply with the new Occupational Health and Safety (OHS) Code for the province, which came into effect April 30, 2004.[243] The OHS Regulation deals primarily with administrative and policy issues related to occupational health and safety. Although the provinces and territories carry most of the responsibility for occupational health, the federal government assumes jurisdiction for its own employees as well as for employees at certain types of work sites, such as nuclear power work stations, banks, and transportation businesses.[244]

A comprehensive federally legislated system to ensure the safe use of hazardous material in the Canadian workplace is the Workplace Hazardous Materials Information System (WHMIS). The WHMIS's purpose is to decrease illness and injury through workplace hazard communication.[245] Many of the requirements and exemptions of WHMIS legislation have been incorporated into the *Hazardous Products Act* and the *Hazardous Materials Information Review Act*.[246] Suppliers, employers, and workers all have responsibilities in the *Hazardous Products Act*. The supplier must label the product or container, and must provide a material safety data sheet (MSDS) to their customers. The employers must provide education and training sessions to employees who are exposed to hazardous products. Employers must also make certain that all controlled products are correctly labelled and that an MSDS is present for each controlled product. The MSDS must provide accurate details on the product's identification, chemical and toxicological properties, hazardous ingredients, and effects on health; it is also expected to reflect measures for personal protection, first aid, and prevention.[247]

The *Workers' Compensation Act* was introduced to protect both employers and employees from work-related injuries and the occurrence of illnesses. Compensation legislation, related to work injury and disease, is in place in all provinces and territories.[248] The agency that deals with compensation in most provinces is the Workers' Compensation Board, which is governed by the *Workers' Compensation Act*.[249] The main thrust of the Workers' Compensation Board is three-fold—it is autonomous, employers pay for the costs, and it determines the benefits allotted to the worker.[250] In making decisions, the Workers' Compensation Board must take into account all relevant facts and circumstances relating to the case before it.

CRITICAL THINKING

What may be some health-related cases that would be submitted to the Workers' Compensation Board to consider?

The Canadian Centre for Occupational Health and Safety (CCOHS) is a federal government agency whose purpose is to support the mission of abolishing Canadian work-related illnesses and injuries. Established in 1978, the CCOHS is governed by a council that represents three key stakeholder groups: the government (federal, provincial, and territorial), employers, and employees. The council mandates the CCOHS's unbiased approach to information dissemination relating to occupational health and safety.[251]

In addition, there are other policies and standards that are applicable to the safety and health of workers. For example, the

Canadian Standards Association (CSA) supports standards development in organizations, trade and industry, government departments in Canada, as well as the global marketplace. The CSA has earned an international reputation for both integrity and technical credibility.[252]

Canada's human rights legislation protects workers and provides for workers' freedom in the workplace. It requires employers to consider individual differences. Workers in both the public (except for some police) and the private sectors have the right to organize and bargain in a collective manner. While the law protects collective bargaining, limitations exist that vary from province to province, such as for some public-sector workers providing essential services.[253]

CRITICAL THINKING

Besides nurses, who else in the public sector provides essential services?

Frequently, organizations ensure that other policies are in place for the health and safety of the worker. One such policy is the sexual harassment policy. Such policies should be clearly written and should include a definition of sexual harassment with examples of unacceptable behaviours. Organizational policies should be clearly indicated by ensuring that procedures exist to allow victims to register complaints and that such complaints will be considered immediately. The prime consideration is to clearly indicate that the mission of the organization is that sexual harassment is not to be tolerated at any level in the organization.[254]

According to Statistics Canada, nurses' work-related injuries cost more than those of the firefighters or police officers who are engaged in high-risk occupations. Such aspects as poor workplace maintenance, inadequate equipment, and supply shortages increase nurses' risk for injury.[255] One of the thrusts in the Canadian Nurses Association Position Statement on Quality Professional Practice Environments for Registered Nurses is that developing and supporting quality professional practice is a shared responsibility by practitioners, employers, governments, regulatory bodies, professional associations, educational institutions, unions, and the public.[256] Others also describe work-related health hazards for nurses.[257–261]

Often occupational hazards are taken for granted. They are seen as part of the job. Employees in laundry and dry-cleaning establishments, for example, suffer hazards of excess heat, humidity, and noise; falls and accidents from slipping on wet floors; back injury and muscle strain from lifting; and circulatory problems from standing. Janitorial workers may have contact with dangerous chemicals in cleaning agents. Asthma is an occupational hazard for animal workers, veterinarians, farmers, bakers, carpenters, welders, and many other workers.

Industrial nurses and safety engineers emphasize wearing protective clothing and using protective equipment. Yet there are problems. The employee may not want to be bothered with cumbersome protective clothing; or the protective clothing and equipment given to a female worker may be too large and heavy and thus be ill-fitting and not protective, because they are designed for the male employee. (A few companies do specialize in protective clothing designed for women.) Hardhats, safety shoes and gloves, and ear muffs that fit improperly may actually contribute to an accidental injury.

To compound the problem of prevention, length of exposure to an industrial substance often determines if it will cause disease or death. The amount of exposure to the worker often depends on the production phase involved. Additionally, each substance appears likely to produce a disease such as cancer in a specific body part; such information becomes available after workers become ill. Gender is also a factor, for some substances affect the reproductive organs of women (or the fetus) but do not affect men. Some substances do not affect the male reproductive organs, but the exposed father's genes may contribute to fetal damage.

Various pollutants and agents are a health hazard. However, accidental injury, gun-related homicide, fire, and explosions are occupational hazards to many workers, including police officers, firefighters, emergency medical workers, and workers in any service establishment that is open during late night or early morning hours. School teachers, staff, and students are at risk for death from homicide (shootings) or fire.

Farming, be it corporate farming or on a smaller scale, or being employed as a farm labourer or migrant worker, is one of the most dangerous occupations. Some of the reasons are as follows:

1. Use of hazardous equipment or machinery that can cause traumatic injury or death if it is not well maintained, if it is incorrectly or hurriedly operated, or in cases of rollover or turnover accidents. Cost of parts may result in not buying protective devices. An accident involving farm machinery may not be detected for many hours, in contrast to an accident in a factory.

2. Exposure to environmental changes or temperature extremes, often drastic, harsh, or sudden, which may contribute to cardiac, respiratory, and vascular diseases.

3. Exposure to herbicides, insecticides, anhydrous ammonia fertilizer (82% ammonia), and other agricultural chemicals that may cause a variety of health problems.

4. Exposure to dust, silage, and manure gases; mould, fungi, and inhaled chemicals; exposure to the carbon monoxide gas from faulty exhaust systems or from working in enclosed areas.

5. Complications from wounds contaminated by soil, manure, or chemicals and from traumatic injuries causing severe blood loss.

6. Effects of consistently long hours of hard work with insufficient sleep, especially during busy seasons of planting and harvest, and stress related to uncertainties that accompany farming as an occupation and dependence on weather conditions.

7. Exposure to excessive machinery noise, causing hearing loss.

8. Effects of not taking time for safety practices and a denial of the need for safety habits or protective shields or clothing; these are the result of heavy workload, sense of pressure and hurry, and cost factors.

Children and elders may be especially vulnerable to the above hazards as they help with chores and farm work beyond their developmental capacity.[262]

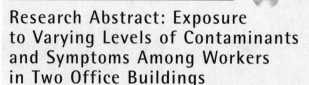

2-3 BONUS SECTION IN CD-ROM

Research Abstract: Exposure to Varying Levels of Contaminants and Symptoms Among Workers in Two Office Buildings

Have you heard of the "sick building syndrome"? In this research abstract the results of a study of two buildings in downtown Montreal with opposite ventilation systems are presented. See what symptoms emerged as a result of this study.

Hazards of the factory or mine can extend beyond the workplace and endanger the workers' families and other residents of the community. Workers carry out dust particles on skin and clothing; wind currents also deposit particles. Even if workers shower before leaving work, the total removal of all dust particles of some chemicals or elements is difficult. As a result, some communities become known for a high incidence of certain types of cancer or skin or respiratory disease.

Table 2–4 summarizes common industrial agents (various substances, elements, or chemicals) and their major known effects. Refer to the endnotes at the end of the chapter for more information.[263–278]

An excessive amount of heat, cold, humidity, sunlight, noise, or vibration is a health hazard in many occupations. Examples are listed below. These hazards are further aggravated by smoking or alcohol or drug abuse in these occupations:[279]

Agriculture	Gasoline station
Airlines	Highway/street construction
Auto mechanics	Laundry
Commercial fishing	Lumbering/sawmill operations
Construction	Meat butchering/wrapping
Cosmetology	Mining
Dry cleaning	Painting
Extermination	Police/security
Factory assembly line production	Post office
Firefighting	Shipping industry
Forestry	Shipyard
Foundry/smelter	Transportation
Garden/nursery	Welding
	Woodworking

Other occupational hazards exist for women and men. Clerical and other workers who regularly use video display terminals and computers have higher stress-related illnesses, more eyestrain, neck and back strain, headaches, and greater emotional burnout.

Knowing that the worker may come in contact with a variety of harmful substances and that presenting symptoms may often seem unrelated to the occupation should help you be more thorough and careful in assessment. Also, as a citizen you can work for enforcement of preventive measures for known hazards and for continued research.

HEALTH CARE AND NURSING APPLICATIONS

Global Responsibility

The environment and people are interdependent. What we do to the environment and how we live affects everyone, eventually worldwide, as we see with destruction of rain forests to obtain their products. What is destroyed cannot be regained, and synthetic development may not be adequate.[280–282]

The size, concentration, and mobility of populations have greatly increased. The spread of diseases, such as HIV/AIDS, Ebola virus hemorrhagic disease, pulmonary syndrome virus, hepatitis C virus, tuberculosis, cholera, dengue fever, diphtheria, Lyme disease, bubonic plague, and yellow fever, has also increased, according to the World Health Organization (WHO). New diseases have emerged in the past 20 years and are a threat to all countries. There are several reasons for new and re-emerging diseases:[283]

- Changes in lifestyle, including overcrowded cities where population growth has outpaced supplies of clean water and adequate housing
- Dramatic increases in national and international travel, whereby a traveller may spread the disease from one country to another before falling ill
- Deterioration of traditional public health activities needed to quickly recognize emerging problems, such as surveillance and diagnostic laboratories
- Antibiotic resistance, so that effective treatment of gonorrhea, staphylococcal infections, dysentery, malaria, and even the simplest infection is difficult
- Existence of unrecognized microorganisms in nature that are as deadly as the Ebola virus and will be distributed as people go into remote areas

Canada has experienced some serious health related outbreaks in recent years, which we'll now look at briefly.

Severe acute respiratory syndrome (SARS) is thought to have arisen in southern China in November 2002.[284] The outbreak of SARS in Canada, especially in Toronto 2003, was dramatic and devastating. The findings of a survey conducted in a large Toronto tertiary-care institution reported that the SARS outbreak had significant psychosocial effects on hospital staff, as well as on their families and their lifestyles. However, these effects differed depending upon one's occupation and perceived risk. The results also indicate the need for strategies to address psychosocial distress and concern and to provide assistance for employees during times of crisis.[285]

Since its arrival in North America in 1999, West Nile virus (WNV) has spread rapidly across the United States and into Canada.[286] The prevention of WNV transmission relies on the elimination of mosquitoes' breeding sites and the use of personal protection.[287] Sayao and her team of researchers reviewed clinical and laboratory information which was obtained from a retrospective review of client hospital and clinical charts. Clients were included in the study if they showed serological evidence of WNV infection. Inclusion criteria also included clinical evidence of aseptic meningitis, encephalomyelitis, cerebellar

TABLE 2–4
Effects of Some Common Industrial Agents on the Worker

Agent	Type of Industry or Occupation	Body Area Affected
Acetaldehyde	Chemical; paint	All body cells, especially brain and respiratory tract
Acetic anhydride	Textile	Exposed tissue damage, especially eye and respiratory tract (ulceration, irritation)
Acetylene	Welding; plastic; dry cleaning	Respiratory tract asphyxiant; explosive, especially when combined with certain substances
Acrolein	Chemical	Skin. Eye. Respiratory tract
Allyl chloride	Plastic	Skin. Respiratory tract. Kidney
Ammonia	Chemical; leather; wool; farmers; refrigeration workers	Eyes. Skin. Respiratory tract (ulceration, irritation)
Anaesthetic gases (leakage from equipment, exhalation of patients)	Surgical nurses; medical, hospital, dental, veterinary workers	Reproductive organs (spontaneous abortions, infertility, congenital abnormalities and cancer, whether male or female exposure) Neurological system (drowsy, irritable, headache) Respiratory tract (infections, cancer) Leucopenia. Lymphoma.
Aniline	Paint; rubber; dye manufacture	Skin. Hematopoietic system. Respiratory system
Arsenic	Mines; smelters; leather; chemical; oil refinery; ship builders; insecticide and pesticide makers and sprayers; pottery workers; agriculture; brass and bronze makers	Skin (ulcerations, cancer) Lung. Liver (cancer) Neurological damage. Gastrointestinal symptoms Reproductive system (birth defects, chromosome alterations); if acute exposure, death in 1 to 7 days
Asbestos	Brake mechanics; mines; textiles; insulation; paint; sheet metal workers; shipyard workers; construction; plastics; pipe fitters; maintenance workers; millers; present on city streets	Respiratory tract (cancer, asbestosis, bronchitis, emphysema). Laryngeal cancer. Gastrointestinal tract (cancer) More harmful to people who smoke
Benzene	Rubber; chemicals; explosives; paints and paint strippers; shoemakers; dye users; office workers; chemists; hospital workers; solvent cleaner users; coke oven workers; furniture finishers; artists; degreasers	Skin. Liver. Brain (carcinogenic). Respiratory system Hematopoietic system (anemia, leukemia). Reproductive system (chromosome mutations in males, menstrual irregularities, stillbirths)

(continued)

TABLE 2-4 *(continued)*
Effects of Some Common Industrial Agents on the Worker

Agent	Type of Industry or Occupation	Body Area Affected
Beryllium	Foundry; metallurgic; aerospace; nuclear; household appliance; production, metal cans; shipbuilding	Skin and eye (inflammation, ulcers). Respiratory tract (acute inflammation and berylliosis, chronic lung infection). Systemic effects on heart, liver, spleen, kidneys
Butyl alcohol	Lacquer; paint	Eye. Skin. Respiratory tract
Cadmium	Smelters; storage battery workers; silver industry; plastics; dental; pigment makers; artists; electrical workers; households (silver cleaner, ice cube trays); plating; alloys	Gastrointestinal tract (irritation, cancer). Reproductive system (decreased sperm count, impotence). Kidney Respiratory tract. Hematopoietic system
Carbon disulphide	Rubber; viscose rayon workers; plastics; soil treaters; wax, glue, or resin makers; medical; laboratory workers; agriculture	Gastrointestinal tract. Cardiovascular. Liver. Kidney. Brain Reproductive system (decreased sperm count, decreased libido, impotence, infertility, menstrual changes, stillbirth, spontaneous abortion)
Carbon tetrachloride	Solvent; dry cleaning; paint; chemical laboratory; household (fire extinguishers)	Skin. Gastrointestinal tract. Liver. Kidney. Bladder Brain. Respiratory tract (irritation and carcinogen)
Chemotherapy (antineoplastic) medications	Medical; nurses	Skin and cornea (irritation, ulcers). Hair loss. Leucopenia. Reproductive system (fetal damage, miscarriage, cancer). Liver and other organs (may be carcinogenic) (some need special handling; effects vary with specific agent)
Chlorine	Industrial bleaching; laundry; chemical industries; swimming pool maintenance	Eyes. Respiratory tract. Skin (irritation, ulcerations, infections, cancer) Skin discolouration (orange)
Chloroform (chlorinated hydrocarbons)	Chemical; plastics; dry cleaners; drug workers; electronic equipment workers; insect control	Heart degeneration. Liver. Kidney. Reproductive system (infertility, male and female). Brain. Skin
Chromium	Chrome plating; chemical; industrial bleaching; glass and pottery; linoleum makers; battery makers; metal cans and coatings	Irritating to all body cells, skin, eye, respiratory tract (cancer, ulcerations), liver, kidney
Cleaning agents, solvents	Maintenance workers; painters; households	Respiratory tract (irritation, allergy, asthma, cancer) Eyes (irritation, ulcers) Skin (ulcers, dermatosis, cancer)
Coal combustion products (soot, tar, coal tar products)	Gashouse workers; asphalt, coal tar, or pitch workers; coke oven workers; mines; plastics; roofers; waterproofers; metal coating workers; ship building	Skin. Respiratory tract. Larynx. Gastrointestinal tract Scrotum. Urinary tract. Bladder (carcinogenic to all areas) Hyperpigmentation of skin

(continued)

TABLE 2–4 *(continued)*
Effects of Some Common Industrial Agents on the Worker

Agent	Type of Industry or Occupation	Body Area Affected
Cotton, flax, hemp, lint	Textile Cigarette smokers especially affected	Respiratory tract (byssinosis–chest tightness, dyspnoea, cough, wheezing; chronic bronchitis)
Creosol	Chemical; oil refining	Denatures and precipitates all cellular protein Skin. Eye. Respiratory Tract. Liver. Kidney. Brain
Dichloroethyl ether	Insecticide; oil refining	Respiratory tract
Dimethyl sulphate	Chemical; pharmaceutical	Eye. Respiratory tract. Liver. Kidney. Brain
Dyes	Dye workers	Urinary bladder (cancer)
Ethylene oxide	Hospital workers (sterilization); workers using epoxyresins	Skin. Eyes (infection, ulcers, burns) Neurological system (drowsy, weak). Leukemia; lymphoma Respiratory tract (dyspnoea, cyanosis, pulmonary edema, cancer) Gastrointestinal tract (vomiting, cancer) Reproductive organs (chromosome damage, spontaneous abortion, fetal damage, infertility in male and female)
Exhaust fumes	Mechanics; gas station and garage workers	Respiratory tract. Urinary bladder (cancer)
Formaldehyde	Laboratory workers; medical (cold sterilization); mechanics; textile workers; home insulators; mobile home owners; households (wet-strength paper towels, permanent-press clothing, foam insulation)	Reproductive tract (gene mutation) Liver. Lung. Skin (infection, ulcers, cancer) Eye, nose, throat (irritation) Neurological system (headache, fatigue, memory loss, nausea)
Freon	Refrigeration; aerosol propellants	Respiratory tract. Cardiovascular system
Fungus, parasites, microorganisms	Food; animal; outdoor workers; clinical laboratory workers	Skin. Respiratory tract (infection, including hepatitis B)
Germicidal agents	Health care providers; maintenance and cleaning workers	Skin (contact allergy, dermatosis)
Hydrogen chloride	Meat wrappers	Respiratory tract (irritation and asthma)
Hydrogen sulphide	Mines; oil wells; refineries; sewers	Respiratory tract (respiratory paralysis in high concentrations). Eye

(continued)

Agent	Type of Industry or Occupation	Body Area Affected
Iron oxide	Mine, iron foundry; metal polishers and finishers	Respiratory tract (cancer). Larynx
Laser, non-ionizing radiation	Health care providers	Eye and skin injury at the point of contact
Latex (natural rubber products)	Health care providers; patients with multiple hospitalizations; maintenance/cleaning workers; workers in industries that manufacture or use latex products; anyone with history of allergy.	Skin hives, contact allergy, when touched by latex. Respiratory tract (rhinorrhea, asthma, chronic sinus infection). Potential for anaphylactic shock.
Lead	Auto; smelters; plumbing; paint; metallurgic; battery workers; paint; plumbers; plastics; pottery; ceramics; gasoline station attendants; electronics; manufacture; shipbuilding; shoemakers; households; exposure in 120 industries	Hematopoietic. Cardiovascular (hypertension) Liver. Kidney. Central nervous system and brain (behavioural change). Muscles; bone. Gastrointestinal tract. Reproductive system (decreased sperm count, chromosome mutation, causes fetal damage or spontaneous abortion during first trimester of pregnancy, infertility in male and female, stillbirth, impotency, menstrual irregularities)
Leather	Leather; shoe	Nasal cavity and sinuses. Urinary bladder (carcinogenic). Larynx
Lye	Households (drain openers, oven and other cleaners)	Eyes (corneal ulceration) Skin (ulcerations) Respiratory tract (irritation)
Manganese	Mine; metallurgic; welders; shipbuilding	Respiratory tract. Liver. Brain
Mercury	Electrical and laboratory workers; dye makers; explosives; drug workers; plastics; paint; pesticide workers; households; exposure in 80 different types of industries	Toxic to all cells. Skin (ulcers, dermatosis, hyper pigmentation). Respiratory tract. Liver Brain damage. Reproductive system (infertility in male and female, spontaneous abortions, birth defects). Reduced vision. Psychic changes Exposure of pregnant women causes congenital defects and retardation in child
Methylene chloride	Paint removers	Respiratory tract (irritant, carcinogen). Skin. Eye. Liver. Brain. Heart. Gastrointestinal tract
Mica	Rubber; insulation	Respiratory tract
Naphthalene	Textile cleaners	Larynx (cancer). Eyes. Lungs.

(continued)

85

TABLE 2-4 *(continued)*
Effects of Some Common Industrial Agents on the Worker

Agent	Type of Industry or Occupation	Body Area Affected
Nickel	Metallurgic; smelter; electrolysis workers	Skin. Respiratory tract (infection and cancer). Reproductive tract
Nitric acid	Chemical industries; electroplaters; jewellers; lithographers	Skin (ulcerations, orange discoloration) Eye (ulcerations)
Nitrobenzene	Synthetic dyes	Skin. Hematopoietic system. Brain
Nitrogen dioxide	Chemical; metal; arc welding; explosives; silos	Eye. Respiratory tract. Hematopoietic system
Organophosphates (pesticides; insecticides)	Agriculture; pesticide manufacturers and sprayers; exterminators	Reproductive system (congenital anomalies) Brain dysfunction and neurological damage (memory loss, disorientation, ataxia, liver and convulsions). Kidney (cancer) Respiratory tract (infections, cancer). Cardiovascular system
Pentachlorophenol	Wood preservative industry	Liver. Kidney. Nervous system. Reproductive system. Carcinogenic to all systems
Petroleum products	Rubber; textile; aerospace; workers in contact with fuel oil, coke, paraffin, lubricants Dry cleaning; diesel jet testers	Skin. Respiratory tract. Larynx. Scrotum. Carcinogenic to all systems. Dermatosis. Hyperpigmentation of skin
Phenol	Plastics	Corrosive to all tissue, liver, kidney, brain Skin (ulceration)
Polyurethane	Plastics and most other industries	Respiratory tract (asthma, cancer) Dermatosis
Printing ink	Printers	Respiratory tract (irritation). Larynx (cancer). Urinary bladder (cancer)
Radiation	Health care providers: doctors, nurses, dentists, radiologists, and x-ray technicians (diagnostic, fluoroscopy, treatment, isotopes), physical therapists (diathermy), microbiologists and laboratory technicians (electron microscope); office workers (some types of computers and office machines); radar systems (police, weather, airport workers); nuclear generating stations; AM, FM, TV broadcasting stations; atomic workers; food workers; fibre workers; households (microwave ovens, some computers)	Reproductive system (chromosome irritation, sterility in men and women, birth defects, impotence, cancer) Hematopoietic system (leukemia) Thyroid (cancer) Other body systems bone and skin (cancer)

(continued)

TABLE 2–4 *(continued)*
Effects of Some Common Industrial Agents on the Worker

Agent	Type of Industry or Occupation	Body Area Affected
Rubber dust	Rubber	Respiratory tract (chronic disease, cancer). Dermatosis.
Silica	Mine; foundry, ceramic or glass production	Respiratory tract (silicosis, pneumoconiosis, emphysema)
Sulphur dioxide	Oil refining; ore smelting; brewery workers; flour bleachers; paper; sulphuric acid workers	Respiratory tract (acute exposure causes laryngospasm, circulatory arrest, death)
Talc dust	Mining	Respiratory tract (cancer). Calcification of pericardium
Tetraethyl lead	Chemical	Hematopoietic system. Brain
Thallium	Pesticide; fireworks or explosives	Skin. Eye. Respiratory and gastrointestinal tracts. Kidney. Brain
Toluene	Metal coatings; rubber; paint; clerical workers; printers; cosmetologists; plastics	Skin. Respiratory tract. Liver. Hematopoietic system. Brain (may cause drunken state and accidents). Reproductive system (infertility, birth defects, chromosome damage in male). Kidneys
Trichloroethylene	Chemical–metal degreasing; contact cement; paint; plastics; upholstery cleaners	Skin. Liver. Kidney. Brain (carcinogen). Cardiac system
Vinyl chloride	Plastic; rubber; insulation; organic–chemical synthesizers; polyvinyl-resin makers	Skin. Respiratory tract (asthma). Cancer in the liver, kidney, spleen, and brain. Reproductive system (chromosome mutation, stillbirth, spontaneous abortion); exposure of pregnant woman to polyvinyl chloride causes defective fetus
Wood products	Furniture	Respiratory tract (asthma). Larynx (cancer).
Zinc	Plating; in brass, bronze, other alloys	Respiratory tract. Neurological system. Hematopoietic system

syndrome, or motor neuronopathy.[288] Three clients received a treatment course of 3 million units IFN alpha-2b, administered by subcutaneous injection once per day for 14 days. The researchers found marked improvement in two patients who received IFN alpha-2b. This finding raised preliminary optimism toward this potential treatment.[289]

Bovine spongiform encephalopathy (BSE), or "mad cow disease," is a progressive fatal disease of the nervous system of cattle.[290] Only two cases of BSE have ever been diagnosed in Canada. The first case was found in 1993 in a beef cow that had been imported from Britain in 1987. The animal carcass and the herd were destroyed and additional measures were taken immediately by the federal government to deal with any risk that Canadian cattle might have been affected. The second case of BSE was reported in May 2003. The animal was condemned to slaughter, so no meat from the carcass entered the food system. The Canadian Food Inspection Agency (CFIA) responded with a comprehensive investigation that tested some 2000 animals, and all test results were negative for BSE. Canada, as well as many other countries, has taken precautions to prevent the introduction and spread of BSE.[291]

Canada is continually assessing international scientific information as it becomes available and modifying policies as required, based on new information.

Personal Responsibility

Consider the environment, the various social institutions, and the population as a complex of interacting, interdependent systems. Environmental problems are a concern to everyone and are of equal consequence to every part of the world. Each of us shares the earth, so we are all responsible for its well-being.

Environmental pollution is our collective fault and requires our collective solutions. A fourfold environmental protection system is useful for continuously identifying, analyzing, and controlling environmental hazards:[292]

1. Surveillance: maintaining awareness of what people and industries are doing to the air, water, and land and of the effect of these actions on health; monitoring exposure
2. Development of criteria for the detection of pollution; detection
3. Research: including data from various records
4. Compliance: getting local government and industry to accept and implement new standards

Citizen Role

An informed public can help establish such a system, but the financial support and legislative and administrative guidance of federal, provincial, and local governments provide the most feasible solutions. Lobby your governments to pass legislation that would protect the environment. Support production of biodegradable products from potato scraps, corn, molasses, beets, and castor oil. These nonpetroleum ingredients can be transformed into a strong, flexible plastic that will degrade completely.

CRITICAL THINKING

What interventions are important to you regarding the environment in promoting the health of individuals and their families?

Refer to Table 2–5 for disposal of hazardous products. See the box entitled "Conservation Solutions" for a summary of conservative strategies.[293–300]

TABLE 2–5
Common Toxic Agents and How to Dispose of Them

Product	Danger	Disposal
Pest-control chemicals (insecticides, mothballs, flea and roach powder, weed killer)	Poisonous, carcinogenic	Offer leftovers to a nursery or garden shop or local business. Pesticides may be accepted by a chemical waste company or regional agricultural agency.
Oil-based paints	Flammable	Call your local health department; ask if it has a policy for disposal of paint (some agencies have free cleanup days). Paint you cannot use can go to a neighbour, friend, or local organization or theatre group.
Solvents (paint thinner, turpentine, rust remover, nail polish remover, furniture stripper)	Flammable and poisonous; respiratory, eye, and skin irritant	Use all of them or give them away. Paint thinner can be reused by letting the liquid set (in a closed jar) until paint particles settle out. Strain off and reuse the clear liquid. Wrap the residue in plastic and put in trash.
Waste motor oil	Poisonous if ingested	Recycle at a gas station or auto service centre.
Car batteries	Corrosive to skin and eyes	Check area gas stations. Some will take old batteries. A few offer cash for them.

As a citizen, you should conserve natural resources to the best of your ability and learn about the environmental pollution in your own area. Campaign the government for minimized waste and for safe disposal of unavoidable waste in communities. Encourage the development of additional burial sites for long-term safety and the monitoring of present sites for escape of wastes.[301,302]

Lifestyle Changes

The box entitled "Conservation Solutions" summarizes activities to conserve resources, reduce pollution, and change lifestyle that can be accomplished by citizens. For some people, following the suggestions means major changes—in shopping, in not carelessly disposing of articles, or in transportation—or it could mean planting a patio or rooftop garden or limiting the number of pets.

Quiet surroundings are a natural resource, too. Make your own quieter through personal habits. Help plan for local recreation sites that offer natural surroundings. Lobby the government for adequate acoustical standards in homes, apartments, hospitals, and industrial buildings and for noiseless kitchen equipment. Participate in local government planning to decrease town and city noise in relation to transportation routes, zoning, and industrial sites.

Support for Conservation

In Canada, the Greenpeace organization, founded in 1971, is an independently funded organization that works to protect the environment. Now it has offices in about 30 countries worldwide. Its mission is to protect biodiversity in all its forms, and prevent the pollution of oceans, land, air, and fresh water. It seeks to end all nuclear threats, and promotes peace, world disarmament, and nonviolence. Public education is an important element of the Greenpeace mandate.[303]

Professional Responsibility

Although health care and nursing responsibilities have been interwoven throughout this chapter, consider that your primary responsibilities are detection through thorough assessment, making suggestions for intervention based on health promotion and prevention of illness, health teaching, and advocacy related to policy development and legislation.

The Canadian Nurses Association (CNA) Policy Statement on a Joint CNA/CMA Position Statement on Environmentally Responsible Activity in the Health Sector states that its purpose is to express the commitment of both the Canadian Nurses Association (CNA) and the Canadian Medical Association (CMA) to accelerate responsible activity toward the environment within the health sector.[304] CNA argues that nurses and physicians, as decision-makers, caregivers, and role models for health behaviour, should not only encourage but implement measures to achieve environmentally responsible activity.[305] These professionals also have the responsibility to encourage international professional bodies and their members to lobby their governments to promote healthy environments. One example of such a cause is the problem of toxic waste disposal in the Third World.

Nurses, physicians, and other health professionals have the prime responsibility to provide leadership in implementing the 4R principle of reduce, reuse, recycle, and recover. All health professionals should feel obligated to re-educate Canadians about maintaining a healthy environment in the workplace and in their communities.

The Canadian Handbook on Health Impact Assessment, Volume 2: Decision Making in Environmental Health Impact Assessment was written by a group of doctors and other professionals, for health professionals—doctors, nurses, environmental health inspectors, and sanitarians. It is possible that such professionals might lack expertise in the area of environmental assessment, but they are asked frequently to provide their perspectives on issues such as the community health impacts of mining developments, landfill sites, or high-voltage lines. This handbook has been prepared for use by other stakeholders who plan and conduct environmental assessments and impact studies in Canada. Examples of such stakeholders include consulting firms in the fields of social science and engineering.[306]

Fraser states that nurses need to have a basic knowledge of environmental threats and their effects on various communities.[307] Nurses must be aware that environmental contaminants may affect the quality of life throughout the life span. People with kidney disease, compromised immune systems or genetic predispositions to slow chemical metabolism react differently to environmental contaminants. In fact, the most vulnerable are children and pregnant women because of their relatively high metabolic rate and caloric demand.[308] The Canadian Nurses Association Position Statement, "The Environment Is a Determinant of Health," notes that acute and chronic diseases, as well as death, are frequently triggered by the contamination of water.[309] In fact, environmental contaminants and health concerns are particularly relevant in cases of asthma, impaired capacity to learn, reduced fertility, and cancers. CNA firmly believes that the quality of health, and thus life, can be improved by minimizing the use of products containing contaminants.[310]

Nurses at each level of nursing instruction need to confront their own attitudes toward the environment and health, and determine ways in which they will help to educate and inform their clients about such matters. Curricula need to reflect health protection, health promotion, and the prevention of illness in rural, northern, and urban dwellings.

CRITICAL THINKING

What types of health-promotion courses dealing with the environment would you develop in your own program of studies? State your rationale.

Assessment and Nursing Diagnosis

Screening for occupational diseases resulting from exposure to contaminants is most accurately done by occupational health nurses and physicians rather than by employees in corporate medical groups. Increasingly, there are improved radiological and blood chemistry diagnostic tests to detect diseases that are related to occupations, including a blood test to detect pesticide contamination. Keep abreast of medical advances.[311–317]

Conservation Solutions

Energy Solutions

- Use **public transportation;** carpool; bike, walk rather than drive a car if feasible.
- Invest in **ample insulation,** weather stripping, and caulking for home and workplace.
- **Use electricity and hot water efficiently.** Buy energy-saving household appliances.
- **Reduce demand for energy** by turning off lights, radio, and television when no one is using them; run dishwasher and washer and dryer only when they have full loads.
- **Make the most of oven heat**—bake foods in batches; turn oven off shortly before baking is finished and use remaining heat to complete the job.
- **Dry clothes outdoors** on a line.
- **Use clothes dryer efficiently;** separate loads into heavy and lightweight items as lighter ones take less time.
- In **winter turn down thermostat** a few degrees, especially at night and when house is empty. In **summer** if using **air conditioning, turn thermostat up a few degrees.** Regularly service the furnace and air conditioner.
- **Close off** and do not heat or cool **unused rooms;** use insulating shades and curtains on cold winter nights and hot summer days.

Food Solutions

- **Eat foods lower on the food chain**—vegetables, fruits, and grains; decrease consumption of meat and animal products.
- **Read the labels on food;** buy foods that have not been heavily processed. Learn which additives are harmful.
- **Support laws that ban harmful pesticides,** drugs, and other chemicals used in food production. Support markets that offer contaminant-free food.
- **Avoid food from endangered environments,** such as rain forests.

Water Solutions

- **Fix leaks** promptly.
- Install sink faucet aerators and **water-efficient showerheads** which use two to five times less water with no noticeable decrease in performance.
- Take showers, not baths, to **reduce water consumption.**
- **Do not let water run** when it is not actually being used while showering, shaving, brushing teeth, or hand washing clothes.
- **Use ultra-low-flush or air-assisted toilets,** saving 60% to 90% water. Composting toilets use no water and recycle organic waste.

- **Buy phosphate-free, biodegradable soaps and detergents;** ask your supermarket to carry them if it does not.
- Do not run the tap until the water is cold to get a drink. Instead, **keep water in a refrigerator bottle.**
- **Economize water** when washing the car, sprinkling the lawn, and removing debris from surfaces; repair leaks.

Toxins and Pollutants Solutions

- Read labels; **buy the least toxic products** available; find out the best disposal methods for toxic products. Use no harmful substitutes.
- Avoid purchasing clothes that require dry cleaning, which uses toxic chlorinated solvents. **Dry clean them only when necessary.**
- **Avoid contact with pesticides** by thoroughly scrubbing or peeling foodstuffs; if possible, maintain your own garden without use of pesticides.
- **Test your home for radon,** especially if you live on the East Coast.
- **Ask your service station to use CFC recovery equipment** when repairing auto air conditioners.
- **Use more energy-efficient cars.**
- **Keep your automobile in top working condition** with a regular tune-up; make sure anti-pollution controls are working properly.
- **Operate your vehicle properly;** do not idle or rev engine; drive at steady pace; obey speed limits.
- **Support legislative initiatives that encourage industry to modify manufacturing processes** to eliminate the production of hazardous wastes and to reuse and recycle wastes when possible.

Waste Reduction and Recycling Solutions

- **Buy products in bulk or with the least amount of packaging.** (A major contributor to acid rain is sulphur dioxide, one of the chemicals used to process virgin paper. In the very low-oxygen environment of the trash dump, paper or plastic may take 40 or more years to degrade.)
- **Buy products that are recyclable,** repairable, reusable, and biodegradable; avoid disposables. (Every three months enough aluminium cans are thrown away to rebuild an entire commercial fleet.)
- **Separate your recyclable garbage** such as newspaper, glass, paper, aluminium, and organic waste if you have a garden. Send to the landfill what cannot be used.
- **Recycle newspapers** through paper drives. Each weekend thousands of trees are made into newspapers that are not recycled.
- **Use recycled products.** Landfills are rapidly being exhausted, and the cost of recycling must be recovered.

- **Buy recycled paper for all uses.** It takes nearly 18 000 kilowatt-hours of electricity to produce 1 tonne of paper from virgin wood pulp. It takes 64% fewer kilowatt-hours (approximately 6500) to produce 1 tonne of recycled paper from waste paper.
- **Recycle used oil** to be re-refined for lubricants.
- If you do not have a **recycle centre,** ask your city council to **establish one.** Find local groups that can use your recyclable materials.
- Urge your area to use **Glasphalt** from recycled glass for parking areas and roadways.

Housekeeping Solutions

- **Use simple substances for cleaning.** An all-purpose cleaner, safe for all surfaces, is 4 litres of hot water, 60 ml sudsy ammonia, 60 ml vinegar, and 15 ml baking soda. After use, wipe surface with water to rinse.
- **Keep drains open by using the following mix** once weekly: 250 ml baking soda, 250 ml salt, 60 ml cream of tartar. Pour 60 ml of the mixture weekly into the drain; follow with a pot of boiling water. If drain is clogged, pour in 60 ml baking soda followed by 120 ml vinegar. Close drain until fizzing stops. Then flush with boiling water.
- **Use low-phosphate or phosphate-free detergents** to wash clothes and dishes.
- **Use natural furniture- and floor-polish products;** such products use lemon oil or beeswax in a mineral oil base.
- **Use nontoxic products to control pests.** Control ants by sprinkling barriers of talcum power, chalk, bone meal, or boric acid across their trails. Control cockroaches by dusting lightly with borax. Control ticks and fleas on pets by applying an herbal rinse. Boil 60 ml of fresh or dried rosemary in a litre of water: Steep herb 20 minutes, strain, and cool. Then sponge on pet. Air-dry.
- **Maintain air circulation and clean ventilation systems** and ducts to remove fungi, mould, pollen, toxic residues, sprays, and other contaminants. Avoid hair spray and cleaning sprays.
- **Manage household hazardous waste:** buy only what is needed; do not store with household products: give unused product to someone else that may be able to

use it rather than disposing of it. Do not pour oil, grease, or hazardous chemicals down the drain.

Tree-Saver Solutions

- **Plant trees;** as trees grow, they remove carbon dioxide from the atmosphere through photosynthesis, slowing build-up of carbon dioxide. (Carbon dioxide causes over 50% of the greenhouse effect.)
- **Plant fast-growing poplar tree hybrids** that suck contamination from soil and groundwater through **phytoremediation,** *a process that stores or metabolizes chemical and releases volatile compounds through leaves.*
- Join efforts to **save forests** from being cleared or burned. When forests are burned, carbon is released, adding to carbon dioxide build-up and global warming.

Preservation of Life and Environment Solutions

- **Do not burn leaves** or garbage; instead, compost organic materials.
- **Do not buy endangered plants,** animals, or products made from overexploited species (furs, ivory, reptile skin, or tortoise shell).
- **Avoid buying wood from the tropical rain forests** unless it was propagated by sustainable tree farming methods.
- **Buy products from companies that do not pollute** or damage the environment.
- **Join, support, and volunteer your time to organizations working on environmental causes.**
- **Contact your elected representatives** through letters, e-mails, calls, or visits to communicate your concerns about conservation and environmental issues.
- **Contact environmental authorities** before using non-native plants for decorative, conservation, or gardening purposes to avoid invasions that kill native plants and destroy habitats.
- **Advocate saving the wetlands,** which help filter pollution out of waterways, protect communities from floods, and sustain fish and wildlife.
- **Use wind turbines to produce energy** for electric power, which avoids pollution and nuclear waste of conventional power plants.

An example of questions usually not asked on standard health history forms that you could use in assessment of the employed client is presented in Figure 2–4 (page 92). Also see the box entitled "Selected Nursing Diagnoses Related to Environmental Considerations" (page 93).

Intervention

Health teaching and advocacy can increase client and community awareness and contribute to prevention of illness from pollutants or hazards. Encourage people to read labels and cur-

rent literature on products. Natural or human-made chemical pollution in soil, water, and food products can produce various adverse effects, ranging from slight health impairments to death.

You may have an opportunity to teach people who earn a living as *pesticide applicators and handlers.* They should *follow the following precautions:*

- Wear rubber or neoprene gloves while handling pesticides to avoid skin contact.
- Keep pesticide-soiled clothing separate from other family laundry.

1. Occupational history (start with last job first).

	COMPANY	DATE EMPLOYED	JOB
(a)	_____	_____	_____
(b)	_____	_____	_____
(c)	_____	_____	_____
(d)	_____	_____	_____

2. In these jobs, have you ever been exposed to:
Excessive radiation or radioactive material? _____
Excessive noise? _____   Excessive heat or light? _____

3. Have you worked in dusty trades? _____
With any specific chemicals? _____
In any vapours or fumes?_____
If your answer is yes to any questions in (2) and (3), please elaborate. _____
_____
_____

4. Has a job ever made you "sick"? _____   If so, which job? _____
Explain how you were sick. _____

5. Have you ever worn any protective equipment or a specific support? _____
If so, what? _____

6. Have you ever had a serious work injury? _____   If so, please describe. _____
_____

7. Have you ever had several minor work injuries? _____   If so, please describe. _____
_____

8. Have you ever applied for, or received, workers' compensation? _____

9. Have you ever had a pension for disability? _____
_____

FIGURE 2–4

Occupational history form.

- Empty all cuffs and pockets before doing laundry so trapped pesticide granules do not dissolve in wash water.
- Wash all clothing daily that is worn while applying pesticides. The longer the garments are stored before laundering, the more difficult it is to remove the pesticide.
- Pre-rinsing is an effective way to dislodge pesticide residue.
- Wash only a few items at a time, and wash for a 12- to 14-minute cycle. Use the recommended amount of heavy-duty detergent. Liquid detergents are more effective than powders in removing oil-based pesticides.
- The hotter the water—preferably 60 degrees C (140 degrees F)—the more effectively pesticide is removed.
- It may be necessary to discard heavily contaminated clothing.
- To remove possible pesticide residues from the washing machine tub, run the washer through a complete cycle using detergent and a full level of hot water.[318]

Another dangerous problem associated with chemical pollution is its possible carcinogenic effect (Table 2–5). Incidence of specific forms of cancer can be higher or 1ower, depending on exposure to specific compounds, a common example being the high incidence of lung cancer in Canada, the United States, and England because of heavy tobacco use. Be aware and knowledgeable about the incidence of chemically produced cancer in your particular locale. Health teaching can then be directed at trying to eliminate or control the responsible carcinogenic chemical.

Encourage the use of protective clothing and sunscreen lotions to prevent overexposure to the sun and potential skin cancer or melanoma (see the "Evidence-Based Practice" box). Prevent overexposure to ionizing radiation by making certain that unnecessary x-ray studies are not taken, by keeping a record of the frequency of such studies, and by using a lead shield when x-ray examinations are given.

Selected Nursing Diagnoses Related to Environmental Considerations

Pattern 1: Exchanging

Risk for Infection
Risk for Injury
Risk for Poisoning
Risk for Late Allergy Response
Late Allergy Response

Pattern 3: Relating

Social Isolation

Pattern 5: Choosing

Health-Seeking Behaviours

Pattern 6: Moving

Altered Health Maintenance

Pattern 7: Perceiving

Powerlessness

Pattern 8: Knowing

Knowledge Deficit

Many of the NANDA nursing diagnoses are applicable to the person who is ill as a result of environmental pollution or hazards, or occupational causes. *Source: North American Nursing Diagnosis Association,* NANDA Nursing Diagnosis Definitions & Classification 1999–2000. *Philadelphia: North American Nursing Diagnosis Association, 1999.*

EVIDENCE-BASED PRACTICE

Predictors of Sun Protection in Canadian Adults

Data from light-skinned respondents of the 1996 National Survey on Sun Exposure & Protective Behaviours who spent more than N minutes per day of their leisure time in the sun ($N = 1027$) were analyzed. Multivariable logistic regression models were developed to identify four types of sun protection behaviour (avoiding the sun between 11 a.m. and 4 p.m., seeking shade, wearing protective clothing, applying sunscreen to the body). The analysis also included data of reports of the use of these four practices in combination.

The results showed the following:

1. At least one protective behaviour was performed by 81% of respondents.
2. Each protective behaviour was practised by between 40% and 48% of individuals.
3. Respondents more likely to perform the behaviours in combination were:
   (a) older individuals,
   (b) women,
   (c) those who wanted a tan,
   (d) those who found sun protection practices inconvenient, or
   (e) forgetful about protection from the sun.
4. Women were less likely than men to wear protective clothing.

5. Older individuals were less likely to report sunscreen use.
6. Individuals with a higher education level were more likely to report wearing protective clothing and applying sunscreen.
7. Respondents reporting a higher income level reported sunscreen use more often.
8. Only 30% of respondents reported always/often employing three or four of the behaviours.
9. Younger adults are less likely to report avoiding the sun during peak hours, seeking shade, and wearing protective clothing.
10. Men, who have a higher incidence of skin cancer, are less likely than women to engage in sun protection.
11. Men tend to report finding sun protection practices inconvenient; and they tend to report a lack of concern about the health effects of excessive sun exposure.

Practice Implications

Canadians need to adopt the use of a greater number of sun protection strategies, especially during peak hours. The results of poor sun protection practices among younger individuals is particularly perilous because sun exposure early in life has been found to be associated with high-risk melanoma and other skin cancers later in adulthood. Therefore, as a health care professional, you are challenged to devise effective means to educate all clients—young people and men in particular—regarding the risks of sun exposure.

Source: Purdue, M.P., Predictors of Sun Protection in Canadian Adults, Canadian Journal of Public Health, *93, no. 6 (2002), 470–474. Used with permission.*

The biochemical response to chemical pollution or radiation can influence the cells in various ways. **Teratogenic** (*producing fetal malformations*) and **mutagenic** (*producing hereditary changes*) are two such changes in cells. Be aware that these changes can occur in both the client and the health care provider who are exposed to radiation, as radiation can also be carcinogenic. Genetic counselling is indicated for couples who have been exposed to radiation. Citizens should know of the possibility for dealing effectively and therapeutically with biochemical changes, whether prenatal or in any other stage of growth and development.[319]

As a professional and as a citizen, you can encourage officials and consumers in your community to develop innovative technologies to cope with the hazardous effects of aspects of our current lifestyle.

Educate the public about current issues influencing health and the environment, including environmental toxins and pollutants, nuclear energy and energy alternatives, resource recovery and recycling, chemical and biologic warfare, and occupational hazards. In the past 100 years disease and death have been reduced because of preventive public health measures in the form of environmental control, such as water and waste management, rodent and insect control, and development of housing codes. Now we are again faced with problems and diseases that have an environmental impact. Prevention can begin with informed consumer groups that have educational and work projects as their goals. It can begin with your responsibility for the client's environment.

Client's Immediate Environment

Besides a feeling of responsibility for the community and physical environment in which the client lives, you also have a responsibility for that individual's immediate environment while receiving health care. The client's *surroundings should constitute a* **therapeutic milieu** *free of hazards and conducive to recovery, physically and emotionally.*

The *client's surroundings* should be clean and adequately lighted, ventilated, heated, and safe. Precautions should always be taken to prevent injury, such as burns from a hot water bottle. Falls should be prevented by removing obstacles and electric cords from walking areas and having the person wear well-fitted shoes and use adequate support while walking. Lock the bed or wheelchair while the client is moving to and from them. In the home be sure that electric cords and scatter rugs are not placed so that the person could fall. Wipe up spilled liquids immediately. Use sterile technique and proper hand washing methods to ensure that you bring no pathogenic organisms to the client. Avoid excessive noise from personnel and equipment to the degree possible. Various pieces of equipment used in client care must be monitored for safe function.

The *aesthetic environment* is also important for rest. Arrange articles on the bedside table in a pleasing manner if the client is unable to do so. Keep unattractive equipment and supplies out of sight as much as possible. Electric equipment should be in proper repair and function. Minimize offensive odours and noise. Place the person's bed or chair by a window or door so that the person can watch normal activity rather than stare at the ceiling or walls. As a nurse, involve yourself in making the entire ward and the clients' rooms look pleasing. Consider colour combinations and the use of drapes, furniture, clocks, calendars, pictures, and various artefacts to create a more homelike atmosphere. The committee in charge of decorating and building should include at least one nurse. You may need to volunteer to ensure that nursing and, indirectly, clients are represented in such programs.

The client's surroundings should not only be safe and attractive, but the *emotional climate of the unit and entire institution affects clients and staff as well.* The client and family are quick to respond and react to the attitudes and manner of the staff. Here are some questions you might ask yourself:

- How do I treat delivery workers who bring gifts and flowers to clients?
- Do I participate in the joy such remembrances bring to the client?
- Do I treat visitors as welcome guests or as foreign intruders?

The emotional climate should radiate security and acceptance. Warmth should prevail that promotes a sense and feeling of trust, confidence, and motivation within the client as he or she and the staff work together to cope with problems. The emotional relationship between the client and the health care staff should help the client reach the goal of maximum health.

In a truly therapeutic milieu, the *staff members also feel a sense of harmony among themselves.* There is mutual trust and acceptance between staff and supervisors, and supervisors recognize work well done by the staff. As a result, staff members feel motivated to continue to learn and to improve the quality of client care. Staff members are not likely to give individualized, comprehensive, compassionate care in an agency where they are not treated like individuals or where their basic needs are not met.

Be aware of environmental pollution in the health care environment. "No smoking" should be the rule. Sometimes there are designated smoking areas outside the building so that employees or visitors who smoke must go outdoors. It is difficult to teach a client the adverse effects of smoking and nicotine when an odour of cigarette smoke hangs on the clothing of the health care worker. Moreover, health care providers benefit from practising what they teach others. Health care providers and clients may also come in contact with agents listed in Table 2–4. Constant vigilance is necessary to detect harmful agents and prevent or reduce their usage. Early assessment of harmful effects to reduce the symptoms and proper interventions for dermatosis, allergens, or other symptoms is essential.

Be aware that sick building syndrome exists. The symptoms clear when the person leaves the building. Vents must be cleaned and furniture arranged so that airflow can be maintained. Fresh air should be circulated indoors. Co-workers should unite to find and correct the problem. There are standards for various settings, and employees and clients have a right to a workplace free of recognized hazards.[320,321]

There are times when the treatment for the client's infection or the therapy modalities may also affect the health care provider—for example, radiotherapy and chemotherapy. Proper precautions should be taken to protect the provider from excess exposure and to protect the client. Follow the guidelines and universal precautions developed by the Centers for Disease Control and Prevention to prevent infection spread. Follow guidelines for handling chemotherapeutic and radioactive materials.

Measures to reduce work-related hazards in health care environments include:

1. Provide safer needle-stick devices and needle disposal containers.
2. Substitute less toxic sterilizing or cleaning substances.
3. Design work and computer systems space with high-efficiency ventilation and high-quality ergonomics to avoid muscle and vision strain.
4. Use work practice controls, such as hand washing, good hygiene, housekeeping measures, and immunization.
5. Use assistive devices for lifting.
6. Provide adequate staffing; create permanent shifts to avoid shift rotation.
7. Use personal protective equipment, such as gloves and equipment that is latex-free, low protein, and powder-free. Wear gowns and respiratory masks. Use lead shields.
8. Provide occupational health and safety training programs.

Joan Petruck, a health and safety coordinator with the East Central Regional Health Authority, in Camrose, Alberta, formed a sharp-injury prevention task team from various health care settings. The mandate of the team was to investigate how and why sharp injuries were occurring, and then to develop a realistic strategy for preventing future injuries. The team worked together from the premise that injuries are both predictable and preventable.[322] One of the changes introduced by the task team was to replace penlets with retractable, disposable lancets. Petruck claims that since retractable lancets were introduced, injuries have been eliminated in the facilities.[323] The team is currently investigating the cost of retractable syringes. They believe these syringes will eliminate both the risk posed by recapping and the danger from needles encountered in the laundry or garbage.[324]

If you are caring for persons in the home, you are limited in the amount of change you can make. You can point out such hazards as electric cords in the walking area, however. You can suggest furniture rearrangement if you think that the person could function more easily with the change. You can put a clock in sight, pull the drapes, or place needed materials within the client's reach, if feasible.

Specific ways of meeting the client's environmental needs also differ for various developmental stages. The components of a therapeutic milieu are different for the baby than for the middle-aged man; however, a safe, secure environment, physically and psychologically, must be present for both. Accurately determining the factors that make up the environment and making appropriate changes may be the first step in promoting health.

It is past time for all of us to ask ourselves some basic questions. How much energy and natural resources do we need to sustain life, to maintain the high standard of living in North America? How much are we willing to pay for benefits that will not poison us with side effects? How does population growth affect the use and abuse of natural resources? Will strictly controlled energy allocation be necessary because people refuse to abide by suggested limits? Must children continue to grow up exposed to all types of hazards in the environment? What more can each of us do personally and professionally to maintain a health-fostering environment?

INTERESTING WEBSITES

AIR QUALITY

http://www.hc-sc.gc.ca/air
Visit Health Canada's Health and Air Quality website to learn more about how air pollution affects us and what you can do to help reduce it. Just follow the links that interest you.

NATURAL RESOURCES CANADA

http://www.oee.nrcan.gc.ca/english/index.cfm
For personal and business use, this site provides information on residential, transportation, commercial, and institutional buildings. The links include Environmental Issues and Impacts, Publications, Data and Analysis, and FAQs.

CLIMATE CHANGE

http://www.ec.gc.ca/climate
This site provides information on the effects of climate change, what we can do, and opportunities for community group work. Climate change is one of the most significant environmental challenges the world has ever faced. Visit this site and learn more.

CANADIAN MEDICAL ASSOCIATION JOURNAL

http://www.cmaj.ca
This online journal provides daily updates on such topics as clinical guidelines, health alerts, drug advisories, and general information.

THE BIOTECHNOLOGY REGULATORY ASSISTANCE VIRTUAL OFFICE

http://bioregulations.gc.ca
Visit this site to find out about various Canadian federal and provincial regulations and guidelines concerning biotechnology in the sectors of agriculture, aquaculture, energy, environment, forestry, health, and mining.

THE CANADIAN NURSES ASSOCIATION

http://www.cna-nurses.ca/cna
The CNA's site provides information on various position statements and articles regarding the environment.

SUMMARY

1. Health and development are adversely affected by air, water, soil, food, noise, and surface pollution.

2. Sources of air pollution are carbon monoxide; sulphur and nitrogen oxide; suspended particles, such as dust, ash, aerosols, and asbestos; tobacco smoke; hydrocarbons; ozone; photochemical smog; acid rain; radioactive substances; formaldehyde; and radon.

3. Sources of water pollution are sewage and pathogenic organisms; plant nutrients; synthetic and inorganic chemicals; sediment; radioactive material; oil spills; and heat from industrial processes.

4. Sources of food pollution include pesticides and food additives such as antibiotics and hormones administered to animals that are produced for food; contaminated water and soil used in food production; and contamination from pathogens during food processing or handling.

5. Noise pollution in the home and workplace produces numerous adverse health and safety effects.

6. Sources of surface pollution include open dumps; landfills; incineration of waste; salvage operations; unsafe disposal of hazardous, pathogenic, or radioactive wastes in the home or workplace; and lead found in soil, the home, and the workplace.

7. Health workers must be aware of various health hazards in the workplace—for the clients and their families, as well as themselves.

8. Health care workers have global, local, personal, and professional responsibilities for promoting health and controlling pollution effects and preventing further hazards to health and development populations.

9. Health care workers must engage in legislative advocacy, public education, public policy changes, and creation of societal resources to foster a healthy environment.

ENDNOTES

1. Thomlinson, E., Environmental Health and Nursing, in M. McIntyre and E. Thomlinson, eds., *Realities of Canadian Nursing: Professional, Practice, and Power Issues*, Lippencott: Williams & Wilkins, 2003.

2. Furgal, C., and P. Gosselin, Challenges and Directions for Environmental Public Health Indicators and Surveillance, *Canadian Journal of Public Health*, 93 (2003), Supplement 1, s5–s8.

3. Furgal and Gosselin, *op. cit.*

4. Shah, C.P. *Public Health and Preventative Medicine in Canada* (5th ed.). Toronto: Elsevier Canada, 2003.

5. Health Canada, *Health Environment: The Health and Environment Handbook for Health Professionals*. Ottawa: Minister of Public Works and Governmental Services Canada, 1998.

6. Thomlinson, *op. cit.*

7. Furgal and Gosselin, *op. cit.*

8. Shah, *op. cit.*

9. von Schirnding, Y.E., Health-and-Environment Indicators in the Context of Sustainable Development, *Canadian Journal of Public Health*, 93 (2002) Supplement 1, s9–s15.

10. Hodge, R. Anthony, and J. M. Justin Longo, International Monitoring for Environmental Health Surveillance. *Canadian Journal of Public Health*, 93 (2002), Supplement 1, s16–s23.

11. Health Canada, *op. cit.*

12. Bill C-32: *The Canadian Environmental Protection Act*, 1999, Website: http://www.ec.gc.ca/CEPARegistry/the_act, March 2004.

13. Health Canada, *Regulations Information Sheet*, Website: http://www.hc-sc.gc.ca/ear_ree/ear_infosheet_e.htm, March 2004.

14. *Ibid.*

15. Environment Canada, *Informing Canadians on Pollution* 2002, Highlights of the 2000 National Pollutant Release Inventory (NPRI).

16. *Ibid.*

17. Environment Canada, *National Pollutant Release Inventory (NPRI)*, Website: http://www.ec.gc.ca/pdb/npri/npri_home_e.cfm, March 2004.

18. Environment Canada, *Informing Canadians on Pollution* 2002, Highlights of the 2000 National Pollutant Release Inventory (NPRI).

19. Dickinson, G., M. Liepner, S. Talos, and D. Buckingham, *Understanding the Law* (2nd ed.). Toronto: McGraw-Hill Ryerson Ltd., 1996.

20. *Ibid.*

21. Shah, *op. cit.*

22. Quebec City Consensus Conference on Environmental Health Indicators, Selected Papers. *Canadian Journal of Public Health* 93 (2002), Supplement 1, s1–s70.

23. Shah, *op. cit.*

24. Health Canada, *Health Environment: The Health and Environment Handbook for Health Professionals*.

25. Environment Canada, *Informing Environmental Decisions: First Steps Towards a Canadian Information System for the Environment*. The Interim Report of the Task Force on a Canadian Information System for the Environment to the Minister of the Environment. Minister of Public Works and Governmental Services, 2001.

26. What Price Clean Up?, *Chemecology*, 22, no.4 (1993), 2–7.

27. Commoner, B., *Making Peace with the Planet*. New York: Pantheon Books, 1990.

28. Shah, *op. cit.*

29. Edwards, P., Climate Change: Air Pollution and Your Health, *Canadian Journal of Public Health*, 92, no. 3 (2001), I1–I12.

30. *Ibid.*

31. *Ibid.*

32. Manfreda, J., M.R. Becklake, M.R. Sears, M. Chan-Yeung, H. Dimich-Ward, H.C. Siersted, P. Ernst, et al., Prevalence of Asthma Symptoms among Adults Aged 20–40 Years in Canada, *Canadian Medical Association Journal*, 164, no. 7 (2001), 995–1001.

33. Boulet, L-P, A. Becker, D. Berube, R. Beveridge, and P. Ernst, Summary of Recommendations from the Canadian Asthma Consensus Report, 1999. *Canadian Medical Association Journal*, 161, no. 11 (1999), Supplement 2.

34. *Ibid.*

35. Manfreda et al., *op. cit.*

36. Boulet, et al., *op. cit.*

37. American Lung Association, *Fact Sheet: Smoking and Pregnancy*, Website: http://lungusa.org/tobacco/pregnancy, September, 1998.

38. Barker, P., and D. Lewis, The Management of Lead Exposure in Pediatric Populations, *Nurse Practitioner: American Journal of Primary Health Care*, 15, no. 12 (1990), 8–10, 12–13, 16.

39. Boezen, H. M., S. C. van der Zee, D. S. Postma, J. M. Vonk, et al., Effects of Ambient Air Pollution on Upper and Lower Respiratory Symptoms and Peak Expiratory Flow in Children, *Lancet*, 353, no. 9156 (March 13, 1999), 874–878.

40. Children at Risk From Ozone Air Pollution—United States, 1991–1993, *Journal of the American Medical Association*, 273 (May 17, 1995), 1484–1485.

41. Davis, R. M., Exposure to Environmental Tobacco Smoke: Identifying and Protecting Those at Risk, *Journal of American Medical Association*, 280, no. 22 (December 9, 1998), 1947–1949.

42. Dejin-Karisson, E., B. S. Hanson, P. Ostergren, et al., Does Passive Smoking in Early Pregnancy Increase the Risk of Small-for-Gestational-Age-Infants?, *American Journal of Public Health,* 88, no. 10 (October 1998), 1523–1527.

43. Environmental Protection Agency, *Children and Secondhand Smoke,* EPA Document Number 402-F-99-003, Washington, D.C.: Environmental Protection Agency, March, 1999.

44. Environmental Protection Agency, *Air Pollution and Water Quality: What Are the Effects of Atmospheric Deposition?,* Website: http://epa.gov/owow/airdep, Environmental Protection Agency, July 1999.

45. Environmental Protection Agency, *Air Pollution and Water Quality: What Is Atmospheric Deposition and How Does It Occur?* Website: http://epa.gov/owow/airdep, Environmental Protection Agency, July 1999.

46. Environmental Protection Agency, *Air Pollution and Water Quality: Where Is the Air Pollution Coming From?,* Website: http://epa.gov/owow, airdep, Environmental Protection Agency, July 1999.

47. Gong, H., Ozone's Ill Effects, *Respiratory Therapy,* 9, no. 5 (August–September 1996), 23–24, 26, 28.

48. He, J., S. Vupputuri, K. Allen, M. R. Prerost, et al., Passive Smoking and the Risk of Coronary Heart Disease—A Meta-analysis of Epidemiologic Studies, *New England Journal of Medicine,* 340, no. 12 (March 25, 1999), 920–926.

49. Van Dongen, C., Environmental Health Risks, *American Journal of Nursing,* 98, no. 9 (1998), 16B, 16D–16E.

50. Von Stackelberg, P., Whitewash: The Dioxin Cover-up, *Greenpeace,* March–April (1989), 7–11.

51. Wagner, G. R., Asbestosis and Silicosis, *Lancet,* 349, no. 9061 (May 3, 1997) 1311–1315.

52. Health Canada, Environment Canada, National Ambient Air Quality Objectives for Ground-Level Ozone. 1999, Part 1. A report by the Federal-Provincial Working Group on Air Quality Objectives and Guidelines. Environment Canada.

53. *Ibid.*

54. Health Canada, *Health Environment: The Health and Environment Handbook for Health Professionals.*

55. Environment Canada, *Air Quality Index, Smog Alerts and 2001 Smog Episodes,* Website: http://www.ene.gov.on.ca/envision/techdocs/4521e_5.pdf, March 2004.

56. *Ibid.*

57. Environmental Protection Agency, *Environmental Effects of Acid Rain,* Website: http://epa.gov/docs/acidrain/effects, Acid Rain Program: Environmental Protection Agency, April 1999.

58. Environmental Protection Agency, *Air Pollution and Water Quality: Where Is the Air Pollution Coming From?,* Website: http://epa.gov/owow, airdep, Environmental Protection Agency, July 1999.

59. Weldon, C., *Introduction to Atmospheric Chemistry,* Website: http://cac.yorku.ca, York University, Toronto, June 15, 1999.

60. Kay, J., Car Sick Country, *Sierra,* July–August, 1999, 42–43, 77.

61. Environment Canada, *Clean Air, Introduction,* 2003, Website: http://www.ec.gc.ca/air/introduction_e.html, March 2004.

62. Kay, J., Car Sick Country, *Sierra,* July–August, 1999, 42–43, 77.

63. McCullagh, M., Linking Practice & Research. Agricultural Workers, *AAOHN,* 46, no. 9 (1998), 465–468.

64. Starr, N. B., Patient Management Exchange. Sun Smarts: The Essentials of Sun Protection, *Journal of Pediatric Health Care,* 13, Part 1, (May–June 1999), 136–138.

65. Environmental Protection Agency, *Air Pollution and Water Quality: What Is Atmospheric Deposition and How Does It Occur?*

66. Environmental Protection Agency, *Air Pollution and Water Quality: Where Is the Air Pollution Coming From?*

67. Is the Earth Heating Up? *National Wildlife,* 33, no. 5 (1995), 5.

68. Weldon, *op. cit.*

69. Environmental Protection Agency, *Environmental Effects of Acid Rain.*

70. Is the Earth Heating Up?

71. Weldon, *op. cit.*

72. Edwards, *op. cit.*

73. Environmental Protection Agency, *Environmental Effects of Acid Rain.*

74. Government of Canada, *The Green Lane, Canada–United States Border Air Quality Strategy, Border Projects,* Website: http://www.ec.gc.ca/press/2003/030623-2_b_e.htm, March 2004.

75. Environmental Protection Agency, *Environmental Effects of Acid Rain.*

76. Schuster, E., and C. Brown, C., eds., *Exploring Our Environmental Connections.* New York: National League for Nursing Press (Public No. 14-2634), 1994.

77. Weldon, *op. cit.*

78. Environment Canada, *Clean Air, Acid Rain,* Website: http://www.ec.gc.ca/air/acid-rain_e.html, March 2004.

79. Bardana, E. J., Jr., Sick Building Syndrome: A Wolf in Sheep's Clothing, *Annals of Allergy and Asthma Immunology,* 79, no. 4 (1997), 283–294.

80. Eisenbud, M., *Environmental Radioactivity: From Natural, Industrial, and Military Sources.* Orlando: Academic Press, 1987.

81. Stomach Cancer in Navahos and Uranium Link Suspected, *The Nation's Health,* July (1987), 9.

82. Wagner, *op. cit.*

83. Bardana, *op. cit.*

84. Buckler, G., The Effect of Indoor Air Quality on Health, *Imprint,* 41, no. 3 (1994), 60–62, 65, 93.

85. Ordin, D., and L. Fine, Editorial: Surveillance for Pesticide-Related Illness: Lessons from California, *American Journal of Public Health,* 85 (1995), 762–763.

86. Redlich, C., J. Sparer, and M. Callen, Sick Building Syndrome, *Lancet,* 349 (9059), (April 5, 1997), 1013–1016.

87. Soine, L., Sick Building Syndrome and Gender Bias: Imperiling Women's Health, *Social Work in Health Care,* 20, no. 3 (1995), 51–65.

88. Thorn, A., The Sick Building Syndrome: A Diagnostic Dilemma, *Social Science Medicine,* 47, no. 9 (1998), 1307–1312.

89. Van Dongen, *op. cit.*

90. Sabo, B. Indoor Air Quality in Canadian Schools, *Canadian Nurse,* 97, no. 2 (2001), 28–31.

91. *Ibid.*

92. Bower, J., *The Healthy House: How to Buy One, How to Build One, How to Cure a "Sick" One.* Bloomington, IN: Healthy House Institute, 1997.

93. Schuster, and Brown, *op. cit.*

94. Brenner, D., *Radon: Risk and Remedy.* New York: W. H. Freeman, 1989.

95. Buckler, *op. cit.*

96. Environmental Protection Agency, *Asbestos Fact Book,* Washington, DC: Office of Public Affairs, May 1986.

97. Environmental Protection Agency, *Sources of Information on Indoor Air Quality: Radon,* Website: http://www.epa.gov/iaq/radon/index.html, July 1999.

98. Little, S.P., F. Lewis, C. Yang, and F.A. Zampiella, Worksite Indoor Air Quality Management, *AAOHN Journal,* 42, no. 6 (1994), 277–283, 296–299.

99. Soine, *op. cit.*

100. Van Dongen, *op. cit.*

101. *Ibid.*

102. *Ibid.*

103. de Groh, Margaret, and Howard I. Morrison, Environmental Tobacco Smoke and Deaths from Coronary Heart Disease in Canada, *Chronic Diseases in Canada,* 23, no. 1 (2002), 13–16.

104. Van Dongen, *op. cit.*

105. Obtaining an Exposure History, *American Family Physician*, 48, no. 3 (1993), 483–485.

106. Van Dongen, *op. cit.*

107. *Ibid.*

108. Calabrese, E., *Biological Effects of Low Level Exposures to Chemicals and Radiation.* Boca Raton, FL: Lewis, 1992.

109. *Cryptosporidium* in Drinking Water, *Missouri Epidemiologist*, XVII, no. 4 (1995), 1, 8.

110. Gallagher, M.M., et al., Cryptosporidiosis and Surface Water, *American Journal of Public Health*, 79, no. 1 (1989), 39–42.

111. Gay, K., *Water Pollution.* New York: Franklin Watts, 1990.

112. Jorgensen, E., ed., *The Poisoned Well: New Strategies for Groundwater Protection.* Washington, DC: Island Press, 1989.

113. Lanyon, L.E., Dairy Manure and Plant Nutrient Management Issues Affecting Water Quality and the Dairy Industry, *Journal of Dairy Science*, 77, no. 7 (1994), 1999–2007.

114. Larson, S., P. Capel, and M. Majewski, *Pesticides in Surface Water: Distribution, Trends, and Governing Factors.* Chelsea, MI: Ann Arbor Press, 1997.

115. Stomach Cancer in Navahos and Uranium Link Suspected.

116. Davies, John-Mark and Asit Mazumder, Health and Environmental Policy Issues in Canada: The Role of Watershed Management in Sustaining Clean Drinking Water Quality at Surface Sources. *Journal of Environmental Management*, 68, no. 3 (2003), 273–286.

117. McQuigge, M., Water: A Clear and Present Danger, *Canadian Journal of Public Health*, 93, no. 1 (2002), 10–11.

118. Raina, P., Pollari, F., Teare, G., Goss, M., Barry, D., and Wilson, J., The Relationship between E. Coli Indicator Bacteria in Well-Water and Gastrointestinal Illnesses in Rural Families, *Canadian Journal of Public Health*, 90, no. 3 (1999), 172–175.

119. Davies, and Mazumder, *op. cit.*

120. Health Canada, *Summary of Guidelines for Canadian Drinking Water Quality*, Website: http://www.hc-sc.gc.ca/hecs-sesc/water/pdf/summary.pdf, April 2004.

121. *Ibid.*

122. *Ibid.*

123. *Ibid.*

124. Environment Canada, Ocean Disposal, Waste Management and Remediation: Atlantic Region, Website: http://www.ns.ec.gc.ca/epb/wastemgmt/dispos.html, March 2004.

125. Gay, *op. cit.*

126. Can You Still Drink the Water? *Environmental Health Perspective*, 102, no. 3 (1994), 286–288.

127. Drinking Water Guidelines, *Environmental Health Perspective*, 102, no. 3 (1994), 271.

128. Gay, *op. cit.*

129. Jorgensen, *op. cit.*

130. Nyren, P., Testing the Waters: The Basics of Water Quality, *Flinn Scientific Inc.*, 95, no. 2 (1995), 1–4.

131. Woo, D.M., and K.J. Vincente, Sociotechnical Systems, Risk Management, and Public Health: Comparing the North Battleford and Walkerton Outbreaks, *Reliability Engineering & System Safety*, 80, no. 3 (2003), 253–269.

132. Thomlinson, *op. cit.*

133. Weldon, *op. cit.*

134. Pip, E., Survey of Bottled Drinking Water Available In Manitoba, Canada, *Environmental Health Perspectives*, 108, no. 9 (2000), 863–866.

135. Manitoba Government, Bill 22, *The Water Protection Act*, 2002, Website: http://www.gov.mb.ca/index.html, April 2004.

136. Environment Canada, *National Environmental Emergencies Contingency Plan*, Website: http://www.ec.gc.ca, April 2004.

137. Boulding, R., *Practical Handbook of Soil, Vadose Zone, and Ground Water Contamination: Assessment, Prevention, and Remediation.* Boca Raton, FL: Lewis Publishers, 1995.

138. Health Canada, *Health Environment: The Health and Environment Handbook for Health Professionals.*

139. Shah, *op. cit.*

140. *Ibid.*

141. Environment Canada, *The Backyard Bug Brigade, Presents Tips on Safe Pest Control*, Website: http://www.ns.ec.gc.ca/epb/factsheets/bkyard_bug/bugs_brch.htm, April 2004.

142. Shah, *op. cit.*

143. Whyatt, R.M., Setting Human Health-Based Groundwater Protection Standards When Toxicological Data are Inadequate, *American Journal of Industrial Medicine*, 18, no. 4 (1990), 505–510.

144. Baker, J.L., Agricultural Chemical Management Practices to Reduce Losses due to Drainage, *American Journal of Industrial Medicine*, 18, no. 4 (1990), 477–483.

145. Bode, L.E., Agricultural Chemical Application Practices to Reduce Environmental Contamination, *American Journal of Industrial Medicine*, 18, no. 4 (1990), 485–489.

146. Geiss, J., and D. Savitz, Home Pesticide Use and Childhood Cancer: A Case-Control Study, *American Journal of Public Health*, 85 (1995), 249–252.

147. Hallenbeck, W.H., *Pesticides and Human Health.* New York: Springer-Verlag, 1985.

148. Lanson, S., J. Kolcher, and R. Frey, Pesticide Poisoning: An Environmental Emergency, *Journal of Emergency Nursing*, 23, no. 6 (1997), 516–517.

149. Maizlish, N., L. Rudolph, and K. Dervin, The Surveillance of Work-Related Pesticide Illness: An Application of the Sentinel Event Notification System for Occupation Risks (SENSOR), *American Journal of Public Health*, 85 (1995), 806–811.

150. O'Malley, M., Clinical Evaluation of Pesticide Exposure and Poisonings, *Lancet*, 349 (9059), (Apr. 19, 1997), 1161–1166.

151. Ordin and Fine, *op. cit.*

152. Pesticides Linked to Cancer, Birth Defects, *Allergy Hotline*, 7, no. 1 (1998), 6.

153. Putting Risk in Perspective: Pesticide Benefits Far Outweigh Risk, *Chemecology*, 19, no. 6 (1990), 2–3.

154. Whyatt, *op. cit.*

155. Dioxins: A Polychlorinated Perplexity, *Health and Environment Digest.* Navarre, NM: Freshwater Foundation, 1990, p. 1.

156. Dioxin's Threat to Human Health, *MOPIRG Reports*, 10, no. 1 (1995), 2.

157. EPA Study Confirms Dioxin Health Threat, *MOPIRG Reports*, 10, no. 1 (1995), 1.

158. Van Dongen, *op. cit.*

159. Von Stackelberg, *op. cit.*

160. Dioxins: A Polychlorinated Perplexity.

161. Dioxin's Threat to Human Health.

162. EPA Study Confirms Dioxin Health Threat.

163. Von Stackelberg, *op. cit.*

164. Dioxins: A Polychlorinated Perplexity.

165. Von Stackelberg, *op. cit.*

166. Weaver, D., Our Global Community and You, *Missouri Resource Review*, Winter–Spring (1990), 18–27.

167. Women Farmworkers Speak Out on Conditions, *The Nation's Health*, April (1993), 10.

168. *Dioxin Pollution in Northern Canada*, Website: http://www.inui-tcircumpolar.com/index.html, April 2004.

169. *Ibid.*

170. Agriculture and Agri-Food Canada, *New Program to Build on Canada's Food Safety and Quality Systems*, Website: http://www.agr.gc.ca/cb/apf/index_e.php, April 2004.

171. Health Canada, Health Environment: *The Health and Environment Handbook for Health Professionals.*

172. Saskatchewan Interactive, *Agriculture Food, Food & Nutrition, Food Additives*, Website: http://interactive.usask.ca, April 2004.

173. *Ibid.*
174. Canadian Cancer Society, *Food Additives and Cancer*, Website: http://www.cancer.ca, April 2004.
175. Saskatchewan Interactive, *Agriculture Food, Food & Nutrition, Food Additives*.
176. Canadian Cancer Society, *Food Additives and Cancer*.
177. Saskatchewan Interactive, *Agriculture Food, Food & Nutrition, Food Additives*.
178. *Ibid.*
179. Canadian Nurses Association, Position Statement, *Food Safety and Security Are Determinants of Health,* Website: http://www.cna-nurses.ca, April 2004.
180. The Royal Society of Canada, *The Future of Food Biotechnology*, Website: http://www.rsc.ca/foodbiotechnology/indexEN.html, April 2004.
181. Canadian Nurses Association, *Position Statement, Food Safety and Security Are Determinants of Health.*
182. Shah, *op. cit.*
183. Canadian Food Inspection Agency, *Contributing to the Quality of Canadian Life*, Website: http://www.inspection.gc.ca/english/corpaffr/publications/prog/agence.shtml, April 2004.
184. Health Canada, *Nutrition Labelling*, Website: http://www.hc-sc.gc.ca/hpfb-dgpsa/onpp-bppn/labelling-etiquetage/index_e.html, April 2004.
185. Gormly, A., *Lifespan Human Development* (6th ed.). Fort Worth: Harcourt Brace College Publishers, 1997.
186. Winston, M., *Nature Wars: People vs. Pests.* Cambridge, MA: Harvard University Press, 1997.
187. Your Health: Hormone Mimics: They're in Our Food, Should We Worry? *Consumer Report,* 63, no. 6 (1998), 52–55.
188. Canada News, *Pest Control Safety Council Formed to Promote Safe, Responsible Use of Pesticides*, Website: http://www.dowagro.com/webapps/search/basicsearch.asp, April 2004.
189. Health Canada, *Health Environment: The Health and Environment Handbook for Health Professionals.*
190. Canada News, *Pest Control Safety Council Formed to Promote Safe, Responsible Use of Pesticides.*
191. Inuit Tapiriit Kanatomi, *Northern Contaminants, Environmental Contaminants,* Website: http://www.itk.ca/english/itk/ departments/enviro/ncp/index.htm, April 2004.
192. *Ibid.*
193. Environmental Protection Agency, *What Are Biopesticides?* Website: http://www.epa.gov/pesticides/biopesticides/whatarebiopesticides.html, August 1999.
194. *Ibid.*
195. Health Canada, *Health Environment: The Health and Environment Handbook for Health Professionals.*
196. *Ibid.*
197. Schuster and Brown, *op. cit.*
198. Bourne, J., The Organic Revolution, *Audubon,* 101, no. 2 (1999), 64–70.
199. Health Canada, *Health Environment: The Health and Environment Handbook for Health Professionals.*
200. Grossman, J., The Quest for Quiet, *Health,* February (1990), 57.
201. Kalb, C., Our Embattled Ears, *Newsweek,* August 25, 1997, 75–76.
202. Sawhill, R., and C. Brown, Pumping up the Volume, *Newsweek,* July 6, 1998, 66.
203. Shah, *op. cit.*
204. Grossman, *op. cit.*
205. Kalb, *op. cit.*
206. Sawhill and Brown, *op. cit.*
207. Shah, *op. cit.*
208. Health Canada, *Canadian Handbook on Health Impact Assessment,* Appendix 1: Examples of Health Risks by Economic Sector, Website: http://www.hc-sc.gc.ca/hecs-sesc/ehas/, April 2004.
209. Shah, *op. cit.*
210. Environment Canada, *The 4Rs: Reduce, Reuse, Recycle, Recover,* Website: http://www.ns.ec.gc.ca/, April 2004.
211. Shah, *op. cit.*
212. Environment Canada, *Atlantic Green Lane—Waste Paper Recycling in Canada*, Website: http://www.ns.ec.gc.ca/, April 2004.
213. Environment Canada, *The 4Rs: Reduce, Reuse, Recycle, Recover.*
214. *Ibid.*
215. *Waste Reduction Week—Canada*, Website: http://www.wrwcanada.com/, April 2004.
216. Cohen, G., and J. O'Connor, *Fighting Toxics: A Manual for Protecting Your Family, Community, and Workplace.* Washington, DC: Island Press, 1989.
217. Eisenbud, *op. cit.*
218. Losi, M.E., C. Amrhein, and W.T. Frankenberger, Environmental Biochemistry of Chromium, *Review of Environmental Contamination Toxicology,* 136 (1994), 91–121.
219. Sticklin, L.A., Strategies for Overcoming Nurses' Fear of Radiation Exposure, *Cancer Practice: A Multidisplinary Journal of Cancer Care,* 2, no. 4 (1994), 275–278.
220. Von Stackelberg, *op. cit.*
221. Shah, C.P. *op. cit.*
222. Industry Canada, *Health Industrial Activities*, Website: http://bravo.ic.gc.ca/biotech/health/htwaste.htm, April 2004.
223. Industry Canada, *Health Industrial Activities.*
224. Crawford, M., *Toxic Waste Sites: An Encyclopedia of Endangered America.* Santa Barbara, CA: ABC-CL10, 1997.
225. McCuen, G., *Nuclear Waste: The Biggest Clean-up in History.* Hudson, WI: GEM, 1990.
226. Ratoff, I., and D.E. Thomsen, Chernobyl May Be Worst Nuclear Accident, *Science News,* 129 (1986), 276.
227. Schuster and Brown, *op. cit.*
228. Flaherty, M., Healthy Planet: Hospitals Learn to Clean-Up Their Act, *Nurseweek,* 12, no. 2 (1999), 1, 6.
229. Schuster and Brown, *op. cit.*
230. *Ibid.*
231. Stewart, M., Nurses Call for Stricter Hospital Pollution Control Prevention, *American Nurse,* 32, no. 2 (1998), 6.
232. *Ibid.*
233. Weir, E., Hospitals and the Environment, *Canadian Medical Association Journal*, 166, no. 3 (2002), 354.
234. Escaf, M. and Shurtleff, R. N., A Program for Reducing Biomedical Waste: The Wellesley Hospital Experience. *Canadian Journal of Infection Control,* 11 (1996), 7–11.
235. Sanborn, M.D., A. Abelsohn, M. Campbell, and E. Weir, Identifying and Managing Adverse Environmental Health Effects: 3. Lead Exposure, *Canadian Medical Association Journal,* 166, no. 10 (2002), 1287.
236. Escaf and Shurtleff, *op. cit.*
237. *Ibid.*
238. Canadian Association of Physicians for the Environment, *Implications for Human Health*, Website: http://www.cape.ca/index.html, April 2004.
239. Wigle, D. *Child Health and the Environment,* New York: Oxford University Press, 2003.
240. Environment Canada, *Informing Canadians on Pollution.*
241. Rogers, B., Is Health Care a Risky Business? *American Nurse,* 31, no. 5 (1997), 5.
242. Shah, *op. cit.*
243. Alberta Government, *Human Resources and Employment, Workplace Health and Safety*, Website: http://investincanada.ic.ca, April 2004.
244. Shah, *op. cit.*
245. Welsh, M., S., M. Lamesse, and E. Karpinski, The Verification of Hazardous Ingredients: Disclosures in Selected Material Safety

Data Sheets. *Applied Occupational and Environmental Hygiene,* 15, no. 5 (2000), 409–420.

246. Health Canada, Product Safety Bureau, *Occupational Health and Safety, Workplace Hazardous Materials Information System,* Website: http://www.ccohs.ca, April 2004.

247. Alberta Government, *Human Resources and Employment, Workplace Health and Safety.*

248. Shah, *op. cit.*

249. Welsh et al., *op. cit.*

250. Shah, *op. cit.*

251. Canadian Centre for Occupational Health and Safety, *Background,* Website: http://www.ccohs.ca/ccohs.html, April 2004.

252. Canadian Standards Association, *Standards,* Website: http://www.csa.ca, April 2004.

253. Canadian Heritage, *Human Rights Program,* Website: http://www.pch.gc.ca, April 2004.

254. Johns, G., and A.M. Saks, *Organizational Behaviour* (5th ed.). Toronto: Addison Wesley Longman, 2001.

255. Baumann, A., L. O'Brien-Pallas, Blythe J. Armstrong-Strassen, R. Bourbonnais, S. Cameron, D. Doran, M. Kerr et al., *Commitment and Care: The Benefits of Health Workplaces for Nurses, Their Patients and the System, a Policy Synthesis.* Canadian Health Research Foundation, Ottawa: Government of Canada, 2001.

256. Canadian Nurses Association, *Position Statement, Quality Professional Practice Environments for Registered Nurses,* Website: http://www.cna-nurses.ca, April 2004.

257. Aiden, L., D. Sloans, and J. Klocinski, Hospital Nurses' Occupational Exposure to Blood: Prospective, Retrospective, and Institutional Reports, *American Journal of Public Health,* 87, no. 1 (1997), 103–107.

258. Bruser, S., Workplace Violence: Getting Hospitals Focused on Prevention, *American Nurse,* 32, no. 3 (1998), 11.

259. Trossman, S., RN Explores Agent Orange's Lasting Effects on Women Vets, *American Nurse,* 31, no. 3 (1999), 24.

260. Van Dongen, *op. cit.*

261. Worthington, K., Workplace Hazards: The Effect on Nurses as Women, *American Nurse,* February 1994, 15.

262. Wright, K., Management of Agricultural Injuries and Illness, *Nursing Clinics of North America,* 18, no. 1 (1993), 253–265.

263. American Lung Association, *op. cit.*

264. Briasco, M.E., Indoor Air Pollution: Are Employees Sick From Their Work? *AAOHN Journal,* 38, no. 8 (1990), 375–380.

265. Del Gaudio, D., and D. Menonna-Quinn, Chemotherapy: Potential Occupational Hazards, *American Journal of Nursing,* 98, no. 11 (1998), 59–65.

266. Egginton, J., Menace of Whispering Hills, *Audobon,* January (1989), 28–35.

267. Health and Safety on the Job, *American Nurse,* September–October, 1997, 1, 12.

268. Henderson, D., Cookware as a Source of Additives, *FDA Consumer,* 16, no. 2 (1982), 11-B.

269. Inh, R.W., and N. Asal, Mortality Among Laundry and Dry Cleaning Workers in Oklahoma, *American Journal of Public Health,* 74, no. 11 (1984), 1278–1280.

270. Ossler, C., Men's Work Environments and Health Risks, *Nursing Clinics of North America,* 21, no. 1 (1986), 25–36.

271. Precautionary Measures in the Preparation of Antineoplastics, *American Journal of Hospital Pharmacy,* September (1980), 1184–1186.

272. Wigle, *op. cit.*

273. Schuster and Brown, *op. cit.*

274. Stewart, *op. cit.*

275. Topf, M., Theoretical Considerations for Research on Environmental Stress and Health, *IMAGE: Journal of Nursing Scholarship,* 26 (1994), 289–294.

276. Bruser, *op. cit.*

277. Williamson, K., et al., Occupational Health Hazards of Nurses, Part II, *IMAGE: Journal of Nursing Scholarship,* no. 3 (1988), 162–168.

278. Trossman, *op. cit.*

279. Inh and Asal, *op. cit.*

280. Byrnes, P., Wild Medicine, *Wilderness,* Fall (1995), 28–33.

281. Schuster and Brown, *op. cit.*

282. WHO Reports on New, Re-emerging Diseases Threatening World Health, *The Nation's Health,* 25, no. 10 (1995), 24.

283. Topf, *op. cit.*

284. Hynes-Gay, P., J. Bennett, A. Sarjoo-Devries, H. Jones, and A. McGeer, Severe Acute Respiratory Syndrome: The Mount Sinai Experience, *Canadian Nurse,* 99, no. 5 (2003), 17–19.

285. Nickell, L.A., E.J. Crighton, C.S. Tracy, H. Al-Enazy, Y. Bolaji, S. Hanjrah, A. Hussain, S. Makhlouf, and R.E.G. Upshur, Psychosocial Effects of SARS on Hospital Staff: Survey of a Large Tertiary Care Institution. *Canadian Medical Association Journal,* 170, no. 5 (2004), 793–798.

286. Canadian Medical Association, West Nile Virus, *Canadian Medical Association Journal,* 168, no. 11 (2003), 1443–1444.

287. Nickell, et al., *op. cit.*

288. Sayao, A-L, O Suchowersky, A Al-Khathaami, B Klassen, N R. Katz, R Sevick, P Tilley, J. Fox, and D. Patry, Calgary Experience with West Nile Virus Neurological Syndrome During the Late Summer of 2003, *Canadian Journal of Neurological Science,* 31, no. 2 (2004), 194–203.

289. Canadian Medical Association, West Nile Virus.

290. Canadian Food Inspection Agency, *Bovine Spongiform Encephalopathy (BSE),* Website: http://www.inspection.gc.ca/english/anima/heasan/disamala/bseesh/bseesbfse.shtml, August 2004.

291. Sayao et al., *op. cit.*

292. Schuster and Brown, *op. cit.*

293. Collins, E., The Perils of Plastic, *Health* (June 1990), 36–37.

294. How Agricultural Nurses Are Improving Safety and Health, *Successful Farming,* April (1995), 64.

295. MacEachern, D., *Save Our Planet.* New York: Dell Trade Paperback, 1990.

296. Obtaining an Exposure History.

297. Wigle, *op. cit.*

298. Schuster and Brown, *op. cit.*

299. Sticklin, *op. cit.*

300. Weaver, *op. cit.*

301. Collins, *op. cit.*

302. Women Farmworkers Speak Out on Conditions.

303. Greenpeace Canada, *About Greenpeace,* Website: http://www.greenpeace.ca, April 2004.

304. Canadian Nurses Association, *Policy Statement, Joint CAN/CMA Position Statement on Environmentally Responsible Activity in the Health Sector,* Website: http://www.cna-nurses.ca, April 2004.

305. Greenpeace Canada, *op. cit.*

306. Health Canada, Environmental Health Assessment Services (EHAS), *Canadian Handbook on Health Impact Assessment,* Website: http://www.hc-sc.gc.ca/hecs-sesc/ehas/publications.htm, April 2004.

307. Canadian Nurses Association, *Policy Statement, Joint CAN/CMA Position Statement on Environmentally Responsible Activity in the Health Sector.*

308. Fraser, Gloria, Environmental Health and Nursing. *Canadian Nurse,* 100, no. 1 (2004), 17–19.

309. Canadian Nurses Association, *Position Statement, The Environment is a Determinant of Health,* Website: http://www.cna-nurses.ca, April 2004.

310. Fraser, *op. cit.*

311. RN's Facing New Dangers at Works, *American Journal of Nursing,* 95, no. 10 (1995), 78, 81.

312. Wigle, *op. cit.*
313. Schuster and Brown, *op. cit.*
314. Precautionary Measures in the Preparation of Antineoplastics.
315. Bruser, *op. cit.*
316. Van Dongen, *op. cit.*
317. Trossman, *op. cit.*
318. Sohn, M., Special Care Is Required with Pesticide Applicator's Clothing, *Union Banner,* May 23 (1990), 11.
319. Schuster and Brown, *op. cit.*
320. Maizlish et al., *op. cit.*
321. Van Dongen, *op. cit.*
322. Petruk, J., Sharp Injuries: Time to Change Our Equipment and Our Attitudes, *Canadian Nurse,* 99, no. 9 (2003), 19–22.
323. Canadian Nurses Association, *Policy Statement, Joint CAN/CMA Position Statement on Environmentally Responsible Activity in the Health Sector.*
324. Sohn, *op. cit.*

Chapter 3

SPIRITUAL AND RELIGIOUS INFLUENCES
ON THE PERSON AND FAMILY

Faith is the soul riding at anchor.

H.W. Shaw

OBJECTIVES

STUDY OF THIS CHAPTER WILL ENABLE YOU TO:

1. Define the terms *religious* and *spiritual* and determine your personal meaning of each.

2. Compare and contrast the major tenets of the Hindu, Sikh, Buddhist, Jainist, Shinto, Confucian, Taoist, Islamic, Jewish, Christian, and North American Indian religions.

3. Differentiate the major tenets of the various branches of Christianity: Roman Catholicism, Eastern Orthodox, various Protestant denominations, and other Christian sects.

4. Gain an overview of the variety of religions in Canada.

5. Discuss how religious beliefs influence the lifestyle and health status of individuals and families.

6. Identify more clearly your religious or spiritual beliefs and explore how they might influence your practice.

7. Discuss your role in helping to meet the spiritual needs of clients and their families.

8. Describe specific nursing measures that can be used to meet the needs of persons with different religious and spiritual backgrounds.

> *Until an illness occurs, the person may give no thought to the meaning of his or her life or spiritual beliefs. But when he or she feels vulnerable and fearful of the future, solace is sought. Religion and spiritual beliefs can provide that solace.*

The attitude that medical science is superior to the spiritual dimension or to religion has affected us all. Yet the spiritual dimension and religion are there as they always have been. Each culture has had some organization to sustain the important rituals and myths of its people. Primitive peoples combined the roles of physician, psychiatrist, and priest.

> *I had the cancer patient visualize an army of white blood cells attacking and overcoming the cancer cells. Within two weeks the cancer had diminished and he was rapidly gaining weight. He is alive and well today.*

Is this a priest or a faith healer talking? No, this is a prominent tumour specialist talking today. An internationally known neurosurgeon says, "In a very real sense, medicine is now—as it has always been—faith healing." Other health providers have seen life return after death. Thus, some health workers are trying to reunite the biopsychospiritual being.

History reveals that in the 5th century A.D., Western society disintegrated and religion and scientific theory split. Through a long process, the two theories are now sharing dialogue. In her manuscript, "Suggestion for Thought," Florence Nightingale attempted to integrate science and mysticism. She felt the universe was an incarnation of a divine intelligence that regulated all things through law.[1] She recognized that humans have spiritual needs; spiritual care enables the person to be conscious of the presence of God, the creator and sustainer of the universe.[2] *Spiritual care has continued to be part of the nursing tradition.*

There has been an increased awareness of the link between health and religion, and the subject is being discussed and researched more openly.[3–7] Pangman states that research on the family has confirmed the importance of spirituality, particularly in those families that have demonstrated the tenacity and ability to cope effectively with stress.[8] A study of 1718 men and women over age 65 suggested that those who attended church at least once weekly were half as likely as nonattenders to have high blood levels of interleukin-6. This protein regulates immune and inflammatory response and the level is elevated in patients who have certain cancers, autoimmune diseases, or heart disease.[9] Other studies show that people who practice religion have a lower incidence of hypertension, depression, and suicide rates.[10,11] Furthermore, persons with high levels of spiritual well-being can better cope with AIDS or chronic illness; and they can care better for clients with AIDS.[12,13] One study showed that church attenders, as compared with non–church attenders, reported better health, more happiness, and longer marriages than did their counterparts.[14]

An interpretive phenomenological study investigated the meaning of the experience of feeling healthy for people living with chronic illness and/or disability. The study was conducted with eight participants living with a variety of different chronic conditions.[15] The results provided a valuable mosaic of themes to express the participant's health experience. One of the themes included acquiring a state of grace whereby the participants attributed their experience of feeling healthy to an awareness of their spirituality and a sense of connectedness, wholeness, harmony, and peacefulness.[16] Another study interviewed 88 adult patients (50% men), who were admitted to a

Canadian tertiary care psychiatry inpatient unit, about their religious beliefs and practices. The results indicated that certain religious practices may protect against severity of symptoms and hospital use, and these practices increase life satisfaction among psychiatric inpatients.[17]

Several articles in medical and nursing journals and in the newspapers have discussed physicians and nurses who pray with their patients. The authors claim that prayer has added to the effectiveness of therapy.[18–22] Recently, several articles have appeared in scholarly journals on the importance of prayer in nursing practice.[23,24] These articles stress that prayer, as well as being a significant practice in most religions, results in comfort; and it sustains coping ability among individuals and their families.

CRITICAL THINKING

What is your personal meaning of a sense of connectedness?

DEFINITIONS

Religion is defined on various levels: *a belief in a supernatural or divine force that has power over the universe and commands worship and obedience; a personal and institutional system of beliefs; a comprehensive code of ethics or philosophy; a set of practices that are followed; a church affiliation; the conscious pursuit of any object the person holds as supreme. In short, religion signifies that a group of people have established and organized practices that are related to spiritual concerns.*

This definition, however, does not portray the constancy and the fervency that can at times underlie religious belief. In every human there seems to be a **spiritual dimension**, *a quality that goes beyond religious affiliation, which strives for inspiration, reverence, awe, meaning, and purpose, even in those who do not believe in any God. The spiritual dimension tries to be in harmony with the universe, strives for answers about the infinite, and especially comes into focus as a sustaining power when the person faces emotional stress, physical illness, or death. It goes outside a person's own power.*

Spirituality is the umbrella for religion. It is the framework for beliefs, values, and rituals. However, spirituality is broader and need not include religious practice. **Spirituality,** according to Chilton,[25] *is an inner strength related to a belief in and sense of interconnection with a greater power.* Native spiritual life is founded on a belief in the fundamental interconnectedness of all natural aspects, all forms of life where primary importance is attached to Mother Earth. The symbol of a circle is significant in Native beliefs; and it is often referred to as the Medicine Wheel.[26] The Medicine Wheel is a powerful and sacred symbol of the universe depicting the circularity of life and the four components of the self: body, mind, emotion, and spirit. The Medicine Wheel incorporates the values, beliefs, and social mores of the traditional Aboriginal culture. Common Native healing practices include shamanism, herbal remedies, and various purification rituals such as smudging and sweat lodges.[27–29]

Some authors subsume spirituality or spiritual needs under cultural traditions or philosophic beliefs; or they describe spirituality as including all positive human qualities. Culture, philosophy, love, and reverence for another person are all *humanizing influences.* The feelings called forth by the consciousness of the presence of a nature higher than human, unconnected with material objects or qualities, are *spiritual influences.*[30]

In the midst of our specialized health care, you have an opportunity to go beyond the dogma to bring together the biopsychospiritual being through the study of the religions, religious symbols, and spiritual values of your clients and their families.

CRITICAL THINKING

How would you define or describe your own spirituality?

WORLD RELIGIONS

Use this information about world religions in assessment, intervention, and teaching of clients and family members. Understanding these beliefs will also help you better understand and work with your co-workers.

Studying world religions poses a semantic difficulty in that an expression in the Chinese-based religion of Confucianism may have no equivalent in the English language. Thus, language has dictated what people think, how they act, and how their religious beliefs are carried out.[31]

Concepts, however, are often basically the same but are rephrased in each religion's own linguistic style. The saying "Love one another as I have loved you" will appear to the Hindu as "This is the sum of religion, do not unto others what causes pain to you"; to the Taoist as "Return goodness for hatred"; and to the Muslim as "No one is a believer unless he desires for his brother what he desires for himself."

Each religion also has other characteristics in common:

- A worldview, a way of perceiving reality; a description of existence and life meaning; assumptions about the universe and life
- Basis of authority or source(s) of power
- A portion of scripture or sacred word
- An ethical code that defines right and wrong
- A psychology and identity so that its adherents fit into a group and the world is defined by the religion
- Aspirations or expectations
- Some ideas about what follows death

See Figure 3–1, "The Golden Rule," for the similarities reflected in the phrase of each religion.[32]

See Table 3-1 for key facts about eight major world religions. For additional information about philosophic and mystical aspects of Hinduism, Buddhism, Islam, Taoism, and Sikhism, see Rice,[33] the descriptions in this chapter, and related references.

HINDUISM
This is the sum of duty:
do not do to others what would
cause pain if done to you.
Mahabharata 5:1517

BUDDHISM
Treat not others in ways
that you yourself would
find hurtful.
The Buddha,
Udana-Varga 5.18

BAHA'I FAITH
Lay not on any soul a load
that you would not wish to
be laid upon you, and
desire not for
anyone the
things you
would not
desire for
yourself.
Baha'u'llah,
Gleanings

CONFUCIANISM
One word which sums up the
basis of all good conduct....
loving-kindness.
Do not do to
others what
you do not
want done
to yourself.
Confucius,
Analects 15.23

ISLAM
Not one of you truly believes
until you wish for others what
you wish for yourself.
The Prophet Muhammad,
13th of the 40 Hadiths of Nawawi

THE GOLDEN RULE

TAOISM
Regard your neighbour's gain
as your own gain, and your
neighbour's loss as your own loss.
Lao Tzu, T'ai Shang Kan Ying P'ien, 213-218

JUDAISM
What is hateful to you,
do not do to your neighbour.
This is the whole Torah;
all the rest is commentary.
Go and learn it.
Hillel, Talmud, Shabbath 31a

SIKHISM
I am a stranger to no one;
and no one is a stranger
to me. Indeed, I am
a friend to all.
Guru Granth Sahib, pg. 1299

JAINISM
One should treat all
creatures in the world
as one would like
to be treated.
Mahavira, Sutrakritanga

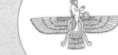

CHRISTIANITY
In everything, do to others
as you would have them
do to you; for this is the
law and the prophets.
Jesus, Matthew 7:12

ZOROASTRIANISM
Do not do unto others
whatever is injurious
to yourself.
Shayast-na-Shayast 13.29

NATIVE SPIRITUALITY
We are as much alive
as we keep the earth alive.
Chief Dan George

UNITARIANISM
We affirm and promote respect
for the interdependent
web of all existence
of which we are a part.
Unitarian principle

FIGURE 3–1

The Golden Rule

Note: This is a reduced version of a 56 × 74 cm four-colour poster available in Canada from Broughton Books, sales@bbroughton.com, and in USA from Pflaum Publishing, service@pflaum.com. Used with permission.

TABLE 3-1
Key Facts about Eight Major World Religions

Religion	Primary Location	Supreme Being	Founder and Date	Historical Leaders	Leadership	Sacred Writings	Holy Places	Some Holy Days
Hinduism	India Sri Lanka	Brahman All reality	No founder 3200 B.C.	Mahatma Gandhi Ramakrishna	Sannyasis (holy men) Guru (preacher)	Vedas Brahmanas Upanishads Great Epics	Benares (city) Ganges (river)	The Mela Holi Festival Dasera Divuli
Judaism	Israel Western Hemisphere	Yahweh (Jehovah or God)	Abraham 1300 B.C.	Moses Amos Micah Other prophets	Rabbis	Torah Talmud	Jerusalem	Rosh Hashanah Yom Kippur Hanukkah Purim Passover
Taoism	China	Jade Emperor Many folk gods	Lao-Tzu (or Lao-Tse) 604 B.C.	Lao-Tse Chuang-Tse 350–275 B.C.	None	Tao-Te-Ching	Kiangsi and many holy mountains	Birthdays of Gods Festival of Souls Autumn Festival
Confucianism	China Japan	Confucius Shang-Ti	Confucius 557 B.C.	Yang Chu Moh Tih	None	NuChin Sau Shu	None	None
Buddhism	India Burma	108 different names	Gautama 560–480 B.C.	Gautama Amitabha	Bhikkhus Monks Nuns Lamas	Dharma (Sutta) Vinaya Abhidhamma	Sarnath Lumbini Buddh-Gaya Kusinara	Perahera Festival in Sri Lanka Wesak (Kason) in May
Christianity	Western Hemisphere	God	Jesus 30 A.D.	John the Baptist, 12 disciples, 4 gospel writers, writers of epistles	Priests Ministers Laymen	Bible Old Testament New Testament	Bethlehem Jerusalem Rome Nazareth	Christmas Good Friday Easter Pentecost
Shinto	Japan	Izanagi (Sky Father) Izanami (Earth Mother)	No founder 6th century A.D.	None	None	Nihongi Kojiki	Mt. Fujiyama	New Year Bon (Festival of Dead) Tenri-Kyo (January)
Islam	Middle East	Allah	Mohammed 570–632 A.D.	Muhammed Husein (grandson) Abu Bakr Omar Othman Ali	None	Quran	Mecca Jerusalem	Ramadan (Sacred Month)

The major world religions can be divided into categories in an attempt to group characteristics even further.[34] The *alpha* group includes Christianity, Judaism, and Islam. All adhere to a Biblical revelation of a supernatural, monotheistic God. People in these religions are "doers." They obey because God commands; they make covenants with God for protection; they have a historical fixed scripture that is canonized for public use, and they often proselytize. The *gamma* group includes Taoism (pronounced "dowism"), Confucianism, and Shintoism. In these religions people believe either that everything is in the being of God or that there is no godhead (still a definite belief). These people try to be in harmony with the world around them. Their most immediate concern is in relationships with others. Scripture is a family affair. They can be characterized as simple in faith, spontaneous, and straightforward in feelings of affection for people, plants, and animals. The final grouping is the *beta* group, which includes Buddhism and Hinduism. These religions have their roots in Indian soil, their worldview is pantheistic, and they teach that everything is in the being of God. Adherents are interested in "being" rather than "doing." They have a collective literature for private devotion. Control of mind and body is desired, as some of the yoga practices show. The beta and gamma groups do not define God as clearly as the alpha group. The beta and gamma groups look inside themselves for answers: common sense rather than commands from God determines good. Salladay contrasts pantheistic with Christian beliefs.[35]

The following discussion presents a more detailed insight into each major world religion through personality sketches. *Each person has a fictitious name and represents not a single person but a composite of knowledge gained from the authors' interviewing, reading, and personal experience.* Although these personalities are presented as acting and thinking in a certain way, remember that the person's culture, family background, and personality affect how that person lives out a religious experience.

Hinduism and Sikhism

Rama tells us that nothing is typically **Hindu** and that anyone who puts religion in neat packages will have difficulty comprehending his outlook. Rama is named after **Ramakrishna,** *the greatest saint of Hinduism of the 19th century.* The history of Rama's religion goes back to approximately 1500 B.C., when the **Vedas**—*divine revelations*—were written. His main religious texts are the **Upanishads,** or *scriptures,* and the **Bhagavad Gita,** *a summary of the former with additions. The most expressive and universal word of God is* **Om,** *or* **Aum.** This word provides the most important auditory and visual symbol in Rama's religion.*

Rama speaks of some of the worship popular in India today: of the family and local deities and of the trinity—**Brahma,** *the*

creator, **Vishnu,** *the preserver and god of love,* and **Shiva,** *the destroyer.*

Rama tells of his own shrine in his home where, in the presence of various pictures of **incarnations** (*human forms of God*) and with incense burning, he meditates. He also thinks of Buddha, Mohammed, and Jesus as incarnations and sometimes reads from the scriptures being inspired by their teachings, although they represent other major religions.

Despite this vast array of deities and the recognition that all religions are valid, Rama believes in one universal concept—**Brahman,** the *Divine Intelligence,* the *Supreme Reality.* Rama believes all paths lead to the understanding that this "reality" exists as part of all physical beings, especially humans. Rama's entire spiritual quest is directed toward uniting his *inner and real self,* the **atman,** with the concept of Brahman. So, although Rama has gone through several stages of desire—for pleasure, power, wealth, fame, and humanitarianism—the last stage, his desire for freedom, for touching the infinite, is his main goal. Figure 3–2 expresses that journey.

Rama is interested in health and illness only as a guide to this goal. He feels that the human love for the body is a cause for illness. He says, for example, that we overeat and get a stomachache. He views the pain as a warning—in this case, to stop overeating. He does not oppose medical treatment if absolutely necessary, but he believes that medicine can sometimes dull the pain and then the person overeats again, thus perpetuating the cause of the problem. Medical or psychiatric help, Rama says, is at best transitory. The cause of the pain must be rooted out.

To avoid dwelling on physical concerns, Rama strives for moderation in eating and in other body functions. He considers only the atman as real and eternal and the body as unreal and finite. The body is a temple, a vehicle, no more. He tries to take care of it so that it will not scream at him because of overindulgence or underindulgence. Rama is a vegetarian. He believes that meat and intoxicants would excite his senses too much. Yet the Hindu diet pattern is flexible; definite rules are not set. If Rama is sick, he tries to bear his illness with resignation, knowing its temporary nature. He believes that the prayer of supplication for body cure is the lowest form of prayer, whereas the highest form is devotion to God. To him, death and rebirth are nearly synonymous, for the atman never changes and always remains pure. He compares the atman to the ocean: as ocean water can be put into various containers without changing its nature, so can the atman be put into various physical and human containers without changing its nature.

Thus, if death is imminent, Rama believes that the body, mind, and senses weaken and become lifeless but that the never-changing atman is ready to enter into a new form of life, depending on the person's knowledge, deeds, and past experiences. Full acceptance of death is encouraged. Death is a friend to be faced bravely, calmly, and confidently.

Rama says that as a devotee of God he is following a *training course* called **yoga.** As a preliminary, however, he must establish certain moral qualifications. He must strive for self-control, self-discipline, cleanliness, and contentment. He must avoid injury, deceitfulness, and stealing. His overwhelming

---

*See the symbol at the beginning of this section. A transliteration of the script is *a, u, m.* It is written in English as *Om,* or *Aum. Om, God,* and *Brahman* are synonymous and mean a *consciousness* or *awareness* rather than a personified being.

GITA IS A WAY OF LIFE

a way of karma—

a way to Moksha

Like a lamp of a steady flame

Not overjoyed by achievements.

Nor dejected by calamities.

One observes the light

and darkness evenly.

Reigning the senses,

Within the reasonable limits

knowing that atma is eternal

unlike physical existence of self—

which changes from time to time,

bound by one's karmas and

controlled by the 'treacherous' mind

But the wise one

bows to the Lord in humility

in the 'wake' of humble surrender

offers karma without desire

For this can only be led by

'Gyana' the light

That enlightens by the practice of

uniting mind and body to a peaceful Omkar.

Unyielding to one's pride & passion

Persisting destructive thoughts,

Undisillusioned by the illusions

of this world as 'Maya'.

Where—what is there is not there

But what doesn't seem to be there (atma) is very

much present

When the veil is unfurled by the light of 'Gyana'

One reaches the Lord even by the feel of His existence—

One opens the path of eternity

—a journey to an empty road

Where the tripti of the desired senses

Have evaporated in the air as the water takes the form

of vapor

It's then that one realizes . . . the blissful state of atma

Vibrating OM ! OM !! OM !! chanting

'Om Namo Bhagawate Vasudevaya. Om!!'

FIGURE 3–2

Gita is a way of life. (Written by A.D. Desai, Boulder, Co.)

desire to reach God can be implemented through one or a combination of the four yoga paths: (1) **inana yoga** through *reading and absorbing knowledge*, (2) **bhakti yoga** through the *devotion of emotion and love*, (3) **karma yoga** through *work dedicated to God*, and (4) **raja yoga** through *psychological experiments on oneself.* Rama combines the first three by reading and memorizing portions of the ancient scriptures, by meditating daily at his shrine, and by dedicating the results of his professional work to God.

Rama mentions that various forms of yoga have spread around the world to form hybrid groups with varied purposes. One branch that has appeared in medical centres is **hatha yoga,** meaning *sun and moon, symbolizing an inner balance that is achieved through muscle and breathing exercises.* Ultimately the body is prepared for meditation through these exercises.

From the bhakti emphasis comes **Sikhism,** founded by Nanak, who was born in 1469. The Sikhs had nine other gurus, or spiritual mentors, who sequentially taught that God was the one and only reality. The fifth guru compiled the scripture. Starting as a pacifist group, the Sikhs evolved to warriors.

Also from bhakti influence the **Hare Krishna** movement has come to North America, starting in 1965 when A.C. Bhaktivedanta came to New York City.[36]

For Rama, religion is not something to be picked up and put down according to a schedule or one's mood. It is a constant and all-pervading part of his life, every value and action, and the life of his country. India's literature and art are witness to this fact. It also influences family life and structure. Basically marriage is for life, and people usually marry someone in the same social level. The husband is treated with respect, and the mother is thought of as ideal. The family is patrifocal; the father usually has final authority. All family members are close. Elders are respected, cared for when they are ill, and considered as experienced models; children and grandchildren seek their wisdom. Children have reverence for both father and mother, and backtalk is unthinkable. Friends are to be treated as brothers and sisters, and visitors are always treated congenially.

Rama will be married soon and gives us some insight into the ceremony and meaning. The traditional Indian wedding customs were formulated more than 5000 years ago. Each ceremony, each occasion, and each ritual has a deep philosophical meaning and purpose. The ceremony is performed in Sanskrit, the most ancient surviving language in the world. It is meant to unite two souls so firmly that after they are married, although their bodies remain separate, their souls merge and become spiritually one. Thus, divorce is unacceptable.[37,38]

First, eight sacred blessings are given. Then the groom is welcomed amidst recitations including the five elements. The bride follows the bridesmaids and groomsmen and is welcomed following an exchange of garlands between bride and groom. The couple declares their union and ties together the ends of scarves that each is wearing. The bride and groom then walk around a fire (purifier), taking seven sacred steps, each signifying vows and promises made to each other. Finally, the rings are exchanged.[39]

CRITICAL THINKING

How effectively do you see yourself as being able to relate comfortably to a person who lives by the teachings of Sikhism?

 ## Buddhism, Jainism, and Shintoism

Umeko Sato is a member of the sect of **Buddhism** called **Soka Gakkai.** This sect is a powerful religion in Japan, with a government party, a university, and a grand temple representing it. This organization, which includes about 10% of Japan's population, known previously as a militant proselytizing group, has toned down this phase and is living more graciously with other sects and creeds. Based on the **Lotus Sutra,** *part of the Buddhist scriptures,* its doctrine advocates the three values of happiness: profit, goodness, and beauty. Sato is attracted by the practicality of the teaching, the mottoes that she can live by, the emphasis on small group study, and present world benefits, especially healing.

Although Sato's beliefs at some points seem in direct contrast to the original Buddhist teachings, she is happy to explain the rich multi-religious tradition that her family has had for generations. She emphasizes that she is affected by the **Confucian** emphasis on the family unit, by Christianity's healing emphasis, by **Shintoism,** the state religion of Japan until 1945, and by Buddhism, which originated about 600 B.C. in India with a Hindu named Siddhartha Gautama.

Currently, approximately 90% of Japan's people adhere both to Buddhism and to Shintoism, although the nation has never been known as devout. Less than 1% are Christian. Another small religion is **Jainism.** The "Jains" hark back to the 6th century B.C., about the same time as Buddha. Their fundamental tenet is **ahimsa,** *a refusal to injure any living thing.* Jains believe every living thing has a soul.

There are two groups of Jains. A small group of approximately 100 are called *sky clad* because they wear no clothes. They renounce clothing and all earthly possessions. The other, larger group is called *white clad* because they wear white clothes. Together the groups contain monks, nuns, laymen, and laywomen who all take vows to guide them in all aspects of daily life.

Although the Jains are found in Japan and other countries, they probably are known best for their bird hospital in Old Delhi, India, which treats 20 000 birds each year.

Gautama, shortly after a historic enlightenment experience, during which he became the Buddha, preached a sermon to his followers and drew on the earth a wheel representing the continuous round of life and death and rebirth. Later, eight spokes were added to illustrate the sermon and to provide the most explicit visual symbol of Buddhism* today. Sato repeats Buddha's four noble truths: (1) life is disjointed or out of balance, especially in birth, old age, illness, and death; (2) the cause of this imbalance is ignorance of one's

own true nature; (3) removal of this ignorance is attained by reaching **Nirvana,** *the divine state of release,* the *ultimate reality,* the *perfect knowledge* via (4) the eightfold path.

The eight spokes of the wheel represent the eightfold path used to reach Nirvana. Sato says that followers subscribe to right knowledge, right intentions, right speech, right conduct, and right means of livelihood, right effort, right mindfulness, and concentration. From these concepts has arisen a moral code that, among other things, prohibits intoxicants, lying, and killing of any kind (which explains why Buddhists are often vegetarians). She further explains that the Mahayana branch of Buddhism took hold in Japan as opposed to the Theravada branch. The **Theravada branch** *emphasizes an intellectual approach through wisdom, people working by themselves through meditation and without ritual.* The **Mahayana branch** *emphasizes involvement with humankind, ritual, petitionary prayer, and concern for one's sibling.* Sato believes that the Mahayana branch provides the happier philosophy of the two, and she tells of the ritual of celebration of Gautama's birthday. But most Japanese believe in **Amitabha Buddha,** *a god rather than a historical figure,* who is replacing the austere image of Gautama as a glorious redeemer, one of infinite light. Also, the people worship **Kwannon,** *a goddess of compassion.*

Sato explains that she cannot omit mention of the *one austere movement within the Mahayana branch,* the **Zen sect.** Taking this example from Gautama's extended contemplation of a flower, Zen followers care little for discourse, books, or other symbolic interpretations and explanations of reality. Hours and years are devoted to meditation, contemplation of word puzzles, and consultation with a Zen master. In seeking absolute honesty and truthfulness through such simple acts as drinking tea or gardening, the Zen student hopes to experience enlightenment. In North America, a version of Buddhism called *Buddhaharma* is emerging. Women and men are considered equal. This group provides meditations for the public on a CD-ROM disk.

Sato next turns to her former state religion, **Shintoism.** Whereas Buddhism produced a solemnizing effect on her country, Shintoism had an affirmative and joyous effect. Emperor, ancestor, ancient hero, and nature worship form its core. Those who follow Shintoism, she says, feel an intense loyalty and devotion to every lake, tree, and blossom in Japan and to the ancestral spirits abiding there. They also have a great concern for cleanliness, a carryover from early ideas surrounding dread of pollution in the dead.

Sato says that her parents have two god shelves in their home. One contains wooden tablets inscribed with the name of the household's patron deity and a symbolic form of the goddess of rice and other texts and objects of family significance. Here her family performs simple rites such as offering a prayer or a food gift each day. In a family crisis, perhaps an illness, the family conducts more elaborate rites, such as lighting tapers or offering rice brandy. The other god shelf, in another room, is the Buddha shelf; and if a family member dies, a Buddhist priest, the spiritual leader, performs specified rituals there.

Sato strongly emphasizes that if illness or impending death causes a family member to be hospitalized, another well

---

*See the symbol at the beginning of this section.

family member will stay at the hospital to bathe, cook for, and give emotional support to the ill person. Sato believes that recovery depends largely on this family tie. If death occurs, Sato will be reminded of the Buddhist doctrine teaching that death is a total nonfunction of the physical body and mind and that the life force is displaced and transformed to continue to function in another form. Every birth is a rebirth, much as in the Hindu teaching; the rebirth happens immediately after death, according to some Buddhists. Others believe that rebirth occurs 49 days after death, during which time the person is in an intermediary state. The difference in quality of death, birth, and existence depends on whether the person lived a disciplined or undisciplined life.

Buddhism teaches the living how to die well. The elderly, or feeble, are to prepare themselves mentally for a state that would be conducive for a good rebirth. The person is to remain watchful and alert in the face of death, to resist distraction and confusion, to be lucid and calm. Distinct instructions are given in what to expect as life leaves the body, as the person enters an intermediary state, and as Nirvana is about to occur.

So, although Sato has grasped a new religious path for herself, her respect for tradition remains.

In giving care to a person with Umeko Sato's background, be aware of the varied religious influences on her life. The sect's emphasis on the here and now, rather than on the long road to Nirvana, may place a high value on physical health so that the person can benefit from the joys and beauty of this life. The person may readily voice impatience with the body's dysfunction. You can also respond to the great concern for cleanliness, the desire to have family nearby, and the need for family rites that are offered for the sick member. Should a family member be dying, you may see some ambivalence. The family member may want to prepare himself or herself in the traditional way, but someone with Sato's background, with emphasis on present world benefits and healing, may deny that there is a valid preparation for death.

 ## Confucianism and Taoism

Wong Huieng is a young teacher in Taiwan simultaneously influenced by **Taoism,** the *romantic and mystical,* and **Confucianism,** the *practical and pragmatic.* To provide insights into these Chinese modes of thinking, although it is more representative of Taoism, Wong Huieng uses the **yin–yang symbol.** * The symbol is a circle, representing **Tao** or the *absolute,* in which two tear shapes fit perfectly into one another, each containing a small dot from the other. Generally **yang** is *light or red,* and **yin** is *dark.* Ancient Chinese tradition says that everything exists in these two interacting forces. Each represents a group of qualities. **Yang** is *positive or masculine— dry, hot, active, moving, and light.* **Yin** is *feminine or negative— wet, cold, passive, restful, and empty.* For example, fire is almost

pure yang and water almost pure yin, but not quite. The *combination of yin and yang constitutes all the dualisms a person can imagine:* day–night, summer–winter, beauty–ugliness, illness–health, life–death. Both qualities are necessary for life in the universe; they are complementary and, if in harmony, good. Yang and yin energy forces are embodied in the body parts and affect food preferences and eating habits.

Huieng translates this symbol into a relaxed philosophy of life: "If I am sick, I will get better. Life is like going up and down a mountain; sometimes I feel good and sometimes I feel bad. That's the way it is." Although educated, she is not interested in climbing up the job ladder, accumulating wealth, or conquering nature. Her goal is to help provide money to build an orphanage in a natural wooded setting.

Huieng thinks of death as a natural part of life, as the peace that comes when the body is worn out. She admits, however, that when her father died, human grief took hold of her. Before his death, her mother went to the Taoist temple priest and got some incense that was to help cast the sickness from his body. After death, they kept his body in the house for the required time, 49 days. The priest executed a special ceremony every seven days. Her mother could cry only one hour daily, from 2:00 until 3:00 in the morning. Now her mother talks through the priest to her father's ghost. Although Huieng regards this practice as superstitious and thinks that painting a picture of a lake and mountain is a more fitting way to erase her grief, she looks at the little yellow bag, containing a blessing from the priest, hanging around her neck, and finds it comforting if not intellectually acceptable.

Now Huieng turns to her practical side and talks about **Confucius,** the *first saint of the nation.* Although **Lao-tzu,** the *founder of Taoism,* is a semi-legendary figure said to have vanished after he wrote the *bible of Taoism,* **Tao-te-ching,** Confucius has a well-documented existence.

Confucius, born in 551 B.C., wrote little. His disciples wrote the **Analects,** *short proverbs, embodying his teachings.* He is revered as a teacher, not as a god. Huieng does not ask him to bless her but tries to emulate him and his teachings, which she has heard since birth. The temple in his memory is a place for studying, not for praying. And on his birthday, a national holiday, people pay respect to their teachers in his memory.

Five important terms in Confucius' teaching are **Jen,** *a striving for goodness within;* **Chun-sui,** *establishing a gentlemanly or womanly approach with others;* **Li,** *knowing how relationships should be conducted and having respect for age;* **Te,** *leading by virtuous character rather than by force;* and **Wen,** *pursuing the arts as an adjunct to moral character.* Huieng stresses that in Li are found the directives for family relationships. So strongly did Confucius feel about the family that he gave directives on proper attitudes between father and son, elder brother and junior brother, and husband and wife. Also, Huieng believes she cannot harm her body because it was given to her by her parents. Her concept of immediate family includes grandparents, uncles, aunts, and cousins. Her language has more words for relationships between relatives than the English language does.

Huieng believes that in caring for her body, she cares for her family, the country, and the universe. Essentially, to her, all people are family.

---

*See the symbol at the beginning of this section.

Important in your understanding of a person with Wong Huieng's background is the dualism that exists in such thinking. Acceptance of the particular version of mysticism and practicality and of the yin and yang forces that are seen as operating within self will help in building a foundation of personalized care.

The person may have more respect for older than younger staff members and may respond well to teaching. There may be a strong desire to attain and maintain wellness. These factors are directly related to the religious teaching; you can use them to enhance care. Additionally, talk slowly to the person if language is an issue. Rely on family members to help you understand the person's feelings. Permit familiar foods. Remember that foods are also divided into appropriate groups for types of illness. Address the person by the proper name. Do not use excessive touch signals unless they are invited. Remember this person may be in awe of health care authority and may be intimidated.

Islam

Omar Ali is *Muslim,* a member of **Islam,** the youngest of the major world religions.* "There is no God but Allah; Muhammad is His Prophet"[†] provides the key to Omar's beliefs. He must say this but once in his life as a requirement, but he will repeat it many times as an affirmation. Muslims believe in a final judgment day when everyone will be judged and sent either to Paradise or to the fire of hell, depending on how justly he or she lived life according to God's laws. They believe everyone, except children before the age of puberty, are responsible for their own good and bad actions and deeds and that no one can intercede on behalf of another.

Omar has also been influenced by 3000-year-old **Zoroastrianism,** *which is a religion of pre-Islamic Iran that* flourishes in Bombay today. Likewise, it was a monotheistic religion even though dualism was also espoused.

Omar is an Egyptian physician whose religious tradition was revealed through Muhammad, born approximately 571 A.D. in Mecca, then a trading point between India and Syria on the Arabian Peninsula. Hating polytheism and paganism in any form, Muhammad recited God's revelation to him as is documented in the **Quran,**[‡] *scriptures.* Omar believes in the biblical prophets, but he calls Muhammad the greatest—the seal of Prophets.

Through the Quran and the **Hadith,** *the traditions,* Omar has guidelines for his thinking, devotional life, and social obligations. He believes he is a unique individual with an eternal soul. He believes in a heaven and hell, and while on earth he wants to walk the straight path.

To keep on this path, Omar prays five times a day: generally on rising, at midday, in the afternoon, in the early evening, and before retiring. Articles needed are water and a prayer rug. Because the Quran emphasizes cleanliness of body, Omar performs a ritual washing with running water over the face, arms, top of head, and feet before each prayer. Omar explains that in the bedridden client this requirement can be accomplished by pouring water out of some sort of receptacle. If a Muslim's entire body is considered ritually unclean, he must wash the entire body. If water is unavailable or the person cannot bathe, clean soil may be used in place of the ritual washing. After this washing, the Muslim needs either a ritually clean cloth or a prayer rug and a clean place to pray. He may not face a dirty area such as the bathroom when making his prayer, even if this area is in the line toward Mecca. The Muslim must physically readjust himself in this case to comply with Islamic regulations. Then, facing Mecca, he goes through a series of prescribed bodily motions and repeats various passages in praise and supplication.

Omar also observes **Ramadan,** *a fast month,*[*] during which time he eats or drinks nothing from sunrise to sunset; after sunset he takes nourishment only in moderation. He explains **fasting** (*abstinence from eating*) as a discipline aiding him to understand those with little food and more importantly, as a submission to Allah. At the end of Ramadan, he enters a festive period with feelings of goodwill and gift exchanges. The sick, the very old, pregnant and lactating mothers, children, and Muslims who require the ingestion or injection of substances throughout the day hours are exempt without penalty from practice of this belief.

Omar has made one pilgrimage to Mecca, another requirement for all healthy and financially able Muslims. He believes the experience created a great sense of brotherhood, for all the pilgrims wore similar modest clothing, exchanged news of followers in various lands, and reviewed their mutual faith. The 12th day of the Pilgrimage month is the **Feast of Sacrifice (Eida-Fita),** when all Muslim families kill a lamb in honour of Abraham's offering of his son to God.

In line with the Quran's teaching, Omar does not eat pork (including such items as bologna, which might contain partial pork products), gamble, drink intoxicants, use illicit drugs, or engage in religiously unlawful sexual practices such as premarital sex, homosexuality, and infidelity. The emphasis on strict moral upbringing—dating, dancing, drinking, and sex outside marriage are forbidden—puts the Muslim on a common ground with conservative Christians. Abstinence from drug use also eliminates many potential health and social problems.

Omar worships no images or pictures of Muhammad, for the prophet is not deified. Nor does he hang or display pictures of any prophet or any god or worship statues or religious symbols. He gives a portion of his money to the poor, for Islam advocates a responsibility to society.

Omar points out that not all Arabs are Muslims and not all Muslims are Arabs. Arabs come from a number of nations

---

*A portion of this section was contributed by Caroline Samiezadé-Yazd, RN, MSN, PNP.

[†]These words are a translation of the sacred calligraphy in the symbol shown at the beginning of this section. The prophet's name is sometimes spelled *Mohammad.*

[‡]Sometimes spelled *Koran.*

---

*Coming during the ninth month of the Muslim year, always at a different time each year by the Western calendar, and sometimes spelled *Ramazan.*

stretching from Morocco to the Persian Gulf. Persons who are Arab Muslims speak Arabic and uphold the tenets of Islam. Omar emphasizes the importance of gaining specific knowledge about their complex social structure. The centrality of religion and the family are closely related and reflect many aspects of health care.

Omar mentions that parts of the basic Islam faith are used by an American-based group commonly known as the **Black Muslims (Nation of Islam).** Known to have stringent, seclusionist rules, the Black Muslims are rapidly increasing in numbers and power. They seem to be moving away from orthodox Islam. Members may not get politically involved; membership is especially appealing to young black men who like the masculine focus, the structure, and the emphasis on self-help and self-esteem.

Omar outlines the ideas of his religion as it applies to his profession. He believes that he can make a significant contribution to health care but that essentially what happens is God's will. Submission to God is the very meaning of Islam. This belief produces a very fluid feeling of time and sense of fatalism. Planning ahead for a Muslim is not a value as it is in Western culture. It is believed that if God's will is defied, the evil eye will appear.

Muslim clients who are ill are excused from many, but not all, religious rules, but many will still want to follow them as closely as possible. Even though in a body cast and unable to get out of bed, a client may want to go through prayers symbolically. The person might also recite the first chapters of the Quran, centred on praise to Allah, which are often used in times of crises. Family is a great comfort in illness, and praying with a group is strengthening, but the Muslim has no priest. The relationship is directly with God. Some clients may seem fatalistic, completely resigned to death, whereas others, hoping it is God's will that they live, cooperate vigorously with the medical program. Muslims do not discuss death openly, because if they did, the client and family may lose all hope and the client could die as a result. Instead, Muslims tend to communicate grief in gradual stages rather than immediately and all at once. Further, they make it a point never to let the affected person lose hope. The family, even in the gravest of situations, will not attempt to prepare for the death even when it is imminent. After death, a body must be washed with running water by a Muslim and the hands folded in prayer. Muslims do not perform autopsies, embalm, or use caskets for burials. Instead, they wrap a white linen cloth around the dead person and place the body into the ground facing Mecca. Knowledge of these attitudes and traditions can greatly enhance your care.

Judaism

Seth Lieberman, strongly influenced by the emphasis on social concern in **Judaism,** is a psychiatrist. In the Jewish community each member is expected to contribute to others' needs according to his or her ability. Jews have traditionally considered their community as a whole responsible for feeding the hungry, helping the widowed and orphaned, rescuing

the captured, and even burying the dead. Jewish retirement homes, senior citizens' centres, and medical centres are witnesses to this philosophy.

Seth cannot remember when his religious instruction began—it was always there. He went through the motions and felt the emotion of the Sabbath eve with its candles and cup of sanctification long before he could comprehend his father's explanations. Book learning followed, however, and he came to understand the fervency with which his people study and live the law as given in the **Torah,** *the first five books of the Bible,* and in the **Talmud,** *a commentary and enlargement of the Torah.* His spiritual leader is the *rabbi.* His *spiritual symbol* is the **menorah.***

His own *entrance into a responsible religious life and manhood* was through the **bar mitzvah,** a ceremony that took place in the synagogue when he was 13. Girls are also educated to live responsible religious lives, and congregations now have a similar ceremony, the **bat mitzvah,** for girls.

Although raised in an Orthodox home, Seth and his family are now members of the Reform sect. He mentions another group, the Conservatives. The **Orthodox** followers *believe God gave the law; it was written exactly as He gave it; it should be followed precisely.* **Reform Jews** *believe the law was written by inspired men* at various times and therefore is *subject to reinterpretation.* Seth says he follows the traditions because they are traditions rather than because God demands it. **Conservatives** *are in the middle, taking some practices from both groups.* Overriding any differences in interpretation of ritual and tradition is the fundamental concept expressed in the prayer "Hear, O Israel, the Lord our God, the Lord is One." Not only is He one, He loves His creation, wants His people to live justly, and wants to bless their food, drink, and celebration. Judaism's double theme might be expressed as "Enjoy life now, and share it with God." Understandably then, Seth's religious emphasis is not on an afterlife, although some Jewish people believe in one. Although Jews have had a history of suffering, the inherent value of suffering or illness is not stressed. Through their observance of the law, the belief of their historical role as God's chosen people, and their hope for better days, Jews have survived seemingly insurmountable persecution.

Seth works with physically, emotionally, and spiritually depressed persons. He believes that often the spiritual depression is unnoticed, misunderstood, or ignored by professional workers. He cites instances in which mental attitudes have brightened as he shared a common bond of Judaism with a client.

He offers guidelines for working with a Jewish person in a hospital or nursing home. Although Jewish law can be suspended when a person is ill, the client will be most comfortable following as many practices as possible.

Every Jew observes the **Sabbath,** *a time for spiritual refreshment, from sundown on Friday to shortly after sundown*

---

*See the symbol at beginning of this section. The seven-branched candelabrum stands for the creation of the universe in seven days, the centre light symbolizes the Sabbath, and the candlelight symbolizes the presence of God in the Temple.

on Saturday. During this period Orthodox Jews may refuse freshly cooked food, medicine, treatment, surgery, and use of radio, television, and writing equipment lest the direction of their thinking be diverted on this special day. An Orthodox male may want to wear a **yarmulke** or *skullcap* continuously, use a *prayer book* called **Siddur,** and use **phylacteries,** *leather strips with boxes containing scriptures,* at weekday morning prayer. Also, the ultra-Orthodox male may refuse to use a razor because of the Levitical ban on shaving.

Some Orthodox Jewish women observe the rite of **mikvah,** *an ancient ritual of family purity.* From marriage to menopause (except when pregnant) these women have no physical or sexual relations with their husbands from 24 hours before menstruation until 12 days later when a ritual immersion in water renders them ready to meet their husbands again.

Jewish dietary laws have been considered by some scholars as health measures: to enjoy life is to eat properly and in moderation. The Orthodox, however, obey them because God so commanded. Food is called **treyfe** (or *treyfah*) if it is *unfit* and **kosher** if it is *ritually correct.*

Foods forbidden are pig, horse, shrimp, lobster, crab, oyster, and fowl that are birds of prey. Meats approved are from those animals that are ruminants and have divided hooves. Fish approved must have both fins and scales. Also, the kosher animals must be healthy and slaughtered in a prescribed manner. Because of the Biblical passage stating not to soak a young goat in its mother's milk, Jews do not eat meat products and milk products together. Neither the utensils used to cook these products nor the dishes from which to eat these products are ever intermixed.

Guidelines for a satisfactory diet for the Orthodox are as follows:

- Serve milk products first, meat second. Meat can be eaten a few minutes after milk, but milk cannot be taken for six hours after meat.
- If a person completely refuses meat because of incorrect slaughter, encourage a vegetarian diet with protein supplements, such as fish and eggs, which are considered neutral unless prepared with milk or meat fat.
- Buy frozen kosher products marked Ⓤ, *K,* or *pareve.*
- Heat and serve food in the original container and use plastic utensils.

Two important holy days are Rosh Hashanah and Yom Kippur. **Rosh Hashanah,** *the Jewish New Year,* is a time to meet with the family, give thanks to God for good health, and renew traditions. **Yom Kippur,** the *Day of Atonement,* a time for asking forgiveness of family members for wrongs done, occurs ten days later. On Yom Kippur, Jews fast for 24 hours, a symbolic act of self-denial, mourning, and petition. **Tisha Bab,** the *day of lamentation,* recalling the destruction of both Temples of Jerusalem, is another 24-hour fast period. **Pesach** or **Passover** (eight days for Orthodox and Conservative, seven days for Reform) *celebrates the ancient Jews' deliverance from Egyptian bondage.* **Matzo,** *unleavened bread,* replaces leavened bread during this period.

The Jewish person is preoccupied with health. Jews are future-oriented and want to know diagnosis, how a disease will affect business, family life, and social life. The Jewish people as a whole are highly educated, and although they respect the doctor, they may obtain several medical opinions before carrying out a treatment plan.

Although family, friends, and a rabbi may visit the ill, especially on or near holidays, they will also come at other times. Visiting the sick is a religious duty. And although death is final to many Jews except for living on in the memories of others, guidelines exist for this time. When a Jewish person has suffered irreversible brain damage and can no longer say a **bracha,** *a blessing to praise God,* or perform a **mitzvah,** *an act to help a fellow,* he or she is considered a "vegetable" with nothing to save. Prolonging the life by artificial means would not be recommended. But until then, the dying client must be treated as the complete person he or she always was, capable of conducting his or her own affairs and entering into relationships.

Jewish tradition says never to leave the bedside of the dying person, which is of value to the dying and the mourners. The dying soul should leave in the presence of people, and the mourner is shielded from the guilt of thinking that the client was alone at death or that more could have been done. The bedside vigil also serves as a time to encourage a personal confession by the dying, which is a *rite of passage* to another phase of existence (even though unknown). This type of confessional is said throughout the Jewish life cycle whenever one stage has been completed. Confessional on the deathbed is a recognition that one cycle is ending and that another cycle is beginning. Recitation of the *Shema* in the last moments before death helps the dying to affirm faith in God and focus on the most familiar rituals of life.

Death, being witnessed at the bedside, helps to reinforce the reality of the situation. Immediate burial and specified mourning also move the remaining loved ones through the crisis period. (Note, however, that if a Jew dies on the Sabbath, he or she cannot be moved, except by a non-Jew, until sundown.) After the burial, the mourners are fed in a meal of replenishment called *se'udat havra'ah.* The step symbolizes the rallying of the community and the sustenance of life for the remaining. Also, Jews follow the custom of **sitting shiva** or *visiting with remaining relatives for one week after the death.*[40]

Judaism identifies a *year of mourning.* The first three days are of deep grief; clothes may be torn to symbolize the tearing of a life from others. Seven days of lesser mourning follow, leading to 30 days of gradual readjustment. The remainder of the year calls for remembrance and healing. During that year a prayer called the mourner's *Kaddish* is recited in religious services. It helps convey the feeling of support for the mourner.[41] At the annual anniversary of death, a candle is burned and special prayers are said.[42]

So from circumcision of the male infant on the eighth day after birth to his deathbed and from the days of the original menorah in the sanctuary in the wilderness until the present day, the followers of Judaism re-enact their traditions. Because many of these traditions remain an intrinsic part of the Jew, even when striving to maintain or regain wellness, the preceding guidelines offer a foundation for knowledgeable care.

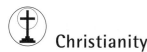 # Christianity

Beth Meyer, a *Roman Catholic,* Demetrius Callas, an *Eastern Orthodox,* and Jean Taylor, a *Protestant,* are Christian nurses representing the three major branches of Christianity. Although **Christianity** divided into Eastern Orthodox and Roman Catholicism in 1054 A.D., and the Protestant Reformation provided a third division in the 16th century, these nurses share some basic beliefs, most importantly that Jesus Christ, as described in the Bible, is God's son. Jesus, born in Palestine, changed "B.C." to "A.D." The details of His 33 years are few, but His deeds and words recorded in the Bible's New Testament show quiet authority, loving humility, and an ability to perform miracles and to visit easily with people in varied social positions.

The main symbol of Christianity is the cross,* but it signifies more than a wooden structure on which Jesus was crucified. It also symbolizes the finished redemption—Christ rising from the dead and ascending to the Father to rule with Him and continuously pervade the personal lives of His followers.

Christians observe **Christmas** as *Christ's birthday;* **Lent** as a *season of penitence and self-examination preceding* **Good Friday,** *Christ's crucifixion day;* and **Easter,** *His Resurrection day.*

Beth, Demetrius, and Jean rely on the New Testament as a guideline for their lives. They believe that Jesus was fully God and fully man at the same time, that their original sin (which they accept as a basic part of themselves) can be forgiven, and that they are acceptable to God because of Jesus Christ's life and death. They believe God is three persons—the Father, the Son, and the Holy Spirit (Holy Ghost), the last providing a spirit of love and truth.

Beth, Demetrius, and Jean differ in some worship practices and theology, but all highly regard their individuality as children of God and hope for life with God after death. They feel responsible for their own souls, the *spiritual dimension of themselves,* and for aiding the spiritual needs of their patients.

Roman Catholic Church

Roman Catholicism, according to Beth, is a religion based on the dignity of the person as a social, intellectual, and spiritual being made in the image of God. She traces the teaching authority of the church through the scriptures: God sent His Son to provide salvation and redemption from sin. He established the Church to continue His work after ascension into heaven. Jesus chose apostles to preach, teach, and guide. He appointed Saint Peter as the Church's head to preserve unity and to have authority over the apostles. The mission given by Jesus to Saint Peter and the apostles is the same that continues to the present through the Pope and his bishops. Beth notes that in the last several years, women in the Roman Catholic Church, both nuns and laywomen, are speaking out more on issues and are asking for more recognition and respect as God's spokespeople.

———————————————————

* See the symbol at the beginning of this section.

Beth believes that the seven **Sacraments** are *grace-giving rites that give her a share in Christ's own life and help sustain her in her efforts to follow His example.* The Sacraments that are received once in life are Baptism, Confirmation, Holy Orders, and usually Matrimony.

Through **baptism,** Catholics believe the *soul is incorporated into the life of Christ and shares His divinity.* Any infant in danger of death should be baptized, even an aborted fetus. If a priest is not available, you can perform the sacrament by pouring water on the forehead and saying, "I baptize thee in the name of the Father, of the Son, and of the Holy Spirit." The healthy baby is baptized some time during the first weeks of life. Adults are also baptized when they convert to Catholicism and join the church.

Confirmation *is the sacrament in which the Holy Spirit is imparted in a fuller measure to help strengthen the individual in his or her spiritual life.* **Matrimony** *acknowledges the love and lifelong commitment between a man and a woman.* **Holy Orders** *ordain deacons and priests.*

The Sacraments that may be received more than once are **Penance** (*confession*), the **Eucharist** (*Holy Communion*), and the **Anointing of the Sick** (*sacrament of the Sick*). Beth believes that **Penance,** *an acknowledgment and forgiveness of her sins in the presence of a priest,* should be received according to individual need even though it is required only once a year by church law. The **Mass,** often called the **Eucharist,** is the *liturgical celebration whose core is the sacrament of the Holy Eucharist.* Bread and wine are consecrated and become the body and blood of Christ. The body and blood are then received in Holy Communion.

The Eucharist is celebrated daily, and all Roman Catholics are encouraged to participate as often as possible; they are required by church law to attend on Sundays (or late Saturdays) and specified holy days throughout the year unless prevented by illness or some other serious reason.

Beth is glad that the Anointing of the Sick has been modified and broadened, and she explains the rite to client and family to allay anxiety. Formerly known as Extreme Unction, or the last rites, this sacrament was reserved for those near death. Now **Anointing of the Sick,** *symbolic of Christ's healing love and the concern of the Christian community,* can provide spiritual strength to those less gravely ill. After anointing with oil, the priest offers prayers for forgiveness of sin and restoration of health. Whenever possible, the family should be present to join in the prayers.

If the client is dying, extraordinary artificial measures to maintain life are unnecessary. At the hour of death, the priest offers Communion to the dying person by means of a special formula. This final Communion is called *Viaticum.* In sudden deaths, the priest should be called and the anointing and Viaticum should be administered if possible. If the person is dead when the priest arrives, there is no anointing, but the priest leads the family in prayer for the person who just died.

Beth divides the Roman Catholic funeral into three phases: the **wake,** *a period of waiting or vigil during which the body is viewed and the family is sustained through visiting;* the **funeral mass,** *a prayer service incorporated into the celebration of the Mass;* and the **burial,** *the final act of placing the person in the ground.* (This procedure may vary somewhat, for some Catholics are now choosing cremation.) The mourners retain the memory of the dead through a Month's Mind Mass, celebrated a month after death, and anniversary masses. Finally, the priest integrates the liturgy for the dead with the whole parish liturgical life.

Beth is convinced that her religious practice contributes to her health. She believes that the body, mind, and spirit work together and that a spirit rid of guilt and grievances and fortified with the strength of Christ's life has positive effects on the body. She believes that suffering and illness are allowed by God because of our disobedience (original sin) but that they are not necessarily willed by God or given as punishment for personal sin.

While in the hospital, a Roman Catholic may want to attend Mass, have the priest visit, or receive the Eucharist at bedside. (Fasting an hour before the sacrament is traditional, but in the case of physical illness, fasting is not necessary.) Other symbols that might be comforting are a Bible, prayer book, holy water, lighted candle, crucifix, rosary, and various relics and medals.

Eastern Orthodox Church

The Eastern Orthodox Church, the main denomination, is divided into groups by nationality. The **Greek Eastern Orthodox faith** is discussed by Demetrius. Each group has the **Divine Liturgy,** the *Eucharistic service,* in the native language and sometimes in English also. Although similar in many respects to the Roman Catholic faith, the Eastern Orthodox faith has no pope. The seven sacraments are followed with slight variations. Baptism is by triple immersion: the priest places the infant in a basin of water and pours water on the forehead three times. He then immediately confirms the infant by anointing with holy oil.

If death is imminent for a hospitalized infant and the parents or priest cannot be reached, you can baptize the infant by placing a small amount of water on the forehead three times. Even a symbolic baptism is acceptable, but only a living being should receive the sacrament. Adults who join the church are also baptized and confirmed.

The **Unction of the Sick** has never been practised as a last rite by the Eastern Orthodox; it is a *blessing for the sick.* Confession at least once a year is a prerequisite to participation in the Eucharist, which is taken at least four times a year: at Christmas, at Easter, on the Feast Day of Saint Peter and Saint Paul (June 30), and on the day celebrating the Sleeping of the Virgin Mary (August 15).

Fasting from the last meal in the evening until after **Communion,** another term for the *Eucharist,* is the general rule. Other fast periods include each Wednesday, representing the seizure of Jesus; each Friday, representing His death; and two 40-day periods, the first before Christmas and the second before Easter.

Fasting, to Demetrius, means that he must avoid meat, dairy products, and olive oil. Its purpose is spiritual betterment, to avoid producing extra energy in the body, and instead to think of the spirit. Fasting is not necessary when ill. Religion should not harm one's health.

Demetrius retains the Eastern influence in his thinking. He envisions his soul as blending in with the spiritual cosmos and his actions as affecting the rest of creation. He is mystically inclined and believes insights can be gained directly from God. He tells of sharing such an experience with a patient, Mrs. A., also Greek Orthodox.

Mrs. A. had experienced nine surgeries to build up deteriorating bones caused by rheumatoid arthritis. She faced another surgery. On the positive side, the surgery promised hope for walking; on the negative, it was a new and risky procedure. Possibly she would not walk; possibly she would not live. Demetrius saw Mrs. A. when he started working at 3:30 p.m. She was depressed, fearful, and crying. Later, at 6:30 p.m., he saw a changed person—fearless and calm, ready for surgery. She explained that she had seen Jesus in a vision, and that He said, "Go ahead with the surgery. You'll have positive results. But call your priest and take Communion first." Demetrius called the priest, who gave her Communion. She went into surgery the next day with supreme confidence. She now walks.

In addition to Communion, other helpful symbols are prayer books, lighted candles, and holy water. Especially helpful to the Orthodox are **icons,** *pictures of Jesus, Mary, or a revered saint.* Saints can intercede between God and the person. One of the most loved is *Saint Nicholas,* a 3rd-century teacher and father figure who gave his wealth to the poor and became an archbishop. He is honoured on Saint Nicholas Day, December 6, and prayed to continuously for guidance and protection.

Every Sunday morning Demetrius participates in an hour-long liturgy. Sitting in an ornate sanctuary with figures and symbols on the windows, walls, and ceiling, facing the tabernacle containing the holy gifts and scripture, Demetrius finds renewal. He recites, "I believe in one God, the Father Almighty, Maker of Heaven and Earth and of all things visible and invisible; and in one Lord Jesus Christ, the only begotten Son of God."

Protestantism

There are many Protestant denominations and sects. Jean Taylor is a member of the *Church of God* (Anderson, Indiana). She identifies the church by its headquarters because there are some 200 independent church groups in North America using the phrase "Church of God" in their title. Her group evolved late in the 19th century because members of various churches felt that organization and ritual were taking precedence over direction from God. They banded together in a drive toward Christian unity, toward recognition that any people who followed Christ's teachings were members of a universal Church of God and could worship freely together.

This example speaks of one of the chief characteristics of Protestantism: the insistence that God has not given any one person or group of persons sole authority to interpret His truth to others. Protestants use a freedom of spiritual searching and reinterpretation. Thus, new groups form as certain persons and their followers come to believe that they see God's teaching in a new and better light. Jean believes that reading the Bible for historical knowledge and guidance, having a minister to teach and counsel her, and relying on certain worship forms are all important aids. But discerning God's will for her life individually and following that will are her ultimate religious goals.

Jean explains that she "accepted Christ into her life" when she was eight years old. This identified her as personally following the church's teaching rather than just adhering to family religious tradition. A later experience, in which the *Holy Spirit gives the person more spiritual power and discernment,* is called **sanctification.**

Jean defines her corporate worship as free liturgical, with an emphasis on congregational singing, verbal prayer, and Scripture reading. A sermon by the **minister,** *the spiritual leader,* may take half the worship period. As with many Protestant groups, two sacraments or ordinances are observed:

(1) baptism (in this case, **believer's,** or **mature, baptism** by *total immersion into water*) and (2) Communion. To Protestants, the bread and wine used in Communion are symbolic of Christ's body and blood rather than the actual elements. One additional ordinance practised in Jean's church and among some other groups is **foot washing,** *symbolic of Jesus' washing His disciples' feet.* These ordinances are practised with varied frequencies.

Because of the **spectrum of beliefs and practices, defining Protestants,** even within a single denomination or sect, is almost impossible (see Table 3-2). Some Protestant groups,

TABLE 3-2
Summary of Major Health Care Implications of Selected Religious Cultures and Subcultures

Religion	Food Preference	Responsibility Related to Client Belief or Need
Hinduism	Vegetarian; no alcoholic beverages; other restrictions conform to sect doctrine; fasting important part of religious practice, with consequences for person on special diet or with diabetes or other metabolic diseases	Medical care is last resort; client considers help will come from own inner resources. Nurse should treat client with respect and convey sense of dignity. Reinforce need for medical care and explain care measures. Client may reject help and be stoic. Assess carefully for pain. Provide privacy. Assist to maintain religious practices. Cleanliness and dietary preferences are important. Certain prescribed rites are followed after death. The priest may tie a thread around the neck or wrist to signify blessing; the thread should not be removed. Immediately after death, the priest will pour water into the mouth of the corpse; the family will wash the body. They are particular about who touches their dead. Bodies are cremated. Loss of limb is considered sign of wrongdoing in previous life.
Buddhism Zen, sect of Buddhist Shintoism, Japan's state religion	Vegetarian; no intoxicants; moderation in eating and drinking	Family help care for ill member and give emotional support. Religion discourages use of drugs; assess carefully for pain. Cleanliness important. Question about feelings regarding medical or surgical treatment on holy days. Prepare for death; help patient remain alert, resist confusion or distraction, and remain calm. Last rite chanting is often practised at bedside soon after death. Contact the deceased's Buddhist priest or have the family make contact.
Islam	No pork and pork-containing products; no intoxicants	Members are excused from religious practices when ill but may still want to pray to Allah and face Mecca. There is no spiritual advisor to call. Family visits are important. Cleanliness is important. After 130 days, fetus is treated as fully developed human. Members maintain a fatalistic view about illness; they are resigned to death, but encourage prolonging life. Patient must confess sins and beg forgiveness before death, and family should be present. The family washes and prepares the body, folds hands, and turns the body to face Mecca. Only relatives or friends may touch the body. Unless required by law, no autopsy and no body part should be removed.

(continued)

TABLE 3-2 *(continued)*
Summary of Major Health Care Implications of Selected Religious Cultures and Subcultures

Religion	Food Preference	Responsibility Related to Client Belief or Need
Black Muslim (Nation of Islam)		There is no baptism. Procedure for washing and shrouding dead and performing funeral rites is carefully prescribed. Cleanliness is important.
Judaism	Orthodox Jews eat only kosher (ritually prepared) foods; milk consumed before meat, or meat eaten six hours before milk consumed; do not eat pig, horse, shrimp, lobster, crab, oyster, birds of prey. Others may restrict diet. Special utensils and dishes for Orthodox. Fasts on Yom Kippur and Tisha Bab; may fast other times but excluded if ill	There is no infant baptism. Baby boy is circumcised on eighth day if Orthodox. Preventative measures, avoiding illness, are important. Members are concerned about future consequences of illness and medication. Some are preoccupied with health; will convey that pain is present and want relief. Nursing measures for pain are important. On Sabbath, Orthodox Jews may refuse freshly cooked foods, medicine, treatment, surgery, and use of radio or television. Orthodox male may not shave. Nurse should avoid loss of yarmulke, prayer books, or phylacteries. Nurse must arrange for kosher or preferred food; food may be served on paper plates. Check consequences of fasting on person's condition. Visits from family members are important. If patient is without family, notify synagogue so other people may visit. Family or friends should be with dying person. Artificial means should not be used to prolong life if patient is vegetative. Confession by dying person is like a rite of passage. Human remains are ritually washed following death by members of the Ritual Burial Society. Burial should take place as soon as possible. Cremation is not permitted. All Orthodox Jews and some Conservative Jews are opposed to autopsy. Organs or other tissues should be made available to the family for burial. Parts of the body are not donated to medical science or removed, even during autopsy. Donation or transplantation of organs requires rabbinical consultation. A fetus is to be buried, not discarded.
Christianity		All will wish to see spiritual advisor when ill and to read Bible or other religious literature and follow usual practices.
Roman Catholic	Nothing special, except fasting or abstaining from meat on Ash Wednesday and Good Friday; some Catholics may fast every Friday and other holy days	Client finds comfort in having rosary, Bible, prayer book, crucifix, medals. Infant baptism is mandatory, and especially urgent if prognosis is poor. Baptism is demanded if aborted fetus may not be clinically dead. For baptismal purposes, death is a certainty only if there is obvious evidence of tissue necrosis. Tell priest if you baptize baby; it is done only once. Inquire about dietary preferences and fasting. Members may want information on natural family planning. The Rite for Anointing of the Sick is mandatory. If the prognosis is poor, the patient or his or her family may request it. In sudden death, priest is called to anoint and administer Viaticum, if possible, or special prayers are said.

(continued)

TABLE 3-2 *(continued)*
Summary of Major Health Care Implications of Selected Religious Cultures and Subcultures

Religion	Food Preference	Responsibility Related to Client Belief or Need
		Amputated limb may be buried in consecrated ground; there is no blanket mandate but it may be required within a given diocese. Donation or transplantation of organs is approved providing the recipient's potential benefit is proportionate to the donor's potential harm.
Orthodox		
Eastern Orthodox (Turkey, Egypt, Syria, Cyprus, Bulgaria, Rumania, Albania, Poland, Czechoslovakia)	Fasting each Wednesday, each Friday, and 40 days before Christmas and Easter; avoid meat, dairy products, and olive oil	Prayer book and icons are important. Infant is baptized if death is imminent. Check consequences of fast days on health; fasting is not necessary when ill. Blessing for the sick (unction) is not last rite but a form of healing by prayer. Last rites are obligatory if death is impending; cremation is discouraged.
Greek	Fasting periods on Wednesday, Friday, and during Lent; avoid meat and dairy products	Prayer book and icons are important. Infant is baptized if death is imminent. Patient prepares by fasting for Holy Communion and Sacrament of Holy Unction. Fasting is not mandatory during illness. Members oppose euthanasia. Every reasonable effort should be made to preserve life until terminated by God. Cremation or autopsies that may cause dismemberment are discouraged. Last rites are administered for the dying.
Russian Orthodox	Fasting on Wednesday, Friday, and during Lent; no meat or dairy products	Prayer book and icons are important. There is no baptism of infant. Check consequences of fasting on health. Cross necklace is important; it should be replaced immediately when patient returns from surgery. Do not shave male patients except in preparation for surgery. Patients do not believe in autopsies, embalming, or cremation. Traditionally, after death, arms are crossed, and fingers are set in a cross. Clothing at death must be of natural fibre so that the body will change to dust sooner.
Protestantism (Many denominations and sects) Baptist	Some groups condemn coffee and tea; most condemn alcoholic beverages; some groups may fast on Sundays or other special days, especially in Black Baptist churches	There is no infant baptism. Client may be fatalistic; may believe illness is punishment from God; and may be passive about care. Inquire about effect of fasting if client is on special diet, is a diabetic, or has disease dependent on dietary regulation.
Brethren (Grace) (Plymouth)	Most abstain from alcohol, tobacco, and illicit drugs	There is no infant baptism. Anointing with oil is done for physical healing and spiritual uplift. There are no last rites.
Church of Christ, Scientist (Christian Scientist)	Avoid coffee and alcoholic beverages	There is no infant baptism. If hospitalized or receiving medical treatment, guilt feelings may be intense. Be supportive. Allow practitioner or reader to visit freely as desired. Use nursing measures to alleviate pain. Patient may refuse blood transfusions as well as intravenous fluids and medication. There are no last rites or autopsy, unless sudden death.

(continued)

TABLE 3-2 *(continued)*
Summary of Major Health Care Implications of Selected Religious Cultures and Subcultures

Religion	Food Preference	Responsibility Related to Client Belief or Need
Church of Christ	Avoid alcoholic beverages	There is no infant baptism. Anointing with oil and laying on of hands are done for healing. There are no last rites.
Church of God	Most avoid alcoholic beverages	There is no infant baptism.
Church of Jesus Christ of Latter Day Saints (Mormon)	Eat in moderation; limit meat; avoid coffee and tea; no alcoholic beverages; avoid use of tobacco	There is no infant baptism, but baptism of dead is essential; living person serves as proxy. Laying on of hands is done for healing. White undergarment with special marks at navel and right knee is to remain on; it is considered a safeguard against danger.
Episcopalian	May fast from meat on Friday	Infant baptism is mandatory, but not for aborted fetus or stillbirth. Patient fasts in preparation for Holy Communion, which may be daily; thus, check effects on disease. Rite for Anointing Sick (last rites) is not mandatory.
Society of Friends (Quakers)	Moderation in eating; most avoid alcoholic beverages and drugs	There is no infant baptism. Health teaching is important. Give explanations about medical technology used in care. Share information about condition as indicated.
Jehovah's Witnesses	Avoid food to which blood is added, e.g., certain sausages and luncheon meats	There is no infant baptism. Members are opposed to blood transfusion. (Hospital administrator or doctor may seek court order to be appointed guardian of child in times of emergency need for blood.) There are no last rites.
Lutheran		Baptize only living infants shortly after birth, by pastor. Communion may be given before or after surgery or similar crisis.
Mennonite	Most avoid alcoholic beverages	There is no infant baptism. Shock therapy, psychotherapy, and hypnotism conflict with individual will and personality.
Methodist		No baptism at birth. Communion may be given before surgery or similar crisis.
Nazarene	Avoid alcoholic beverages	There is no need to baptize infant. Stillborn is buried. Laying on of hands is done for healing. There are no last rites.
Pentecostal	Avoid alcoholic beverages	There is no infant baptism. Prayer, anointing with oil, laying on of hands, speaking in tongues, shouting, and singing are important for healing of patient.
Unitarian/Universalist		Infant baptism is not necessary. Cremation is preferred to burial. Check before calling clergy to visit.
Seventh-Day Adventists	Vegetarian (no meat) or lacto-ovo-vegetarian (may eat milk and eggs but not meat); pork and fish without fins and scales prohibited; avoid coffee and tea; avoid alcoholic beverages	There is no infant baptism. Health measures, prevention, and health education are important. Some believe in divine healing and anointing with oil. Avoid administering narcotics and stimulants. Use nursing measures for pain; medication is last resort. Check on food preferences. Sabbath is Friday sundown until Saturday sundown for most groups. Client may refuse medical treatment and use of secular items, such as television, on Sabbath.

retaining their initial emphasis on individual freedom, have allowed no written creed, but expect members to follow an unwritten code of behaviour. Jean does suggest some guidelines, however. She lists some of the *main Protestant bodies* in North America, beginning with the most formal liturgically and sacramental, the *Protestant Episcopal* and *Lutheran* churches. The in-betweens are the *Presbyterians, United Church of Christ, United Methodists,* and *Disciples of Christ (Christian Church).* The liturgically freest and the least sacramental are the *Baptists* and *Pentecostals.* Bibby states that the established Roman Catholic and Protestant churches continue to monopolize the religion market. The Anglican and the United Church of Canada remain powerful religious corporations that are well established and have many followers.[43]

Among these groups, some of the opposing doctrines and practices are as follows: living in sin versus living above sin; predestination versus free will; infant versus believer's baptism; and loose organization versus tightly knit organization. Some uphold **fundamental precepts,** *holding to the Scriptures as infallible,* whereas others uphold **liberal precepts,** *using the Scriptures as a guide, with various interpretations for current living.* Recently, liberal and conservative Christians have become even more divided by subjects such as abortion, same-sex relationships, and what constitutes morality. The groups on the right, while proclaiming their absolute stands, have not exhibited the tolerance, forgiveness, or freedom of conscience that is part of Christianity, notes one Lutheran pastor.[44]

With this infinite variety, Jean believes that learning the individual beliefs of her Protestant client is essential. When and if a client wants Communion, if an infant should be baptized, and what will be most helpful spiritually to the patient—these factors are learned by careful listening. Generally Jean believes that prayer, a scriptural motto such as "I can do all things through Christ who gives me strength" (Philippians 4:13) or a line from a hymn can give strength to a Protestant. Some patients will also want anointing with oil as a symbolic aid to healing.

Jean has discovered that there are wide differences in Protestantism, sometimes even within the same denomination, about the theology and rituals of death. Some Protestant theologies have come to grips with the realities and meaning of death; others block authentic expression of grief by denying death and focusing on "If you are a Christian, you won't be sad."

Some Protestants view death as penalty and punishment for sins; others see death as a transition when the soul leaves the body for eternal reward; and still others view death as an absolute end. All agree that death is a biological and spiritual event, a mystery not fully comprehended.

Rituals surrounding death vary widely. Some churches believe that the funeral service with a closed casket or memorial service with no casket present is more of a testimony to the joy and victory of Christian life than the open-casket service. Others believe that death is a reality to face instead of deny and that viewing the dead person promotes the grief process and confrontation with death in a Christian context.

Jean believes that, for most Protestants, the minister represents friendship, love, acceptance, forgiveness, and

understanding. His or her presence seems to help the dying face death with more ease. She also believes that Protestants are becoming more active in ministering to the bereaved through regularly scheduled visits during the 12 to 18 months after the funeral, although there are no formal rituals.

Special Religious Groups of Interest

Practices or beliefs unique to certain groups should be part of every health provider's knowledge.

Seventh-Day Adventists rely on Old Testament law more than do other Christian churches. As in Jewish tradition, the Sabbath is from sundown Friday to sundown Saturday. Like the Orthodox Jew, the Seventh-Day Adventist may refuse medical treatment and use of secular items such as television during this period and prefer to read spiritual literature. Diet is also restricted. Pork, fish without scales and fins, tea, and coffee are prohibited. Some Seventh-Day Adventists are **lacto-ovo-vegetarians:** *they eat milk and eggs but no meat.* Tobacco, alcoholic beverages, and narcotics are also avoided. Because Adventists view the body as the "temple of God," health reform is high on their list of priorities and they sponsor health institutes, cooking schools, and food-producing organizations. They are pioneers in making foods for vegetarians, including meat-like foods from vegetable sources. Worldwide they operate an extensive system of more than 4000 schools and 400 medical institutions and are active medical missionaries.[45] Much of their inspiration comes from Ellen G. White, a 19th-century prophet who gave advice on diet and food and who stressed Christ's return to earth.

The **Church of Jesus Christ of Latter-Day Saints (Mormon)** takes much of its inspiration from the **Book of Mormon,** *translated from golden tablets found in what is now the U.S. by the prophet Joseph Smith.* The Mormons believe that this book and two others supplement the Bible. Every Mormon is an official missionary. There is no official congregational leader, but a **seventy** and a **high priest** *represent successive steps upward in commitment and authority.*

Specific beliefs are that the dead can hear the Gospel and can be baptized by proxy. Marriage in the temple seals the relationship for time and eternity; families are forever and essential for one's eternal destiny. This celestial marriage permits husband and wife to become gods. This process, called *exaltation,* or *eternal progression,* allows the pair to populate other worlds by having newly created human souls as their offspring. The church believes in a whole-being approach and provides education, recreation, and financial aid for its members. A health and conduct code called *Word of Wisdom* prohibits tobacco, alcohol, and hot drinks (interpreted as tea and coffee) and recommends eating, though sparingly and with thankfulness, herbs, fruit, meat, fowl, and grain, especially wheat.

The Mormon believes that disease comes from failure to obey the laws of health and from failure to keep the other commandments of God; however, righteous persons sometimes become ill simply because they have been exposed to microorganisms that cause disease. They also believe that by faith the righteous sometimes escape plagues that are sweeping the land and often, having become sick, the obedient are restored to full physical well-being by the gift of faith. There is no restriction on the use of medications or vaccines and there is no restriction on the use of blood or blood components.[46]

The two groups just discussed (the Seventh-Day Adventists and the Church of Jesus Christ of the Latter Day Saints) generally accept and promote modern medical practices. The next two groups, Jehovah's Witnesses and Church of Christ, Scientist, hold views that conflict with the medical field.

The first group, **Jehovah's Witnesses,** refuses to accept blood transfusions. Their refusal is based on the Levitical commandment, given by God to Moses, declaring that no one in the House of David should eat blood or he or she would be cut off from his or her people, and on a New Testament reference (in Acts) prohibiting the tasting of blood. Every Jehovah's Witness is a minister. The people who belong to Jehovah's Witnesses engage in door-to-door proselytizing, worship in Kingdom Halls, and try to sell their magazines *Awake* and the *Watchtower* to the public.[47] Today, they are most widely known for their refusal to accept blood transfusions—even when their own lives, or those of their children, are at stake.[48] However, some articles have spoken out in criticism of the Watchtower Society Blood Policy.[49]

The second group, **Church of Christ, Scientist (Christian Scientists),** turn wholly to spiritual means for healing. Occasionally they allow an orthopedic surgeon to set a bone if no medication is used. Parents do not allow their children to undergo a physical examination for school; to have eye, ear, or blood pressure screening; or to receive immunizations. In addition to the Bible, Christian Scientists use as their guide Mary Baker Eddy's *Science and Health with Key to the Scriptures,* originally published in 1875. The title of this work indicates an approach to wholeness, and those who follow its precepts think of God as Divine Mind, of spirit as real and eternal, and of matter as unreal illusion.

Christian Scientists are not against doctors in the health care delivery system. They exercise their own autonomy regarding treatment in any given situation. However, they generally choose to rely on spiritual healing because they have seen its effectiveness in the experience of their own family and fellow church members.[50]

One religious group, the Mennonites, has retained its lifestyle, geographic solidarity, and theological unity. Mennonites believe that each person is responsible before God to make decisions based on his or her comprehension of the Bible.[51] The Mennonite faith encompasses a wide range of cultural circumstances, which are more responsible for differences among individual Mennonites rather than for the relatively uniform basic theology.[52] For example, regarding health care practices, there is no religious ritual to be applied unless that client asks for one which is personally meaningful.[53]

In Canada, the **Mennonites** settled mainly in southern Ontario and the western provinces, where they maintained their religious practices.[54] The Mennonites generally emphasize plain ways of dressing, living, and worshipping. They do not believe in going to war, swearing oaths, or holding offices that require the use of force. Many of them farm the land, while some are inclined toward service professions. They are well known for

their missionary efforts. Another group, the **Amish,** split from the Mennonites. Amish people believe that the body is the temple of God and that people are the stewards of their bodies. Their belief is that medicine and health care should always be used with the understanding that it is God who heals.[55]

CRITICAL THINKING

What may be some barriers to health care for the Amish people?

Choquette, in his book *Canada's Religions,* explains how globalization has generated much religious diversity in society. Further, Canada's largely Christian heritage has been transformed into both a multi-ethnic mosaic and a pluralistic society.[56] He claims that the alternative religions, with their two components of *new religious movements* and *new religions,* may be classified into two categories. The first category is composed of those religious movements that are rooted in traditional mainstream religions—Aboriginal spiritualities included—which continue to teach the fundamental doctrines of that religion. Such religions include Christian Scientists, Mormons, and Jehovah's Witnesses. Others, of similar organization, include the following.

The **North American Indian religions** developed for centuries with very little influence from outside the continent. Power, Supreme Being, guardian spirits, totems, fasting, visions, **shamanism** (*belief in a priest who can influence good and evil spirits*), myth telling, and ritualism are all part of a wide-ranging belief system. The geographic location of the tribal group influenced its belief system. Aboriginals of the Far North, Northeast Woodlands, Southeast Woodlands, Plains, Northwest Coast, California, the Intermountain Region, and the American Southwest make up the main tribal divisions.

All belief systems have certain features in common: (1) **spirit world**—a *dimension that permeates life but is different;* (2) a **Supreme Being**—*God who represents other lesser deities;* (3) a **culture hero**—a *spirit who competes with the Great Spirit and who sometimes is a trickster;* (4) spirits and ghosts, such as atmospheric spirits (wind) or underworld powers (snakes); (5) guardian spirits acquired by visions seen during fasting; (6) medicine men and medicine societies; (7) ritual acts, such as the Sun Dance; and (8) prayers and offerings. Harmony or spiritual balance is what North American Indians want to achieve in their relations with the supernatural powers.

Many Canadians and Americans have learned the practice of **yoga.** The term yoga is a form of activity designed to harness its practitioners to knowledge of the divine. Yoga refers to the various paths leading to spiritual liberation.[57] The **Baha'i faith** is a monotheistic religion led by an elected body called the Universal House of Justice. The faithful practise daily personal devotions, annual fasts, missionary activity, and regular communal gatherings; and they celebrate annual feast days.[58] Baha'i members believe that the main purpose of marriage is the procreation of children; and to have children is the highest physical honour of people's existence.[59] The Baha'i are encouraged to seek out competent medical care, follow the advice of those in whom they have confidence, and pray.[60]

Canada's **Pentecostals**, while remaining diversified, became part of the mainstream of evangelical Protestantism. In fact, some of the key Pentecostal ideas made inroads into several Christian churches, including the Roman Catholic Church. Pentecostalism has spread globally. This means it can no longer be closely identified with fundamentalist Protestantism.[61]

The **Hare Krishna** is the eighth and the most famous incarnation of the god Vishnu and is the object of much devotion by the Hindu faithful. Devotees are encouraged to proselytize and to chant in the street.[62]

The second category of the new religions is that of religions that seem to be concerned with creating a new doctrine, a new revelation, or a new truth—frequently combined with elements drawn from a variety of traditions and cultures.[63] These new religions include some North American Aboriginal religions, Scientology, and New Age. Reason and Scripture have insignificant importance in new religions as sources of truth.[64] These new religions, even though there is a rapid turnover in membership, exert a significant impact in the West, and particularly in Canada. The **Native American Church** has spread with a desire to preserve Aboriginal people's ancestral lifestyle and customs. By consuming peyote (a stimulant from cacti), the devotees achieve an altered state of consciousness that they consider to be a religious experience.[65]

Meanwhile, the Church of Scientology originated from the writings of Hubbard. He coined a new vocabulary that became part of **Scientology**. A few of his concepts are engram, reactive mind, clear, auditing, and analytical mind. Scientology has been criticized, and has faced a number of lawsuits, in Canada and elsewhere.[66]

The New Age, although the movement itself may be in decline, has had tremendous influence on contemporary culture. The followers of the **New Age** recognize a wide range of movements, customs, beliefs, and objects. Unlike most formal religions, it has no holy text, formal clergy, dogma, creed, or central organization.[67] It stands apart from Judaism and Christianity. In its monistic tradition, New Age is in the company of the occult sciences—spiritualism, Eastern religions, and psychology, each having imparted an influence on its growth.[68] Choquette explains that one of the New Age's foundational components is modern psychology whose focus is on the inner self. This focus is the awareness of self, and the awareness of one's divinity that replaces conversion, while personal transformation replaces salvation. New Age dismisses religion as irrelevant and invites individuals to look inside themselves for wholeness and divinity. The best-known symbol of the New Age is the crystal. Crystals are embraced by New Age individuals who consider them as instruments of transformation and healing,[69] believing that they assist in healing by restoring the natural harmony between the physical and etheric (or spiritual) bodies.[70]

CRITICAL THINKING

How does the practice of health promotion affect someone who is a follower of the New Age?

3–1 BONUS SECTION IN CD-ROM

The African-American Church

This section provides a brief insight into spirituality from the historical perspective for African Americans. It mentions adaptations of religious practices of the dominant culture and how the church became a spiritual, social, and psychological source of support to the black family.

Other Spiritual Movements

Agnosticism and Atheism

This chapter has concentrated so far on worship of God, the divine or other positive spirits, with an emphasis on traditional teaching. Some people live by ethical standards, considering themselves as either **agnostic**, *incapable of knowing whether God exists*, or **atheistic**, *believing that a God does not exist.*

Wright[71] discusses ethical principles that must be practised with all people as follows:

1. **Beneficence:** *the duty to do no harm.* Give of self wholeheartedly in interactions with patients because this positive action is beneficial.

2. **Nonmalfeasance:** *constraint from doing harm to another.* Judging that another's beliefs can be harmful. However, you can share your beliefs in a nonjudgmental way as you provide care in the spiritual dimension.

3. **Autonomy:** *the right of patient self-determination.* Assess what patients desire regarding spiritual care and avoid imposing your own ideas on the patient.

4. **Advocacy:** *actively assisting the patient in exercising autonomy.* Help the patient find meaning, hope, and clarification of personal beliefs and values.

3–2 BONUS SECTION IN CD-ROM

Other Spiritual Movements: New Age, Cults, and Devil or Satan Worship.

The New Age movement, frequently mentioned in the media a few years ago, is considered. New Age preoccupation with God as All, or God is Everything, leads to a brief discussion of cults and their popularity in the 1970s. The relationship of Devil or Satan worship, as a cult, is explained.

Other Trends in the Spiritual Dimension

One trend that has not only been popular but is an important treatment modality for addictions is the 12-step program (originally developed by Alcoholics Anonymous). Such programs help individuals overcome several types of addictions and help to build spiritual strength. This approach refers to "God" but may view God as a higher power, deity, spiritual force, or even collective power of the group.[72]

CRITICAL THINKING

As a health professional how can you approach an individual who is a substance abuser and inform him or her about either Alcoholics Anonymous or Narcotics Anonymous?

3–3 BONUS SECTION IN CD-ROM

Other Trends in the Spiritual Dimension: Voodoo Illness and Its Trends

Did you know that what formerly was known as "voodoo" is now called "spiritualism"? This section explains voodoo illness and even relates the trend to university and college campuses.

Profile of Changing World Religions in Canada

It is important to note that religious diversity has been increasing in Canada since the 1960s. Most of this shift has been attributed to the changing source of immigration in the country.[73] The 2001 Census reports that Canada is still predominantly Roman Catholic and Protestant.[74] The largest religious group in Canada is Roman Catholic. Religions of Asian origin have grown, and the number of Canadians who reported being affiliated with religions such as Islam, Hinduism, Sikhism, and Buddhism has increased substantially. Within the Orthodox denominations—the two largest being Greek Orthodox and Ukrainian Orthodox, slight declines have occurred. However, the numbers of two other Orthodox churches—the Serbian Orthodox and Russian Orthodox, have more than doubled. A slight increase of individuals of Jewish faith has occurred. There was also an increase in the number of people reporting "no religion" in Canada. This group accounted for 16% of the population in 2001, compared to 12% a decade earlier.[75] It is important to note that on average, the people who reported they had no religion were younger than the general population.

Many Canadian scholars, theologians, and writers have contributed to a comprehensive view of religions in contemporary Canada.[76–81] Each has contributed significantly toward understanding religious patterns and the belief systems that affect individual, as well as family, views and practices in everyday life.

Choquette claims that during the second half of the twentieth century a number of diverse worldviews and theologies appeared in Canada.[82] The descriptions of the world that accompany these views and theologies reflected not only

radically different views of the East and West but growing diversity within Catholic, Protestant, and Orthodox Christians. The increased visibility of Aboriginal religion also occurred at that time. Above all, the fundamental worldview put forth by the religions of the East constituted a radically new element in Canadian society.[83] In two of his earlier books,[84,85] Bibby claimed a steep descent in religious involvement and interest by Canadians. Now, in his more recent book *Restless Gods*, Bibby indicates that significant signs exist of renewed religious interest—both inside and outside churches.[86] Bibby also explains that acceleration has occurred in the spiritual quest of Canadians, specifically since the 1980s.

One of the results from the Project Canada 2000 Survey indicated that generally Canadians have an interest in spirituality; and a solid majority indicate that they have spiritual needs. More than half see themselves as spiritual.[87] Fay states that social justice, interfaith ecumenism, Native people, and Canadian women are meaningful dynamics in today's Roman Catholic Church.[88] He goes on to say that in order to enrich the Catholic community, women, the marginalized, and Native people, given an opportunity, will help to energize, universalize, and organize the church in the 21st century.[89]

Finally, Stackhouse indicates that the significant confluence of Canadian evangelicalism occurred as Canadian culture steadily became less influenced by traditional Christianity.[90] Recently, a number of religious organizations have turned to computer technology to disseminate their message. In fact, 5% of the national television audience tunes in to religious television.[91] The current popularity of media ministries and the high levels of recent immigration will together result in a diversification of the religious profile of Canadian societies in the years to come.[92]

The growing presence of diverse religions constitutes a shift in political, social, and cultural life in Canada. Choquette claims that Canada's new immigrants have not only given the country a more religious outlook but have contributed to the development of a society much more open to change and difference.[93]

HEALTH CARE AND NURSING APPLICATIONS

You can use the foregoing concepts—basic beliefs, dietary laws, ideas of illness and health, body, spirit, mysticism, pragmatism, pain, death, and family ties—as a *beginning*. Even more basic than understanding these concepts is respecting your client as a person with spiritual needs who has a right to have these needs met, whether or not he or she has formal religious beliefs. You are not expected to be a professional spiritual leader, for which lengthy training and experience would be required. You can, however, assist clients in their journey. *You are the transition, the key person between the client and spiritual help.*

There are several books available for nurses that detail spiritual care giving, including *Spiritual Care Nursing: Theory, Research and Practice*[94] and *Spiritual Care in Nursing Practice*.[95] Both books explore the meaning of spirituality and the world of spiritual care. Each book can be used to assist the nurse in applying the concepts of spirituality to clients and their families. The *Journal of Christian Nursing* is a helpful resource. In particular, the Summer 1999 issue is totally devoted to the connection between faith and health.

CONTROVERSY DEBATE

You are a registered nurse who has worked on a palliative care unit for five years. Joan, who recently graduated as a registered nurse, has been partnered with you by the nurse unit manager (NUM). As a result of a brief meeting with the NUM, you and Joan have agreed to work each shift together first, for orientation purposes, and secondly, so you can assess Joan's work performance and provide feedback information to both Joan and the NUM. You like Joan, and it appears that the two of you might become friends. However, one evening Joan informs you that her feelings were hurt a few months ago by certain members of her church. Joan shares with you how she has come to believe that institutionalized forms of worship do not promote spiritual growth, and that actually she doesn't really see spirituality as an identifiable entity. She states that she avoids making referrals to chaplains and clergy for her dying patients. She says she firmly believes she is acting in the clients' best interest when she bypasses chaplains and clergy. She asks you not to share her beliefs and actions on spirituality with anyone on the unit because she thinks that most of the professionals on the unit might be "overly involved with religion." You have a deep conviction to your own faith and you consider yourself a spiritual person. Tomorrow is your first meeting with the NUM to review Joan's work performance.

1. What will you do with the information that Joan has shared with you regarding her views on religion and spirituality?
2. What will you say to the NUM regarding Joan's performance and convictions?
3. What do you consider to be the best way for you to approach Joan on the matter? What other realistic alternatives exist for you?

Assessment

Although you can learn much from selecting points in the case study found in this chapter, you can also refer to Table 3-2 (see pages 115–118), and to the questions posed in Table 3-3 and Table 3-4. However, each of these is only a basis to begin your quest to provide holistic care to clients and their families.

CRITICAL THINKING

What single concept derived from this chapter so far stands out for you as most meaningful as you think about providing spiritual care to your clients and their family members?

TABLE 3-3
Questions for Spiritual Assessment

1. What is your concept of God? What is your God like? (Or, what is your religion? Tell me about it.)
2. Do you believe that God or someone is concerned for you?
3. Who is the most important person to you? Is that person available?
4. Has being sick (what has been happening to you) made any difference in your feelings about God? In the practice of your faith? If it has, could you explain how it has changed?
5. Do you believe that your faith is helpful to you? If it is, how? If it is not, why not?
6. Are there any religious beliefs, practices, of rituals that are important to you now? If there are, could you tell me about them? May I help you carry them out by showing you where the chapel is? By telling the dietary department about your vegetarian preference? By allowing you specific times for prayer or meditation?
7. Is there anything that would make your situation easier? (Such as a visit from the minister, priest, rabbi, or chaplain? Someone who would read to you? Time for reading your religious book or praying? Someone to pray with you?)
8. Is prayer important to you? (If so, has being sick made a difference in your practice of praying?) What happens when you pray?
9. Do you have available religious books or articles such as the Bible, prayer books, phylacteries, or a crucifix that mean something to you?
10. What are your ideas about illness? About life after death?
11. Is there anything especially frightening or meaningful to you right now?
12. If these questions have not uncovered your source of spiritual support, can you tell me where you do find support?

Robert Coles[96] recounted anecdotes from Hopi, Christian, Muslim, Jewish, agnostic, and atheist children. His conclusion was that they all have an immediacy of spiritual issues in their lives. An adolescent or young adult caught up in sorting out various facets of learned idealism and trying to fit them into more realistic daily patterns may temporarily discard religious teaching. He or she may reject the guidance of a spiritual leader because that person is associated with the parents' beliefs; yet the adolescent is nevertheless searching and needs guidance. An elderly person suffering the grief of a recently lost mate may repeatedly question how a God of love could allow this loss. Some physiologically mature people are not religiously mature; they may expect magic from God. The spiritually maturing individual experiences the fruits of faith in God in behavioural terms of love, trust, and security. The external spiritual stimuli of God's word, sacraments, and relationships with other believers create an inner peace and love through which the person experiences God within and then

TABLE 3-4
Religious and Spiritual Assessment Questionnaire

1. Are religious or spiritual issues important in your life?
   - ☐ Yes
   - ☐ Somewhat
   - ☐ No

2. Do you believe in God or a Supreme Being?
   - ☐ Yes
   - ☐ No

3. Do you believe you can experience spiritual guidance?
   - ☐ Yes
   - ☐ No

   If so, how often have you had such experiences?
   - ☐ Often
   - ☐ Occasionally
   - ☐ Rarely
   - ☐ Never

   Are you committed to it and actively involved?
   - ☐ Yes
   - ☐ Somewhat
   - ☐ No

4. How important was religion or spiritual belief to you as a child and adolescent?
   - ☐ Important
   - ☐ Somewhat Important
   - ☐ Unimportant

5. Are you aware of any religious or spiritual resources in your life that could be used to help you overcome your problems?
   - ☐ Yes
   - ☐ No

   If "yes," what are they?

   _____
   _____
   _____
   _____
   _____
   _____

6. Do you believe that religious or spiritual influences have hurt you or contributed to some of your problems?
   - ☐ Yes
   - ☐ No

   If "yes," briefly explain how.

   _____
   _____
   _____
   _____
   _____

This questionnaire contributed by Sylvia Adams, MSN, RNC, and Pamela Talley, MSN, RN, CS, CSAC.

reaches out to others in supporting relationships. Yet, most elders, at a time when they are attending fewer organized religious functions, seem to have greater inner spiritual strength.

Furthermore, realize that people can use the same religious terms differently; *saved, sanctified, fell out, slain by the spirit,* and *deathbed conversion* all connote religious experiences. You should listen carefully, and you may have to ask questions to determine accurately the individual person's meaning.

Spiritual beliefs and beliefs about purpose in life and life after death are important dimensions of high-level wellness. Beliefs are related to feelings about self-worth, goals, interactions with others, philosophy of life, interpretations of birth, life events, and death. The value and meaning of life are not judged by its length but by the purpose for which the person lives, the principles by which he or she lives, the reflection about a being greater than the self, and the love and joy obtained from relationships with others. All of these factors may directly affect health status.

Assessment for spiritual needs of any client, not just the terminally ill or dying, should be part of the nursing history. **Spiritual need** is defined as *lack of any factor necessary to establish or maintain a dynamic, personal relationship with God, or a higher being, as defined by the individual.* Four areas of concern can be covered later in the interview as part of assessment after the client feels safe with the nurse in the therapeutic relationship. The following are the assessment areas:

- Person's concept of God or deity
- Person's source of strength and hope
- Significance of religious practices and rituals
- Perceived relationship between spiritual beliefs and current state of health

During this part of the assessment, be prepared for any answer. The agnostic or atheist may answer with as much depth and meaning from his or her perspective as someone with a specific religious background. The person who is part of a formal religion may not answer freely, reserving such conversation for the spiritual leader or hesitating until the nurse is better known to the client.

When determining medical background, such as drug or food allergies, you could also ask about religious dietary laws, special rituals, or restrictions that might be an important part of the client's history. Recording and helping the client follow beliefs could speed recovery.

Perhaps *you could share with the chaplain the responsibility for asking questions related to spirituality as you give client care.* No specific set of questions will be right for every client, but the questions in Table 3-3 or Table 3-4 might draw helpful responses as you assess and diagnose in the spiritual realm.

Be sure to look for the person's strengths, not weaknesses. Remember that you must not preach or reconstruct. Allow the client to assume his or her own spiritual stance.

Because your relationship with the person may be of short duration, be sure to document well the results of this interview. Later, when you or others care for the client, you should watch for religious needs that may be expressed through nonreligious language. You must again let the client know what options are open for spiritual help. If you hide behind hectic activities and procedures, you may lose a valuable opportunity to aid in health restoration.

You can now relate your understanding of social class and cultural differences obtained from Chapter 1 to comprehend more fully the religious and cultural differences related in this chapter. Review both chapters and take time to reflect on how you can apply the various concepts and belief systems presented regarding the different groups in regions throughout Canada.

3-4 BONUS SECTION IN CD-ROM

Assessment and Intervention with the African-American Client

This table presents a concise and comprehensive list of 23 professionally oriented suggestions for health care professionals to follow when interacting with an African-American client.

Religion influences behaviour and attitudes toward:

- Work: whether you work to expiate sin, because it is there to do, or because of a conviction that it is a God-given right and responsibility
- Money: whether you save money to deny yourself something, buy on an instalment plan, buy health insurance, consider money the root of all evil, or believe that it should be used for the betterment and development of persons and society
- Political behaviour: ideas about the sanctity of the Constitution, effects of Communism, importance of world problems, spending abroad versus spending for national defence, school or residential desegregation, welfare aid, and union membership
- Family: kinds of interaction within the family, honouring of parents or spouse, children, or siblings
- Childrearing: interest in the child's present and future, attitudes toward punishment or rewards for behaviour, values of strict obedience as contrasted with independent thinking, or how many children should be born
- Right and wrong: what is sin, how wrong is gambling, drinking, birth control, divorce, smoking, and abortion

Consider how essentially the same situation can be diversely interpreted by two teenagers of different faiths. One, a Fundamentalist Protestant, may spend an evening dancing and suffer crushing guilt because she participated in supposed sinful acts. The other, a Jewish teenager, may participate in the same activity and consider it a religiously based function. Your knowledge of and sensitivity to such differences are important, for essentially similar kinds of decisions—right and wrong as religiously defined—will be made about autopsy, cremation, and organ transplants. Furthermore, although religious bodies may hand down statements on these issues, often the individual person alters the group's stand while incorporating individual circumstances into the decision.

Ideally, religion provides strength, an inner calm and faith with which to work through life's problems. But you must be prepared to see the negative aspect. To some, religion seems to add guilt, depression, and confusion. Some may blame God for making them ill, for letting them suffer, or for not healing them in a prescribed manner. One Protestant believed she had made a contract with God: if she lived the best Christian life she could, God would keep her relatively well and free from tragedy. When an incurable disease was diagnosed, she said, "What did I do to deserve this?" Another Protestant, during her illness, took the opposite view of her contract with God. She said, "I wasn't living as well as I should and God knocked me down to let me know I was backsliding."

Healing, too, has varied meanings. Some will demand that God provide a quick and miraculous recovery, whereas others will expect the process to occur through the work of the health team. Still others combine God's touch, the health providers' skill, and their own emotional and physical cooperation. Some even consider death as the final form of healing.

Sometimes you must deal with your own negative reactions. Your medical background and knowledge may cause you dismay at some religious practices. For instance, how will you react as you watch a postoperative Jehovah's Witness client die because she has refused blood? Basically they prefer to die. Should you dictate otherwise? You may need to think through and discuss such situations with a spiritual leader.

CRITICAL THINKING

What conflicts could arise in the health care delivery system because of different beliefs and values held by individuals?

Nursing Diagnosis

The spiritual needs of clients have become a part of the evolving nursing diagnosis system of classification under the value–belief category of the North American Nursing Diagnosis Association. **Spiritual distress,** *when the person experiences or could experience a disturbance in the belief system that is his or her source of strength,* is the main diagnostic category. This problem may be related to not being able to practise certain spiritual rituals; or it may be caused by a conflict between one's spiritual beliefs and the health regimen.[97] Another diagnostic category is "potential for enhanced spiritual well-being."[98] The strengths of clients and their families must be assessed in order to write wellness nursing diagnoses.[99] Stolte argues that the outcomes of health promotion should fulfill the goals of increased well-being and self-actualization. The careful assessment of the client's general lifestyle can provide a pattern of healthy behaviours that can become the client's strengths.[100]

Other issues may be present also. For example, clients may question their belief system, may be discouraged or despairing, may feel spiritually empty, or may be ambivalent, first asking for spiritual assistance, then rejecting it. On the other hand, the client may be at peace within and accept his or her diagnosis with calm. Clients may desire prayer from a nurse to help them thank God for their life.

As nurses become more attuned to these situations, perhaps meeting the client's spiritual needs will not be unattached from other care. At the same time, the spiritual dimensions must be thought of as something in addition to the psychosocial dimension. Specific measures must be taken for spiritual care—measures which are not necessarily included in psychosocial care. One study showed that nursing educators were using only psychosocial intervention for spiritual care.[101] Olson and her researchers conducted a study to identify the extent to which the spiritual dimension was addressed in Canadian university undergraduate nursing curricula. The results indicated that some educators view the spiritual dimension as part of the psychosocial dimension. These researchers concluded that it is time to seriously engage in dialogue about the spiritual dimension in nursing education because there appears to be conceptual confusion in the area.[102]

It is interesting to note the concept of spirituality addressed in other health care disciplines. For example, a study was conducted to examine the manner and extent to which Canadian occupational therapy education addressed the concept of spirituality. Results indicated that although Canadian occupational therapy programs address spirituality in their curricula, the importance focused on the concept is low.[103] Grabovac and Ganesan surveyed 16 psychiatry residency programs in Canada to determine to which psychiatry related religion and spirituality training is being made available. Their findings indicated that most Canadian programs offer minimal instruction on issues pertaining to religion, spirituality and psychiatry. These researchers propose a ten-session lecture series, with outlines, designed to introduce residents in psychiatry to religious and spiritual issues as they pertain to clinical practice.[104]

Intervention

The Canadian Holistic Nurses Association (CHNA), a recognized interest group of the Canadian Nurses Association (CNA), emphasizes the development of holistic nursing practice.[105] The main goal of CHNA is to further the development of holistic nursing practice to ensure that professional health maintenance and health promotion care are available to the people of Canada.[106] The objectives of the CHNA include the following: to promote CNA Nursing Practice Standards of provinces

---

NARRATIVE VIGNETTE

You are beginning your final year of studies as a student nurse in the Baccalaureate Nursing Degree Program. You have been asked to be a teaching assistant (TA) for the Introduction to Nursing Care course being taught at the first-year level of the program. While reviewing your TA responsibilities with you, the course leader asks you, as a senior student, to share with her your opinion on what you believe to be the more important aspects that first-year nursing students should realize about spirituality. Because the course leader knows that health care professionals conduct numerous teaching/learning experiences after graduation, she is also interested in learning what you believe, from a learner's point of view, to be effective approaches to take in teaching spirituality.

Reflect for a few minutes on what you believe to be important early in one's health care career regarding spirituality. Think about the teaching/learning methods used when you were taught spirituality.

1. What teaching/learning approaches would you prefer to have experienced regarding spirituality?

2. How will you respond to the course leader?

   a. What do you believe to be the more important aspects of spirituality for early-career health care professionals?

   b. What are the more effective approaches to use in teaching spirituality?

Spiritual Distress

Susan Santini is a 40-year-old, middle-class bank president. She lives in a small town with her husband and four children. She also deals in real estate, works with civic and Roman Catholic church groups, and is developing an advertising company. She seems constantly busy. She discusses business over lunch and competes with friends when playing golf or bridge.

One evening she started having severe chest pain. She was taken in an ambulance to a metropolitan hospital 120 kilometres away where a specialist successfully performed triple-bypass surgery.

For the first time in her life, Susan was stopped. She was away from family and friends and was confined. Good and bad memories flooded her mind. She began to evaluate her activities, her emphasis on material gain and competition, how her children were growing so fast, how her religious activities were superficial, and how, without skilled surgery, she might have died.

At first she tried being jovial with the staff to strike out these new and troubling thoughts. But she could not sleep well. She was dreaming about death in wild combinations with her past life. She began to mention these dreams, along with questions about how the surgery would affect her life span, diet, and activities. She mentioned a friend who seemed severely limited from a similar surgery. She also said she was worried about the problems her teenagers were beginning to face and about her own ability to guide them properly.

The staff members never forced Susan to express more than she wished but answered the questions and asked her if she would like to see the chaplain since her own priest was not available. Susan agreed. An appointed nurse then informed the chaplain of Susan's physical, emotional, and spiritual history to date. In the course of several sessions the chaplain helped Susan work through a revised philosophy of life that put more emphasis on spiritual values, family life, and healthy use of leisure.

QUESTIONS

1. If the chaplain was unable to come to Susan, because, let's say, he had suffered a heart attack, what could the nurse do to address Susan's spiritual needs?
2. What barriers might the nurse encounter when endeavouring to provide spiritual care to Susan and her family?
3. If you were Susan's nurse, to what sources of information could you turn to learn more about addressing spiritual needs?

and territories as applicable; to promote holistic nursing practice, education, research, and administration; and to adhere to the CNA Code of Ethics for Nurses.[107]

Spirituality is an integral part of *holistic health.* In a study that indicated spiritual perspectives, hope, acceptance, and self-transcendence showed connectedness and a positive outcome when viewed together.[108] There is a qualitative difference between giving spiritual care and supporting another person by sharing transcendent human qualities. Florence Nightingale described spiritual care as that which enables a person to be conscious of the presence of God, who is the creator and sustainer of the universe. Karns stated that nurses can only cooperate in spiritual care; they cannot give it. She explained that the highest form of spiritual care in the Christian tradition is to help the person be in a position to be conscious of God's touch and the presence of the Holy Spirit. To do that, the nurse must have had such an experience. *Thus, spiritual care will differ from person to person, for the Christian and non-Christian, for the believer and agnostic or atheist.*[109]

In nursing, a few scholars, such as Wright, describe the ethical, professional, and legal responsibilities for spiritual care,[110] and Meyeroff, Van Hofwegen, Hoe Harwood, and Drury present the development of spiritual nursing interventions to restore meaning in the lives of clients and their families.[111]

CRITICAL THINKING

What personal characteristics and qualities do you have that enable you to provide good spiritual care? (You might want to refer to Pesut[112] for some ideas.)

Several other authors write about how prayer and faith enable them to better implement the nursing process and give holistic care—physical, emotional, sociocultural, and spiritual. Some say that when they pray, the tasks go more smoothly. Others say that when they pray with patients, they benefit as much as do the patients.[113–115] Others describe the barriers to giving spiritual care.[116,117] Wallace[118] writes about one family's effort to incorporate a holistic approach to care. When staff learned about the patient as he had been, staff became more responsive. The patient's recovery for three years was viewed as a miracle by all. Wright in her clinical work with families claims that her goal and obligation is to alleviate or heal emotional, physical, or spiritual suffering.[119]

Role of Faith Communities in Intervention
Churches or faith communities contribute to health promotion. * *Churches have been a refuge for people of all faiths throughout the centuries, and they have been and still are a major centre for health promotion.*

Westberg[120] said, "The church is a healing community… engaged in keeping people well" (p. 189), which was accomplished by particular qualities found in a faith community that were not usually present in the modern scientific medical model of health services. The qualities were the power of group dynamics, inspirational experiences, and caring fellow humans. These qualities were further defined as:

1. Inspirational worship experiences that gave people faith and hope
2. Opportunities for individuals to be part of a greater community of like-minded people

*This section contributed by Frances Atkins, PhD, MS(N), RN, CS.

3. Continuing education in many areas
4. Singing with others
5. Retreat experiences for meditation and prayer
6. Summer camping for the whole family
7. Daycare centres for children and elders
8. Opportunities for volunteering time and money

Four qualitative case studies conducted in a community of 5000 people in four mainstream Christian denominations, which did not have a parish nurse, reported all the qualities identified by Westberg except the summer camping for the whole family and daycare centres for elders.[121] Outcomes from integrating the studies of the original four cases indicated that participants experienced spiritual, mental, emotional, and physical health as a result of their church attendance, faith and prayer, friendships and fellowship, moral and religious teachings, youth groups, and community service. Members saw the need and shared the responsibility for providing the healing community that was engaged in keeping people well.[122]

Faith communities have contributed to health promotion in two ways, by the generic nature of the faith community and by intentional, planned activities to address health issues in the faith community and in the larger community beyond the faith community.

Faith communities are excellent settings for health promotion.[123] In fact, faith communities are considered to be competent in the spiritual area, a fact which is often overlooked in secular health promotion programs. In Canada, greater attention is being given to different ways individuals and their families can take responsibility of their own well-being. Churches have begun to reclaim their heritage of providing for people's health-related needs—spiritual, physical, mental, social, emotional, and cultural.[124] For example, healthy child development is one determinant of health that can be focused on particularly well in a faith community.[125] These realizations cause one to wonder how the parish nurse relates to faith communities.

The concept of parish nursing began in Europe, arrived in the United States in the mid-1980s, and spread to Canada less than a decade later, as early as 1992.[126] A parish nurse, known sometimes as a faith community nurse, is a registered nurse who has specialized knowledge and is hired and acknowledged by a faith community to provide intentional health promotion ministry.[127] In fact, parish nursing is practised from a holistic framework that promotes the health of the whole person.[128] With specialized knowledge in health promotion, parish nurses capitalize on the strengths of individuals and their families. A parish nurse relates to faith communities as well as to the broader community when informing and connecting individuals and their families to resources that address the determinants of health.[129]

In order to practise safely and effectively in health ministry, the Canadian Association for Parish Nursing Ministry has developed Parish Nursing Core Competencies for Basic Parish Nurse Educational Programs along with five standards of practice for parish nursing ministry: facilitation of spiritual care, health promotion, collaboration, advocacy and professional accountability.[130,131]

CRITICAL THINKING

Compare the roles of a parish nurse in an urban community to those of a parish nurse in a rural community.

Guidelines for Intervention
Certain *norms for providing spiritual care* must be followed:

- Do not impose personal beliefs on clients or families. A sickbed or deathbed is not a proper time for proselytizing.
- Respond to the person out of his or her own background. Use knowledge about that background, but avoid acting on stereotypes (e.g., "all Catholics believe this" or "all Hindus do this").
- If you cannot give the spiritual support being asked for by the person, enlist someone who can.

Spiritual support can be given to the *ill and dying person* in various ways. Your warmth, empathy, and caring human relationship are essential. Respect for the person's beliefs, willingness to discuss spiritual matters, and providing for rituals and sacraments of religion are important. Be open to religious and philosophic beliefs other than your own. You may be uncomfortable discussing spiritual matters, yet for the client, you will try to overcome personal reluctance to discuss spiritual concerns. Often the intimacy of spiritual concerns is discussed by the client during the intimacy of physical care. Helping the person ask questions and seek solutions does not mean that you have to supply the answers.

With the *dying client,* the aspects of spiritual support considered most helpful are (1) calling the person directly by name, (2) talking directly to the person (realize everything may be heard by the dying person), and (3) supporting the family by staying with them as they say goodbye. Let family members know they can touch their dying loved one, offer your condolences, and offer to help them in any appropriate way.

Spiritual care of the *psychiatric patient* is often overlooked. Assessment must determine whether the person is describing a religious delusion, something most people would consider false, such as "I am Jesus Christ" or "I am Mohammed," or stating conflicts between religious beliefs and rituals and the current situation or feelings. Such statements may sound like and be labelled as delusions, but the *nursing diagnosis of spiritual distress* would be more appropriate. The spiritual components that you can address through listening and counselling are the person's sense of not being loved by others, of having no meaning or purpose in life, and of feeling unforgiven or not being able to forgive another. These issues take time to resolve; referral to clergy may be indicated.

Interventions for the person who makes delusional statements include the following:

- Understand that what sounds delusional to you and contrary to your religious beliefs may have been religious fact taught to the person. For example, some religions teach that mental illness is demonic possession.
- Convey acceptance of the need for the delusion while you state that you do not agree with it.

- Do *not* argue with the person's belief; state doubt about the belief if it is obviously unrealistic.
- Respond to the feelings or themes presented in the statements rather than to the exact words. For example, in response to "I am God," you may say, "I sense you are saying you want to be important."
- Avoid abstract discussion about religion or the delusional statements.
- Restate core beliefs that the person is conveying, such as, "You are special to God."

Be alert to subtle clues that indicate desire to talk about spiritual matters, need for expressions of love and hope, desire for your silent presence, and acceptance of behaviour when the client labels self as bad.

Communication between health care providers and pastoral care representatives is essential. You can fill that gap. Such rapport can mean that the *whole* person is served rather than segmented parts. Chaplains are especially helpful to clients and to nurses when they assist with the expression of anger, death, and grief. You and the chaplain, however, need to know what to expect from each other; there is no substitute for talking about these expectations and agreeing on strategies.

CRITICAL THINKING

What are some reasons for nurse–chaplain consultation?

Nine combinations of patient behaviour that call for conferring with, or referring to, a spiritual leader, unless contraindicated by the care plan, are:

1. Withdrawn, sullen, silent, depressed
2. Restless, irritable, complaining
3. Restless, excitable, garrulous, wants to talk a lot
4. Shows, by word or other signs, undue curiosity, anxiety about self
5. Takes turn to worse, critical, terminal
6. Shows conversational interest, curiosity in religious questions, issues; reads scripture
7. Specifically inquires about chaplain, chapel worship, scripture
8. Has few or no visitors; has no cards, flowers
9. Has had, or faces, particularly traumatic or threatening surgical procedure

With all these aspects to consider, a *team approach* that includes the client, family, health care providers, and chaplain or other spiritual leader is imperative. Assist in preparing the client for chapel service or seeing that the Sabbath ritual is carried out. Work with the team to provide the important factors, be they rituals, diet, quiet, group work, various articles, or family relationships.

Validate the appropriateness of proposed interventions with the client; for example, ask if the person wishes you to pray with him or her about the concerns that have been voiced. The person can then accept or reject your offer.

Consider the milieu. If a client is confined to a room, you can prepare a worship centre or shrine by arranging flowers, prayer book, relics, or whatever other objects have spiritual meaning.

You should *keep one or more calendars of various religious holidays.* The Eastern Orthodox Easter usually does not coincide with the Roman Catholic and Protestant Easter. Jewish holidays usually do not fall on the same dates of the Western calendar in successive years. Remember, also, that holidays are family days and that ill people separated from the family at such times may be especially depressed.

Maintain a list of available spiritual leaders, know when to call them, and know how to prepare for their arrival. If a client cannot make the request, consult with the family. One woman said, "If my sister sees a priest, she will be sure she is dying." Once a health care provider took the initiative to call an Eastern Orthodox priest who, unfortunately, represented the wrong nationality; the client's main source of comfort was to have come from discussion and prayers in the native language.

As you *prepare the client and the setting for a spiritual leader,* help *create an atmosphere* that reflects more than sterile procedure. Privacy has previously been emphasized by drawing curtains and shutting doors. Although acceptable to some, this approach may produce a negative response in others. Perhaps more emphasis should be given to cheerful surroundings: sunshine, flowers, lighted candles, openness, and participation by family and staff in at least an introductory way. Perhaps the client and spiritual leader could meet outdoors in an adjoining garden. The Shintoist and Taoist would especially benefit from the aesthetic exposure. If the client is a child on a prolonged hospitalization, a special area might be designated for religious instruction.

Brief the spiritual leader on any points that might provide special insight and be sure that the client is ready to receive him or her. Prepare any special arrangements, such as having a clean, cloth-covered tray for Communion. Guard against interruption by health care providers from other departments who may be unaware of the visit. Finally, incorporate the results of the visit into the client's record.

CRITICAL THINKING

What experience have you had with spiritual care leaders?

Many will benefit from the sacraments, the prayers, scripture reading, and counselling given by the spiritual leader, but others will want to rely on their own direct communication with God. The Zen Buddhist, Hindu, Muslim, and Friend (Quaker) might be in the latter category. All may want reading material, however. Most will bring their sacred book with them, but if they express a desire for more literature, offer to get it. Some hospitals furnish daily and weekly meditations and a Bible.

Occasionally it may be helpful to give scripture references for various stated spiritual needs. For example, reference to love and relatedness can be found in Psalm 23; reference to forgiveness in Matthew 6:9–15; reference to meaning and purpose in Acts 1:8.

If you feel comfortable doing so, you can at times say a prayer, read a scripture, or provide a statement of faith helpful to the client. If not comfortable in providing this kind of spiritual care, you can still meet the client's spiritual needs through respectful conversation, listening to the client talk about beliefs, referral to another staff member, or calling one of the client's friends who can bolster his or her faith. If spiritual leaders are not available, you could organize a group of health workers willing to counsel with or make referrals for clients of their own faiths.

Shared prayer, if it is accepted by the client, counteracts the loneliness of illness or dying by offering the person intimacy with a Supreme Being and another person without the need for confession. It can be a means of bringing both human and divine love. It holds transcendent qualities and conveys both present and future hope. Prayer can focus on the conditions or emotions that the client is unable to talk about, allowing the person to handle the matter or vent in another way. Prayer should promote closeness, through closed eyes and hands that touch. Prayer should not strip the person of defences. Nor should prayers be recited as a way to avoid the person or avoid questions raised by the person.

Use of life review can foster developmental, emotional, and spiritual maturity (not only in the elder and dying person). Encourage the person to reminisce about past life experiences. Memories can be pleasurable or painful, but recalling them with a skilled listener can help resolve those ridden with shame, guilt, anger, or other feelings. Past sources of strength can also be identified, and sometimes they are useful in the present situation. (Refer to Chapter 14.) Music can also be used to lift depression, convey calm, stimulate hope and joy, and promote physical and mental healing.

Counselling and mental and spiritual methods can be combined to help the client heal hurtful or traumatic memories, forgive self or others, work through unresolved grief, promote healing within self, and establish healthier relationships with others. You may refer to spiritual leaders or a counsellor to assist you with these aspects. Do not overlook needs not overtly expressed.

Atheists should not be neglected because they do not profess a belief in God. They have the same need for respect as everyone else and may need you to listen to fears and doubts. Moreover, just as health teaching is often omitted for health care providers who are clients, so is spiritual guidance often omitted for spiritual leaders who are clients. You must recognize that each person, regardless of religious stand or leadership capacity, may need spiritual help.

Various groups refuse medical or hospital treatment for illness, including members of Fundamentalist or Holiness groups, Jehovah's Witnesses, Amish, and Christian Scientists. Realize that if adults refuse treatment for themselves or their children, they are not deliberately choosing death. They are rejecting something objectionable, based on their beliefs. Nurses may teach nutritional therapy or various stress-management or relaxation techniques. Sometimes parents accept the services of a home health nurse, even though they refuse hospital and formal medical treatment.

Although a hospital setting has been used as a point of reference throughout this chapter, you can improvise in your setting—nursing home, hospice, school, industry, clinic, home, or other health centre—to provide adequate spiritual assistance.

You may give spiritual care via the Internet, as described by one rabbi.[132] But most people may prefer a more personal contact. One author, however, describes studies that revealed that the more time persons spent at their computer keyboards, the more depressed, socially isolated, and lonely they became. The chat room and Internet acquaintances do not consistently take the place of direct contact with living people.[133]

Table 3-2 (see pages 115–118) summarizes interventions for many of the religions discussed in this chapter.

Research in Spiritual Care

More research on spirituality and health is being done. However, how to assess and intervene and exactly what constitutes spiritual care needs further research. Yet, there are obstacles to carrying out a scientific study that is theologically sound (i.e., in keeping with the beliefs and needs of the person). Further, there is no effective way to determine if an intervention, such as prayer, is equally effective regardless of who is saying the prayer or the situation in which prayer is said.

The article by O'Mathuna[134] discusses the importance of and problems with research on prayer and healing. Hudson[135] writes of the observed results of a hospital chaplain working with patients. The patient's sense of hope, renewed motivation to live, and unexpected recovery are all outcomes that are real. Atkins[136] discusses how progress has occurred in refining research and presents findings of a multi-case study research design.

Research with Nurses
In a research study, "Spiritual Care Interventions by Psychiatric Nurses" (using 300 professional, registered, hospital-based psychiatric nurses in Missouri), the most commonly recalled interventions were psychosocial rather than spiritual.* Therapeutic communication or use of self ranked first; being cheerful and kind and use of touch were the most common interventions after that. The respondents were least comfortable doing specific spiritual care interventions such as praying with the patient or family, discussing God, and reading scripture to the patient. Although use of spiritual interventions was low, the nurses' attitudes toward doing them were positive. If obstacles, such as lack of time, unfavourable institutional policy, and lack of basic and in-service nursing education about spiritual care, were removed, the nurses reported they would provide spiritual care. The majority of the nurses believed spiritual care was the responsibility of every nurse and the right of every patient, and that it provides holistic care. The core problem underlying these findings was that the majority of nurses in the study did not see the spiritual dimension as separate and distinct from the physical and psychosocial

---

*Sections on Research with Nurses and Evaluation were contributed by Elaine Cox, RN, MSN (R).

dimensions and this was reflected in their behaviours.[137] The findings by Cox with psychiatric nurses were similar to the findings in a study with oncology nurses.[138]

CRITICAL THINKING

What nursing research findings could you include when caring for your clients and their families?

Evaluation

Exactly what aspects of spiritual care can be evaluated are difficult to determine. Evaluation of spiritual care interventions can best be analyzed by using both objective and subjective criteria, with spiritual well-being as the major criterion. The following questions with positive answers indicate a direction toward that criterion. Does this intervention: (1) bring peace or unity;[139] (2) provide a source of help, comfort, relief, or strength;[140] (3) promote transcendent values such as meaning, purpose, love, relatedness, and forgiveness of self, God, and others;[141] (4) decrease or alleviate symptoms, such as anxiety, withdrawal, helplessness, agitation, crying, hostility, guilt, shame, depression, and nonforgiveness;[142] (5) bring integration to the personality;[143] (6) help the person to cope and solve problems;[144] and (7) promote hardiness, hope, and intrinsic spiritual values?[145] The above would provide evidence of spiritual well-being. These questions can be measured on a continuum of 1 to 10, answered by both nurse and patient. Objective measures alone are inadequate, as the patient must realize the positive value of the outcome for continuing reinforcement and success.

EVIDENCE-BASED PRACTICE

Health within Illness: Experiences of Chronically Ill/Disabled People

The concept of health within illness is beginning to gain recognition in nursing. Although there has been little research to explore and describe this phenomenon, a recent study investigated the meaning of the experience of feeling healthy for people living with a chronic illness and/or disability. The results of that study provide the basis for this box.

An interpretive phenomenological study was undertaken with eight participants living with a variety of different chronic conditions. The results provide a rich mosaic of themes describing the participants' health experiences. These themes include (1) honouring the self; (2) seeking and connecting with others; (3) creating opportunities; (4) celebrating life; (5) transcending the self; and (6) acquiring a state of grace. The significance of these results is that they provide for a reconceptualization of health and illness. Such a reconceptualization calls for a transformation in nursing practice from a problem focus and deficit perspective, to one that focuses on the client's capacity and the promotion of health and healing.

Discussion

The results of this study are "phenomenologically informative" in that they provide guidance for understanding and promoting the health experience for people with chronic conditions. These research findings have been presented in workshops to people with chronic illnesses/disabilities, and the majority of these workshop participants say that they recognize many similarities between the study participants' experiences and their own. The author of the report, Dr. Elizabeth Lindsey, states however that some caution should be introduced here. This study, she asserts, is only one representation of health within illness. No claim should be made that all ill people with chronic conditions have similar experiences. Dr. Lindsey goes on to say that if the researcher asks about the illness experience, he or she will probably explore with the participants their experience of the illness. In contrast, if the researcher asks about the experiences of health within illness, the results are necessarily very different.

Practice Implications

1. If nurses in clinical practice focus their questions and their care on problem identification and illness experience, they are likely to be aware of only dimensions of the client's experience.

2. Nurse educators and practitioners need to become sensitized to the phenomenon of health within illness. Medicine and nursing have traditionally focused on problem identification and on the alleviation of symptoms and of cure. Health professionals should abandon this problem orientation and adopt an approach that focuses on people's capacities.

3. Nurse educators must relinquish their emphasis on teaching students to investigate client problems and needs and to consider other forms of client management that provide opportunities for the promotion of health and well-being. Such a shift is not merely a shift in orientation, but a fundamental transformation in philosophical perspective.

4. As nurses adopt a caring and health-promoting stance, they expand their own potential for promoting health and healing. This potential could be experienced on a personal and professional level. Not only will clients be provided the opportunity to expand their health potential, but the nurse might also experience the power of this caring and health-promoting potential. Such a transformation will help facilitate the health and healing capacities for both nurses and clients.

Source: Lindsey, E., Health within Illness: Experiences of Chronically Ill/Disabled People, Journal of Advanced Nursing, 24 (1996), 465–472. Used with the permission of Blackwell Science Ltd.

Outcomes that we must strive for are those that (1) enhance trust, (2) allow people to carry on spiritual practices not detrimental to health, (3) decrease feelings of anxiety and guilt, and (4) cause satisfaction with their spiritual condition. To ensure these responses, spiritual care should be considered part of quality assurance. Sister Rosemary Donley suggests that this incorporation—with the addition of more mystery and more grace—will help foster support for poor, minority, and very rich people, that is, those who are sometimes blamed for their illnesses.[146]

INTERESTING WEBSITES

CANADIAN RELIGIONS

http://www.forces.gc.ca/hr/religions/engraph/religions_toc_e.asp

From Baha'i and Buddhism through Christianity in Canada to Judaism, Sikhism, and Alternative Spirituality, this site provides information, book lists and insights into Canada's religions.

STATISTICS CANADA'S OVERVIEW OF RELIGION

http://www12.statcan.ca/english/census01/Products/Analytic/companion/rel/canada.cfm

Head to this site for extensive information on religion from Statistics Canada using census data.

RELIGIONS OF NEWFOUNDLAND AND LABRADOR

http://www.ucs.mun.ca/~hrollman/

Religion, society, and culture in Newfoundland and Labrador as presented by Dr. Hans Rollmann, Department of Religious Studies, Memorial University of Newfoundland, provides information in depth on the religions of Newfoundland and Labrador.

SUMMARY

1. Spirituality and the spiritual dimensions are inherent in all people, regardless of the presence of beliefs.
2. You will care for clients who adhere to beliefs different from your own.
3. The major world religions are Hinduism, Sikhism, Buddhism, Jainism, Shintoism, Confucianism, Taoism, Islam, Judaism, and Christianity.
4. Wide religious diversity exists in Canada today.
5. Some religious groups of interest are Seventh-Day Adventists; Church of Jesus Christ of Latter-Day Saints (Mormon); Jehovah's Witnesses; Church of Christ, Scientist (Christian Scientist); Mennonites; and Amish.
6. Alternative religions are divided into two components—religious movements and new religions.
7. You can practise in every health care setting principles of spiritual care based on concepts presented in this chapter.
8. Faith communities are ideal to promote health in individuals and their families.

9. You can now engage in life-long learning about your own and others' beliefs to enable you to assess, plan, and provide holistic care to clients and their families.

ENDNOTES

1. Macrae, J., Nightingale's Spiritual Philosophy and Its Significance for Modern Nursing, *IMAGE, Journal of Nursing Scholarship,* 27, no. 1 (1995), 8–14.
2. *Ibid.*
3. Begley, S., Science Finds God, *Newsweek,* July 20, 1998, 46–51.
4. Making a Place for Spirituality, *Harvard Health Letter,* 23, no. 4 (1998), 1–3.
5. Rubin, M., The Healing Power of Prayer, *Journal of Christian Nursing,* 16, no. 3 (1999), 4–7.
6. Study Finds Link Between Religion and Healthy Stable Immune Systems, *St. Louis Post-Dispatch,* October 3, 1997, A1.
7. Toth, J., Faith in Recovery: Spiritual Support After an Acute MI. *Journal of Christian Nursing,* 9, no. 4 (1992), 29–30.
8. Pangman, V.C. Canadian Perspectives: A Canadian Context of Spirituality. In Perri J. Bomar, ed. *Promoting Health in Families: Applying Family Research and Theory in Nursing Practice* (3rd ed., pp. 208–209). Philadelphia: Saunders Publishing, 2004.
9. Making a Place for Spirituality.
10. Can Religion Be Good Medicine? *The Johns Hopkins Medical Letter,* 10, no. 9 (1998), 3.
11. Koenig, H., How Does Religious Faith Contribute to Recovery from Depression, *The Harvard Mental Health Letter,* 15, no. 8 (1999), 8.
12. Chilton, B., Recognizing Spirituality, *IMAGE: Journal of Nursing Scholarship,* 30, no. 4 (1998), 400–401.
13. O'Neill, D., and E. Kenny, Spirituality and Chronic Illness, *IMAGE: Journal of Nursing Scholarship,* 30, no. 3 (1998), 275–280.
14. Hering, M., Believe Well, Live Well, *Focus on The Family,* September (1994), 1–4.
15. Lindsey, Elizabeth, Health within illness: Experiences of chronically ill/disabled people, *Journal of Advanced Nursing,* 24 (1996), 465–472.
16. *Ibid.*
17. Baetz, M., D.B. Larson, G. Marcoux, R. Bowen, and R. Griffin, Canadian Psychiatric Inpatient Religious Commitment: An Association with Mental Health, *Canadian Journal of Psychiatry,* 47, no. 2 (2002), 159–166.
18. Anderson, B., and A. Steen, Spiritual Care, Reflecting God's Love to Children, *Journal of Christian Nursing,* 12, no. 1 (1995), 12–17.
19. Easton, K., and J. Andrews, Nursing the Soul: A Team Approach, *Journal of Christian Nursing,* 16, no. 3 (1999), 26–29.
20. Plante, P., Formula for a Miracle, *Journal of Christian Nursing,* 16, no. 3 (1999), 34–35.
21. Rubin, *op. cit.*
22. Wallace, J., Jr., and T. Forman, Religion's Role in Promoting Health and Reducing Risk Among American Youth, *Health Education and Behavior,* 25 (1998), 721–741.
23. Johnston Taylor, E., Prayers, Clinical Issues and Implications, *Holistic Nursing Practice,* 17, no. 4 (2003), 179–188.
24. Cavendish, R., B. Kraynyak, L. Konecny, and M. Lanza, Nurses Enhance Performance Through Prayer, *Holistic Nursing Practice,* 18, no. 1 (2004) 26–31.
25. Chilton, *op. cit.*
26. Bopp, J., M. Bopp, L. Brown, and P. Lane, Jr., *The Sacred Tree.* Lethbridge: Four Worlds International Institute for Human and Community Development, 1984.
27. *Ibid.*
28. Mullin, J., L. Lee, S. Hertwig, G. Silverthorn, Final Journey: A Native Smudging Ceremony, *Canadian Nurse,* 97, no. 9 (2001), 20–22.

29. Compton, B.R., and B. Galaway. *Social Work Processes.* Pacific Grove, CA: Brooks/Cole, 1994.

30. Karns, P.S., Building a Foundation for Spiritual Care, *Journal of Christian Nursing,* 6, no. 5 (1991), 11–13.

31. Braswell, G.J., *Understanding World Religion* (rev. ed.). Nashville, TN: Broadman & Holman, 1994.

32. Statistics Canada, *2001 Census: Analysis Series, Religions in Canada,* Website: http://www.12.statcan.ca/English/census01/Products/Analytic/companion/rel/pdf/96F0030XIE2001015.pdf, July 2004.

33. Rice, E., *Eastern Definitions.* Garden City, NY: Doubleday & Company, 1978.

34. Braswell, *op. cit.*

35. Salladay, S.A., World Views Apart: Nursing Practice and New Age Therapies, *Journal of Christian Nursing,* 6, no. 4 (1991), 15–18.

36. Eck. D., *Roots in Who Are They?* Los Angeles: Bhaktivedanta Book Trust, 1982.

37. Interview: Desai, A.D., Boulder, Colorado, Nov. 26, 1998.

38. Interview: Desai, B., Boulder, Colorado, May 5, 1997.

39. Interview: Desai, D. and A., Wedding at Boulder, Colorado, May 17, 1997.

40. Kushner, H., *When Bad Things Happen to Good People,* New York: Schocken Books, 1989.

41. *Ibid.*

42. *Ibid.*

43. Bibby, R.W., *Restless Gods: The Renaissance of Religion in Canada.* Toronto: Stoddart, 2002.

44. Weber, G., A Radical Religious Crusade, *St. Louis Post-Dispatch,* February 22 (1995).

45. Braswell, *op. cit.*

46. Andrews, M.M., and P.A. Hanson., Religion, Culture, and Nursing, in M.M. Andrews and J.S. Boyle, eds., *Transcultural Concepts in Nursing Care* (4th ed, pp. 432–469). Philadelphia, Lippincott, 2003.

47. Choquette, *op. cit.*

48. *Ibid.*

49. Muramoto, O., Jehovah's Witnesses and artificial blood. *Canadian Medical Association Journal,* 164, no. 7 (2001), 969.

50. Andrews and Hanson, *op. cit.*

51. *Ibid.*

52. *Ibid.*

53. *Ibid.*

54. Kulig, J.C., and C. McCaslin, Health care for the Mexican Mennonites in Canada, *Canadian Nurse,* 94, no. 6 (1998), 34–39.

55. Wenger, A.F., and M.R. Wenger. The Amish, in L.D. Purnell and B.J. Paulanka, eds., *Transcultural Health Care: A Culturally Competent Approach* (2nd ed., pp. 54–67). Philadelphia, F.A. Davis Company, 2003.

56. Choquette, *op. cit.*

57. *Ibid.*

58. *Ibid.*

59. Andrews and Hanson, *op. cit.*

60. *Ibid.*

61. Choquette, *op. cit.*

62. *Ibid.*

63. Bibby, Reginald W. *Fragmented Gods: The Poverty and Potential of Religion in Canada.*

64. Choquette, *op. cit.*

65. *Ibid.*

66. Choquette, *op. cit.*

67. Ontario Consultants on Religious Tolerance, *New Age Spirituality,* Website: http://www.religioustolerence.org/newage.htm, July 2004.

68. Choquette, *op. cit.*

69. *Ibid.*

70. *Ibid.*

71. Wright, K., Professional, Ethical, and Legal Implications for Spiritual Care in Nursing, *IMAGE: Journal of Nursing Scholarship,* 30, no. 1 (1998), 81–83.

72. Stafford, T., The Hidden Gospel of the 12 Steps, *Christianity Today,* 35, no. 8 (1991), 14–19.

73. Statistics Canada, 2001 Census: Analysis Series, Religions in Canada, 2003.

74. *Ibid.*

75. *Ibid.*

76. Choquette, R., *Canada's Religions.* Ottawa: University of Ottawa Press, 2004.

77. Bibby, R.W., *Fragmented Gods: The Poverty and Potential of Religion in Canada.* Toronto: Stoddart, 1987.

78. Bibby, R.W., *Unknown Gods: The Ongoing Story of Religions in Canada.* Toronto: Stoddart, 1993.

79. Bibby, R.W., *Restless Gods: The Renaissance of Religion in Canada.*

80. Fay, Terence J., *A History of Canadian Catholics.* Montreal: McGill-Queen's University Press, 2002.

81. Stackhouse, J.G., Jr., *Canadian Evangelicalism in the Twentieth Century: An Introduction to its Character.* Toronto: University of Toronto Press, 1993.

82. Choquette, *op. cit.*

83. *Ibid.*

84. Bibby, *Fragmented Gods: The Poverty and Potential of Religion in Canada.*

85. Bibby, *Unknown Gods: The Ongoing Story of Religions in Canada.*

86. Bibby, *Restless Gods: The Renaissance of Religion in Canada.*

87. *Ibid.*

88. Fay, *op. cit.*

89. *Ibid.*

90. Stackhouse, *op. cit.*

91. Macionis, J.J., and L.M. Gerber, *Sociology* (4th ed.). Toronto: Pearson Education Canada, 2002.

92. *Ibid.*

93. Choquette, *op. cit.*

94. Taylor, E.J., *Spiritual Care: Nursing Theory, Research, and Practice,* Upper Saddle River, NJ: Prentice Hall, 2002.

95. Mauk, K.L., and N.K. Schmidt. *Spiritual Care in Nursing Practice.* Philadelphia: Lippincott Williams & Wilkins, 2004.

96. Coles, R., *The Spiritual Life of Children.* Boston: Houghton Mifflin, 1991.

97. Piles, C., Providing Spiritual Care, *Nurse Educator,* 15, no. 1 (1990), 36–41.

98. Chilton, *op. cit.*

99. Stolte, K.M. *Wellness: Nursing Diagnosis for Health Promotion.* Philadelphia: J. B. Lippincott Co., 1996.

100. *Ibid.*

101. Piles, *op. cit.*

102. Olson, J.K., P. Paul, L. Douglass, M.B. Clark, J. Simington, and N. Goddard, Addressing the Spiritual Dimension in Canadian Undergraduate Nursing Education. *Canadian Journal of Nursing Research,* 35, no. 3 (2003), 94–107.

103. Kirsh, B.D., S. Antolikova, and L. Reynolds, Developing Awareness of Spirituality in Occupational Therapy Students: Are Our Curricula Up to the Task? *Occupational Therapy International,* 8, no. 2 (2001), 119–125.

104. Grabovac, A., and S. Ganesan, Spirituality and Religion in Canadian Psychiatric Residency Training. *Canadian Journal of Psychiatry,* 48, no. 3 (2003), 171–175.

105. Petersen, B., The Mind–Body Connection. *The Canadian Nurse,* 92, no. 1 (1996), 29–31.

106. Canadian Holistic Nurses Association, *Philosophy and Objectives,* Website: http://mypage.direct.ca/h/hutchings/chna.html, July 2004.

107. *Ibid.*

108. Haase, J, T. Britt, D. Coward, N. Leidy, and P. Penn, Simultaneous Concept Analysis of Spiritual Perspective, Hope, Acceptance, and Self Transcendence, *IMAGE, Journal of Nursing Scholarship,* 24, no. 2. (1992), 141–145.
109. Karns, *op. cit.*
110. Wright, *op. cit.*
111. Meyerhoff, H., L. van Hofwegen, C. Hoe Harwood, M. Drury, and J. Emblen, Emotional Rescue: Spiritual Nursing Interventions. *Canadian Nurse,* 98, no. 3 (2002) 21–24.
112. Pesut, B., The Development of Nursing Students' Spirituality and Spiritual Care-Giving. *Nurse Educator Today,* 22 (2002), 128–135.
113. Chilton, *op. cit.*
114. Plante, *op. cit.*
115. Rubin, *op. cit.*
116. Hurley, J., Breaking the Spiritual Care Barrier, *Journal of Christian Nursing,* 16, no. 3 (1999), 8–13.
117. Sumner, C., Recognizing and Responding, *American Journal of Nursing,* 98, no. 1 (1998), 26–30.
118. Wallace, N., My Name is Jim? Do You Know Me? *Journal of Christian Nursing,* 16, no. 3 (1999), 36–37.
119. Wright, L.M., Suffering and Spirituality: The Soul Of Clinical Work with Families. *Journal of Family Nursing,* 3, no. 1 (1997), 3–14.
120. Westburg, G., The Church as "Health Place," *Dialog,* 27, no. 3 (1988), 189–191.
121. Atkins, F., *Church Members' Views About Healing and Health Promotion in Their Church: A Multi-Case Study.* Unpublished doctoral dissertation. St. Louis: St. Louis University, 1997.
122. Westburg, *op. cit.*
123. Buijs, R., and J. Olson, Parish Nurses Influencing Determinants of Health. *Journal of Community Health Nursing,* 92, no. 1 (2001), 13–23.
124. Martin, L.B., Parish Nursing: Keeping Body and Soul Together. *The Canadian Nurse,* 92, no. 1 (1996), 25–28.
125. Atkins, *op. cit.*
126. Canadian Association for Parish Nursing Ministry, *Historical Perspective of Parish Nursing in Canada,* Website: http://www.capnm.ca/historical_overview.htm, July 2004.
127. Clark, M., and Olson, J. *Nursing within a Faith Community: Promoting Health in Time of Transition.* Thousand Oaks, CA: Sage, 2000.
128. Simington, J., J. Olson, and L. Douglass, Promoting Well-Being within a Parish. *The Canadian Nurse,* 92, no. 1 (1996), 20–34.
129. Atkins, *op. cit.*
130. Canadian Association for Parish Nursing Ministry, *Guide for Parish Nursing Core Competencies,* Website: http://www.capnm.ca/core_competencies.htm, July 2004.
131. Simington, *op. cit.*
132. Goldstein, N., My Online Synagogue, *Newsweek,* September 14, 1998, 16.
133. Adler, J., 800,000 Hands Clapping, *Newsweek,* June 13 (1994), 46–47.
134. O'Mathuna, D., Prayer Research: What Are We Measuring? *Journal of Christian Nursing,* 16, no. 3 (1999), 17–21.
135. Hudson, T., Measuring the Results of Faith, *Hospitals and Health Networks,* September 20, 1996, 23–28.
136. Westburg, *op. cit.*
137. Cox, E., *Spiritual Interventions by Psychiatric Nurses.* Unpublished master's thesis, St. Louis University, 1995.
138. Are RNs Reluctant Spiritual Caregivers? *American Journal of Nursing,* 95, no. 8 (1995), 12–13.
139. Stoll, R., Essence of Spirituality. In Carson, V., ed., *Spiritual Dimensions of Nursing Practice.* Philadelphia: W.B. Saunders, 1989.
140. Toth, *op. cit.*
141. Piles, *op. cit.*
142. Cox, *op. cit.*
143. Peterson, E., and K. Nelson, How to Meet Your Client's Spiritual Needs, *Journal of Psychosocial Nursing,* 25, no. 5 (1987), 35–39.
144. Mickley, J., K. Soeken, and A. Belcher, Spiritual Well-Being, Religiousness, and Hope Among Women with Breast Cancer. *IMAGE, Journal of Nursing Scholarship,* 24, no. 4 (1992), 267–272.
145. Stoll, *op. cit.*
146. Donley, Sr. R., Spiritual Dimensions of Health Care: Nursing's Mission, *Nursing and Health Care,* 12, no. 4 (1991), 178–183.

Part 2

BASIC CONCEPTS RELATED TO THE DEVELOPING PERSON AND FAMILY UNIT

CHAPTER 4

THE FAMILY: BASIC UNIT FOR THE DEVELOPING PERSON

CHAPTER 5

OVERVIEW: THEORIES RELATED TO HUMAN DEVELOPMENT

CHAPTER 6

THE DEVELOPING PERSON: PRINCIPLES OF GROWTH AND DEVELOPMENT

Chapter 4

THE FAMILY: BASIC UNIT FOR THE DEVELOPING PERSON

When we speak of "family" each of us reaches into our store of images and experiences to give meaning to the term. In every culture there are fundamental roles fulfilled by the family. And the family instils values, the sense of what is important, what is worth preserving, protecting <u>and, if necessary, fighting for.</u>

Marlene Brant Castellano (2002). Aboriginal Family Trends, Section 4. Reprinted from the Vanier Institute of the Family's website at www.vifamily.ca. Used with permission.

OBJECTIVES

STUDY OF THIS CHAPTER WILL ENABLE YOU TO:

1. Define *family* and discuss the family as a system and the implications for the developing person.

2. Assess various theoretical approaches for studying the family.

3. Describe the purposes, tasks, roles, and functions of the family and their relationship to the development and health of its members.

4. Compare family adaptive mechanisms and their purposes.

5. List stages of family life and developmental tasks for the establishment, expectancy, parenthood, and disengagement stages.

6. Determine your role in helping the family achieve its developmental tasks.

7. Relate the impact of feelings about the self and childhood experiences on later family interaction patterns.

8. List and describe the variables affecting the relationship between parent and child and general family interaction, including single parent, stepparent, and adoptive families.

9. Compare and contrast ways in which your family life has influenced your present attitudes about family.

10. Analyze the influence of 20th-century changes on family life and childrearing practices in Canada, the United States, and other countries.

11. Predict how a changing culture may affect the development and health of the family system.

12. Practise therapeutic communication methods to be used when working with a family or other clients.

13. Analyze characteristics and phases of a therapeutic relationship with a client such as the family.

14. Assess a family, constructing a genogram and using criteria listed in the chapter, to formulate a nursing diagnosis and plan of care.

15. Evaluate your role and various measures and resources to use in promoting physical and emotional health of a family in various situations.

It's an uncanny feeling—to suddenly know that I am answering my son's question with the same words—even the same tone—as my father used with me 30 years ago.

...

Even though I have a happy, successful marriage, two loving children, a nice home, and a profession in which I feel competent, I constantly fight a feeling of inferiority. A contributing factor must be that my parents never encouraged or complimented me. When I took a test, they emphasized the 2 wrong, not the 98 right.

...

I always admired my aunt. If my cousin, her son, had told her he wanted to build a bridge to the moon, she would have furnished the nails.

These three people are speaking of aspects of a social and biological phenomenon that is often taken for granted: the family. So strongly can this basic unit affect our development and health that we may live successfully or unsuccessfully because of its influence. Much that the person learns about loving, coping, and the various aspects of life is first learned in the family unit.

Some form of family exists in all human societies. Culture, not biology, determines family organization.[1] Between society and the individual person, the family exists as a primary system and social group, for most people share many of life's experiences with the family. Thus the family has a major role in shaping the person; it is a basic unit of growth, experience, adaptation, health, or illness.

The traditional family persists as a norm in the imagination, but today norms hardly exist, with the fragility of marriage, the high incidence of divorce (and remarriage), the many styles of family life, the diversity of roles held by members, and the increasing number of homeless families. Thus today's children are being shaped differently—sometimes negatively—by the family unit. For many youngsters, the pain of family life, a changing family scene, having no permanent home, and being separated from other family members are compounded by poverty and neglect.

This chapter is not an exhaustive study of families or family life. Rather, it is an overview of the various forms, stages, and functions of contemporary families and of how you can use this knowledge. Although various aspects of the family are discussed separately, keep in mind that family purposes, stages of development, developmental tasks, and patterns of interaction are all closely interrelated, all influenced by historical foundations, and all continually evolving into new forms. Thus the *family should be viewed as a system, affected by the culture, the environment, religious-spiritual dimensions, and other variables, which in turn affect the person and society.*

DEFINITIONS

Families may have difficulty in maintaining the characteristics proposed in these definitions. Your support, teaching, and counselling may assist them in promoting and maintaining health.

Family

The **family** *is a small social system and primary reference group made up of two or more persons living together who are related by blood, marriage, or adoption or who are living together by agreement over a period of time.* The family unit is *characterized by face-to-face contact; bonds of affection, love, loyalty, emotional and financial commitment; harmony; simultaneous competition and mutual concern; a continuity of past, present, and future; shared goals and identity; and behaviours and rituals common only to the specific unit.*[2]

The **family** may also be defined as *domestic partners, people who have chosen to share each other's life in an intimate and committed relationship of mutual caring.* This definition permits the extension of legal benefits usually accorded traditionally married heterosexuals, such as health and life insurance and pension benefits, property rights, hospital and prison visitation rights, and bereavement leave to homosexual or same-sex families or unmarried partners.

Many headlines declare the demise of the family. However most of us live, or have lived in a family unit. A family may exist in one of several forms—traditional, common-law, blended, lone-parent, or same-sex family.[3] We define our own family. The data from the 2001 Canadian Census clearly indicates that the family, while in transition, endures as society's oldest and most basic indestructible institution.[4]

CRITICAL THINKING

Give your own definition of a family.

Family may be defined, and viewed, differently by various cultures. Aboriginal families are adopting a variety of forms. For example, the extended family networks on reserves and in rural communities continue to contribute toward a stable point of reference—especially for younger members, even though they may relocate while pursuing education and career opportunities. The nuclear family, two-generation families consisting of parents and children, is steadily becoming the unit of family organization. Because Aboriginal community membership is becoming increasingly more heterogeneous in ethnic origin and cultural practices, a vigorous movement exists to conserve and revitalize traditional languages, teachings, and ceremonial practices. Spontaneous and self-directed ways to heal from the effects of trauma, past and present, constitute the most promising sign of what the future holds for Aboriginal families.[5] Healing circles have been adopted as preventative, supportive, and rehabilitative measures in dealing with family violence.[6] Brenda Many Fingers found in her study that elders appear to be an invaluable source of inspiration for better living.[7] Due to the growing interdependence of individuals, families, and communities, efforts by the individual must be complemented by collective efforts to offset many of the structural disadvantages which Aboriginal families experience. The fact of these structural disadvantages is made evident in statistics regarding income, education, and health. It is important to note that different challenges exist between subgroups of the Aboriginal population. A common theme prevails, however, in Aboriginal community effort: Institutions that collaborate with families to protect children, provide quality education, promote and restore health, and prevent disease must be responsive to the culture and identity of Aboriginal citizens.[8] According to Brant Castellano, a strong movement exists to re-establish Aboriginal control of public services, including health, education, and justice.[9]

The family is a group whose members rely on each other for daily services. With the family, the person can usually let down his or her guard and be more himself or herself than with other people. The family comprises a household (or cluster of households) that persists over years or decades and that is characterized by value, role, and power structures; communication patterns; affective socialization, family coping, and health care functions; and developmental stages and tasks.[10]

Internal and external structures exist in a family. **Internal structure** *includes family composition, rank order, subsystems, and boundary.* **External structure** *includes culture, religion, social class status and mobility, environment, and extended family.* **Instrumental function** *refers to how routine activities of daily living are handled.* **Expressive function** *refers to nonverbal and verbal communication patterns, problem-solving roles, control aspects, beliefs, alliances, and coalitions.*

Healthy families are characterized by (1) a sense of togetherness that promotes capacity for change; (2) a balance between mutual and independent action on the part of family members; (3) availability of nurturance and resources for growth and sustenance; (4) stability and integrity of structure; (5) adaptive functioning; and (6) mastery of developmental tasks, leading to interdependence, progressive differentiation, and transformation to meet the requisites for survival of the system.[11]

Sometimes families live together daily. Sometimes the adult partners are employed in different geographic areas, or one member is hospitalized or in prison. They maintain contact by telephone, correspondence, and visits. In the two-career family the partners share the same residence on weekends or on a consistent basis. These families carry out their functions and characteristics in their own unique way.

Family Composition

The family takes several forms. Table 4-1 defines traditional, as well as nontraditional family forms, such as the *same-sex,* or *homosexual family,* who may be childless, have custody of and care for biological children from a previous heterosexual marriage, or have adopted children. Alternately, lesbian women may, through artificial insemination or one-time contact with a selected man, bear a child, and the other woman in the relationship also takes on the parenting role, clearly acknowledging that she is not the mother; or the gay couple may contract with a woman to carry a baby to term for them. The homosexual who has had a biological child is now more frequently exerting custody, visiting, and care-taking rights and responsibilities with the child after establishment of the same-sex relationship. Various authors describe the same-sex family.[12–16] The family may comprise a childless couple; siblings, especially in middle or late life; friends in a commune; or a man and woman living together without being married, with or without children. In Canada, changes in legislation are becoming more open for same-sex couples to choose a legal marriage. As a result, many of these couples are lining up waiting to walk to the altar and sign on the dotted line.[17] The Courts of Appeal in Ontario, British

Columbia, and Quebec have directed that marriage be open to same-sex couples. In 2003, Prime Minister Martin announced that the federal government would draft legislation to legally recognize the union of same-sex couples, but, at the same time, attend to the freedom of churches and religious organizations not to perform marriages against their beliefs.[18] The prime minister indicated that the draft legislation would be referred to the Supreme Court of Canada to ensure its constitutionality.[19]

CRITICAL THINKING

What legal rights and spousal benefits, if any, are in place in your province or territory for lesbian and gay families?

The family may also be a *series of separate but interrelated families.* The middle-aged parents are helping the adolescent and young adult offspring to be emancipated from the home while simultaneously caring for increasingly dependent parents and sometimes up to four pairs of grandparents plus older aunts and uncles (see Chapter 13).

The family group may be a **psychologically extended family** in which *people who are not biologically related consider themselves as siblings, "adopted" parent, child, aunt, uncle, or grandparent-in-spirit.* Further, related or unrelated family members may not live under the same roof.

Present-day mobility of people, ease of communication over distance, freedom to evolve and think independently, freedom to develop in ways less restricted by strong or rigid ethnic or cultural mores, and ease of transportation allow families in Canada and in the United States to be geographically distant, yet emotionally close and often quite involved with each other, to the point of giving assistance.

Regarding divorce, the 2001 Canadian Census claims that the most appropriate way to measure the divorce rate is to compare the number of divorces to the number of marriages that occurred in the year that the couple married. Based on that premise, the Canadian rate is currently 31–36%.[20] The average "age" of a marriage at a divorce is 13.7 years with the highest rate of divorce resulting after five years of marriage.[21]

People are beginning to realize that divorce does not necessarily improve life; the allure of creativity, growth, and expanding oneself emotionally through divorce is not necessarily realistic. Some families speak of trying harder, resolving to stay committed to each other in times of conflict.

OVERVIEW OF FAMILY THEORETIC APPROACHES

Theoretic approaches to the study of families include developmental, structural-functional, interactional, role, family systems, and crisis theories (Table 4-2). Refer to endnotes at the end of the chapter for more extensive explanation.[22–26]

TABLE 4–1
Types of Family Composition

1. **Nuclear family:** Mother, father, child(ren).
2. **Extended family:** Nuclear plus other relatives of one or both spouses. Relatives of the nuclear family may or may not live with the nuclear family. May include great-grandparents and great-great-grandparents.
3. **Single-parent family:** Mother or father, living with either biological or adopted children, possibly tied emotionally but not legally to a partner.
4. **Stepfamily:** One divorced or widowed adult with all or some of his or her children and a new spouse with all or some of his or her children, and often, also, the children born to this union so that parents, stepparents, children, and stepchildren (or stepsiblings) live together.
5. **Patrifocal/patriarchal family:** Man has main authority and decision-making power.
6. **Matrifocal/matriarchal family:** Woman has main authority and decision-making power.
7. **Same-sex/homosexual family:** Gay or lesbian partners live together.
8. **Single state:** Never married, separated, divorced, widowed.

TABLE 4–2
Summary of Major Family Theories and Approaches

Family Theory	Definition of Family	View of Person	Approach/Focus
Developmental theory: compilation of several frameworks	*Series of interacting personalities, intricately organized into paired positions (father, husband, daughter, sister); norms for reciprocal relations prescribe role behaviour for each position; predictable natural history designated by stages*	Person is a member of group; each new member adds to complexity of interaction.	**Study family** in terms of role behaviours for each family life-cycle stage, along with the changing ages of each person; study quality and type of interaction as age and member composition of family changes. **Focus:** Analyze developmental needs and tasks of each family life-cycle stage; analyze family behaviours and changing developmental tasks and role expectations in terms of increasing complexity, analyze children, parents, and family units as a whole. Cultural influences at each stage of family life cycle are considered.
Structural-functional theory: focus on family as a system	*Social system open to outside influences and transactions; maintains boundaries by responding to demands of system or acting under family constraints, passively adapting to external forces rather than acting as an agent of change in itself*	Person is seen as reactive in fulfilling roles and as having status in the social system.	**Study family** in relation to other social structures or social systems and in terms of roles. **Focus:** Determine how family patterns are related to other institutions and overall society; study family functions (reproduction, socialization of children, provision of physical needs, economics).
Interactional theory: reflection of role theory and psychodynamic theory	*Defined in terms of individual members, a unity of interacting personalities with assigned position and roles, expectations, and norms of behaviour, seen as closed unit with little relationship to outside institutions, associations, or cultures*	Person is seen as fulfilling roles and as an interacting being. Messages sent by members to each other have multi-level meanings.	**Study family** in terms of overt interactions, fulfillment of interacting roles and ways of communicating. **Focus:** Analyze roles, interstatus relations, authority matters, and action taking communication processes, conflicts, problem solving and decision making. Teach most effective communication methods.

(continued)

TABLE 4–2 *(continued)*
Summary of Major Family Theories and Approaches

Family Theory	Definition of Family	View of Person	Approach/Focus
Role theory: life is structured according to roles that are ascribed or assumed by the person in interaction with others; roles are learned through socialization	*Defined in terms of members' role interaction;* roles contribute in the following way to the family unit: Circumscribe behaviour Define social position, responses, and expectations Influence group associations Are purpose of interaction Provide norms for the family or group	Person is seen in terms of roles, which are specialized or shared and depend on sex, age, social norms, status, and ability to complement. Roles change through development and negotiation, which depend on flexibility, stability, and congruence of expectations. Person experiences role reciprocity, being complemented, or strain. **Role reciprocity:** *mutual exchange; sharing affects decision making and cohesion;* personal and family needs met; high mutual dependence in division of labour; potential for growth; commitment to family and reducing conflict **Role complementarity:** *family members differentiate and define roles in relation to each other;* opportunity for growth; sometimes not a sense of mutual-gratification; can confirm identity of one at expense of other; if rigid roles, transitions are difficult **Role strain:** *occurs when individuals have difficulty meeting others' or own expectations and the obligations of the role and is manifested as:* 1. **Role conflict:** *unclear, incomplete, contradictory elements in role; performing one role makes it impossible to perform another;* conflicting norms 2. **Role overload:** *must consider impact of distribution of power;* the greater the control over negotiation of roles, the more the person	**Study family** in terms of role interactions, differentiation, allocation, role change, and role strain. **Focus:** Analyze role reciprocity, complementarity, and strain.

(continued)

TABLE 4-2 (continued)
Summary of Major Family Theories and Approaches

Family Theory	Definition of Family	View of Person	Approach/Focus
		can avoid role strain; *person with less power assumes more unwanted burdens; person with more power has less dependency needs and can make role demands.*	
Family systems theory	*Integral unit in society, made up of parts or members, with individual and family characteristics that are interacting and interdependent. Maintain equilibrium by developing repetitive techniques of interaction.*	Person is member of system and subsystem.	**Study family** as a whole unit; sum of whole is greater than its parts or subsystems. **Focus:** Analyze family's adaptive process, exchange between members and subsystems, and decision making, transactions, bargaining, cooperative, and coercive processes. Examine rules of family organization, patterns of interaction, traditions, whether boundaries are open and flexible or closed, and interaction with other systems.
Crisis theory	*Family made up of members who individually experience hazardous events*	Problems or illness of one member is expressed in conflict or problems of that family. All family members are affected by inability of one to cope.	Brief therapy **Study family** in terms of crisis impact on all, rather than just one. **Focus:** Analyze present situation. Identify role and conflicts, general coping skills. Avoid blame; focus on perception and reality. Specific tasks are to be mastered. Alternate plans for coping are attempted until effective ways to reduce tension and disorganization are found. Ways to handle future crisis are explored. Therapist uses a variety of cognitive, educational, behavioural, and communication approaches to help family cope with crisis and become more functional.

PURPOSES, TASKS, ROLES, AND FUNCTIONS OF THE FAMILY

Knowledge of the following sections will enhance assessment, health promotion intervention, teaching, referral, and advocacy. Family structure, roles, and responsibilities have been influenced by communications technology, globalization of economy, globalization of marketing, and bio-genetic engineering, and the resulting social changes, leading to a hurried culture.[27] The demands of time have entered into our contemporary descriptions of family life. Daly states that it is almost pure madness to think of families living without sophisticated scheduling tools.[28] The forces shaping this continuous growing pace are the following:

- *Changing family form.* The dual-earner family is the dominant family form, and it faces heavy demands in negotiating time for its members. Many such families, as well as other family forms, have too many responsibilities and not enough time.[29] Even as the Canadian population ages, the demand on families in their role as caregivers will rise.
- *Increasing effects of technology.* Technology has accelerated the family's lifestyle along many avenues. One such avenue is the growing impatience and the desire for immediate results brought on by beepers, cell phones, and even microwave ovens, to name a few.
- *Increasing workload.* Daly argues that the culture of overwork has flourished in our society. Families are working more hours than ever before; and they are playing less.[30] This scarcity of available time to relax is felt not only by the adult members in the family, but by children as well.

Frederick claims that 15- to 17-year-old students report feeling anxious when their time is limited; and when they need more time they cut back on sleep.[31]

In Canada and other industrialized nations, balancing paid work and family activities is a pivotal issue that must be explored. Hall and Callery conducted a study, utilizing the grounded theory method, to explain how dual-earner couples manage work and family life. The analysis of data produced a substantive theory whose outcomes, processes, and strategies offer opportunities for health professionals to influence individual and family development and viability.[32]

Purposes and Tasks of the Family

The family is still considered responsible for the child's growth and development and behavioural outcomes; indeed, the family is a cornerstone for the child's competency development. Because the family is strongly influenced by its surrounding environment and the child itself, the family should not bear full blame for what the child is or becomes. The family is expected to perform the tasks listed below. *The tasks may be basically the same for most types of family composition, but how they are manifested often is related to the type of family structure:* nuclear, extended, single-parent, same-sex, patrifocal, or matrifocal. *Culture of the family group (racial, ethnic, geographic, socioeconomic, religious) also influences how the following tasks are achieved.* **Basic tasks** are as follows:

- Provide for physical safety and economic needs of its members and obtain enough goods, services, and resources to survive.
- Create a sense of family loyalty and a mentally healthy environment for the family's well-being.

NARRATIVE VIGNETTE

Your neighbours and friends, Janet and Abe, along with their two school-age children, who are highly active in school and community activities, constitute a dual-earner family. Last evening Janet called you and related that things are getting difficult for her at work. It seems that she is working longer hours this year, and she is finding it increasingly more difficult to juggle her time satisfactorily between work and family life. Janet wants to inform her supervisor that her (Janet's) mother has just been hospitalized and that she needs some time off work to care for her mother. However, Janet knows that her supervisor is also under heavy pressure due to recent lay-offs in the business. Janet, realizing that you know her supervisor well, asked you to speak to the supervisor in support of Janet's upcoming request for time away from work. You listened to Janet last

evening, but told her, as a friend, that you were exhausted and would call her back this evening. You would like to help Janet, but you remember her habit of being late for appointments and her increasing anxiety about the daily activities of her family.

As a lone parent yourself, with two preschool children, you are also very busy balancing your nursing duties and family life.

As a health professional:

1. How will you respond to Janet?
2. In what ways can you help her to cope with the many issues she faces?

To help you to respond to these questions, see Hall and Callery (2003).[33]

■ Help members to develop physically, emotionally, intellectually, and spiritually and to develop a personal and family identity.

■ Foster a value system built on spiritual and philosophic beliefs and the cultural and social system that is part of the identity.

■ Teach members social skills and to communicate effectively their needs, ideas, and feelings and to respect each other.

■ Provide social togetherness through division of labour and performance of family and gender roles with flexibility and cooperation.

■ Reproduce and socialize the child(ren), teaching values and appropriate behaviour, providing adult role models, and fostering a positive self-concept and self-esteem in the child(ren).

■ Provide relationships and experience within and without the family that foster security, support, encouragement, motivation, morale, and creativity.

■ Help the members to cope with crises and societal demands; create a place for recuperation from external stresses.

■ Maintain authority and decision making, with the parents representing society to the family as a whole and the family unit to society.

■ Promote integration into society and the ability to use social organizations for special needs when necessary.

■ Release family members into the larger society—school, church, organizations, work, and governmental system.

■ Maintain constructive and responsible ties with the neighbourhood, school, and broader community.[34]

The family often has difficulty in meeting these tasks and needs assistance from external resources. The family's ability to meet its tasks depends on the maturity of the adult members and the support given by the social system—nursing and health care, educational, work, religious, social, welfare, governmental, leisure outlets, and other resources in the community. The family that is most successful as a unit has a working philosophy and value system that is understood and lived, uses healthy adaptive patterns most of the time, can ask for help and use the community services available, and develops linkages with nonfamily units and organizations.[35]

Roles of the Family

The family assigns **roles,** *prescribed behaviours in a situation,* in a way similar to society at large. In society there are specialists who enforce laws, teach, practise medicine, and fight fires. In the family there are:

1. Performance roles: breadwinner, homemaker, handyman (or handywoman), the expert, political advisor, chauffeur, and gardener.

2. Emotional roles: leader, nurturer, protector, healer, arbitrator, scapegoat, jester, rebel, dependent, "sexpot," and "black sheep."

3. Members may fill more than one role. The fewer people there are to fulfill these roles, as in the nuclear family, the greater the number of demands placed on one person. If a member leaves home, someone else takes up his or her role. Any member of the family can satisfactorily fulfill any role in either category unless he or she is uncomfortable in that role. They enjoy sharing roles; working together to get the tasks done without worrying about what is man's or woman's work.

The emotional response of a person to the role he or she fulfills should be considered. Someone may perform the job competently and yet dread doing it. Changes in performance roles also necessitate emotional changes (e.g., in the man who takes over household duties when his wife becomes incapacitated).

The child learns about emotional response to roles in the family while imitating adults. The child experiments with various roles in play. The more pressure put on the child by the parents to respond in a particular way, the more likely that child is to learn only one role and be uncomfortable in others, as evidenced by the athletic champion who may be a social misfit. The child becomes less adaptive socially and even within the family as a result.

Exercising a capacity for a variety of roles, either in actuality or in fantasy, is healthy. The healthy family is the one in which there is opportunity to shift roles intermittently with ease. Through these roles family functions are fulfilled.

CRITICAL THINKING

What are the various roles in your family?

Functions of the Family as a Social System

The *family meets the criteria of a system because it functions as a unit* to:

1. Fulfill its purposes, roles, and tasks.

2. Provide shelter, stability, security, and a setting for nurturance and growth.

3. Provide opportunity to experiment with the dynamics and role behaviours required in a system.

4. Provide a support system for individual members.

5. Adapt in order to meet individual needs and prepare its members to participate in the social system.

The *organization of a family system is hierarchal,* although it may not be directly observable. The usual family hierarchies are built on kinship, power, status, and privilege relationships that may be related to individual characteristics of age, sex, education, personality, health, strength, or vigour. We can infer a hierarchy by observing each person's behaviour and communication. For instance, who talks first? Last? Longest? Who talks to whom? When? Where? About what? If one family member consistently approaches the staff about the client's health care, he or she probably holds an upper position in the family and has the task of being the "expert." Your attempt to communicate with family members may meet with resistance if the communication inadvertently violates the family communication hierarchy.[36]

Hierarchal relations in the family system determine the role behaviour of family members. These hierarchal role relationships typically have great stability, and ordinarily family members can be counted on to behave congruently with their roles. When there are differences in behaviour from situation to situation, they are almost inevitably in response to the family's expectations for that particular situation or circumstance.[37] Families develop a system of balanced relationships. Roles and relationships are based on reciprocal interaction, with each member of the family contributing to the total unit in a unique and functional way.

Family functions cover the physical, affectionate or emotional, social, and spiritual dimensions. Most families agree generally with the functions described below. For example, Jones[38] found that there was no significant difference between deaf and hearing parents' perceptions of family function and that they agreed on seven of ten items ranked as most important.

Physical functions of the family are met by the parents' *providing food, clothing, and shelter, protection against danger, and provision for bodily repairs after fatigue or illness, and reproduction.* In some societies these physical needs are the dominant concern. In Western societies many families take them for granted.

Affectional functions are equally important. Although many traditional family functions such as education, job training, and medical care are being absorbed by other agencies, *meeting emotional needs and promoting adaptation and adjustment are still two of the family's major functions.* The family is the primary unit in which the child tests emotional reactions. Learning how to react and maintain emotional equilibrium within the family enables the child to repeat the pattern in later life situations. The child who feels loved is likely to contract fewer physical illnesses, learn more quickly, and generally have an easier time growing up and adapting to society.

A healthy family has several dominant characteristics:

1. All persons are seen as unique, developing, and worthy of respect.
2. When a disturbing situation arises, members understand that many factors were involved—people were not simply trying to be difficult.
3. Members accept that change is continuous.
4. Members share their thoughts and feelings with a minimum of blame and feel good about each other and themselves.

Other important attitudes are:

- The feeling of unity between man and woman and separateness from their families of origin
- An ability to invest in the marriage to a greater degree than in other relationships
- A feeling of balance or harmony, for perfect equality is probably impossible
- A movement from a romantic "falling in love" to a warm, loving, companionable, accepting relationship
- An ability to maintain variety and frequent interactions with each other

Social functions of the modern family include *providing social togetherness, fostering self-esteem and a personal identity tied to family identity, providing opportunities for observing and learning social and sexual roles, accepting responsibility for behaviour, and supporting individual creativity and initiative.* The family gives a name to the infant and hence indicates a social position or status in relation to the immediate and kinship-group families. Simultaneously, each family begins to transmit its own version of the cultural heritage and its own family culture to the child. Through this process, the child learns to share family values.[39]

Thus *socialization is a primary task of the parents,* for they teach the child about the body, peers, family, community, age-appropriate roles, language, perceptions, social values, and ethics. The family also teaches about the different standards of responsibility society demands from various social groups.

The **spiritual function** to raise the child to be a moral person with a belief system of some kind is now discussed less frequently in texts. The authors believe parents have such a responsibility (see Chapter 3).

The parent generation educates by literal instruction and by serving as models. Thus the child's **personality,** *a product of all the influences that have and are impinging on him or her,* is greatly influenced by the parents.

CRITICAL THINKING

What aspects of family culture would an Inuit family transmit to their children?

FAMILY ADAPTATION

The following information can be used in assessment and in health promotion. You can teach healthy adaptive patterns, assess for unhealthy or abusive patterns, and use interventions discussed throughout the chapter.

Adaptive responses in the family represent the *means by which it maintains an internal equilibrium so that it can fulfill purposes and tasks, deal with internal and external stress and crises, and allow for growth of individual members.* Some capacity for functioning may be sacrificed to control conflict and aid work as a unit. But the best functioning family keeps anxiety and conflict within tolerable limits and maintains a balance between effects of the past and new experiences. In the same ways that other social systems adjust, the family system must adjust as well.[40]

Ideally, the family achieves equilibrium by talking over problems and finding solutions together. Humour, problem solving, flexibility, nonsense, shared work, and leisure all help relieve tension.

Successful and happy people define their most important priority as the spouse and the family; the business or career comes second. Each spouse or partner is a comforter, listener, companion, and counsellor to the other, supportive and fully committed. The partners or spouses may wish to set aside one night a week, or a month, to be only with each other, sharing uninterrupted time and activity. Each parent may wish to have a day date with each child monthly, spending time together at lunch, shopping, or in some mutually favourite activity.

Adaptive Mechanisms in Family Life

Various types of internal family coping strategies have been discussed. Strategies that extend outside the family include (1) seeking information, (2) maintaining links with the extended family or with people or agencies in the community, (3) using self-help groups or informal or formal support networks, and (4) seeking spiritual support.[41]

Dysfunctional or ineffective coping strategies used by families during stressful times include denial of problems, exploitation or manipulation of one or more family members, abuse of or violence toward children or adult members, use of authoritarianism or threats, changing to ineffective customs or traditions or family myths, use of alcohol or drugs, and abandonment of the family by one member through separation, divorce, or suicide.[42] Family response to stressors and conflict between the spouses or the parents and children affect the personality development and behaviour of children and adolescents and may contribute to illness, such as hyperactivity or behavioural acting out.[43,44]

Emotional conflicts in the family may be avoided, minimized, or resolved through scapegoating, coalitions, withdrawal of emotional ties, repetitive verbal or physical fighting, and use of family myths, reaction formation, compromise, and designation of a family healer. Two or more of these mechanisms may be used within the same family. If these mechanisms are used exclusively, however, they become defensive and are unlikely to promote resolution of the conflict, so that the same issue arises repeatedly.

Scapegoating or Blaming

Scapegoating or blaming involves labelling one member as the cause of the family trouble and is expressed in the attitude, "If it weren't for you...." Or one member may offer himself or herself as a scapegoat to end an argument by saying, "It's all my fault." Such labelling controls the conflict and reduces anxiety, but it prevents communication that can get at the root of the problem. Growth toward resolution of the problem is prohibited.

Coalitions or Alliances

Coalitions or alliances may form when some family members side together against other members. Antagonisms and anger result. Eventually the losing party tries to get control.

Withdrawal of Emotional Ties

Loosening the family unit and reducing communication may be used to handle conflict, but then the family becomes rigid and mechanized. Family members are also likely to seek affection outside the family so that the home becomes a hotel with everyone superficially nice.

Repetitive Fighting

Verbal abuse, physical battles, loud complaints, curses, or accusations may be used to relieve tension and allow some harmony until the next round. The fight may have the same theme each time stress hits the family. The healthy family allows some "blowing up" as a release from everyday frustrations, but it does not make a major case out of every minor incident or temporary disagreement.

Family Myths or Traditional Beliefs

These myths or beliefs can be used to overcome anxieties and maintain control over others, as illustrated in the following statements: "Children are seen, not heard." "We can't survive if you leave home." "Talking about feelings will cause loss of love." In contrast, the healthy family members encourage growth and creativity rather than rigid control.

Reaction Formation

Reaction formation is seen in a family in which there is superficial harmony or togetherness. Traumatic ideas are repressed and transformed into the opposite behaviour. Everybody smiles, but nobody loves. No one admits to having any difficulties. Great tension is felt because true feelings are not expressed.

Resignation or Compromise

Temporary harmony may occur when someone gives up or suppresses the need for assertion, affection, or emotional expression to keep peace. The surface calm eventually explodes when unmet needs can no longer be successfully suppressed.

Designation of One Person as Family Healer

This mechanism involves using a "wise one" (most often in the extended family), "umpire," a minister, storekeeper, bartender, or druggist to arrange a reconciliation between dissenting parties. A variant of the healer role is that of the family "counsellor," who assists family members to cope with their stress.

The Aboriginal community is undergoing a cultural, traditional, and spiritual renewal. The inclusion of tradition and culture in Aboriginal healing practices has facilitated the means for Aboriginal people to seek out healing. They view healing as a celebration of survival and triumph over one's human condition.[45] In the Aboriginal community, one of the roles of the elder is that of a healer. An elder's wisdom is seen as coming from deep within his or her being; and it reaches to the roots of the past to help link contemporary peoples with their ancestors and their traditions.[46] It is important to realize that to the Aboriginal people, family has a relatively broad meaning. Family encircles an extended network of grandparents, aunts, uncles, and cousins.[47] In essence, family and community represent the same network of resources.

CRITICAL THINKING

How do Aboriginal traditional practices differ from your own family healing practices?

Maladaptation

Signs of strained or destructive family relationships include the following:[48,49]

- Lack of understanding, communication, and helpfulness between members, resulting in unclear roles and conflict

- Each family member alternately acting as if the other did not exist or harassing through arguments
- Lack of family decision making and lines of authority
- Parents' possessiveness of the children or the mate
- Children's derogatory remarks to parents or vice versa
- Extreme closeness between husband and his mother or family or the wife and her mother or family
- Members not maintaining individuality, being too close or enmeshed or too distant with each other
- Parent being domineering about performance of household tasks
- Few outside friends for parents or children
- Scapegoating or blaming each other for difficulties
- High level of anxiety or insecurity present in the home
- Lack of creativity and stability
- Pattern of immature or regressive behaviour in parents or children
- Boundaries between generations not maintained; children carrying out parental roles because of parent's inability to function, illness, or abandonment

You may find yourself in the role of family healer. Help the family to develop harmonious ways of coping and avoid the protector or omnipotent role. Several texts give in-depth information pertinent to assessment of and intervention with families.[50–55]

STAGES OF FAMILY DEVELOPMENT

You have a critical role in assisting families to prepare for and work through the tasks of each family stage. Like an individual, the family has a developmental history marked by predictable crises. The developmental crises are normal, but they are also disturbing or frightening because each life stage is a new experience. The natural history of the family is on a continuum: from courtship to marriage or cohabitation; choosing whether to have children; rearing biological or adoptive offspring, or thinking about assisted human reproduction if there are concerns conceiving. Then allowing teenagers and young adults to find their own niche in society to either continue their studies, or find employment and establish homes of their own. In later life, the aging parents or grandparents are a couple once again, barring divorce or death. The nurturing of spouse or children goes on simultaneously with a multitude of other activities: work at a job or profession, managing a household, participation in church and community groups, pursuit of leisure and hobbies, and maintaining friendships and family ties. Or the person may decide to remain single but live with a person of the same or opposite sex; then the purposes, tasks, and roles of family life must also be worked out.

Tables 4-3, 4-4, 4-5, and 4-6 summarize the main stages of the family and major concerns or tasks for each stage, including establishment, courtship and engagement, expectant parenthood, and disengagement.[56–59] These tasks are also discussed in Chapters 7 through 14.

Initial or Establishment Stage

Courtship and **engagement** precede establishment of the family unit. In the **establishment stage**, *the couple establishes a home of its own; the main psychological tie is no longer with family of orientation (parental family)* (Table 4-3). Readiness for marriage in Canadian and U.S. societies is discussed in relation to young adulthood in Chapter 12.

Today families may choose to have no children, one child and adopt others, or two or three children instead of a larger family. They may even consider assisted reproductive technology as a means of conceiving. Some people are wise enough to know that children do not automatically bring happiness to a marriage. Children bring happiness to parents who want them and who are selfless enough to become involved in the adventure of rearing them.

Expectant Stage

The **expectant stage**, or *pregnancy*, is a developmental crisis; many domestic and social adjustments must be made. The couple (or the single mother and her significant other) is learning new roles and gaining new status in the community. Attitudes toward pregnancy and the physical and emotional

---

TABLE 4-3
Establishment Stage of Family

Courtship and Engagement

Become better acquainted with your partner, including values, expectations, and life ways.

Contend with pressures from parents or relatives about partner selection.

Resolve to mutually give up some autonomy and retain some independence.

Become free of parental domination.

Prepare for marriage, including mutually satisfying sexual patterns.

Establishment

Commit self to the partner, usually through marriage.

Establish own home and life patterns.

Focus psychological tie and lifestyle with partner.

Work out differences in expectations and patterns of communication, daily living, and sexual relations.

Establish and resolve conflicts related to a budget.

Work on establishing philosophy of life for the family unit that incorporates each partner's personal philosophy.

Determine whether or not to have children (biological or adopted) and desired number and spacing of children.

Discuss meaning of being a parent: fulfillment, responsibility, selfless need to rear children.

Stage ends when woman becomes pregnant or couple decides not to have children and works out living patterns.

TABLE 4-4
Expectant Stage of Family

Woman is pregnant; prenatal care is essential.

Couple incorporates idea of baby into thinking and planning for future and learns new roles.

Couple resolves feelings about pregnancy (desired, expected, not desired, unexpected) and impact on lifestyle and plans.

Woman experiences changing emotions and physical changes; more preoccupied with self and body; less interested in surroundings; has fears and fantasies about baby and childbirth.

Man must work through his feelings related to changes in the pregnant woman; his pride, guilt, fears, and fantasies related to childbirth; sense of virility; and ambivalence about demands of fatherhood.

Couple reworks sexual relationship.

Couple makes decisions about attending childbirth education classes and labour and delivery experience.

Woman prepares to be a mother; needs extra support from partner, family, and others.

Man prepares to be a father; needs extra support from family and others.

Couple discusses childrearing, discipline plans, and desires and resolves differences of opinion.

CASE SITUATION

Wan, and his now 34-year-old Japanese-Canadian wife, Oniki, immigrated to Canada a few years ago. Initially, Wan was happy that Oniki was pregnant with their first child. Lately, however, he has been behaving in a somewhat stressed manner, presumably about the coming baby; but he says he is hoping for a boy. At the clinic he informs you shyly that he has to be the provider and fears that he will not have much time to devote either to Oniki or to the baby. Both sets of future grandparents, who recently arrived to stay in Canada, are delighted that Oniki is pregnant.

1. According to the Steinberg, Kruckman, and Steinberg study on "Reinventing Fatherhood" in Japan and Canada, what is meant in this case by a "reciprocal cultural" barrier?

2. What may be some other challenges experienced by Wan that should be considered in order to assist him in his adjustment to his role of fatherhood?

3. What can you say, and do, to assist Wan as he adapts to his role as a father?

See Steinberg, Kruckman, and Steinberg (2000)[68] and Leininger (2002).[69]

status of the mother and father (and of significant others) affect parenting abilities. Now the couple thinks in terms of family instead of a pair (Table 4-4).

The woman may initially dislike being pregnant because it interferes with her personal plans, or she may feel proud and fulfilled.

Becoming a father is a critical stage in adult life. The man experiences a variety of feelings on learning of the pregnancy, feelings that change during the pregnancy. The reality of the pregnancy increases with time. Concerns identified by fathers are caring for the infant, adequacy as a father, financial security, and the baby's effect on the marital dyad.[62,63]

Historically, men have been known as providers. Traditionally, men had to spend much time outside the home providing for the family in terms of economic security. Now, Dubeau argues, the pendulum has swung in the other direction; and men are becoming not only affectionate, but caring, fathers.[64] Presently, fathers are emotionally involved in rearing, caring for, and communicating with their children. A paucity of literature and research exists on the experiences of men who take on the primary caregiving of children. More research and scholarly articles are needed, however, to assist health professionals to gain more knowledge in this field.

One area that is important to examine, mainly due to the increased rate of immigration to Canada, is the role of immigrant fathers. Steinberg, Kruckman, and Steinberg conducted a transnational study of Japanese and Canadian families.[65] Their results suggest that the social meaning of

fatherhood has been transformed, justifying the presence of the father in the household as a result of shifting extended family domestic structures, economic conditions, and the empowerment of women. The findings indicated other significant patterns. For example, Canadian fathers participate in labour and delivery to a higher degree than Japanese fathers.[66] Leininger, in writing about Japanese Americans and culture care, addresses important cultural information about the Japanese worldview, cultural values, and other pertinent issues.[67] As Canadian authors, we believe that the study of acculturation and value changes is important for health professionals to provide quality health care to the family.

For additional information about prenatal influences on the mother and baby, see Chapters 6 and 7. Information about parenting and developmental tasks for the expectancy phase is also presented in Chapter 12. Several authors give further information on the fathers' reactions and responsibilities.[70–72]

The family that prepares for adoption of a child does not have the tasks associated with the physical aspects of pregnancy, but it does have to accomplish the other tasks of readiness.

Parenthood Stage

In the **parenthood stage,** there is *birth or adoption of a child,* and the couple assumes a status that it will never lose as long as each has memory and life—that of parent. The *stages of parenthood* are summarized in Table 4-5.

TABLE 4-5
Parenthood Stage of Family

Parenthood/Expansion

Birth of child(ren), adoption, or foster care of child(ren) creates status of parent.

Expansion may occur if couple decides not to have children but couple does incorporate others' children into unit, parent groups of children, develop psychologically extended family, or become stepparents.

Parents recognize they are single most important influence on child.

No set patterns to parenthood in North America; parents rely on own uniqueness, wisdom, and skills; how their parents raised them; and current available information.

Experience **honeymoon stage**, or time following birth, when they feel excited about new relationship but also uncertain about meaning of parental love. Parent–child attachment is beginning.

Adjust to changes in lifestyle created by new baby; less freedom for own pursuits; 24-hour responsibility.

Work through **tasks** of becoming a parent **with birth of each child**, as follows:[60]

- Provide for the physical and emotional needs of the child, conveying love and security freely, regardless of the child's appearance or temperament
- Reconcile conflicting roles: wife–mother, husband–father, worker–homemaker or family man, and parent–citizen
- Accept and adjust to the demands and stresses of parenthood, learning or relearning basics of child care, adjusting personal routines and needs to meet the child's needs, and trying to meet the spouse's needs as well
- Provide opportunities for the child to master competencies expected for each developmental stage, to allow the child to make mistakes and learn from them, to restrict the child reasonably and constantly for safety, and to attain the emotional developmental tasks described by Erikson[61]
- Share responsibilities of parenthood and together make necessary adjustments in space, finances, housing, lifestyle, and daily routines that are healthy for the family (meals and sleep)
- Maintain a satisfying relationship with spouse emotionally, sexually, intellectually, spiritually, and recreationally, while maintaining a personal sense of autonomy and identity
- Feel satisfaction from being competent parents and the parenting experience but maintain contacts with relatives and the community
- Provide socialization experiences to help the child make the emotional shift from family to peers and society so that the child can become a functioning citizen
- Refine the communication system and relationships with spouse, children, and others and permit offspring to be autonomous after leaving home

See self as steward, guide, helping friend, and standard setter for child.

Invest in creative potential of offspring by nurturing, educating, protecting; offer freedom and promote autonomy without abandoning.

Parenthood/Consolidation

Active in role of mother and father, socialization and education of child(ren).

Continue to work on developmental tasks.

Concern with family planning, additional children or none.

Deal with problems in family, community, church, school, and immediate social sphere.

Participate in various ways with extended family and in community, school, church; activities and organizations for child(ren).

Accept and enjoy challenges, rewards, and responsibilities of childrearing.

Invest time, energy, and resources together to bring quality to relationship with child.

Avoid excess pressure on child(ren), such as controlling and possessiveness, neglect, and too little guidance.

Parenthood/Contraction

Change in parent–child family; let go of responsibilities, last child leaves home permanently.

Change in relationships (let go of responsibility) with members of psychologically extended family, for whom the couple feels ties or responsibilities, but who are not offspring.

Encourage and assist *autonomy and independence* in offspring or those for whom couple had responsibility.

Focus less on concept of self as parent, reworking self-concept as parent and person.

Assume new roles, responsibilities, and leisure activities.

TABLE 4-6
Disengagement or Contraction Stage of Family

Couple reworks sense of separateness from child(ren);
   new focus on couple unit and time for each other.

Woman may enter workforce if not previously employed.

Make readjustments if offspring return home for a time,
   with or without partner and child(ren), related to
   space, tasks, rules, roles (see Table 4-3).

Engage in retirement planning.

Prepare for death of spouse and self.

Resolve deaths, losses, and changes that occur in extended
   family and with friends.

At some point, role reversal with child(ren), parents need
   assistance with life tasks.

How the parents care for and discipline the child is influenced considerably by the following:

1. Parents' own maturity.
2. How they were cared for as children (as shown by studies on child abuse).
3. Their feelings about self; culture, social class, and religion (see Chapters 1 and 3).
4. Their relationship with each other.
5. Their perceptions of and experiences with children and other adults.
6. Their values and philosophy of life.
7. Life stresses that arise.

Moreover, the historical eras in which the parents were reared and in which they are now living and the prominent social values of each era subtly influence parental behaviour. Parents should rethink their priorities when they have children. Parents must invest time in such a way that it brings quality to their relationship with the child. Children need the encouragement of doing things and talking through things with adults.[73,74] As the children mature and leave home, the parents must rework their self-concepts as parents and people.

Disengagement or Contraction Stage

The last, or **disengagement or contraction, stage** occurs *when children leave and the partners must rework their separateness* (Table 4-6). This is often a time for maximum contact between the partners, especially when retirement occurs. Rosenthal and Gladstone, who studied demographic trends in present-day families, state that women who were born around 1850 had their last child when they were about 40 years old; meanwhile women who were born around 1955 had their last child when they were 26.[75] Due to the present rate of increase of life expectancy, it is more possible for women who were born around 1955 to experience what is known as the empty nest syndrome.[76] The women's age when the last child leaves

home could be around 50 to 56 years of age. However, the 2001 Canadian Census claims that young men aged 20 to 24 comprise the majority of adult children living at home, with 64% in the nest.[77] Do women experience the empty nest syndrome—that is, isolation, grief, or depression—when their last child leaves home? The answer may be somewhat variable depending upon the context of the family.

Sometimes teenage or young adult offspring return with children of their own because of divorce, economic problems, or other crises, so that grandparents may become involved in raising the grandchildren. Inwood states that the demands of parenting young children may affect the physical and emotional reserves of grandparents, which, in turn, can present many challenges.[78] Health professionals can be instrumental in first assessing the grandparent's health care needs, and second, informing them of resources in the community that might provide support for them.

The aged parents or other relatives may be unable to continue to live independently and are included in the household of middle-aged offspring. Consequently, the tasks, functions, roles, and hierarchical relationships of the family must be reworked. Space and other resources must be reallocated. Time schedules for daily activities may be reworked. Privacy in communication, use of possessions, and emotional space must be ensured. Old parent–child conflicts and ideas about who is boss and how rules are set and discipline is accomplished may resurface and should be discussed and worked through. These families can benefit from counselling; your guidance may be crucial. The middle-aged family is more fully discussed in Chapter 13.

CRITICAL THINKING

How can you help a mother who is experiencing the empty nest syndrome?

Table 4-7 lists suggestions for adult children and their parents to make living together more harmonious.[79]

Family Interaction

Family interaction is a *unique form of social interaction based on a set of intimate and continuing relationships. It is the sum total of all the family roles being played within a family at a given time.*[80] Families function and carry out their tasks and lifestyles through this process.

Family therapists, psychiatrists, and nurses are giving increased attention to the emotional balance in family **dyads** or *paired role positions*, such as husband and wife or mother and child. They have noted that a shift in the balance of one member of the pair (or of one pair) alters the balance of the other member (or pair). The birth of a child is the classic example. Dyads and emotional balance also shift in single-parent and stepparent families.[81–83]

Interaction of the husband and wife or of the adult members living under one roof is basic to the mental, and sometimes physical, health of the adults and to the eventual health

TABLE 4–7
Guidelines for Parents When Young Adult Offspring
Move Back Home

1. Remember what it was like when a new baby came home. No matter how beloved the child, disruptions are bound to occur. Realize that another relative's homecoming will be the same.

2. Everyone involved should remember whose house it is.

3. Realize that no matter how many years sons or daughters have been away, family procedures do not change. Mom may still be critical. Dad may be constant advice giver. Expect it.

4. Talk about resentments. Discuss problems if you think it will help.

5. Parents may say offspring are grown up. But that does not mean they believe it. Still, they cannot exert the same authority with a 30- or 40-year-old as with a youngster.

6. Offspring and elderly parents must be flexible. It is unfair to expect the middle-agers who are "hosts" to change their household and life routines too much.

7. Even if parents refuse money, adult offspring should insist on paying something, no matter how minimal. Otherwise, the offspring are reinforcing the idea that parents are taking care of them. Elderly parents can also contribute financially most of the time.

8. When grandchildren are involved, set rules about who is in charge. To decrease dependency, babysitters should be hired when possible. Then family members do not feel obligated or constrained.

9. Determine length of the adult offspring's stay. It need not be a precise date, but future plans about leaving the home should be explicitly stated.

10. Both adult offspring and older relatives should share responsibilities if possible. But do not upstage mom or dad; for example, if mom loves cooking, do not make her feel useless by taking over in the kitchen.

11. Space permitting, privacy is important. The relative who has lived on his or her own is probably used to time and space alone.

12. Middle-agers should resist meddling in the affairs of either offspring or parents. They can advise. But grown offspring need to think for themselves, and older relatives expect to make their own decisions.

13. Realize that the living situation may be temporary. Living together may not be ideal for anyone. But some parents and offspring or middle-agers and their parents become closer during such periods.

of the children. Two factors strongly influence this interaction: (1) the sense of self-esteem or self-love of each family member and (2) the different socialization processes for boys and girls.[84,85]

Importance of Self-Esteem

The most important life task for each person—to feel a sense of self-esteem, to love the self and have a positive self-image—evolves through interaction with the parents from the time of birth onward and, in turn, affects how the person interacts in later life with others, including spouse and offspring. You can help family members realize the importance of respecting and loving one another and help them work through problems stemming from the low self-esteem of a family member.[86–89]

Influence of Childhood Socialization

The second crucial influence on interaction between adults in the family is the difference in socialization processes for boys and girls. These differences exist, even in our changing society. In some cultural groups, the differences are obvious, including among people in mainstream society who may deny they socialize boys and girls differently. The girl may be loved simply because she exists and can attract, as shown by the admiration pretty little girls receive. The girl may be taught to be subtle, for such behaviour is part of her attraction. The boy may be loved for what he can do and become; he must prove himself. Boys, especially from school age on, are given less recognition than girls for good looks and much recognition for what they can do.[90–94] You can help the couple to recognize the effect of their process of socialization on their children and assist them in working through misunderstandings.

CRITICAL THINKING

What effects did your culture have upon your socialization process during your formative years?

Variables Affecting Interaction between the Child and Adult

Each critical period in the child's development reactivates a critical period in the parent. Demands made on the parent vary with the age of the child. The infant needs almost total and constant nurturance. Some parents thrive during this period and depend on each other for support. Other parents feel overwhelmed by the infant's dependency because their own dependent needs are stimulated but unmet. The baby's cry and behaviour evoke feelings of helplessness, dependency, and anger associated with their unacceptable dependency needs and feelings and then guilt and fatigue. The toddler struggles with individuality and autonomy, exploring and vacillating between dependency and independency. The parents may enjoy this explorative, independent behaviour of the child, even though the toddler leaves the parent feeling tired and frustrated. Parents who have difficulty caring for the dependent infant may do very well with the independent preschooler or adolescent, or the reverse may be true. With your intervention, support, and teaching, the parent may be able to resolve personal conflicts and move to a more advanced level of integration as he or she works with the developing child.[95]

Long before the child learns to speak, sensory, emotional, and intellectual exchanges are made between the child and other family members. Through such exchanges, and later with words, the child receives and tests instructions on how to consider the rights of others and how to respond to authority. The child also learns how to use language as a symbol, how to carry out certain routines necessary for health, how to compete, and what goals to seek. The games and toys purchased for and played with the child, the books selected and read, and the television programs allowed can provide key learning techniques.

Ordinal position and sex of the children, presence of an only child or of multiple births, of an adoptive child, or stepchild, all affect individual experiences within family, influence strategies to secure parental favour, and alter family dynamics and experiences.

Parents tend to identify with their children and to treat them according to how they were treated as children. A parent can identify best with the child who matches his or her own sibling position. For example, a man from a family of boys may not know how to interact with a daughter and may not empathize with her. In the process of identifying with the parent, the child picks up many of the parent's characteristics, especially if the child is the oldest or lone child. Using family constellation theory, Hoopes and Harper[96] and Sulloway[97] describe features of each child in a family, based on sex and ordinal position, how the child feels about and interacts with people, and which ordinal position spouse he or she will most happily marry.

Ordinal Position of the Child

Birth order is important to development. Table 4-8 lists characteristics of children in first, middle, and last ordinal positions, as well as of the only child. *Siblings, both same and opposite sex, have an important influence on each other as buddies, bullies, or heroes, and the early relationship often affects the adult relationship.* Whether the child has male or female siblings also affects personality development.[98,99] For example, second-born boys with an older sister are more feminine or empathic and nurturing than those with an older brother. If two siblings are more than six years apart, they tend to grow up like only children.[100]

As you counsel parents who plan for or have only one child, emphasize the need for peer activity and the danger of too much early responsibility and pressure.

Family with a Large Number of Children

The nuclear family with more than three or four children is less frequently seen now than in the past. The last-born child may be less wanted than the first- or middle-born, although parents feel more skilled and self-confident in rearing the younger children. Large families have advantages. Of necessity, the children learn thrift and conservation of resources and material goods. Members know the hot water supply is not unlimited, that food is not to be wasted, and that toys and clothing can be recycled. Children learn to share time, space, and possessions. In a loving home, they have not only their parents' love but also that of siblings, a listening ear, respect, support, compassion, and help. If the parent does not have time to read to the three-year-old, the older sibling does. He

or she gains more experience in reading, gains increased self-esteem from being helpful, and learns responsibility and caring. Each child learns cooperation, compromise, and tolerance and how to handle peer pressure. The effort, work, expense, and self-denial of having a large family can be offset by the rewards of watching children grow and develop and by a sense of contribution to the generations to come.

Your teaching and support can influence how well parents cope with responsibility of a large family.

Multiple Births

The increased use of assisted reproductive technology, as well as the increased frequency of multiple births, has had profound impacts on the family and Canadian society.[101] Twins or other multiple births have considerable impact on family interaction. If ovulation has been inhibited with contraceptive pills or if certain infertility drugs are used, multiple births are more likely to occur. Multiple fetuses in uteri create many problems for the parents in relation to the health of the mother and babies, financial strain, ethical decisions if certain embryos may not live, and family relationships. The needs and tasks of these parents will differ from the parents who have a single birth. Your suggestions and support in engaging others to assist the family can influence how well the parents cope with their responsibility.

Because multiple births are often premature, the first four or five months are very demanding on the parents in terms of the amount of energy and time spent in child care; this means that the parents have less energy and time for each other or other children. The mother should have help for several months or longer if there are more than two babies, from the husband, a relative, friend, or neighbour. Financial worries and concern about space and material needs may also intrude on normal husband–wife relationships or on relationships with other children.

Although books discourage the mother of twins from breastfeeding or using alternate breast- and bottle-feeding, the mother may be able to breastfeed both twins successfully by alternating breastfeeding with bottle-feedings. The babies will not necessarily be poor breast-feeders with this arrangement.

You can suggest shortcuts in, or realities about, care that will not be detrimental to twin babies and that will give the parents more time to enjoy them. Each can be given a total bath every other day instead of daily. Heating bottles before feeding is not necessary. Multiple offspring should be fun as well as work. Encourage the parents of twins (or other combinations of multiple offspring) to perceive the babies as individuals and to consider the long-term consequences of giving them similar-sounding names, dressing them alike, and expecting them to behave alike. Inform parents about the different resources in Canada, such as Multiple Births Canada (MBC), whose vision is to improve the quality of life for multiple birth individuals and their families across Canada. MBC provides support, advocacy, research, and education.[102] Another support network is Mom2Many.com—Parents of Multiples across Canada, which provides parents with various resources and information.[103] One example of the type of

TABLE 4–8
Influence of Ordinal Position on Child

Firstborn Children

1. Are most likely to be wanted
2. Enjoy advantages until second child comes along
3. Are subject to greater parental expectations for achievement in school, work at home, and adult success
4. Begin to speak earlier in life
5. Demonstrate higher intellectual achievement
6. Are more achievement-oriented and responsible
7. Are more goal-directed, plan better, and experience fewer frustrations
8. Identify more with parents than with peers
9. Are more dominant with siblings and peers
10. Have stronger superego or conscience, more self-discipline, and inner direction
11. Are more socially insecure
12. Engage in less risk-taking
13. Tend to have responsible leadership or high-level positions and be successful in adulthood

Middle Children

1. Are more difficult to characterize because of variety of positions in family
2. Receive less of the parents' time
3. Are praised less often
4. Are less stimulated toward achievement
5. Learn to compromise, handle conflict, and be adaptable because they are caught between jealousy of older sibling and envy of younger sibling
6. Develop sense of humour as adaptive mechanism
7. Learn double or triple roles and are prepared for more relationships in adulthood because of sibling coalitions
8. May succeed in role of mediator or negotiator in adulthood

Youngest Children

1. Benefit from parents' experience with childrearing
2. Tend to identify more with peer group than with parents
3. Are less tense, more affectionate, more good-natured, possibly to gain parental attention and sibling acceptance
4. Are popular with peers
5. Are more flexible in thinking
6. Have fewer expectations for household tasks or school achievement from parents
7. Are more dependent in relationships

Only Child

1. Resemble first-born children
2. Experience greater parental pressure for mature behaviour and achievement
3. Learn to fill many roles because fewer family members have more demands
4. May be forced to assume roles prematurely without adequate preparation
5. Are more mature, cultivated, serious, and goal-oriented than peers who have siblings
6. Are more assertive, responsible, and independent
7. May be adept at various roles but lack self-confidence
8. Are usually intellectually superior, curious, creative with rich fantasy life, and academically successful
9. May feel lonely but able to entertain self and find satisfaction in personal pursuits because of parental demands
10. Demonstrate superiority in use of language
11. Do not usually share feelings and experiences with someone close
12. Learn less about coping with jealousy, envy, and sibling rivalries and sharing adult attention than peers with siblings
13. Learn less about intimate interactions with opposite or same-sex peers
14. Develop into a well-adjusted, capable adult rather than the stereotype of spoiled, selfish child

information supplied is that on April 7, 2004, Canada became the first country to ban the selling, reselling, advertising, and importing of baby walkers.

Multiple-birth children usually are closer than ordinary siblings. These children have lived with each other from before birth so experiences are different from that of having various aged siblings. Parents often force one to be older and one to be younger in behaviour, but it is difficult for the one to play role of "older" because neither has the advantage of extra years of experience over the other, who is developmentally on the same level. With fraternal twins, authority preference of parents tends to determine what age ranks the girl and the boy will be ascribed. In contrast, identical twins meet the world as a pair; it is difficult to imagine life without each other. It takes longer to separate in adolescence and adulthood (they may not, emotionally or physically). Each tends to seek multiple-birth persons as friends or mates.[104]

Siblings of a multiple birth usually are more detached from other siblings, even from parents, than each other. Multiple-birth children may each receive less parental affection and communication because parents have less time to devote to each child. Thus they are often slower to talk and many have slower intellectual growth unless parents work to prevent it.[105,106] Yet the bond and sharing that occurs between twins or multiple-birth individuals can have positive effects on development as well. The sense of security and identity and the ability to share may be stronger, and these people have a unique empathy and ability to switch roles that enhances interpersonal relationships.[107]

CRITICAL THINKING

What can you do to help a multiple-birth family from the Yukon who is seeking information on multiple births?

Sex of the Child

Sex also influences development within the family.[108] In most cultures, a higher value is placed on male than on female children. Actually, in some cultures only a boy's birth is welcomed or celebrated, and the family's status is partially measured by the number of sons. A family with several girls and no boys may perceive another baby girl as a disappointment. The girl may discover this attitude in later years from overhearing adult conversations, and she may try to compensate for her sex and gain parental affection and esteem by engaging in tomboy behaviour and later assuming masculine roles.

If a boy arrives in a family that hoped for a girl, he may receive pressure to be feminine. He may even be dressed and socialized in a feminine manner. If the boy arrives after a family has two or three girls, he may receive much attention but also the jealousy of his sisters. Often he will grow up with three or four "mothering" figures (some may be unkind) and in a family more attuned to feminine than to masculine behaviour. Developing a masculine identity may be more difficult for him, especially if there is no male nearby with whom to relate. The girl who arrives in a family with a number of

boys may also receive considerable attention, but she may have to become tomboyish to compete with her brothers and receive their esteem. Feminine identity may be difficult for her.

You can help parents understand how their attitude toward their own sexuality and their evaluation of boys and girls influence their relationship with their children. Emphasize the importance of encouraging the child's unique identity to develop.

Adopted Child

The adopted child may suffer some problems of the only child. In addition, the adopted child may have to work through feelings about rejection and abandonment by the biological parents versus being wanted and loved by the adoptive parents. The child should be told that he or she is adopted as early as the idea can be comprehended. Usually by the preschool years he or she can incorporate the idea of being a wanted child. Explanations will have to be repeated and expanded in the years ahead.

Adopted children bring their own genes, birth experiences, biological family ties, and often an extensive life history to their adoptive family. The adoptive family is not the same as a biological family. Both adoptive parents and adopted children tend to feel that they have less control over their situation than other families. Adoptive parents and adopted children are both likely to have experienced a sense of loss. It is not unusual for the adoptive child to seek his or her own biological parents in late adolescence or young adulthood, especially if the child was old enough to remember both parents when adopted, even when the adoptive parents are truly considered the parents. This search may be a threat to adoptive parents, or the adoptive parent(s) and biological mother may feel secure enough to even assist the offspring in the search.

Major determinants of the child's adjustment and development are the adoptive parents' personal qualifications, their marital harmony, their love of the child, their ability to communicate with the child about the adoptive process, their acceptance of the child as is, and the child's having friends. Factors not predictive of adjustment are socioeconomic status; occupational status; presence or absence of biological siblings; and the parents' age, health, religion, or experience with children.[109,110]

The definition of "suitable" adoptive parents has been liberalized. The adoptive parent may be a man, a homosexual couple, an infertile couple, or a relative. Additionally, today's couples consider adoption even if they have their own children. Some believe they have a responsibility and enough love to provide a home for an existing child rather than add to the total population. Others are single or older persons who want to offer love and security to a child.

In Canada, each provincial government has a designated office that is responsible for adoptions, and each office has specific procedures for adoptions.[111] The process of adoption is carried out through either a public or private agency. Public domestic adoption refers to any adoption arranged by a public, or government, agency. It is important to note that the focus of a public adoption is on meeting the needs of the child rather then on satisfying the needs of the adoptive couple.[112]

Usually, no costs are involved in adopting through a public agency. In the private system, there is a longer waiting period especially for a healthy newborn. Biological mothers who are seeking to have a child put up for adoption find the private system easier to deal with and more responsive to their needs. However, social workers and psychologists now consider that giving up a child for adoption can be psychologically damaging for both the mother and child.[113] Additional information is available from http://www.canadaadopts.com.

Recently, the number of foreign adoptions has increased, mainly because couples tend to be highly motivated to be parents and babies are quite readily available from abroad.[114] Many couples are also concerned about the conditions of war, extreme poverty, or the exploitation of children. The guidebook *How to Adopt Internationally* was designed by Jean and Heino Erichsen to provide couples with the information they need. To note the list of features in the book, refer to http://www.internationaladoption.ezhoster.com.

You may have an opportunity to educate adults about the opportunity for adopting an older child with special needs or a foreign-born child, or to work with adoptive parents, who also have needs.

Adoption of a child with special needs involves four phases: (1) commitment of adults and child, (2) honeymoon or placement period, (3) storm period, and (4) adaptation and adjustment. The phases do not abruptly begin and end; each phase builds on the preceding phase and sometimes reversals occur. The phases, along with thoughts, emotions, and activities accompanying each phase, are summarized in Table 4-9. The adoptive process can terminate at any point. If termination is necessary, both sides—the family and child—need help to understand what happened and to understand that no one person is responsible. Future adoption procedures are enhanced if proper guidance is given with the first failure.[115]

Stresses to adoptive families include the following:[116–120]

- The parents may worry about the child's heredity.
- The parents choose to be parents; hence they are highly motivated to parent and invest considerable expense and time.
- The parents see themselves as a chosen group because someone thought they should be good parents; the chosen group idea leads to problems such as difficulty in setting limits, increased stress in parenting role, and oversensitivity to problems in the child.
- Infertile couples may have feelings of hostility or inferiority that are projected on the child; the child is a constant reminder of their inability to conceive.
- The adopted child or adolescent may project normal feelings of anger onto "adoptive" parents; parents may think normal developmental problems are a fact of adoption.
- If one child is adopted and one is biological, favouritism, insufficient rewards to the adoptive child, or competition between children may result.
- Sanctions and regards for role performance differ from those for biological parents (e.g., the company may not have maternity leave for adoptive parents; there is little emotional support for adoptive parents in society).
- Role autonomy is lacking. Adoptive parents need someone (e.g., extended family, adoption agency) to agree with them that they will be good parents but need someone else to bear a child. These requirements inject dependence into a role considered independent, which may undermine parental confidence.
- Community or school attitudes may be negative; one's "own" child is spoken of as a biological child. The child encounters these attitudes of distinguishing between "real" and "adoptive," which undermines the sense of belonging and can drive a wedge between parents and child.

Adoption is a unique way of building families. These families are different from other families because of the circumstances that bring people to adoption and because of the way adoption continues to affect their lives.[121–122] If the adoption was biracial or international, cultural differences must be acknowledged. The adopted child must be given opportunities to learn about his or her cultural background.

Adoptive parents, adoptive children, and adoptive family dynamics are different from birth parents, birth children, and birth family dynamics. Sometimes these differences generate problems within a family, and sometimes the adoption becomes the focus of other conflicts or unresolved family issues. Changes

---

CONTROVERSY DEBATE

Question of Adoption

You work as a nurse counsellor at a recently opened fertility clinic in a small town. The other health professional in the clinic is a social worker, who is scheduled to begin work in a few weeks. Today, a childhood friend, June, telephoned to arrange a counselling session with you, as her counsellor and friend. She informs you that she will bring her husband Jay to the session. You have agreed to see this couple because there is no other office in town to which you might refer them. During the brief telephone conversation, you learn that they have been transferred here from the city, but they must return to the city in a few days to pack their belongings and complete arrangements for the move. She relates that for a couple of years she has been taking physician-prescribed fertility drugs, but she has not been able to conceive. She advises you that Jay seems to strongly favour assisted human reproduction technology, while she really wants to adopt either a disabled child or a child from a foreign country. From the telephone conversation you have become quite certain that Jay is not interested in adoption and that June wants to adopt a child.

Both June and Jay are scheduled to see you for counselling in your office tomorrow morning.

1. In what ways can you be therapeutically present to both June and Jay?
2. How can you help this couple to cope with, and to adapt to, the stressors they seem to be experiencing?

TABLE 4-9
Adoptive Process of a Child with Special Needs

Phases	Thoughts and Emotions	Activities
Commitment of Adults and Children	*Adults* make general decision to adopt (stage 1), leading to decision to adopt specific child(ren) (stage 2).	*Adults* prepare for adoption through dialogue with helpful people and agencies and sometimes attend sessions on adoption given by adoption agency.
"Courting stage"	*Child* expresses desire for adoption (stage 1), leading to decision on specific family (stage 2).	*Child* is counselled for potential adjustment by adoption agency staff. Visits are arranged and made between potential family and child. All members involved (including existing children in family) get to know each other.
Placement	*Parents* are on an "emotional high"; excitement.	Household routines are altered to accommodate child. Limit setting is minimal. Parent(s) meet child's whims.
"Honeymoon period" (child comes to live with parents)	*Child* is excited but somewhat scared. "Can I trust these people?" "Will they send me away when I don't act my best?"	*Child* is put on best behaviour. Sometimes parents' show of affection for child is not accepted because of child's past negative parenting.
"Storm period"	*Parents* are tired of permanent houseguest, feel anger, disappointment and guilt, and displace these feelings on each other and the child. They may wish the child would leave. *Child* can no longer keep up good behaviour but wants to be loved and accepted. *Parents* may feel sense of failure. They may have expected too much of themselves and child and now may strike out at each other and other family members. Spouses may be jealous of time and energy mate gives to child. *Child* may think, "They don't want me. What's going to happen to me?" and may live with anticipatory grief, fears of rejection, and insecurity, based on past hurts. Parents and child test each other.	*Parents* treat child or other family members with decreasing tolerance for behaviour not in family norm. *Child* may have tantrums, run away, or try to reject parents before they reject him or her. If the outcome is positive, the *parents* will use problem solving, limit setting with flexibility, sense of humour, ongoing empathy and caring, supportive others, and community resources.
Adaptation and Adjustment Phase (Equilibrium Occurs)	*All* believe they can live and work together; mutual trust is growing; family feels fused as a unit and able to handle frustrations and crisis.	Parents are consistent with child. *Parents* and *child* can attend to outside interests without threatening family status.

"Adults" and "child" are used in this table; however, only one adult may be adopting (single parent), and more than one child may be adopted.

Intervention Guidelines for Therapy with Adoptive Families

- Conventional treatment may not work well with adoptive families.
- Adoptive parents need validation as parents and of their decision to adopt.
- Adoptive parents must be included in therapeutic interventions to empower them further and to reinforce the adoptive commitment.
- In treating child-rooted problems, often the job will be to help parents modify their expectations.
- A child cannot successfully mourn the past and integrate it into the present circumstances if preoccupied with emotional survival. Developing a sense of safety and security is of paramount importance.
- Child-rooted barriers can come from unfinished emotional business, attachment disorders, or poor preparation for adoption.
- Adult-rooted barriers may stem from unfinished business, marital problems, or individual pathologies.
- Environmental barriers include lack of support or active disapproval from the extended family or the broader community.
- Any assessment is useful only if the assessed family accepts it as valid.
- In deciding to terminate an adoption that is not working, one must be committed to preserving the family's integrity, yet open to the removal of the child as a viable option.
- When an adoption is terminated, avoid judgment about reasons for its failure. Plans for adoption of another child should not be made until grief over the loss is resolved.

in the nature of adoptions have meant that more adoptive families have been seeking professional assistance and that professionals are having to consider the kinds of services the families may need and how to deliver them. The box entitled "Intervention Guidelines for Therapy with Adoptive Families" summarizes therapy considerations.[123,124]

Stepchild

Both adults and children experience loss and disruption, psychologically, socially, and economically, and changed life patterns and roles with each restructuring cycle of the family—divorce, custody battles, remaining a single parent with the child(ren), choosing to live unmarried with a partner or remarriage, and possibly another divorce and remarriage. The resulting combinations of people may never be a "blended family." Further, the adjustment may never be fully made; at best, it is likely to take several years for all involved. The child may express a desire for the biological parents to reunite for years after a divorce, even if the union was abusive and dysfunctional.[125–128]

The stepchild grieves and mourns the loss of a biological parent from death or divorce and must also deal with problems associated with integration into a new family unit. The stepchild may have conflicting feelings of loyalty to the natural parent

and to the stepparent, thinking that acceptance of the stepparent is rejection of the natural parent. The stepchild may also feel rejected by his or her remarried natural parent, seeing the stepparent as a rival for the parent's attention. Further, when there are stepsiblings, jealousy, conflict, and hate may be dominant feelings in the offspring. More on the stepparent family follows in the next section.

There is great need to educate parents, family members, lawyers, and judges about the impact of divorce and conflict on children. Public assistance programs and ensuring support from the father are critical to reduce effects of poverty on divorced women who are awarded child custody.

FAMILY LIFESTYLES AND CHILDREARING PRACTICES

There is no single type of contemporary Canadian or U.S. family, but the lifestyles of many correspond to the factors discussed in this section, including family structure, family cultural pattern, and the impact of the 20th century. These factors, in addition to those already discussed, influence family interaction. An understanding of them will assist you in family care.

Family Structure

Childrearing and family relationships are influenced primarily by family structure. The biological and reproductive unit considered typical in North America is the mother–father–child group. Traditionally, the parents were married, had established a residence of their own, were viewed (along with their children) as an integral social unit, and lived in an intimate, monogamous relationship.

In many situations, however, a child may grow up in a family that differs from the typical one. Some cultures believe it takes a village (or a whole community) to raise a child. In some cultures or families, an aunt, uncle, or grandparent may be a continuing member of the household unit; one or the other parent may be absent because of death, divorce, illegitimacy, military service, or occupation involving travel. The children may not suffer long-lasting effects, yet most studies show children fare better emotionally, and usually physically and economically, in homes with both biological parents, regardless of parents' education, race, or social status.[129,130]

Single-Parent Family

The *single-parent family* is becoming increasingly more common. In fact, Lynn states that one of the most notable changes in Canadian families over the past three decades is the increase in single-parent families.[131] Although death, or being born to a single parent, may cause the child to have only one parent, divorce of the natural parent is the more common reason. If the parents are divorced, the family may have experienced considerable disruption before the break-up. Sometimes the single-parent family is a planned event. A woman, lacking a suitable partner but wanting to be a mother, will choose to have a child by artificial insemination; or a single man or woman may choose to adopt a child. Regardless of the reason for the situation, some of these families have undergone a considerable change in lifestyle and often encounter considerable stress, including financial strain and sometimes even poverty. Other families appear to survive. Many of the children whose parents live in separate households are not only spending time with but are being cared for by both parents on a weekly basis.[132]

Children living in the single-parent household often exhibit more adaptability, responsibility, and maturity than do their peers. However, the child who lives with the parent of the opposite sex may have more difficulty with adjustment to the divorce or death of the other parent, or to the remarriage of the parent, than if the child lived with the same-sex parent. Inappropriate social behaviour, difficulty with identity formation, depression, and poorer school performance may be manifested by the child. If there always was only one parent, the child may have evolved behaviour and roles appropriate to the partner, regardless of the child's sex. This may also create later developmental problems.[133–135]

Often a series of open discussions concerning the changed lifestyle, along with support from relatives, friends, and other single-parent families, enhances the problem-solving abilities of these persons. Family members may need professional help if they exhibit symptoms of more extreme dysfunction, grieving, or prolonged "acting-out" behaviours. The family may also need information about various community resources. A major concern for single-parent families is financial strain or poverty, especially for the woman, because of wage inequities, difficulty with divorce settlements and child support, or lack of financial preparation in the case of parental death.[136] However, some studies suggest that, while there is less family money available, women are better financially and have more money at their disposal than they had within a marriage.[137]

Ford-Gilboe not only describes the strengths of single-parent families, but compares these strengths to those of two-parent families. This study presents families' explanations of the effect of self-identified strengths on health.[138] Her findings indicate that although structural differences exist between the single-parent and the two-parent family, the nature and pattern of strengths are found to be more alike than different between these two groups. In essence, these findings challenge the stereotypical views of single-parent families that emphasize vulnerability and problematic issues and exclude their strengths.[139]

Stepfamilies

The proportion of stepfamilies in Canada is lower than that in the United States due to lower rates of divorce and remarriage in Canada.[140] In the 2001 Canadian Census, stepfamilies were not counted in a formal manner. Participants were asked to list their stepsons and stepdaughters as "sons" or "daughters."[141]

The number and variety of relationships are greater in stepfamilies than in nuclear, nondivorced families. Church states that in many instances there are no terms for some of the multiple relationships. For example, let's enter Heather's life for a moment. As a result of living with Harry, Heather has increased the number of her relationships. What does she call herself in relation to Harry's ex-wife, Sybil?[142] In her study, Church found that many women who become stepmothers have no idea of the complications brought about by such a family.[143]

Although many stepfamilies are harmonious, they can pose problems for a variety of reasons. One reason is that couples who form stepfamilies after a divorce have many problems to solve (e.g., financial problems) even before the new family begins. Another reason is that most of the problems associated with stepfamilies have, at their source, the quality and quantity of changes a child must make in the new family. Adapting to new parents and new siblings may cause confusion and turbulence for a child. Even if the child gets along with the new siblings, he or she may feel in competition with near-strangers for the affection of his or her parent.[144]

Church states that increasing our acceptance of stepfamilies is important. On the positive side, the stepfamily can offer more choice of kin and a greater freedom in defining roles. Church also claims that we can use stepfamilies to assist us in examining some of our unexamined beliefs of how a family should act.[145]

CRITICAL THINKING

What effect does the media have on childrearing practices?

4-1 BONUS SECTION IN CD-ROM

Stepparent Family

In this bonus section on stepparents and the families they suddenly create, you will find further insights regarding this special kind of family. All is not always pleasant. You will read about the stages of fantasy and reality. A table shows the characteristics and tasks in stepfamilies; and you will be able to experience some of the problems that children encounter in stepfamilies.

Another type of family structure has been termed **apartners,** or as some investigators have termed, **"living apart together" (LAT) couples.**[146] *Rather then getting married, a couple, who may have children by a previous marriage, might choose to maintain separate residences, take care of their own children, professional life, and everyday affairs; but they might share special times with each other on a regularly scheduled basis.* Personal time and freedom, coupled with intimacy, are what the participants say they seek. Gay or lesbian couples may also have this arrangement, often because of social constraints rather than choice. It is necessary to point out that this arrangement is not just for young adults who may have children. For older individuals, a LAT arrangement may be an adequate arrangement whereby they can keep their own households, if they wish, and still have the relationship they desire.[147]

Single Person Family

The **single state** (never married, separated, divorced, or widowed) is another family structure. Today in both Canada and the United States more individuals are choosing singlehood than was the case in the past. Society now views being single an option rather than a deviant lifestyle. Some would apply family developmental tasks to this person; however, it is no longer considered necessary to marry and bear children to be fulfilled and accomplished. The following are some advantages of being single:[148,149]

- *Privacy:* Being able to think and create in a peaceful atmosphere without interruption
- *Time:* Being able to travel, cultivate talents and interests, entertain and be entertained, and follow intellectual pursuits
- *Freedom:* Being able to choose and make decisions, form friendships, use time as desired, depend on self, have a healthy narcissism
- *Opportunity:* Being able to extend borders of friendship, develop skills and knowledge, enjoy geographic moves or job mobility and success (e.g., the single person is often preferred for certain jobs or positions)

Many single adults claim that personal freedom is one of the major advantages of being single.[150] Nowadays, in Canada many singles hold values that are more individualistic than family oriented. Such individualistic values may intensify the longer the person remains unmarried. Currently, there seems to be less parental pressure to marry directed toward young sons and daughters, despite the fact that some parents reflect disappointment when intimate relationships do not result in marriage. Middle-aged divorced women who have a flourishing career may tend to look with skepticism at marriage, viewing it as a bad bargain once they have gained financial and sexual independence. One of the greatest challenges encountered by single people is the development of strong social networks to provide positive adjustments and satisfactions.[151]

CRITICAL THINKING

What do you see as the main components of a satisfying single life?

Stepgeneration Parents

The **stepgeneration family** develops when *the next generation (grandparents or great-grandparents) become the parenting people because the mother will not, does not, cannot, or should not care for her offspring.* Many children live in households (sometimes five-generation) that are headed by one or both grandparents or great-grandparents. Circumstances that lead the grandparent generations to provide care for the grandchildren transcend race and economic level and reflect a number of factors that create instability in family life. The elder generation may provide a home to both grandchildren and great-grandchildren and their parent(s) if:

1. The parental generation is unemployed or in financial difficulty.
2. There has been separation, divorce, or death of one of the parents.
3. One or both parents are physically or mentally ill.

4. One or both parents are abusing or addicted to alcohol or drugs.
5. Physical, emotional, or sexual abuse of the child has occurred.
6. One or both parents are imprisoned or have abandoned the child.

How well the situation works depends on the degree of respect, love, and communication shown; how clearly rules are set and enforced in the home; who takes responsibility for child care and home maintenance tasks; and legal and financial problems for the family unit. In a stable home, all generations can benefit from each other and learn to appreciate each other. In a home with conflict, each person may carry scars. Some conflicts will be inevitable as the children and grandparent generations each grow older and have different needs. Yet, the grandparents can have real peace of mind as they realize their contribution to the young ones, which offsets the sense of burden that comes with the tasks of caring for young children. In Canada, several organizations offer assistance to grandparents who are caregivers (see the box entitled "Canadian Organizations for Grandparent Caregivers").[152–154] The real concern is that the grandparents may become ill or die before the child is reared. Most grandparents realize that the physical and emotional care and moral and spiritual guidance they give may prevent the grandchild from repeating the pattern into which the child was born.

Canadian Organizations for Grandparent Caregivers

- Cangrands: http://www.cangrands.com/groups.htm
- Grandparents Support Groups in Canada: http://www.grandparentagain.com/community/support_canada.html

Family Size

Canadians have fewer children now than they did in earlier decades.[155] For example, in the early 20th century women gave birth to an average of 3.5 children; in the latter part of the 20th century the figure was 1.5 children.[156] The portrait of the family taken by the census at the outset of the 21st century indicates a continuation of many changes occurring in the family. The proportion of "traditional" families—dad, mom, and the kids—is continuing to decline, partially as a result of a much lower fertility rate. Regarding same-sex couples, there were more male same-sex couples than female, but more female same-sex couples had children living with them.[157]

The *small family system, with one to three or four children* has the following features:

1. Emphasis is on planning (the number and the frequency of births, the objectives of childrearing, and educational possibilities).
2. Parenthood is intensive rather than extensive (great concern is evidenced from pregnancy through every phase of childrearing for each child).
3. Group actions are usually more democratic.
4. Greater freedom is allowed individual members.[158]

The child or children in the small family usually enjoy advantages beyond those available to children in large families of corresponding economic and social level, including more individual attention. On the other hand, these children may retain emotional dependence on their parents, grow up with extreme pressure for performance, and retain an exaggerated notion of self-importance.

The *large family, generally thought of as one with six or more children,* is not a planned family as a rule. Parenthood is commonly extensive rather than intensive, not because of less love or concern but simply because parents must divide their attention more ways. In the very large family, emphasis is on the group rather than on the individual member. Conformity and cooperation are valued above self-expression. Discipline in the form of numerous and stringent rules frequently is stressed, and there is a high degree of organization in the activities of daily living.

Family Cultural Pattern

The ways of living and thinking that constitute the intimate aspects of family group life constitute the **family cultural pattern.** The family transmits the cultural pattern of its own ethnic background and class to the child, together with the parents' attitudes toward other classes. It becomes the responsibility of the health professional to be aware of their own beliefs and attitudes about families and cultures in order to provide quality care. Dicicco-Bloom and Cohen claim that cultural competence is a significant aspect of health care delivery.[159]

Influence of 20th-Century Changes

Shift from an Agrarian to a Complex Technologic Society
This paradigm shift has produced dramatic changes for the North American family. A greater percentage of children now survive childhood than in 1900, and a higher percentage of mothers survive childbirth. Some marriages occur at an earlier age. Some women marry at a later age than in former generations because they first pursue a career or profession. These young adults believe they can manage both; typically, the husband-to-be encourages the young woman to be as committed to her profession as she is to him. Fewer children are born to most parents, they are spaced closer together, and more first children are born to parents in their late thirties or early forties. There is an increasing number of women who are single mothers by choice, whether they are teenagers or in their late thirties or early forties. Middle-aged couples now typically have more years together after their children are grown and leave home. Because of an increased life expectancy, families now have more living relatives than formerly, especially elderly relatives, for whom the family may have responsibility.

Other Trends Related to Living in a Complex Industrial and Information Society
Families live primarily in urban or metropolitan areas; more families than ever are homeless or at risk for homelessness. More women work outside the home. The woman who formerly stayed home and was the "homemaker" has also gone through several changes. Now modern conveniences make tasks easier. The woman who stays home today concentrates more on "mothering" and she may receive considerable criticism.[160] Her outside activities may include volunteer work so she can control her hours and feel she has prime time at home, yet is also making significant contributions outside the family unit. Or the father may be the house parent because he has an office in the home or is the unemployed member who thereby assumes child and home care responsibilities. Family members are becoming better educated. Family incomes may be unstable; acquisition of personal housing and equipment sought early in the marriage is not always possible. Greater individual freedom exists. Sexual mores are changing, with trial and serial marriages. Value changes and different patterns of living apparently are the norm.

The emphasis on the nuclear family-kinship group has been replaced by acceptance of other types of family forms. Cheal claims that a shift has occurred toward a more diverse family, expanding a sense of individuality and personal autonomy. He claims that post-modernism has had an influence on family life.[161] One such influence can be realized with the study of families regarding their appreciation of pluralism or diversity.[162] Because North Americans are so mobile and are increasingly living in smaller homes or apartments, or in townhouses or condominiums, many ties with kin other than the immediate family are loosened or at least geographically extended. Sometimes close friends become "the family." Yet many North Americans strengthen kinship ties through e-mail, telephone calls, and holiday and vacation visits. Religious influences affect family ties. For example, Jews and European Catholics, with their many family traditions, are generally more embedded in a network of relatives than are white Protestants. The four- and five-generation family and great-grandparent–great-grandchild (as well as grandparent–grandchild) relationships are gaining the attention of researchers.

Yet there are other trends to counter technology, anonymity, the sense of being treated as an impersonal object, and societal and family violence. There is a growing body of knowledge available to parents and to family members, for almost any type of situation. There are more parenting classes. There is more emphasis on the need for tenderness and warmth in relationships and the importance of meeting psychosocial rather than materialistic needs. Promoting the maximum potential of each family member and preventing or breaking the cycle of family abuse and violence are of great concern. Health promotion rather than treatment of illness is considered important socially and economically.

CRITICAL THINKING

In what ways do families address the challenges facing them today?

Rapid Change
Rapid change is a fact of life that families must acknowledge. Medical, pharmacologic, and scientific advances in birth technology and all other areas of health, the increased number of single-parent families, the growing emphasis on the civil and

economic rights of minority groups, and the women's liberation movement are only a part of the cultural expansion of this time. As people live longer, older people will divorce, remarry, or cohabitate. Those who lack healthy emotional roots within their nuclear families, who have few or no kinship ties, who cannot adjust to rapid change, and who have little identity except as defined by job and income are more likely to become depressed, alcoholic, unfaithful to a mate, or divorced.[163,164] Today's changing social environment makes it increasingly difficult for a parent to be certain of his or her identity. How, then, is he or she to provide emotional roots for the child?

Childrearing Practices in Canada and the U.S.

There is no one traditional pattern, only the general concern that children develop "normally." Cham claims that good child care allows for the fact that each family and child is unique. That is, each child and family has their own social, physical, and developmental needs.[165] Parents are encouraged through culture, education, and the mass media to use whatever the dominant childrearing theory is at the time. With each new wave of "knowledge," and through media influence, parents are bombarded by conflicting reports. Often the change in theory application occurs during the same parental generation, so that parents do not trust their own judgment, and considerable inconsistency results. The inconsistency, rather than the theory, probably creates the main problems in childrearing. Sometimes parents strive to avoid rearing their children as they were reared but nevertheless do so unwittingly because of the permanency of enculturation. Children are often given approval and disapproval for their behaviour. Research continues to show that children who experience consistent love, attention, and security will grow up to be adults who can better survive change and stressors, with self-reliance, optimism, and identity intact.[166,167]

Aboriginal cultures in Canada have allocated a significant role to the extended family regarding childrearing. Even if the child's grandparents, or other relatives, do not actively partake in caring for the child, they give advice on the child's welfare.[168] The recent move to Aboriginal self-government has been met by a growing self-respect, and many communities have taken over education and child welfare services.[169]

CRITICAL THINKING

What effects do the media have on childrearing practices?

Father's Role

The father's role is being reconsidered, and he is more active in child care than in the past.[170–174] Still, the mother is primarily responsible for the crying baby and young child care. The infant is often trained in privacy, individualism, and independence by childrearing practices. Fear of "spoiling" the infant if he or she is held too much or responded to spontaneously still exists. Thus the infant may develop behavioural extremes to get needs met.

Daycare centres or babysitters, who are usually not relatives, continue to be important in child care. Daycare centres

provide care for the child, and are a business for the owners.[175] What happens if the mother and parent-surrogate differ greatly about childrearing practices? The child generally acknowledges the authority of parents or at least the mother, but parent-surrogates affect him or her nevertheless. Any adult who is with the child reinforces behaviour in the child that conforms to the adult's own standard of behaviour. The child conforms to the adult's desires to gain approval. If the parent-surrogate acts in a way contrary to the values of the parents, both parents and child probably will be distressed.

Renewed Focus on the Family

Certainly, the health of a nation, and the world, depends on the health of the family. In fact, Health Canada supports Aboriginals in their recognition of children as the nation's most valuable resource.[176] North American adults recognize that family life is difficult to maintain; there is renewed emphasis on making changes. There is more talk about family values, including members of Generation X, many of whom grew up in families of divorce and stepfamilies.[177] The key is for families to make sacrifices in their economic lifestyle to make time for each other and their children. To maintain a marriage and raise children takes much time. Business can promote family values by providing opportunities for flex-time and using the home as the workplace. When it is feasible, and by providing paternity as well as maternity leave, the father who is at home for one or two weeks with the new mother and baby provides necessary nurturing and help with child care and household tasks. There must be more media and cultural emphasis on the real freedom that comes from fulfilling duties to the spouse and our children, rather than from pursuing personal pleasures.[178,179]

It is important to consider the strengths of families in today's society. Schlesinger claims that despite the diversity in the patterns of family development and function, it is possible to define common aspiration, common needs, and common obligations of Canadian families. He goes on to say that it is necessary to understand these common elements that cut across different patterns of family formation and function, if we are to learn how to deal in a constructive manner with that diversity and lend support to the families in Canada.[180]

Family Life Around the World

In the past 20 years, *Britain's* families have struggled with rising rates of divorce, remarriage, lone parenting, mobility, and increasing cohabitation. Often both parents work. In some areas state education begins at age four, but older family members or private institutional care are typically used for young children of working parents. Even afternoon tea, designed for family time, is gradually disappearing. Marriage seminars and literature and films supporting family life are popular as young families work to commit themselves to each other and their children.[181]

In the multicultural society of *Australia,* marriages and children are valued, although families are experiencing an increasing rate of divorce. The impact of divorce is seen in schoolchildren adjusting to visitation rights as well as in participation in church and social life. Teens are becoming more unsettled in behaviour and more Western in appearance. The church has dropped some of the strong moral stands it took in the 1950s and 1960s; religious education in schools has had to fight for existence. Home schooling, typical in the Outback, is increasing in urban areas. Conflicts between generations over the old and new ways are common. Family life in urban areas differs considerably from family life in sparsely settled rural areas, on the huge ranches in the Outback, or for the Aborigines. Yet amidst the harshness of the sunburnt country is seen a gentleness in families.[182]

In *Latin America,* from Mexico to the tip of Chile, a common family characteristic is that the mother is the core of the family. Yet, family life is changing drastically in some countries. For example, in Mexico, there are about 4000 requests for divorce daily; 40% of children live with divorced parents; and 25% of children are raised by single mothers. During the past 15 years, there has been an increasing rate of murder, abortions, suicide, and substance-addicted and runaway youths. There is renewed effort by the government, churches, and educational institutions to emphasize family life.[183]

In *Costa Rica,* a small, democratic Central American country, the economy flourishes, and it offers some of the best health care and educational possibilities in Latin America. Religion is important. The typical Costa Rican family is composed of five to seven members, often including grandparents or other relatives. The father has traditionally been the sole breadwinner while the mother stayed home to care for the children. Urbanization and industrialization, however, are changing the concept of family; there is less emphasis on family relations and more emphasis on employment, even for mothers. Many social problems seen in Canada and the United States are now seen in Costa Rica. There is a new concern about social and family issues and solutions.[184]

In *Italy, Germany,* and *France,* family life is valued. A meal is cooked, not popped in the microwave. The family sits around the dinner table and converses. Young families with children stroll through the park on Sunday afternoon. Attitudes toward childrearing differ from those in North America. Parents motivate children by fear and humiliation, in contrast to encouragement, which is commonly used in North America. As a result, the offspring are more likely to feel insecure and hostile, which can spill over to how they relate to their own family and children. In Western Europe, there is greater emphasis on cohabitation before marriage, more open display of nudity, and declining church attendance. Thus, we see a combination of old customs and new morality, which will influence family development.[185]

In *Russia,* the family is considered the primary unit of society, just as in other countries. Under Communism, other maxims of official propaganda diminished the emphasis on family. Crime rates and unemployment soar; wages are below living minimum. The birth rate is falling as the abortion rate escalates. Often young families live in small apartments with the parents because of the housing shortage. Both parents work because of economic necessity; older members help with child care. Biblical principles have always been present, even under Communism. There are rapid and great social changes now. With the fall of Communism, parents are demonstrating renewed interest in the now available religious books and television programs to help them continue to teach moral principles.[186]

Africa is made up of many countries, cultures, and lifestyles. Traditional culture is family-oriented; the extended family has undergirded tribal society for centuries. In urban areas of South Africa, husbands commute to work, and the materialism and lack of family time seen in Western societies are evident. In the Black townships of South Africa, the legacy of apartheid has split families for generations. Children live with grandparents while parents work the mines in far-off locales. Husbands live in single-sex hostels with minimal facilities. New relationships may be started; families are destroyed. Progress, materialism, high population growth, and the influence of Western culture have precipitated a massive influx of families from the country to the city; three generations are crowded into small living quarters. Because of employment and school conditions, parents and children may see little of each other. In some countries, drought, famine, migrations, and war have disrupted all life patterns and caused massive numbers of deaths, leaving no trace of a family and countless orphaned children or single survivors in a family. Whether families are black, white, or socially mixed, the turbulent political and social issues continue to dominate and affect family life negatively.[187]

In *Japan,* Westernization has taken its toll. An overly efficient, stressful work environment and focus on economic success has had its effect. Fathers may work in a remote location with no opportunity for family life for months at a time. Both husbands and wives are tempted to be unfaithful. Fathers die suddenly in their forties from overwork (*karoshi*). There is renewed emphasis on the family unit, with construction of larger dwelling units so that extended families can live together with less crowding. Employers are beginning to refocus on the value of family and the importance of a male role model in the home for children.[188]

CRITICAL THINKING

In the light of so many languages and cultures in Canada, how can a health professional cope with language differences?

HEALTH CARE AND NURSING APPLICATIONS

The family as the basic unit for the developing person and health cannot be taken for granted. Although family forms have changed and will continue to change, each person, to develop healthfully, needs some intimate surroundings of human concern. "No man is an island."

You will frequently encounter the entire family as your client in the health care system, regardless of the setting. Increasingly, the *emphasis is on health promotion of the family.*[189,190] *You may be asked to do family-centred care, to nurse the client and the family, or to do "family therapy." Yet you will not be able to care for the family even minimally unless you understand the family system and the dynamics of family living presented in this chapter.*

Rapid change, increasing demands on the person, technologic progress, and other trends mentioned seem to isolate people. Many families are not aware of the forces pulling them apart. More than ever, they need one place in their living where they can act without self-consciousness, where the pretences and roles demanded in jobs, school, or social situations can be put aside. The living centre should be a place where communication takes place with ease; where each knows what to expect from the other; where an intimacy exists that is based on nonverbal messages more than verbal; and where a person is accepted for what he or she is. The family may need your help in becoming aware of disruptive forces and maladaptive patterns, and in learning ways to promote an accepting home atmosphere.

Communication and Relationship Principles Basic to Client Care

Communication is the heart of the nursing process and health care, for it is one of the primary methods used to accomplish specific and general goals with many different kinds of people. It is used in assessing and understanding the client and family and in intervention. Communication helps people express thoughts and feelings, clarify problems, receive information, consider alternate ways of coping or adapting, and remain realistic through feedback from the environment. Essentially the client learns something about the self, how to identify health needs, and if and how he or she wishes to meet them.

Analysis of your communication pattern will help you improve your methods. Realize that you cannot become skilled in therapeutic communication without supervised and thoughtful practice. As you talk with another, however, do not get so busy thinking about a list of methods that you forget to focus on the person. Your keen interest in the other person and use of your personal style are essential if you are to be truly effective. To be effective while communicating with the person or family, use simple, clear words geared to the person's intelligence and experience. Develop a well-modulated tone of voice. Be attuned to your nonverbal behaviour. Basic methods for conducting purposeful, helpful communication, along with their rationales, are listed in Table 4-10. These communication methods are used in the interview during assessment, goal setting, and intervention with a family or individual client, well or ill, in any setting. Table 4-11 lists guidelines for an effective interview. Table 4-12 lists barriers to effective communication and interviewing.[191–195]

The quality of any response depends on the degree of mutual trust in the relationship. Techniques can be highly successful, or they can be abused, depending on your attitude at the time, the other person's interpretation, and how they are used. Facilitative techniques are stepping stones to better understanding, an understanding that nurtures the trust, relationship, and expression of feeling. There must be a feeling of caring, or safety and security in your company, and a feeling that you want to help the person help him- or herself. By

---

EVIDENCE-BASED PRACTICE

Symptom Experiences: Perceptual Accuracy between Advanced-Stage Cancer Patients and Family Caregivers in the Home Care Setting

A convenience sample of 98 dyads composed of advanced-stage heterogeneous cancer patients and their caregivers completed the Memorial Symptom Assessment Scale in the home care setting on a one-time basis. This scale is a 32-item Likert-type scale for assessing the presence, frequency, severity, and distress arising from symptoms in cancer patients.

The results showed that:

1. There was a confirmation of trends previously described in related studies where, for example, caregivers tend to overreport on symptom experiences.
2. The degree of absolute difference between patient and caregiver responses was normally around 1 unit (on a theoretical range of 0 to 4 units).
3. Levels of patient–caregiver agreement were better on more concrete questions related to symptom frequency, severity, and distress than on broad questions related to the presence of a symptom.

4. Patients and caregivers achieved better levels of agreement on physical versus psychological symptoms.

Practice Implications

1. Family caregivers can provide reasonable proxy or complementary reports on patient symptom experiences of frequency, severity, and distress.
2. Family caregivers have greater difficulty in achieving high levels of accuracy on psychological versus physical symptoms.
3. For psychological symptoms, health care professionals need to carefully interpret the information provided by family caregivers because the bias to overestimate was more pronounced for ratings on psychological symptoms.
4. It is advisable that professional providers verify caregivers' perceptions on psychological or emotional symptoms by eliciting feedback directly from patients whenever possible.

Source: Lobchuk, M.M., and L.F. Degner, Symptom Experience: Perceptual Accuracy between Advanced-Stage Cancer Patients and Family Caregivers in the Home Care Setting, Journal of Clinical Oncology, *20, no. 16 (2002), 3495–3507. Used with permission.*

TABLE 4-10
Effective Communication Methods and Their Rationale

Communication Method	Rationale
Be accepting in nonverbal and verbal behaviour (does not mean agreement with person's words or behaviour).	All behaviour is motivated and purposeful. Promotes climate in which person feels safe and respected. Indicates that you are following the person's trend of thought and encourages further talking while you remain nonjudgmental.
Use thoughtful silence at intervals, while continuing to look at and focus on person.	Indicates accessibility to mute, withdrawn, or depressed person. Encourages person to talk and set own pace. Gives both you and client time to organize thoughts. Aids consideration of alternate courses of action; provides opportunity for explanation of feelings; gives time for contemplation. Conserves energy and promotes relaxation in physically ill person.
Use "I" and "we" in proper context; **call person by name and title, as preferred.**	Strengthens identity of person in relation to others.
State **open-ended, general, leading statements or questions;** "Tell me about it." "What are you feeling?"	Encourages person to take the initiative in introducing topics and to think through problems. May gain pertinent information that you would not think to ask about because client has freedom to pursue feelings and ideas important to him or her.
Ask **related or peripheral questions** when indicated: "And what else happened?" "You have four children. What are their ages?"	Explores or clarifies pertinent topic. Adds to database. Encourages person to work through larger or related issues and to engage in problem solving. Explores subject in depth without appearing to pry. Helps person see implications, relationships, or consequences. Helps keep communication flowing and person talking.
Encourage description of feelings: "Tell what you feel."	Helps person identify, face, and resolve own feelings. Validates your observation. Deepens your empathy and insight.
Place described events in time sequence: "What happened then?" "What did you do after that?" "And then what?"	Clarifies how event occurred or explains relationships associated with given event. Places event in context or manageable perspective. Helps identify recurrent patterns or difficulties or significant cause–effect relationships.
State your observations about the person: "You appear ...," "I sense that you ...," "I notice that you...."	Acknowledges client's feelings, needs, behaviour, or efforts at a task. Offers content to which person can respond. Encourages comparisons or mutual understanding of client's behaviour. Validates your impressions. Helps person notice own behaviour and its effects; encourages self-awareness. Reinforces behaviour. Adds to person's self-esteem.
State the implied, what client has hinted, or a feeling that you sense may be a consequence of an event.	Expresses acceptability of feeling or idea. Clarifies information. Conveys your attention, interest, and empathy. May be used as subtle form of suggestion for action.
Paraphrase; translate into your own words the feelings, questions, ideas, key words of other person: "I hear you saying ...," "You feel ...."	Indicates careful listening and focus on client. Encourages further talking. Validates and summarizes what you think client has said. Conveys empathy and understanding. Indicates that person's words, ideas, feelings, opinions, or decisions are important. Promotes integration of feelings with content being discussed.
Restate or repeat main idea expressed by client.	Conveys interest and careful listening or desire to clarify a vague point. Helps to reformulate certain statements or to

(continued)

TABLE 4-10 *(continued)*
Effective Communication Methods and Their Rationale

Communication Method	Rationale
	emphasize key words to help client recognize less obvious meanings or associations.
Clarify: "Could you explain that further?" "Explain that to me again."	Indicates interest and desire to understand. Helps the person become clearer to him- or herself. Encourages exploration of subject in depth or of meaning behind what is being said.
Make reflective statement, integrating feelings and content.	Indicates active listening and empathy. Synthesizes your perceptions and provides feedback to client. Shares your perception of congruity between person's statements and other behaviour. Provides client with new ways of considering ideas, behaviour, or a situation. Identifies and encourages understanding of latent meanings.
Suggest collaboration and a cooperative relationship.	Offers to do activities **with, not for or to** person. Encourages person to participate in identifying and appraising problems. Involves person as active partner in care. Tells person you are available and interested. Provides reassurance.
Offer information; self-disclose by sharing own thoughts and feelings briefly, if appropriate.	Makes facts available whenever client needs or asks for them. Builds trust; orients; enables decision making. Reduces client's anxiety, frustration, or other distressing feelings that hinder comfort, recovery, or realistic action. Helps client focus on deeper concerns.
Encourage evaluation of situation.	Helps client appraise quality of his or her experience and consider people and events in relation to own and others' experience and values. Assists person in determining how others affect him or her, and personal effect on others. Promotes understanding of own situation and avoidance of uncritically adopting opinions, values, or behaviour of others.
Encourage formulation of plan of action.	Conveys that person is expected to be active participant in own care. Helps person consider alternate courses of action. Helps person plan how to handle future problems.
Voice doubt; present own perceptions or facts; **suggest alternate line of reasoning:** "What gives you that impression?" "Isn't that unusual?" "I find that hard to believe." Respond to underlying feeling.	Promotes realistic thinking. Helps person consider that others do not perceive events as he or she does nor do they draw the same conclusions. May reinforce doubts person already has about an idea or course of action. Avoids argument. May help to gradually reduce delusion. Conveys acceptance that delusion is the client's reality; acknowledges the communication.
Seek consensual validation of words; give definition or meaning when indicated.	Ensures that words being used mean the same to both you and client. Clarifies ideas for you and client as client defines meaning for self. Avoids misunderstanding. May help to reduce autistic, self-centred thinking.
Summarize; condense what speaker said, using speaker's own words.	Synthesizes and emphasizes important points of dialogue. Helps both you and client leave session with same ideas in mind. Emphasizes progress made toward self-awareness, problem solving, and personal development. Provides sense of closure.

Source: Murray, R., and M. Huelskoetter, Psychiatric/Mental Health Nursing: Giving Emotional Care *(3rd ed.). Norwalk, CT: Appleton & Lange, 1991.*

TABLE 4-11
Guidelines for an Effective Interview

Method	Rationale
1. **Wear clothing that conveys the image of a professional and is appropriate for the situation.** Consider wearing casual clothing without excessive adornment instead of a uniform when working in the school, home, occupational setting, or community clinic.	1. Consider expectations the interviewee may have of you. In some cases he or she will respond more readily to your casual dress; at other times the person may need your professional dress as part of the image to help him or her talk confidentially.
2. **Avoid preconceived ideas, prejudices, or biases.** Avoid imposing personal values on others.	2. Acceptance of client promotes feeling of self-respect and security and promotes more accurate assessment.
3. **Control the external environment** as much as possible. This is sometimes difficult or impossible to do, but try to minimize external distractions or noise, regulate ventilation and lighting, and arrange the setting.	3. Minimize discomfort, external distractions, and sense of distance. Comfort factors show respect to client and promote expression of feelings.
4. **Arrange comfortable positions** for yourself and the client.	4. Full attention can be given to the interview.
5. **Establish rapport.** Create a warm, accepting climate and a feeling of security and confidentiality.	5. The person feels free to talk about what is important to her or him.
6. **Use a vocabulary on the level of awareness or understanding of the person.** Avoid professional jargon or abstract words. **Be precise in what you say.**	6. Convey respect for and respond to the interviewee's level of understanding or health condition. Convey that you want the client to understand the meaning of what you say and that you consider the client as part of the health care team.
7. **Begin by stating and validating with the client the purpose of the interview.** Either you or the interviewee may introduce the theme. You may start the session by briefly expressing friendly interest in the everyday affairs of the person, but avoid continuing trivial conversation. Maintain the proposed structure.	7. The client realizes the importance of the interview and that she or he is taken seriously and will be listened to. Client does not confuse interview with social event.
8. **Say as little as possible to keep the interview moving.** Ask questions that are well-timed, open-ended, and pertinent to the situation.	8. This pattern allows the person to place his or her own style, organization, and personality on the answers and on the interview. Getting unanticipated data can be useful in assessment. Questions that bombard the person produce unreliable information. Open-ended sentences usually keep the person talking at her or his own pace. Careful timing of your messages, verbal and nonverbal, allows time for the interviewee to understand and respond and increases accuracy and meaning of response.
9. **Avoid asking questions in ways that elicit socially acceptable answers.**	9. The interviewee often responds to questions with what he or she thinks the interviewer wants to hear, either to be well thought of, to gain status, or to show that she or he knows what other people do and what is considered socially acceptable.
10. **Ask questions beginning with "What . . . ?" "Who . . . ?" and "When . . . ?"** to gain factual information.	10. Words connoting moral judgments are not conducive to a feeling of neutrality, acceptance, or freedom of expression. The "How" question may be difficult for the person to answer because it asks, "In what manner . . . ?" or "For what reason . . . ?" and the individual may lack sufficient knowledge to answer. The "Why" question asks for insights that the person should not be expected to give.
11. **Be gentle and tactful when asking about home life or personal matters.** If a subject meets resistance, change the topic; when the anxiety is reduced, return to the matter for further discussion. Be alert to what the person omits or avoids, "forgets" to mention, or deliberately refuses to discuss.	11. What you consider common or usual information may be considered very private by some. Matters about which it would be tactless to inquire directly can often be arrived at indirectly by peripheral questions. Remember, what the person does not say is as important as what is said.

(continued)

TABLE 4–11 *(continued)*
Guidelines for an Effective Interview

Method	Rationale
12. **Be an attentive listener.** Show interest by nodding, responding with, "I see," etc. Remain silent and control your responses when another's comments evoke a personal meaning and thus trigger an emotional response in you. While the person is talking, find the nonverbal answers to the following: What does this experience mean? Why is this content being told at this time? What is the meaning of the choice of words, the repetition of key words, the inflection of voice, the hesitant or aggressive expression of words, the topic chosen? Listen for feelings, needs, and goals. Listen for what is not discussed. Do not answer too fast or ask a question too soon. If necessary, learn if the words mean the same to you as to the interviewee. Explore each clue as you let the person tell his or her story.	12. Careful listening conveys respect, promotes self-esteem and a sense of security and safety, and aids assessment. It is an important intervention tool.
13. **Carefully observe nonverbal messages for signs of anxiety, frustration, anger, loneliness, or guilt.** Look for feelings of pressure hidden by the person's attempts to be calm. Encourage the free expression of feelings, for feelings often bring facts with them. Focus on emotionally charged topics when the person is able to share deep feelings.	13. Nonverbal behaviour is often the key to the message and is usually not under the client's voluntary control or in his or her awareness. Nonverbal behaviour often conveys more directly the feelings. Ventilation of feeling is the key resolution of many emotional difficulties and opens the door to new data as well as increased understanding and insight in the client.
14. **Encourage spontaneity.** Provide movement in the interview by picking up verbal leads, clues, bits of seemingly unrelated information, and nonverbal signals from the client. If the person asks you a personal question, redirect it to him or her; it may be the topic he or she unconsciously (or even consciously) wishes to speak about.	14. Movement of the interview gives you understanding about the person, her or his behaviour, needs, health, illness, and relationships. Only occasionally will it be pertinent for you to answer personal questions. Sometimes brief self-disclosure will help the interviewee feel comfortable and elicit additional data. Be sure to disclose such information for the benefit of the client, not yourself.
15. **Indicate when the interview is terminated,** and terminate it graciously if the interviewee does not do so first. Make a transition in interviewing or use a natural stopping point if the problem has been resolved, if the information has been obtained or given, or if the person changes the topic. You may say, "There is one more question I'd like to ask," or "Just two more points I want to clarify," or "Before I leave, do you have any other questions, comments, or ideas to share?"	15. The client feels more secure with structure. Avoid social conversation or a feeling in the client that you lack skill. Skillful and distinct termination prevents you from feeling manipulated by the client's prolonging of the interview.
16. **Keep data obtained in the interview confidential and share this information only with the appropriate and necessary health team members,** leaving out personal assumptions. If you are sharing an opinion or interpretation, state it as such, rather than have it appear to be what the other person said or did. The person should be told what information will be shared and with whom and the reason for sharing.	16. Show respect for the individual. Confidentiality is the client's right and your responsibility.
17. **Evaluate the interview.** Were the purposes accomplished?	17. Evaluate yourself in each situation. Recognize that not everyone can successfully interview everyone. Others may see you differently from the way you see yourself. Validation with someone who is a skilled interviewer is helpful.

Source: Murray, R., and M. Huelskoetter, Psychiatric/Mental Health Nursing: Giving Emotional Care *(3rd ed.). Norwalk, CT: Appleton & Lange, 1991.*

TABLE 4-12
Barriers to Effective Communication

1. Conveying your feelings of anxiety, anger, judgment, blame, ambivalence, condescension, placating approach, denial, isolation, lack of control, or lack of physical or emotional health.

2. The appearance of being too busy, of not having time or desire to listen, of not giving sufficient time for an answer, or of not really wanting to hear.

3. Not paying attention to what is being said verbally and nonverbally; rehearsing what you plan to say as the other is talking; filtering (listening selectively); trying to second-guess the other person (mind-reading); daydreaming while the other talks.

4. Using the wrong vocabulary—vocabulary that is abstract or intangible, or full of jargon, slang, or implied status; talking too much; or using unnecessarily long sentences or words out of context.

5. Failing to understand the reason for the person's reluctance to make a message clear.

6. Making inappropriate use of facts, twisting facts, introducing unrelated information, offering premature interpretation, wrong timing, saying something important when the person is upset or not feeling well and thus unable to hear what is really said.

7. Making glib statements, offering false reassurance by saying, "Everything is OK."

8. Using clichés, stereotyped responses, trite expressions, and empty or patronizing verbalisms stated without thought, such as "It's always worse at night," "I know," "You'll be OK," or "Who is to say?"

9. Expressing unnecessary approval, stating that something the person does or feels is particularly good, implies that the opposite is bad.

10. Expressing undue disapproval, denouncing another's behaviour or ideas, implies that you have the right to pass judgment, and that he or she must please you.

11. Giving advice; stating personal experiences, opinions, or value judgments; giving pep talks; telling another what should be done.

12. Requiring explanations, demanding proof, challenging or asking "Why . . . ?" when the person cannot provide a reason for thoughts, feelings, and behaviour and for events.

13. Belittling the person's feelings (equating intense and overwhelming feelings expressed by the client with those felt by everyone or yourself) implies that such feelings are not valid; that he or she is bad; or that the discomfort is mild, temporary, unimportant.

Source: Murray, R., and M. Huelskoetter, Psychiatric/Mental Health Nursing: Giving Emotional Care *(3rd ed.). Norwalk, CT: Appleton & Lange, 1991.*

using therapeutic principles, you will help the person and family identify you as someone to whom ideas and feelings can be safely and productively revealed.

CRITICAL THINKING

When you have experienced family problems, what methods have you tried to resolve them?

You may find the following *guidelines helpful in evaluating your communication methods.* Do you:

- Examine the purpose of your communications?
- Consider the total physical and human setting?
- Plan your communication, clarifying ideas and seeking consultation?
- Analyze the methods used and their effectiveness?
- Identify hidden meanings as well as the basic content of the message you conveyed?
- Support communication with actions?
- Follow up communication to determine if your purpose was accomplished?

The **therapeutic or helping relationship or alliance,** or therapeutic nurse–client relationship, is a *purposeful interaction over time between an authority in health care and a person, family, or group with health care needs, with the focus on needs of the client, being empathic, and using knowledge.* The therapeutic relationship/alliance must be differentiated from mere association. Social contact with another individual, verbal or nonverbal, may exercise some influence on one of the participants and needs may be met. But inconsistency, nonpredictability, or partial fulfillment of expectations often results. *Characteristics of social relationships, which are not helpful between therapists and clients, are as follows:*

- The contact is primarily for pleasure and companionship.
- Neither person is in a position of responsibility for helping the other.
- No specific skill or knowledge is required.
- The interaction is between peers, often of the same social status.
- The people involved can, and often do, pursue an encounter for the satisfaction of personal or selfish interests.
- There is no explicit formulation of goals.
- There is no sense of accountability for the other person.
- Evaluation of interactions does not concern personal effectiveness in the interaction.

Phases of the therapeutic relationship/alliance were first researched and formulated by a nurse, Hildegard Peplau.[196] The phases are: (1) orientation, establishment, or initial phase, (2) identification phase, (3) working or exploitation phase, and (4) termination or resolution phase. Certain behaviours and feelings, for both the nurse/helper and client/patient are typical of these phases (Table 4-13). Because of the nature of mutual participation in a therapeutic relationship, mutual behaviours are also noted in Table 4-13.[197–201]

TABLE 4-13
Phases of the Helping Relationship

Orientation Phase (Problem-defining phase)

Nurse Behaviours

- Initiates interaction:
  - Introduces self
  - Meets client as a stranger
  - Knows client from prior admission/contact
  - Listens to client's/family's perception of problem or expectations
  - Responds to client's expressed need or emergency
  - Establishes rapport with client
  - Demonstrates acceptance
  - Explains own role to person/family
- Establishes contract (verbal or written):
  - Explains nature of relationship
  - Schedules time, duration, and place of interview
  - Discusses goals of relationship/expectations of relationship
  - Explains commitment of nurse to client
  - Discusses issues of confidentiality
  - Discusses parameters of relationship and termination
  - Gathers information from person or family
  - Becomes better acquainted with person/family
- Collaborates with patient to analyze situation and establish goals:
  - Validates whether care plan matches client's impression of problem
  - Focuses client's energy on the task/responsibilities to be accomplished
  - Acts as a resource to person and/or family
  - Refers person and/or family to services within the agency
  - Continues assessment
- Demonstrates therapeutic emotional response:
  - Demonstrates empathy
  - Demonstrates unconditional positive regard
  - Demonstrates trustworthiness to client
  - Examines own thoughts, feelings, expectations, and actions

- Describes and clarifies personal attitudes about caring for client
- Describes and clarifies client's reactions to nurse
- Identifies person's transference and own countertransference feelings and behaviours
- Demonstrates ability to control countertransference behaviour
- Reduces anxiety/tension in the relationship through use of communication and relationship principles

Patient/Client Behaviours

- Meets nurse as a stranger
- Describes perceived need(s)
- Unable to identify need for assistance
- Seeks assistance
- Describes expectations of nurse and/or reactions based on experiences
- Asks questions about role, care plan, agency
- Tests parameters of relationship with a variety of behaviours or questions
- Demonstrates comfort with nurse
- Responds to trust demonstrated by nurse behaviour
- Demonstrates trust in the nurse
- Settles into helping environment
- Identifies specific problems to be explored within context of relationship (indicates end of phase)

Mutual Behaviours

- Identify and define existing problems
- Clarify facts
- Make decisions about assistance needed
- Develop goals and care plan
- Validate that implementation of a care plan meets expectations

Identification Phase

Nurse Behaviours

- Promotes sense of security in person/family
- Continues assessment; becomes better acquainted with client
- Listens attentively and on deeper level
- Discusses confidentiality issues with person/family
- Provides opportunities for increasing self-care and independence in client and decreasing helplessness
- Continues interventions as indicated
- Provides suggestions, information, and educational materials
- Provides experiences for client to release anxiety and tension feelings
- Assists client to focus on goals, coping with problems, and treatment

- Demonstrates therapeutic emotional response:
  - Demonstrates deeper level of empathy
  - Demonstrates unconditional acceptance
  - Maintains separate identity
  - Identifies patient's transference and own countertransference feelings/behaviour
  - Demonstrates ability to control countertransference behaviour
  - Identifies discomfort with patient's dependency on nurse
  - Accepts patient's dependency behaviour

(continued)

TABLE 4-13 *(continued)*
Phases of the Helping Relationship

Patient/Client Behaviours

- ❑ Responds selectively to nurse who is perceived as most helpful:
  - ❑ Describes nurse as significant, own nurse, or capabilities of nurse
  - ❑ Imitates selected nurse's behaviours, behavioural or verbal patterns
  - ❑ Describes or demonstrates positive transference feelings/behaviour
  - ❑ Demonstrates dependency on and identification with nurse
- ❑ Participates in clarifying problem(s)
- ❑ Demonstrates diminishing testing behaviour
- ❑ Responds to nurse's care, interventions
  - ❑ Follows nurse's suggestions, teaching
  - ❑ Works closely (participates) with nurse in interventions
  - ❑ Demonstrates increased attention to goals or treatment tasks
- ❑ Maintains continuity between sessions by following assignments, tasks, attending to process

- ❑ Describes understanding of purpose of interview sessions
- ❑ Changes appearance, self-care behaviour in a positive direction
- ❑ Discloses and explores deeper feelings, more intimate behaviour, or information about self/family:
  - ❑ Describes feeling of belonging in care setting
  - ❑ Describes diminishing feelings of helplessness and hopelessness
  - ❑ Describes increasing self-esteem and optimism about ability to deal with problems

Mutual Behaviours

- ❑ Explore mutually deeper feelings, needs, and goals
- ❑ Describe feelings of trust in each other
- ❑ Move emotionally closer to each other
- ❑ Clarify each other's perceptions and expectations, depending on past experiences
- ❑ Continue development of care plan

Working Phase

Nurse Behaviours

- ❑ Continues assessment:
  - ❑ Encourages client to express feelings and thoughts
  - ❑ Gains deeper understanding of person/family
  - ❑ Listens carefully; client does more talking than nurse
  - ❑ Evaluates problems and goals and redefines as necessary
- ❑ Helps client overcome resistance to change
- ❑ Assists client, as necessary, with tasks and meeting goals
- ❑ Intervenes, using communication principles:
  - ❑ Offers support, as patient works on problems at his or her own pace
  - ❑ Reflects and gives feedback to client
  - ❑ Explores areas of client's life that cause problems, underlying needs, and dysfunctional behaviour patterns
  - ❑ Confronts incongruities in client's verbal and nonverbal behaviour and life patterns in a way that does not threaten client
  - ❑ Explores possible causes for client's behaviour
  - ❑ Clarifies possible solutions, resources, options with client
  - ❑ Discusses the meaning of changes in client's behaviour
  - ❑ Interprets meaning of client's behaviour in a way that client can accept and use the information to change behaviour, gain new self-view
- ❑ Promotes client's development: emotional, interpersonal, and behavioural:
  - ❑ Assists client in developing healthy methods to reduce anxiety
  - ❑ Provides opportunities for client to become more independent and interdependent

- ❑ Facilitates behavioural change in person/family
- ❑ Deals with particular behaviour that is presented by the person/family
- ❑ Deals with therapeutic impasse when it occurs
- ❑ Discusses strengths and positive factors in person/family
- ❑ Supports, instils optimism, conveys hope, and reinforces positive directions in client's behaviour
- ❑ Teaches client as needs emerge, pertinent to life situation and illness:
  - ❑ Teaches effective interpersonal behaviour patterns
  - ❑ Teaches problem-solving skills
  - ❑ Teaches about medication regimen and other aspects of illness/treatment
  - ❑ Accepts that client may not follow nurse's suggestions/teaching
- ❑ Discusses approaching discharge and rehabilitation plans:
  - ❑ Initiates discharge and rehabilitation plans and specific measures
  - ❑ Involves family in treatment and rehabilitation
  - ❑ Teaches patient's family about their role in rehabilitation and recovery of patient
  - ❑ Accepts that patient's family may not consider or follow nurse's suggestions or teaching
- ❑ Demonstrates therapeutic emotional response:
  - ❑ Demonstrates deeper empathy
  - ❑ Continues to convey attitudes of acceptance, concern, and trust
  - ❑ Controls countertransference feelings

(continued)

TABLE 4-13 *(continued)*
Phases of the Helping Relationship

Patient/Client Behaviours

- ❑ Maintains relationship with nurse
- ❑ Describes feelings of trust in and acceptance by nurse
- ❑ Fluctuates between dependency and independency
- ❑ Demonstrates increasing ability to establish own goals:
  - ❑ Demonstrates increasing assertiveness and self-reliance in self-care and goal attainment
  - ❑ Insists on doing tasks in his or her own way
  - ❑ Appears manipulative at times
  - ❑ Demonstrates attention-seeking and self-centred behaviour at times
- ❑ Participates increasingly in decision making about own welfare, treatment, rehabilitation, and post-discharge plans
- ❑ Demonstrates progressive responsibility for self, self-reliance, and independence
- ❑ Utilizes services and resources offered by the nurse and health team that meet his or her needs:
  - ❑ Makes demands on nurse and other health care members
  - ❑ Pursues helpful resources
  - ❑ Demonstrates taking advantage of all available resources, based on personal needs and interests
  - ❑ Carries out assignments between sessions
- ❑ Demonstrates increasingly more open and effective communication skills:
  - ❑ Describes willingness to accept help while recognizing own strengths, abilities, and limits
  - ❑ Describes sense of hope and self-confidence about own potential
  - ❑ Discusses belief that what is explored in sessions can be applied to life situations
- ❑ Considers, integrates, and acts on interpretations given by nurse
- ❑ Describes feeling of being integral part of helping environment
- ❑ Describes some control over situation as services are given by others
- ❑ Describes a progressively developing sense of identity
- ❑ Demonstrates increasingly the signs of physical and emotional health or a higher level of functioning:
  - ❑ Demonstrates increasing ability to cope with situations
  - ❑ Functions optimally in more situations
  - ❑ Demonstrates increasing self-initiation and self-direction in behaviour
  - ❑ Demonstrates increasing skills in interpersonal relationships and problem-solving
  - ❑ Changes behaviour patterns with significant people in a positive direction
  - ❑ Demonstrates sources of inner strength or new problems as new problems or challenges arise
  - ❑ Describes feelings of wellness and readiness for approaching discharge

Mutual Behaviours

- ❑ Examine together the relationship and its meaning
- ❑ Collaborate as partners in meeting health care goals
- ❑ Utilize multidisciplinary team members in various facets of intervention and rehabilitation plans
- ❑ Demonstrate progression toward resolution/termination phase
- ❑ Formulate discharge and rehabilitation plans/goals

Termination Phase

Nurse Behaviours

- ❑ Continues to demonstrate empathy and caring for the client
- ❑ Sustains relationship as long as client demonstrates need
- ❑ Plans for discharge and termination of relationship with client:
  - ❑ Validates client's strengths and progressively positive coping mechanisms
  - ❑ Explores impending separation and discharge
  - ❑ Discusses anticipation of client developing and maintaining new relationships
  - ❑ Shares feelings about separation and termination in an appropriate way with person/family
- ❑ Teaches measures to help person prevent further illness and maintain self-care
- ❑ Promotes interaction between person and family
- ❑ Discusses community resources or networks that could be utilized by person/family

- ❑ Resolves feelings of separation, guilt, or uncertainty related to client's progress or ability to function, misplaced sense of responsibility, countertransference

Patient/Client Behaviours

- ❑ Demonstrates fewer or diminished symptoms
- ❑ Demonstrates defensive manoeuvres that are meant to delay discharge and termination:
  - ❑ Does not keep interview appointments
  - ❑ Is sarcastic or hostile to nurse
  - ❑ Accuses nurse of using client as a guinea pig to deflect awakening pain of past separations
  - ❑ Denies relationship had any impact
  - ❑ Demonstrates regressive behaviour
  - ❑ Demonstrates increasing dependency
  - ❑ Describes lack of confidence in ability to manage post-discharge

(continued)

TABLE 4-13 *(continued)*
Phases of the Helping Relationship

❑ Describes feelings of being pushed out by nurse or health care system	**Mutual Behaviours**
❑ Does not meet nurse at final established session	❑ Discuss what was accomplished in therapy, goals set and accomplished
❑ Demonstrates or describes that needs have been met and goals accomplished:	❑ Examine uncertainty about patient's ability to manage after discharge
❑ Demonstrates improved social functioning	❑ Explore resolution of illness and treatment
❑ Demonstrates being independent of helping person	❑ Plan together how the client will continue to interact and manage life's patterns and stresses
❑ Explores feelings about impending separation and discharge:	❑ Utilize community resources as necessary
❑ Explores past unresolved separations	❑ Discuss feelings to each other about separation
❑ Describes feelings about being cared for and cared about	❑ Resolve issue of gift giving if client gives gift to nurse
❑ Indicates verbally and/or behaviourally that he or she is ready for discharge:	❑ Resolve mourning process that is part of separation and termination
❑ Demonstrates more adaptive mechanisms of behaviour	❑ Demonstrate more mature behaviour as result of relationship
❑ Describes increased self-esteem, self-confidence, and significance to others	❑ Terminate relationship; links are dissolved, each feeling other phases has been successfully completed
❑ Describes hope for the future	
❑ Demonstrates or describes an integration of behaviour and ability to live independently	
❑ Maintains behavioural and communication changes	

The relationship will be therapeutic when the nurse or helper uses a *caring, client-centred approach.* Establishing and maintaining a relationship or counselling another does not involve putting on a façade of behaviour to match a list of characteristics. Rather, both you and the client will change and continue to mature. As the helper, you are present as a total person, blending potentials, talents, and skills while assisting the client to come to grips with needs, conflicts, and yourself. The capacity to be a helping person is strengthened by a genuine desire to be responsible and sensitive to another person. In addition, experience with a variety of people will increase your awareness of others' reactions and feelings, and the feedback you receive from others will teach you a great deal on both the emotional and cognitive levels.

Characteristics of a helping person in a humanistic approach with a client are described in Table 4-14.[202,203] These characteristics were first combined into a total approach by Carl Rogers, and they are considered basic to a professional therapeutic relationship or alliance, and to any counselling or educational role.

Your use of therapeutic communication and a client-centred approach will move you through the relationship with a family or individual. However, *certain constraints* may be experienced if you are not careful about your feelings and behaviours. Table 4-15 describes constraints or problems commonly encountered as you work closely with a family member or unit.[204–208]

Family Assessment

In doing a family assessment, ask questions related to family structure and develop a **genogram,** *a diagram of family members*

and their characteristics and processes[209] (Figure 4–1, page 174). Also, determine communication patterns and relationships, family health, access to health care, occupational demands and hazards, religious beliefs and practices, childrearing practices, participation in the community, and support systems. When you work with the family unit, the information in Figure 4–2 (page 175) will help you assess the family's lifestyle and needs. Other criteria are listed in the box entitled "Criteria for Assessing Healthy Families" (page 176).

The Calgary Family Assessment Model (CFAM) developed by Wright and Leahey is a multidimensional model that incorporates developmental, structural, and functional theory and is based on systems—communication, cybernetics, change theory foundation, as well as postmodernism and biology of cognition. Wright and Leahey claim that CFAM consists of three major categories of structure, development, and function. Further, each category comprises several subcategories and the nurse decides which subcategories should be included in the assessment of the family (see Figure 4–3, page 177).

CRITICAL THINKING

In what way are you able to obtain data regarding a family's emotional communication?

Formulation of Nursing Diagnoses

In a general hospital setting, where you are including the family unit as part of your care of the client, your nursing diagnoses may be general, or family issues may be included in the client's nursing diagnoses. For example, you may state your nursing diagnoses as follows:

■ Anxiety in client related to lack of family contact

TABLE 4-14
Characteristics of a Helping Relationship

Respectful: Feeling and communicating an attitude of seeing the client as a unique human being, filled with dignity, worth, and strengths, regardless of outward appearance or behaviour; being willing to *work* at communicating with and understanding the client because he or she is in need of emotional care

Genuine: Communicating spontaneously, yet tactfully, what is felt and thought, with proper timing and without disturbing the client, rather than using professional jargon, façade, or rigid counsellor or nurse role behaviours

Attentive: Conveying an active listening to verbal and nonverbal messages and an attitude of working with the person

Accepting: Conveying that the person does not have to put on a façade and that the person will not shock you with his or her statements; enabling the client to change at his or her own pace; acknowledging personal and client's feelings aroused in the encounter; to "be for" the client in a nonsentimental, caring way

Positive: Showing warmth, caring, respect, and agape love; being able to reinforce the client for what he or she does well

Strong: Maintaining a separate identity from the client; withstanding the testing

Secure: Permitting the client to remain separate and unique; respecting his or her needs and your own; feeling safe as the client moves emotionally close; feeling no need to exploit the other person

Knowledgeable: Having an expertise based on study, experience, and supervision

Sensitive: Being perceptive to feelings; avoiding threatening behaviour, responding to cultural values, customs, norms as they affect behaviour; using knowledge that is pertinent to the client's situation, being kind and gentle

Empathic: Looking at the client's world from his or her viewpoint; being open to his or her values, feelings, beliefs, and verbal statements; stating your understanding of his or her verbal or nonverbal expressions of feelings and experiences

Nonjudgemental: Refraining from evaluating the client moralistically, or telling the client what to do

Congruent: Being natural, relaxed, honest, trustworthy, and dependable, and demonstrating consistency in behaviour and between verbal and nonverbal messages

Unambiguous: Avoiding contradictory messages

Creative: Viewing the client as a person in the process of becoming, not being bound by the past, and viewing yourself in the process of becoming or maturing

Source: Murray, R., and M. Huelskoetter, Psychiatric/Mental Health Nursing: Giving Emotional Care (3rd ed.). Norwalk, CT: Appleton & Lange, 1991.

- Family's denial of client's disease and of need for special diet and hygiene measures related to lack of understanding on the part of the family

Examples of a nursing diagnosis may be derived from some of the material presented earlier in the chapter. Using family systems theory, you may state your nursing diagnoses in the following manner:

- Family system insufficiently open to internal (or external) environment; related to inability of members to express feelings (or impaired ability to interact with neighbours)
- Impaired communication processes in family system that are related to power struggles
- Family goals and functions are unmet; related to disorganized lifestyle patterns of members
- Dysfunctional family system; related to limited communication between family members, including extended family

Or you may state your nursing diagnoses as follows:

- Impairment in fulfilling family functions and activities related to inadequate material resources
- Impaired intrafamily interactions and lack of communication related to abusive behaviour between spouses
- Disruptive family interpersonal relationships related to power conflicts and lack of closeness

Using a genogram, you may state your nursing diagnoses as follows:

- Altered family relationships related to mourning of death of parent (or divorce, remarriage, or coalitions between stepchildren against wife, children, or death of another family member)
- Unachieved family goals related to inability of family to use environmental resources

TABLE 4-15
Constraints in the Helping Relationship

- **Certain limits exist for you, the helper, and for the client. Relationship means involvement and commitment;** it takes time. The client's dependency may create demands for extra time or responsibility. You will have to consider feelings and needs, meet important demands, and set limits whenever necessary.
- **The client may not be willing to change sufficiently to resolve the problem.** The person may not be able to give up his or her discomforts because these may be a core part of his or her identity.
- **As the helper, you may experience the phenomenon of countertransference**—*an unconscious, inappropriate emotional response to the client as if he or she were an important figure in your life, or unconsciously based in past unresolved experiences with key people in your life.* The helpful measure in this situation would be to respond to the client realistically as he or she really is. Countertransference works in much the same ways as transference does for the client. You relate to the client based on your feelings toward someone from the past.

If you are *experiencing countertransference*, you may have *any of the following reactions.*

1. Overidentify with the client; you exert pressure on the person to act a certain way or to improve.
2. Attempt to make the person over in your own image.
3. Invite gifts or favours, dependence on the client's praise or affection.
4. Offer excessive reassurance or help that is not really necessary.
5. Feel a need to impress the client.
6. Wish to be the client's child, grandchild, or younger sibling may occur with older people, especially if they actually resemble your parents, grandparents, or siblings.
7. Realize thoughts wander from the client, or the client's words trigger unrelated thoughts.
8. Focus repetitively on one aspect or way of looking at the person's behaviour or statements. Be attentive to the client's verbal and nonverbal behaviour.
9. Defend interactions with the patient to others. Ignore behaviour; show lack of objectivity about the behaviour, or focus on one aspect of behaviour.
10. Be impatient with or have guilt about the client's lack of progress, insensitivity to or lack of empathy for his/her needs, or feelings of being unable to help.

11. Experience conflicting feelings of intense affection, dislike, defensiveness, indifference, fear, or angry sympathy with the person.
12. Feel overconcern about the person between sessions or have an overemotional reaction to the client's troubles, believing no one else can care for the person as well as you can.
13. Experience sexual or aggressive fantasies about the client.
14. Experience dreams about the client; be preoccupied with the client when awake.

Countertransference can be overcome through guidance from a supervisor and a willingness to examine your personal behaviour and comments.

- **You may feel anger toward the client.** Your anger may be a reaction to his or her overt behaviour and your fear of acting that way. Your anger may be a counterreaction to the client's anger that is related to something else but is directed toward you. You can stop the cycle by recognizing your own feelings as well as the helplessness felt by the client, by talking with him or her to determine possible sources of anger, and by avoiding either a hostile or too sweet response. Do not joke about anger in yourself or the client and do not reject or punish the client for anger. Make sure that you are not the cause of anger because of actions that demean, aggravate, or neglect him or her. If the person arouses anger in you, seek help from a skilled colleague to work through possible reasons for your anger, to talk about how you demonstrate anger in your behaviour, and to explore how to handle such feelings.
- **You may think you are the only person who can care for the client** or that you can solve all of the problems. Such a feeling of omnipotence is unfounded.
- **You may have difficulty with dependence and independence within a relationship.** You may want to have others depend on you. Therefore, you do things for the client that he or she can do. Such smothering discourages independent behaviour. On the other hand, you may not be able to tolerate the person's dependency, clinging, helplessness, or need for total assistance. Seek help to work through your own feelings.
- **If you joke or tease in a harsh or belittling manner, if you use jestful sarcasm, if you laugh at the client's appearance or behaviour, if you play childish games to get him or her to cooperate or be pleasant, or if you use her or him as a scapegoat,** you will be the cause of the client's anger, hate, despair, hopelessness, and finally complete withdrawal and regression.

You will think of other ways to formulate nursing diagnoses so that the statements are meaningful to you and to other nurses. Refer also to the box entitled "Selected Nursing Diagnoses Related to Family Nursing" (page 178) for other statements of nursing diagnoses that may apply to the family.

It is essential to note that every family has strengths and weaknesses. Family strengths are the cornerstone that assists the family to cope with times of transition and change.[210] In the literature, common threads in healthy families seem to be open communication, an environment that nurtures and

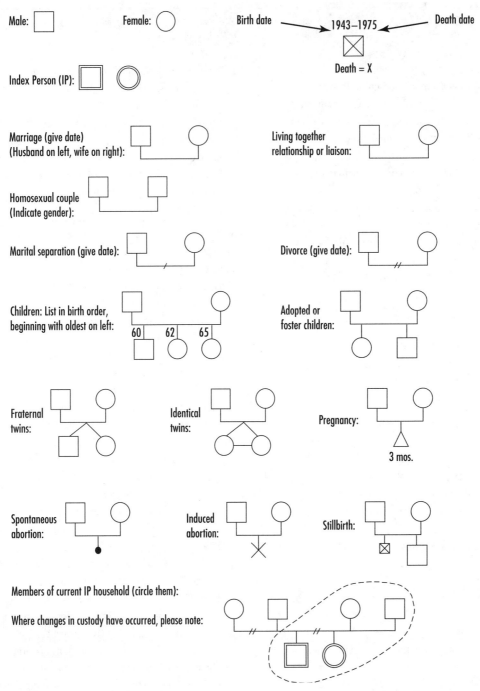

FIGURE 4–1

Genogram format. Symbols to describe basic family membership and structure (include on genogram significant others who lived with or cared for family members; place them on the right side of the genogram with a notation about who they are). Religion, education, or ethnic origin can be written in by oldest generation or other units. Health problems are noted by person.

sustains individual family members as well as the family unit, specific yet flexible definition of roles, and ability to express warmth, intimacy, and humour.[211] Several wellness diagnoses that would reflect family strengths include:

- Progressive sharing by family members of thoughts, feelings, and perceptions
- Analyzing issues together and mutual problem solving that recognizes individual and family needs
- Mutual love, trust, and respect for all family members[212]

CRITICAL THINKING

In what ways can you develop insight into a family's strengths in order to develop a wellness diagnosis?

Formulation of Goals and a Plan of Care

The primary *goal* in working with families is to use yourself and your assessment in a way that allows the family to (1) bring issues into the open, (2) gain a new awareness, (3) learn new

Meeting of Physical, Emotional, and Spiritual Needs of Members
- Ability to provide food and shelter
  Space management as regards living, sleeping, recreation, privacy
  Crowding if over 1.5 persons per room
  Territoriality or control of each member over lifespace
  Access to laundry, grocery, recreation facilities
  Sanitation including disposal methods, source of water supply, control
    of rodents and insects
  Storage and refrigeration
  Available food supply
  Food preparation, including preserving and cooking methods,
    (stove, hotplate, oven)
  Use of food stamps and donated foods as well as eligibility for
    food stamps
  Education of each member as to food composition, balanced
    menus, special preparations or diets if required for a specific
    member
- Access to health care
  Regularity of health care
  Continuity of caregivers
  Closeness of facility and means of access such as car, bus, cab
  Access to helpful neighbours
  Access to phone
- Family health
  Longevity
  Major or chronic illnesses
  Familial or hereditary illnesses such as rheumatic fever, gout, allergy,
    tuberculosis, renal disease, diabetes mellitus, cancer, emotional illness,
    epilepsy, migraine, other nervous disorders, hypertension, blood diseases,
    obesity, frequent accidents, drug intake, pica
  Emotional or stress-related illnesses
  Pollutants that members are chronically exposed to such as air, water,
    soil, noise, or chemicals that are unsafe
- Neighbourhood pride and loyalty
- Job access, energy output, shift changes
- Sensitivity, warmth, understanding between family members
  Demonstration of emotion
  Enjoyment of sexual relations
    Male: Impotence, premature or retarded ejaculation, hypersexuality
    Female: Frigidity (inability to achieve orgasm), enjoyment of sexual
      relations, feelings of disgust, shame, self-devaluation; fear of injury,
      painful coitus
    Menstrual history, including onset, duration, flow, missed periods and
      life situation at the time, pain, euphoria, depression, other difficulties
- Sharing of religious beliefs, values, doubts
  Formal membership in church and organizations
  Ethical framework and honesty
  Adaptability, response to reality
  Satisfaction with life
  Self-esteem

Childrearing Practices and Discipline
- Mutual responsibility
  Joint parenting
  Mutual respect for decision making
  Means of discipline and consistency
- Respect for individuality
- Fostering of self-discipline
- Attitudes toward education, reading, scholarly pursuit
- Attitudes toward imaginative play
- Attitudes toward involvement in sports
- Promotion of gender stereotypes

Communication
- Expression of a wide range of emotion and feeling
- Expression of ideas, concepts, beliefs, values, interests
- Openness
- Verbal expression and sensitive listening
- Consensual decision making

Support, Security, Encouragement
- Balance in activity
- Humour
- Dependency and dominance patterns
- Life support groups of each member
- Social relationship of couple: go out together or separately; change
    since marriage mutually satisfying; effect of sociability
    patterns on children

**Growth-Producing Relationships and Experiences within and
without the Family**
- Creative play activities
- Planned growth experiences
- Focus of life and activity of each member
- Friendships

Responsible Community Relationships
- Organizations, including involvement, membership, active participation
- Knowledge of and friendship with neighbours

Growing with and through Children
- Hope and plans for children
- Emulation of own parents and its influence on relationship with children
- Relationship patterns: authoritarian, patriarchal, matriarchal
- Necessity to relive (make up for) own childhood through children

Unity, Loyalty, and Cooperation
Positive interacting of members toward each other

Self-Help and Acceptance of Outside Help in Family Crisis

FIGURE 4–2

Family assessment tool.

ways to facilitate balance in the family system, and (4) fulfill family functions in more healthful ways. Having diagnosed a dysfunctional pattern within a family system, your specific goal in conjunction with the family is to determine what changes can be effected to create a more constructive pattern.

Short-term goals could be stated as follows:

- Family system will convey support to the ill member through daily visits and empathic conversation.

Criteria for Assessing Healthy Families

- Ability to provide for the physical, emotional, social, and spiritual needs of the family
- Ability to be sensitive to the needs of family members
- Ability to listen and communicate effectively
- Ability to provide trust, support, security, affirmation, and encouragement
- Ability to initiate and maintain growth-producing relationships and experiences inside and outside the family
- Demonstration of mutual respect for family and others
- Commitment to teach and demonstrate moral code
- Concern for family unity, loyalty, and interfamily cooperation
- Capacity to use humour and to share leisure time with each other, to enjoy each other
- Commitment to strong sense of family where rituals and traditions abound
- Ability to perform roles flexibly and share responsibility
- Ability to maintain balance of interaction and privacy among the members
- Ability for self-help and helping other family members, when appropriate
- Ability to use crisis or seemingly injurious experience as a means of growth
- Ability to grow with and through children
- Capacity to maintain and create constructive and responsible community relationships in the neighbourhood, school, town, and local and provincial/state governments and to value service to others.

Sources: Friedman, M., Bowden, V., and Jones, E. Family Nursing: Research, Theory and Family Practice (5th Ed.). Upper Saddle River: Prentice Hall, 2003; and Mellott, R., Enhancing Intimacy, Boulder, CO: Career Track, 1994.

- Family members will be able to describe special dietary needs and other self-care measures essential to client recovery.
- Family member (specific person) will demonstrate correct techniques for rehabilitative care of client.
- Family members will admit each person's contribution to disruptive communication and lifestyle patterns.
- Family members will formulate a contract for 20 minutes of conversation each day, during which feelings can be expressed honestly and without argument (e.g., fear, blame, scapegoating, and derision).
- Husband and wife will discuss dominance and submission patterns and ways to share in decision making.
- Family system will use a community agency (name specific one) as a support while adjusting to changes produced by (a specific family problem).

Long-term goals are appropriate if you will be working with a family over time. Such goals could include the following.

- Family system will accurately identify key issues that contribute to hostile communication and withdrawal of members from participation in family life.
- Family members will practise daily (for an increasing amount of time) communication methods that promote cohesion.

- Parents will discuss and adhere consistently to effective disciplinary measures for children.
- Nuclear family will re-establish harmonious relationships with extended family.
- Spouse will be less authoritarian in interactions with partner and children.
- Husband and wife will contribute toward completion of daily activities related to homemaking, instead of using illness to escape these family functions.
- Husband will avoid seductive behaviour toward his daughter and relate affectionately toward his wife.

You will write goals specific to the family systems with which you are working. Perhaps the examples given will stimulate your thinking.

Intervention

You can help families understand some processes and dynamics underlying interaction so that they, in turn, learn to respect the uniqueness of the self and of each other. Certainly members in the family need not always agree with each other. Instead, they can learn to listen to the other person about how he or she feels and why, accepting each person's impression as real for self. This attitude becomes the basis for mutual respect, honest communication, encouragement of individual fulfillment, and freedom to be. There is then no need to prove or defend the self.

Once the attitude "we are all important people in this family" is established, conflicts can be dealt with openly and constructively. Name calling and belittling are out of place. Families need to structure time together; otherwise individual schedules will allow them less and less time to meet. Parents need to send consistent messages to their children. To say "don't smoke" while immediately lighting a cigarette is hardly effective.

Times of communication are especially necessary when children are feeling peer pressure; children, moreover, should be praised for what they do right rather than reprimanded for what they do wrong. Children need structure but should be told the reason for the structure if they are old enough to comprehend. As you help the family achieve positive feelings toward and with each other, you are also helping them to fulfill their tasks, roles, and functions. Review the adaptive mechanisms of families described in this chapter.

The Calgary Family Intervention Model (CFIM) highlights three types of family interventions that focus on cognitive, affective, and behavioural levels of family functioning and involve teaching and counselling.[213] For example, family nursing interventions focusing on the cognitive level intend to provide the family with fresh ideas about how family members communicate with each other.[214] The choice of interventions utilized depends on how the family perceives the issue at hand, and interventions should be developed to address the family's perception and beliefs in relation to issues of how members interact with one another.[215]

CRITICAL THINKING

What interventions can you develop to change a family's affective domain of functioning?

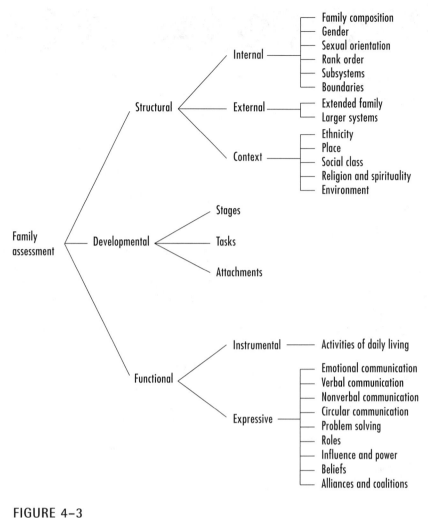

FIGURE 4–3

Branching diagram of CFAM.

Source: Wright, L.M., and M. Leahey, Nurses and Families: A Guide to Family Assessment and Intervention *(3rd ed.), Philadelphia: F.A. Davis, 2000, p. 68.* Used with permission.

The person's health problems, especially emotional ones, may well be the result of the interaction patterns in childhood or in the present family. Knowledge of the variables influencing family interaction—parents' self-esteem and upbringing, number of siblings, person's ordinal position in the family, cultural norms, family rituals—help you assist the person in talking through feelings related to past and present conflicts. Sometimes helping the person understand these variables in relation to the spouse's upbringing and behaviour can be the first step in overcoming current marital problems.

You may assist families to cope with crises or various unexpected disorganizing events, such as illness and natural disasters. Table 4-16 summarizes steps in crisis intervention or brief therapy.

You may help families explore and resolve ethical dilemmas related to their decisions about use of newer technology for getting pregnant or dealing with an adoptive child. Technology that allows infertile couples to become pregnant with in vitro fertilization may also cause parents to face major ethical dilemmas as they determine which of the fertilized embryos should be transplanted into the uterus and which should be frozen for future use. Exploration of feelings and implications is essential.

You may explore with the family the decision to use sperm donors who are paid for their service for artificial insemination. The donor should be carefully screened for a family history of inherited diseases and for current pathogens such as human immunodeficiency virus (HIV). Because some infections, such as HIV, are present long before they may be detected (as long as ten years), transmission of this disease via insemination may occur. The donor is also screened in terms of race, intelligence quotient, physical characteristics, and health. Recipients may choose the baby's gender. Some women become pregnant after the first insemination; others require several or many inseminations.

Selected Nursing Diagnoses Related to Family Nursing

Pattern 2: Communicating

Impaired Verbal Communication

Pattern 3: Relating

Impaired Social Interaction
Social Isolation
Altered Role Performance
Altered Parenting
Risk for Altered Parenting/Infant/Child Attachment
Sexual Dysfunction
Altered Family Processes
Parental Role Conflict
Altered Sexuality Patterns

Pattern 4: Valuing

Spiritual Distress
Potential for Enhanced Spiritual Well-Being

Pattern 5: Choosing

Ineffective Individual Coping
Impaired Adjustment
Defensive Coping
Ineffective Denial
Ineffective Family Coping: Disabling
Ineffective Family Coping: Compromised
Family Coping: Potential for Growth
Potential for Enhanced Community Coping
Decisional Conflict
Health-Seeking Behaviours

Pattern 6: Moving

Diversional Activity Deficit
Impaired Home Maintenance Management
Altered Health Maintenance
Ineffective Breastfeeding
Effective Breastfeeding
Altered Growth and Development

Pattern 7: Perceiving

Chronic Low Self-Esteem
Situational Low Self-Esteem
Personal Identity Disturbance
Unilateral Neglect
Hopelessness
Powerlessness

Pattern 8: Knowing

Knowledge Deficit

Pattern 9: Feeling

Dysfunctional Grieving
Anticipatory Grieving
Risk for Violence: Directed at Others
Risk for Self-Mutilation
Post-Trauma Syndrome
Anxiety
Fear

Source: North American Nursing Diagnosis Association, NANDA Nursing Diagnoses Definitions & Classification 1999–2000. *Philadelphia: North American Nursing Diagnosis Association, 1999.*
Many of the NANDA nursing diagnoses are applicable to the ill individual in the family unit.

Hiring a surrogate mother—a woman to become pregnant and bear the baby for the family—must also be carefully explored because of implications for the surrogate mother and her feelings, consequent feelings of the childrearing family, and legal issues.

Other decisions may not be as difficult but are key to future family development and relationships, for example, helping adoptive parents relate with their child, or the homosexual family explain "coming out" to the children from an earlier marriage. These parents must be prepared to explain the child's origins when the child asks and to help the child understand that there are many kinds of families. We do not yet know the consequences, developmentally and emotionally, for children who are raised without guidance from the opposite sex or who are raised by only one parent. Your assessment, exploration, and teaching with such families are important.

More research is needed in all of these areas. To help families explore values and ethical principles, you must *first* explore and resolve these issues within yourself. You cannot give another *the* answer; you can use therapeutic communication skills to enable clients to find their own answers.

You are not a specialized family counsellor, although with advanced educational preparation you could do family therapy. But you can often sense lack of communication in a family. Through *use of an empathic relationship and effective communication, teaching, and crisis therapy,* you can encourage family members to talk about their feelings with one another and assist in the resolution of their conflicts. Help them become aware of the need to work for family cohesiveness, just as they would work at a job or important project. Refer them to a family counselling service if the problems are beyond your scope. Your work with them should also help them better use other community resources, such as private family or psychiatric counselling or family and children's services.

One family self-help resource can be the formation of a group of four or five complete family units (including stepfamily, single-parent, cohabitation, or traditional units) who contract to meet together over an extended period for shared educational experiences that concern relationships within

TABLE 4-16
Family Crisis Intervention to Assist Families with Coping

1. Encourage family to identify the stressor or hazardous life event.
2. Assess family's interpretation of event and its real impact.
3. Determine family's usual and current coping abilities and resources to handle the event.
4. Assess family's level of functioning as a whole and function of individual members.
5. Assist family members in communicating with each other.
6. Encourage all family members to be involved in finding a solution(s) or resources.
7. Be supportive but encourage the family to mobilize its own resources and extended family or community resources.
8. Empower families by indicating their strengths, reinforcing positive behaviour, helping them make sense of the event, and promoting a sense of being normal.
9. Explore how to prevent and cope with future stressful experiences.
10. Teach coping strategies, ways to prevent or minimize future stressors, stress management, and lifestyle alterations.
11. Recognize members at risk for violence and intervene as necessary.
12. Either continue longer-term therapy, if needed, with the family unit or members or refer them to ongoing therapy as necessary.

their families. This setting provides a positive approach and affirms family members because a commitment is made for all persons—no matter what their age—to have both power and input into the group.

Table 4-17 summarizes intervention measures for counselling or educating families to promote their health.

Role of the Nurse in Well-Baby Care

You may care for well babies and mothers in a variety of settings—clinic, hospital, home, or doctor's office. Your actions contribute significantly to their health.

Prenatal Care

Prenatal care for the mother and her partner may include physical assessment, teaching healthful practices for mother and baby, listening to mother vent frustrations or share fears, counselling her during periods of depression or uncertainty, and sharing her happy feelings about becoming a mother. You may conduct childbirth classes for mother and father so that they can better understand changes occurring in the mother and the nutrition and hygiene necessary during pregnancy; know what to expect during labour, delivery, and postpartum; and prepare for an active role during birth. A maternity nursing book will give adequate detail to help you do prenatal

assessment and care and intrapartum and postpartum assessment and intervention.

If the mother-to-be is unwed, you may also try to work with the father-to-be, if both are willing. The father-to-be needs help in talking about his feelings and needs to support the mother, if they are compatible. He may also seek sex education.

To help the unwed parents and break the cycle for future generations, we must gain a better understanding of the unwed father. Do not perceive him as irresponsible or having taken advantage of an innocent girl. The relationship between the unwed mother and the father is not necessarily a hit-and-miss affair but often meaningful to both. If the parents-to-be are adolescents, they may realize that a new life has been created as a result of their actions. They may want to act in a responsible way. They may be concerned about the child's well-being.[216]

The unwed father can be encouraged to stand by the unmarried mother. Often he feels proud of fathering; he has proven his masculinity. The long-term consequences of having a child are such, however, that alternate solutions regarding the future of the child should be thoroughly explored with and by both partners. Alternatives include marriage, placing the child for adoption, or assumption by either parent or the grandparents of the responsibility for caring for and rearing the child. The man needs help in understanding how and why he became a father and the serious implications for the mother, the child, and himself.

Adolescents may admit that their sexual experiences were unsatisfactory, leaving them depressed, guilty, and scared. The good relationship with the girlfriend may have begun to deteriorate when sexual relations were started. Pregnancy comes as a shock to both. They may have known about contraceptives, but their use may have been sporadic, if at all, for some people believe that the spontaneity and sincerity of the sexual act are lessened by such preparations.[217]

Sex education must relate to the values of interpersonal relations and concern for others if it is to be successful. The implications and responsibilities of sexual behaviour must be discussed with the teenagers. The difference between teenage love and a more mature relationship between people who are ready to meet the problems and responsibilities of adulthood should be discussed.[218]

Parents of the unwed teen father must be involved in helping their son; communication between the boy and parents should be maintained or re-established. In addition, parents should assert themselves in helping the boy take responsibility for his actions and assist the boy in the case of marriage.

Efforts to prevent unwed pregnancies must be directed to improving and strengthening family life and developing a better respect for the father's role in the family. Fathers can help adolescent sons by talking with and listening to them, by being slow to judge, by taking them to the office so the youth can see how the father earns a living, and by being a role model in relating maturely to the spouse and other women. Fathers can create an atmosphere in which the sons will want to talk about emerging sexual feelings and experiences.[219] If

TABLE 4-17
Summary of Intervention Measures

1. **Develop a therapeutic relationship.** Establish rapport and trust between yourself and the family by being open to the family structure or system and the cultural values and norms that are manifested. Use therapeutic communication principles. Use the family's language, but be a model for clear, effective communication. Remember the trust, influence, and impact that you have on the family unit. Be empathic, supportive, and impartial as you give feedback to the family. Thus you will enable the family members to identify and modify patterns that cause dysfunction and discomfort.

2. **Identify issues with the family.** Subjective issues are what the family members perceive as problem areas. Objective issues are what you see as limits or problems. Have each family member list or identify problems and areas for change. Refrain from challenging or questioning the accuracy of anyone's values or statements of problem areas. Do not side with any one particular member. Encourage family members also to explore those areas that you see as dysfunctional.

3. **Encourage and assist members in their communication skills,** to listen to one another, to talk kindly, and to clarify their own perceptions and the feelings, thoughts, and behaviours of the others. You gently confront and are a mirror for the family members so that they can gain increased understanding of themselves as a unit. As they learn to talk honestly to one another, members will have less need to deny the pain they feel or deny hurtful behaviours practised in family living.

4. **Establish a teaching plan for the family unit if it is appropriate,** either for the client as a member of the family or for the family as a whole. Help each one to find appropriate resources in the external environment as well as to identify personal strengths for managing a situation. Encourage the family to find ways to adapt the lifestyle or home situation to manage an illness or crisis better.

5. **Determine willingness of family members to participate in counselling and change.** Keep in mind that families, according to systems theory, strive to maintain their balance and are frightened and ambivalent about negotiating and enacting change. Have each member participate in defining the problem and in making the decision for change to enable family members to feel more in control of what is occurring and more willing to participate. Even so, some members may continue to be resistant to change during counselling or may choose not to participate at all. It is essential for you to remain objective, reassuring, and supportive. Considerable theoretical knowledge, communication skill, and supervised practice are necessary before you will be able to work with deep, long-term, or complex problems; resistant behaviour; power struggles; or coalitions.

6. **Negotiate a contract as to the goals for treatment.** (See Chapter 5 for guidelines for contracting.) Identify with the family one or two goals that are crucial to work toward to begin to achieve some happiness and smoother function. Later, other goals may be added to the list. It is better to set small achievable goals that the family perceives as worthwhile than to inhibit family change through an extensive list of statements. Remember that the behaviour of any one family member is a symptom of a problem in the family system.

7. **Negotiate a contract about specific behavioural changes that can be accomplished** and that will encourage family members to interact or behave in ways that break dysfunctional patterns or rigid structures. Assist members to disagree constructively and to contract with one another for change. Help the family to anticipate problem areas, work through alternatives, and explore consequences of the alternatives.

8. **Be patient.** Do not expect great change. The family may change its behaviour, but only to the point that is comfortable and tolerable to all. Regression to previous patterns will occur. Your consistent kindness and encouragement may be the main factors in the family coping with stressors or crises, adjusting daily routines to the needs of an ill member, or staying with therapy and trying to modify behaviour.

---

the adolescent son comes from a home where no father is present, the mother can work at listening to and discussing problems and feelings with the son. She may also be able to foster a bond between the son and another male member of the family.

CRITICAL THINKING

A pregnant 15-year-old informs you that she is frightened of being pregnant. How can you help her to overcome her fears?

Childbirth Education Classes

If you conduct childbirth and parenting education classes, try to interview each couple in their home early in the pregnancy, by the fourth month if possible, to observe their relationship and determine their response to pregnancy. Their response may be different and more honest in their own home than in class. During the classes, include opportunities for both men and women to talk about their feelings or problems they feel are uniquely theirs. Provide anticipatory guidance about the couvade syndrome. (Couvade is a primitive custom in which the husband of a woman who is in childbed, actually goes to bed himself and suffers a symbolic parturition.) Avoid pushing the father into participation and provide support for him. *Focus childbirth education on the known benefits to the baby and parents and not on overromanticized and dramatic statements about improved marital relationships. Educate both parents about family planning so that future pregnancies can be mutually planned.* Refer either partner, or both, to psychological counselling when necessary, especially if antisocial behaviour is seen or if there has been fetal loss.

Labour and Delivery

During labour and delivery, the nurse gives necessary physical care, may act as a coach for the mother, or may support the father as he assists his wife. Flexibility in hospital routines for obstetric patients is usually possible and contributes to the parents' sense of control.

The physician and nurse, or nurse-midwife, can work as a team with the expectant couple. In some facilities the nurse-midwife assumes primary responsibility for the family unit. Whenever a mother delivers, she has the right to capable, safe care by qualified caretakers. Home deliveries can be carefully planned and safe. Hospital deliveries can be more homelike. Maternity centres now provide families anticipating a normal childbearing experience with antepartum care that is educational in nature; labour and delivery in a homelike setting (but with adequate equipment); discharge to home whenever it is safe for mother and baby; and follow-up care by public health nurses in the home during the postpartum course. The labour and delivery rooms can be designed to accommodate the presence of the father or family during delivery and be less traumatic (less cold, with less intense lights) for the newborn. After the birth, the infant can remain with the mother, and the newborn's physical examination can be done in her presence with the father present. Childbirth should be a positive, maturing experience for the couple. Expectant parents have the right and responsibility to be involved in planning their care with the health team and to know what is happening. Cultural beliefs should be recognized, respected, and accommodated whenever possible. A positive childbearing experience contributes to a healthy family unit.

Postpartum Period

Because of short hospital stays after delivery of the baby (6 to 48 hours), you may not be able to give the traditional essential physical or emotional postpartum care. Instead, the care will be delivered in the home by the family, with the continuing support and assistance from a home health nurse or maternal–child advanced practice nurse who is a consultant.

Realize that various cultural groups may have specific traditional rituals that will also be done. The postpartum period is considered a cold, or yin, period. Practices related to balance of heat and cold, such as avoiding cold and contact with water, avoiding conflict in relationships, ambulation, dietary norms, and rituals to overcome what is considered the state of pollution of mother and baby after birth are described by Horn.[220]

The following guidelines must be taught to the family member(s) who will be caring for the new mother and baby or carried out by the nurse in the home. In the early postpartum period, assess mother and baby. Facilitate the mother's physical care; assist her as necessary, even if she looks well and able. Mother needs to be mothered to enhance attachment between mother and baby. Listen to the mother's (and father's) concerns; answer questions; support maternal and paternal behaviour. In a nonthreatening way, teach the parents how to handle the baby. Help them begin to unlearn preconceived ideas about the baby and to perceive self and the baby positively. If the mother is breastfeeding, teaching and assistance are necessary. After the initial "taking in" period of having received special care and attention, the mother moves to the "taking hold" stage, in which she is able to care for the child.[221]

The interaction between the infant and primary caretaker is crucial. The mothering person helps the baby feel secure and loved, fosters a sense of trust, provides stimulation, reinforces certain behaviour, acts as a model for language development, and trains the baby in basic learning strategies. In turn, maternal behaviour is influenced by baby's cries, coos, smiles, activity, and gazes and by how well baby's behaviour meets the mother's expectations.

Your significant contribution to the family unit is to promote attachment between parents and baby, encourage continuing contacts between the family and health professionals so that adequate health and illness care are received, and encourage parents to meet the baby's needs adequately. You can help the parents feel good about themselves and the baby.

You can be instrumental in continuing new trends in care to make the hospital or clinic environment more homelike, while providing safe, modern care.

Continued Care in the Postpartum Period

During the *six or eight weeks after delivery,* the mother needs assistance with child care and an opportunity to regain her former self physically and emotionally. The father also needs support as he becomes involved in child-care responsibilities. In the nuclear or single-parent family, the parent may struggle alone. Continued visits by a home health nurse may be useful. Some communities have a crisis line for new parents. You may be able to suggest services or help the parent think of people who could be helpful.

As you assess the mother's functioning, consider her physical and emotional energy, support systems, and current level of parenting activity. If she apparently is not caring adequately for the child, assess for anemia, pain, bleeding, infections, lack of food or sleep, drug use, or other medical conditions that would interfere with her activity level and feelings of caring. Depression and postpartum blues are difficult to differentiate. In depression the mother is immobilized and is unable to do basic care for herself or the baby. With postpartum blues from hormonal shifts and the crisis of parenthood, she may cry but cares for the baby's physical needs. Depression has a longer course and should be medically treated. The new mother usually has enough energy to do only top-priority tasks: eating, sleeping, baby care, and essentials for other family members.

The mother's support system is crucial for her energy maintenance, both physical and emotional. She needs direct support and assistance with daily tasks, plus moral support, a listener, a confidant. Support comes from personal and professional sources—the partner, parents, friends, other relatives, and the nurse, doctor, social worker, or pastor. Negative attitudes from others can drain emotional energy. Actual parenting skills can be manifested in various ways: touching, cuddling, a tender, soft voice tone, and loving gazes. Additional information about parents' feelings and the parenting process is described in Chapter 7.

If the baby is progressing in normal fashion, focus on the mother's needs and concerns. Help her find nonprofessional support systems that can assist her when the professional is unavailable or that can help with child care. In addition to concern over child care, we must help the mother grow developmentally. Helping her stay in good physical and emotional health ensures better parenting.

Certain *behaviour patterns in parents strongly suggest a disturbed parent–child relationship and future problems in parenting,* for example, if the parent:

- Is unable to talk about feelings, fears, and sense of responsibility for the child
- Makes little effort to secure information about the baby
- Consistently misinterprets or exaggerates either positive or negative information about the baby
- Receives no practical support or help from family or friends, and community resources are lacking
- Is unable to accept and use help offered

You may be instrumental in suggesting *certain procedures that can be used to promote the parent–child relationship:*

- Permit the mother to see and touch the baby as soon as possible, preferably in the delivery room.
- Permit the mother's involvement in the baby's care as soon as possible.
- Provide an atmosphere that encourages questions.
- Encourage parents to talk with each other, family members, and friends, using others for support.
- Recognize that parents' excessive questions, demands, and criticisms are a reaction to stress and not personal attacks on the professional worker or hospital.
- Arrange for the father to visit the baby before discharge, calling him about the baby's progress at intervals when he is unable to visit.
- Encourage the parents to handle the baby and do the baby's care before discharge; teach about baby care as necessary while the parents are engaged in care of their baby.

In addition, observe the interactions and relationship between the parents or between the mother and other members of the family. It will be difficult for the mother to remain caring if she is abused. A father who is abusive to the mother—verbally, physically, or emotionally—may become abusive to the child at some point. Chapters 6, 7, and 8 and other references can be helpful.[222,223]

Care of Families with a Chronically Ill or Special-Needs Child

Families who have a child with chronic illness or a special-needs child with developmental disabilities or chronic physical or emotional illness experience a number of stressors in addition to the physical, emotional, and social burdens and financial costs of continuing care. Parents may feel like they want collaboration and control, but have no control over the care of and treatment consequences for their child, depending on the health care providers' approaches to the child and family. Some families passively depend on the professional providers for all directions. Parents experience a sense of loss, chronic sorrow, and ongoing grief and mourning related to the ideal or normal child they expected, as they adapt their expectations to fit the real child they have. Ongoing physical care and guidance problems are constant reminders of developmental lag, that the child will not achieve certain developmental tasks and will remain dependent on someone, perhaps for life. There are continual, lifelong adjustments to the child and care. Parents worry about the child's care and quality of life in the future when they are unable to continue care. All family members react to the time and energy demands of a special-needs child, realizing that means less time and energy for each other or themselves. All family members will realize the effects of the financial drain on the previous standard of living. Financial stress includes more than cost of care; it also includes loss of employment or educational opportunities when a parent must either stop or reduce these activities because of child-care demands. McNeil examined the experience of fathers who have a child with juvenile rheumatoid arthritis. His findings indicated that based on the nature of fathers' experience and the extent of their involvement, more attention by health care practitioners to fathers' adaptation is warranted.[224]

Marital stress occurs as parents negotiate parental roles and responsibilities, time, energy, and finances and reconcile career-versus-family demands. Career mobility, especially related to geographic moves, may occur because of dependence on a specific treatment agency or team or the employer's insurance plan. Divorce in families with special-needs children is not unusual.

Families with special-needs children need a social support system to maintain family stability and care adequately for the child. Social support may include an extended family, close friends, religious affiliation, parents of other children with special needs, and access to empathetic professionals. Extra effort is often needed to encourage these parents to participate in self-help or other groups, because they often do not develop or maintain social contacts and so become more isolated. A family with adequate finances, which has lived in a community long enough to have developed contacts and friendships and have a car and telephone and which has a good understanding of and collaboration with the health care system will fare better than a family without any or all of these characteristics.

Health care professionals can develop family support groups to provide:

■ Education about the diagnosis and how to cope with and treat it

■ A place where parents can discuss their feelings and concerns and receive acceptance and empathy as they grieve losses in the situation

■ Information about available services and resources in the community

■ Assistance with fulfilling role responsibility and demand

■ Assistance to parents to become advocates for their children in negotiating for services, education, and favourable legislation

■ Social functions to reduce the sense of isolation the families may feel

Table 4-18 provides telephone numbers of organizations that can provide information for families with special-needs children.

Parent Education

To combat the problems associated with the high adolescent birth rate, some junior and senior high schools are establishing creative programs in parenthood education. Some hospi-

TABLE 4-18 Telephone Numbers for Special Needs Information	
Canadian National Institute for the Blind	1-416-486-2500
Canadian Diabetes Association	1-800-226-8464
Kidney Foundation of Canada	1-800-361-7494
Arthritis Society	1-416-979-7228
Canadian Down Syndrome Society	1-403-270-8291
Canadian Haemophilia Society	1-514-848-0503
Canadian Mental Health Association	1-416-484-7750
Canadian Paraplegic Association	1-613-723-1033
Children's Wish Foundation of Canada	1-613-247-9457
Disabled Peoples' International	1-204-287-8010
Epilepsy Canada	1-514-845-7855
Heart and Stroke Foundation of Canada	1-613-569-4361
Multiple Sclerosis Society of Canada	1-416-992-6065
Muscular Dystrophy Association of Canada	1-416-488-0030
Canadian Cystic Fibrosis Foundation	1-800-378-2233
Canadian Society of the Investigation of Child Abuse	1-403-289-8385
Fetal Alcohol Syndrome World Canada	1-416-465-7766
Canadian Institute of Child Health	1-613-230-8838
Spina Bifida and Hydrocephalus Association of Canada	1-800-565-9488

tals and health clinics are initiating specialized prenatal and postnatal services for the adolescent mother and her at-risk infant. You can initiate nontraditional programs in your own community.

Some health care agencies have established programs to help adolescent mothers become more effective parents. The adolescent mother who decides to keep her baby needs all the family and outside help she can get. She may fear that whatever personal ambitions she has will be thwarted by the baby. Unmarried and unprepared for employment, she finds it almost impossible to make her own way in the world. Anger, frustration, and ignorance hamper her ability to attach to and appropriately care for the baby. Repeated pregnancies, child neglect and abuse, and welfare dependency often occur.

Formation of a mothers' or parents' group, including women and men of various ethnic origins and income brackets, can provide parent education and support and foster talking about feelings. Also educate parents about using community resources.

Our work with the mother may prevent maternal deprivation, insufficient interaction between mother and child, conditions under which deprivation or even abuse develops, and negative effects on the child's development.

Working with Adoptive Families

You can help the adoptive parents in their adjustment. Assure them that attachment develops over time. Help them think through how and when to tell the child that he or she is adopted so that the child understands and is not traumatized. Help the parents anticipate how they will help the child cope when the child is taunted by peers about being adopted. Help them realize that the adopted child will probably seek answers to many questions when he or she gets older. Who were the parents? What is their cultural, racial, or ethnic background? Their ages, occupations, interests, appearance? Why was he or she relinquished? What are the medical facts surrounding heredity and birth? Help parents realize that these questions do not mean that the child does not love them. Various articles supply information on adoption procedures, stresses encountered, and how to make adoption a success.[225–229]

Working with Stepfamilies

The guidelines already discussed will be useful to you as you help the single-parent family or stepfamily adjust to its situation. The single-parent family can be referred to a local chapter of Parents Without Partners if the person seeks support from peers. Do not rush in with answers for these families until you have heard their unique problems. Acknowledge their strengths; help them formulate their own solutions. Often a few sessions of crisis therapy will be sufficient. Several references give further information.[230–232]

Family Care Throughout the Life Cycle

You may be called on to assist families as they meet various developmental crises throughout the life cycle: school entry of the child, the adolescent period, children leaving home, divorce, retirement, death of a member. Your goal is health promotion and primary disease prevention. Your intervention early in the family life cycle may help establish a positive health trend in place of its negative counterpart. The care you give to young parents lays the foundation for their children's health. You may also find yourself becoming an advocate for families in relation to legislation that affects families and child care.

Another way to improve the family as an institution is from within. Parents should teach their children not just to get ahead but to serve, to cooperate, and to be kind. We can teach our children to believe that family ties are the most rewarding values, that social, cultural, and community activities can be deeply satisfying, and that the gratification from income and jobs is not the main priority.[233–235]

Our excessive competitiveness is being passed on to our children as parents try to produce "super kids." Misplaced educational pressure is likely to produce lopsided development and an aversion to schooling. To diminish the competitive atmosphere in schools, grades and examination could be dropped. Excessive competitiveness overlaps with excessive materialism. In most parts of the world, materialism is balanced by spiritual values (e.g., dedication to God in Islamic countries, dedication to the nation in Israel, dedication to the family in Greece). By contrast, in Canada and the United States many children get their values—materialism, competitiveness, and brutality—from television, video games, or the Internet. In turn, rates for violent crime are shockingly high. Parents should demand good programs from media producers and forbid their children's watching violence and sordid sex. It is no wonder some youths panic at finding they have no supporting beliefs and turn to extremist cults and lifestyles and that the rate of teenage suicide has tripled in the past 20 years.[236–238]

Parents can make a profound difference by teaching spiritual values—helpfulness, cooperation, generosity, love—throughout childhood. Two-year-old children can be encouraged to help set the table and then be thanked and praised. Teenagers can be expected to work in hospitals and to tutor younger children. Such jobs should not be presented as distasteful. Children enjoy taking on adult jobs when they are presented as opportunities and efforts are appreciated.[239]

Just as vital is a family atmosphere in which parents treat each other and their children with respect and affection and smile. The best forum is still mealtime and the family meeting. When teenagers first give excuses why they cannot make it to a meal, parents should say very positively, "We like to have the whole family get together." Parents should avoid talking down to children and having the attitude that being older makes them right, but they can still be very clear about their beliefs and expectations.[240,241]

Parents must give careful attention to the topic of sex. We have done well to overcome the shame that used to surround sex; but in declaring sex more wholesome and natural, we have mistakenly ignored its tenderness, generosity, and intensely spiritual aspects. We have failed to instil that the impulse in idealistic youths to save intimacy for the ultimate partner has existed for centuries and has contributed to creativity in all the arts.[242]

When parents are asked questions about sexual matters by two-, three-, and four-year-old children, they should advance from anatomy and physiology to emphasize the loving and caring aspects of sex and marriage. An even greater influence on children is their parents' behaviour toward and commitment to a partner and their admiration and respect for one another. Joking and disparaging remarks about marriage should be avoided. Parents can suggest that if young people want to claim the right to sexual freedom, they should be aware of the responsibilities. If a youthful marriage soon ends in divorce, parents can point out that no marriage succeeds by itself but must be continually cultivated, like a garden. It is wise to look for openings to discuss these topics when children are 9, 10, or 11 years of age. When they are 13 years old and beyond, they think their parents are hopelessly old-fashioned and consider peer opinions as the only truth.[243,244]

You have a role as educator and advocate as well as health care provider. You can assist parents as they guide children toward meeting developmental needs and cooperation for the common good. You can assist adults to be mature parents who present a positive model for the future of the family and society.

INTERESTING WEBSITES

THE VANIER INSTITUTE OF THE FAMILY

http://www.vifamily.ca
Established in 1965 under the patronage of their Excellencies Governor-General Georges P. Vanier and Madame Pauline Vanier, the Vanier Institute is a national, charitable organization dedicated to promoting the well-being of Canadian families. It is governed by a volunteer board with regional representation from across Canada.

DADS CANADA

http://www.dadscan.org
The Dads Canada site is a gateway helping to identify individuals (researchers, professionals), organizations, and institutions interested in promoting fatherhood in Canada. This information is presented for all provinces and territories across the country.

CANGRANDS

http://www.cangrands.com/
The CANGRANDS site welcomes all grandparents and family members who are raising grandchildren or extended family members. The organization's aim is to promote, support, and assist families in maintaining or re-establishing family ties—especially between grandchildren and grandparents and extended families.

MULTIPLE BIRTHS CANADA

http://www.multiplebirthscanada.org/
This organization exists to improve the quality of life for multiple birth individuals and their families. With an extensive

network of local chapters, health care professionals, and organizations.

CANADA ADOPTS

http://www.canadaadopts.com/

This site aimed at adoptive parents is backed by a support team of professionals specializing in adoption, infertility, social justice, law, education, New Media, Web design, marketing, advertising, and journalism.

CANADIAN CHILD CARE FEDERATION

http://www.cccf-fcsge.ca

The CCCF's mission is to improve the quality of child care services for Canadian families. This site includes news about child care in Canada and information about publications for parents and child care practitioners. For a partial list of provincial child care organizations, click on "Affiliates."

SUMMARY

1. There are various types of family structures and systems.
2. You will care for clients who may come from a family background quite different from your own family system in structure and dynamic relationships.
3. People who come from the same type of family structure—matrifocal or homosexual, for example—will be different from each other.
4. All families, regardless of structure, share similar developmental tasks.
5. Family relationships and dynamic processes and the extent to which developmental tasks are met within the family are a major influence on development and health.
6. You will practise principles of family-centred care, based on concepts in this chapter, in every health care setting.
7. Engage in life-long learning about your own and other family systems to assess, plan, and provide comprehensive care to the client and family.

ENDNOTES

1. Seifert, K., R. Hoffnung, and M. Hoffnung, *Lifespan Development*. Boston: Houghton Mifflin, 1997.
2. Beavers, R., and R. Hampson, *Successful Families: Assessment and Intervention*. New York: W.W. Norton, 1990.
3. Canadian Health Network, *Canadian Families*, Website: http://www.canadian-health-network.ca, May 2004.
4. *Ibid.*
5. Vanier Institute of the Family, *Contemporary Family Trends, Aboriginal Family Trends*, Website: http://www.vifamily.ca/library/cft/aboriginal.html, May 2004.
6. Dion Stout, M., with C.R. Bruyere, Stopping Family Violence: Aboriginal Communities Enspirited, in J.R. Ponting, ed., *First Nations in Canada: Perspectives on Opportunity, Empowerment, and Self-Determination* (pp. 273–288). Toronto: McGraw-Hill Ryerson, 1997.
7. *Treaty 7 Community Study: Violence and Community Stress*. Ottawa: Royal Commission on Aboriginal Peoples, 1994.
8. Vanier Institute of the Family, *Contemporary Family Trends, Aboriginal Family Trends*.
9. *Ibid.*
10. Friedman, M., V. Bowden, and E. Jones, *Family Nursing: Research, Theory and Family Practice* (5th ed.). Upper Saddle River: Prentice Hall, 2003.
11. Smilkstein, G., The Cycle of Family Function: A Conceptual Model for Family Medicine, *Family Practitioner*, 11 (1980), 223.
12. Bozett, F., ed., *Gay and Lesbian Parents*. New York: Preager, 1987.
13. Bozett, F., ed, Social Control of Identity by Children of Gay Fathers, *Western Journal of Nursing Research*, 10, no. 5 (1988), 550–565.
14. Gordon, T., *Parent Effectiveness Training*. New York: Peter H. Wyden, 1970.
15. Harris, M., and P. Turner, Gay and Lesbian Parents, *Journal of Homosexuality*, 12, no. 2 (1986), 101–113.
16. Papalia, D., S. Olds, and R. Feldman, *Human Development* (9th ed.). Boston: McGraw–Hill, 2004.
17. Canadian Health Network, *Canadian Families*.
18. Canadian Department of Justice, *Reference to the Supreme Court of Canada*, Website: http://www.canada.com/, May 2004.
19. *Ibid.*
20. Canadian Health Network, *Canadian Families*.
21. *Ibid.*
22. Broderick, C.B., *Understanding Family Process: Basics of Family Systems Theory*. Newbury Park, CA: Sage, 1993.
23. Friedman, *op. cit.*
24. McFarlane, A., A Nursing Reformulation of Bowen's Family Systems Theory, *Archives of Psychiatric Nursing*, 2 (1988), 319–324.
25. Smoyak, S.A., General Systems Model: Principles and General Applications. In Reynolds, W., and Cormack, D. Eds., *Psychiatric and Mental Health Nursing: Theory and Practice*. New York: Chapman & Hall, 1990, pp. 133–152.
26. Whall A., *Nursing Approach to Family Therapy*. New York: Brady, 1994.
27. Vanier Institute of the Family, *It Keeps Getting Faster: Changing Patterns of Time in Families*, Website: http://www.vifamily.ca, May 2004.
28. *Ibid.*
29. *Ibid.*
30. *Ibid.*
31. Frederick, J.A. *As Time Goes By . . . Time Use by Canadians*. Ottawa: Ministry of Supply and Services and Statistics Canada, 1995. Cat. No. 89-544-XPE.
32. Hall, W.A., and P. Callery, Balancing Personal and Family Trajectories: An International Study of Dual-Earner Couples with Pre-school Children. *International Journal of Nursing Studies*, 40, no. 4 (2003), 401–412.
33. *Ibid.*
34. Duvall, E., and B. Miller, *Marriage and Family Development* (6th ed.), New York: Harper & Row, 1984.
35. *Ibid.*
36. Papalia, *op. cit.*
37. *Ibid.*
38. Jones, E., Deaf and Hearing Parents' Perceptions of Family Functioning, *Nursing Research*, 44, no. 2 (1995), 102–105.
39. Anderson, M., The Mental Health Advantages of Twinship, *Perspectives of Psychiatric Care*, 23, no. 3 (1985), 114–116.
40. Friedman, *op. cit.*
41. *Ibid.*
42. *Ibid.*
43. Family Aggression May Compound Hyperactivity in Children, *The Menninger Letter*, 3, no. 11 (1995), 6–7.
44. Parental Work Load Affects Adolescents, *The Menninger Letter*, 3, no. 11 (1995), 6.
45. Dion Stout with Bruyere, *op. cit.*
46. *Ibid.*
47. Canada, *Report of the Royal Commission on Aboriginal Peoples, Vol. 3 Gathering Strength*. Royal Commission on Aboriginal Peoples. Minister of Supply and Services, Ottawa, 1996.

48. Friedman, *op. cit.*

49. Wachtel, E., and P. Wachtel, *Family Dynamics in Individual Psychotherapy: A Guide to Clinical Strategies.* New York: Guilford Press, 1986.

50. Bee, H., Boyd, D. and P. Johnson, *Lifespan Development* (Canadian ed., Study Edition). Toronto: Pearson Education Canada, 2005.

51. Friedman, *op. cit.*

52. Betta, R., and Musi, D., Families South of the Border: Mexico—Trading Its Values, *Focus on the Family,* July (1995), 6.

53. Papalia, *op. cit.*

54. Whall, *op. cit.*

55. Wright, L., and M. Leahey, *Nursing Families: A Guide to Family Assessment and Intervention* (3rd ed.). Philadelphia: F.A. Davis, 1999.

56. Bettelheim, B., *A Good Enough Parent: A Book on Child-Rearing.* New York: Alfred A. Knopf, 1987.

57. Broderick, C.B., *Understanding Family Process: Basics of Family Systems Theory.* Newbury Park, CA: Sage, 1993.

58. Duvall and Miller, *op. cit.*

59. Wright and Leahey, *op. cit.*

60. Duvall and Miller, *op. cit.*

61. Erikson, E., *Childhood and Society* (2nd ed.), New York: W.W. Norton, 1963

62. Papalia, *op. cit.*

63. Wright and Leahey, *op. cit.*

64. Vanier Institute of the Family, *Contemporary Family Trends, Portraits of Fathers,* Website: http://www.vifamily.ca/, May 2004.

65. Steinberg, S., L. Kruckman, and S. Steinberg. Reinventing Fatherhood in Japan and Canada. *Social Science & Medicine,* 50, no. 9 (2000), 1257–1272.

66. *Ibid.*

67. Leininger, M. Japanese Americans and Culture Care, in M. Leininger and M.R. McFarland, eds., *Transcultural Nursing: Concepts, Theories, Research & Practice* (3rd ed, pp. 453–463). New York: McGraw-Hill, 2002.

68. Steinberg et al., *op. cit.*

69. Leininger, *op. cit.*

70. Vanier Institute of the Family, *Contemporary Family Trends, Portraits of Fathers.*

71. Steinberg et al., *op. cit.*

72. Papalia, *op. cit.*

73. Bauer, G., American Family Life Worth Expecting, *Focus on the Family,* July (1994), 2–3.

74. Bettelheim, *op. cit.*

75. Vanier Institute of the Family, *Contemporary Family Trends, Grandparenthood in Canada,* Website: http://www.vifamily.ca/, May 2004.

76. Statistics Canada, Health Statistics Division, *Health Reports,* 12, no. 3. Minister of Industry, 2001.

77. Canadian Health Network, *Canadian Families.*

78. Inwood, S. Family Ties: Grandparents Raising Grandchildren, *Canadian Nurse,* 98, no. 4 (2002), 21–25.

79. Kahana, E., D. Biegel, and M. Wykle, *Family Caregiving Across the Lifespan.* Thousand Oaks, CA: Sage, 1994.

80. Duvall and Miller, *op. cit.*

81. Bozett, F., and S. Hanson, Eds. *Fatherhood and Families in Cultural Context.* New York: Springer, 1991.

82. Gordon, *op. cit.*

83. Visher, E., and J. Visher, *Old Loyalties, New Ties: Therapeutic Strategies with Stepfamilies.* New York: Brunner/Mazel, 1988.

84. Bettelheim, *op. cit.*

85. Smalley, G., Advice You Can Bank On, *Focus on the Family,* February, 1997, 2–4.

86. Bettelheim, *op. cit.*

87. McManus, M., Become a Marriage Saver, *Focus on the Family,* July 1996, 5–7.

88. Mellott, R., *Enhancing Intimacy,* Boulder, CO: Career Track, 1994.

89. Wright and Leahey, *op. cit.*

90. Bettelheim, *op. cit.*

91. Mellott, *op. cit.*

92. Gordon, *op. cit.*

93. Papalia et al., *op cit.*

94. Wright and Leahey, *op. cit.*

95. Bettelheim, *op. cit.*

96. Hoopes, M., and J. Harper, *Birth Order Roles and Sibling Patterns in Individual and Family Therapy.* Rockville, MD: Aspen, 1987.

97. Sulloway, F., Birth Order and Personality, *Harvard Mental Health Letter,* 14, no. 3 (1997), 5–7.

98. Hoopes and Harper, *op. cit.*

99. Sulloway, *op. cit.*

100. Hoopes and Harper, *op. cit.*

101. Wen, S.W. Multiple Birth Rate in Health Canada. In Health Canada, *Canadian Perinatal Health Report.* Ottawa: Minister of Public Works and Government Services Canada, 2003.

102. Multiple Births Canada, Website: http://www.multiplebirthscanada.org/, May 2004.

103. Mom2many—Parents of Multiples Across Canada, Website: http://www.mom2many.com/, May 2004.

104. Hoopes and Harper, *op. cit.*

105. Papalia et al., *op cit.*

106. Peplau, H., Basic *Principles of Patient Counseling* (2nd ed.). Philadelphia: Smith Kline & French Laboratories, 1969.

107. Anderson, *op. cit.*

108. Bettelheim, *op. cit.*

109. Ritchie, C., Adoption: An Option Often Overlooked, *American Journal of Nursing,* 89, no. 9 (1989), 1156–1157.

110. Smit, E., Unique Issues of the Adopted Child, *Journal of Psychosocial Nursing,* 34, no. 7 (1996), 29–36.

111. International Adoption—Canada, Website: http://www.canada.com, May 2004.

112. Canada Adopts, Website: http://www.canadaadopts.com, May 2004.

113. Baker, M. *Families: Changing Trends in Canada* (4th ed.). Toronto: McGraw-Hill Ryerson, 2001.

114. Ward, M. *The Family Dynamic: A Canadian Perspective* (3rd ed.). Toronto: Nelson Thomson Learning, 2002.

115. Brockhaus, J., and R. Brockhaus, Adopting a Child With Special Needs: The Legal Process, *American Journal of Nursing,* 82, no. 2 (1982), 291–294.

116. Nieman, B., Home Away From Home, *Newsweek,* November 11, 1998, 14.

117. Schaffer, J., and C. Londstrum, *How to Raise an Adopted Child.* New York: Crown, 1989.

118. Sieg, K., Growing Up a Foster Kid, *Newsweek,* October 26, 1998, 20.

119. Smit, *op. cit.*

120. Worthington, R., Family Support Networks: Help for Families of Children with Special Needs, *Family Medicine,* 24, no. 1 (1992), 141–144.

121. Ritchie, *op. cit.*

122. Schaffer and Londstrum, *op. cit.*

123. *Ibid.*

124. Smit, *op. cit.*

125. Bee et al., *op cit.*

126. Center for the Future of Children, *The Future of Children: Children and Divorce,* 4, no. 1 (1994), 1–247.

127. Gordon, *op. cit.*

128. Webster, P., and A. Herzog, Effects of Parental Divorce and Memories of Family Problems in Relationships Between Adult Children and Their Parents, *Journal of Gerontology: Social Sciences,* 50B, no. 1 (1995), 823–834.

129. Mellott, *op. cit.*

130. Webster and Herzog. *op. cit.*

131. Lynn, M.M., Single-Parent Families, in M.M. Lynn, ed., *Voices: Essays on Canadian Families* (2nd ed., pp. 32–33). Toronto: Thomson Nelson, 2003.

132. *Ibid.*

133. Ford-Gilboe, M., Family Strengths, Motivation, and Resources as Predictors of Health Promotion Behavior in Single-parent and Two-parent Families. *Research in Nursing,* 20, no. 3 (1997), 205–217.

134. McLanahan, S., and G. Sandefur, *Growing up With a Single Parent.* Cambridge, MA: Harvard University Press, 1994.

135. Reder, N., Single Parents/Dual Responsibilities, *The National Voter,* 39, no. 1 (1989), 9–11.

136. *Ibid.*

137. Lynn, *op. cit.*

138. Ford-Gilboe, M. Dispelling Myths and Creating Opportunity: A Comparison of the Strengths of Single-Parent and Two-Parent Families, *Advances in Nursing Science,* 23, no. 1 (2000), 41–58.

139. *Ibid.*

140. Church, E. Kinship and Stepfamilies, in M. Lynn, ed., *Voices: Essays on Canadian Families* (2nd ed.). Toronto: Thomson Nelson, 2003, pp. 32–33.

141. Statistics Canada, Census Operations Division, *2001 Census Handbook,* Minister of Industry, 2003.

142. Church, *op. cit.*

143. *Ibid.*

144. McDaniel, S.A., and L. Tepperman, *Close Relations: An Introduction to the Sociology of Families, Brief Edition.* Toronto: Prentice Hall, 2002.

145. Church, *op. cit.*

146. Mikan, A., and A. Peters. Couples Living Apart, *Canadian Social Trends,* Summer, 2003, Statistics Canada. Cat. No. 11-008.

147. *Ibid.*

148. Bee et al., *op. cit.*

149. Papalia et al., *op cit.*

150. Santrrock, J.W., A. MacKenzie-Rivers, K.H. Leung, and T. Malcomson. *Life-Span Development* (1st Canadian ed.). Toronto: McGraw-Hill Ryerson, 2003.

151. Riedmann, A., M.A. Lamanna, and A. Nelson. *Marriages and Families* (1st Canadian ed.). Toronto: Nelson Thomson Learning, 2003.

152. Vanier Institute of the Family, Contemporary Family Trends, Grandparenthood in Canada, 2003.

153. Inwood, *op. cit.*

154. Cangands, Website: http://www.cangrands.com/, June 2004.

155. Canadian Health Network, *Canadian Families.*

156. *Ibid.*

157. Statistics Canada, *2001 Census: Families and Households Profile, Website:* http://www12.statcan.ca/, March 2004.

158. Springer, K., Spaced-Out Siblings, *Newsweek,* May 17, 1999.

159. Dicicco-Bloom, B., and D. Cohen. Home Nurses: A Study of the Occurrences of Culturally Competent Care. *Journal of Transcultural Nursing,* 14, no. 1 (2003), 25–31.

160. Greenberg, P. Stay–Home Moms Need Support, Not Bad Mouthing, *American Family Association Journal,* May, 1998, 20.

161. Cheal, D. The One and the Many: Modernity and Post-Modernity. In C.J. Richardson, ed., *Family Life: Patterns and Perspectives* (p. 52–53). New York: McGraw-Hill, 1996,

162. Wright, L.M. and M. Leahey. *Nurses and Families: A Guide to Family Assessment and Intervention* (3rd ed.). Philadelphia: F. A. Davis Company, 2000.

163. Boxx, T., and G. Quenlivan, *The Cultural Context of Economics and Politics.* Baltimore: University Press of America, 1994.

164. Papalia et al., *op cit.*

165. Chan, E. Child Care: A Holistic And Family-Centred Approach. *Transition,* 31, no. 4 (2002), 6–9.

166. Bettelheim, *op. cit.*

167. Papalia et al., *op cit.*

168. Ward, *op. cit.*

169. Das Gupta, T. Families of Native People, Immigrants, and People of Colour, in N. Mandell and A. Duffy, eds., *Canadian Families: Diversity, Conflict, and Change* (2nd ed., pp. 146–147) Toronto: Harcourt Brace Canada, 2000.

170. Vanier Institute of the Family, Contemporary Family Trends, Portraits of Fathers.

171. Bee et al., *op cit.*

172. Bettelheim, *op. cit.*

173. Gordon, *op. cit.*

174. Papalia et al., *op cit.*

175. Nieman, *op. cit.*

176. Health Canada, *Aboriginal People,* Website: http://www. hc-sc.gc.ca/.

177. Hamilton, K., and L. Wengert, Down the Aisle, *Newsweek,* July 10, 1998, 54–57.

178. Bauer, *op. cit.*

179. McManus, *op. cit.*

180. Vanier Institute of the Family, *Contemporary Family Trends, Strengths in Families: Accentuating the Positive,* Website: http:// www.vifamily.ca/, June 2004.

181. Booth, J., British Families: Loss of a Stiff Upper Lip? *Focus on the Family,* July (1995), 5.

182. Shepherd, E., The Multicultural Families Down Under, *Focus on the Family,* July (1994), 13.

183. Betta and Musi, *op. cit.*

184. Rodriguez, R., Families South of the Border: Costa Rica—Paradise Lost? *Focus on the Family,* July (1995), 6–7.

185. Stuart, W., European Families: Old Customs, New Morality, *Focus on the Family,* July (1995), 10.

186. Borisov, B., Russian Families Caught in a Wave of Changes, *Focus on the Family,* July (1994), 11.

187. Taylor, M., and J. Gardner, African Families: Turbulent Times Ahead, *Focus on the Family,* July (1994), 12.

188. Iida, C., Is the Sun Setting on the Family, *Focus on the Family,* June (1994), 14.

189. Hartrick, G., A.E. Lindsey, and A. Hills, Family Nursing Assessment: Meeting the Challenge of Health Promotion, *Journal of Advanced Nursing,* 20, no. 1 (1995), 85–91.

190. Wright and Leahey, *op. cit.*

191. Hutchins, D., and C. Cole, *Helping Relationships and Strategies* (2nd ed.). Belmont, CA: Brooks/Cole, 1992.

192. Murray, R., and M. Huelskoetter, *Psychiatric/Mental Health Nursing: Giving Emotional Care* (3rd ed.). Norwalk, CT: Appleton & Lange, 1991.

193. Peplau, H., *Interpersonal Relations in Nursing.* New York: G.P. Putnam's Sons, 1952.

194. *Ibid.*

195. Rogers, C., *Client-Centered Therapy.* Boston: Houghton Mifflin, 1951.

196. Peplau, *op. cit.*

197. Forchuk, C., Peplau's Theory: Concepts and Their Relations, *Nursing Science Quarterly,* 4, no. 2 (1991), 54–59.

198. Forchuk, C., and B. Brown, Establishing a Nurse–Client Relationship, *Journal of Psychosocial Nursing,* 27, no. 2 (1989), 30–34.

199. Murray and Huelskoetter, *op. cit.*

200. Peplau, *op. cit.*

201. *Ibid.*

202. Murray and Huelskoetter, *op. cit.*

203. Rogers, *op. cit.*

204. Bauer, *op. cit.*

205. Murray and Huelskoetter, *op. cit.*

206. Peplau, *op. cit.*

207. *Ibid.*

208. Rogers, *op. cit.*

209. Starkey, P., Genograms: A Guide to Understanding One's Own Family System, *Perspectives of Psychiatric Care,* 14, nos. 5 and 6 (1987), 164–173.

210. Stolte, K.M. *Wellness: Nursing Diagnosis for Health Promotion,* Philadelphia: Lippincott, 1996.

211. *Ibid.*

212. *Ibid.*

213. Mellott, *op. cit.*

214. Crawford, J.A., and M.A. Tarko. Family Communication, in P.J. Bomar, ed., *Promoting Health in Families: Applying Family Research and Theory to Nursing Practice* (3rd ed., pp. 162–174). Philadelphia: Saunders, 2004.

215. *Ibid.*

216. Papalia et al., *op cit.*

217. *Ibid.*

218. *Ibid.*

219. *Ibid.*

220. Horn, B., Cultural Concepts and Postpartal Care, *Journal of Transcultural Nursing,* 2, no. 1 (1990), 48–51.

221. Wright and Leahey, *op. cit.*

222. Holtzworth-Monroe, A, Marital Violence, *The Harvard Mental Health Letter,* 12, no. 2 (1995), 4–6.

223. Papalia et al., *op cit.*

224. McNeill, T. 2004. Fathers' Experience of Parenting a Child with Juvenile Rheumatoid Arthritis, *Qualitative Health Research,* 14, no. 4 (2004), 526–545.

225. Brockhaus and Brockhaus, *op. cit.*

226. Ritchie, *op. cit.*

227. Schaffer and Londstrum, *op. cit.*

228. Sieg, *op. cit.*

229. Smit, *op. cit.*

230. Hammond, T., and C. Deans, A Phenomenological Study of Families and Psychoeducation Support Groups, *Journal of Psychosocial Nursing,* 33, no. 10 (1995), 7–12.

231. Visher and Visher, *op. cit.*

232. Whall, *op. cit.*

233. Bettelheim, *op. cit.*

234. Duvall and Miller, *op. cit.*

235. Kahana et al., *op. cit.*

236. Bettelheim, *op. cit.*

237. Kahana et al., *op. cit.*

238. Parental Work Load Affects Adolescents.

239. Bettelheim, *op. cit.*

240. *Ibid.*

241. Duvall and Miller, *op. cit.*

242. Bozet and Hanson, *op. cit.*

243. Bettelheim, *op. cit.*

244. Papalia et al., *op cit.*

Chapter 5

OVERVIEW: THEORIES RELATED TO HUMAN DEVELOPMENT

No theory explains everything about the person.

Ruth Beckmann Murray

OBJECTIVES

STUDY OF THIS CHAPTER WILL ENABLE YOU TO:

1. Examine major theoretic perspectives for understanding the developing person.

2. Describe selected physiologic theories about aspects of the developing person.

3. Discuss ecologic theory as it applies to the developing person.

4. Analyze major psychological developmental theorists, according to their views about the developing person.

5. Compare and contrast major concepts of behavioural, psychoanalytic and neo-analytic, cognitive, existential, and humanistic theories.

6. Differentiate major concepts between stress and crisis theories.

7. Apply concepts from at least three theories of development in care of the client.

PROGRESSION OF STUDY OF HUMAN DEVELOPMENT

Human development has been described for millennia. During the 18th century, the "nature versus nurture" argument began. The child was considered to be a little adult, the product either of heredity or environment. Gradually the child was seen as different from the adult. By the 19th century, study of the child was beginning to be more systematic. The science of **psychology,** *the study of human behaviour,* developed in the later 1800s, led people to better understand themselves by learning about child behaviour. Theories about human behaviour were being developed. The rise of Protestantism, with its emphasis on responsibility for self and others, led adults to feel more responsible for how the child developed into an adult. With the Industrial Revolution, children became more important to their parents. Gradually, child education occurred outside of the home. Until the 20th century, study of child development and advice in child care was not based on the scientific method but on biases and folklore.

As the 20th century progressed, theories about human behaviour were developed, and study was expanded to include the child and adult and later the adolescent and different stages of adulthood, including young and middle adulthood. As people are living longer, the elderly have become a focus, and several stages of older adulthood have been described.

Presently, the life span is studied as persons continue to develop or undergo change—physically, emotionally, cognitively, spiritually, and socially. Dying is seen as the last developmental phase, the final attempt to come to terms with self, others, and life in general. The study of the changes made by the individual and the family unit throughout the life span is the focus of this book. By learning more about ourselves and others, including how people respond to surrounding influences to meet basic needs, we hope to help people become better able to meet their individual potential and, in turn, create a better world.

Theories that are used to explain the developing person and the person's behaviour use either a biological, ecologic-social, or psychological basis. Although we focus on the psychological theories, a brief explanation of biological and ecologic-social theories is given. The psychological theories are divided according to their emphases: behaviourism, analytic, cognitive, and humanistic. Theorists who focus on these various psychological theories have been grouped according to similarity of theories.

Keep in mind that any theory explains an aspect of the person. *The whole person is best understood when several theories are combined to explain the person's total development.* The theories have been developed by one or several methods for studying people. Use the theories described in this chapter in assessment, goal-setting, and interventions for health promotion.

CRITICAL THINKING

Before reading this chapter, consider, for a moment, any theories of human development that come to your mind.

Although this chapter focuses on an overview of theories of human development, it is important to note that health promotion of the individual and the family throughout the life span is also pertinent. Therefore, it seems appropriate to outline and to address briefly the theoretical frameworks pertinent to health promotion.

Nutbeam and Harris state that four theories have been influential on the practice of health promotion. These theories are (1) the health belief model, (2) the theory of reasoned action, (3) the trans-theoretical (stages of change) model, and (4) the social cognitive theory.[1] The main thrust of these theories is that they explain health behaviour and health behaviour change by focusing on the individual. The health belief model is designed to explain health behaviour by understanding better beliefs about health first, from the individual and the families, and regarding the relative costs and benefits of strategies to protect and improve health. The major assumption underlying the theories of reasoned action, developed by Ajzen and Fishbein, is that people are usually rational and will make predictable decisions—particularly in those circumstances that are well defined. The reasoned action model is based on the assumption that the intention to act is the most immediate determinant of behaviour and all other variables influencing behaviour will be mediated through behavioural intention. The transtheoretical (stages of change) model, developed by Prochaska and DiClimente, is based on the premise that behaviour change is a process, not an event, and that individuals have different levels of motivation or readiness to change. The social cognitive theory has evolved from social leaning theory and is one of the most widely applied theories for health promotion because it addresses both the underlying determinants of health as well as methods to promote change. Many researchers have contributed to the social cognitive theory, but one of the most influential contributors has been Albert Bandura. These four theories are becoming increasingly important to know in the implementation of health promotion because health professionals' demands are calling for theory-based decisions.

BIOLOGICAL THEORIES

Basic to the person is his or her anatomic and physiologic structure and function. Various areas of the brain control functions and influence development and behaviour. The mind represents a range of brain functions—simple to complex, including physical, sensory, cognitive, and affective functions. The brain controls behaviour—how we perceive, think, feel, behave, act, and interact. The two halves of the brain are mutually involved in all high levels of psychological functioning. Each hemisphere functions independently in perception, learning, and memory (see Table 5-1); however, consciousness and the conscious self are single and unified, mediated by brain processes that span both hemispheres. Consciousness is an active integral part of the cerebral process; it exerts control over the biophysical and chemical activities at subordinate levels.[2]

The huge quantity and vast range of sensory information that is transmitted to the cerebral cortex and the way in which the brain sorts, classifies, organizes, and interprets sensory information; handles input and output; considers expectations, past experiences, and other sources of information; and sends messages throughout the body are beyond the capability of any computer system. Research on the physiologic basis for behaviour has gained sophistication with advancing technology in studying the complexity of the brain and nervous system, endocrine and immune functions, and physiologic responses in a variety of situations. These findings affect current beliefs about health, normality, and development. In the following discussion, theories related to genetic, biochemical, and neurophysiologic factors are covered briefly. For comprehensive study, refer to the chapter's endnotes.[3–5] Also, Chapters 6 through 14 present physiologic factors that affect the person.

Genetic Factors

Understanding of the role of genetic factors has been derived historically from studies focusing on pedigree descriptions, incidence of abnormalities in generations of families, and more recently, in direct visual examination of chromosomes and biochemical analyses of genetic material and enzymatic processes.[6] As molecular biology, neurobiology, and study of genes and DNA through the Human Genome Project continue to advance, there is a growing tendency to see all human behaviour, whether it is a craving for chocolate, generosity, or sexual addiction, only in genetic terms.[7,8]

The Mendelian Law of Inheritance states that a dominant gene for a trait or characteristic in at least one parent will cause, on the average, 50% probability that any child (of those parents) will inherit it. If both parents have the dominant gene, 75% of their children will inherit the trait. When the trait is attributed to a recessive gene, the offspring does not inherit it unless the gene was received from both parents. If the gene was received from only one parent, the offspring is not affected but will probably pass on the gene to a child (the grandchild). If the spouses are **heterozygous** for a recessive gene (*both received the same gene type from only one of their parents*), 25% of the children probably will be affected. If the spouses are **homozygous** for the recessive gene (the *same gene type was received from both of their parents*), all the children probably will inherit the trait or characteristic.[9,10]

The genetic system has several levels of complexity. For example, each neuron is genetically assigned to produce certain neurotransmitters. Genes also produce many kinds of receptors for each neurotransmitter. A single cell may respond differently to the same receptor at different times, for unknown reasons. When a neuron learns or is altered by experiences, there is a radical change in its surface proteins as well as in the receptors. Thus, environment and experience can alter genetic predisposition.[11]

To isolate environmental factors from genetic effects, researchers have used several methodological designs, such as the family resemblance method, the twin study method, and a combination of the two. The family resemblance method looks for similarity between a person with a disorder and his or her relatives.

The twin study method relies on differences between **monozygotic twins** (*from a single ovum and therefore identical*) and between **dizygotic twins** (*from two ova fertilized by two sperm and therefore not identical, i.e., fraternal twins*). For example, one study indicates the correlation for depressive symptoms is highest among identical twins. Twin studies indicate that there is a stable predisposition to temperament and that environment of the child contributes little to adult depression.[12,13] However, recent stressful events were a powerful predictor for onset of illness in those genetically predisposed. Genetic factors may alter the person's response to the depression-inducing effect of stressors such as the death of a close relative, assault, severe marital problems, and divorce.[14] Monozygotic twins have been found to resemble each other more in mood level and lability than dizygotic twins. Research is also being done on identical and fraternal twins reared apart.[15] For example, one recent Canadian study was

TABLE 5-1
Right Brain–Left Brain Information Processing Differences

Mode	Left Brain (Controls Right Side of Body)	Right Brain (Controls Left Side of Body)
Thinking	Time bound Rational, logical, sequential or linear, analytical, interpretive Synthesis of sensory input Spirituality	Space bound Concrete, appears irrational Artistic Intuitive; holistic
Language	Hearing words Writing words Voice recognition Reading Speech comprehension Verbal memory	Metaphoric Singing songs Face and form recognition Draw figures Body image
Mathematics	Algebraic functions, adding, subtracting, multiplying, dividing	Geometric, spatial, relational
Problem solving	Focus on specifics Breaks problems into parts, linear, sequential Details	Focus on generalities Grasps problem in totality Grasps relational dimensions Patterns
Organizational	Action mode: primed to manipulate environment Focal attention Heightened boundary perception Object-oriented Dominance of formal over sensory	Receptive mode: primed to take in environment Diffuse attention Boundary fusion Dominance of sensory over formal
Interactional	Controlled, consistent Explicit, directed, objective, judgmental, evaluative	Emotive Affect-laden Tacit Tolerant of ambiguity, subjective Nonjudgmental, noncritical
Operational	Figures things out in stepwise order One idea follows another Comfortable with precise connotations, right/wrong Computer-like functions Memory for verbal and auditory stimuli	Makes leaps of intuition Creativity Pattern recognition and relationships form basis of ideas Comfortable with alternatives and multiple explanations, nonlinguistic stimuli

conducted to examine the correlation between genetic liabilities for alcohol and drug misuse with perceptions of the social environment of the family of origin and the classroom. In Vancouver, a mail-out survey collected data from monozygotic and dizygotic twin pairs using newspaper advertisements and media stories. The researchers concluded that genotype–environment correlations (in particular, moral-emphasis in the home) appear to be important in the development of substance misuse.[16]

CRITICAL THINKING

What other twin studies have you found to have interesting results?

There has been recent interest in the study of the respective contributions of environmental and genetic influences to an individual's body fat in order to control the "epidemic" of obesity. A study was conducted at Toronto's York University to estimate the degree of familial resemblance in anthropometric indicators and fat distribution. Examples of anthropometric indicators include body mass index, skin folds, and waist circumference. The results suggested that in this sample of 327 Caucasian participants from 102 nuclear families, the role of genes explains at least part of the heritability.[17]

Simonen and her colleagues conducted a study on familial aggregation of physical activity levels in the Quebec Family Study. They investigated 696 subjects from 200 families of the Quebec Family Study. The findings suggested that physical activity is represented by a significant degree of familial resemblance. Physical inactivity has a slightly higher heritability level than does moderate to strenuous physical activity or total physical activity phenotypes. These researchers also found that the pattern of familial correlations suggests that shared familial environmental factors, along with genetic factors, are important in accounting for the familial resemblance in physical activity levels.[18]

The Mendelian law explains the occurrence of many physical traits such as eye colour and height and may explain certain physiologic charactcristics; *however, the Mendelian law does not fully explain emotional or mental development and does not include social, moral, or spiritual development.*

Specific genes cannot be linked with specific kinds of behaviour until the behaviour is precisely defined, which has not been done, in contrast to linking a gene with a specific disease, such as cystic fibrosis, which has been done.[19]

Genes determine a foundation for reaction or predisposition; the exact behavioural expression depends on many prenatal, parental, and postnatal influencing factors. For example, a specific chromosomal aberration, such as the presence of an extra chromosome, is directly related to Down syndrome, with resultant limited intellectual function. Yet the intellectual achievement may be lower than the inherited capacity if the person receives inadequate education, and the achievement may be somewhat higher than indicated by early testing when a loving family and appropriate education coexist to develop fully the inherited potential.[20]

Or, consider the quest for a genetic basis for sexual orientation. Sexual fantasies and arousal, homosexuality, bisexuality, and heterosexuality all lie on a continuum and may be outwardly expressed by the same person at different times in his or her life. Mood, environment, emotional attachments, and the person–culture interaction all are important in sexual arousal and sexual behaviour. To isolate the human gene(s) for sexual orientation, it would be necessary to identify genes for all these factors.[21,22]

Thus, **polygenic** inheritance, the *combination or interaction of many genes acting together to produce a behavioural characteristic,* is believed to be a factor if certain characteristics or behavioural defects occur. Environmental effects contribute to the person's development of genetic potential from the moment of conception.[23–25]

Hegele claims that in familial hypercholesterolemia (FH), early coronary heart disease (CHD) is a complex trait resulting from a large monogenic component of susceptibility due to elevated low-density lipoprotein (LDL).[26] Not all subjects, however, with a LDLR gene mutation suffer from early coronary heart disease. In fact, the environment plays a large role in modulating the expression of the genetic susceptibility to coronary heart disease.[27]

The Healthy Heart Kit is a brochure sponsored by Health Canada, Population and Public Health Branch (PPHB), in partnership with the College of Family Physicians of Canada, Health and Social Services (Montreal), and the Heart and Stroke Foundation of Canada and Quebec. This brochure helps individuals understand cholesterol and its impact on heart disease.[28] For example, it informs the individual of the nature of both "good" cholesterol, called HDL (high-density lipoprotein), and "bad" cholesterol, LDL (low-density lipoprotein). The LDL tends to block arteries. Furthermore, the desirable cholesterol levels, measured in millimoles per litre, or mmol/L for short, are provided in the handbook. The ideal level of LDL for people with heart disease is less than 2.5 mmol/L. In addition, the brochure informs individuals of ways to control their blood cholesterol regarding diet and exercise. It also emphasizes "no smoking" and following doctors' orders on prescription medication.[29] All provinces and territories have Heart and Stroke Foundation offices, which supply other useful and informative resources.

CRITICAL THINKING

What differences do you observe in the content of pamphlets among the provinces and territories?

A study was conducted to determine the diagnostic performance characteristics of HNF1A genotyping for diabetes and impaired glucose tolerance (IGT) in Oji-Cree Aboriginal people in Canada.[30] The researchers had identified a private HNF1A mutation, G319S, which was associated strongly with type 2 diabetes in the Oji-Cree. The HNF1A S319 allele occurred in less than 40% of the Oji-Cree who had diabetes, and was linked with a younger age at onset of diabetes, adolescent-onset type 2 diabetes, and changes in plasma lipoproteins. All subjects in this study were genotyped for the HNF1A G319S mutation. The results indicated that the most specific genetic test yet reported for the prediction of a common multifactor disease by considering present-day standards of clinical epidemiology in molecular genetics is the HNF1A genotype. The result of a positive test had particular diagnostic value in the Oji-Cree. That is, a subject with HNF1A S319 was certain of having diabetes or IGT by age 50. On the other hand, a subject without HNF1A S319 had a decreased risk, compared with the age specific prevalence, but was not totally risk-free. It is important to note that HNF1A S319 was not the only relevant factor for diabetes in the Oji-Cree. It was found that subjects without HNF1A S319 were still at some risk for diabetes or IGT.[31]

Young, Reading, Elias, and O'Neil reviewed the published literature on type 2 diabetes mellitus from the past two decades, and focused on the First Nations people in Canada. (They excluded the Inuit and Métis, as diabetes is not a serious health problem for the Inuit, and little data exists for the Métis.) These investigators conclude that the current health and social effects of the disease are considerable and that genetic interactions are likely the cause.[32]

Virtually every disease has a genetic component based on a specific gene or gene mutation. Research with molecular

CASE SITUATION

Ted Smith, a 40-year-old husband, and father of three young children, is a sales manager with a well-known computer company. A few years ago Ted was diagnosed with coronary heart disease (CHD). His father died of a heart attack a few months ago. Over the last few weeks Ted has mentioned several times to his wife, Sharon, that he has been experiencing "chest heaviness." He attributes this discomfort to work stress and assures Sharon that it will likely pass when business picks up. Sharon, however, is worried that Ted frequently eats packaged snacks and drinks a lot of canned drinks and coffee while "on the run" between appointments. Ted's usual twice-weekly stop at the gym for his work-out has been neglected now for almost a year. With these observations in mind, Sharon has convinced Ted to stop at the Walk-In Clinic to check out the chest heaviness symptom.

You are a clinical nurse specialist at this clinic. When Ted arrives you conduct the initial assessment. Sharon shares her concerns and observations about Ted with you. Ted then consults with the doctor, who recommends that he have his blood cholesterol checked. Ted makes arrangements with the lab to have his blood drawn for blood cholesterol. In a few days, the lab sends you his results of the three types of cholesterol and the triglycerides. You particularly notice that Ted's LDL reading is high—that is, above 4.0 mmol/L. You know that Ted will return for the results of his blood cholesterol by the end of the week.

1. What is your understanding of blood cholesterol levels?
2. According to the *Healthy Heart Kit*, is Ted's LDL level borderline high, or high? (See http://www.healthyheartkit.com.)
3. What health promotion strategies would you plan with Ted at this time?

techniques is helping us understand genetic contributions (the specific chromosomal regions) to such diseases as Alzheimer's disease, hypertension, diabetes, various cancers, heart and kidney diseases, and some mental illness or brain diseases. In the future, a genetic profile will be developed for each child at birth. However, genetic predisposition or causation is not immutable. Environmental factors can modify and affect the expression of a specific gene or gene mutation. For example, even though an individual has a very strong genetic susceptibility to coronary heart disease (CHD), personal decisions and actions to modify the environment will have an effective impact on the unfavourable genetics in CHD.[33] Health professionals can play a significant role in promoting a healthy lifestyle through screening methods and teaching risk reduction measures to individuals and their families.

A prime component of the Human Genome Project is the effort to construct a detailed map of human DNA and the genes that guide the development of a human being from a fertilized egg cell. Another interest of the project is the examination of the ethical, legal, and social implications of this recently discovered genetic knowledge. Also included within the mandate of the project is the development of policy options for public consideration regarding this genetic research strategy. The genome is the sum total of genes carried by all 46 chromosomes in the human being.[34,35] It is estimated that 60% of Canadians will experience during their life span an illness with some form of genetic component. Genetic technologies hold the potential to assist a large majority of Canadians.[36] In fact, the combined effects of recent and anticipated genetics research hold the potential to redefine medicine within the lifetime of many Canadians. Actually, the recent plethora of knowledge of individual susceptibility to diseases raises questions about the types of related ethical issues, including the need to protect the privacy and safety of individuals and to outlaw the use of genetic information in the place of employment.[37] It is important not only to educate all health care professionals with the tools and knowledge they need to navigate this complex terrain, but to build a climate of understanding and acceptance of genetic innovation in the community and society in general.[38]

CRITICAL THINKING

What is your understanding of Parkinson's disease and its management? See Guttman et al. (2003).[39]

Genome Canada is a not-for-profit corporation whose aim is to develop and to implement a national strategy to genomics and proteomics in Canada. With financial assistance from the federal government, Genome Canada has established five genome centres across the country.[40] Together with these centres and other partners, Genome Canada invests and manages large-scale research projects in important areas such as agriculture, environment, fisheries, forestry, health, and new technology.[41]

As a matter of interest, in April 2004 the I.H. Asper Clinical Research Institute, at the St. Boniface General Hospital in Winnipeg, hosted Canada's first national, travelling, bilingual exhibition on DNA and genomics. It was called "The Geee!"[42] You may wish to check whether or not this innovative exhibit continues to be hosted in Canada.

CRITICAL THINKING

Will knowledge of the human genome lead to the development of a repair manual for the human body?

As a partner with Genome Canada, the Ontario Genomics Institute (OGI) is dedicated to developing new preventative measures, diagnostics, and treatments that will affect the lives of people in Ontario and globally.[43] One of the projects, funded jointly by Genome Canada, the Canadian Cystic Fibrosis Foundation, and the National Institutes of Health, is the mapping and isolation of genes that influence the severity of disease in cystic fibrosis. The leaders of this project are Lap-Chee Tsui and Peter Druie of Toronto's Hospital for Sick Children.[44]

Reproductive screening can be conducted for carriers of autosomal recessive diseases, such as cystic fibrosis, in order to provide information to the partners, which they might use regarding decisions about family planning. However, careful counselling is necessary with carrier screening to make certain that individuals comprehend the limitations of testing and the implications of results.[45] Wilson and his associates assessed the role of cystic fibrosis testing within the Canadian health care system. They recommended that in pregnancy, CF testing should be indicated for individuals who may be at increased risk for CF because of family history or clinical manifestations, and prior to CF screening, each province/territory should review the ethnic diversity of its reproductive population to ensure that CF screening would be appropriate. The screening of all women for CF carrier status during pregnancy could not be recommended at this time.[46]

CONTROVERSY DEBATE

Reproductive Screening

In a classroom debate your colleagues are discussing reproductive screening tests. The situation at hand pertains to Jean, a pregnant young woman who has advised the nurse that both she and her partner are carriers of cystic fibrosis (CF). Based on the Mendelian Law of Inheritance, you understand that there are four possibilities to combine genes from parents who are both carriers. Carriers will have both a dominant normal gene (N) for CF, *and* a recessive gene (c) for CF. Each parent's gene pool for CF will be represented as (Nc). The CF gene combination possibilities for the offspring of these parents are as follows:

1. N/N (Normal), no CF in offspring

2. N/c (Carrier), no CF in offspring

3. N/c (Carrier), no CF in offspring

4. c/c (Disease), shows Cystic Fibrosis in offspring.

You can predict that there is a 25% probability that the child will have CF.

1. What is your position on reproductive screening for this couple?

2. If pregnant women who are carriers of other autosomal recessive diseases wish to pay for reproductive screening, would you, as a health professional, support and lobby for their cause?

The Human Genome Project (HGP), launched in the United States in the late 1980s, is a research effort to create a genomic map to provide precise information about the structure, organization, and characteristics of human DNA. This information provides a basic set of inherited instructions for the development and functioning of every human being. Scientists seek to obtain an unprecedented understanding of health and disease, life and death.[47]

As a result of biotechnology, another industry, **bioinformatics,** *a field that focuses on the storage and retrieval of biological information from a database in a biologically meaningful way,* is developing. The new research and computerized information is important; it is equally essential to remember that genetics *alone* cannot explain human behaviour.[48,49]

Practice applications are apparent because of the rapidly advancing knowledge about genetics and health care, and requests for genetic services will be affected. The Canadian Nurses Association Position Statement on The Role of the Nurse in Reproductive and Genetic Technologies states that nurses will be called on to play a critical role in advocating the availability of helpful information. Nurses will be essential in encouraging public participation in developing policies about a number of highly significant issues. Some of the issues in which the nurses will play key roles include assisted human reproduction, genetic testing, genetic therapy, genetic enhancements, the human genome project, and privacy concerns—as well as human cloning.[50] Even though the role of genetics in human health is complex, nurses are well situated to play an important role in genetics in their various practice settings.[51] In order to do so, nurses must take the responsibility to become knowledgeable about this rapidly changing field, and help clients make well-informed decisions about the risks and benefits of assisted human reproduction, and genetic testing.

A two-year grant project, "Managing Genetic Information: Policies for U.S. Nurses," was funded by the Center for Human Genome Research at the National Institutes for Health and was coordinated by the American Nurses Association's Center for Ethics and Human Rights. The purpose of the project was to collect data about how genetic information can be used in practice and ethical, legal, and social concerns related to genetic engineering and services. There are a number of practice implications, including the need to:[52–54]

- Obtain a genetic history as part of assessment.
- Explain diagnostic tests related to genetic-based disease and the meaning of positive and negative results.
- Provide emotional support to persons with genetic disorders and to their families.
- Offer genetic screening and testing to those who do not request it.
- Address ethical issues related to expansion of genetic information, such as reproductive issues, individual rights, confidentiality, and treatment issues.
- Learn about gene therapy, gene transfer, rationale, and constraints.
- Realize that genetic tests can tell the client if she or he carries the disease but do not predict if the person will eventually be diagnosed with the disease.
- Teach that with positive genetic findings, environmental or other events may have to occur before a disease, such as cancer or depression, is manifested.
- Teach that with negative genetic findings, not having a gene for a disease does not mean that the disease will not occur for other reasons.
- Explain that knowledge that the client has a defective gene does not mean prevention or treatment is available related to the disease or that the disease course can be altered.
- Counsel the client if he or she feels guilt about having the flawed gene.

- Advocate for the client with genetic predisposition to disease in relation to employment and health insurance coverage.
- Teach that the person may not want, and has a right not to have, genetic testing.

In summary, two principles explain how differences in heredity may exert influence. The **Principle of Differential Susceptibility** suggests that *individual differences in heredity exist that make people susceptible to the influence of certain environments.* Given different experiences, a person with certain hereditary potential would develop in different ways. For example, the person with hereditary predisposition to schizophrenia would be likely to develop the disease if raised in a certain kind of environment. The **Principle of Differential Exposure** suggests that *inherited characteristics cause differing reactions from people, which in turn affect or shape the personality of the individual.* For example, body build, facial structure, and presence or absence of overall physical attractiveness result primarily from inheritance. People perceive, judge the actions of, and react more favourably to physically attractive children than to less attractive children. Over time, reactions of others contribute to formation of the self-concept, positive or negative feelings about self, and a sense of competency or incompetence that may affect behaviour toward others or general performance. Excessive negative reaction from others may predispose to abnormal behaviour and even mental illness if the stress is great enough.[55,56]

Much remains unknown about the manner and extent to which early individual differences result in later personality differences, and the extent to which early transactions between parents and child either enhance or obscure genetic characteristics. Intellect, emotions, societal factors, values, and learned life patterns are crucial to consider in health promotion.[57,58]

CRITICAL THINKING

What assessment tool would you use to gather information about factors important to consider for health promotion?

Biochemical Factors

Research on the relationship between biochemical factors and behaviour involves the areas of neurochemistry and hormones.

Neurochemistry is implicated in some behavioural development. The amount of biogenic amines, especially the **neurotransmitters,** *chemicals involved in transfer or modulation of nerve impulses from one cell to another,* apparently is related to mood. Acetylcholine, norepinephrine, dopamine, serotonin and GABA are important neurotransmitters in the brain and are involved in such emotional states as arousal, fear, rage, pleasure, motivation, exhilaration, sleep, and wakefulness. Brain opioids and peptides aid in control of pain and maintain a euphoric mood. Such behaviour, in turn, affects reactions of others, especially parents, to the child, and the child's moods may affect childrearing behaviour.

Hormonal factors, based on changes in the endocrine system during stress or endocrine system disorders, may contribute to certain behaviours. Steroid hormones are increased during stress behaviour, which in turn may interfere with normal developmental processes physically and cognitively.[59] Excess steroid hormone intake (prescribed for illness or to build muscles and strength in athletes) causes mental as well as physical problems. The person may develop depression, elation, aggression, paranoia, hallucinations, delusions, or psychosis. The mental disorders disappear after discontinuation of the drug, although it may take some time.[60] The pineal gland secretes the hormone melatonin, which increases when darkness falls and appears to keep the mind synchronized with the outside world. An imbalance may be linked to inducing sleep and melancholia. Various benefits attributed to melatonin, such as protecting cells from damage, boosting the immune system, preventing aging, and extending life, have been claimed but are unproven.[61]

Thyroid dysfunction, such as hypothyroidism or autoimmune thyroiditis, which results in thyroid atrophy, may cause signs and symptoms that match the criteria for depression: fatigue, constipation, vague aches and pains, feeling cold, poor memory, anxiety, and low mood. Eventually, the person may manifest confusion, cognitive impairment, and psychosis. Hyperthyroidism may manifest as anxiety, irritability, restlessness, euphoria, or mild manic disorder.[62] As a matter of interest, Liu, Semenciw, Ugnat, and Mao examined the time trends in thyroid cancer incidence in Canada by the following variables: age, time period, and birth cohort between 1970 and 1996. Their findings indicated that increases in thyroid cancer incidence in Canada may be associated with more intensive diagnostic activities and change in radiation exposure in childhood and adolescence. In addition, temporal changes in reproductive factors among young women may explain some of the gender differences observed.[63]

Excess cortisol production may manifest as depression or mania, confusion, and eventually, psychosis. Hypocortisolism may result in apathy, fatigue, and depression.[64]

The hormone estrogen appears to play a role maintaining and possibly improving memory in encoding, storing, and retrieving data. Women taking estrogen therapy show significantly more activity in brain areas associated with memory than women on a placebo.[65]

Biochemical differences exist between persons and can be identified. What is not clear is whether the biochemical changes precede, and thus contribute to, abnormal behaviour, or result from changes that occur interpersonally or socially as a result of the person's abnormal behaviour. The person in acute or short-term stress or crisis may have an abnormal level of a neurotransmitter as a result of normal feelings precipitated by and related to the event, yet that person is not predetermined to be, or does not become, mentally ill.[66]

Neurophysiologic Factors

Neurophysiologic factors mediate all physiologic processes and behaviour via the nervous system; however, neurophysiologic factors in behaviour and personality development are inconclusive. Some specific motor and speech functions and various sensations in different body parts can be traced to specific brain areas.

Localization of brain function means that *certain areas of the brain are more concerned with one kind of function than* *another.* It does not imply that a specific function is mediated by only one brain region. Specific brain function requires the integrated action of neurons located in many different brain regions.

Specialized functions of brain regions are as follows:[67–71]

I. Cerebral cortical lobes
   A. Frontal—planning and movement: aggression
   B. Parietal—somatic sensation
   C. Temporal—hearing, memory, learning, and emotion
   D. Occipital—vision
   E. Major association cortices
      1. Prefrontal cortex—highest brain functions
      2. Limbic cortex—memory, emotion, motivation of behaviour
      3. Parietal-temporal-occipital—higher sensory function, language
      4. Premotor association cortex—planning of action and initiation of movement (damage affects execution of movement)
      5. Parietal-temporal-occipital association cortex—links information from the senses that is necessary for perception (damage causes deficit in body image and spatial relations, aphasia, agnosia, and astereognosis)
      6. Limbic association cortex, composed of the medial and ventral surfaces of the frontal lobe, the medial surface of the parietal lobe, portions of the temporal lobe, the orbital-frontal cortex, the cingulate region, the anterior tip of the temporal lobe, and the parahippocampal region, receives from higher-order sensory areas and projects to other critical regions and the prefrontal cortex; orbital-frontal portion concerned with motivation and emotional behaviour; temporal lobe concerned with memory;[72] basal ganglia involved in how we handle habits and physical skills;[73,74] amygdala associated with fear and anxiety

Linkage of the hypothalamus, limbic system, and cerebral cortex maintains homeostasis directly by regulating the endocrine and autonomic nervous systems and indirectly by regulating emotions and drives, including sexual preference, and any pleasure, by acting through the external environment. Hypothalamic integration of cardiovascular and respiratory function, motor and endocrine responses, combined with forebrain suppression of emotional responses, mediates emotional behaviour. The limbic system is the seat of emotion and is involved in affective and cognitive function and motivation, feelings, and behavioural homeostasis. Further, it is especially prone to pathology because neurotransmitter effects are rapid and the neuromodulatory effects are slow.[75]

Motivated behaviour can be regulated by factors other than tissue needs, including learned habits and subjective pleasurable feelings. Central reward circuitry or the central reward system (CRS) is located within the limbic system. It is not fully known how the CRS mediates and registers reward or reinforcement, but it is responsible for the pleasure response.[76]

Scientists have found severe depletion of key cells in the brains of people who died with depressive illness. Study of brain tissue of seven people with depression or manic depression showed that 40% to 90% of glial cells in the anterior cingulate in the prefrontal cortex were gone. Glial cells support other cells and provide growth factors and nutrients to neurons. Brains of people who were not depressed did not show this. Studies have shown reduced blood flow in this area of patients who have depression and manic depression that does not go away with treatment.[77]

Children apparently are born with a predisposition to be outgoing or quiet, and there may be a chemical predisposition to seeking danger or high risk. Yet neurophysiology does not supply all the answers. A supportive environment may cause further development of certain neurophysiologic rudiments and promote further development of the neurophysiologic processes that are manifested: thus environment helps to produce a well-adjusted child. A hostile home environment, especially in early life, produces the opposite result.

Immunologic Factors

The *immune system* functions to protect the body against disease; it recognizes and distinguishes foreign substances, such as bacteria, toxins, and cancer, from the body's own tissue. Immune suppression and stimulation are both necessary at different times to maintain health. At times the system responds excessively and destroys normal tissues. The system's function is closely interrelated with the central nervous system, endocrine system, perceptions, and behaviour.

A chronic inflammatory autoimmune collagen disease resulting from disturbed immune regulation that causes exaggerated production of autoantibodies is systemic lupus erythematosus (SLE).[78] In Manitoba, Peschken and Esdaile conducted the first study to examine the prevalence, disease course, and survival of patients with SLE. They studied a population of 120 000 North American Indians (NAI) and contrasted the results to those found in the non-Indian population. The researchers concluded that the prevalence of the disease was increased twofold in the NAI population. Further, NAI patients had higher SLE Disease Activity Index (SLEDAI) scores at the time of diagnosis. The NAI patients exhibited more frequent vasculitis and renal involvement. They also required more treatment later in the disease trajectory, accumulated more damage following diagnosis, and had increased fatality.[79]

A number of disorders can cause serious, often lifethreatening, alterations within the body's immune system. The one disorder that profoundly increases the anxiety level within the individual, family, and community is human immunodeficiency virus (HIV), and the subsequent development of acquired immunodeficiency syndrome (AIDS).[80] Canadians are at the forefront of the response to HIV/AIDS, and they continue to expand their involvement through collaborative initiatives at the local, regional, national, and international levels.[81]

EVIDENCE-BASED PRACTICE

How People with HIV/AIDS Manage and Assess Their Use of Complementary Therapies: a Quantitative Analysis

The results of this study provide a qualitative analysis of the practical concerns that people with HIV/AIDS have with regard to their use of complementary therapies. The authors cite studies that have identified therapies and activities most often used by people with HIV/AIDS—aerobic exercise, prayer, massage, needle acupuncture, meditation, support groups, visual imagery, breathing exercises, spiritual activities, and nonaerobic exercise. In-depth semi-structured interviews were conducted with a diverse group of 46 people with HIV/AIDS. An inductive grounded approach was used to collect and analyze the data. There were five central concerns: (1) selecting which therapies to use, (2) judging which therapies work, (3) combining Western medicine with complementary therapies, (4) assessing the safety of complementary therapies, and (5) dealing with the barriers to the use of complementary therapies. A better understanding of the practical dimensions of complementary therapy use highlights the treatment and care issues that people with HIV/AIDS face and offers insights into the role that nurses might play in addressing some of these issues.

Nursing Implications

1. Health care professionals can represent an important source of information, but respondents typically drew on other resources.

2. Many health care professionals with whom they have contact do not seem to posses enough knowledge about or interest in complementary therapies to provide them with much advice.

3. Nurses can play an important role in assisting those people with HIV/AIDS who wish to take a complementary approach to health care.

   a.   They can inform themselves about the dominant complementary approaches, and they can encourage other health care providers to do so.

   b.   Nurses can play a supportive role with patients and physicians alike in encouraging a more open dialogue with regard to the broad range of health care approaches that people with HIV may be employing.

   c.   Nurses can play an important role in linking patients to community supports that will help actively involve them in making informed decisions about possible strategies for managing their health and in overcoming barriers to accessing the care they desire.

4. Health care professionals, and nurses in particular, can play a critical role as a resource and form of support for people with HIV/AIDS who are dealing with the practical challenges of integrating different types of health care options, both complementary therapies and Western medical treatments.

Source: Gillett, J., D. Pawluch, and R. Cain. How People with HIV/AIDS Manage and Assess their Use of Complementary Therapies: A Qualitative Analysis, Journal of the Association of Nurses in AIDS Care, *13, no. 2 (2000), 17–27.*

CRITICAL THINKING

What initiatives are being taken in your province/territory to combat HIV/AIDS?

The field of psychoneuroimmunology has shown the connections between stress in the environment and physical and emotional health. Certain mechanisms, not yet fully understood, produce greater physical health when there is emotional well-being. The stress of rapid or unexpected change can negatively affect health.

Maturational Factors

The maturational view emphasizes the emergence of patterns of development of organic systems, physical structures, and motor capabilities under the influence of genetic and maturational forces. Because of an inherent predisposition of the neurological, hormonal, and skeletal-muscular systems to develop spontaneously, *physiologic and motor development occurs in an inevitable and sequential pattern in children throughout the world.* The growth of the nervous system is critical in this maturation,

unless the normal process is inhibited by severe environmental, physiologic, and emotional deprivation.[82]

Sex differences may be inherent for some characteristics. For example, women generally have a greater response to the intuitive and analytic side of the brain, whereas men have a greater response to the spatial side of the brain. Yet many characteristics are the result of sociocultural influences; women from certain cultures may demonstrate characteristics common to men in other cultures. Sex differences are described in Chapters 10 to 14.

Biological Rhythms

Biorhythms are *self-sustaining, repetitive, rhythmic patterns established in plants, animals, people, and seasonal-environmental events.* These daily or monthly biological cycles affect a number of physical functions, such as blood cell, blood glucose, and hormone levels; body temperature; heartbeat; blood pressure; renal and gastrointestinal function; sleep; and muscular strength and coordination. Mental skills and emotional changes are also apparently affected. Biological rhythm is unique to the individual and may be recorded through

(1) interview, (2) a detailed diary recording quantitative information about body process and subjective experiences, and (3) autorhythmometry, in which the person records and rates physiologic processes and mood.[83,84] Biological rhythms are discussed in Chapter 12.

Biological Deficiencies

Biological stressors, such as certain kinds of foods, lack of food or malnutrition, medications, and lack of sleep, may change behaviour and the course of development. These factors are discussed further in Chapters 6 and 14.

ECOLOGIC THEORIES

Ecology is a *science that is concerned with the community and the total setting in which life and behaviour occur.* A basic ecologic principle is that the continuity and survival of a person depend on a deliberate balance of factors influencing the interactions between the family or person and the environment.

Family is dependent on the resources and groups in the community to survive and continue its own development and to nurture adequately development of offspring. Further, climate, terrain, and natural resources affect family lifestyle and development and behaviour of family members. The neighbourhood may adversely affect development, especially if the person is reared in a family that lives in a deteriorating neighbourhood or in an area with poor schools, inadequate housing, and a high crime rate. Excessively crowded housing may create stresses within the family that contribute to sleep deprivation, bickering, incest, or other abuse, which, in turn, affect developmental progress in all spheres of the person. Job loss because of a changing community and the resultant financial problems may affect health care practices and nutrition and, in turn, physical growth and emotional security.

Urbanization, rapid social changes, social stressors, discrimination, unemployment, poor housing, inadequate diet and health care, poverty, feelings of **anomie** (*not being part of society*), and negative self-image all contribute to stress and developmental difficulties in the vulnerable, immature person or in one without an adequate support system.[85]

There are four theories about how neighbourhoods affect behaviour:

1. *Contagion model.* People follow the example of others in their neighbourhood or immediate community. Part of this model includes the social control model, where adults are enforcers who keep children off the streets and out of trouble; police help maintain order; high-socioeconomic-status adults act as behavioural role models because they show that success is possible if one works hard and behaves appropriately.

2. *Relative deprivation model.* High-socioeconomic-level neighbours and affluence shown in mass media provoke resentment in the poor; the poor feel a greater need to create a deviant subculture if they live nearer to the affluent than the poor.

3. *Neighbours-are-irrelevant model.* People base their decisions and actions on their own circumstances and long-term interests, not on what neighbours consider acceptable; however, rational behaviours are usually restricted to choosing among familiar alternatives. Even in the poorest neighbourhoods, a youth can find a friend who stays out of trouble and stays in school. In affluent neighbourhoods, some youth get into trouble.

4. *Neighbours-do-not-matter-but-neighbourhoods-do model.* Individuals in the neighbourhood may not matter, but institutions such as schools and resources such as health care facilities do matter. Authorities often treat youth differently based on where they live.[86]

Sociologic variables, including family socioeconomic level and position in the community, and the prestige related to birth, race, age, cultural ties, and power roles affect development, behaviour, and adaptation of the person and family. Certain behaviours may be expected from a person because of age, sex, race, religion, or occupation. The individual may experience role conflicts and developmental problems when there are discrepancies between norms and values and the demands of age, sex, occupation, or religion.[87]

Cultures vary in their definitions of normal and abnormal behaviour; cross-cultural comparisons of developmental norms are difficult. Theorists in each culture describe their research findings about normal child or adult characteristics or behaviour based on norms of their culture and their cultural bias. For example, a research study was conducted to explore arthritis management strategies among Chinese immigrants in Calgary and to assess factors that impacted on these strategies. The findings illustrated that disease management strategies among Chinese immigrants are not only affected by the disease itself but also by personal and cultural strategies. In fact, these factors suggest helpful guidelines to providing culturally sensitive care, which, in turn, can lead to greater satisfaction and well-being for Chinese immigrants with arthritis.[88]

CRITICAL THINKING

What question might you ask an Inuit client about his or her health beliefs and practices?

5-1 BONUS SECTION IN CD-ROM

Research Abstract: Genetic and Environmental Influences on Cardiovascular Disease Risk Factors in Adolescents

Twin studies are always interesting. When such studies are longitudinal in nature, they are even more interesting. Here the cardiovascular disease risk factors in adolescents are studied and the implications for practice involve children.

Geographic moves may create many adjustments for the person as he or she attempts to meet norms of the new community. Developmental problems and dysfunctional behaviour may occur among those who migrate.[89] Persons who move often as children may never form "chumships" or close relationships later in adulthood; however, the mobile family and individual do learn coping skills that help them adjust to unfamiliar or stressful situations.

DeWit explored the relationship between the number of geographic moves before the age of 16 and the timing of onset of drug use, as well as the progression to drug-related problems. The data was obtained from 3700 young adults aged 18 to 35 years participating in the 1990–1991 Ontario Mental Health Supplement, a large random-probability survey of the residents in Ontario. The significant results indicated positive relationships between moving and early initiation of illicit drugs, such as marijuana, hallucinogens, and crack/cocaine, and the illicit use of prescribed drugs. The relationship between moving and measures of alcohol use/problems (onset of first drink, onset of any alcohol-related problems) were either weak or nonsignificant. However, important sex differences were found. A statistically significant relationship was found between moving and early drug use initiation. It was also established that progression occurred primarily among males. DeWit urges that future research is needed (1) to discover why drug use appears to be a more common response to relocation among boys, and (2) to test for possible mediating factors linking relocation with the onset of drug use as well as moderating influences.[90]

CRITICAL THINKING

After reading about the study conducted by DeWit,[91] what are your thoughts on why drug use appears to be a more common response to relocation among boys than among girls?

One view of an individual's psychological problems is the result of some personal circumstances, such as deficient achievement of developmental tasks, immaturity, character defect, or maladjustment. An alternate view is to see the individual problems as stemming from social causes. The broad economic, political, cultural, and social patterns of our society and particular subcultures can be viewed as determinants of individual developmental responses. Then the community is the place to begin making changes if individual dysfunction is to be decreased.[92] Chapters 1 through 4 discuss cultural, environmental, religious, spiritual, and family variables, and Chapters 7 through 14 present the interrelationship of these variables on the person.

Systems Perspective: General Systems Theory Applied to Behaviour

First proposed by von Bertalanffy,[93] general systems theory presents a comprehensive, holistic, and interdisciplinary view. This theory proposes that the family, individual, various social groups, and cultures are systems. Nothing is determined by a single cause or explained by a single factor. Nothing can be studied as a lone entity, be it the environment; various sociocultural components; political-legal, religious, educational, and other social institutions or organizations; the person, family, group, or community; or the health care delivery organization. All have interrelating parts, and all components interact with each other.[94–96] An interconnectedness or interrelationship exists at and between every system level. A complementarity exists between parts of a system.

A **system** is an *assemblage, unit, or organism of interrelated, interdependent parts, persons, or objects that are united by some form or order into a recognizable unit and that are in equilibrium.*[97–102]

Synergy exists, meaning that *the whole is greater than the sum of the parts or units.* Within a system, **subsystems** exist as *smaller units within the whole,* such as spouses and children in the family, or the mental health clinic within the larger health care centre. **Suprasystems** *refer to the large environment or community.* All systems need energy and activity to maintain self. Input of energy allows **differentiation,** *the tendency for the system to advance or mature to a higher level of complexity and organization.*[103]

The elements or components that are common to all systems are listed in Table 5-2. A given entity is not a system unless these characteristics are present.[104–108]

People satisfy their needs within social systems. The **social system** is a *group of people joined cooperatively to achieve common goals, using an organized set of practices to regulate behaviour.*[109] The person occupies various positions and has defined roles in the social system. The person's development is shaped by the system; in turn, people create and change social systems.[110,111] Other social systems are the family, church, economic systems; politico-legal and educational institutions; and health care agencies.

All living organisms (i.e., every person) comprise an open social system. Change occurs constantly within and between the system and other systems. An **open system** is *characterized by the ability to exchange energy, matter, and information with the environment to evolve into higher levels of heterogeneity, organization, order, and development.*[112,113] Physically, there is a *hierarchy of components,* such as cells and organ systems. Emotionally, there are levels of needs and feelings. Cognitively, a person has memories, knowledge, and cognitive strategies. Socially, the person is in a relative rank in a hierarchy of prestige roles, such as boss, worker, adult, or child. Spiritually, the person may orient his or her life in terms of an inner awareness.[114] The *boundaries or environment,* such as one's skin, the limits set by others, social status, home, and community, influence the person's *needs* and *goal achievement.* To remain healthy, the person must be able to *communicate* and must have *feedback.* A constant *exchange of energy and information* must exist with the surrounding specified environment if the system is to be open, useful, and creative. If this *information or energy exchange does not occur,* the system becomes a **closed system** and ineffective, and disorganization, disease, and sometimes death result.

Linkage *occurs when two systems exchange energy across their boundaries.*[115] Industry, the church, or the health agency, for example, draws energy from its linkage to the family. In

TABLE 5-2
Elements and Characteristics of a System

Element	Definition/Example
Parts	*The system's components that are interdependent units.* None can operate without the other. Change in one part affects the entire unit. The person as a whole system is composed of physical, emotional, mental, spiritual, cultural, and social aspects. Physically, he or she is composed of the body systems—neurological, cardiovascular, and so on. The health agency is one part of the health care system, and it, in turn, is composed of parts: physical plant, employees, clients, departments that give services.
Attributes	*Characteristics of the parts* such as temperament, roles, education, age, or health of the person or family members.
Information/communication	*Sending of messages and feedback, the exchange of energy,* which varies with the system but is essential to achieve goals. A system has input and output with the environment.
Feedback	*Monitoring of internal and external responses to behaviour* (output) that allows the system to readjust or change if needed.
Equilibrium	*Steady state or state of balance that is maintained through adaptive, dynamic, self-regulating processes,* and information input, transformation, output, and feedback.
Boundary	A *barrier or area of demarcation that limits or keeps a system distinct from its environment and within which information is exchanged.* The skin of the person, home of the family, or walls of the health agency each constitutes a boundary. The boundary is not always rigid. Relatives outside the home are part of the family. The boundary may be an imaginary line, such as the feeling that comes from belonging to a certain racial or ethnic group.
Organization	The *formal or informal arrangement of parts to form a whole entity so that the organism or institution has a working order that leads to an established hierarchy, rules, or customs.* The person is organized into a physical structure, basic needs, cognitive stages, and achievement of developmental tasks. Hierarchy in the family or health agency provides organization that is based on power (ability to control others) and responsibility. Nursing care may be organized into primary or team nursing, which is a way of differentiating services. The specialization of medical practice is also a way of organizing care. Organization in an institution is also maintained by norms, roles, and customs that each member must follow.
Goals	*Purposes of or reasons for the system to exist.* Goals may be *long term or short term.* Goals include survival, development, and socialization of the individual member of the family or contributions to society.
Environment	The *social and physical world outside the system, boundaries, or the community in which the system exists.* The person's or family's environment may be a tribal enclave, farm, small town and surrounding area, or an urban neighbourhood and surrounding city. Environment of a health care system may be the city in which the agency is located or may extend to other regions for a major urban medical centre.
Evolutionary processes	*Changes within the person and the environment, proceeding from simple to complex,* occur at all times, in all systems. The person undergoes changes in physical, psychological, and social growth throughout the life span, within certain parameters.

return, industry is willing to contribute to family welfare funds, the United Way, mental health campaigns, or ecologic improvements. The church maintains its role as prime defender of family stability. The health agency sets standards of health care and refines policies and procedures based on feedback from consumers, employees, and accrediting bodies.

Each person and family you care for is a system interacting with other systems in the community. Development and function are greatly affected by the interdependence and interrelationships of each component part and by all other surrounding systems. Best and his associates claim that although there is general agreement about the complex interplay among individual-, family-, organizational-, and community-level factors, as they affect health outcomes, a gap exists between health promotion research and practice. They suggest a few critical steps to close this gap: (1) investing in networks that promote, support, and sustain ongoing discussion and the sharing of experience; (2) finding common ground in an approach to community partnering; and (3) gaining consensus on the proposed integrating framework.[116]

Family systems theory has been derived from general systems theory. Relationships that exist between family members constitute a system, and a reaction in one family member is followed by a predictable reaction in others. The smallest stable relationship system within a family or social system is the *three-person system* or *triangle*. When a two-person relationship is unstable and anxiety increases, that relationship becomes uncomfortable. When the level of intensity reaches a certain level, the twosome involves a vulnerable third person. Often the issue is an emotional one. With the involvement of the third person, the level of anxiety decreases as it shifts from one to the other of the three relationships in the triangle. The triangle becomes more flexible and stable than that of the twosome. Further, the threesome has a higher tolerance of anxiety; and it is capable of handling more of life's stresses. The same emotional patterns are then repeated, so that family members develop fixed, often unchanging, roles in relation to each other.[117–120]

CRITICAL THINKING

What family situation can you think of whereby a twosome would triangulate someone new into the emotional issue at hand?

Ecologic Systems Theory

Bronfenbrenner has formulated **ecologic systems theory,** to describe *how the person's development is influenced by a broad range of situations and from interactive and overlapping contextual levels,* as follows:

1. **Microsystems.** *Face-to-face physical and social situations that directly affect the person,* such as family, schoolroom, workplace, church, peers, and health services.

2. **Mesosystems.** *Connections and relationships among the person's microsystems.*

3. **Exosystems.** *Settings or situations that indirectly influence the person,* such as the extended family, friends of the family, neighbours, spouse's workplace, mass media, legal services, the local government, and community agencies and organizations.

4. **Macrosystems.** *Sociocultural values, beliefs, and policies that provide a framework for organizing our lives and indirectly affect the person* through the exosystem, mesosystem, and microsystem.[121]

PSYCHOLOGICAL THEORIES

A number of psychological theories have been formulated to explain human development, behaviour, and personality. A theorist who follows one perspective may disagree with another theorist from the same perspective. For example, some behaviourists would disagree with B.F. Skinner on some points. Further, no theorist or group of theorists has all the answers about human behaviour, development, or learning. Realize that often theorists who sound very different in their theory may be stating basically similar concepts.

BEHAVIOURAL THEORY

Overview

Behaviourists *adhere to stimulus-response conditioning theories.* This scientific approach to the study of the person generalizes results from animal experiments to people. The **neo-behaviourists**—*contemporary behavioural theorists and the theorists in this school who have changed their ideas*—obtain data for laws of behaviour by observing the human's behavioural response to stimuli. The person is considered in terms of component parts. *The focus is on isolated, small units of behaviour or parts of behavioural patterns that are objectively observed and analyzed from the perspective of nonmental, physiologic associations.*

View of the Human

Behavioural theorists view the living organism as a self-maintaining mechanism. Because the *focus is on physiologic processes and identifiable aspects of the person, subjective, unobservable, unique, and inner aspects of the human are not studied.* There are no concepts that explain self-concept; ideas; emotions such as love, joy, sadness, and anger; the meaning in a situation; memory; understanding; insight; empathy; the person initiating and being an active agency in his or her behalf; or variety in human behaviour. The person is explained by overt behaviour or physiologically, not in abstractions. There are no biases except for past conditioning. The learner or the client is considered deficient, which results in *activity or behaviour* called **learning.** Rest or cessation of behaviour follows reward.[122,123]

View of Education and Therapy

The goals of education and treatment are to (1) control the person's behaviour; (2) help the person become more efficient and realistic, as defined by others in the environment; (3) move toward a goal set by external standards; and (4) create learning by forming bonds, connections, or associations. Responses that are appropriate are rewarded and therefore are stamped in to form habits.[124,125]

The teacher, health care provider, or therapist is at the centre of and in control of the educational or treatment process. The learner or client is passive. Programmed or computerized instruction is considered efficient education, with the teacher functioning as a reinforcer to help the learner achieve behavioural objectives.

Behavioural theorists propose that maladaptive behaviours are reinforced and learned. A treatment approach is to identify factors in the environment or in prior learning that must be modified to change the problem behaviour. A problem with this approach is that the person who is elderly or a member of a minority group and feels powerless may feel he or she is being manipulated, that something is being done to rather than with the person, or being done for rather than allowing the person to do for self. Further, who defines which behaviour is maladaptive, the client or the therapist? What the therapist considers maladaptive, such as hypervigilance, may be adaptive for the client's life situation. To change that behaviour would make the client more vulnerable to harm. Also, the approach may seem too superficial or simplistic. The person may develop different symptoms to express the underlying problem or pathology, the person may resist behaviour change, or the person may not return to the therapist after the initial visit because he or she felt misunderstood.

Behavioural Theorists

Early Theorists
Ivan Pavlov laid the foundations for the behavioural school. He was a Russian physiologist and pharmacologist of the mid–19th century who wrote about psychic processes during his study of salivation and flow of digestive juices in dogs. His experiments established **classical conditioning:** *An unconditioned or new stimulus is presented with a stimulus that is already known just before the response to the conditioned familiar stimulus. The organism learns to respond to a new stimulus in the same way it responded to a familiar stimulus.* Associations are shifted from one stimulus to another, with the same response being made to the substituted stimuli.[126]

John B. Watson is considered the founder of **behaviourism.** His experiments showed that fears and phobias could result from classical conditioning in childhood and could, in turn, be unlearned in adulthood.[127]

Some *present-day relaxation methods used by health care providers are based on classical conditioning.* The client is trained to respond to a therapist's direction by relaxing a muscle group; music is then played while the therapist gives directions for relaxing. Later the person is able to respond automatically by relaxing when music plays.[128] Classical conditioning is also used in the Lamaze preparation for childbirth or other kinds of childbirth education classes.

Thorndike: S-R Bond Theory, or Connectionism
E. Thorndike was the most dominant figure in American psychology for much of the 20th century. From experiments with cats, he formulated a theory of learning called **S-R (stimulus-response) bond theory,** or **connectionism,** which affected every educational facility directly, and many psychiatrists and mental health facilities at least indirectly. Thorndike's theory implies that, through **instrumental conditioning,** *a specific response is linked with a specific stimulus, and the response is followed by a reward or is instrumental in bringing about reinforcement.*

Thorndike is best known for three laws, which are paraphrased and applied as follows:[129]

1. **Law of readiness.** *When the person is ready to perform or learn, it is satisfying to do so.* It is annoying not to be able to act when a state of readiness exists or when action is demanded but there is no readiness. In education and therapy, the readiness level of the person toward action, learning, or behavioural change must be assessed and is considered essential for results.

2. **Law of effect.** *When a connection is made between a stimulus and response and is accompanied by a satisfying state of affairs, the connection is increased.* If a person is ready to respond, the response is itself pleasurable, and the response will be fixed or learned. When working with the client, the teaching–learning situation should be satisfying, pleasurable, or harmonious, rather than boring, harsh, or conflictual, in order for the person to follow through with directions or suggestions.

3. **Law of exercise (repetition).** *Whenever a connection is made between a stimulus and a response, the connection's strength is increased.* The more times a stimulus-induced response is repeated or the person performs an activity, the longer it will be retained in behaviour.

Repetition is important to provide an opportunity to give reinforcement. Behaviour that is not rewarded would become boring and be discontinued. Repetition, however, may be considered excessive by the learner, and too much repetition of an idea in therapy may cause resistance to carrying out directions.[130]

One of Thorndike's secondary laws, **associative shifting,** or **stimulus substitution,** is now considered important by all behaviourists. The law states that *any response can be linked with any stimulus;* the person's purposes or thoughts have nothing to do with learning. This is an example of *automatic behaviour,* which all people use in certain situations, although such behaviour would be inappropriate elsewhere. The social courtesies are an example. If too much behaviour undergoes associative shifting, the behaviour may be inappropriate; the person may be considered emotionally ill.[131,132]

Other ideas and principles proposed by Thorndike remain in use today. He advocated reward of acceptable behaviour (strengthening a connection) rather than punishment of undesirable behaviour. The **principle of set or attitude** states that *the person's attitude or mental set guides learning and behaviour change; the response is set or determined by enduring adjustment patterns* that result from being reared in a certain environment or culture. Certainly the client who has an attitudinal set against counselling or a specific treatment is unlikely to benefit by it.

Skinner: Operant Conditioning Theory

Skinner is well known for his operant conditioning theory, which used animal studies and built on the theories of Watson and Thorndike. According to Skinner, **behaviour** is an *overt response that is externally caused and is controlled primarily by its consequences.* The environmental stimuli determine how a person alters behaviour and responds to people or objects in the environment. Feelings or emotions are the accompaniments or result, not the cause of behaviour. Innate or hereditary reflexes activate the internal glands and smooth muscles, but reflexive behaviour accounts for little of human behaviour.[133,134]

Learning is a *change in the form or probability of response as a result of conditioning.* **Operant conditioning** is the *learning process whereby a response (operant) is shaped and is made more probable or frequent by reinforcement.* **Transfer** is an *increased probability of response in the future.* A set of acts are called *operant responses* because *they operate on the environment and generate consequences.* The important stimulus is the one immediately *following* the response, not the one preceding it.

Operant conditioning occurs in most everyday activities, according to Skinner. People constantly cause others to modify their behaviour by reinforcing certain behaviour and ignoring other behaviour. During development, people learn to balance, walk, talk, play games, and handle instruments and tools because they are reinforced after performing a set of motions, thereby increasing the repetition of these motions. Social and ethical behaviours are learned as people are reinforced to continue them through their reinforcing of others for the same behaviours. Operant reinforcement improves the efficiency of behaviour, whether the behaviour is appropriate or inappropriate. Any attention, even if negative, reinforces response to a stimuli.[135–142]

CRITICAL THINKING

In what ways do you see operant conditioning used in your practice?

Positive reinforcement occurs when the *presence of a stimulus strengthens a response;* **negative reinforcement** occurs when *withdrawal of a stimulus strengthens the tendency to behave in a certain way.* A positive reinforcer is food, water, a smile, or a pleasant, friendly interchange with another person. A negative reinforcer consists of removing painful stimuli. Skinner's theory emphasizes positive reinforcement.[143] He rejected use of negative reinforcement or aversive control, contending that this merely produces escape or avoidance behaviour. A **reinforcement schedule** is a *pattern of rewarding behaviour at fixed time intervals, with a fixed number of responses between reinforcements.* Reinforcement does not strengthen a specific response, but rather it tends to strengthen a general tendency to make the response, or a class of responses, in the future. Thus trial-and-error learning does not exist.[144–150]

Punishment *consists of presenting a negative stimulus or removing a positive one.* Experiments show that punishment does not reduce a tendency to respond. Apparently, reward strengthens behaviour because the response is stamped in. Punishment does not weaken behaviour, however, because the response cannot be stamped out. **Extinction,** *letting a behavioural response die by not reinforcing it,* is preferred instead of punishment for breaking habits. Extinction is a slower process than reinforcement in modifying behaviour.[151] Operant reinforcement covers most human behaviour. Imitative behaviour is an example. It arises over time because of discriminative reinforcement. A person waves to someone because of the reinforcement, not because of the stimulus of the other person's hand waving. Differentiation of responses improves motor skills. The person selects a motion because it was reinforced. In this process, reinforcement must be immediate.[152] **Behaviour modification** is the *deliberate application of learning theory and conditioning, thereby structuring different social environments to teach alternate behaviours and to help the person gain control over behaviour and environment.* **Shaping** (the *gradual modification of behaviour by breaking complex behaviour into small steps and reinforcing each small step that is a closer approximation to the final desired behaviour*) also achieves behavioural change.[153,154]

Recently, Garry Martin and Joseph Pear of the University of Manitoba wrote an authoritative and widely used text, *Behavior Modification: What It Is and How to Do It.*[155] This text, with highly accessible format and hands-on experience, relates principles to applications in everyday situations. These experiences include clinical, home, school, and work settings. In this text, which is widely used in both Canada and the U.S., Martin and Pear explain that shaping is the development of a new behaviour by the successive reinforcement of closer approximations and the extinguishing of preceding approximations of the behaviour. They explain four factors that influence the effectiveness of shaping. In one interesting example we meet Frank, who retired early at 55, and, as an admitted "couch potato," decided, on the advice of his doctor, to begin a regular exercise program. Frank, who had never been active in his life, decided he would jog one kilometre daily. After a couple of attempts he became discouraged and returned to his couch potato routine. He had expected too much; but a friendly neighbour suggested he use shaping. The factors influencing shaping, according to Martin and Pear, are as follows:[156]

1. *Specify the final desired behaviour.* In Frank's case the final desired behaviour was jogging one kilometre each day. Because this distance might have been too great for Frank to accomplish successfully, a shorter, more easily attainable distance would be better to select.

2. *Choose a starting behaviour.* Frank's neighbour encourages him to lace on his runners and walk around the outside of his house each day, as a start. On successful completion of this starting behaviour, the neighbour praises Frank for his good effort. He arranges to meet Frank the next day to do it again as a step toward the half-kilometre jog objective which, with the neighbour's guidance, Frank selected. It is important that, throughout the shaping steps, the activity and the successive approximations be enjoyable and attainable.

3. *Choose the shaping steps.* Frank's neighbour assists Frank in outlining the behaviours to approximate the final behaviour—jogging half a kilometre per day. Behaviours

---

NARRATIVE VIGNETTE
Shaping

You are trying to help a college friend, Judy, to lose 5 kg. Judy tells you that she eats a great number of chocolates each day, and that she is considering the low-carbohydrate diets she has read about in magazines. You recall, however, that in your psychology class the concept of behaviour modification seemed appealing to you, and that eating fruits instead of chocolates might be good for Judy. Together, you and Judy

decide that through the process of shaping, she will seek to eat more fruits (and consequently lose 5 kg).

1. What is Judy's final desired behaviour?
2. What might be a starting behaviour for Judy?
3. List the shaping steps through which Judy might progress toward her desired behaviour.

---

such as walking around the outside of the house, followed by walking around the block, and so forth, constitute successive approximations to the desired behaviour. So, when Frank walks around the house several times, the neighbour reinforces that approximation. Then, when Frank has progressed to walking around the block several times, the neighbour again reinforces that approximation. The shaping procedure continues while Frank progresses through the step of jogging, say, 10 strides followed by walking 20 steps. A next step might be that of jogging 100 strides followed by walking 100 steps, until he reaches the desired behaviour (also referred to as the terminal behaviour). The final desired behaviour is jogging half a kilometre each day.

In behaviour modification, the behaviour first must be reinforced each time it occurs. Once the desired response has been established and maintained by a continuous reinforcement schedule (i.e., each time the desired response is seen, it is reinforced), the next step is to switch to an **intermittent schedule of reinforcement,** *whereupon reinforcement is contingent on increasingly multiple emissions of the desired behaviour.* After this, occasional reinforcement will keep the desired behaviour going. Behaviour that has been maintained by an intermittent schedule of reinforcement or partial reinforcement is highly resistant to extinction.[157,158]

The aim of behavioural therapy is maximum benefit for the client and society, but behaviour therapy is exclusively reliant on the therapist's judgment and goals for the client.

Sometimes aversive methods (e.g., seclusion) are used to change behaviour. The purpose is not punishment but time out, as in allowing a tantrum to run its course, without accidental reinforcement and without triggering similar behaviour in other people. Strategies of punishment and deprivation, which are standard techniques in childrearing, are examples of using Skinner's principles of behaviour modification. Some parents do not question sending a child to bed without a meal as punishment, and parents may even be criticized by other parents if they do not spank their children for naughty behaviour.

Operant techniques include the following:

■ **Time out.** *Seclusion for examination of behaviours*
■ **Assertion training.** *Using role playing, modelling, feedback, and social reinforcers to change communication patterns*

■ **Token economies.** *Rewards or payments for behaviour improvement that are applied to an entire unit of patients*
■ **Social skills training.** *Rehearsal of appropriate social behaviours*

Operant conditioning is used in many situations, including to:

■ Replace undesirable behaviours of normal or developmentally disabled children
■ Reduce abnormal or self-destructive behaviour
■ Train parents, teachers, probation officers, and nurses to be more efficient in their roles
■ Reduce specific maladaptive behaviours such as stuttering, tics, poor hygiene, and messy eating habits
■ Control physical symptoms through biofeedback

Figure 5–1 illustrates how development is viewed by learning theorists. Table 5-3 lists key terms and definitions, with examples.

Wolpe: Desensitization Theory

Joseph Wolpe uses Skinner's principles in deconditioning of anxiety or desensitization of phobias or other behaviours. When treating symptoms of fear by desensitization, the person is helped to relax completely. Then, over many sessions, the person is presented with progressively more threatening stimuli related to the feared situation and is instructed to remain simultaneously relaxed. Then the person is asked to think of the feared object but to stop thinking about it if he or she feels uneasy.[159]

The major criticism of Wolpe's therapy is that only the symptom and not the underlying problem is treated. Therefore, **symptom substitution,** *another maladaptive behaviour replacing the extinguished behaviour,* will occur.[160]

Behavioural Contract

Use a contract with your client in your practice. A **verbal or written contract** is an *explicit mutual agreement between you and the client that defines the nature of your relationship, your mutual expectations, and the different but equal responsibilities toward a common goal, and accountability for the outcome.* Terms in the contract include the **target behaviour** that is to be changed, appointment time and place, or the specific care activities and their timing that are involved. Tentative duration

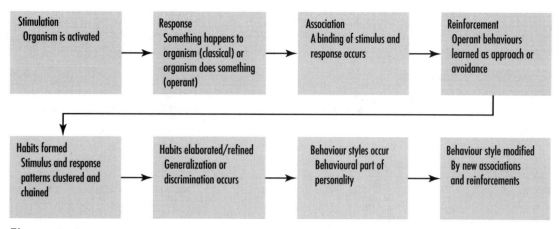

Figure 5–1

Development as viewed by learning theorists. Stimuli from inside or outside the organism are reinforced (positively or negatively) and on a particular schedule that determines their force and strength. Habits develop. The response processes of generalization and discrimination elaborate these habits and modify them. Effective habits are equated with effective development. This force rarely speaks about the whole organism but rather about situationally determined behaviours.

TABLE 5-3
Selected Terminology Pertaining to Application of Behavioural Theory

Term	Definition	Example
Respondent conditioning	*Pairing a neutral stimulus with a nonneutral stimulus until the person learns to respond to the neutral stimulus as to the nonneutral stimulus*	Baby learns to "love" a sibling (nonneutral stimulus) because the sibling shakes a rattle and offers other toys (neutral stimulus) while cooing, touching, and smiling at baby.
Operant conditioning	*Rewarding or punishing a response until the person learns to repeat or avoid that response in anticipation of positive or negative consequences*	Preschooler returns toys to the toy box at the end of the day because he remembers the consequences: doing so is followed by ten minutes of time with the parent; failure to do so results in sitting alone in his room for five minutes.
Positive reinforcement	*Rewarding desired behaviour to maintain that behaviour*	Parent buys a desired item for the child who earns an A in a course.
Negative reinforcement	*Removing an aversive stimulus in response to behaviour, which maintains that behaviour*	Parent allows the child to forgo household tasks if he complains when asked to do them, yet the child receives an allowance weekly.
Extinction	*Suppressing behaviour by removing reinforcers that are maintaining the behaviour*	Parent does not give the child who complains about doing household tasks the allowance at the end of the week and explains why.
Punishment	*Suppressing an undesirable behaviour by using an aversive stimulus in response to the person's behaviour*	Parent spanks the child for running into the street.

(continued)

TABLE 5-3 *(continued)*
Selected Terminology Pertaining to Application of Behavioural Theory

Term	Definition	Example
Time-out	*Suppressing maladaptive behaviour by removing the subject to a neutral environment, void of reinforcements when the behaviour is manifested*	Parent makes the four-year-old child sit facing a corner for five minutes after hitting a sibling.
Generalization	*Transferring a conditioned response from the conditional stimulus to another stimulus*	Child who is bitten by a dog fears all animals.
Systematic desensitization	*Pairing an anxiety-causing stimulus with an induced state of relaxation to extinguish fearful behaviour*	Parent remains with the child who has been bitten by a dog when the child is in the vicinity of animals, gradually helps the child to relax, and eventually to pet a very friendly dog.
Discrimination	*Responding only to a specific stimulus*	Toddler learns via punishing encounters with mother that playing in water in the bathtub is acceptable and playing in the water in the toilet is not.
Escape behaviour	*Initiating a response to escape an unpleasant or aversive stimulus*	Adolescent brings the parents a gift when returning late from a weekend with a friend.
Avoidance learning	*Arranging responses to avoid exposure to an aversive stimulus*	Adolescent verbally refuses the offer and walks away from the person offering a marijuana joint after a bad experience with it.
Chaining	*Developing complex behaviour by focusing on the individual components of the behaviour; this is done in a backward fashion*	Schoolchild learns to clean his room with the parent instructing and assisting with each step of the task and then verbally repeating in reverse order the steps after the task is finished.
Shaping	*Reinforcing successive approximations or small units of a desired response until that behaviour is gradually achieved*	Parent teaches the child to clean his room by praising him for doing every step of the process—vacuuming the rug, dusting each piece of furniture, and so on.
Fading	*Removing gradually the reinforcement given to the person*	Parent gives less and less verbal approval to the schoolchild for doing assigned household tasks.
Satiation	*Providing excessive amount of reinforcer, which causes loss of effectiveness*	Chocolate candy is reward for behaviour. Child is given extra candy and loses desire for candy and for behaviour change.
Token	*Object that serves as general reinforcer; may be exchanged for other reinforcers*	Client earns tokens for helpful behaviour on unit, exchanges 10 tokens for trip to Science Museum.
Contingency	*Relationship between behaviour to be changed and activities or consequences following behaviour*	Condition a desired response or suppress maladaptive response by drawing up contract indicating rewards and punishments contingent on or related to responses in the contract.

of treatment, specific contributions of other professionals, and fees, if any, are included in the contract. The contract should be evaluated periodically by the health care provider and client to be sure that each is meeting the contract terms and goals, and the terms should be changed when necessary. If an aspect of a contract is broken by the client, do not become judgmental. Renegotiate the terms.[161]

PSYCHOANALYTIC AND NEO-ANALYTIC THEORIES

Knowledge of genetics, developmental levels, and effects of internal stimuli, unconscious processes, social relationships, and environmental context are all used to understand, assess, and treat the person.

Overview

Psychoanalytic theorists include those who adhere to psychoanalytic and neo-analytic theories. These theorists generally believe *data for study about the person come from within the developing person, observation of interpersonal relationships, and knowledge of the impact of social units, norms, and laws on the person. Data from unconscious processes, early development, and the past are used to understand present behaviour and goal direction.* This group of theorists studies the person more comprehensively and as a social being, *using experimentation, objective observation, and self-report methods.* These theorists give us a helpful view of causation and provide a way of dealing with developmental and behavioural problems.[162]

View of the Human

Reality is external and interpersonal—what people agree on. The person is a social organism with a developmental past on which to build and a level of readiness that influences or contributes to learning and behaviour. *The person has maturational and social needs that affect development, learning, and behaviour; he or she seeks social role satisfaction and reacts to social values and symbolic processes.* The person internalizes societal rules to gain approval, can understand cause-and-effect relationships and complex abstract issues, is capable of insight and emotions, and initiates action and makes choices. The person is seen as a reactive being responding to stimuli that are usually sociosexual in nature. The goal of behaviour is seen as reduction of symbolic or internal needs or tension.[163,164]

View of Education and Therapy

The goal of developmental guidance and discipline is to help the person become an adaptive, effective social being, aware of and responsive to social reality and patterns. The person has to learn and follow socially prescribed values, customs, and norms to fit into society. Development, learning, and behaviour are also influenced strongly by the person's developmental level, personal history, cognitive processes and intellect, and intrapsychic processes.[165,166]

The health care provider, teacher, or therapist is the central figure, a social role model who directs the client. Emphasis is on the person, even in the younger years, understanding self and his or her behaviour. Increased insight promotes development and maturation. If the person is not ready to learn or change behaviour, the parent, teacher, or another acts as an external motivator or facilitator of readiness to change. Rewards are given through approval, affiliation, and various verbal and nonverbal methods. Learning and behaviour change also are self-reinforcing to the person.[167,168]

Psychoanalytic and Neo-Analytic Theorists

The **psychoanalytic theory** or perspective is divided into two groups: psychoanalytic and neo-analytic. The writings of Freud, Sullivan, Erikson, and Jung are discussed in this chapter. They are known as *"stage theorists"* because they emphasize that people develop in sequential stages. Other current stage theorists are George Vaillant, Roger Gould, Gail Sheehy, and Daniel Levinson. Their concepts and theories are discussed in Chapters 12 and 13 on young adulthood, middle age, and later maturity. The neo-analytic theorists reinterpreted Freud's psychoanalytic theory in formulating their theories. Sullivan further developed new emphases in his interpersonal theory. Erikson, in his epigenetic theory, expanded understanding of normal developmental stages and tasks throughout the life span, emphasized sociocultural influences to a greater degree, and saw the person as capable of emotional growth throughout life.

Psychodynamic Perspective
The **psychodynamic perspective** is concerned with the *inner and unconscious processes of the person—drives, needs, motivations, feelings, and conflicts.* Most of the neo-analytic theorists have paid less attention to biology.[169]

Freud: Psychoanalytic Theory. Sigmund Freud, a Viennese neurologist, developed psychoanalytic theory, the first psychological theory to include a fully developed explanation of abnormal behaviour. He gave biological factors little emphasis but used the medical model of emphasizing pathology and symptoms.

Freud's *theory of personality* seems complicated, because it *incorporates many interlocking factors.* Major components are psychic determination; psychic structures of the id, ego, and superego; primary and secondary process thinking; the conscious–unconscious continuum; libido or psychic energy; behaviour, anxiety, and defence mechanisms; transference; and psychosexual development. Some of his theory is discussed here and referred to in the chapters on childhood. Table 5-4 summarizes these concepts.[170]

Anxiety is the *response of tension or dread to perceived or anticipated danger or stress and is the primary motivation for behaviour.* There are two types of anxiety-provoking situations. Anxiety may be caused by excessive stimulation that the person cannot handle, of which birth is the prototype experience. Anxiety may also rise from intrapsychic or unconscious conflicts, unacceptable wishes, unknown or anticipated events,

TABLE 5-4
Summary of Freud's Theory of Personality

Psychic determination	All behaviour determined by prior thoughts and mental processes
Psychic structures of the personality	**Id**—*Unorganized reservoir of psychic energy;* furnishes energy for ego and superego
	Consists of instinctual forces, primitive biological drives, and impulses necessary for survival
	Operates on **pleasure principle** (*seeking of immediate gratification and avoidance of discomfort*)
	Discharges **tension** (*increased energy*) through reflex physiologic activity and **primary process thinking** (*image formation, drive-oriented behaviour, free expression of feelings and impulses, inability to distinguish between reality and non-reality; dream-like state*)
	Ego—*Establishes relations with environment through conscious perception, feeling, action*
	Controls impulses from id and demands of superego
	Operates on **reality principle** (*external conditions considered and immediate gratification delayed for future gains that can be realistically achieved*)
	Controls access of ideas to conscious
	Appraises environment and reality
	Uses various mechanisms to help person feel emotionally safe
	Guides person to acceptable behaviour
	Directs motor and all cognitive functions
	Assists with **secondary process thinking** (*delayed or substitute gratification; realistic thoughts; conscious processes; cognitive strategies*)
	Superego—*Represents internalized moral code based on perceived social rules and norms; restrains expression of instinctual drives; prevents disruption of society*
	Active and concrete in directing person's thoughts, feelings, actions
	Made up of two systems:
	Ego ideal—*Perfection to which person aspires; corresponds to what parents taught was good*
	Conscience—*Responsible for guilt feelings; corresponds to those things parents taught were bad*
Conscious–unconscious continuum	**Conscious**—*All aspects of mental life currently in awareness or easily remembered*
	Preconscious—*Aspects of mental life remembered with help; not currently in awareness*
	Unconscious—*Thoughts, feelings, actions, experiences, dreams not remembered; difficult to bring to awareness; not recognized*
	Existence inferred from effects on behaviour
Instincts (drives)	Basic force in personality and behaviour
	Inborn psychological representation or wish of inner somatic source of excitation
	Kinds of instincts: self-preservation, preservation of species, life, death; life and death instincts in conflict
Libido (sexuality)	*Sexual or psychic energy arising from hidden drives or impulses involved in conflict*
	Desire for pleasure, sexual gratification
	Not limited to biology or genital areas; includes capacity for loving another, parental love, and preservation of species
Anxiety	*Response to presence of unconscious conflict, tension, or dread; perceived or anticipated danger; and stress—primary motivation for behaviour*
	Basic source is the unconscious, related to loss of self-image
	Psychic energy accumulates if anxiety not expressed; may overwhelm ego controls; panic may result
	Kinds of anxiety: (1) neurotic—id–ego conflict; (2) realistic—in response to real dangers in world; (3) moral anxiety—id–superego conflict
	Managed by direct action, coping strategies, or unconscious defence mechanisms

(continued)

TABLE 5-4 *(continued)*
Summary of Freud's Theory of Personality

Transference	*Phenomenon of investing libido in another object; projection of feelings, thoughts, and wishes onto therapist, who represents significant person from the past (usually the parent); and based on unconscious and repressed material and is therefore not realistic or appropriate to the situation*
Primary process	*Thought processes based in the id and unconscious; thought processes are drive-oriented, unable to distinguish between reality and non-reality, primitive, illogical, labile, and without synthesis; thought processes are related to instinctual impulses, obtaining self-pleasure, and to free expression of feelings and impulses; opposite thought processes may coincide; process carried out through pictorial, concrete images or dreams*
Secondary process	*Realistic, conscious thought processes based in the ego and occurring in normal waking life; association of ideas subject to reality conditions and conform to ethical and moral laws; instinctual impulses cannot obtain gratification because of ego and superego constraints; process based on use of words, cognitive strategies, and delayed or substitutive gratification*
Cathexis	*Energy responsible for behaviour*

superego inhibitions and taboos, and threatened loss of self-image. Anxiety at the mild level is probably always present when the person is awake; but it can escalate to panic levels. If anxiety cannot be managed by direct action or coping strategies, the ego initiates unconscious defences by warding off awareness of the conflict to keep the material unconscious, to lessen discomfort, and to maintain the self-image. Because everyone experiences psychological danger, the use of defence mechanisms clearly is not a special characteristic of maladaptive behaviour. Such mechanisms are used by all people, either singly or in combination, at one time or another, and are considered adaptive.[171] Commonly used ego adaptive (defence) mechanisms are summarized in Table 5-5 and described throughout the text in relation to the developmental era during which they arise.

Freud proposed five stages of psychosexual development and contended that personality was formed by age five. The stages in psychosexual development, each resolved in turn, are summarized in Table 5-6 and are referred to throughout the text.

Freud's ideas about psychosexual development are undoubtedly the most controversial aspects of his theory. His theory continues to influence thought and research, especially in Western cultures, in relation to development and therapy of the ill person.[172] Recently, feminist scholars have begun to reassess Freud's theory, recognizing the value of his ideas and their applicability to understanding men and women, boys and girls.[173]

CRITICAL THINKING

What may be some criticisms of Freud's theory?

Major Neo-Analytic Theorists

Neo-Freudians or Neo-analysts follow Freud's theory in general but disagree with or have modified some of the original propositions. They *maintain the medical model and share the view of intrapsychic determinism as the basis for external behaviour. Some take into account the social and cultural context in which the person lives.* Harry Stack Sullivan, Erik Erikson, and Carl Jung are described briefly; Sullivan and Erikson are referred to throughout the text.

Sullivan: Interpersonal Theory of Psychiatry. Harry Stack Sullivan[174] formulated the interpersonal theory of psychiatry. The theory focuses on relationships between and among people, in contrast to Freud's emphasis on the intrapsychic sexual phenomena and Erikson's focus on social aspects. Experiences in major life events are the result of either positive or negative interpersonal relationships. Personality development is largely the result of the mother–child relationship, childhood experiences, and interpersonal encounters. There are two basic needs: satisfaction (biological needs) and security (emotional and social needs).

Sullivan used the following biological principles to understand the person's development:[175]

■ **Principle of communal existence.** *A living organism cannot survive if separated from the necessary environment for survival.* For example, the embryo must have the correct intrauterine environment to live, and the baby must have love and human contact to become socialized or human.

■ **Principle of functional activity.** *Functional or physiologic activities and processes affect the person's interaction with the environment.*

■ **Principle of organization.** *The person is systematically arranged physically and emotionally and within society and this organization enables function.*

An important principle for the study and care of people is the **One-Genus Postulate**, which states *we are all more simply human than otherwise, hence more similar than different in basic needs, development, and in the meaning of our behaviour.*

TABLE 5-5
Ego Adaptive or Defence Mechanisms

Compartmentalization	*Separation of two incompatible aspects of the psyche from each other to maintain psychological comfort;* behavioural manifestations show the inconsistency. **Example:** The person who attends church regularly and is overtly religious conducts a business that includes handling stolen goods.
Compensation	*Overachievement in one area to offset deficiencies, real or imagined, or to overcome failure or frustration in another area.* **Example:** The student who makes poor grades devotes much time and energy to succeed in music or sports.
Condensation	*Reacting to a single idea with all of the emotions associated with a group of ideas;* expressing a complex group of ideas with a single word or phrase. **Example:** The person says the word *crazy* as a shorthand expression for many types of mental illness and for feelings of fear and shame.
Conversion	*Unconscious conflicts are disguised and expressed symbolically by physical symptoms* involving portions of the body, especially the five senses and motor areas. Symptoms are frequently not related to innervations by sensory or motor nerves. **Example:** The person is under great pressure on the job; awakes at 6 A.M. and is unable to walk but is unconcerned about the symptom.
Denial	*Failure to recognize an unacceptable impulse or undesirable, but obvious thought, fact, behaviour, conflict, or situation, or its consequences or implications.* **Example:** The alcoholic person believes that he or she has no problem with drinking even though family and work colleagues observe the classic signs.
Displacement	*Release or redirection of feelings and impulses on a safe object or person as a substitute for that which aroused the feeling.* **Example:** The person punches a punching bag after an argument with the boss.
Dissociation	*Repression or splitting off from awareness of a portion of a personality or of consciousness;* however, repressed material continues to affect behaviour (compartmentalization). **Example:** A client discusses a conflict-laden subject and goes into a trance.
Emotional isolation	*Repression of the emotional component of a situation, although the person is able to remember the thought, memory, or event,* dealing with problems as interesting events that can be rationally explained but have no feelings attached. **Example:** The person talks about the spouse's death and details of the accident that caused it with an apathetic expression and without crying or signs of grieving.
Identification	*Similar to and the result of introjections; unconscious modelling of another person so that basic values, attitudes, and behaviour are similar to those of a significant person or group, but overt behaviour is manifested in an individual manner.* (Imitation is not considered a defence mechanism per se, but imitation usually precedes identification. Imitation is consciously copying another's values, attitudes, movements, etc.). **Example:** The adolescent over time manifests the assertive behaviour and states ideas similar to those that she admires in one of her instructors, although she is unaware that her behaviour is similar.
Introjection	*Symbolic assimilation of or process of taking in attitudes, behaviour, wishes, ideals, or values of significant person into the ego and/or superego* (a part of identification). **Example:** The client talks about how much she or he helps other people with their problems.

(continued)

TABLE 5-5 *(continued)*
Ego Adaptive or Defence Mechanisms

Projection	*Attributing one's unacceptable or anxiety-provoking feelings, thoughts, impulses, wishes, or characteristics to another person.* **Example:** The person declares that the supervisor is lazy and prejudiced; work colleagues note that this person often needs help at work and frequently makes derogatory remarks about others.
Rationalization	*Justification of behaviour or offering a socially acceptable, intellectual, and apparently logical explanation for an act or decision actually caused by unconscious or verbalized impulses. Behaviour in response to unrecognized motives precedes reasons for it.* **Example:** A student fails a course but maintains that the course was not important and that the grade can be made up in another course.
Reaction formation	*Unacceptable impulses repressed, denied, and reacted to by opposite overt behaviour.* **Example:** A married woman who is unconsciously disturbed by feeling sexually attracted to one of her husband's friends treats him rudely and keeps him at a safe distance.
Regression	*Adopting behaviour characteristic of a previous developmental level; the ego returns to an immature but more gratifying state of development in thought, feeling, or behaviour.* **Example:** The person takes a nap, curled in a fetal position, on arriving home after a stressful day at work.
Repression	*Automatic, involuntary exclusion of a painful or conflictual feeling, thought, impulse, experience, or memory from awareness.* The thought or memory of the event is not consciously perceived. **Example:** The mother seems unaware of the date or events surrounding her child's death and shows no emotions when the death is discussed.
Sublimation	*Substitution of a socially acceptable behaviour for an unacceptable sexual or aggressive drive or impulse.* **Example:** The adolescent is forbidden by her parents to have a date until she graduates from high school. She gives much time and energy to editorial work and writing for the school paper. The editor of the school paper and the faculty advisor are males.
Suppression	*Intentional exclusion of material from consciousness.* **Example:** The husband carries the bills in his pocket for a week before remembering to mail in the payments.
Symbolization	*One object or act unconsciously represents a complex group of objects and acts,* some of which may be in conflict or unacceptable to the ego; external objects or acts stand for any internal or repressed desire, idea, attitude, or feeling. The symbol may not overtly appear to be related to the repressed ideas or feelings. **Example:** The husband sends his wife a bouquet of roses, which ordinarily represents love and beauty. But roses have thorns; his beautiful wife is hard to live with, but he consciously focuses on her beauty.
Undoing	*An act, communication, or thought that cancels the significance or partially negates a previous one;* treating an experience as if it had never occurred. **Example:** The husband purchases a gift for his wife after a quarrel the previous evening.

Sullivan postulated that people experience events in the following three modes:

1. **Prototaxic mode of experiencing.** *Experiences that occur in infancy before language symbols are acquired or the first time a person experiences an event that is difficult to describe in words.*

2. **Parataxic mode of experiencing.** *Experiences characterized by symbols used in a private (autistic) way; encompasses*

fantasy, magical thinking, and lack of cause-and-effect thinking that is seen in children and adults.

3. **Syntaxic mode of experiencing.** *Experiences of preadolescence, adolescence, and adulthood characterized by consensual validation, whereby persons communicate with each other using language or symbols that are mutually understood.* This mode of experiencing begins during the "chum"

TABLE 5-6
Freud's Stages of Psychosexual Development: Libidinal Extension

Stage (years)	Major Body Zone	Activities	Extension to Others
Oral (0–1½)	Mouth (major source of gratification and exploration)	Security—primary need Pleasure from eating and sucking Major conflict—weaning Incorporation (suck, consume, chew, bite, receive)	Sense of *We*—no differentiation or extension Sense of *I* and *Other*—minimum differentiation and total incorporation Beginning of ego development at 4–5 months
Anal (1½–3)	Bowel (anus) and bladder source of sensual satisfaction, self-control, and conflict (mouth continues in importance)	Expulsion and retention (differentiation, expelling, controlling, pushing away) (Incorporation still is used.) Major conflict—toilet training	Sense of *I* and *Other*—separation from other and increasing sense of *I* Beginning control over impulses
Phallic (4–6)	Genital region—penis, clitoris (mouth, bowel, and bladder sphincters continue in importance).	Masturbation Fantasy Play activities Experimentation with peers Questioning of adults about sexual topics Major conflict—Oedipus complex, which resolves when child identifies with parent of same sex (Mastery, incorporation, expulsion, and retention continue.)	Sense of *I* and *Other*—fear of castration in boy Sense of *I* and *Other*—strengthened with identification process with parents Sense of *Other*—extends to other adults
Latency (6–puberty)	No special body focus	Diffuse activity and relationships (Mastery, incorporation, expulsion, and retention continue.)	Sense of *I* and *Other*—extends out of nuclear family and includes peers of same sex
Genital (puberty and thereafter)	Penis, vagina (mouth, anus, clitoris)	Develop skills needed to cope with the environment Full sexual maturity and function (Mastery, incorporation, expulsion, and retention continue.) Addition of new assets with each stage for gratification Realistic sexual expression Creativity and pleasure in love and work	Sense of *I* and *Other*—extends to other adults and peers of opposite sex

stage in the school-age child or thereafter. The differences between these models are due to the crucial role of language in experience and development and are described further in Chapters 7, 9, and 10.

Sullivan implied that the need to avoid anxiety and the need to gratify basic needs are the primary motivations for behaviour. His **concept of anxiety** states that *anxiety has its origin in the prolonged dependency of infancy, urgency of biological and emotional needs, and how the mothering person meets those needs. Anxiety is the result of uncomfortable interpersonal relationships, is the chief disruptive force in interpersonal relationships, is contagious through empathic feelings, and can be relieved by being in a secure interpersonal relationship.*[176]

The **self-system** is the *internal organization of experiences that exists to defend against anxiety and to secure necessary security.* One aspect of the self-system is known as *good-me, bad-me,* and *not-me,* which refers to feelings about the self that begin to form in infancy.[177]

Erikson: Epigenetic Theory of Personality Development. Erik Erikson[178] formulated the epigenetic theory based on the principle of the unfolding embryo: anything that grows has a ground plan out of which parts arise. Each part has its time of special ascendancy until all parts have arisen to form a functional whole. Thus each stage of development is the base for the next stage. A result of mastering the developmental tasks of each stage is virtue or a feeling of competence, or direction.

His theory explains step-by-step unfolding of emotional development and social characteristics during encounters with the environment. Erikson's psychosexual theory enlarges on psychoanalytic theory because it is not limited to historical era, specific culture, or personality types; encompasses development through the life span and is universal to all people; and acknowledges that society, heredity, and childhood experiences all influence the person's development.[179]

The following are basic principles of his theory, based on cross-cultural studies:[180]

- Each phase has a specific developmental task to achieve or solve. These tasks describe the order and sequence of human development and the conditions necessary to accomplish them, but actual accomplishment is done at an individual pace, tempo, and intensity.
- Each psychosexual stage of development is a developmental crisis because there is a radical change in the person's perspective, a shift in energy, and an increased emotional

vulnerability. During this peak time, the potential in the personality comes in contact with the whole environment, and the person has some degree of success in solving the crucial developmental task of the specific era. How the person copes with the task and crisis depends on previous developmental strengths and weaknesses.

- The potential inherent in each person evolves if given adequate chance to survive and grow. Anything that distorts the environment essential for development interferes with evolution of the person. Society attempts to safeguard and encourage the proper rate and sequence of the unfolding of human potential so that humanity is maintained.
- Each developmental task is redeveloped, reworked, and redefined in subsequent stages. Potential for further development always exists.
- Internal organization is central to development. Maturity increases as the tasks of each era are accomplished, at least in part, in proper order.

Erikson proposed eight stages of development and described the developmental task of crisis for each stage (Figure 5–2). They are described in Chapters 7 through 14 in relation to each developmental era. His theory is widely accepted and used in understanding the developing person and in administering nursing care.

CRITICAL THINKING

If an eight-year-old child is not able to resolve his or her developmental tasks at the expected stage, what may be the consequences for the child?

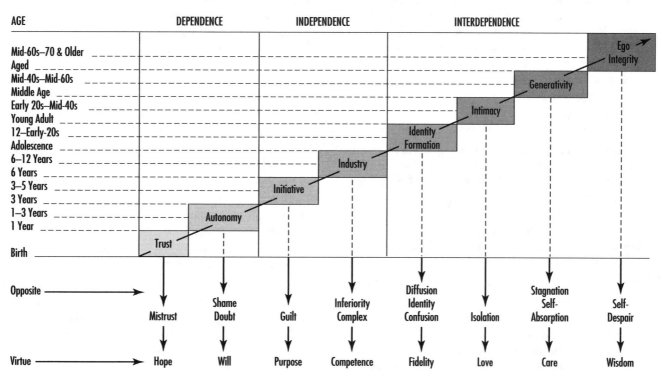

Figure 5–2

Erikson's eight stages of the person.

Jung's Theory. Carl Jung, another neo-analytic theorist, proposed the following assumptions about personality structure:[181]

1. The ego or **consciousness** includes *awareness of self and the external world.*

2. The **persona** is the *image or mask presented to the outer world,* depending on the roles of the person.

3. The **shadow** consists of *traits and feelings that cannot be admitted to the self;* it is the opposite of ego or self-image.

4. The **anima** and **animus** in the personality refer to the *characteristics traditionally considered feminine and masculine.* Each person has both characteristics or is androgynous or bisexual—with the feminine, nurturing, feeling side and the masculine, logical, assertive side. Socialization forces the person to overemphasize gender characteristics so that the opposite aspect of the person is not usually fully developed.

5. The unconscious is composed of two layers:
   a. The **personal unconscious** is unique, *contains all the repressed tendencies and feelings that build over the lifetime,* and *includes the shadow and some of the anima or animus.*
   b. The **collective unconscious** is *inherited and shared by all humankind and is composed of archetypes, or innate energy forces and organizing tendencies.* Archetypal images are unknowable and are found in myths, art, dreams, and fantasies throughout the world and include the image of earth mother, wise old man, and death, the witch, rebirth, and God. The archetypes influence the nature and growth of other parts of the personality. They are essentially unknowable, like instincts or innate perceptual tendencies.

6. Self is the most important archetype, our unconscious centredness, wholeness, and meaning. It is an inner urge to balance and reconcile the opposing aspects of our personalities, represented in drawings of **mandalas,** *figures in which all sides are perfectly balanced around a centre point.*

7. **Individuation** is the unattainable goal pursued by the self, which *involves finding the unique way, achieving a measure of psychic balance while separating self from social conformity to goals and values.*

8. There are two basic personality types or tendencies:
   a. **Introversion** refers to being *inner-reflective; caught up in one's inner state, fears, hopes, and feelings.* The introvert hesitates in relationships, is more secure in his or her inner world, and takes pleasure in activities that can be done alone.
   b. The **extrovert** confidently *engages in direct action and starts interactions with others.* The extrovert moves outward toward the world and prefers activities with people.

To Jung, life is a series of periods identified by different energy uses. Early childhood years were not emphasized in this developmental theory. The first period, until age 35 or 40, is a time of outward expansion. Maturational forces direct the growth of the ego and unfolding of capacities. After age 40, the person undergoes a transformation and looks for meaning in personal activities. With increasing age, there is increasing reflection. Jung's theory is referred to again in the chapters on adulthood. His theory is gaining wider acceptance in the understanding of the developing adult.

COGNITIVE THEORY AND THEORISTS

Cognitive theorists can be divided into four groups:

1. Beck's cognitive theory
2. Behavioural-cognitive theorists
3. Social learning theorists
4. Cognitive development theorists

Cognitive theory *deals with the person as an information processor and problem solver.* The cognitive perspective is concerned with internal processes but emphasizes how people attempt to acquire, interpret, and use information to solve life's problems and to remain normal or healthy. It emphasizes conscious processes, present thoughts, and problem-solving strategies. The cognitive perspective has grown out of new directions in learning and psychodynamic theories. Relationships among emotions, motivations, and cognitive processes are being studied.

Cognitive Theory of Beck

Aaron Beck originated cognitive theory and therapy. His premise was that psychological problems may result from repetitive, automatic distorted or dysfunctional patterns of thinking, which have evolved from faulty learning, making incorrect inferences on the basis of inadequate or incorrect information, and not distinguishing adequately between imagination and reality (Table 5-7). Unrealistic thinking may be attributed to enduring negative attitudes (low self-esteem, hopelessness, and helplessness) about self, the world, and the future. The idiosyncratic, angry, or distorted thought patterns may become activated by life stresses, yet the responses are automatic or based on past experiences, usually developed early in life and formed by relevant experience.[182,183]

Cognitive therapy is a short-term, structured therapy involving an active collaboration between the client and therapist toward achieving the therapy goals. It is usually conducted on an individual basis but may also be used with groups. The *goals of therapy* are to:

1. Help the person identify erroneous beliefs in relation to stressful events or behaviours.

2. Help the person look at these thoughts, compare them with objective evidence, and correct distortions.

3. Give feedback to the person about the accuracy of the new thoughts.

4. Allow and encourage the person to rehearse new cognitions in therapy and at home.

Cognitive therapy helps the patient to use problem-solving techniques to identify distorted thoughts, to correct dysfunctional thoughts, and to learn more realistic ways to formulate the experiences. The health care provider or therapist serves as a teacher or guide in the process and is nonjudgmental, objective, and empathetic. Questioning rigid beliefs and attitudes guides the person to refocus problems, alter errors in thinking, and rehearse new behaviour patterns.[184,185]

TABLE 5–7
Definitions of Cognitive Distortions

Distortion	Definition
All-or-nothing thinking or dichotomous thinking	*Seeing events in black-and-white categories;* if performance falls short of perfect, the self is a total failure.
Overgeneralization	*Seeing a single negative event as a never-ending pattern of defeat.*
Mental filter or selective inattention	*Focusing on a single negative detail exclusively so that vision of all reality becomes darkened;* interpreting situation or life on basis of one incident.
Disqualifying the positive	*Rejecting positive experiences by insisting they "don't count" for some reason or other.* In this way a negative belief that is contradicted by everyday experiences is maintained.
Jumping to conclusions or arbitrary inference	*Making a negative interpretation even though there are no definite facts that convincingly support the conclusion;* holding to beliefs without supporting evidence.
Mind reading	*Arbitrarily concluding that someone is reacting negatively to the self* and not checking this out.
The fortune teller error	*Anticipating that things will turn out badly,* and feeling convinced that prediction is an already established fact.
Magnification (catastrophizing) or minimization	*Exaggerating the importance of things* (such as a goof-up or someone else's achievement), *or inappropriately shrinking things until they appear tiny* (own desirable qualities or the other person's imperfections). This is also called the "binocular trick."
Emotional reasoning	*Assuming that negative emotions necessarily reflect the way things really are:* "I feel it, therefore it must be true."
Should statements	*Trying to motivate self with "shoulds" and "should nots." "Musts" and "oughts" are also offenders.* The emotional consequence is guilt. Directing "should" statements toward others creates feelings of anger, frustration, and resentment.
Labelling and mislabelling	*An extreme form of overgeneralization.* Instead of describing the error, a negative label is attached to self: "I'm a loser." When someone else's behaviour rubs the wrong way, attaching a negative label to him: "He's a louse." Mislabelling involves describing an event with language that is highly coloured and emotionally loaded.
Personalization	*Seeing self as the cause of some negative external event for which there was no responsibility.*

Behavioural-Cognitive Theorists

Two theorists, Albert Ellis and William Glasser, are part of this group, and each has formulated a therapy approach based on his beliefs about people's needs and behaviour.

Ellis: Rational-Emotive Therapy. Ellis developed rational-emotive therapy (RET), a cognitive-behavioural therapy that includes a here-and-now or existential focus. *The basic premises of RET are*:[186]

- The person is the centre of his or her universe and has an enormous amount of potential control over what he or she feels and does and can change behaviour.
- All people have a basic set of values and assumptions that govern much of life. After assumptions are made, subsequent rational and irrational thinking and behaving can be specified, understood, and worked with. Negative self-talk about these values and assumptions is the cause of much misery.

- All people want to be happy and free from unnecessary pain and can learn to overcome biological handicaps and various idiosyncrasies.
- People want to live in and get along with members of a social group and can learn to overcome manifestations of hurt, self-depreciation, rejection, and depression.
- People want to relate closely with a few selected members of the group.
- People are not disturbed by the things that happen to them but by their view of these things.

Behaviours that support these basic values are rational; those that interfere with achieving happiness and valuing achievement are irrational.

The *goal of RET* is creation of personal autonomy through a philosophic and educative approach. The person must understand that the universe is neither for nor against him or her and that there are no absolute values by which to live. There are five criteria for rational thinking that are guides for determining whether a thought is rational or irrational and should be accepted by the self:[187]

1. **Objective reality.** This really happens; it is a fact.
2. **Life-preserving.** What is rational will not take life.
3. **Goal-producing.** Action and thoughts that assist in meeting personal goals.
4. **Significant personal conflict.** Person must determine how much conflict he or she will take and how to prevent this conflict.
5. **Significant environmental conflict.** Person must determine if his or her behaviour will cause great problems with others (e.g., rejection or punishment). If problems with others are prevented, conflict is prevented.

The health care provider or therapist is active and collaborates with the client in a carefully structured, time-limited therapy that focuses on specific problem areas or issues. The therapist may use a combination of behavioural and cognitive techniques, such as relaxation, thought stopping, assertiveness training, self-instruction, internal dialogues, and problem solving related to perceptions.

The person is taught to state the problem and feelings in response to the problem, challenge the thoughts through self-talk, and apply the five criteria for rational thinking. If the thought does not meet four out of the five criteria, it is irrational. The person then imagines self in a real situation that is positive and continues to hold that image until he or she can think and act in a more positive way, and thus feel more positive.[188]

Glasser: Reality Therapy. William Glasser is the founder of reality therapy, which derives its name from the insistence on dealing with behaviour in the real world rather than with a client's subjective interpretation of feelings and thoughts. Reality therapy can be used with people of any age and with any problem. Similar problems are handled in the same manner.[189]

Glasser believes that all humans, in addition to survival, have a need to:

- Be loved, accepted, and belong
- Feel respected and worthwhile to self and others

- Be competent, achieve, and gain status, recognition, and power
- Have fun and enjoyment
- Have freedom, independence, and autonomy

Behaviour is the attempt to reduce the difference between what we want and what we have. When needs are not met, the person acts differently, irresponsibly, or in a way that is called mental illness. The person's behaviour will get him or her into trouble, and behaviour, not feelings, is the key. It is the person's choice whether or not to act responsibly or to feel miserable. Yet the person is suffering because she or he cannot meet her or his needs and wants involvement with another person.

The *goal of therapy* is to develop a sense of responsibility defined as the ability to satisfy one's own needs without interfering with the needs of others, while behaving responsibly. The therapeutic problem is to get the client to abandon what may be called the "primitive pleasure principle" and to adopt long-term, wise pursuit of pleasure, satisfaction, joy, and happiness, which the reality principle implies.[190]

The most effective ways for the therapist to use the involvement-commitment process is to remember the following points:

1. A single experience with definition of a problem, involvement, and satisfaction of the person's needs does not guarantee responsible behaviour in the next experience of a similar nature.
2. Responsible behaviour is not necessarily generalized by the client and applied in a cognitive way.
3. The therapist's demands for behavioural standards may be unrealistic for the client.
4. The client may find ways of satisfying his or her psychological needs without using responsible behaviour.
5. Behaviour changes slowly: thus, the therapist or client should never give up[191]

Social Learning Theorist: Bandura
Albert Bandura's social learning theory states that learning occurs without reinforcement, conditioning, or trial-and-error behaviour because people can think and anticipate consequences of behaviour and act accordingly. This theory emphasizes:

1. That cognitive processes, modelling, environmental influences, and the person's self-directed capacity all contribute to development, learning, and behaviour.
2. The importance of vicarious, symbolic, and self-regulatory processes in psychological functioning.
3. The capacity of the person to use symbols, represent events, analyze conscious experience, communicate with others at any distance in time and space, and plan, create, imagine, and engage in actions of foresight.

The person does not simply react to external forces: he or she selects, organizes, and transforms impinging stimuli and thus exercises some influence over personal behaviour. *Bandura's model of causation involves the interaction of three components: (1) the person, with cognitive, biological, and other internal events that affect perceptions and actions, (2) external environment, and (3) behaviour* (Figure 5–3).[192–194]

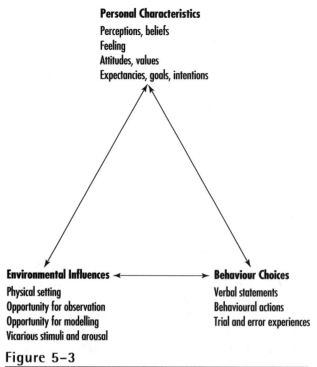

Personal Characteristics

Perceptions, beliefs
Feeling
Attitudes, values
Expectancies, goals, intentions

Environmental Influences

Physical setting
Opportunity for observation
Opportunity for modelling
Vicarious stimuli and arousal

Behaviour Choices

Verbal statements
Behavioural actions
Trial and error experiences

Figure 5–3

Bandura's concept of reciprocal determinism

Human nature is characterized as a vast potential that can be fashioned by knowledge and skill that results from direct and vicarious experience into a variety of forms of development and behaviour within biological limits. The level of psychological and physiologic development restricts what can be acquired at any given time.[195]

The person may be motivated by ideas or fantasies of future consequences or by personal goal-setting behaviour. If the person wants to accomplish a certain goal and there are distractions from the task, the person visualizes how he or she will feel when the goal is attained. After evaluating their behaviour, people usually respond to their own behaviour and tend to persist until the behaviour or performance meets the goal.[196]

Bandura[197] proposes that learning occurs through **modelling,** *imitation of another's behaviour. Four interacting mental processes must be present:*

1. *Attention.* The learner must perceive the model.

2. *Memory.* The learner must encode the information obtained from observing the model in a form that can be used at a later time.

3. *Motor control.* The learner must be able to use this coded information to guide his or her own actions.

4. *Motivation.* The learner must have some reason or inducement to perform the modelled actions.

These processes must be involved in behaviour that depends on information gained from the environment. Learning is achieved primarily through interactions with other people. Social rewards such as praise and acceptance help motivate and reinforce such learning as well as simple observation of other people. Bandura asserts that people learn and, thereby, modify their cognitive constructs throughout life as they interact with others. The person acts on the environment (and the environment on the person) in a continuous lifelong process.[198,199]

According to his theory, much of our daily behaviour is learned by modelling and the perceptions that form in the process. Imitation is one of the most effective forms of learning. Babies learn to speak by imitating the sounds of their parents; older children learn a number of behaviours by watching teachers, parents, or peers. People learn how to be normal or abnormal. Maladaptive behaviour arises from modelling when the child imitates abnormal parental behaviour. Bandura's research also shows the power of watching television on people's behaviour and that for some people the model of aggressive behaviour will cause later acting-out behaviour. This research is discussed further in Chapter 10.

CRITICAL THINKING

What behaviours have you learned through the modelling of others?

Bandura also identified self-efficacy as a mediator in behaviour. Self-efficacy is a judgment about one's ability to organize and execute action and to accomplish a certain level of performance in a situation. Self-efficacy is based on mastered experiences, vicarious experiences or observation of other people doing the behaviour, verbal persuasion from another to adjust behaviour, and physiologic states, or internal cues that are evidence of the capability or deficit. Bandura also described the importance of giving information, rather than just fear-producing statements, to motivate change.[200,201]

Bandura's research combines aspects of behavioural and psychodynamic theories and is pertinent to understanding certain aspects of the developing person. His theory is pertinent to nursing and health care, especially the educational role.[202–208]

Cognitive Development Theorist: Piaget

Jean Piaget[209–221] formulated the theory of cognitive development. The bulk of his research was concerned with the child's thinking at particular periods of life and with studying differences among well children of a specific age. He believed that development is neither **maturational,** an *unfolding of the innate growth process,* nor **learning,** an *accumulation of experiences.* Rather, development is an active process resulting from **equilibration,** an *internal force that is set in motion to organize thinking when the child's belief system develops sufficiently to contain self-contradictions.*

Four factors interact within the person to stimulate mental development:[222]

1. Maturation of the nervous and endocrine systems, which provides physical capabilities

2. Experience involving action, with a consequent discovery of properties of objects

3. Social interaction with opportunity to observe a wide variety of behaviours and gain direct instruction and to receive feedback about individual performance

4. An internal self-regulation mechanism that responds to environmental stimuli

Intelligence is an adaptive process by which the person modifies and structures the environment to fit personal needs and also modifies self in response to environmental demands.

By interaction with the environment, the person constructs reality by assimilation, accommodation, and adaptation. **Assimilation** is *taking new content and experiences into the mind or cognitive structure.* **Accommodation** is the *revising, realigning, and readjusting of cognitive structure to take into account the new content.* **Adaptation** is the *change that results from the first two processes.* Piaget emphasizes the innate, inborn processes of the person as the essential force to start the process of equilibration or cognitive growth. Cognitive development proceeds from motor activity to interaction with the wider social world. Finally, cognitive development arrives at abstract ideas. Development is seen as solidly rooted in what already exists, and it displays continuity with the past. Adaptations do not develop in isolation; all form a coherent pattern so that the totality of biological life is adapted to its environment. The theory focuses on development of intellectual capacities with little reference to emotional or social development.[223–236]

The thinking process is explained by schematic mental structures of pictures formed in response to stimuli. A **schema** is a *cognitive structure, a complex concept encompassing both motor behaviour and internalized thought processes. A schema involves movement of the eyeballs, paying attention, and the mental picture that is formed as a result of the sensory process.* Thinking eventually involves using combinations of mental pictures, forming concepts, internalizing use of language or subvocal speech, drawing implications, and making judgments. When these internal actions become integrated into a coherent, logical system, they are considered logical operations. The schemata that are developed and the specific levels of function are unique to each person and, in turn, structure future learning. Learning is determined by (1) what is observed, (2) whether new information is fit into old schemata accurately or in a distorted way, and (3) how much increase in competence results from the encounter or experience.[237–250]

Piaget divided human development into four periods: sensorimotor, preoperational, concrete operations, and formal operations. Table 5-8 is a summary of the periods. In each stage, the person demonstrates interpretation and use of the environment through certain behaviour patterns. These periods are discussed with development of the infant, toddler, preschooler, schoolchild, adolescent, and adult. You will find these stages pertinent to determining mental development of the person and corresponding educational approaches and activities.[251–265]

Information Processing; Neo-Piagetian Theory

This neo-Piagetian *approach does not propose stages of cognitive development but, like Piaget, sees people as active thinkers about their world.* People learn by becoming efficient at processing information rather than through equilibration. These theorists *study mental processes underlying intelligent behaviour; perception, attention, memory, and problem solving; and how people acquire, transform, and use sensory information through active manipulation of symbols or mental images.* They look at the

mind as a computer. Practice enables learning, since there is a limit to the number of schemes a person can keep in mind. *With practice, an idea or skill becomes automatic, which frees the person to learn additional information and do more complex problem solving.* These theorists believe learning does not occur in demarcated stages but is more gradual and continuous. However, this theory neglects study of creativity, motivation, and social interaction as they relate to cognitive development.[266,267]

According to this theory, information is taken from the environment, through the senses, and held in memory: the first memory storage. If the person pays attention, the information is transferred to the short-term memory storage. The short-term memory can only hold about seven pieces of information at a time, so the information is either forgotten or processed to the long-term memory storage. To save information at this third level, organizing and hearing it is necessary. Retrieval may be difficult. As the child grows older, information is processed more efficiently and comprehensively. The child develops **metacognition**, *an awareness of how to think and learn, and an understanding of self as a learner.* Thus, a knowledge base is developed through the life span. However, knowledge is specialized, depending on the information and skills accumulated.[268]

Moral Development Theorists
Kohlberg's Theory of Moral Development. Lawrence Kohlberg formulated a theory of moral development. Moral development is related to cognitive and emotional development and to societal values and norms and is divided into stages by Kohlberg.[269–273]

Moral reasoning focuses on ten universal values: punishment, property, roles and concerns related to affection, roles and concerns related to authority, law, life, liberty, distribution of justice, truth, and sexual behaviour. A conflict between two or more of these universal values necessitates a moral choice and its subsequent justification by the individual, requiring systematic problem solving and other cognitive capabilities.[274–279]

Kohlberg theorized that a person's moral reasoning process and behaviour develop through stages over varying lengths of time. Each stage is derived from a prior stage and is the basis for the next stage. *Each moral stage is based or dependent on the reason for behaviour and shows an organized system of thought by which the person is consistent in the level of moral judgment.* The person is considered in a specific stage when the same level of reason for action is given at least half the time. More advanced logical thinking is needed for each successive moral stage. One criterion of moral maturity, the ability to decide autonomously what is right and caring, is lacking in the preconventional and conventional levels because in each level the person is following the commands of authority figures. If the person's cognitive stage is at the stage of concrete operations, according to Piaget, the person is limited to the preconventional or conventional levels of moral reasoning. Even the person in the stage of formal operations may not be beyond the conventional level of moral maturity. Kohlberg found that 50% of

TABLE 5–8
Summary of Piaget's Theory of Cognitive Development

Period	Age	Characteristics
Sensorimotor Period		
Stage 1: Use of reflexes	0–1 month	Behaviour innate, reflexive, specific, predictable to specific stimuli **Example:** sucking, grasping, eye movements, startle (Moro reflex)
Stage 2: First acquired adaptations and primary circula reactions	1–4 months	Initiates, prolongs, and repeats behaviour not previously occurring Acquires response to stimulus that creates another stimulus and response Modifies innate reflexes to more purposeful behaviour; repeated if satisfying Learns feel of own body as physiologic stabilization occurs **Example:** Looks at object, reaches for it, and continues to repeat until vision, reaching, and mouthing are coordinated
Stage 3: Secondary circular reactions	4–8 months	Learns from unintentional behaviour Motor skills and vision further coordinated as infant learns to prolong or repeat interesting act Interest in environment around self Explores world from sitting position Assimilates new objects into old behaviour pattern Behaviour increasingly intentional **Example:** Looks for object that disappears from sight; continues to drop object from different locations, which adult continues to pick up
Stage 4: Coordination of secondary schema acquisition of instrumental behaviour, active search for vanished objects	8–12 months	Uses familiar behaviour patterns in new situation to accomplish goal Differentiates objects, including mother from stranger (stranger anxiety) Retains memory of object hidden from view Combines actions to obtain desired, hidden object; explores object Imitates others when behaviour finished Develops individual habits Cognitive development enhanced by increasing motor and language skills
Stage 5: Tertiary circular reactions and discovery of new means by active experimentation	12–18 months	Invents new behaviour not previously performed Uses fewer previous behaviours Repeats action without random movements Explores variations that occur when same act accomplished Varies action deliberately as repeats behaviour Uses trial-and-error behaviour to discover solution to problem Differentiates self from object and object from action performed by self; increasing exploration of how objects function Invents new means to solve problems and variation in behaviour essential to later symbolic behaviour and concept formation
Stage 6: Internal representation of action in external world	18–24 months	Pictures events to self; follows through mentally to some degree Imitates when model out of sight Forms mental picture of external body, of body in same space with another object, and of space in limited way Uses deliberate trial and error in solving problems
Preoperational Period		
	2–7 years	Internalizes schemata of more and more of the environment, rules, and relationships Forms memories to greater extent Uses fantasy or imitation of others in behaviour and play Intermingles fantasy and reality Uses words to represent objects and events more accurately; symbolic behaviour increases

(continued)

TABLE 5-8 *(continued)*
Summary of Piaget's Theory of Cognitive Development

Period	Age	Characteristics
		Egocentric *(self-centred in thought)*—focuses on single aspect of object and neglects other attributes because of lack of experience and reference systems, which results in false logic
		Follows rules in egocentric way; rules external to self
		Is static and irreversible in thinking; cannot transform from one state to another (e.g., ice to water)
		Develops story or idea while forgetting original idea so that final statements disconnected, disorganized; answer not connected to original idea in monologue
		Tries logical thinking; at times sounds logical but lacks perspective so that false logic and inconsistent, unorganized thinking result
		Is magical, global, primitive in reasoning
		Begins to connect past to present events, not necessarily accurate
		Links events by sequence rather than causality
		Deals with information by recall; begins to categorize
		Is **anthropomorphic** *(attributes human characteristics to animals and objects)*
		Unable to integrate events separated by time, past to present
		Lacks reversibility in thinking
		Unable to anticipate how situation looks from another viewpoint
Preconceptual stage	2–4 years	Forms images or preconcepts on basis of thinking just described
		Lacks ability to define properly or to denote hierarchy or relationships of objects
		Constructs concepts in global way
		Unable to use time, space, equivalence, and class inclusion in concept formation
Intuitive stage	4–7 years	Forms concepts increasingly; some limitations
		Defines one property at a time
		Has difficulty starting definition but knows how to use object
		Uses transductive logic (from general to specific) rather than deductive or inductive logic
		Begins to classify in ascending or descending order; labels
		Begins to do seriation; reverses processes and ordinality
		Begins to note cause-effect relationships
Concrete Operations Period		
	7–11 years (or beyond)	Organizes and stabilizes thinking; more rational
		See interrelationships increasingly
		Does mental operations using tangible, visible references
		Able to **decentre** *(sees other perspectives; associates or combines events; understands reversibility [e.g., add–subtract, ice–water transformation])*
		Recognizes number, length, volume, area, weight as the same even when perception of object changes
		Develops conservation as experience is gained with physical properties of objects
		Arranges objects in order of size and other characteristics
		Fits new objects into series
		Understands simpler relationships between classes of objects
		Distinguishes between distances
		Understands observable world, tangible situations, time, and tangible space
		Retains essential idea when perceiving conflicting or unorganized data
		Recognizes rules as essential; perceives mutually agreed on standards
		Is less egocentric except in social relationships

(continued)

TABLE 5-8 *(continued)*
Summary of Piaget's Theory of Cognitive Development

Period	Age	Characteristics
Formal Operations Period		
	12 years and beyond	Manifests adult like thinking
		Not limited by own perception or concrete references for ideas
		Combines various ideas into concepts
		Coordinates two or more reference systems
		Develops morality of restraint and cooperation in behaviour
		Uses rules to structure interaction in socially acceptable way
		Uses probability concept
		Works from definition or concept only to solve problem
		Solves problem mentally and considers alternatives before acting
		Considers number of variables at one time
		Links variables to formulate hypotheses
		Begins to reason deductively and inductively instead of solving problem by action
		Relates concepts or constructs not readily evident in external world
		Formulates advanced concepts of proportions, space, destiny, momentum
		Increases intellectual ability to include art, science, humanities, religion, and philosophy
		Is increasingly less egocentric

late adolescents and adults are capable of formal operations thinking, but only 10% of these adults demonstrated the postconventional level in stages 5 and 6. Thus the person moves through stages, but few people progress through all six stages. Table 5-9 shows the three levels and six stages. *Kohlberg added a seventh stage of moral reasoning shortly before his death. This stage moves beyond considerations of justice and has more in common with self-transcendence and faith* explained in religious and Eastern philosophies. He asked: Why be moral? He believed the answer was to achieve a cosmic perspective, a sense of unity with the cosmos, nature, or God. This perspective enables the person to see moral issues from a universal whole, seeing that everything is connected. Moral development is discussed in relation to each developmental era in Chapters 7 through 14.[280–284]

CRITICAL THINKING

Who in the world, in your opinion, may have progressed to the postconventional stage? State your rationale.

Development of moral judgment is stimulated whenever (1) the educational process intentionally creates cognitive conflict and disequilibrium so that the person can work through inadequate modes of thinking, (2) the person has opportunity for group discussion of values and can participate in group decision making about moral issues, and (3) the person has opportunity to assume responsibility for the consequences of behaviour.[285] Kohlberg's theory has application to nursing, education,[286] and family counselling.[287]

Gilligan's Theory of Moral Development. Gilligan's research on moral development has focused on women in contrast to Kohlberg's focus on men. Gilligan found that moral development proceeds through three levels and two transitions, with each level representing a more complex understanding of the relationship of self and others and each transition resulting in a crucial re-evaluation of the conflict between selfishness and responsibility. Women define the moral problem in the context of human relationships, exercising care, and avoiding hurt. In Gilligan's studies, women's moral judgment proceeded from initial concern with survival, to a focus on goodness, to a principled understanding of others' need for care. Table 5-10 summarizes the three levels and two transitions of moral development proposed by Gilligan.[288–290]

The care focus proposed by Gilligan is concerned with issues of abandonment, and the theory values ideals of attention and response to need. Some people may combine both Kohlberg's and Gilligan's perspectives and incorporate them into their moral development, such values as honesty, courage, and community, which are implied in Kohlberg's postconventional level. More research in all age groups, men and women, and all races and ethnic groups is needed to understand moral development fully.

Friedman[291] tested Gilligan's claim that men and women differ in moral judgments. College students read four traditional moral dilemmas and rated the importance of 12 considerations for deciding how the protagonist should respond. There were no reliable sex differences on moral reasoning. Sex-typed personality measures also failed to predict individual differences in moral judgments.

TABLE 5-9
Progression of Moral Development

Level	Stage
Preconventional	
The person is responsive to cultural rules of labels of good and bad, right or wrong. Externally established rules determine right or wrong actions. The person reasons in terms of punishment, reward, or exchange of favours.	I. *Punishment and Obedient Orientation* Fear of punishment, not respect for authority, is the reason for decisions, behaviour, and conformity. *Good* and *bad* are defined in terms of physical consequences to the self from parental, adult, or authority figures. The person defers to superior power or prestige of the person who dictates rules ("I'll do something because you tell me and to avoid getting punished"). Average age: toddler to 7 years
Egocentric focus	II. *Instrumental Relativist Orientation* Conformity is based on egocentricity and narcissistic needs. The person's decisions and behaviour are usually based on what provides satisfaction out of concern for self: something is done to get something in return. Occasionally the person does something to please another for pragmatic reasons. There is no feeling of justice, loyalty, or gratitude. These concepts are expressed physically ("I'll do something if I get something for it or because it pleases you"). Average age: preschooler through school age
Conventional	
Person is concerned with maintaining expectations and rules of the family, group, nation, or society. A sense of guilt has developed and affects behaviour. The person values conformity, loyalty, and active maintenance of social order and control. Conformity means good behaviour or what pleases or helps another and is approved.	III. *Interpersonal Concordance Orientation* A. Decisions and behaviour are based on concerns about others' reactions; the person wants others' approval or a reward. The person has moved from egocentricity to consideration of others as a basis for behaviour. Behaviour is judged by the person's intentions ("I'll do something because it will please you or because it is expected"). B. An empathic response, based on understanding of how another person feels, is a determinant for decisions and behaviour ("I'll do something because I know how it feels to be without; I can put myself in your shoes"). Average age: school age through adulthood (Most North American women are in this stage.)
Societal focus	IV. *Law-and-Order Orientation* The person wants established rules from authorities, and the reason for decisions and behaviour is that social and sexual rules and traditions demand the response. The person obeys the law just because it is the law or out of respect for authority and underlying morality of the law. The law takes precedence over personal wishes, good intentions, and conformity to group stereotypes ("I'll do something because it's the law and my duty"). Average age: adolescence and adulthood (Most men are in this stage; 80% of adults do not move past this stage.)
Postconventional	
The person lives autonomously and defines moral values and principles that are distinct from personal identification with group values. He or she lives according to principles that are universally agreed on and that the person considers appropriate for life.	V. *Social Contract Legalistic Orientation* The social rules are not the sole basis for decisions and behaviour because the person believes a higher moral principle applies such as equality, justice, or due process. The person defines right actions in terms of general individual rights and standards that have been agreed on by the whole society but is aware of relativistic nature of values and opinions. The person believes laws can be changed as people's needs change. The person uses freedom of choice in living up to higher

(continued)

TABLE 5-9 *(continued)*
Progression of Moral Development

Level	Stage
	principles but believes the way to make changes is through the system. Outside the legal realm, free agreement and contract are the binding elements of obligation ("I'll do something because it is morally and legally right, even if it isn't popular with the group"). Average age: middle age or older adult. No more than 20% of North Americans achieve this stage.
Universal focus	**VI.** *Universal Ethical Principle Orientation* Decisions and behaviour are based on internalized rules, on conscience rather than social laws, and on self-chosen ethical and abstract principles that are universal, comprehensive, and consistent. The rules are not concrete moral rules but instead encompass the Golden Rule, justice, reciprocity, and equality of human rights, and respect for the dignity of human beings as individual persons. Human life is inviolable. The person believes there is a higher order than social order, has a clear concept of civil disobedience, and will use self as an example to right a wrong. The person accepts injustice, pain, and death as an integral part of existence but works to minimize injustice and pain for others ("I'll do something because it is morally, ethically, and spiritually right, even if it is illegal and I get punished and even if no one else participates in the act"). Average age: middle age or older adult. (Few people attain or maintain this stage. Examples of this stage are seen in times of crisis or extreme situations.)

Source: Data used here are based upon Kohlberg, L., ed., Collected Papers on Moral Development and Moral Education, *Cambridge, MA: Moral Educational Research Foundation, 1973; Kohlberg, L., Moral Stages and Moralization: The Cognitive Developmental Approach, in Lickona, T., ed.,* Moral Development and Behavior, *New York: Holt, Rinehart, & Winston, 1976, pp. 31–53; Kohlberg, L., Recent Research in Moral Development, New York: Holt, Rinehart, & Winston, 1977; Kohlberg, L., The Cognitive-Developmental Approach to Moral Education, in Scharf, P., ed., Readings in Moral Education, Minneapolis: Winston Press, 1978, pp. 36–51.*

TABLE 5-10
Gilligan's Theory of Moral Development

Level	Characteristics
Orientation of Individual Survival Transition 1: From Selfishness to Responsibility	*Concentrates on what is practical and best for self;* selfish; dependent on others Realizes connection to others; thinks of responsible choice in terms of another as well as self
Goodness as Self-Sacrifice Transition 2: From Goodness to Truth	*Sacrifices personal wishes and needs to fulfill others' wants* and to have others think well of her; feels responsible for others' actions; holds others responsible for her choices; dependent position; indirect efforts to control others often turn into manipulation through use of guilt; aware of connectedness with others. *Makes decisions on personal intentions and consequences of actions rather than on how she thinks others will react;* takes into account needs of self and others; wants to be good to others but also honest by being responsible to self; increased social participation; assumes more responsibilities.
Morality of Nonviolence	*Establishes moral equality between self and others; assumes responsibility for choice in moral dilemmas;* follows injunction to hurt no one, including self, in all situations; conflict between selfishness and selflessness; judgment based on view of consequences and intentions instead of appearance in the eyes of others.

Sources: The data used here are based upon Gilligan, C., In a Different Voice: Women's Conceptualization of Self and of Mortality, Harvard Educational Review, *47, no. 4 (1977), 481–517; Gilligan, C., In a Different Voice: Psychological Theory and Women's Development. Cambridge, MA: Harvard University Press, 1982; Gilligan, C., and D. Attanucci, Two Moral Orientations: Gender Differences and Similarities,* Merrill-Palmer Quarterly, *34, no. 3 (1988), 332–333.*

EXISTENTIAL AND HUMANISTIC THEORIES

Overview

Existential and humanistic psychologies acknowledge the dynamic aspect of the person but emphasize the impact of environment to a greater degree.

Existentialism has its roots in philosophy, theology, literature, and psychology and *addresses the person's existence in a hostile or indifferent world and within the context of history.* It is phenomenological in nature; the context, uniqueness, and ever-changing aspects of events are considered. Existentialism regards human nature as unexplainable but emphasizes freedom of choice, responsibility, and satisfaction of ideals, the burden of freedom, discovery of inner self, and consequences of action. *Themes addressed* include suffering, death, despair, meaninglessness, nothingness, vacuum, isolation, anxiety, hope, self transcendence, and finding spiritual meaning. The transcendence of inevitable suffering, anxiety, and alienation is emphasized.[292–294]

Humanism *emphasizes self-actualization, satisfaction of needs, the individual as a rule unto himself or herself, the pleasure of freedom, and realization of innate goodness and creativity.*[295] *Humanism shares the following assumptions with existentialism:* uniqueness of the person, potential of the person, and necessity of listening to or studying the person's perceptions, called the *phenomenological approach.*

Both existentialists and humanists seek to answer the following questions:

1. What are the possibilities of the person?
2. From these possibilities, what is an optimum state for the person?
3. Under what conditions is this state most likely to be reached? These disciplines strive to maximize the individuality and developmental potential of the person.[296–299]

Because all behaviour is considered a function of the person's perceptions, *data for study of the person are subjective and come from self-reports,* including (1) feelings at the moment about self and the experience, (2) meaning of the experience, and (3) personal values, needs, attitudes, beliefs, behavioural norms, and expectations. Perception is synonymous with reality and meaning. The person has many components—physical, physiologic, cognitive, emotional, spiritual, cultural, social, and familial—and cannot be adequately understood if studied by individual components. All behaviour is pertinent to and a product of the phenomenal or perceptual field of the person at the moment of action. The **phenomenal field** is the *frame of reference and the universe as experienced by the person at the specific moment (the existential condition).*[300,301]

View of the Human

The person is *viewed as a significant and unique whole individual in dynamic interaction with the environment and in the process of becoming.* In addition, the person is seen as *holistic, with organizational complexity, more than the sum of the parts.* The person is constantly growing, changing, expanding perceptual processes, learning, developing potential, and gaining insights. Every experience affects the person, depending on the perceptions. The person is never quite the same as he or she was even an hour or day earlier. The goals of the creative being are growth, feeling adequate, and reaching the potential. The person is active in pursuing these goals. Basic needs are the maintenance and enhancement of the self-concept and a sense of adequacy and self-actualization.[302–304]

Reality is internal; the *person's reality is the perception of the event* rather than the actual event itself. No two people will view a situation in exactly the same way. *Various factors affect perception:*

1. The sensory apparatus and central nervous system of the person.
2. Time for observation.
3. Opportunities available to experience events.
4. The external environment.
5. Interpersonal relationships.
6. Self-concept.

What is most important to the person is conscious experience, what is happening to the self at a given time. The person is aware of social values and norms but lives out those values and norms in a way that has been uniquely and personally defined.[305]

Perceptions are crucial in influencing behaviour. Of all the perceptions that exist for the person, none is more important than those held about the self and the personal meaning and belief related to a situation. *Self-concept* is learned as a consequence of meaningful interactions with others and the world and has a high degree of stability at its core, changing only with time and opportunity to try new perceptions of self.

The *truly adequate person* sees self (and others) as having dignity, integrity, worth, and importance. Only with a positive view of self can the person risk trying the untried or accepting the undefined situation. The person can become self-actualized only through the experience of being treated as an adequate person by significant others. This person is open to all experiences, develops trust in self, and dares to recognize feelings, live life fully, and express uniqueness. The person feels a sense of oneness with other people, depending on the nature of previous contacts.

View of Education and Therapy

Education and therapy are:

1. Growth-oriented rather than controlling.
2. Rooted in perceptual meaning rather than facts.
3. Concerned with people rather than things.
4. Focused on the immediate rather than the historical view of people.
5. Hopeful rather than despairing.

The goals of education and therapy are the same goals as those of the person: full functioning of the person, ongoing development, meeting the individual's potential, and movement toward self-actualization. Education and therapy are a process, not a condition or institution, and through the process the person achieves effective behaviour. The basic tenets of freedom and responsibility are essential focal points in this approach.[306–312]

Characteristics of the learner or client are as follows:

1. Is unique, has dignity and worth.
2. Brings a cluster of understandings, skills, values, and attitudes that have personal meaning.
3. Presents total self as sum of reactions to previous experiences and cultural and family background.
4. Wants to learn that which has personal meaning; learns from experience.
5. Wants to be fully involved; learning involves all dimensions of person.
6. Believes finding the self is more important than facts.[313]

The health care provider, teacher, or therapist is a unique, whole person with a self-concept that directly affects the philosophy and style of teaching or counselling. He or she does not consider self as central. Instead she or he is learner- or client-centred. Each sees the self as using the personality as an instrument, acting as a permissive facilitator, and providing a warm, accepting, supportive environment that is as free from threat and obstacles as possible. The teacher or therapist provides an enriched environment and a variety of ways for the person to perceive new experiences and to learn. The teacher or therapist realizes that all people need to be perceived and related to as empathic, cooperative, forward-looking, trustworthy, and responsible. These theorists reject the traditional, pessimistic, or mechanical view of people.[314–320]

Humanistic psychology emphasizes the natural tendency of all people, regardless of age or stage of life, to strive for self-actualization. Treatment approaches promote increased self-esteem and positive self-concept, problem solving to achieve goals, and helping the person achieve optimal functioning through a supportive therapeutic relationship characterized by warmth, nonpossessive caring, and validation of the person's worth and dignity. Martin claims that the therapist's characteristics contribute to successful outcomes.[321]

Existential and Humanistic Theorists

Maslow: Theory of Motivation and Hierarchy of Needs

Maslow studied normal people and mental health in contrast to other developmental and personality theorists. One of his most important concepts is **self-actualization,** the *tendency to develop potentialities and become a better person,* and the need to help the person achieve the sense of self-direction implicit in self-actualization. Implicit in this concept is that people are not static but are always in the process of becoming different and better.[322,323]

The needs that motivate self-actualization can be represented in a hierarchy of relative order and predominance. The basic needs, always a consideration in client care, are listed in Table 5-11.

Maslow's study of self-actualizing people refutes Freudian theory that the human unconscious, or id, is only bad or

dangerous. In self-actualizing people, the unconscious is creative, loving, and positive.

Although *Maslow ranked these basic human needs from lowest to highest, they do not necessarily occur in a fixed order.* The physiologic and safety needs (deficiency needs), however, are dominant and must be met before higher needs can be secured. Personal growth needs are those for love and belonging, self-esteem and recognition, and self-actualization. The highest needs of self-actualization, knowledge, and aesthetic expression may never be as fully gratified as those at lower levels. Individual growth and self-fulfillment are a continuing, lifelong process of becoming.[324]

To motivate the person toward self-actualization, there must be freedom to speak, to pursue creative potential, and to inquire; an atmosphere of justice, honesty, fairness, and order; and environmental stimulation and challenge.

Carl Rogers: Theory on Self-Concept and Person-Centred Therapy

Carl Rogers is, along with Maslow, one of the leaders of humanistic-existentialist psychology. He questioned several traditional concepts of science and developed a perspective on personality with a *focus on self-concept.* Self-actualization is also a key concept in his theory. Rogers assumed that the person sees self as the centre of a continually changing world and that he or she responds to the world as it is perceived. The person responds as a whole in the direction of self-actualization. The ability to achieve self-understanding, self-actualization, and perception of social acceptance by others is based on experience and interaction with other people. The person who, as a child, felt wanted and highly valued is likely to have a positive self-image, be thought well of by others, and have the capacity to achieve self-actualization. Optimal adjustment results in what Rogers called the fully functioning person. The fully functioning person accepts self, avoids a personality façade, is genuine and honest, is increasingly self-directive and autonomous, is open to new experiences, avoids being driven by other people's expectations or the cultural norms, and has a low level of anxiety.[325–331]

CRITICAL THINKING

What should a parent or significant caregiver do to help a child build his or her self-concept?

The person also has an *ideal self,* an idea of what he or she wishes to be, which may or may not be congruent with the "real" self. When a discrepancy develops between the "ideal" self and the "real" self, a state of tension and confusion occurs. Feelings of unworthiness may produce anxiety and defensive psychological reactions.[332,333]

Each person is basically rational, socialized, and constructive.[334] Behaviour is goal-directed and motivated by needs. Unlike the intrapsychic and interpersonal theorists, *Rogers states that current needs are the only ones the person endeavours to satisfy.*[335–337]

Rogers identifies neurotic and psychotic people as those whose self-concept and experiences do not match up. They are

TABLE 5-11
Maslow's Theory of Hierarchy of Needs

Needs*	Characteristics
Physiologic	Requirements for oxygen, water, food, temperature control, elimination, shelter, exercise, sleep, sensory stimulation, and sexual activity met
	Needs cease to exist as means of determining behaviour when satisfied, re-emerging only if blocked or frustrated
Safety	Able to secure shelter
	Sense of security, dependency, consistency, stability
	Maintenance of predictable environment, structure, order, fairness, limits
	Protection from immediate or future danger to physical well-being
	Freedom from fear, anxiety, chaos, and certain amount of routine
Love and belonging	Sense of affection, love, and acceptance from others
	Sense of companionship and affiliation with others
	Identification with significant others
	Recognition and approval from others
	Group interaction
	Not synonymous with sexual needs, but sexual needs may be motivated by this need
Esteem from others	Awareness of own individuality, uniqueness
	Feelings of self-respect and worth and respect from others
	Sense of confidence, independence, dignity
	Sense of competence, achievement, success, prestige, status
	Recognition from others for accomplishments
Self-actualization	Acceptance of self and others
	Empathetic with others
	Self-fulfillment
	Ongoing emotional and spiritual development
	Desire to attain standards of excellence and individual potential
	Use of talents, being productive and creative
	Experiencing fully, vividly, without self-consciousness
	Having peak experiences
Aesthetic	Desire for beauty, harmony, order, attractive surroundings
	Interest in art, music, literature, dance, creative forms
Knowledge and understanding	Desire to understand, systematize, organize, analyze, look for relations and meanings
	Curiosity; desire to know as much as possible
	Attraction to the unknown or mysterious

Needs are listed in ascending order. Physiologic needs are most basic, and self-actualization is highest level of needs.

Sources: Maslow, A., The Farther Reaches of Human Nature. New York: Viking Press, 1971; Maslow, A., Towards a Psychology of Being (2nd ed.). New York: D. Van Nostrand, 1968.

afraid to accept their own experiences as valid, so they distort them, either to protect themselves or to win approval from others. A therapist can help them give up the false self that has been formulated.[338,339]

Rogers's *technique of person-centred therapy* brings about behavioural change by conveying complete acceptance, respect, and empathy for the client. The therapist neither provides interpretations nor gives advice. Providing this high degree of acceptance allows the person to meet basic needs that should have been met in childhood by significant people, to incorporate into the self-structure threatening feelings that were previously excluded, and to become aware of unconscious material that is controlling life. Recently, Rogers has given the therapist a more active role that includes sharing emotions and feelings in an interchange with the client. *Chapter 4 discusses use of Rogers's technique as it can be applied to the nurse–client relationship.*[340,341]

STRESS AND CRISIS THEORIES

Stressors and crises are a part of development throughout the life span and do affect health. An understanding of stress and crisis theories is essential for health promotion assessment, and interventions.

Two theories describe how a person responds to stressors, both routine and severe, and to overwhelming events. *The Theory of Stress and General Adaptation Syndrome,* as formulated by Seyle, *described the physiologic adaptive response to stress,* the everyday wear and tear on the person;[342–348] however, continued studies show that the stress response has emotional, cognitive, and sometimes social effects as well. *Crisis theory was formulated to explain how people respond psychologically and behaviourally when they cannot cope adequately with stressors,* but crises or overwhelming events also have physical effects. The two theories together explain a range of adaptive responses, for stress response always occurs in crisis to some extent, although not every stressor constitutes a crisis.

Theory of Stress Response and Adaptation

Stress Response and Adaptation Syndrome

Stress is a *physical and emotional state always present in the person, one influenced by various environmental, psychological, and social factors but uniquely perceived by the person and intensified in response when environmental change or threat occurs internally or externally and the person must respond.* The manifestations of stress are overt and covert, purposeful, initially protective, maintaining equilibrium, productivity, and satisfaction to the extent possible.[349–356]

CRITICAL THINKING

What are some stressors you are encountering today? How are you coping with them?

The person's survival depends on constant mediation between environmental demands and adaptive capacities. Various self-regulatory physical and emotional mechanisms are in constant operation, adjusting the body to a changing number and nature of internal and external stressors, agents, or factors causing intensification of the stress state. **Stressors** (*stress agents*) encompass a number of types of stimuli (Table 5-12).[357] **Eustress** is the *stress that comes with successful adaptation and that is beneficial or promotes emotional development and self-actualization.* It is *positive stress,* an optimum orientation to life's challenges coupled with the person's ability to regulate life and maintain optimum levels of stress for a growth-promoting lifestyle.[358,359] A moderate amount of stress, when regulatory mechanisms act within limits and few symptoms are observable, is constructive. **Daily hassles** are the *repeated and chronic strains of everyday life.* Daily hassles have a negative effect

TABLE 5–12
Stimuli That Are Stressors

Physical: excessive or intense cold or heat, sound, light, motion, gravity, or electrical current

Chemical: alkalines, acids, drugs, toxic substances, hormones, gases, or food and water pollutants

Microbiologic: viruses, bacteria, moulds, parasites, or other infectious organisms

Physiologic: disease processes, surgery, immobilization, mechanical trauma, fever, organ hypo- or hyperfunction, or pain

Psychological: anticipated marriage or death, imagined events, intense emotional involvement, anxiety or other unpleasant feelings, distortions of body image, threats to self-concept, others' expectations of behaviour, rejection by or separation from loved ones, role changes, memory of negative past experiences, actual or perceived failures

Developmental: genetic endowment, prematurity, immaturity, maturational impairment, or the aging process

Sociocultural: sociocultural background and pressures, inharmonious interpersonal relationships, demands of our technologic society, social mobility, changing social mores, job pressures, economic worries, childrearing practices, redefinition of sex roles, or minority status

Environmental: unemployment, air and water pollution, overcrowding disasters, war, or crime

on both somatic health and psychological status.[360] **Distress** is *negative, noxious, unpleasant, damaging stress* that results when adaptive capacity is decreased or exhausted.

What is considered a stressor by one person may be considered pleasurable by another. The amount of stress in the immediate environment cannot be determined by examining only the stressor or source of stress. *Certain principles, however, apply to most people:*[361–368]

- **The primary response to a stressor is behavioural.** When an event or situation is perceived as threatening, the person reacts in intensity and scope to meet the threat; physiologic impact is secondary.
- **The impact is cumulative.** Most stressors in the environment occur at levels below that which would cause immediate physical or emotional damage.
- **Circumstances alter the impact or harm done by a stressor.** The social and emotional context of an event and the attitude and previous experiences of the person are as important as the physical properties of the stimuli.
- **People are remarkably adaptable.** Each person has evolved a normal range of response or a unique pattern of defence. What may at first be considered uncomfortable or intolerable may eventually be perceived as normal routine. The immediate impact of a stressor is apparently different from long-term or indirect consequences, which are more difficult to detect.

- **Various psychological or social factors can ease or exaggerate the effects of a stressor.** If a stressor is predictable, it will not be as harmful as an unpredictable one. If the person feels in control of the situation or can relate positively or directly to the stressor, the effects are less negative. For example, the person in a noisy environment suffers less startle reaction if sudden noises come regularly and are anticipated. Those who work in a noisy environment without the ability to control the noise show low frustration tolerance, uncooperative behaviour, and more errors on reading and arithmetic problems. Studies also show less stress response when people feel control and actually have control over a stressful environment.

- **There are definite low points when stressors are poorly tolerated.** Time of day affects stress response. For example, in most people, hydrocortisone secretion normally peaks in the early morning and decreases through the day, until it is almost undetectable at night. Although diurnal rhythms vary from person to person, stressors may be better tolerated early in the day.

- **Conditioning is an important protection.** The person whose heart, lungs, and skeletal muscles are conditioned by exercise can withstand cardiovascular and respiratory effects of the alarm stage better than someone who leads a sedentary life.

- **Responses to stress throughout life are both local and general.**

The **local adaptation syndrome,** typified by the inflammatory response, is the *method used to wall off and control effects of physical stressors locally.* When the stressor cannot be handled locally, the *whole body responds to protect itself and ensure survival in the best way possible through the* **general adaptation syndrome.** The general body response augments body functions that protect the organism from injury, psychological and physical, and suppresses those functions nonessential to life. The general adaptation syndrome is characterized by alarm and resistance stages and, when body resistance is not maintained, an end stage, exhaustion.[369–375]

General Adaptation Syndrome

The **alarm stage** is an *instantaneous, short-term, life-preserving, and total sympathetic nervous system response* when the person consciously or unconsciously perceives a stressor and feels helpless, insecure, or biologically uncomfortable. This stage is typified by a "fight-or-flight" reaction.[376,377] Perception of the stressor—the alarm reaction—stimulates the anterior pituitary to increase production of adrenocorticotropic hormone (ACTH). The adrenal cortex is stimulated by ACTH to increase production of glucocorticoids, primarily hydrocortisone or cortisol, and mineral corticoids, primarily aldosterone. Catecholamine release triggers increase sympathetic nervous system activity, which stimulates production of epinephrine and norepinephrine by the adrenal medulla and release at the adrenergic nerve endings. The alarm reaction also stimulates the posterior pituitary to release increased antidiuretic hormone.[378–385] *Generally, the person is prepared to act, is more alert, and is able to adapt* (Figures 5–4 and 5–5).

Physiologically, the responses that occur when the sympathetic nervous system is stimulated are shown in Figure 5–6.[386–393]

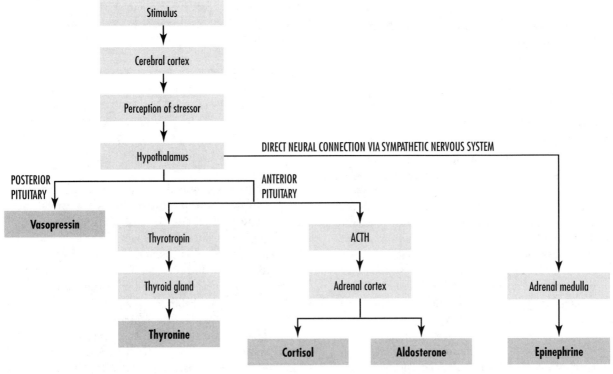

Figure 5–4

Neuroendocrine response to stress.

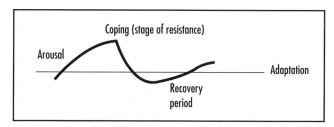

Figure 5–5
Reaction pattern in acute stress.

To complicate assessment, there are times when *parts of the parasympathetic division of the autonomic nervous system are inadvertently stimulated during a stressful state because of the proximity of sympathetic and parasympathetic nerve fibres.* With intensification of stress, opposite behaviours are then observed. They are shown in Figure 5–7.[394,395]

Lazarus identified three psychological stages that occur during the alarm stage: threat, warning, and impact. The psychological processes that occur when the stress stage is intensified begin with appraisal of the threat or potential degree of harm (warning). This process is cognitive and affective and involves perception, memory, thought, and a feeling response to the

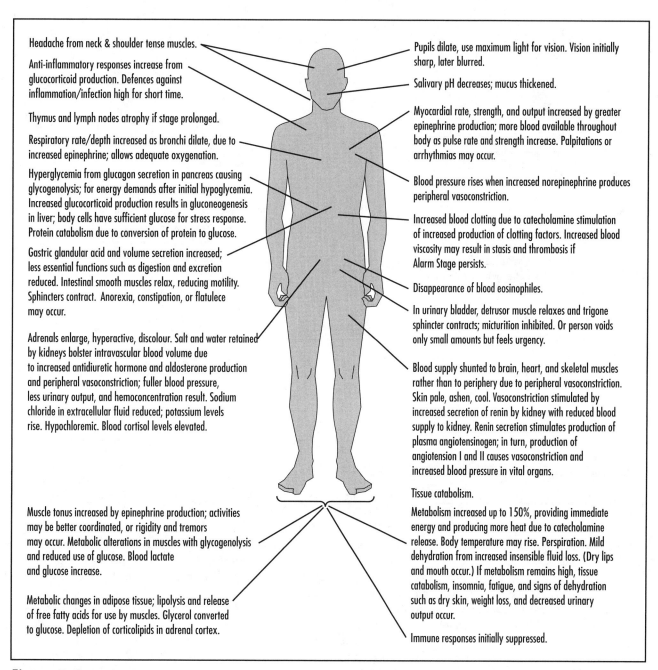

Figure 5–6

Alarm stage, General Adaptation Syndrome: physiologic responses to sympathetic nervous system stimulation.

Source: Murray, R., and M. M. Huelskoetter, Psychiatric/Mental Health Nursing: Giving Emotional Care *(3rd ed.). Stamford, CT: Appleton & Lange, 1991, p. 336.*

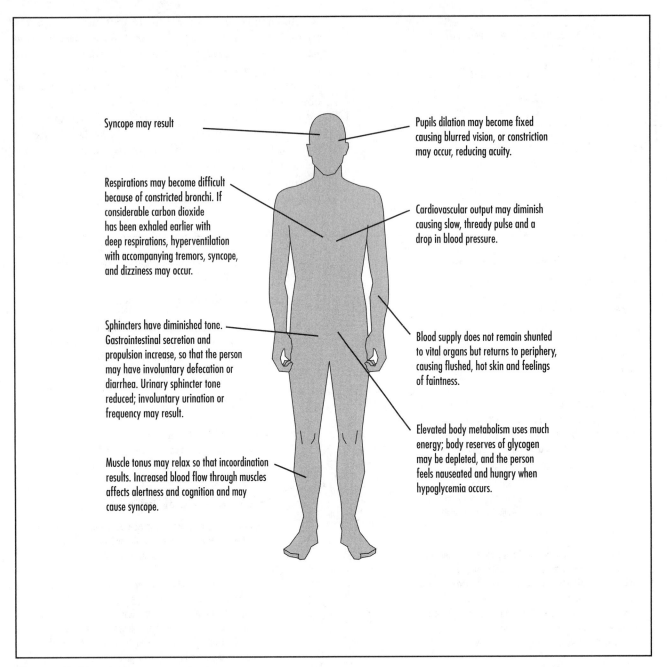

Syncope may result

Pupils dilation may become fixed causing blurred vision, or constriction may occur, reducing acuity.

Respirations may become difficult because of constricted bronchi. If considerable carbon dioxide has been exhaled earlier with deep respirations, hyperventilation with accompanying tremors, syncope, and dizziness may occur.

Cardiovascular output may diminish causing slow, thready pulse and a drop in blood pressure.

Sphincters have diminished tone. Gastrointestinal secretion and propulsion increase, so that the person may have involuntary defecation or diarrhea. Urinary sphincter tone reduced; involuntary urination or frequency may result.

Blood supply does not remain shunted to vital organs but returns to periphery, causing flushed, hot skin and feelings of faintness.

Elevated body metabolism uses much energy; body reserves of glycogen may be depleted, and the person feels nauseated and hungry when hypoglycemia occurs.

Muscle tonus may relax so that incoordination results. Increased blood flow through muscles affects alertness and cognition and may cause syncope.

Figure 5–7

Alarm stage, General Adaptation Syndrome: physiologic responses to parasympathetic nervous system stimulation.

Source: Murray, R., and M. M. Huelskoetter, Psychiatric/Mental Health Nursing: Giving Emotional Care *(3rd ed.). Stamford, CT: Appleton & Lange, 1999, p. 337.*

meaning of the impact of the threat, such as anxiety, fear, anger, guilt, or shame.[396]

The **stage of resistance** is the *body's way of adapting, through an adrenocortical response, to the disequilibrium caused by the stressors of life.* Because of the adrenocortical response, increased use of body resources, endurance and strength, tissue anabolism, antibody production, hormonal secretion, and changes in blood sugar levels and blood volume sustain the body's fight for preservation. Body response eventually returns to normal.

The tissue tranquilizers released help us adapt passively to stimuli, and the enzymes and blood cells released attack pathogens. Moderate anxiety is felt; habitual ego defences are unconsciously used. Responses eventually return to normal when stressors diminish or when the person has found adaptive mechanisms that meet emotional needs and physical demands.[397–404]

If biological, psychological, or social stresses, alone or in combination, occur over a long period without adequate relief, the stage of resistance is maintained. *With continued stressors, the person becomes distressed and manifests objective and subjective emotional, intellectual, and physiologic responses, as shown in Figures 5–8 and 5–9.*[405–412]

Protective factors *modify, ameliorate, or alter the person's response to stressors and to a potentially maladaptive outcome.*

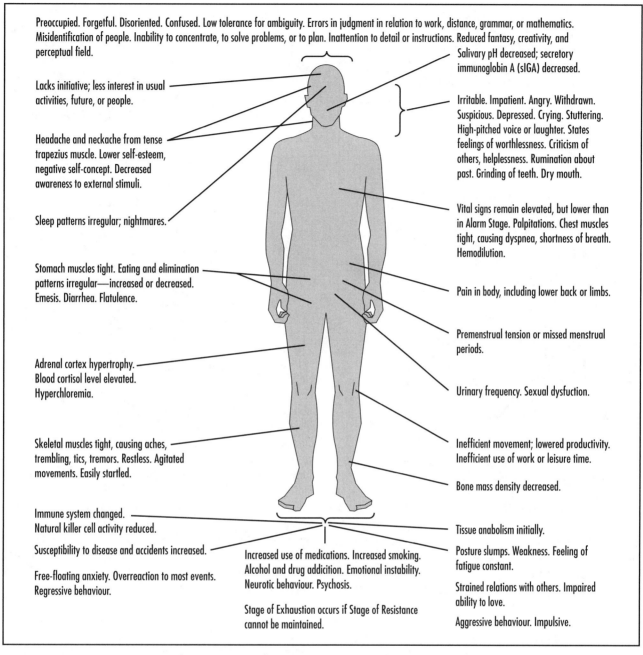

Preoccupied. Forgetful. Disoriented. Confused. Low tolerance for ambiguity. Errors in judgment in relation to work, distance, grammar, or mathematics. Misidentification of people. Inability to concentrate, to solve problems, or to plan. Inattention to detail or instructions. Reduced fantasy, creativity, and perceptual field.

Lacks initiative; less interest in usual activities, future, or people.

Headache and neckache from tense trapezius muscle. Lower self-esteem, negative self-concept. Decreased awareness to external stimuli.

Sleep patterns irregular; nightmares.

Stomach muscles tight. Eating and elimination patterns irregular—increased or decreased. Emesis. Diarrhea. Flatulence.

Adrenal cortex hypertrophy. Blood cortisol level elevated. Hyperchloremia.

Skeletal muscles tight, causing aches, trembling, tics, tremors. Restless. Agitated movements. Easily startled.

Immune system changed. Natural killer cell activity reduced.

Susceptibility to disease and accidents increased.

Free-floating anxiety. Overreaction to most events. Regressive behaviour.

Salivary pH decreased; secretory immunoglobin A (sIGA) decreased.

Irritable. Impatient. Angry. Withdrawn. Suspicious. Depressed. Crying. Stuttering. High-pitched voice or laughter. States feelings of worthlessness. Criticism of others, helplessness. Rumination about past. Grinding of teeth. Dry mouth.

Vital signs remain elevated, but lower than in Alarm Stage. Palpitations. Chest muscles tight, causing dyspnea, shortness of breath. Hemodilution.

Pain in body, including lower back or limbs.

Premenstrual tension or missed menstrual periods.

Urinary frequency. Sexual dysfuction.

Inefficient movement; lowered productivity. Inefficient use of work or leisure time.

Bone mass density decreased.

Tissue anabolism initially.

Posture slumps. Weakness. Feeling of fatigue constant.

Strained relations with others. Impaired ability to love.

Aggressive behaviour. Impulsive.

Increased use of medications. Increased smoking. Alcohol and drug addiction. Emotional instability. Neurotic behaviour. Psychosis.

Stage of Exhaustion occurs if Stage of Resistance cannot be maintained.

Figure 5–8

Stage of resistance, General Adaptation Syndrome: signs of emotional, intellectual, and physiologic distress.

Source: Murray, R., and M. M. Huelskoetter, Psychiatric/Mental Health Nursing: Giving Emotional Care *(3rd ed.). Stamford, CT: Appleton & Lange, 1991, p. 338.*

They include such factors as positive temperament; intelligence; ability to relate well to others; participation in achievements; success in school or the job; family support, closeness, and safe family environment; and extended family, friends, and teachers.[413]

The **stage of exhaustion** occurs when the *person is unable to continue to adapt to internal and external environmental demands.* Physical or psychic disease or death results, because the body can no longer compensate for or correct homeostatic imbalances (Figure 5–9). Manifestations of this stage are similar to those of the alarm stage except that all reactions first intensify and then diminish in response and show no ability to return to an effective level of function. Frequent or prolonged General Adaptation Syndrome response triggers disease through adrenocortical hypertrophy, thymolymphatic atrophy, elevated blood glucose, ulceration of the gastrointestinal tract, reduced tone and fibrosis of tissues, and vasoconstriction.[414,415]

Health care providers are concerned with promoting the resistance stage and preventing or reversing the exhaustion stage, whether through drugs, bed rest, medical treatments, crisis intervention, psychotherapy, or social action. Ideally you

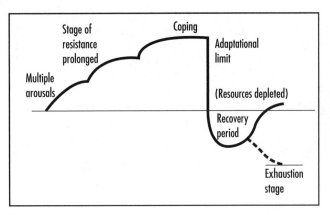

Figure 5-9

Reaction pattern in chronic stress.

Source: Adapted from Seyle, H., The Stress Concept Today, in Kutash, I.C., and Schlesinger, L.B. eds., Handbook on Stress and Anxiety. New York: Jossey-Bass, 1980, pp. 127–144.

TABLE 5-13 Positive Coping Strategies	
Affiliation:	Seek help and support from others.
Altruism:	Dedicate self to meet the needs of others.
Anticipation:	Prepare by thinking of future problems, realistic solutions, and consequences.
Assertiveness:	Express one's feelings and thoughts directly.
Humour:	Recognize the amusing aspects of a situation; maintain the ability to laugh.
Self-Observation:	Reflect on one's thoughts, feelings, motivations, and behaviour, and respond appropriately to self-evaluation.

should identify potential stressors that the person might encounter and determine how to alter the stressors or best support the person's adaptive mechanisms and resources physically, emotionally, and socially, because the person will respond as an entity to the stressors. The relationship of stress to life crises or changes must be considered whenever you are doing health promotion measures or intervening with the ill person.[416]

Although responses to stressful situations vary, anxiety is a common one. Other responses include the adaptive mechanisms described in Table 5-5 and Table 5-13.

The **mind–body relationship,** the *effect of emotional responses to stress on body function and the emotional reactions to body conditions,* has been established through research and experience. Emotional factors are important in the precipitation or exacerbation of nearly every organic disease and may increase susceptibility to infections. Stress and emotional distress, including depression, may influence function of the immune system via central nervous system and endocrine mediation.

Apparently adrenocortical steroid hormones are immunosuppressive. Recurring or chronic emotional stress has a cumulative physiologic effect and eventually may produce chronic dysfunction, such as hypertension or gastric ulcers. The dynamics involve repression of certain feelings such as rage or guilt, fooling the mind into thinking the feelings have disappeared. But the body's physiologic functions respond to the feelings or perception of the effect (stressor).[417–427] *When physical or organic symptoms appear, or disease results from feeling states, the process is called* **psychosomatic** *or* **psychophysiologic.** *The opposite process, feeling states of depression or worry in response to physical states, is called* **somatopsychic.**

MacPherson, Enns, and McWilliams, researchers from Winnipeg, investigated increased neuroticism and self-criticism in association with the presence, versus absence, of post-traumatic stress disorder (PTSD) in a nationally representative sample of adults who experienced a traumatic stressor. They concluded that self-criticism, and especially the broad personality domain of neuroticism, may represent

robust psychological dimensions associated with the presence of PTSD. Further, these psychological dimensions are likely to be as important to assess as more commonly assessed variables, such as personal and familial psychiatric history.[428]

The field of **psychoneuroimmunology** *focuses on the links between the mind, brain, and immune system.* This is a newer perspective of the mind–body relationship in psychophysiologic causation of illness. Research shows that the immune system responds to the mind.[429]

Use of positive adaptive mechanisms, such as compensation, identification, and sublimation (described in Table 5-5), and positive coping strategies (described in Table 5-13), as well as visualization, imagery, and positive thinking, all promote a health response in the immune system. All of these strategies also help to handle stressors.[430]

Crisis Theory

Definitions and Characteristics

Crisis is *any temporary situation that threatens the person's self-concept, necessitates reorganization of the psychological structure and behaviour, causes a sudden alteration in the person's expectation of self, and cannot be handled with the person's usual coping mechanisms.*[431,432]

Crises always involve change and loss. Either the changes or losses that occur result in the person's inability to cope, or as a result of the crisis, the person is no longer the same. He or she will have to change behaviour to remain adaptive and functional, and in the process, loss will be felt. Resolution of the crisis and growth mean that something is lost even while something else is gained.

During crisis, the person's ordinary behaviour is no longer successful—emotionally, intellectually, socially, or physically. The person may refer to a crisis as a "tough time" or speak of the lack of coping ability by saying, "I'm at the end of my rope. I can't manage anymore." The usual coping skills or adaptive mechanisms do not work in the situation; old habits and daily patterns are disturbed. Thus, the person feels motivated to try new behaviour to cope with the new situation. Although behaviour during crisis is inadequate or inappropriate to the present situation and may be different from normal, it should not be considered pathologic. For example, rage or bitterness or prolonged crying by a usually jovial person may be an emotional release that paves the way for problem solving.[433]

The crisis may also reactivate old, unresolved crises or conflicts, which can impose an additional burden to be handled at the present time. The crisis is a turning point; however, it operates as a second chance for resolving earlier crises or for correcting faulty problem solving. The time of crisis serves as a catalyst or opportunity for growth emotionally. Readjustment of behaviour occurs; if all goes well, a state of equilibrium or behaviour that is more mature than the previous status results. On the other hand, because of the stress involved and the felt threat to the equilibrium, the person is also more vulnerable to regression and emotional or physical illness. The outcome—either increased, the same level of, or decreased maturity, or illness—depends on how the person handles the situation and on the help others give. Encountering and resolving crisis is a normal process that each person or family faces many times during a lifetime.[434]

Not all persons facing the same hazardous event will be in a state of crisis, but *some events or situations are viewed as a crisis by all persons,* of any age, in that some behavioural adjustment must be made by anyone facing that situation. *Crises also vary in degree;* a situation may be perceived as major, moderate, or minimal in the degree of discomfort caused and in the amount of behavioural change demanded. A person may view minimal crises as stressful life situations, but the objective observer would see that the individual is ineffective in coping.

CRITICAL THINKING

What life events do you see as more stressful than others?

Crisis differs from transition. **Transition** refers to a *passage or movement from one state or place to another that occurs over time, involving changes that can be managed.*[435]

Types of Crises

Crises are divided into two categories: (1) developmental, maturational, or normative, and (2) situational, accidental, or catastrophic.[436,437] **Developmental crises** *occur during transition points, those periods that every person and family experience in the process of biopsychosocial maturation.* Examples are school entry, puberty, graduation, marriage, pregnancy, childbirth, menopause, retirement, and death. These are times in development when new relationships are formed and old relationships take on new aspects. There are new expectations of the person, and certain emotional tasks must be accomplished to move on to the next phase of development. The onset of the developmental or maturational crisis is gradual because it occurs as the person moves from one stage of development to another. The crisis resolves when the individual succeeds in new age-level behaviours; disruption does not last for the entire developmental phase.[438]

There are *three main reasons why someone may be unable to make role changes necessary to prevent a maturational crisis:*[439,440]

1. The person may be unable to picture self in a new role. Roles are learned, and adequate role models may not exist.

2. The person may be unable to make role changes because of a lack of intrapersonal resources (e.g., inadequate communication skills); the realization that, with life passing, certain goals will not be achieved; or the lack of past opportunities to learn how to cope with crises because of overprotection.

3. Others in the social system may refuse to see the person in a different role. For example, when the adolescent tries to move from childhood to the adult role, the parent may persist in keeping him or her in the child role.

Several factors help the person adjust to a new life era: (1) desire for a change and boredom with present experiences, (2) agenda for a life course—present versus future plans, (3) accomplishments in the present era, (4) past success in coping with turning points, (5) group support in meeting turning points, and (6) examples of how peers have coped with similar situations. The more clear-cut the cultural definitions, the less frightening is the future situation, because the person has models of behaviour and can prepare in advance for change.

Situational crisis *is an external event or situation, not necessarily a part of normal living, often sudden, unexpected, and unfortunate that looms larger than the person's immediate resources or ability to cope and thereby demands a change in behaviour.* Life goals are threatened; tension and anxiety are evoked; unresolved problems and crises from the past are reawakened. The amount of time taken for healthy or unhealthy adaptation to occur usually ranges from one to six weeks, although resolution may take longer. A situational crisis may occur at the same time as a developmental crisis.

Situational crises include natural disasters, such as hurricane, tornado, earthquake, and flood; loss through separation, divorce, or death of a loved one; loss of one's job, money, or valued possessions; and a job change. Additions to the family, such as an unwanted pregnancy; return of a prisoner of war, a deserter, or someone taken as a hostage; adoption of a child; and remarriage resulting in a stepparent and stepsiblings, also can cause a change in lifestyle and are potential crises. Illness, hospitalization, or institutionalization; a power struggle on the job; a sudden change in role responsibilities; and a forced geographic relocation are other examples. Rape, suicide, homicide, and imprisonment can also be classified as this type of crisis.

Crisis always involves a sense of loss. Developmental and situational events that involve loss, in reality or symbolically, are listed in Table 5-14.[441,442]

Phases of Crisis

All crises require a sudden and then a later restructuring of biopsychosocial integration before normal function can be restored. The phases involved are (1) shock, followed closely by general realization of the crisis; (2) defensive retreat; (3) acknowledgment and mourning; and, finally, (4) adaptation or resolution.[443,444]

TABLE 5-14
Loss Situations That Contribute to Crises

1. Period of weaning in infancy; learning to wait
2. First haircut, even when it involves pride and anticipation
3. Period of increasing locomotion, exploration, and bowel and bladder control and resultant loss of dependency
4. Loss of baby teeth, baby possessions, toys, clothes, or pets
5. Change in the body, body image, self-concept, and self-attribute with ongoing growth and development
6. Change in body size and shape and in feelings accompanying pregnancy and childbirth; loss of body part or function, external or internal, through accident, illness, or aging
7. Departure of children from the home when they go to school or marry
8. Menopause and loss of childbearing functions
9. Loss of hearing, vision, memory, strength, and other changes and losses associated with old age
10. Changes and losses in relationships with others as the person moves from childhood to adulthood—loss of friends and lovers; separation from or death of family members; changes in residence, occupation, or place of business; promotions and graduations
11. Losses with symbolic meanings, such as the loss of a symptom that attracted others' attention; a loss or change that necessitates a change in body image; or "loss of face," honour, prestige, or status
12. Loss of home due to natural disaster or relocation projects; loss of possessions or money
13. Loss experienced with divorce or incapacitation of a loved one

Table 5-15 presents the feelings and behaviours that may be experienced by the person during the phases of crisis. These behaviours are normal when a crisis is encountered and you must be aware of that fact in your assessment.[445,446] Grief and mourning processes are discussed further in Chapter 13.

Table 5-16 summarizes factors that influence how the person, family, or community will react to and cope with crisis and, thereby, the crisis outcome.[447–450]

The family unit undergoes essentially the same phases of crisis and manifests similar reactions as the designated client, although the intensity and timing may be different for each person. Furthermore, members of the family in crisis interact with each other, compounding the crisis reaction and creating more intense or complex behavioural responses. Roles are disorganized; expectations of self, other family members, and outsiders change; and individual needs intensify. All families have problems, and all families have ways of managing them, successfully or otherwise.

Crisis events for the family include the developmental and situational crises previously discussed, which can also be categorized as follows:[451,452]

- ■ **Dismemberment.** Medical emergencies; loss of family member through death, divorce, separation, marriage, or geographic move.
- ■ **Accession.** *Addition of family member through birth, adoption, marriage, or foster placement, or older relative moving into the home.*
- ■ **Demoralization.** *Loss of morale in the family unit* through delinquency, legal problems, economic problems, job loss, child or spouse abuse, certain illnesses such as AIDS, crimes, or events that cause alienation from the community or carry a social stigma.
- ■ **A combination of the above.**

Various factors influence how prone a group or community is to crisis:[453,454]

1. Personal strengths, characteristics, and level of need satisfaction of its members
2. Social and economic stability of family units or groups versus social and economic inequities among ethnic, racial, or socioeconomic groups
3. Adherence to versus rebellion against social norms by families and groups
4. Adequacy of community resources to meet social, economic, health, welfare, and recreational needs of individuals and families
5. Geographic, environmental, and climatic resources and characteristics that surround the group or community

The community is also affected by natural disasters, such as floods, tornadoes, hurricanes, earthquakes, volcanic eruptions, and blizzards; by disasters resulting from advances in our civilization, such as chemical or radiation spills and electrical blackouts; and by disasters for which humans are responsible, such as snipings in a schoolyard or restaurant, fire, and war. Reactions of a community to any of these disasters will be influenced by the factors listed in Table 5-17.[455–458]

A group in crisis demonstrates:

- ■ Acute unmanageable anxiety that interferes with daily function
- ■ Sudden alteration in perceptions of meaning, purpose, and goals—a turning point
- ■ Sudden disruption in cognitive, emotional, or physical alterations

Communities in crisis have characteristics in common with individuals and groups in crisis. The most immediate social consequence of a disaster is disruption of normal social patterns and services; the community is socially paralyzed. Furthermore, one disaster such as a chemical spill may contribute to another disaster, such as an explosion or fire.

In a major disaster, about 75% to 90% of the victims will be in shock; this is followed by the phase of defensive retreat, in response to warnings of disaster, orders of evacuation, destruction of homes, and disruption of water, electricity, heat, food supplies, communication, traffic, and transportation. Furthermore, there is potential inability of the health agencies to care for the injured and ill because of manpower and supply shortages or damage. In addition to individual

TABLE 5–15
Individual Reactions in the Crisis Phases

Phase and Duration	Feelings	Cognitive Manifestations	Physical Symptoms	Interpersonal/Social Behaviour
Initial Impact; Shock (duration of 1 to 24–48 hours)	Anxiety. Helplessness. Chaos. Overwhelmed. Hopeless. Incomplete. Detached. Despair. Depersonalized. Panic. Self-concept threatened. Self-esteem low. Anguish may be expressed by silent, audible, or uncontrollable crying *Developmental Crisis* Response more gradual. Feelings less intense. May feel anxiety, frustration, lack of confidence, discouragement, imperfection, unfamiliarity with self, loss of self-control as realizes new responsibilities. Cannot move emotionally into next stage or change life perception.	Altered sensorium. Disorganized thinking. Unable to plan, reason logically, or understand situation. Impaired judgment. Preoccupation with image or hallucination of last object/person	Somatic distress. May suffer physical illness or injury and ignore symptoms. Shortness of breath. Choking. Sighing. Hyperventilation. Weakness. Fatigue. Tremors. Anorexia. Lump in throat or abdomen. Respiratory or other infection may develop	Disorganized behaviour. Habitual or automatic behaviours used unsuccessfully. Withdrawn. Docile. Hyperactive. May appear overtly as if nothing happened or may be unable to carry out routine behaviour. Lacks initiative for daily tasks. May need assistance meeting basic needs. Very suggestible, even if contrary to values or well-being *Developmental Crisis* May try to do more than is biologically or emotionally realistic. Unable to achieve behaviour appropriate to role or to change inappropriate behaviour in relationships
Denies Retreat (duration of hours to weeks)	May feel tense and inadequate, but usually feels as if nothing is wrong because of use of repression and defence mechanisms. Apathetic or euphoric. Feelings displaced onto other objects	Tries habitual coping mechanisms unsuccessfully. States nothing is wrong. May try to redefine problem unrealistically. Fantasizes about what could be done, how well past problems handled. Avoids thinking about event. May be disoriented. Maintains rigid thinking. States same ideas over and over. May be unable to devise alternate courses of action or predict effects of behaviour. Denies through rationalization cause for situation	Denies symptoms including presence of physical illness	Tries habitual behaviours and defence mechanisms unsuccessfully. May seek support of others indirectly. Usually withdraws from others. Superficial response. May avoid reality with overactivity. Resistant to change suggested by others. Unwilling to initiate new behaviour. Ineffective, disorganized behaviour. May be unable to maintain daily activities, work performance, or social roles. Denies through demands, complaints, or projections of inadequacy

(continued)

235

TABLE 5-15 *(continued)*
Individual Reactions in the Crisis Phases

Phase and Duration	Feelings	Cognitive Manifestations	Physical Symptoms	Interpersonal/Social Behaviour
		Developmental Crisis Denies that physical, emotional, or role changes are occurring or that different behaviour is expected; behaviour reflects earlier developmental stage; developmental tasks not worked out or met		
Acknowledgment of Reality (duration varies)	Tension and anxiety rise. Loneliness. Irritable. Depressed. Agitated. Apathetic. Self-hate. Low self-esteem. Grief–mourning occurs. Gradually self-satisfaction increased. Self-concept becomes more positive. Gains self-confidence in ability to cope	Becomes aware of facts about change, loss, event. Asks questions about situation. Slowly redefines situation. Attempts problem solving. May be disorganized in thinking. Trial-and-error approach to problems. Gradually perceives alternatives. Makes appropriate plans. Gives up undesirable goals. Validates personal experiences and feelings. Coping skills improved	Symptoms may reappear or intensify. New symptoms may occur. May somatize feelings. Gradually regains physical health	Exhibits mourning behaviours. Gradually demonstrates appropriate behaviours and resumes roles. Uses suggestions. Tries new approaches. Greater maturity demonstrated
Resolution Adaptation, Change (duration of mourning and crisis work may be 6–12 months)	Painful feelings integrated into self-concept and sense of maturity. New sense of worth. Firm identity. Gradual increase in self-satisfaction about mastery of situation. Gradual lowering of anxiety. Does not feel bitter, guilty, or ashamed	Perceives crisis situation in positive way. Integrates crisis event into self. Problem solving successful. Discusses feelings about event. Organizes thinking and planning. Redefines priorities. Does not blame self or others. Remembers comfortably and realistically pleasures and disappointments of last relationship.	Functions at optimum level	Discovers new resources. Uses support systems and resources appropriately. Resumes status and roles. Strengthens relations with others. Adaptive in relationships. Lifestyle may be changed. Initiates measures to prevent similar crisis if at all possible

Note: Temporary retreat emotionally, mentally, and socially is adaptive and protective from perceived stress and loss and overwhelming anxiety. Allows time to gradually realize what has happened. Avoids debilitating effects of high anxiety or panic. Initially person fluctuates between the phases of Defensive Retreat and Acknowledgment of Reality.

Table 5-16
Factors Influencing the Outcome of Crisis

1. **Perception of the event.** If the event (or the implications or consequences of it) threatens the self-concept; conflicts with the value system, self-expectations, or wishes for the future; contributes to a sense of shame or guilt; or is demoralizing or damaging to self, family, or personal objects, the situation is defined as hazardous. The perception of the event is reality for the person or family, regardless of how others might define reality. How the event is perceived depends in large measure on past experience.
2. **Degree of perceived dependency on a lost object.** This is also crucial; the greater the dependency, the more difficult the resolution of loss.
3. **Physical and emotional status.** This includes level of health, amount of energy present, age, genetic endowment, and biological rhythms of the person or family, or the general well-being of the community. Working through crisis takes considerable energy.
4. **Coping techniques or mechanisms and level of personal maturity.** If adaptive capacities are already strained, or if the stress is overwhelming, the person will cling to old habits or existing defences, and behaviour will very likely be inappropriate to the task at hand. The person or family who has met developmental tasks all along and who perceives self as able to cope will adapt more easily in any crisis. The group or community that has mechanisms, policies, or procedures defined and in operation to cope with the unexpected event or disaster can better meet the crisis.
5. **Previous experiences with similar situations.** The person, family, or group needs to learn to cope with stress, change, and loss. If past crises were handled by distorting reality or by withdrawing, when similar crises arise, burdens of the prior failure will be added to the problem of coping with the new situation. Unresolved crises are cumulative in effect. The most recent crisis revives the denial, depression, anger, or maladaptation that was left unsettled from past crises. If the person, family, or group successfully deals with crises, self-confidence and self-esteem will thereby be increased, and future crises will be handled more effectively.
6. **Realistic aspects of the current situation.** These include personal, material, or economic losses, the extent to which group ties or community services are interrupted, and changes in living pattern or family life necessitated by the loss.
7. **Cultural influences.** How the person is trained and socialized in the home to solve problems and meet crisis situations; the use of religious, cultural, or legal ceremonies or rituals to handle separation or loss and facilitate mourning; expectations of how the social group will support the person or family during crisis; and the method established by the community to provide help—all influence present behaviour.
8. **Availability and response of family and close friends, community groups, or other helping resources, including professional persons.** The less available the environmental or emotional support systems are to decrease stress or buttress the coping response, the more hazardous the event will be. The family system, by its influence on development of self-concept and maturity, can increase or decrease the person's vulnerability to crisis.

Table 5-17
Factors That Influence Community Response to Disasters

1. **Element of surprise versus preparedness.** If warnings are not given about an impending crisis—or if warnings are given without an action plan—panic, shock, denial, and defensive retreat are more likely to occur.
2. **Separation of family members.** Children are especially affected by separation; the family should be evacuated from a disaster area as a unit.
3. **Availability of outside help,** such as the sending of food, shelter, and workers.
4. **Leadership.** Someone must make decisions and give directions. Usually the police, Red Cross and Civil Defence workers, military, or professionals in a community are seen as authoritative persons. Coordination of the activities of all of those groups is essential to deliver services and avoid chaos.
5. **Communication.** Public information centres have to be established to avoid rumour, provide reassurance and direction, and ensure that all citizens get information about coping measures, evacuation, reconstruction, rehabilitation, and available financial aid. Otherwise citizens will later be bitter and suspicious when some learn that others benefited more than they did.
6. **Measures taken to help reorientation.** Communication networks lay the foundation for re-identification of individuals into family and social groups and for registration of survivors.
7. **Presence of plans for individuals and social institutions to cope with disaster,** including evacuation of a population from a stricken area if necessary. Emergency plans focus on the following concerns:
   a. Preservation of life and health through rescue, triage, inoculation, and treatment of the injured
   b. Conservation and distribution of resources, such as shelter, water, food, and blankets
   c. Conservation of public order by police surveillance to prevent looting and further accidents or injuries
   d. Maintenance of morale through dispatching of health and welfare workers to the disaster scene
   e. Administration of health services

reactions, an atmosphere of tension, fear, confusion, and suspicion exists; facts are distorted and rumours are rampant. Normal functioning is reduced because businesses, vital services, schools, and recreational areas may be closed. Yet, one may see all available community service providers, such as police officers, firefighters, construction workers, city planners, Red Cross volunteers, medical personnel, and corporation executives, cooperating to assist in rescue, cleanup, and restoration of services and a sense of normality. Although some people are in shock or denial, a proportionate few will display altruism and heroic behaviour. There will be a few who take advantage of the chaos to loot and steal, and a few businesses may profiteer.

Response to external emergencies is often quicker than the response to internal stresses or crises. About 10% to 25% of the victims remain reality-oriented, calm, and able to develop and implement a plan of action. These people often are those with advanced training; however, these people may experience the crisis phases later.

HEALTH CARE AND NURSING APPLICATIONS

Table 5-18 summarizes how the theories discussed in this chapter can be applied in nursing and health care practice.

Table 5-18 Health Promotion Implications of Selected Theories	
Theorist/Theory	Practice Implications
General Systems Theory	1. Consider self as an individual system as well as part of other systems.
	2. Consider client (individual, family, group, or community) as part of a system in implementing nursing process.
	3. Consider client in totality and the relationships and interactions between parts: physiologic, psychological, spiritual, and sociocultural. Dysfunction in one part affects all parts.
	4. Client, as a system, has definite range for absorption, processing, and retention of stimuli. Avoid overstimulation or deprivation of stimuli. Assess needs and intervene accordingly.
	5. Help client determine resources and supportive systems that will maintain or return function and wellness.
Skinner's Operant Conditioning Theory	1. In teaching or therapy, follow the guidelines previously described for a behaviour modification program.
	2. The general procedure for behaviour modification is to:
	a. Plan what behaviour is to be established; plan what is to be taught and at what specific time. Objectives are specific. Follow the teaching or treatment plan explicitly.
	b. Determine available reinforcers. Feedback from physical sensations, excelling over others, or the teacher's affection—all may reinforce. The only way to determine whether a consequence is rewarding is to observe its effect on the behaviour associated with it.
	c. Identify the responses that can be made by the person.
	d. Plan how reinforcements can be efficiently scheduled so the behaviour will be repeated. Reinforcements must immediately follow the desired behaviour.
Freud's Psychoanalytic Theory	1. Insight into own behaviour can add to personal maturity and understanding of others.
	2. Constructs of id, ego, superego, conscious–unconscious continuum, manifestations of anxiety and defence mechanisms, and psychosexual development are useful in assessment and therapy.
	3. All behaviour is meaningful; outer behaviour may hide inner need or conflict.
	4. Use knowledge of psychosexual development to teach parents about norms and meaning of child's behaviour.
	5. Transference and resistance must be worked through in therapy.
Sullivan's Interpersonal Theory	1. One Genus Postulate basic to nursing practice with clients from all settings and backgrounds.
	2. Assess developmental stage and task; teach family about normal development and development of self-system.
	3. Promote syntaxic rather than parataxic mode of experiencing through intervention.
	4. Promote positive experiences for client so that "good-me" or positive self-concept can develop.

(continued)

Table 5-18 *(continued)*
Health Promotion Implications of Selected Theories

Theorist/Theory	Practice Implications
Erikson's Epigenetic Theory	1. Assessment of and insight into own stage of development. 2. Use knowledge of eight stages and psychosexual tasks in assessment, therapy, and teaching parents about child development. 3. Help clients and staff realize that emotional development is lifelong process and that society influences health and behaviour.
Jung's Theory	1. Assessment of personality tendencies. 2. Promote self-acceptance, including masculine and feminine characteristics. 3. Assist person in finding unique self, balance spirituality. 4. Promote reflection, finding meaning of life.

Beck's Cognitive Theory	1. Facilitate person's recognition of how thoughts influence emotions through questions, examples, examination of person's self-conversation.
	2. Facilitate person's recognition of irrational beliefs by having person tell what would happen if belief actually was true; enumerate reasons for problems created by the belief.
	3. Facilitate person's recognition that rational beliefs influence emotional or physical distress by systematically exploring situations related to feelings of inadequacy, helplessness, aloneness, depression, or anger. Sort out facts in a supportive way.
	4. Facilitate person's efforts to revise and contradict irrational beliefs through alternative self-messages, homework assignments, role-play, rehearsal, and invalidation of distorted belief.
	5. Restructuring experience with person helps him or her recognize and revise unrealistic expectations and negative self-conversations, reduce sensitivity to other's response, and interact more flexibly and effectively.
	6. Therapy lasts about six months and is divided into stages:
	  a. Eliciting and answering automatic thoughts
	  b. Discovering and testing underlying assumptions
	  c. Cognitive restructuring
	7. Basis for improvement is in change of basic philosophy of the person, not necessarily in removal of present symptoms.
	8. Therapist is active in confronting person; person is expected to do homework assignments.
	9. Therapist is to act as role model for person; as an authoritative, scientific helper who is highly trained and rational, and to show unconditional positive regard for the person.

Ellis's Rational Emotive Therapy	1. Facilitate person's recognition of how thoughts influence emotions and how the person can control own behaviour. 2. Facilitate person's recognition of basic values and assumptions that govern life. 3. Facilitate person's recognition of irrational thoughts and negative self-talk, and how these contribute to emotional pain. 4. Facilitate person's ability to identify the five criteria for rational thinking. 5. Facilitate person's efforts to revise and contradict irrational beliefs and perceptions of events. 6. Teach relaxation techniques, control of thoughts, assertive communication, self-instruction, internal self-talk, and problem-solving methods to strengthen realistic perceptions, rational thoughts, and personal autonomy. 7. Teach person to hold a positive image and act on that image until the person feels more positive. 8. Therapy is weekly and short term, but may last two years, and focuses on specific current problem.
Glasser's Reality Therapy	1. Assess current needs, problems, and unrealistic behaviour. 2. Assess strengths and capacity for change.

(continued)

Table 5-18 *(continued)*
Health Promotion Implications of Selected Theories

Theorist/Theory	Practice Implications
	3. Explore discrepancy between needs and wants of client.
	4. Develop specific plan for client to meet needs.
	5. Elicit commitment from client to follow plan.
	6. Determine if plan works.
	7. Revise plan if unable to achieve prior plan; avoid negative reaction or blame.
	8. Continue encouragement and plan revision until behaviour changes, needs are met, and person acts realistically and responsibly.
Bandura's Social Learning Theory	1. Your appearance and behaviour are a model for client.
	2. Determine who significant adults were in the person's life and who role models were.
	3. In teaching, demonstrate desired self-care behaviour.
	4. Recovered person visiting an ill client can serve as model for rehabilitation and a normal life (e.g., person with mastectomy, colostomy, amputation, alcoholism).
	5. Demonstrate nurturing approaches or discipline methods to child client so that parents can learn effective childrearing methods.
	6. Nurse–client relationship is a behavioural model of trust and interpersonal relations for the client.
Piaget's Theory of Cognitive Development	1. Teach parents about process of child's cognitive development and the implications for education, purchase of toys, and interactions.
	2. Assess cognitive stage of client as basis for planning content and presentation in teaching sessions.
	3. Assess cognitive development to determine language and abstraction level to use in therapy.
	4. Use knowledge of cognitive development in play therapy.
Kohlberg's Theory of Moral Development/Gilligan's Theory of Moral Development	1. Assess own level of moral development.
	2. Assess client's level of moral development when working with children, adolescents, or adults.
	3. Through your modelling, clarification, explanation, and validation, contribute to client's moral development.
Existential Theory	1. Each person is in charge of own destiny; each person is primary agent of change and is responsible for own future. Destiny is not in hands of others.
	2. In therapy, be concerned with basic conflicts that are outgrowths of confrontation with existence—death, freedom, helplessness, loss, isolation, aloneness, anxiety, and meaninglessness—and promote reflection about these life issues.
	3. Nurse is facilitator who understands and accepts the person as being and becoming. Main themes of therapy are self-awareness, self-determination, search for meaning, and relatedness.
	4. In therapy, assist person in learning how to confront self, how behaviour is viewed by others, how others feel about own behaviour, and how behaviour contributes to opinions about self.
	5. In therapy, assist person to learn how to change; give support to reduce anxiety, low self-esteem, and loneliness.
	6. Help person move to self-actualization and achieve maximum potential.
Maslow's Theory of Motivation and Hierarchy of Needs	1. Assessment can be done around hierarchy of needs. Planning and intervention must consider need hierarchy and priorities in care.
	2. Person is a unified whole, not divided into components of needs.
	3. Higher-level needs can be met simultaneously with some lower-level needs.
	4. Concepts of needs and motivation can be used in teaching and therapy. By meeting needs of client on one level, you can help client mature and feel motivated to meet growth needs.

(continued)

Table 5-18 *(continued)*
Health Promotion Implications of Selected Theories

Theorist/Theory	Practice Implications
Carl Rogers's Theory on Self-Concept and Client-Centred Therapy	1. Assess own self-concept and self-actualization needs prior to counselling clients. 2. Assess client's self-concept; promote positive experiences and contribute to development of positive self-concept. 3. In therapy, assume as much as possible client's frame of reference to perceive world as she or he does. 4. Be accepting, warm, genuine, and empathic to help client discover self and mature.
Stress and Adaptation Theory	1. Assess physical, emotional, and cognitive manifestations of stress response. 2. Assess level of anxiety. 3. Determine stage of adaptation. 4. Teach stress management methods. 5. Counsel as necessary. 6. Intervene as necessary to prevent exhaustion stage.
Crisis Theory/Crisis Intervention (Brief Therapy)	1. Assess anxiety level, feelings, and perceptions of client. 2. Assess presence of emotional and physical symptoms. 3. Determine whether person is suicidal or homicidal. 4. Explore support system and usual coping patterns. 5. Clarify crisis event, its onset and impact. 6. Provide comfort measures for client. 7. Help client work through feelings about situation. 8. Develop plan with client to resolve crisis; develop alternative options to achieve goal. 9. Reinforce strengths and healthy adaptive patterns. 10. Involve client in decisions and working on specific tasks. 11. Help person establish necessary social relationships; assist person in seeking and accepting help. 12. Refer as necessary for additional services.

INTERESTING WEBSITES

HUNTINGTON SOCIETY OF CANADA

http://www.hsc-ca.org

On this site you will find information about Huntington disease, the many ways the Huntington Society works to support the needs of people with the disease, and opportunities to support the organization's work.

THE HOSPITAL FOR SICK CHILDREN

http://www.sickkids.on.ca

Affectionately called "Sick Kids," this is one of the largest pediatric academic health science centres in the world, with an international reputation for excellence in health care, research, and teaching.

GENOME CANADA

http://www.genomecanada.ca

This is the primary funding and information resource relating to genetics and proteomics in Canada. To date, Genome

Canada has invested more than $379 million across Canada. It has established five genome centres across the country and has a main objective to ensure that Canada becomes a world leader in genomics and proteomics research.

SUMMARY

1. Various theories describe aspects of the developing person; no theory describes all dimensions (physiologic, emotional, cognitive, cultural, social, moral, spiritual) of development.

2. Biological theories include study of genetics, biochemistry, neurophysiology, immunology, maturational factors, biological rhythms, and biological deficiencies.

3. Ecologic theories include study of sociologic variables, culture, geographic environments, and systems such as the family, school, community, and organization.

4. Behavioural theories study behaviour that is learned or modified through various kinds of conditioning and shows a measurable outcome.

5. Psychoanalytic and neo-analytic theories include study of the intrapsychic processes, emotional life stage, and interpersonal development of the person; and the effect

of these dimensions on behaviour of the person, family unit, or the broader society.

6. Cognitive theories include study of the stages of the person's cognitive development, the person as an information processor and problem solver, and effects of modelling or imitation on behaviour.

7. Moral theories study how the person learns to incorporate societal and philosophical norms into behaviour and the relationship of moral to cognitive and emotional behaviour.

8. Existential and humanistic theories study the needs, self-concept, and dynamic aspects of the person's existence and development within the self and in relation to the environment or society.

9. Stress and crisis theories study the person's responses to routine, severe, and overwhelming events; the local and general adaptation syndromes and phases of response to various types of crisis explain the reactions of the person to unexpected, situational, or developmental events.

10. The theories presented in this chapter form the basis for various approaches for therapy, nursing, and health care.

ENDNOTES

1. Nutbeam, D., and E. Harris, *Theory in a Nutshell* (2nd ed.). Toronto: McGraw-Hill, 2004.

2. Sperry, R., Forebrain Commissurotomy and Conscious Awareness, in Travarthen, C., ed., *Brain Circuits and Functions of the Mind.* New York: Cambridge University Press, 1990, pp. 371–388.

3. Kandel, E., J. Schwartz, and T. Jessell, eds., *Principles of Neural Science* (3rd ed.). New York: Elsevier, 1991.

4. Kendler, K., E. Walters, K. Truett, et al., Sources of Individual Differences in Depressive Symptoms: Analysis of Two Samples of Twins and Their Families. *American Journal of Psychiatry,* 51 (1994), 1605–1614.

5. Panksepp, J., The Neurochemistry of Behavior, *Annual Review of Psychology,* 37 (1986), 77–107.

6. Papalia, D., S. Olds, and R. Feldman, *Human Development* (7th ed.). Boston: McGraw-Hill, 1998.

7. Lashley, F., Thinking About Genetics in New Ways, *IMAGE: Journal of Nursing Scholarship,* 29, no. 2 (1997), 202.

8. Medina, J., Genetic Study of Human Behavior. Its Progress and Limitations, *Harvard Mental Health Letter,* 12, no. 10 (1996), 4–6.

9. Papalia et al., *op. cit.*

10. Rogers, J., Yellow Skies, Blue Trees? *Newsweek,* November 30, 1998, 14.

11. Medina, *op. cit.*

12. Kendler et al., *op. cit.*

13. Talon, J., Brain Study Finds Depression Clue; A Severe Depletion of Key Support Cells, *NAMI Advocate,* January–February, 1998, 20.

14. Kendler, K., et al., Stressful Life Events, Genetic Liability, and Onset of an Episode of Major Depression in Women, *American Journal of Psychiatry,* 152 (1995), 833–842.

15. Papalia et al., *op. cit.*

16. Jang, K.L., P.A. Vernon, W.J. Livesley, M.B. Stein, and H. Wolf, Intra- and Extra-Familial Influences on Alcohol and Drug Misuse: A Twin Study of Gene-Environment Correlation. *Addiction,* 96 (2001) 1307–1318.

17. Katzmarzyk, P.T., R.M. Malina, L. Perusse, T. Rice, M.A. Province, D.C. Rao, and C. Bouchard, Familial Resemblance in Fatness and Fat Distribution. *American Journal of Human Biology,* 12, no. 3 (2000), 395–404.

18. Simonen, R.L., L. Perusse, T. Rankinen, T. Rice, D.C. Rao, and C. Bouchard, Familial Aggregation of Physical Activity Levels in the Quebec Family Study. *Medicine and Science in Sports and Exercise,* 34 (2002), 1137–1142.

19. Medina, *op. cit.*

20. Papalia et al., *op. cit.*

21. Is DNA Destiny? Genetic Discoveries Raise Women's Expectations—and Tougher Questions, *Women's Health Advocate Newsletter,* 2, no. 9 (1995), 1, 7–8.

22. Medina, *op. cit.*

23. Bee, H., *Lifespan Development* (2nd ed.). New York: Longman, 1998.

24. O'Connor, C., Are We More Then the Sum of Our Genes?, *Washington University Outlook,* Fall, 1997, 10–15.

25. Papalia et al., *op. cit.*

26. Hegele, R.A, Environmental Modulation of Atherosclerosis End Points in Familial Hypercholesterolemia. *Atherosclerosis Supplements,* 2, no. 3 (2002), 5–7.

27. *Ibid.*

28. Health Canada, *The Healthy Heart Kit, Controlling your Blood Cholesterol,* 2002, Website: www.healthyheartkit.com, April 2004.

29. *Ibid.*

30. Hegle, R.A., H. Cao, A.J.G. Hanley, B. Zinman, S.B. Harris, and C.M. Anderson, Clinical Utility of HNF1A Genotyping for Diabetes in Aboriginal Canadians. *Diabetes Care,* 23, no. 6 (2002) 775–778.

31. *Ibid.*

32. Young, T.K., J. Reading, B. Elias, and J.D. O'Neil, Type 2 Diabetes Mellitus in Canada's First Nations: Status of an Epidemic in Progress, *Canadian Medical Association Journal,* 163, no. 5 (2000), 561–566.

33. Hegele, *op. cit.*

34. Pranke, P., Fetal Development, in M.A Hogan and R.S. Glazebrook, eds., *Maternal-Newborn Nursing* (pp. 77–80). Upper Saddle River, NJ: Prentice-Hall, 2003.

35. Shah, C.P. *Public Health and Preventative Medicine in Canada* (5th ed.). Toronto: Elsevier Canada, 2003.

36. Ontario Report to Premiers, *Genetics and Gene Patenting: Charting New Territory in Healthcare,* Website: www.health.gov.on.ca/english/public/pub/ministry_reports/geneticsrep02/genetics.html, April 2004.

37. Shah, *op. cit.*

38. *Ibid.*

39. Guttman, M., S.J. Kish, and Y. Furukawa, Current concepts In The Diagnosis and Management of Parkinson's Disease. *Canadian Medical Association Journal,* 168, no. 3 (2003), 293–301.

40. Genome Canada, *About Genome Canada,* Website: http://www.genomecanada.ca, April 2004.

41. *Ibid.*

42. Genome Canada, *Media,* Website: http://www.genomecanada.ca, April 2004.

43. Ontario Genomics Institute, *OGI Backgrounder,* Website: http://www.ontariogenomicsinstitute.ca, April 2004.

44. Ontario Genomics Institute Annual Report 2002/2003, Competition II. Mapping and Isolation of Genes Influencing Severity of Disease in Cystic Fibrosis. 21.

45. Hockenberry, M.J., D. Wilson, M.L. Winkelstein, and N.E. Kline, *Wong's Nursing Care of Infants and Children,* Seventh Edition. St Louis: Mosby, 2003.

46. Wilson, R.D., G. Davies, V. Desilets, G.J. Reid, D. Shaw, A. Summers, P. Wyatt et al., Cystic Fibrosis Carrier Testing in Pregnancy in Canada. *Journal of Obstetrics and Gynaecology Canada,* 24, no. 8 (2002), 644–651.

47. Bee, *op. cit.*

48. Coccaro, E., The Biology of Aggression, *Scientific American: Science & Medicine,* 2, no. 1 (1995), 38–47.

49. Is DNA Destiny?
50. Canadian Nurses Association, *Position Statement, The Role of the Nurse in Reproductive and Genetic Technologies*, Website: http://www.cna-nurses.ca, May 2004.
51. Cox, S.M., Human Genetics, Ethics, and Disability, in J.L. Storch, P. Rodney, and R. Starzomski, eds., *Toward a Moral Horizon: Nursing Ethics for Leadership and Practice* (pp. 378–379). Toronto: Pearson Education Canada, 2004.
52. Is DNA Destiny?
53. O'Rourke, K., Genetic Testing: Ethical Issues, *Ethical Issues in Health Issues in Health Care,* 16, no. 9 (1995), 1–2.
54. Survey Assesses RN Management of Genetic Information, *The American Nurse,* January–February (1995), 27.
55. Murray, R.B., and M. Huelekoetter, *Psychiatric/Mental Health Nursing: Giving Emotional Care* (3rd ed.). Norwalk, CT: Appleton-Lange, 1991.
56. O'Connor, *op. cit.*
57. De Longis, A., S. Folkman, and R. Lazarus, The Impact of Daily Stress on Health & Mood: Psychological and Social Resources as Mediators, *Journal of Personality and Social Psychology,* 54 (1988), 486–495.
58. O'Connor, *op. cit.*
59. Papalia et al., *op. cit.*
60. *Ibid.*
61. Bronfenbrenner, U., Ecological Systems Theory, in R. Vast, ed., *Annals of Child Development; Vol. 6. Six Theories of Child Development: Revised Formulations and Current Issues.* Greenwich, CT: JAI Press, 1989.
62. Papalia et al., *op. cit.*
63. Liu, S., R. Semenciw, A-M Ugnat, and Y. Mao, Increasing Thyroid Cancer Incidence in Canada, 1970–1996: Time Trends and Age-Period-Cohort Effects. *British Journal of Cancer,* 85, no. 9 (2001), 1335–1339.
64. Papalia et al., *op. cit.*
65. *Ibid.*
66. *Ibid.*
67. Giancola, P., and A. Zeichner, Neuropsychological Performance on Tests of Frontal Lobe Functioning and Aggressive Behavior in Men, *Journal of Abnormal Psychology,* 103 (1994), 832–835.
68. Horker, F., Mapping the Brain, *Washington University School of Medicine Outlook,* 29, no. 1 (1992), 10–14.
69. Kandel et al., *op. cit.*
70. Kelly, J., and J. Dodd, Anatomical Organization of the Nervous System, in Kandel, E., Schwartz J., and Jessell, T. eds., *Principles of Neural Science.* New York: Elsevier, 1991, pp. 273–282.
71. Kupferman, I., Hypothalamus and Limbic Systems: Motivation, in Kandel, E., J. Schwartz, and Jessell, T. eds., *Principles of Neural Science* (3rd ed.). New York: Elsevier, 1991, pp. 750–760.
72. Kelly and Dodd, *op. cit.*
73. Giancola and Zeichner, *op. cit.*
74. Horker, op. cit.
75. Furth, H.G., and H. Wachs, *Thinking Goes to School: Piaget's Theory in Practice.* New York: Oxford University Press, 1975.
76. Kupferman, *op. cit.*
77. Talon, *op. cit.*
78. Young Johnson, J. *Handbook for Brunner and Suddarth's Textbook of Medical Surgical Nursing* (10th ed.). Philadelphia: Lippencott Williams & Wilkins, 2004.
79. Peschken, C.A., and J.M. Esdaile, Systematic Lupus Erythematosus in North American Indians: A Population Based Study. *Journal of Rheumatology,* 27, no. 8 (2000), 1884–1891.
80. Hockenberry et al., *op. cit.*
81. Health Canada, *Canada's Report on HIV/AIDS,* Website: www.hc-sc.gc.ca/hppb/hiv_aids/report03/, May 2004.
82. Seifert, K., R. Hoffnung, and M. Hoffnung, *Lifespan Development.* Boston: Houghton Mifflin, 1997.
83. Murray and Huelekoetter, *op. cit.*
84. Papalia et al., *op. cit.*
85. *Ibid.*
86. Beck, A.T., and M.E. Weisharr, *Suicide Risk Assessment and Prediction.* Philadelphia: Hogrefe & Huber, 1990.
87. Seifert et al., *op. cit.*
88. Zhang, J., and M.J. Verhoef, Illness Management Strategies Among Chinese Immigrants Living with Arthritis, *Social Science & Medicine,* 55, no. 10 (2002), 1795–1802.
89. Papalia et al., *op. cit.*
90. DeWit, D. J., Frequent Childhood Geographical Relocation: Its Impact on Drug Use Initiation and the Development of Alcohol and Other Drug-Related Problems Among Adolescents and Young Adults, *Addictive Behaviors,* 23, no. 5 (1998), 623–634.
91. *Ibid.*
92. Papalia et al., *op. cit.*
93. Von Bertalanffy, L., *General System Theory.* New York: George Braziller, 1968.
94. Anderson, R., and I. Carter, *Human Behavior in the Social Environment.* Chicago: Aldine, 1974.
95. Berrien, K., *General and Social Systems.* New Brunswick, NJ: Rutgers University Press, 1968.
96. Smoyak, S., Changing American Families, in Hoekelman, R., S. Friedman, N. Nelson, and H. Seidel, eds., *Primary Pediatric Care* (2nd ed.). St. Louis: Mosby, 1992.
97. Anderson and Carter, *op. cit.*
98. Berrien, *op. cit.*
99. Loomis, C.P., *Social Systems.* New York: D. Van Nostrand, 1960.
100. Smoyak, *op. cit.*
101. Von Bertalanffy, L., The History and Status of General Systems Theory, in G. Klir (ed.), *Trends in General Systems Theory.* New York: Wiley, 1972.
102. Von Bertalanffy, L., *General System Theory.*
103. Papalia et al., *op. cit.*
104. Anderson and Carter, *op. cit.*
105. Berrien, *op. cit.*
106. Loomis, *op. cit.*
107. Von Bertalanffy, The History and Status of General Systems Theory.
108. Von Bertalanffy, L., *General System Theory.*
109. Berrien, *op. cit.*
110. Anderson and Carter, *op. cit.*
111. Loomis, *op. cit.*
112. Anderson and Carter, *op. cit.*
113. Lilly, L., and R. Guanci, Applying Systems Theory, *American Journal of Nursing,* 95, no. 11 (1995), 14–15.
114. Wright, L.M., and M. Leahey, *Nurses and Families: A Guide to Family Assessment and Intervention* (3rd ed.). Philadelphia: F.A. Davis Company, 2000.
115. Anderson and Carter, *op. cit.*
116. Best, A., D. Stokols, L.W. Green, S. Leischow, B. Holmes, and K. Bucholz, An Integrative Framework for Community Partnering to Translate Theory into Effective Health Promotion Strategy. *The Science of Health Promotion,* 18, no. 2 (2003), 168–176.
117. Lilly and Guanci, *op. cit.*
118. McFarlane, A., A Nursing Reformulation of Bowen's Family Systems Theory, *Archives of Psychiatric Nursing,* 2 (1988), 319–324.
119. Smoyak, *op. cit.*
120. Wright and Leahey, *op. cit.*
121. Bronfenbrenner, *op. cit.*
122. Murray and Huelekoetter, *op. cit.*
123. Patterson, C. and C. Watkins, *Theories of Psychotherapy* (5th ed.). New York: HarperCollins, 1996.
124. O'Rourke, *op. cit.*
125. Patterson and Watkins, *op. cit.*

126. *Ibid.*

127. *Ibid.*

128. *Ibid.*

129. Murray and Huelekoetter, *op. cit.*

130. Patterson and Watkins, *op. cit.*

131. Murray and Huelekoetter, *op. cit.*

132. Patterson and Watkins, *op. cit.*

133. Skinner, B.F., *Walden Two.* New York: Macmillan, 1948.

134. Skinner, B.F., *Cumulative Record* (3rd ed.). New York: Appleton-Century-Crofts, 1972.

135. Murray and Huelekoetter, *op. cit.*

136. Skinner, B.F., *The Behavior of Organisms.* New York: Appleton-Century-Crofts, 1938.

137. Skinner, *Walden Two.*

138. Skinner, B.F., *Science and Human Behavior.* New York: Macmillan, 1953.

139. Skinner, B.F., Behaviorism at Fifty. *Science,* 140 (1963), 951–958.

140. Skinner, B.F., *Contingencies of Reinforcement: A Theoretical Analysis.* New York: Appleton-Century-Crofts, 1969.

141. Skinner, B.F., *Beyond Freedom and Dignity.* New York: Alfred A. Knopf, 1971.

142. Skinner, *Cumulative Record.*

143. *Ibid.*

144. Murray and Huelekoetter, *op. cit.*

145. Skinner, *The Behavior of Organisms.*

146. Skinner, *Walden Two.*

147. Skinner, Behaviorism at Fifty.

148. Skinner, *Contingencies of Reinforcement: A Theoretical Analysis.*

149. Skinner, *Beyond Freedom and Dignity.*

150. Skinner, *Cumulative Record.*

151. Murray and Huelekoetter, *op. cit.*

152. *Ibid.*

153. *Ibid.*

154. Rimm, R.C., and J.C. Masters, *Behavior Therapy Techniques and Empirical Findings.* New York: Academic Press, 1979.

155. Martin, G. and J. Pear. *Behavior Modification: What It Is and How to Do It* (7th ed.). Englewood Cliffs, NJ: Prentice-Hall, 2003.

156. *Ibid.*

157. Murray and Huelekoetter, *op. cit.*

158. Rimm and Masters, *op. cit.*

159. Murray and Huelekoetter, *op. cit.*

160. *Ibid.*

161. *Ibid.*

162. De Longis et al., *op. cit.*

163. Murray and Huelekoetter, *op. cit.*

164. Patterson and Watkins, *op. cit.*

165. Murray and Huelekoetter, *op. cit.*

166. Patterson and Watkins, *op. cit.*

167. Murray and Huelekoetter, *op. cit.*

168. Patterson and Watkins, *op. cit.*

169. Murray and Huelekoetter, *op. cit.*

170. *Ibid.*

171. *Ibid.*

172. Hartmann, H., *Essays on Ego Psychology.* New York: International Universities Press, 1964.

173. Papalia et al., *op. cit.*

174. Sullivan, H.S., *The Interpersonal Theory of Psychiatry.* New York: W.W. Norton, 1953.

175. *Ibid.*

176. *Ibid.*

177. *Ibid.*

178. Erikson, E., *Childhood and Society* (2nd ed.). New York: W. W. Norton, 1963.

179. *Ibid.*

180. *Ibid.*

181. Storr, A., *The Essential Jung.* Princeton, NJ: Princeton University Press, 1983.

182. Murray and Huelekoetter, *op. cit.*

183. Patterson and Watkins, *op. cit.*

184. Murray and Huelekoetter, *op. cit.*

185. Patterson and Watkins, *op. cit.*

186. Murray and Huelekoetter, *op. cit.*

187. *Ibid.*

188. *Ibid.*

189. *Ibid.*

190. *Ibid.*

191. *Ibid.*

192. Bandura, A., Regulation of Cognitive Processes Through Perceived Self-efficacy. *Developmental Psychology,* 25 (1989), 729–735.

193. Bandura, A., Social Cognitive Theory, in Vasta, R., ed., *Annals of Child Development: Six Theories of Child Development: Revised Formulations and Current Issues.* Greenwich, CT: Jai Press, 1989, pp. 1–60.

194. Bandura, A., Social Cognitive Theory of Self-Regulation, *Organizational Behavior and Human Decision Processes,* 50 (1991), 248–287.

195. Bandura, A., *Social Learning Theory.* Morristown, NJ: General Learning Press, 1977.

196. *Ibid.*

197. *Ibid.*

198. Bandura, A., *Social Foundations of Thought and Action: A Social Cognitive Theory.* Englewood Cliffs, NJ: Prentice-Hall, 1986.

199. Bandura, Regulation of Cognitive Processes Through Perceived Self-efficacy.

200. Bandura, *Social Foundations of Thought and Action: A Social Cognitive Theory.*

201. Bandura, Regulation of Cognitive Processes Through Perceived Self-efficacy.

202. Bandura, *Social Learning Theory.*

203. Bandura, *Social Foundations of Thought and Action: A Social Cognitive Theory.*

204. Bandura, Regulation of Cognitive Processes Through Perceived Self-efficacy.

205. Bandura, Social Cognitive Theory.

206. Bandura, A., Social Cognitive Theory of Moral Thought and Action, in Kurtines, W., and Gerwitz J., eds., *Handbook of Moral Behavior and Development.* Hillsdale, NJ: Lawrence Erlbaum, 1991, pp. 45–103.

207. Bandura, Social Cognitive Theory of Self-Regulation.

208. Patterson and Watkins, *op. cit.*

209. Piaget, J., *The Child's Conception of Physical Causality.* London: Kegan Paul, 1930.

210. Piaget, J., *The Moral Judgment of the Child.* New York: Free Press of Glencoe, 1948.

211. Piaget, J., *Play, Dreams, and Imitation in Childhood.* New York: W. W. Norton, 1951.

212. Piaget, J., *The Child's Conception of the World,* London: Routledge and Kegan Paul, 1951.

213. Piaget, J., *Judgment and Reasoning in the Child.* London: Routledge and Kegan Paul, 1951.

214. Piaget, J., *The Origins of Intelligence in Children.* New York: W. W. Norton, 1963.

215. Piaget, J., *Six Psychological Studies.* New York: Random House, 1967.

216. Piaget, J., *Biology and Knowledge.* Chicago: University of Chicago Press, 1971.

217. Piaget, J., *Psychology and Epistemology.* New York: Orion Press, 1971.

218. Piaget, J., *Understanding Causality.* New York: W. W. Norton. 1974.

219. Piaget, J., *The Grasp of Consciousness.* Cambridge, MA: Harvard University Press, 1976.

220. Piaget, J., and B. Inhelder, *The Psychology of the Child.* New York: Basic Books, 1969.

221. Piaget, J., and B. Inhelder, *The Origin of the Idea of Chance in Children*. New York: W. W. Norton, 1975.
222. Piaget and Inhelder, *The Psychology of the Child*.
223. Piaget, *The Child's Conception of Physical Causality*.
224. Piaget, *The Moral Judgment of the Child*.
225. Piaget, *Play, Dreams, and Imitation in Childhood*.
226. Piaget, *The Child's Conception of the World*.
227. Piaget, *Judgment and Reasoning in the Child*.
228. Piaget, *The Origins of Intelligence in Children*.
229. Piaget, *Six Psychological Studies*.
230. Piaget, *Biology and Knowledge*.
231. Piaget, *Psychology and Epistemology*.
232. Piaget, *Understanding Causality*.
233. Piaget, *The Grasp of Consciousness*.
234. Piaget and Inhelder, *The Psychology of the Child*.
235. Piaget and Inhelder, *The Origin of the Idea of Chance in Children*.
236. Wadsworth, B., *Piaget's Theory of Cognitive and Affective Development* (5th ed.). New York: Longman, 1996.
237. Bandura, Social Cognitive Theory of Moral Thought and Action.
238. Piaget, *The Child's Conception of Physical Causality*.
239. Piaget, *The Moral Judgment of the Child*.
240. Piaget, *Play, Dreams, and Imitation in Childhood*.
241. Piaget, *The Child's Conception of the World*.
242. Piaget, *Judgment and Reasoning in the Child*.
243. Piaget, *The Origins of Intelligence in Children*.
244. Piaget, *Six Psychological Studies*.
245. Piaget, *Biology and Knowledge*.
246. Piaget, *Psychology and Epistemology*.
247. Piaget, *Understanding Causality*.
248. Piaget, *The Grasp of Consciousness*.
249. Piaget and Inhelder, *The Psychology of the Child*.
250. Piaget and Inhelder, *The Origin of the Idea of Chance in Children*.
251. Furth, H.G., and H. Wachs, *Thinking Goes to School: Piaget's Theory in Practice*. New York: Oxford University Press, 1975.
252. Piaget, *The Child's Conception of Physical Causality*.
253. Piaget, *The Moral Judgment of the Child*.
254. Piaget, *Play, Dreams, and Imitation in Childhood*.
255. Piaget, *The Child's Conception of the World*.
256. Piaget, *Judgment and Reasoning in the Child*.
257. Piaget, *The Origins of Intelligence in Children*.
258. Piaget, *Six Psychological Studies*.
259. Piaget, *Biology and Knowledge*.
260. Piaget, *Psychology and Epistemology*.
261. Piaget, *Understanding Causality*.
262. Piaget, *The Grasp of Consciousness*.
263. Piaget and Inhelder, *The Psychology of the Child*.
264. Piaget and Inhelder, *The Origin of the Idea of Chance in Children*.
265. Wadsworth, *Piaget's Theory of Cognitive and Affective Development*.
266. Bee, *op. cit.*
267. Papalia et al., *op. cit.*
268. Seifert et al., *op. cit.*
269. Kohlberg, L., ed., *Collected Papers on Moral Development and Moral Education,* Cambridge, MA: Moral Educational Research Foundation, 1973.
270. Kohlberg, L. Moral Stages and Moralization: The Cognitive Developmental Approach, in Lickona, T., ed., *Moral Development and Behavior*. New York: Holt, Rinehart, & Winston, 1976, pp. 31–53.
271. Kohlberg, L. *Recent Research in Moral Development*. New York: Holt, Rinehart, & Winston, 1977.
272. Kohlberg, L. The Cognitive-Developmental Approach to Moral Education, in Scharf, P., ed., *Readings in Moral Education*. Minneapolis: Winston Press, 1978, pp. 36–51.
273. Kohlberg, L. and E. Turiel, Moral Development and Moral Education, in Lesser, G.S., ed., *Psychology and Education Practice*. Chicago: Scott, Foresman, 1971.
274. Kohlberg, *Collected Papers on Moral Development and Moral Education*.
275. Kohlberg, Moral Stages and Moralization: The Cognitive Developmental Approach.
276. Kohlberg, *Recent Research in Moral Development*.
277. Kohlberg, The Cognitive-Developmental Approach to Moral Education.
278. Kohlberg and Turiel, *op. cit.*
279. Rest, J., The Legacy of Lawrence Kohlberg, *Counseling and Values,* 32, no. 3 (1988), 156–162.
280. Kohlberg, *Collected Papers on Moral Development and Moral Education*.
281. Kohlberg, Moral Stages and Moralization: The Cognitive Developmental Approach.
282. Kohlberg, *Recent Research in Moral Development*.
283. Kohlberg, The Cognitive-Developmental Approach to Moral Education.
284. Kohlberg and Turiel, *op. cit.*
285. Kohlberg, The Cognitive-Developmental Approach to Moral Education.
286. *Ibid.*
287. Rest, *op. cit.*
288. Gilligan, C., In a Different Voice: Women's Conceptualization of Self and of Mortality, *Harvard Educational Review,* 47, no. 4 (1977), 481–517.
289. Gilligan, C., *In A Different Voice: Psychological Theory and Women's Development*. Cambridge, MA: Harvard University Press, 1982.
290. Gilligan, C., and D. Attanucci, Two Moral Orientations: Gender Differences and Similarities, *Merrill-Palmer Quarterly,* 34, no. 3 (1988), 332–333.
291. Friedman, W., et al., Sex Differences in Moral Judgments: A Test of Gilligan's Theory, *Psychology of Women Quarterly,* 7, no. 1 (1987), 87.
292. Frankl, V., *Man's Search for Meaning*. New York: Washington Square Press, 1967.
293. Frankl, V., *The Unheard Cry for Meaning*. New York: Washington Square Press, 1978.
294. Travelbee, J., *Interpersonal Aspects of Nursing*. Philadelphia: F.A. Davis, 1971.
295. *Ibid.*
296. Maslow, A., *Motivation and Personality* (2nd ed.). New York: Harper & Row, 1970.
297. May, R., *Psychology and the Human Dilemma*. New York: D. Van Nostrand, 1967.
298. Middleton, J., Existentialist as Helper? *Canadian Psychiatric Nursing,* 20, no. 3 (1979), 7–8.
299. Travelbee, *op. cit.*
300. Maslow, A., *The Farther Reaches of Human Nature*. New York: Viking Press, 1971.
301. Travelbee, *op. cit.*
302. Maslow, A., *Towards a Psychology of Being* (2nd ed.). New York: D. Van Nostrand, 1968.
303. Maslow, *The Farther Reaches of Human Nature*.
304. Travelbee, *op. cit.*
305. Maslow, *The Farther Reaches of Human Nature*.
306. Murray and Huelekoetter, *op. cit.*
307. Rogers, C., *Client-Centered Therapy*. Boston: Houghton-Mifflin, 1951.
308. Rogers, C., *On Becoming a Person*. Boston: Houghton-Mifflin, 1961
309. Rogers, C., *Freedom to Learn*. Columbus, OH: Charles E. Merrill, 1969.
310. Rogers, C., *On Encounter Groups*. New York: Harper & Row, 1970.
311. Rogers, C., A Theory of Personality, in Millan, T., ed. *Theories of Psychopathology*. Philadelphia: W.B. Saunders, 1973.
312. Rogers, C., *Way of Being*. Boston: Houghton Mifflin, 1980.

313. Rogers, *Client-Centered Therapy.*
314. Murray and Huelekoetter, *op. cit.*
315. Rogers, *Client-Centered Therapy.*
316. Rogers, *On Becoming a Person.*
317. Rogers, *Freedom to Learn.*
318. Rogers, *On Encounter Groups.*
319. Rogers, A Theory of Personality.
320. Rogers, *Way of Being.*
321. Osachuk, T.A.G. and S.L. Cairns, Relationship Issues, in D.G. Martin and A.D. Moore, eds., *First Steps in the Art of Intervention* (pp. 19, 21). Pacific Grove: Brooks/Cole, 1995,
322. Maslow, *Towards a Psychology of Being.*
323. Maslow, *The Farther Reaches of Human Nature.*
324. Maslow, *Motivation and Personality.*
325. Murray and Huelekoetter, *op. cit.*
326. Rogers, *Client-Centered Therapy.*
327. Rogers, *On Becoming a Person.*
328. Rogers, *Freedom to Learn.*
329. Rogers, *On Encounter Groups.*
330. Rogers, A Theory of Personality.
331. Rogers, *Way of Being.*
332. Murray and Huelekoetter, *op. cit.*
333. Rogers, *Client-Centered Therapy.*
334. Rogers, *On Encounter Groups.*
335. Murray and Huelekoetter, *op. cit.*
336. Rogers, *Client-Centered Therapy.*
337. Rogers, *On Becoming a Person.*
338. Murray and Huelekoetter, *op. cit.*
339. Rogers, *Client-Centered Therapy.*
340. Murray and Huelekoetter, *op. cit.*
341. Rogers, *Client-Centered Therapy.*
342. Seyle, H., Stress Syndrome, *American Journal of Nursing,* 65, no. 3 (1965), 97–99.
343. Seyle, H., *Stress Without Distress.* Philadelphia: J.B. Lippincott, 1974
344. Seyle, H., Implications of Stress Concept, *New York State Journal of Medicine,* October (1975), 2139–2145.
345. Seyle, H., Forty Years of Stress Research: Principal Remaining Problems and Misconceptions, *Canadian Medical Association Journal,* 115 (July 3, 1976), 53–56.
346. Seyle, H., *The Stress of Life* (rev. ed.). New York: McGraw-Hill, 1976.
347. Seyle, H., Stress and the Reduction of Distress, *Primary Cardiology,* 5, no. 8 (1979), 22–30.
348. Seyle, H., The Stress Concept Today, in Kutash, I.C., and Schlesinger, L.B. eds., *Handbook on Stress and Anxiety.* New York: Jossey-Bass, 1980, pp. 127–144.
349. Murray and Huelekoetter, *op. cit.*
350. Seyle, Stress Syndrome.
351. Seyle, *Stress Without Distress.*
352. Seyle, Implications of Stress Concept.
353. Seyle, Forty Years of Stress Research: Principal Remaining Problems and Misconceptions.
354. Seyle, *The Stress of Life.*
355. Seyle, Stress and the Reduction of Distress.
356. Seyle, The Stress Concept Today.
357. Murray and Huelekoetter, *op. cit.*
358. Seyle, *Stress Without Distress.*
359. Seyle, Stress and the Reduction of Distress.
360. De Longis et al., op. cit.
361. Murray and Huelekoetter, *op. cit.*
362. Seyle, Stress Syndrome.
363. Seyle, *Stress Without Distress.*
364. Seyle, Implications of Stress Concept.
365. Seyle, Forty Years of Stress Research: Principal Remaining Problems and Misconceptions.
366. Seyle, *The Stress of Life.*
367. Seyle, Stress and the Reduction of Distress.
368. Seyle, The Stress Concept Today.
369. Seyle, Stress Syndrome.
370. Seyle, *Stress Without Distress.*
371. Seyle, Implications of Stress Concept.
372. Seyle, Forty Years of Stress Research: Principal Remaining Problems and Misconceptions.
373. Seyle, *The Stress of Life.*
374. Seyle, Stress and the Reduction of Distress.
375. Seyle, The Stress Concept Today.
376. Seyle, Stress Syndrome.
377. Seyle, The Stress Concept Today.
378. Murray and Huelekoetter, *op. cit.*
379. Seyle, Stress Syndrome.
380. Seyle, *Stress Without Distress.*
381. Seyle, Implications of Stress Concept.
382. Seyle, Forty Years of Stress Research: Principal Remaining Problems and Misconceptions.
383. Seyle, *The Stress of Life.*
384. Seyle, Stress and the Reduction of Distress.
385. Seyle, The Stress Concept Today.
386. Murray and Huelekoetter, *op. cit.*
387. Seyle, Stress Syndrome.
388. Seyle, *Stress Without Distress.*
389. Seyle, Implications of Stress Concept.
390. Seyle, Forty Years of Stress Research: Principal Remaining Problems and Misconceptions.
391. Seyle, *The Stress of Life.*
392. Seyle, Stress and the Reduction of Distress.
393. Seyle, The Stress Concept Today.
394. Murray and Huelekoetter, *op. cit.*
395. Seyle, Forty Years of Stress Research: Principal Remaining Problems and Misconceptions.
396. Lazarus, R., *Psychological Stress and the Coping Process.* New York: McGraw-Hill, 1966.
397. Murray and Huelekoetter, *op. cit.*
398. Seyle, Stress Syndrome.
399. Seyle, *Stress Without Distress.*
400. Seyle, Implications of Stress Concept.
401. Seyle, Forty Years of Stress Research: Principal Remaining Problems and Misconceptions.
402. Seyle, *The Stress of Life.*
403. Seyle, Stress and the Reduction of Distress.
404. Seyle, The Stress Concept Today.
405. Murray and Huelekoetter, *op. cit.*
406. Seyle, Stress Syndrome.
407. Seyle, *Stress Without Distress.*
408. Seyle, Implications of Stress Concept.
409. Seyle, Forty Years of Stress Research: Principal Remaining Problems and Misconceptions.
410. Seyle, *The Stress of Life.*
411. Seyle, Stress and the Reduction of Distress.
412. Seyle, The Stress Concept Today.
413. Murray and Huelekoetter, *op. cit.*
414. Seyle, Stress Syndrome.
415. Seyle, Implications of Stress Concept.
416. Murray and Huelekoetter, *op. cit.*
417. Groër, M., Psychoneuroimmunology, *American Journal of Nursing,* 91, no. 8 (1991), 33.
418. Murray and Huelekoetter, *op. cit.*
419. Robinson, L., Stress and Anxiety, *Nursing Clinics of North America,* 25, no. 4 (1990), 935–943.
420. Seyle, Stress Syndrome.
421. Seyle, *Stress Without Distress.*
422. Seyle, Implications of Stress Concept.

423. Seyle, Forty Years of Stress Research: Principal Remaining Problems and Misconceptions.

424. Seyle, *The Stress of Life.*

425. Seyle, Stress and the Reduction of Distress.

426. Seyle, The Stress Concept Today.

427. Sullivan, *op. cit.*

428. Cox, B.J., P.S.R. MacPherson, M.W. Enns, and L.A. McWilliams, Neuroticism and Self-Criticism Associated With Posttraumatic Stress Disorder in a Nationally Representative Sample. *Behaviour Research and Therapy,* 42, no.1 (2003), 105–114.

429. Groër, *op. cit.*

430. *Ibid.*

431. Caplan, G., *Principles of Preventive Psychiatry.* New York: Basic Books, 1964.

432. Fink, S., Crisis and Motivation: A Theoretical Model, *Archives of Physical Medicine and Rehabilitation,* 48, no. 11 (1967), 592–597.

433. Murray and Huelekoetter, *op. cit.*

434. *Ibid.*

435. Schumacher, K., and A. Meleis, Transitions: A Central Concept in Nursing, *IMAGE: Journal of Nursing Scholarship,* 26, no. 2 (1994), 119–127.

436. Hoff, L.A., *People in Crisis: Understanding and Helping.* (3rd ed.). Redwood City, CA: Addison-Wesley, 1987.

437. De Longis et al., *op. cit.*

438. Murray and Huelekoetter, *op. cit.*

439. Hoff, *op. cit.*

440. Murray and Huelekoetter, *op. cit.*

441. Hoff, *op. cit.*

442. Murray and Huelekoetter, *op. cit.*

443. Fink, *op. cit.*

444. Murray and Huelekoetter, *op. cit.*

445. Fink, *op. cit.*

446. Murray and Huelekoetter, *op. cit.*

447. Caplan, *op. cit.*

448. Fink, *op. cit.*

449. Hoff, *op. cit.*

450. Murray and Huelekoetter, *op. cit.*

451. Hoff, *op. cit.*

452. Murray and Huelekoetter, *op. cit.*

453. Hoff, *op. cit.*

454. Murray and Huelekoetter, *op. cit.*

455. Hoff, *op. cit.*

456. Lindermann, E., Symptomology and Management of Acute Grief, *American Journal of Psychiatry,* 101 (1944), 141–148.

457. Murray and Huelekoetter, *op. cit.*

458. Weeks, S., Disaster Mental Health Services: A Personal Perspective, *Journal of Psychosocial Nursing,* 37, no. 2 (1999), 14–18.

Chapter 6

THE DEVELOPING PERSON: PRINCIPLES OF GROWTH AND DEVELOPMENT

Nothing has a stronger influence on their children than the unlived lives of their parents.

Carl Jung

OBJECTIVES

STUDY OF THIS CHAPTER WILL ENABLE YOU TO:

1. Define growth, development, and related terms.

2. Explore general insights into and principles of human behaviour.

3. Examine various influences that have an effect on the developing person: prenatal variables involving father, mother, and fetus; variables related to childbirth; early childhood variables, including child abuse; sociocultural experiences; and environmental factors.

4. Relate information in this chapter to yourself as a developing person.

5. Apply knowledge from this chapter when assessing the person through the life span.

6. Teach the person and family about factors that influence development of self or offspring, when appropriate.

Developmental theory, the study of the person throughout the life span, centres on certain principles of the person's growth and development. Although growth and development are usually thought of as a forward movement, of a kind of adding on such as increase in height and weight or the self-actualizing personality, the model can also apply to reversal, decay, deterioration, or death. Three kinds of reversals occur: (1) loss of some part, such as occurs with catabolism (changing of living tissue into wastes or destructive metabolism), (2) purposefully changing behaviour when it is no longer useful, and (3) death.[1]

Growth and development are generally characterized by the following:[2]

- Direction, goal, or end state
- Identifiable stage or era
- Forward progression, so that once a stage is worked through, the person does not return to the same position
- Increasing specialization
- Causal forces that are either genetic or environmental
- Potentialities and capabilities for various behaviours and achievements

DIMENSIONS OF TIME

Use theory about time dimensions, assumptions about behaviour, and principles of growth and development in assessment and health promotion interventions. This theory is applicable to all age eras.

Lifetime or chronologic age is frequently used as an index of maturation and development but is only a rough indicator of the person's position on any one of the numerous physical or psychological dimensions. Furthermore, the society is a reference point for understanding the behaviour; what is appropriate for a 14-year-old individual in one society is not in a different society.

Social time, or *social expectations of behaviour for each age era,* is not necessarily synchronous with biological timing. Neither chronologic age nor maturational stage is itself a determinant of aging status but only signifies the biological potentiality on which a system of age norms and age grading can operate to shape the life cycle.[3]

Historical time shapes the social system, and the social system creates a changing set of age norms and a changing age-grade system that shapes the person's life cycle. **Historical time** refers to a *series of economic, political, and social events that directly shape the life course of the person and long-term processes,* such as industrialization and urbanization, which create the social cultural context and changing definitions of the phases of the life cycle.[4]

A group of people born at a certain calendar time (cohort) has, as a group, a particular background and demographic composition so that most of the people of that specific age or generation will have similar experiences, level of education, fertility and childrearing patterns, sexual mores, work and labour force participation patterns, value systems, leisure patterns, religious behaviour, consumer behaviour, and ideas about life generally.[5]

Social time is prescribed by each society in that all societies rationalize the passage of lifetime, divide life into socially relevant units, and transform calendar or biological time into social time. Thus age grading occurs; the life cycle consists of a succession of formally age-graded, descriptive norms. Duties, rights, and rewards are differentially distributed to age groups. In societies in which division of labour is simple and social change is slow, a single age-grade system becomes formalized, and family, work, religious, and political roles are allocated. A modern, complex, rapidly changing society, which has several or overlapping systems of age status, has some tasks and roles that are tied to chronologic age and some that are more fluid or less defined. In every society there is a time to be a child and dependent, a time to be educated to whatever level is needed, a time to go to work, to form a partnership, to have a family, to retire, and to die. The members of the society have a general consensus about these age expectations and norms, although perceptions may vary somewhat by age, sex, or social class. Patterns of timing can play an important role with respect to self-concept and self-esteem, depending on the person's level of awareness about his or her fit to social age norms and the rigidity in the culture. The young are more likely to deny that age is a valid criterion by which to judge behaviour. Middle-aged and older adults, who see greater constraints in the age-norm system than do the young, have learned that to be too far ahead or behind in one's developmental stage involves negative consequences. Many of the major marks in the life cycle are ordered and sequential and are social rather than biological, and their time is socially regulated.[6-9]

This book is organized along chronologic lines, with the life cycle divided into different periods rather than having content organized around a topical approach. The person's life is divided into the following chronologic stages; the prenatal period (from the moment of conception to birth); infancy (birth to one year); toddler hood (one to three years); preschool (three to six years); school years (six to 12 years); adolescence (12 to 20 or 25 years); young adulthood (20 or 25 to 45 years); middle age (45 or 50 to 65 or 70 years); and late maturity (65 or 70 years and older). *The divisions are somewhat arbitrary because it is difficult to assign definite ages; individual lives are not marked off so precisely.*

The study of development is not merely a search for facts about people at certain ages. The study involves finding *patterns* or *general principles* that apply to most people most of the time.

People are often at one level in one area of development and at another level in another area. For example, an 11-year-old girl may have begun to menstruate—an activity that marks her physical transition from childhood to puberty—before she has outgrown many childish feelings and thoughts. A 48-year-old man who took several years to find his career direction, who married in his thirties, and who became a father in his forties may in many important psychological ways be in the young adulthood period. On the other hand, his 49-year-old neighbour who settled early on a professional direction and into family life may already be a grandfather and may act and feel more like a middle-aged man. Furthermore, individual differences among people are so great that they enter and leave these age periods at different times of life. People are aware of their own timing and are quick to describe themselves as "early," "late," or "on time" regarding developmental tasks.

Ideal **norms,** *standards* or *expectancies,* for different behaviours vary among different groups of people. The entire life cycle is speeded up for the poor and working classes, who tend to finish their education earlier than middle- or upper-class people, to take their first jobs sooner, marry younger, have children earlier, reach the peak of their careers earlier, and become grandparents earlier. These differences are related to financial needs that make it imperative for poor and working-class people to get paying jobs earlier in life. People from more affluent backgrounds can pursue their educations for a longer time, can use young adulthood to explore options, and then delay becoming financially independent and beginning a family.

CRITICAL THINKING

In what ways has the Information Age changed the concept of social time?

PRINCIPLES OF GROWTH AND DEVELOPMENT

Definitions

Certain words are basic to understanding the person and are used repeatedly. They are defined below for the purpose of this book.

Growth refers to *increase in body size or changes in structure, function, and complexity of body cell content and metabolic and biochemical processes up to some point of optimum maturity.*[10] Growth changes occur through incremental or replacement growth. **Incremental growth** refers to *maintaining an excess in growth over normal daily losses from catabolism, seen in urine, feces, perspiration, and oxidation in the lungs.* Incremental growth is observed as increases in weight or height as the child matures. **Replacement growth** refers to *normal refills of essential body components* necessary for survival.[11] For example, once a red blood cell (erythrocyte) has entered the cardiovascular system, it circulates an average of 120 days before disintegrating, when another red blood cell takes its place.[12] Growth occurs through **hypertrophy,** *increase in the size of cellular structures,* and **hyperplasia,** *an increase in the number of cells.*[13] Growth during the fetal and infancy periods is achieved primarily through hyperplasia, which is gradually replaced by hypertrophic growth. Each body organ has its own optimum period of growth. Body tissues are most sensitive to permanent damage during periods of the most rapid hyperplastic growth.

Development is the *patterned, orderly, lifelong changes in structure, thought, feelings, or behaviour that evolve as a result of maturation of physical and mental capacity, experiences, and learning and results in a new level of maturity and integration.*[14] Development should permit the person to adapt to the environment by either controlling the environment or controlling responses to the environment. Developmental processes involve interplay among the physiologic characteristics that define the person; the environmental forces, including culture, that act on him or her; and the psychological mechanisms that mediate between them. Psychological processes include the person's perception of self, others, and the environment, and the behaviours he or she acquires in coping with needs and the environment. Development combines growth, maturation, and learning and involves organizing behaviour.

A **developmental task** is a *growth responsibility that arises at a certain time in the course of development, successful achievement of which leads to satisfaction and success with later tasks.* Failure leads to unhappiness, disapproval by society, and difficulty with later developmental tasks and functions.

Maturation refers to the *emergence of genetic potential for changes in form, structure, complexity, integration, organization, and function, physically and mentally.*[15]

Biological age is the *level of physical growth and development and how the body functions over time.* **Psychological age** *is the person's perception of aging processes.* **Social age** *refers to society's expectations of the person at a specific age or stage.*[16] **Chronologic age** is the *time since birth* and is not always identical to the other ages.

Learning is the *process of gaining specific knowledge or skill and acquiring habits and attitudes as a result of experience, training, and behavioural changes.* Maturation and learning are interrelated. No learning occurs unless the person is mature enough to be able to understand and change his or her behaviour.[17]

CRITICAL THINKING

What may be some health issues for an individual who has failed to work through his or her developmental tasks?

General Principles of Development

The following statements apply to the overall development of the person.

Childhood is the foundation period of life. Attitudes, habits, patterns of behaviour and thinking, personality traits, and health status established during the early years (the first five determine to a large extent how successfully the person will continue to develop and adjust to life as he or she gets older). Early patterns of behaviour persist throughout life, within the range of normalcy.[18]

Development follows a definable, predictable, and sequential pattern and occurs continually through adulthood. Each person progresses through similar stages, but the age for achievement varies because achievement depends on inherent maturational capacity interacting with the physical and social environment. The different areas of growth and development—physical, mental, emotional, social, and spiritual—are interrelated, proceed together, and affect each other; yet these areas mature at their own pace. The stages of development overlap, and the transition from one stage to another is gradual.[19]

Growth and development are continuous, but they occur in spurts rather than in a straight upward direction. At times the person will appear to be at a standstill or even regress developmentally.

Growth is usually accompanied by behaviour change. As the child matures, he or she retains earlier ways of behaving, but there will be a developmental revision of habits. For example, the high-activity infant becomes a high-activity toddler or adult, but the object of the activity changes from diffuse interests to concentrated play to work. The young child's temperament is a precursor of later behaviour, although the

person is adaptable and changes throughout life. Behaviour changes also occur because of others' reactions and expectations, which change as the person matures physically.

Human behaviour has purpose or is goal directed. Therefore, the behaviour is commonly preceded by imagining the desired result. The person visualizes the future and tries to bring it about. Behaviour is directed to meeting needs and goals.

When one need or goal is met, the person has energy to pursue another need, interest, or goal. Behaviour changes direction, but it does not come to an end.

Critical periods in human development *occur when specific organs and other aspects of a person's physical and psychosocial growth undergo marked rapid change and the capacity to adapt to stressors is underdeveloped. During these critical periods when tremendous demands are placed on the person, the individual has an increased susceptibility to adverse environmental factors* that may cause various types and degrees of negative effects. For example, implantation is a critical period, and at certain times during pregnancy certain substances are more likely to damage fetal structures.[20,21] The form of the brain is established by the 12th week of gestation. Critical periods of brain growth are during early formation (organogenesis) from the third to ninth weeks of gestation; during brain growth spurt from 12 to 20 weeks of gestation; and during the time of rapid neuronal additions from 30 to 40 weeks of gestation and during the first 18 to 24 months after birth. Exposure of the nervous system to a teratogen during these time frames may affect specific brain regions that are growing the most rapidly at that time. During adolescence the rapid physical growth may negatively affect social relationships or feelings about self. Middle or old age may be another critical period.[22,23]

If appropriate stimuli and resources are not available at the critical time or when the person is ready to receive and use particular stimuli for the development of a specific psychomotor skill, the skill may be more difficult to learn later in the developmental sequence. Learning of any psychomotor skill, however, is also influenced by sociocultural factors; the extent to which any skill is influenced by genetics, environmental opportunity, cultural and family values and patterns, and emotional status is not fully known.

Mastering developmental tasks of one period is the basis for mastering the next developmental era, physically and emotionally. Certain periods exist when the task can be best accomplished and the task should be mastered then; if the time is delayed, the person will have difficulty in accomplishing the task. Each phase of development has characteristic traits and a period of equilibrium when the person adjusts more easily to environmental demands and a period of disequilibrium when he or she experiences difficulty in adjustment. Developmental hazards exist in every era. Some are environmental and interfere with adjustment; others come from within the person.[24–26]

Progressive differentiation of the self from the environment results from increasing self-knowledge and autonomy. The young child first separates as an object apart from mother. Gradually he or she becomes less dependent emotionally on the parents. As the child matures into adulthood, an increase in cognitive development enables more control over behaviour. The person can think and act on his or her own and becomes more and more autonomous.

The developing person simultaneously acquires competencies in four major areas: physical, cognitive, emotional, and social. **Physical competency** includes *various motor and neurological capacities* to attain mobility and manipulation and care for self physically. **Cognitive competency** includes *learning how to perceive, think, solve problems, and communicate thoughts and feelings* that, in turn, affect emotional and social skills. **Emotional competency** includes *developing an awareness and acceptance of self as a separate person, responding to other people and factors in the environment because others have been responsive to him or her, coping with inner and outer stresses, and becoming increasingly responsible for personal behaviour.* **Social competency** includes *learning how to affiliate securely with the family first and then with various people in various situations.* These four competencies constantly influence one another. Health of one domain or the extent of competency affects the other domains or competencies. Lack of care or stimulation in any one area inhibits development of the other three areas. Repetition and practice are essential to learning. Rewarded behaviour is usually repeated. The person optimally uses personal assets, inner resources, competencies, and abilities to keep energy expenditures at a minimum while focusing toward the achievement of a goal.[27,28]

Readiness and motivation are essential for learning to occur. Hunger, fatigue, illness, pain, and the lack of emotional feedback or opportunity to explore inhibit readiness and lower motivation.[29]

Many factors contribute to the formation of permanent characteristics and traits, including the child's genetic inheritance, undetermined prenatal environmental factors, family and society when he or she is an infant and young child, nutrition, physical and emotional environment, and degree of intellectual stimulation in the environment.

Progressive differentiation of the self from other people and the environment, the **Principle of Development toward Self-Knowledge and Autonomy,** is made apparent with the individual's increasing self-awareness and emergent self-concept. The young child achieves increasing ability to perceive himself or herself as an initiator of action on the environment and an increasing ability to regulate his or her own behaviour, to think and act in an individual and unique way, and to become more autonomous. The ability to be autonomous and interdependent is reworked throughout life.[30,31]

CRITICAL THINKING

What are some situations that might increase the likelihood of a negative developmental outcome for the individual?

Principles of Growth

Several principles of growth are emphasized in the following pages, but the primary determinant of normal growth is the development of the central nervous system, which, in turn, governs or influences other body systems.

The **Principle of Readiness** states that the *child's ability to perform a physical task depends not only on maturation of neurological structures in the brain but also on the maturation of the muscular and skeletal systems.*[32] Until a state of physiologic readiness is reached, the child cannot perform a function, such as toilet training, even with parental training or planned practice.

The **Principle of Differentiation** means that *development proceeds from simple to the complex; homogeneous to heterogeneous; and general to specific.*[33] For example, movement from *simple to complex* is seen in mitotic changes in fetal cell structures as they undergo cell division immediately after ovum fertilization by a sperm.[34] All human embryos are anatomically female for the first six weeks of life; only through the action of testosterone does the male embryo develop between the 6th and 12th weeks of life. Androgens or steroids administered prenatally can "masculinize" a genetic female brain.[35] *Differentiation from simple to complex* motor skill is seen after birth as the baby first waves his or her arms and then later learns to control finger movements. The general body configurations of males and females at birth are much more similar than during late adolescence, thus indicating *movement from homogeneity to heterogeneity.* The mass of cells in the embryo is at first homogeneous, but the limbs of the five-week-old embryo show considerable differentiation as the elbow and wrist regions become identifiable and finger ridge indentations outline the progressive protrusion of future fingers from the former paddle-shaped arm bud.[36] *General to specific* development is observed in motor responses, which are diffuse and undifferentiated at birth and become more specific and controlled later. Baby first moves the whole body in response to a stimulus; later he or she reacts with a specific body part.[37,38] The behaviour of the child becomes more specific to the person or situation with increasing age.

The **Cephalocaudal, Proximodistal, and Bilateral Principles** all indicate that *major physical and motor changes invariably proceed in three bipolar directions.* **Cephalocaudal** *(head to tail)* means that the *upper end of the organism develops with greater rapidity than and before the lower end of the organism.* Increases in neuromuscular size and maturation of function begin in the head and proceed to hands and feet. For example, a comparison of pictures of a five-week-old embryo during a period of several days clearly shows the extensive head growth, caused mainly by development of the brain, accompanied by further elongation of the body structure from head to tail. Further, auditory, visual, and other sensory mechanisms in the head develop sooner than motor systems of the upper body. At the same time, the arm buds, first appearing paddle shaped, continue to change in shape and size more rapidly than do the lower limbs. After birth the infant will be able to hold the head erect before being able to sit or walk.[39,40] **Proximodistal** *(near to far)* means that *growth progresses from the central axis of the body toward the periphery or extremities.* **Bilateral** *(side to side)* means that the *capacity for growth and development of structures is symmetric;*[41,42] growth that occurs on one side of the body occurs simultaneously on the other.

The **Principle of Asynchronous Growth** focuses on *developmental shifts at successive periods in development.* A comparison of pictures of persons of different ages indicates that the young child is *not* a "small adult"; the proportional size of the head to the chest and of the torso to the limbs of younger and older persons is vastly different. Length of limbs in comparison to torso length is smaller in the infant than the schoolchild and greater in the aged than the adolescent because of the biological changes of aging.

The **Principle of Discontinuity of Growth Rate** refers to the *different rate of growth changes at different periods during the life span.* The *whole* body does not grow as a total unit simultaneously. Instead, various structures and organs of the body grow and develop at different rates, reaching their maximum at different times throughout the life cycle. For instance, in its rudimentary form the heart and circulatory system begin to function during the third week of embryonic life, continue to mature slowly compared with the rest of the body, and after the age of 25 years remain fairly constant in size. Before birth the head is the fastest growing body part. The brain grows and develops according to a different pattern; this vital organ grows very rapidly during fetal life and infancy, reaching 80% of its maximum size at the age of two years. Full growth is seen at approximately six years of age.[43] Body growth is rapid in infancy and adolescence and relatively slow during school years.

All body systems normally continue to work in unity throughout the life span. Some physiologic characteristics, such as oxygen concentration in the blood, remain fairly stable throughout life. Others, such as body temperature, undergo minor changes, depending on age, hormonal balance, or time of day. Some characteristics such as pulse rate and fluid intake that are affected by changes in body surface, organ size, or maturity change markedly during the life cycle.[44,45] Age-related changes occur at varying chronologic periods. Structural deterioration usually precedes functional decline. Some organs and systems deteriorate more rapidly than others. In late life, the capacity for adaptation changes and finally decreases. Before death, decline or deterioration usually affects most structural and many functional centres in the aged person.[46,47]

The study of growth and development processes must focus on the complete continuum of the life cycle—from conception through death—to acquire a comprehensive understanding of the complexity of these processes and how these principles are activated throughout the life span.

LIFE-SPAN DEVELOPMENTAL PSYCHOLOGY

Life-span developmental psychology encompasses the study of the individual from conception to old age.[48] As you probably know, development is not completed at adulthood but extends across the life span. Lindenberger and Baltes claim that across the life span, adaptive processes such as acquisition, maintenance, transformation, and attrition all take place in the psychological structures and functions of the individual.[49] As a result, the ontogenesis of mind and behaviours in the individual's development involves the following constructs:

■ *Lifelong:* Development spans the years from conception to old age. Each stage has its own unique experiences and none is more important than the others.

■ *Dynamic:* Development involves much change throughout the years as well as a series of challenges. Development is always being constituted by gains and losses. Many individuals maximize their gains to minimize their losses.

■ *Multidimensional:* Development consists of connections and interplays among the physical, cognitive, social, psychological, and spiritual dimensions, each of which varies in its rate of development.

■ *Multifunctional:* Many abilities of the individual throughout the life span can either be improved upon or redirected. For example, cognitive performance may be portrayed as the combined outcome of biological and cultural systems of influence.

■ *Nonlinear:* The progression of development in many instances is either circular or reversible in nature, depending upon cultural contexts and age-related changes. For example, parental roles may change from that of childrearing to contending with an empty nest syndrome.

These constructs can serve as a framework for the study of life-span development. A central theme in life-span psychology concerns malleability. Most significant is the optimization of psychological functioning and behaviour throughout all phases of life. For example, the effects of cohort, historical period, and environmental differences on age changes and differences in cognitive performance are indications of malleability.[50]

Research that is informed by life-span psychology is intended to generate knowledge about three components of individual development: (1) inter-individual similarities (regularities) in development; (2) inter-individual differences in development; and (3) intra-individual plasticity (malleability) in development. The joint attention directed toward each of these components, and the specification of their age-related interplays, creates not only the conceptual but the methodological foundations of developmental psychology.[51]

This brief introduction to life-span developmental psychology will help you to examine more closely individuals and their families throughout the life span, as you find them in diverse cultures. The understanding you will attain will undoubtedly help you to recognize the importance of health promotion and disease prevention so that you might help to enhance the quality of life in the young as well as the old.

CRITICAL THINKING

Give a few examples of how development is influenced by both biology and culture throughout the life span.

DEVELOPING PERSON: PRENATAL STAGES AND INFLUENCES

Use the following information in prenatal assessment, teaching, other health promotion measures, and advocacy for public policy related to health.

The Beginning

The cell, the basis for human life, is a complex unit. Refer to an anatomy or physiology text for review of cell structure and function. This chapter presents a brief overview of the prenatal period as the beginning of life. For in-depth study of the biological differences of the male and female, the reproductive process, including fertilization and development of the unborn child in utero, inheritance patterns, and the process of labour and delivery, refer to an anatomy and physiology[52] or developmental text[53] and to a maternity nursing text.[54,55]

All body cells have 22 pairs of rod-shaped particles, nonsex **chromosomes** (*autosomes*), and a pair of sex chromosomes. The biological female has two X chromosomes; the biological male has one X and one Y chromosome. Each of the chromosomes contains approximately 20 000 *segments strung out like lengthwise beads* called **genes.** The genes, apparently located according to function, are made up of deoxyribonucleic acid (DNA), which processes the information that determines the makeup and specific function of every cell in the body. The genes play a major role in determining hereditary characteristics.[56,57]

The female reproductive cycle is more regular and is easier to observe and measure than the male reproductive cycle.[58,59] In contrast to the normal ovulatory cycle, spermatogenesis normally occurs in cycles that continuously follow one another.

Approximately 14 days after the beginning of the menstrual period, fertilization may occur in the outer third of the fallopian tube. The sperm cell from a male penetrates and unites with an **ovum** (*egg*) from a female to form a *single-cell* **zygote.** The sperm and ovum, known as **gametes** (*sex cells in half cells*), are produced in the reproductive system through **meiosis,** a *specialized process of cell division and chromosome reduction.*[60,61]

A newborn girl has approximately 400 000 immature ova in her ovaries; each is in a **follicle,** or *small sac.* **Ovulation,** the *expelling of an ovum from a mature follicle in one of the ovaries,* occurs approximately once every 28 days in a sexually mature female.[62,63]

Spermatozoa, much smaller and more active than the ovum, are produced in the testes of the mature male at the rate of several hundred million a day and are ejaculated in his semen at *sexual climax* (**orgasm**). For fertilization to occur, at least 20 million sperm cells must enter a woman's body at one time. They enter the vagina and try to swim through the **cervix** (*opening to the uterus*) and into the fallopian tube. Only a tiny fraction of those millions of sperm cells makes it that far. More than one may penetrate the ovum, but only one can fertilize it to create a new human. The sex of the baby is determined by the pair of sex chromosomes; the sperm may carry either an X or Y chromosome, resulting in either a girl (XX zygote) or a boy (XY zygote). Thus *the man determines the sex of the baby.*[64,65]

Spermatozoa maintain their ability to fertilize an egg for a span of 24 to 90 hours; ova can be fertilized for approximately 24 hours. Thus, there are approximately 24 to 90 hours during each menstrual cycle when conception can take place. If fertilization does not occur, the spermatozoa and ovum die. Sperm cells are devoured by white blood cells in the woman's body; the ovum passes through the uterus and vagina in the menstrual product.[66,67]

Multiple births may occur. For example, with twins, two ova are released within a short time of each other; if both are fertilized, fraternal (*dizygotic or two-egg*) **twins** will be born. Created by different eggs and different sperm cells, the twins are no more alike in their genetic makeup than other siblings. They may be of the same or different sex. If the ovum divides in two after it has been fertilized, **identical** (*monozygotic or one-egg*) **twins** will be born. At birth, these twins share the same placenta. They are of the same sex and have exactly the same genetic heritage; any differences they will later exhibit are the result of the influences of environment, either before or after birth. Other multiple births—triplets, quadruplets, and so forth—result from either one or a combination of these two processes.[68,69]

Multiple births have become more frequent in recent years as a result of the administration of certain fertility drugs that spur ovulation and often cause the release of more than one egg. The tendency to bear twins apparently is inherited and more common in some families and ethnic groups than in others. Twins have a limited intrauterine space and are more likely to be premature and of low birth weight. They therefore have a lower rate of survival at birth.[70] Mariano and Hickey claim that Canadian women are two-and-a-half times more likely to have triplets, quadruplets, or even quintuplets today than 20 years ago.[71] Thirty to 50% of the world's twin pregnancies and at least 75% of triplet pregnancies occur in industrialized countries in women using fertility treatments.[72] Reasons for multiple births include increasing maternal age and the use of fertility drugs and other reproductive technologies.[73]

CASE SITUATION

Sue, age 35, comes to the clinic for an appointment with a nurse clinician. She informs the nurse that she and her partner, after a second cycle of in vitro fertilization and embryo transfer, just received news from the gynecologist that she is expecting a multiple birth—possibly triplets. Sue and her partner have two young adopted children at home, and she is quite anxious about how she will manage to care for the multiples as well as the rest of the family. She is wondering if she should expect annoying bouts of "morning sickness," and whether or not they are more intense with a multiple pregnancy. Sue also states that she learned from a neighbour that the risk is higher for preterm delivery with a multiple pregnancy.

1. What would be the nurse's response regarding Sue's concern about "morning sickness"?

2. What are the risk factors specific to multiple pregnancies? How could the nurse counsel Sue?

3. What health promotion strategies could the nurse consider for Sue in caring for herself and her family both now and after delivery?

In Canada, Bill C-6 (An Act Respecting Assisted Human Reproduction and Related Research) became law in March 2004. This law prohibits human cloning and other unacceptable activities, while protecting the health and safety of Canadians who use assisted human reproduction (AHR). Furthermore, this law provides controls for AHR-related research and will lead to the establishment of the Assisted Human Reproduction Agency of Canada, which will be responsible for licensing, inspecting, and enforcing activities controlled under the act.[74]

After either single or multiple fertilization, the zygote travels to the uterus for implantation or imbedding in the uterine wall. Progesterone secretion has prepared the uterus for the possible reception of the fertilized ovum. The continued secretion of ovarian estrogen and progesterone develops the uterus for the nine-month nurturance of the developing embryo and fetus in pregnancy. Continued secretion of estrogen during this period increases the growth of the uterine muscles and eventually enlarges the vagina for the delivery of a child. Continued secretion of progesterone during pregnancy serves to keep the uterus from prematurely contracting and expelling the developing embryo before the proper time. In addition, progesterone prepares the breast cells in late pregnancy for future milk production.[75]

Stages of Prenatal Developmental

Life in utero is usually divided into three stages of development: germinal, embryonic, and fetal. The **germinal stage** lasts *approximately ten days to two weeks after fertilization.* It is characterized by rapid cell division and subsequent increasing complexity of the organism and its implantation in the wall of the uterus. The **embryonic stage,** *from two to eight weeks,* is the time of rapid growth and differentiation of major body systems and organs. The **fetal stage,** *from eight weeks until birth,* is characterized by rapid growth and changes in body form caused by different rates of growth of different parts of the body.[76,77]

The fetus is a very small but rapidly developing human being who is influenced by the maternal and external environment and to whom the mother responds, especially when fetal movement begins. Table 6–1 summarizes some major milestones in the sequential development of the **conceptus,** the *new life that has been conceived;* however, *being precise about the exact timing is difficult.*[78–82]

TABLE 6–1
Summary of the Sequence of Prenatal Development

Time Period after Fertilization	Developmental Event
Germinal Stage	
30 hours	First division or cleavage occurs.
40 hours	Four-cell stage occurs.
60 hours	**Morula,** *a solid mass of 12 to 16 cells;* total size of mass not changed because cell decrease in size with each cleavage to allow morula to pass through lumen of fallopian tube. Ectopic pregnancy within fallopian tube occurs if morula is wedged in lumen.
3 days	Zygote has divided into 32 cells; travels through fallopian tube to uterus.
4 days	Zygote contains 70 cells. Morula reaches uterus; forms a **blastocyst,** *a fluid-filled sphere.*
4½–6 days	Blastocyst floats in utero. **Embryonic disk,** *thickened cell mass from which baby develops,* clusters on one edge of blastocyst. Mass of cells differentiates into two layers: (1) **ectoderm,** *outer layer of cells* that become the epidermis, nails, hair, tooth enamel, sensory organs, brain and spinal cord, cranial nerves, peripheral nervous system, upper pharynx, nasal passages, urethra, and mammal glands; (2) **endoderm,** *lower layer of cells* that develops into gastrointestinal system, liver, pancreas, salivary glands, respiratory system, urinary bladder, pharynx, thyroid, tonsils, lining of urethra, and ear.
6–7 days	**Nidation,** *implantation of zygote* into upper portion of uterine wall, occurs.
7–14 days	Remainder of blastocyst develops into the following: (1) **Placenta,** a *multi-purpose organ connected to the embryo by the umbilical cord* that delivers oxygen and nourishment from the mother's body, absorbs and the embryo's body wastes, combats internal infection, confers immunity to the unborn child, and produces the hormones that (a) support pregnancy, (b) prepare breasts for lactating, and (c) stimulate uterine contractions for delivery of the baby. Placenta circulation is evidenced by 11 to 12 days. (2) **Umbilical cord,** *a structure that contains two*

(continued)

TABLE 6–1 *(continued)*
Summary of the Sequence of Prenatal Development

Time Period after Fertilization	Developmental Event
	umbilical arteries and an umbilical vein and connects embryo to placenta. It is approximately 55 cm long and 3.8 cm in diameter. Rapid cell differentiation occurs. (3) **Amniotic sac,** *a fluid-filled membrane that encases the developing baby,* protecting it and giving it room to move.
2–8 weeks	Period during which embryo firmly establishes uterus as home and undergoes rapid cellular differentiation, growth, and development of body systems. This is a *critical period when embryo is most vulnerable to deleterious prenatal influences.* All development birth defects occur during *first trimester (3 months)* of pregnancy. If embryo is unable to survive, a **miscarriage** or **spontaneous abortion,** *expulsion of conceptus from the uterus, occurs.*
Embryonic Stage	
15 days	Cranial end of elongated disk has begun to thicken.
16 days	**Mesoderm,** the *middle layer,* appears and develops into dermis, tooth dentin, connective tissue, cartilage, bones, muscles, spleen, blood, gonads, uterus, and excretory and circulatory systems. Yolk sac, which arises from ectoderm, assists transfer of nutrients from mother to embryo.
19–20 days	Neural fold and neural grove develop. Thyroid begins to develop.
21 days	Neural tube forms, becomes spinal cord and brain.
22 days	Heart, the first organ to function, initiates action. Eyes, ears, nose, cheeks, and upper jaw begin to form. Cleft palate may occur if development is defective.
26–27 days	Cephalic portion (brain) of nervous system formed. Leg and arm buds appear. Stubby tail of spinal cord appears.
28 days	Crown to rump length, 4–5 mm.
30 days	Rudimentary body parts formed. Limb buds appear. Cardiovascular system functioning. Heart beats 65 times per minute; blood flows through tiny arteries and veins. Lens vesicles, optic cups, and nasal pits forming. By end of first month, new life has grown more quickly than it will at any other time in life. Swelling in head where eyes, ears, mouth, and nose will be. Crown to rump length, 7–14 mm.
31 days	Eye and nasal pit developing. Primitive mouth present.
32 days	Paddle-shaped hands. Lens vesicles and optic cups formed.
34 days	Head is much larger relative to trunk. Digital rays present in hands. Feet are paddle-shaped. Crown to rump length, 11–14 mm.
35–38 days	Olfactory pit, eye, maxillary process, oral cavity, and mandibular process developing. Brain has divided into three parts. Limbs growing. Beginning of all major external and internal structures. Crown to rump length, 15–16 mm.
40 days	Elbows and knees apparent. Fingers and toes distinct but webbed. Yolk sac continues to (1) provide embryologic blood cells during third through sixth weeks until liver, spleen, and bone marrow assume function; (2) provide lining cells for respiratory and digestive tracts; (3) provide cells that migrate to gonads to become primordial germ cells.
42 days	Crown to rump length, 21–23 mm.
50 days	All internal and external structures present. External genitalia present but sex not discernible; yolk sac disappears, incorporated into embryo; limbs, hands, feet formed. Nerve cells in brain connected.
55–56 days	Eye, nostril, globular process, maxilla, and mandible almost completely formed. Ear beginning to develop.

(continued)

TABLE 6–1 *(continued)*
Summary of the Sequence of Prenatal Development

Time Period after Fertilization	Developmental Event
8 weeks	Stubby end of spinal cord disappears. Distinct human characteristics. Head accounts for half of total embryo length. Brain impulses coordinate function of organ systems. Facial parts formed, with tongue and teeth buds. Stomach produces digestive juices. Liver produces blood cells. Kidney removes uric acid from blood. Some movement by limbs. Weight, 1 g. Length, 2.5–3.75 cm.

Fetal Stage

Time Period after Fertilization	Developmental Event
9–40 weeks	Remainder of intrauterine period spent in growth and refinement of body tissues and organs.
9–12 weeks	Eyelids fused. Nail beds formed. Teeth and bones begin to appear. Ribs and vertebrae are cartilage. Kidneys function. Urinates occasionally. Some respiratory-like movements exhibited. Begins to swallow amniotic fluid. Grasp, sucking, and withdrawal reflexes present. Sucks fingers and toes in utero. Makes specialized responses to touch. Moves easily but movement not felt by mother. Reproductive organs have primitive egg or sperm cells. Sex distinguishable. Head one-third of body length. Weight, 30 g. Length, 7.5–9 cm at 12 weeks.
13–16 weeks	Much spontaneous movement. Sex determination possible. **Quickening,** *fetal kicking or movement,* may be felt by mother. Moro reflex present. Rapid skeletal development. Meconium present. Uterine development in female fetus. **Lanugo,** *downy hair,* appears on body. Head one-fourth of total length. Weight, 120–150 g. Length, 20–25 cm. Foetus frowns, moves lips, turns head; hands grasp, feet kick. First hair appears. Ova formed in female.
17–20 weeks	New cells exchanged for old, especially in skin. Quickening occurs by 17 weeks. Vernix caseosa appears. Eyebrows, eyelashes, and head hair appear. Sweat and sebaceous glands begin to function. Skeleton begins to harden. Grasp reflex present and strong. Permanent teeth buds appear. Fetal heart sounds can be heard with stethoscope. Weight, 360–450 g. Length, 30.5 cm.
21–24 weeks	Extrauterine life, life outside uterus, is possible but difficult because of immature respiratory system. Fetus looks like miniature baby. Mother may note jarring but rhythmic movements of infant, indicative of hiccups. Body becomes straight at times. Fingernails present. Skin has wrinkled, red appearance. Alternate periods of sleep and activity. May respond to external sounds. Weight, 720 g. Length, 35.5 cm.
25–28 weeks	Jumps in utero in synchrony with loud noise. Eyes open and close with waking and sleeping cycles. Able to hear. Respiratory-like movements. Respiratory and central nervous systems sufficiently developed; some babies survive with excellent and intensive care. Assumes head-down position in uterus. Weight, 1200 g.
29–32 weeks	Begins to store fat and minerals. Testes descend into scrotal sac in male. Reflexes fully developed. Thumb-sucking present. Mother may note irregular, jerky, crying-like movements. Lanugo begins to disappear from face. Head hair continues to grow. Skin begins to lose reddish colour. Can be conditioned to environmental sounds. Weight, 1362–2270 g. Length, 40.5 cm.
33–36 weeks	Adipose tissue continues to be deposited over entire body. Body begins to round out. May become more or less active because of space constriction. Increased iron storage by liver. Increased lung development. Lanugo begins to disappear from body. Head lengthens. Brain cells number same as at birth. Weight, 2800 g. Length, 46–60 cm.
37–40 weeks	Organ systems operating more efficiently. Heart rate increases. More wastes expelled. Lanugo and vernix caseosa disappear. Skin smooth and plump. High absorption of maternal hormones. Cerebral cortex well-defined; brain wave patterns developed. Skull and other bones becoming more firm and mineralized. Continued storage of fat and minerals. Glands produce hormones that trigger labour. Ready for birth. Weight, 3200–3400 g. Length, 51–53 cm. Baby stops growing approximately 1 week before birth.

Table 6–2 summarizes physiologic changes in the woman during pregnancy.[83–87]

Prenatal Influences on Development

Heredity

Genetic information is transmitted from parents of offspring through a complex series of processes. The *basic unit of heredity* is the **gene.** Each cell in the human body contains about 100 000 genes, which are made up of DNA. DNA carries the biochemical instructions that tell the cells how to make the proteins that enable them to carry out specific body functions. Each gene is located in a definite position in the rod-shaped **chromosome.** Twenty-three pairs of chromosomes in the human germ cells divide into two gametes by meiosis, giving to each of these mature germ cells (female ovum and male spermatozoon) one-half the genetic material necessary for producing a new individual.[88–90]

At conception, the single-celled zygote has all the biological information necessary to develop into a baby through the process of **mitosis,** *a process whereby the cells divide in half over and over.* Each cell, except the **gamete** (*sex chromosomes X or Y*), is identical to the original zygote in normal development.[91–93]

Congenital malformations, *physical or mental disabilities* that occur before birth for a variety of reasons, are discussed in the following pages. However, sometimes disease or defects are **genetic,** *the result of dominant or recessive transmission of abnormalities in the genes or chromosomes.* An example is **fragile X syndrome,** *which involves an abnormal fragile section of DNA at a specific location on the X chromosome.* This is a sex-linked inherited disorder; the female is usually a carrier, the male is more likely to demonstrate the effects. It is estimated that 5% to 7% of all mental retardation is caused by this syndrome.[94] Recessive genes may cause inherited diseases, such as cystic fibrosis, sickle-cell anemia, muscular dystrophy, phenylketonuria (PKU) disease, and Tay-Sachs disease.[95]

An example of a congenital but not inherited disorder is **Down syndrome** (**trisomy 21**) *in which the child has three of the chromosome 21 instead of the normal two.* Various factors contribute to the chromosomal break and are discussed in later sections. The level of mental retardation varies.

CRITICAL THINKING

In what ways can you help a family with a Down syndrome infant to cope?

An inherited predisposition to a disorder may also interact with an environmental factor before or after birth and lead to expression of the disorder. Some abnormalities or diseases that are inherited appear months or years later.[96,97]

There may be a long-term factor in inheritance that is just beginning to be recognized as a result of research with women of childbearing age and their offspring who have lived through harrowing experiences such as the Holocaust, been a victim of war atrocities, survived life as a refugee, or been through less catastrophic experiences. Trauma can cause such intense genetic scrambling in a survivor that the child inherits the same stress-related abnormalities.

Furthermore, the sense of danger, anxiety, and uncertainty that lives on in the family affects the biological system of the child. Thus, the gene for a predisposition has to be "turned on" by an outside force before it can do its job, but the offspring's behaviour reflects the stresses that its mother lived through. High levels of stress activate a variety of genes, including those involved in shyness, panic disorder, and schizophrenia, some of the diseases that can occur in offspring.

However, hereditary factors do not by themselves fully determine what the person will become. There is a **reaction range,** *a range of potential expression of a trait* (e.g., *weight*), *that depends on environmental conditions.* Then, there are some traits, such as eye colour, that are so strongly programmed by genes that they are **canalized,** that is, *there is little variance in their expression.*[98,99]

Genetic endowment with respect to any trait may be compared to a rubber band. The rubber band may remain unstretched because of environmental influences and remain dormant. Or the rubber band may be stretched fully, causing the person to excel beyond what seems his or her potential. The person in later maturity, for example, has had many years of changing environmental influences; what he or she has become is no doubt an expression of innate genetic potential, environmental supports, and the wisdom to take advantage of both.[100–103]

An example of the positive effects of nurture or environment has been found in research on shyness. There is a genetic predisposition to shyness; however, the child can be helped to overcome this by parents who, in some cases, were also shy when they were young children. The parent can help the child face threatening situations, especially those involving people, and reduce anxiety. The child can be encouraged to interact with a variety of adults, play with children, and be around pets and other animals. If this is begun in infancy, by age four less than 20% of shy children are still shy. The competent parent can teach the child how to overcome the predisposition, and research over time shows that such children have become competent adults socially, often leaders.

Thus, judgments cannot be made at birth. Whatever the genetic background, the child deserves the opportunities to master the trait, turn the trait into an advantage, or learn how to cope with the trait.

Parental Age

The age of the mother and father and number of previous pregnancies affect the health of the fetus:

■ In Canada, the birth rate among older teenagers is decreasing, but is considerably higher than that of younger adolescents.[104] The age-specific live birth rate among females age 14 or younger declined steadily from 1.9 per 1000 females in 1991 to 0.9 per 1000 females in 2000.[105] This higher rate among older teenagers is partially a result of the increased likelihood that they will be married, cohabiting, or sexually active if unmarried, compared with their younger peers.[106] Pregnancy during the teen years, especially before age 17, is associated with infants who are premature, of low birth weight, with neurological defects, with higher mortality rates during the first year, and with more developmental problems during preschool and school years.

TABLE 6-2
Summary of Major Physiological Changes in Woman during Pregnancy

Physiological Characteristics	Change Related to Pregnancy
Weight	First trimester: increases by 0.9 to 1.8 kg. Second and third trimester: increases by 0.36 to 0.45 kg per week.
Skin	Warmed by increased blood flow. **Linea nigra:** *dark vertical line from sternum to symphysis pubis.* Stretch marks on abdomen with increasing **chloasma:** *dark brown patches on face or over bridge of nose.*
Musculoskeletal System	Centre of gravity changes, tilting pelvis forward, causing lower back pain. Fatigue and aches caused by increasing weight in abdomen and breasts.
Cardiovascular System	First trimester: blood volume increases gradually. 6-8 weeks: may hear systolic ejection murmur on auscultation. Heart displaced upwards and to the left by rising diaphragm. Orthostatic hypotension during pregnancy because blood pools in lower limbs; varicose veins and hemorrhoids are common. 14-20 weeks: pulse gradually increases by 10 to 15 beats per minute; cardiac output increases 30% to 50%. Last half of pregnancy: drop in colloid osmotic pressure shifts fluid into extra vascular space, causing edema in lower limbs. 32-34 weeks: blood volume increases to 40% to 50% above baseline; 40 weeks: blood volume gradually declines.
Respiratory System	Diaphragm rises and waistline expands even before enlarging uterus exerts much upward pressure. 24th week: thoracic rather than abdominal breathing; mild dyspnoea; nasal mucosa swells as a result of higher estrogen level; nasal stuffiness, epistaxis (nosebleeds) common. Costal ligaments relax because of rising estrogen levels; chest can expand and deeper breathing for increasing oxygen requirements. Respiratory rate increases slightly. Respiratory volume increases 26%, decreasing alveolar carbon dioxide concentration, compensated respiratory alkalosis. Alkalosis facilitates diffusion of nutrients to and wastes from the fetus through placenta.
Renal System	Kidneys excrete additional bicarbonate to compensate for drop in alveolar carbon dioxide concentration. Second trimester: increase in renal plasma flow (35%) and glomerular filtration rate (50%); both drop in late pregnancy. Urinary stasis caused by enlarging uterus and increasing blood volume.
Gastrointestinal System	First trimester nausea and vomiting resulting from increased human chorionic gonadotropin and estrogen. Gastric reflux as uterus enlarges and progesterone relaxes smooth muscle. Reduced bowel sounds; intestinal transit time increases, causing better nutrient absorption and constipation.
Hematological System	Second trimester: physiologic anemia with hemoglobin level and hematocrit slightly lower, proportionate to increased plasma volume. White blood cell count increases during pregnancy. Platelets remain normal.
Reproductive System	Uterus enlarges 20 times normal size to hold fetus, placenta, and amniotic fluid. 12th week: uterus expands out of pelvis into abdominal cavity. 16th week and after: supine position causes uterus to compress vena cava and iliac veins, decreasing blood flow to uterus and lower extremities (left lateral position recommended for sleeping). Vagina: pH more acid in mucus, which acts as barrier against infection to uterus. Breasts begin to feel full and tingly at second month; gradually enlarge as number and size of milk ducts and lobules increase; breast may leak colostrum.

Pregnant teens are more likely to have inadequate income, poor diet, and inadequate prenatal care.[107-111]

■ A baby born to a woman who has had three or more pregnancies before age 20 is less likely to be healthy.[112,113]

■ In recent years, the proportion of women who delay childbearing to later in life has increased markedly in Canada.[114] This delay may be associated with adverse outcomes not only for the infant but for the mother as well. As a woman's age increases, her risk of having a baby with Down syndrome also increases.[115] Antepartum complications associated with delayed childbearing include increased risks of spontaneous abortion, gestational diabetes, hypertension, pre-eclampsia, placenta previa, and prenatal hospital admission.[116] Further labour and delivery complications that arise with advanced maternal age include malpresentation, fetal distress, prolonged labour, operative deliveries, and postpartum hemorrhage.[117,118]

■ The more pregnancies a woman has had, the greater the risk to the infant. Maternal physiology cannot support many pregnancies in rapid succession, and as age increases, the ability to cope with the stresses of pregnancy decreases.[119-121]

■ When fathers are age 40 or older, they are at risk because sperm cells have divided so many times that there are more opportunities for errors. Anomalies linked to autosomal dominant mutations include Down syndrome, dwarfism, bone malformations, and Marfan's syndrome.[122-124]

CRITICAL THINKING

What do you believe the rate of live births to teen mothers would be in Nunavut?

Prenatal Endocrine and Metabolic Functions

Fetal growth and development are dependent on maternal endocrine and metabolic adjustments during pregnancy. The placenta helps to provide necessary estrogens, progesterone, and gonadotropin to sustain pregnancy and trigger other endocrine adjustments that involve primarily the pituitary, adrenal cortex, and thyroid. Fetal endocrine function is regulated independently from the mother, but endocrine or hormonal drugs, such as birth control pills, progestin, diethylstilbestrol (DES), androgens, and synthetic estrogen, that are given to the mother may produce undesirable effects in the fetus.[125-129]

Animal research indicates that later sexual characteristics and behaviour may be affected by administration of or presence or absence of sex hormones during fetal development. *The fetal period is the first critical period for sexual differentiation.* Although the fetus has a chromosomal combination denoting male or female, the fetus must be exposed to corresponding hormones during pregnancy. If the male fetus is insensitive to androgen (a hormone that promotes male sex characteristics) and exposed to large amounts of estrogen (a feminizing hormone), the child may possess many female characteristics.[130-132] Testicular inductor substance causes production of fetal androgens that suppress anatomic precursors of the oviducts and ovaries and, in turn, cause the

male genital tract to develop during the seventh to twelfth weeks. The male embryo's testosterone offsets the maternal hormone influences. Unless androgens are present, the external genitalia of the fetus will appear female regardless of the chromosomal pattern. Estrogens are released in the genetically female embryo and are necessary for the fetus to develop female genitalia. Likewise, inspection of the external genitalia of a newborn female may show abnormal fusion of the labia and enlargement of the clitoris caused by an androgen agent taken by the mother early in her pregnancy.[133]

The second critical period for sexual differentiation occurs just before or after birth, when sex typing of the brain may occur. Testosterone may influence the hypothalamus so that a noncyclic pattern for release of pituitary hormones, the gonadotropin, will occur in males and a cyclic pattern of gonadotropin release will occur in females.[134]

Fetal and placental growth, nourishment, waste excretion, and total function are dependent on the adequacy of the mother's metabolism.[135,136]

Maternal hyperglycemia or diabetes promotes transfer of excessive glucose across the placenta to the fetus, stimulating fetal insulin secretion, a potent growth factor.[137-139] The diabetic mother is at high risk, as is her fetus. These infants have three to four times the incidence of congenital malformations as in the general population.[140] The metabolic stress of fetal hyperinsulinism continues to increase anomalies, such as congenital malformations and disorders of fetal growth and pulmonary development. The metabolic stress of fetal hyperinsulinism apparently contributes to increased anomalies (e.g., obesity of the newborn).[141-143] Many fetal metabolic defects can now be diagnosed.[144] Congenital heart defects are the most common.[145,146] Careful regulation of maternal glycemia through therapy with insulin and diet is often warranted.[147] As most of the anomalies occur in the first few weeks of pregnancy, strict glycemia control beginning before conception appears to be mandated.

Maternal Nutrition

Nutrition is a most important variable for the maintaining of fetal health and for the prevention of prenatal and intrapartum complications. In fact, the physiological changes of pregnancy call for extra nutrients and energy to meet the demands of the expanding blood supply and factors. These other factors include: the growth of maternal tissues, a developing fetus, and the loss of maternal tissues at birth, as well as preparation for lactation.[148] Women, even before pregnancy, should follow *Canada's Food Guide to Healthy Eating* (available at Health Canada's website at www.hc-sc.gc.ca/hpfb-dgpsa/onpp-bppn/food_guide_rainbow_e.html). These guidelines organize foods into four major food groups: (1) grain products, (2) vegetables and fruits, (3) milk products, and (4) meat and alternatives. These guidelines give direction regarding the amount and selections of foods which individuals need each day. The *Food Guide* recommendations are flexible enough to be adapted for age, gender, activity level, and pregnancy.[149]

As a matter of interest, the *Food Guide* has many strengths, including simplicity, flexibility, visual appeal, widespread awareness, and consistency with current science. A draft plan to revise the *Food Guide* was developed early in

2004. The revised *Food Guide* will be an even more useful tool for Canadians, as it promotes a pattern of eating based on meeting nutrient needs, promoting health, and minimizing the risk of nutrition-related disease.[150] A *Cultural Adaptation of Canada's Food Guide to Healthy Eating* exists for use by culturally diverse individuals and families. This guide features culturally specific foods and full-colour illustrations (see the Interesting Websites section at the end of the chapter). A *Northwest Territories Food Guide* is also available and may be accessed on the Web through the Health Canada website.

The Dietary Reference Intakes (DRIs) are a comprehensive set of nutrient reference values for healthy populations that can be utilized to assess and plan diets.[151] They are based on the amount of vitamins, minerals, and other substances (such as fibre) that an individual needs—not only to prevent deficiencies, but to lower the risk of chronic disease. The DRIs were established by Canadian and American scientists through a review process overseen by the National Academy of Sciences, which is an independent, nongovernmental body.[152] Health Canada uses the DRIs in policies and programs that benefit the health and safety of Canadians.

CRITICAL THINKING

Who are the users of the Dietary Reference Intakes (DRIs)?

(Check the Web for the Using the Dietary Reference Intakes, at the Health Canada site.)

Regarding gestational weight gain and pregnancy outcomes, current recommendations suggest weight gain ranges based on pre-pregnancy Body Mass Index (BMI). The BMI is an index of weight-to-height (kg/m^2). The BMI is the most useful indicator to date of health risks associated with overweight and underweight individuals:[153]

- *Pre-pregnancy BMI under 20:* Low pre-pregnancy weight is a critical determinant of intrauterine growth retardation and premature birth. Pregnant women with a low pre-pregnancy BMI should be referred to a registered dietician/nutritionist for dietary assessment and counselling. The weight gain by the woman should be monitored each visit.[154]
- *Pre-pregnancy BMI between 20 and 27:* Healthy-weight women are at lowest risk for giving birth to either a low-birth-weight baby or a high-birth-weight baby. Women with pre-pregnancy weight in this range should gain between 11.5 kg and 16.0 kg overall, or approximately 0.4 kg per week during the second and third trimesters.[155]
- *Pre-pregnancy BMI above 27:* Women with a high BMI are more likely to develop gestational diabetes mellitus and to give birth to high-birth-weight infants, defined as over 4000 g. Although mean birth weights have been increasing, the differences between the proportions of babies over 4000 g in the First Nations population and the general population remains significant.[156] Pregnant women with a BMI over 27 should be referred to a registered dietician/nutritionist for dietary assessment and counselling.[157] Encourage women to gain between 7.0 and 11.5 kg overall, approximately 0.3 kg per week. A suggestion can be made for them to optimize the quality of eating patterns rather than to "diet" to restrict weight gain.[158]

TABLE 6-3
Guidelines for Gestational Weight Gain Ranges (1, adapted from the IOM)

BMI Category*	Recommended Total Gain	
	kg	lb.
BMI >20	12.5–18.0	28–40
BMI 20 – 27	11.5–16.0	25–35
BMI >27	7.0–11.5	15–25

Canadian BMI categories for Healthy Weights, established in 1988 by Health Canada, correspond closely although not exactly to the BMI categories used by the United States Institute of Medicine (IOM).

(1). IOM categories for BMI are low: <19.8; normal/healthy: 19.8–26; high: >26–29. These guidelines do not apply to multiple gestations.

Refer to Table 6–3 for guidelines for gestational weight gain ranges.

CRITICAL THINKING

What may be some contributing factors for the occurrence of high BMI rates among First Nation mothers?

Scientists know that at least 60 nutrients are basic to maintenance of healthy growth and development.[159,160] Lack of these nutrients may contribute to the following:

1. Depressed appetite in the mother.
2. Disease in the mother and in the baby.
3. Low birth weight.
4. Infant prematurity.
5. Congenital malformation.
6. Intrauterine growth retardation (IUGR), with consequent lower number of brain cells, mental retardation.
7. Infant mortality.[161–163]

For example, anemic mothers have average lower-birth-weight infants than nonanemic mothers.[164] During the first two months of pregnancy, the developing embryo consists mostly of water; later more solids in the form of fat, nitrogen, and certain minerals are added. Because of the small amount of yolk in the human ovum, growth depends on nutrients obtained from the mother.[165] Although nutritional requirements for the embryo/fetus are quantitatively small during the first trimester, nutritional deprivations can negatively impact placental structure and the ultimate birth weight. For example, lack of vitamin A, as well as folate and iron, is linked to growth retardation, whereas supplements of calcium and magnesium may increase birth weight and length of gestation.[166] As for folate, evidence suggests that a daily supplement containing folic acid (a form of folate) is important to be taken during the periconceptual period. Folic acid reduces the risk of neural tube defects.[167] It is important to note that taking a supplement containing folic acid does not preclude the need to eat a healthy diet in accordance with *Canada's Food Guide to Healthy Eating*. In 1998, Health Canada made the addition of folic acid to flour and bread mandatory.[168]

CRITICAL THINKING

What are alternate food sources of folic acid?

Caloric and *protein* intake are of particular importance. Calories are needed for cell multiplication, and protein is believed to be primarily related to enlargement of these cells. Therefore, failure of the cells to receive sufficient protein and calories during critical periods of growth can lead to slowing down and ultimate cessation of the ability of these cells to enlarge, divide, and develop specialized functions. Lack of protein also affects later intellectual performance. Further, sufficient calories from fats and carbohydrates are needed so that protein is not used for energy.[169,170]

Caloric requirements for pregnant woman suggest that women should increase daily energy intake by approximately 100 kcal (400 kj) in the first trimester and 300 kcal (1300 kj) in the second and third trimesters. Of course, energy requirements depend on basal metabolic rate and activity patterns, which vary markedly between individuals.[171] Normally, women in the first trimester gain between 1.0 and 3.5 kg. Women who lose weight during the first trimester should be carefully assessed. Women with large weight gain, particularly those women with a pre-pregnancy BMI over 27, should be assessed. Their weight gain should be approximately 0.3 kg per week. For women with a BMI under 20, larger weight gains in the first trimester may be desirable.[172] It is important to emphasize that most women can achieve normal weight gain by following *Canada's Food Guide to Healthy Eating*, and by emphasizing nutrient-dense and lower-fat food choices. After the first trimester, the weight gain is usually steady and increased, indicating a gain of lean and fat tissues.[173] Patterns of either weight gain or loss must be evaluated thoroughly throughout the pregnancy.

Notably, low maternal weight at conception and little weight gain during pregnancy are associated with delivering a child who has low birth weight (less than 2500 g). Low birth weight is associated with neonatal morbidity, mortality, and developmental problems.[174] Excessive gestational weight gain may be associated with high birth weight (defined as more than 4000 g). The possible consequences of gestational weight gain and high birth weight may include prolonged labour and birth, induced hypertension, gestational diabetes, birth asphyxia, birth trauma, caesarean birth, and increased risk of perinatal mortality.[175,176]

Protein requirements are 1.5 g/kg of body weight daily for the pregnant woman, compared with the usual 1 g/kg daily.

More protein is needed for growth and repair of the fetus, placenta, uterus, and breasts and for increased maternal blood volume. High-protein diets have not demonstrated improvement in birth weight and are not recommended prenatally.[177]

Minerals, especially *calcium* and *phosphorus,* follow protein as the next most essential requirement. Calcium is deposited mostly in the fetus during the last month of gestation; a good supply (1000 to 1300 mg/day) must be stored from the early months of pregnancy to meet the demand for skeletal development and to minimize the depletion of maternal reserves.[178,179] Vitamin D is also essential. When the diet does not provide sufficient calcium and vitamin D, and sun exposure is limited, effort must be directed at increasing the dietary intake of these nutrients. Vitamin D is needed for calcium absorption.[180] Calcium and vitamin D supplements may be necessary for some women. The best sources of calcium are dairy products: milk, cheese, and yogurt.[181]

The recommended intake of phosphorus, sodium, zinc, iodine (via iodized salt), magnesium, potassium, and fluoride remains essentially unchanged during pregnancy. Substantial decreases in minerals can predispose the offspring to debilitating conditions; for example, profound zinc deficiency can cause dwarfism and prevent brain development, and severe iodine deficiency can lead to endemic cretinism, characterized by multiple severe neurological defects and inadequate physical and mental growth. Most diets that supply sufficient calories for appropriate weight gain also supply adequate minerals if iodized salt is used. Salt should not be restricted unless edema develops.

Iron intake should be doubled by supplementation *during pregnancy because the maternal blood volume may double* as a result of increases in both plasma and erythrocytes. In addition, almost one-fourth of the maternal iron is transferred to the placenta and fetus. These iron requirements are more prominent during the last two trimester periods of gestation.[182–184] Supplementation with 30 mg is recommended during the second and third trimesters.[185] Iron is beneficial during the last three to four months of pregnancy in building and protecting maternal reserves and preventing iron deficiency anemia, which predisposes the newborn to growth retardation, being underweight, and congenital defects. Most diets will not supply enough iron for the pregnant woman, and most women have only a marginal iron store in the body before pregnancy. For optimal absorption, take iron on an empty stomach or with juice, rather than with a meal. Too much iron can interfere with zinc absorption.[186–188]

NARRATIVE VIGNETTE
High Gestational Weight Client

Jean is four months pregnant with her first child. Her pre-pregnancy BMI was high (over 27). Since her last visit to the prenatal clinic she has gained weight—more than the recommended 0.3 kg per week. She informs you that she "hates milk" and that she has been drinking milkshakes as a source of calcium.

1. What nutritional counselling does Jean need?
2. What better sources of calcium can you suggest for Jean?
3. What risks of high gestational weight gain, and a possible high-birth-weight baby, might you share with Jean?

Folic acid supplementation is used to prevent fetal malformations, especially neural tube defects, and maternal anemia. Health Canada indicates that abundant folic acid needs to be available in early gestation while the neural tube is closing—from 21 to 28 days after conception.[189] Folic acid (folate) is also necessary to build new cells and genetic material and to prevent growth retardation.[190] A supplement containing 0.4 mg in conjunction with the folate present in balanced diets can help reduce the risk of neural tube defects (NTD) among women with no family history of NTD. A folic acid supplement taken throughout pregnancy will help to meet the additional needs for fetal development.[191]

An adequate intake of *vitamins* acquired through foods affects normal metabolism. Vitamin and mineral supplements are necessary but should not be substituted for food.[192,193] Extra intake of *Vitamins B_{12} and B_6* is needed for the extra plasma demands during pregnancy. *Vitamin B_6* also helps protein to make new body cells. Extra intake of the *B vitamins, thiamine, riboflavin, and niacin,* are needed to use the energy from food eaten.[194]

The requirement for *vitamin C* increases by one third; a reasonable diet can supply this amount. Large doses of vitamin C can interfere with vitamin B_{12} absorption and metabolism.[195] As a vitamin C source, orange juice should be taken in moderation because of the emetic effect related to hyperacidity.

Effects of inadequate nutrition are most severe for the pregnant adolescent, who herself has growth requirements. Nutritional deficiencies of the mother during her own fetal and childhood periods contribute to structural and physiologic difficulties in supporting a fetus. Improvement of the pregnant woman's diet when she has previously been poorly nourished does not appreciably benefit the fetus. *The fetus apparently draws most of its raw materials for development from maternal body structure and lifetime reserves.*[196–199] You have a significant role in teaching proper nutrition to children and adolescents.

The small or growth-retarded fetus and premature infant has a much greater illness and death rate compared with its normal counterpart. The long-term cost of some survivors illuminates the importance of prevention and prediction of pregnancies with fetal growth problems. **Better education and nutrition to promote healthy pregnancies and use of ultrasound to safely monitor and manage cases at risk can improve pregnancy outcomes.**[200] Ultrasound assesses gestational age, fetal size, fetal structure, and fetal function.[201]

It is important for pregnant women to include a sufficient amount of the essential fatty acids linoleic and alpha-linolenic acid (one of the omega-3 fatty acids) in their daily diets. Omega-3 fatty acids are important to ensure neural and visual function development in the fetus.[202]

CRITICAL THINKING

What is a source of omega-3 fatty acid?

Anemia. The effects of maternal anemia on the fetus are less clear than those on the mother. Anemia denotes a decrease in the oxygen-carrying capability of the blood, which is directly related to a reduction in hemoglobin concentration and number of red blood cells. The normal mean hemoglobin is 140g/L (SD 20g/L) for women. Clients whose hemoglobin count falls two standard deviations (SD) below the mean should be considered anemic.[203]

Iron deficiency anemia (IDA) accounts for 75% of all the anemia diagnosed during pregnancy. The extra iron requirements of pregnancy are needed for the fetus and placenta and to expand the maternal hemoglobin mass.[204,205] The developing fetus may not suffer severe ill effects of the mother's decreased iron supply if its own hemoglobin production is maintained at a normal level (i.e., if the placental source of iron is of sufficient amounts for the fetus to establish and maintain normal hemoglobin levels).[206] Willows and her colleagues assessed the prevalence of anemia and the associated risk factors among nine-month-old Cree infants in Northern Quebec. They found that iron-deficiency anemia is highly prevalent among the James Bay Cree infants.[207] Another study was conducted with Inuit infants in Nunavik, the northern part of the province of Quebec. These results indicated that iron-deficiency anemia was a problem in Inuit infants as young as six months of age. The researchers concluded that breastfed infants were better protected against iron deficiency anemia than were infants fed cow's milk or low-iron formula.[208]

Sickle cell anemia in the mother, associated with sickle cell disease, which is seen predominantly among blacks, may show a number of negative effects on the developing fetus. Changes in the mother's pathophysiologic state may lead to intrauterine growth retardation, premature labour, a reduction of 250 to 500 g in average birth weight, and even stillbirth, related to the "sickling" or clumping of misshaped erythrocytes within the placental vascular system.[209–213]

Pica. One nutritional tradition is pica—a craving to eat nonfood substances, such as clay, unprocessed flour, cornstarch, laundry starch, coal, soap, toothpaste, mothballs, petrol, tar, paraffin, wood, plaster, soil, chalk, charcoal, cinders, baking powder, baking soda, powdered bricks, and refrigerator frost scrapes. Pica is common in children and women of all cultures who are hungry, poor, malnourished, and desire something to chew.[214–216] Pica is a concern, first, because nonfood items may displace nutritious foods, and secondly, toxic or parasitic substances may be consumed.[217] Pica is usually associated with iron deficiency, whether anemia is the cause or the cause is unknown. Certainly pica interferes with normal nutrition by reducing appetite and can be harmful to baby and mother. Some types of clay interfere with the absorption of iron, zinc, and potassium.[218–222] Women who practise pica are often ashamed of the compulsion and hesitate either to admit to the practice or to share their concern.[223]

CRITICAL THINKING

What may be some health-promoting strategies for women with pica?

Environmental Hazards to the Fetus: Teratogenic Effects
Teratogen. A teratogen is an environmental substance or agent that interrupts normal development and causes malformation.

Teratogenesis is development of abnormal structures. Teratogenesis is time-specific; the stimulus is nonspecific; timing is more important than the nature of the insult or negative stimulus. The first trimester is the most critical. Development is characterized by a precise order; the timing, intensity, and duration of insult, injury, teratogen, or abnormal stimulus or event is important for the consequence. Teratogenic agents affect genes in several ways: (1) genes cease protein production so that development ceases, (2) genes fail to complete the development they have begun, or (3) excess growth of part of the organism occurs.[224,225]

Prominent environmental factors that have potential for damaging the fetus include radiation; chemical wastes; contaminated water; heavy metals, such as lead; some food additives; various pollutants; chemical interactions; nicotine from smoking tobacco; pica; medicinal and nonmedicinal drugs; alcohol; maternal and paternal infections; and maternal stress. The timing of fetal contact with a specific teratogen is a crucial factor (see Figures 6–1 and 6–2). Susceptibility to teratogens, in general, decreases as organ formation advances.[226] For instance, a teratogen introduced into the system of an embryo between three and eight weeks of gestation, when principal body systems are being established, is likely to do much more harm than if it came in contact with the same conceptus during the third or eighth month. During the implantation period when the fertilized ovum lies free within the uterus and uses uterine secretions as its nutrition source, teratogens can cause spontaneous abortion of the embryo or severe birth defects.

Once implantation has occurred (seven or eight days after fertilization), the embryo undergoes very rapid and important transformations for the next four weeks. The sequence of embryonic events shows that each organ (brain, heart, eye, limbs, and genitalia) undergoes a critical stage of differentiation at precise times. For example, during the third week, teratogens can harm basic structures of the heart and central nervous system. During the individual critical periods, the embryo is highly vulnerable to teratogens, producing specific gross malformations. Each teratogen acts on a selected aspect of cellular metabolism.[227–231] Even during the third trimester, fetal cerebral vascular reaction to certain teratogens can be detrimental.[232–234]

There is no evidence that congenital malformations will always be produced when a teratogen is present, for the embryo has the inherent capacity to replace damaged cells with newly formed cells. However, the higher the dose (intensity), the more harmful influences that are present, and the longer the exposure, the greater the chance that the baby will be harmed and that the harm will be more severe than if dose and duration are less. Further, the biogenetic vulnerability of the mother and infant influence the effects of a teratogen.[235]

In many malformations, a genetic predisposition combined with a teratogen is required to produce an abnormality.[236] A substance can have adverse effects on the central nervous system but not on normal development of limbs. A teratogen may cause a variety of gross anomalies; a few show a preferential action on specific organs. For example, thalidomide anomalies are characterized by skeletal malformation; no other form of growth retardation is noted.[237–240]

A complicated interplay exists among the father, mother, offspring, and teratogen. In addition to the critical period of developmental stage and genetic susceptibility, the degree to which a teratogen causes abnormalities depends on its dosage, absorption, distribution, metabolism, physical state of the mother, and excretion by the separate body systems of mother and fetus. A teratogen that enters a mother's system also enters the system of her developing child, meaning that the so-called *placental barrier is practically nonexistent.*[241–243]

External Environmental Factors. Prenatally, environmental teratogens may interfere with the development of the embryo or fetus directly or may cause hormonal, circulatory, or nutritional changes in the mother that in turn damage the organism. Examples include the following:[244–252]

- Excess heat, soaks in hot tubs, or sauna baths in early pregnancy, which may cause fetal neural-tube defects
- High levels of noise
- Crowding and the consequent stressors
- Radiation from multiple sources at work or from diagnostic tests—most procedures cause low-level fetal x-ray exposure if performed accurately, but the pregnant woman should inform diagnosticians
- Ultraviolet light from excessive sun or a sunlamp
- Air, water, and soil pollutants, including lead, mercury, and pesticides or chemicals
- Trace minerals or chemicals linked to the work setting
- Chemicals and drugs in food
- Chemotherapeutic (anti-neoplastic) medications

Depending on dosage, radiation can be responsible for cell destruction that is linked to embryonic death, gross malformations, growth retardation, and an increased risk of malignancy in later life.[253]

Occupational hazards include transfer of drugs and chemicals from the male to the female during intercourse—an action that later can negatively affect fertilization or implantation or, if the woman is already pregnant, can have teratogenic effects on the developing person. For example, decreased sperm count and infertility are related to paternal exposure to dibromochloropropane (DBCP).[254] Paternal exposure to toxic agents is most likely to result in male infertility or spontaneous abortions. Anaesthetic gases, vinyl chloride exposure, chloroprene, or other hydrocarbons have all been connected to spontaneous abortions. Lead present in the environment directly increases sperm abnormalities, induces male infertility, and facilitates spontaneous abortion through either affected sperm or indirect contamination.[255] Persistent environmental contaminants, such as dioxin and polychlorobiphenyls (PCBs), alter the activities of several different hormones.[256]

CRITICAL THINKING

In what ways can paternal exposure to toxins cause birth defects? (Check Community Health Services.[257])

Occupational hazards may also include the effects of physical effort or activity. In a study in southern Sweden

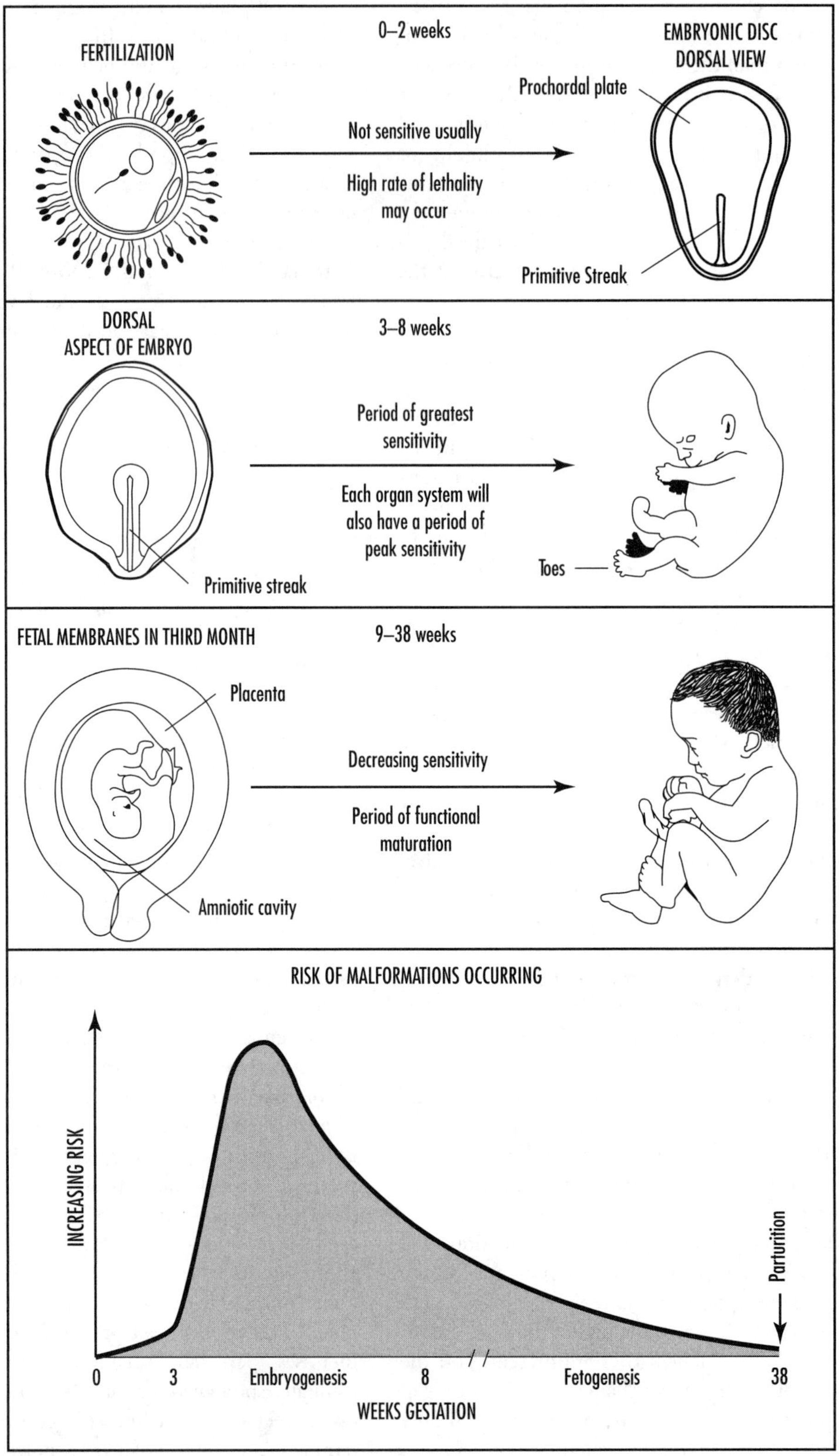

FIGURE 6-1

Periods of susceptibility to teratogens.

Source: Sadler, T.W., Langman's Medical Embryology (5th ed.). Baltimore: Williams & Wilkins, 1985.

comparing pregnant manual workers with nonmanual workers, there were no differences in outcomes of pregnancy.[258] However, a survey of 1470 nurses found that strenuous working conditions, occupation fatigue, and long working hours may be associated with a greater risk of premature birth.[259]

Certain kinds of jobs may also predispose to spontaneous abortion because of contact with chemicals. For example, women who work with chemicals used in manufacturing semiconductor chips have about twice the rate of miscarriage as other female workers. There is no conclusive evidence that

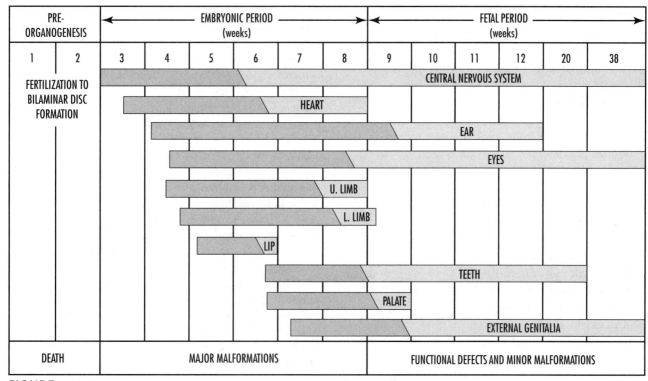

FIGURE 6–2

Susceptibility of organ systems to teratogens. Solid bars denote highly sensitive periods.

Source: Sadler, T.W., Langman's Medical Embryology *(5th ed.) Baltimore: Williams & Wilkins, 1985.*

physical activity via employment promotes preterm birth and low birth weight, although causes could include prolonged standing, long working hours, high speed, bending, and lifting heavy objects. Health care providers should be sensitive to the presence of occupational fatigue associated with workload during pregnancy.[260–263]

Contaminants that are passed from mother to baby during the prenatal period can alter a child's immune system, increasing the risk of cancer, infectious disease, and autoimmune disorders. Exposure to agricultural pesticides and industrial chemicals can cause abnormalities in the reproductive system, causing infertility. Playing in lead-contaminated dust can disrupt brain development, causing attention and learning disorders, and possibly aggressive and antisocial behaviour.[264] Studies of the effects of pesticides in agricultural regions show a higher rate of birth defects in the children of both farming and nonfarming families.[265]

Rates of brain tumours and leukemia in children have been steadily increasing for the past 25 years. Toxic exposure during certain critical periods of pregnancy may cause genetic damage. Then, as the child's immune system develops by around age two, the damaged cell causes leukemia. Social mobility may also be a factor. A child who enters a new community encounters a new array of infectious agents. The immune system working to defend itself may produce a bad cell that multiplies out of control, causing cancer. Chlorinated solvents and domestic pesticides are also associated with brain cancers.[266]

Low-level exposure to industrial chemicals, such as PCBs and the organophosphate and carbonate pesticides, can alter brain development; other pesticides, industrial chemicals,

plastic food containers, and plastic toys can be a hazard because many synthetic chemicals mimic and disrupt the body hormones that are involved in development. PCBs were banned in 1976, but they persist and are still evident in the environment and are stored in the body fats of animals and humans.[267,268] Ayotte and his research team conducted a study to investigate factors influencing plasma PCB levels in Inuit infants during their first year of life. One of their findings indicated that exposure to these lipophilic compounds, through breastfeeding, has a major and long-lasting influence on the offspring's body burden.[269] That is, the infants were affected by the PCBs in breast milk.

Mercury, like lead, has major implications for health of the mother and offspring. Mercury-contaminated water results from medical wastes, industrial by-products, incinerator emissions, and dumpsite leakage. Inorganic mercury converts to the more harmful organic form, methyl mercury, which is absorbed by fish and then consumed by humans. When ingested during pregnancy, nervous system impairment, compromised immune function, and a congenital syndrome similar to cerebral palsy may occur.[270]

Smoking Tobacco. The Canadian Tobacco Use Monitoring Survey (CTUMS) results from the first half of 2003 indicate that the prevalence rate of smoking among youth 15–19 years has dropped below 20% for the first time.[271] The trend among Canadians over age 15 years who reported that they smoke has continued to track slightly downwards. Not only are fewer Canadians smoking, but they are smoking fewer cigarettes (15.7 cigarettes per day).[272] However, we must continue informing the public about the harmful effects of smoking.

Smoking is associated with numerous detrimental effects:

- Decreased maternal pulmonary function; increased carbon monoxide levels[273–275]
- Vasoconstriction in mother, reducing blood flow to fetus[276–278]
- Abnormal bleeding during pregnancy[279–281]
- Decreased fetal oxygen, lower oxygen tension, and fetal apnea or hypoxia from nicotine and cotinine transfer through placenta[282,283]
- Reduced fetal hemoglobin from carbon monoxide that crosses placenta[284,285]
- Higher percentage of spontaneous abortions, stillbirths, and preterm or premature births (decreased gestational age)[286–290]
- Structural defects, cleft palate, limb malformations[291]
- Lower birth weight (less than 2.5 kg or 5.5 pounds), as number of cigarettes smoked daily increase[292–296]
- Higher perinatal mortality for infant at every level of birth weight[297,298]
- Increased possibility of sudden infant death syndrome (SIDS)[299–301]
- Later growth retardation in child related to carbon monoxide effects[302–306]
- Slight retardation in learning skills (reading, mathematics) in child[307,308]
- Increased respiratory disease, pneumonia, bronchitis, and allergy in infancy and childhood[309–311]
- Decreased physical and social development in young children of mothers who smoke 10 or more cigarettes daily[312]
- Childhood cancer linked to prenatal smoking by mother or exposure to smoking by others (passive smoking)
- Poor attention span, hyperactivity, slower perceptual-motor and linguistic development, learning difficulties, and minimal brain dysfunction in school-age children[313–319]

Although data on smoking related to pregnancy are usually collected via self-report, a more accurate method is to measure the cotinine level in either maternal or umbilical serum. Although the mother's level of antenatal attachment to the fetus is a significant predictor of her decrease in alcohol consumption, such a relationship is not found for smoking cessation, suggesting that psychological and physiologic dependence on nicotine may override the effect of an emotional attachment of pregnant woman to her developing fetus.[320] The evidence clearly shows the association between smoking and pregnancy outcomes. Ideally, women should stop smoking prior to conception. Maximum reduction of risk is believed to occur if the women who smoke quit smoking by 16 weeks gestation. However, quitting smoking at any stage of gestation is advisable.[321]

Johnson and her colleagues conducted a study with women who quit smoking during pregnancy and who gave birth at one of five hospitals. These participating women were interviewed six months after delivery and were assessed using biochemical methods to determine their smoking status.[322] The objective of the study was to test a program developed to prevent smoking relapse in the postpartum period by comparing the rates of continuous smoking abstinence, daily smoking, and smoking cessation self-efficacy in treatment and control groups. The researchers concluded that smoking cessation interventions centring on the prenatal period have failed to achieve long-term abstinence. These same researchers continue to claim that interventions can be strengthened if they are extended into the postpartum period.[323]

A Canadian Nurses Association position statement on tobacco—*The Role of Health Professionals in Smoking Cessation*—was developed cooperatively across many health care professional disciplines. Because health professionals are in a unique position to assist smokers, this position statement focuses on smoking cessation as part of a comprehensive strategy.[324] The relapse rate is very high due to two powerful variables—the addictive nature of tobacco, and social pressures on the smoker. However, most smokers attempt to quit several times before they finally succeed.[325]

Health education for pregnant smokers increases the rate of quitting; counselling and information are effective and cost beneficial.[326] Smoking cessation programs range from self-help to structured interventions. For males, cigarette advertisements continue to link smoking with virility; however a growing body of research links smoking with lowered birth weight as well as reduced sperm count and abnormal sperm shape.[327,328] Large doses of marijuana smoke produce the same effect. This may explain why men who smoke have higher infertility rates.[329,330]

CRITICAL THINKING

What steps can a nurse take to develop a smoking cessation program in the community?

Drug Hazards to the Fetus: Teratogenic Effects

New drugs are almost never tested in pregnant women to determine the effects on the fetus. As a result, most drugs are not labelled for use in pregnancy. Many agents may cause toxic rather than teratogenic effects.[331] All of a woman's medications should be reviewed by her physician with regard to the optimal dosage.[332] The Motherisk site (http://www.motherisk.org) is an up-to-date source for evidence-based information about the safety or risk of drugs during pregnancy.[333]

CRITICAL THINKING

What health promotion strategies would you use for a pregnant client who is using an antidepressant called lorazepam?

6-1 BONUS SECTION IN CD-ROM

Drugs That Cross the Placenta

The placenta acts like a sieve, not a barrier. A handy list of medications to avoid, unless medically prescribed, starts this section. A comment on certain cytotoxic drugs follows; and a similar treatment of sex hormones and oral contraceptives follows. Sedatives, barbiturates, and opiates are considered as well.

Drug Abuse and Addiction. During pregnancy, drug abuse and addiction continue to manifest themselves as major psychosocial and physical problems for both mother and child. Substances commonly abused during pregnancy, taken individually or in combination, are known to have multiple effects on the developing person, on the outcome of pregnancy, and on neonatal neurobehaviour.[334] Infants exposed to addictive drugs in utero throughout pregnancy are at great risk for a higher rate of congenital malformations, obstetric complications, and perinatal mortality.[335–338]

These *addictive* drugs include amphetamines, barbiturates, cocaine (includes "crack" and "ice," potent and purified versions), ethchlorvynol (Placidyl), heroin, meperidine hydrochloride (Demerol), methadone, morphine, pentazocine hydrochloride (Talwin), propoxyphene hydrochloride, phencyclidine (known as "angel dust") (PCP), tetrahydrocannabinol (THC) (or marijuana), and methamphetamine.[339] Drugs that act on the central nervous system are often lipophilic and have relatively low-molecular-weight characteristics, which facilitate crossing of the so-called placental–fetal blood–brain barrier.[340] Some drugs can be metabolized by the fetal liver and placenta; however, these metabolites are water soluble.[341,342]

Marijuana, when used by the mother, affects the embryo, fetus, and the child after birth. Low birth weight, premature delivery, small size for gestational age, and various malformations, including chromosomal abnormalities, occur more often than the norm. At birth, the baby is likely to have a depressed Apgar score (see Chapter 7) and neuromuscular abnormalities. Following birth, weight loss is accelerated. There has been a linkage found with acute lymphoblast leukemia in the young child.[343]

Addictive drugs, such as cocaine, heroin, morphine, and codeine, affect mother and baby because they (1) affect the mother's overall health and nutrition, (2) often interfere with motivation to obtain prenatal care, and (3) interfere with blood flow to the placenta by means of vasoconstriction and increasing uterine contractibility. *Cocaine, the most devastating,* acts peripherally to inhibit nerve conduction and prevent norepinephrine uptake at nerve terminals, increasing norepinephrine levels, with subsequent vasoconstriction and abrupt rise in blood pressure. This effect is greater than with use of opiates. The drugs cause a *high incidence of obstetric complications* such as:[344–350]

1. Hypertension
2. Spontaneous abortion
3. Lack of sufficient maternal weight gain
4. Intrauterine growth retardation
5. Toxemia
6. Abruptio placenta
7. Shorter gestation period, premature birth
8. Stillbirth, breech delivery
9. Postpartum hemorrhage

These drugs cause a *high incidence of the following complications at birth and in the* **neonatal** *(newborn) period*:[351–358]

1. Fetal growth retardation
2. Lower birth weight
3. Shorter body length
4. Smaller head circumference
5. Cardiopulmonary abnormalities
6. Tachycardia and hypertension, causing cerebrovascular hemorrhage; computed tomographic (CT) scan of the neonate can confirm presence of acute focal cerebral infarction
7. Perceptual and motor impairments that continue long-term to affect the child's learning.

Use of cocaine, in its various forms, continues to increase and includes women of childbearing age (from teens to 40s), and people of all socioeconomic levels, especially the middle class and wealthy. Koren states that exposure to cocaine, determined by hair analysis, is associated with extensive perinatal risk. In fact, if cocaine exposure were not detected through hair tests, most of the cocaine-exposed infants would not only have perinatal complications, but would go home to be looked after by drug-dependent mothers, further increasing their health risk.[359]

CRITICAL THINKING

Who is at liberty to use the Motherisk Laboratory for Drug Exposure at the Hospital for Sick Children?

Children exposed to cocaine in the fetal state have an abnormally high incidence of "severe" physical and emotional problems, including the following:

- Brain shrinkage or cerebral atrophy
- Learning difficulties; impaired attention span
- Impaired orientation; decreased ability to orient to auditory and visual stimuli
- Growth retardation
- Severe impairments in motor movements, including simple movements such as eating, dressing, and non-nutritive sucking
- Irritability, impulsivity
- Tremors
- Sensitivity to sounds
- Disrupted rapid eye movement (REM) sleep patterns, affecting personality
- Various social personality difficulties
- Permanent physical and mental damage as a result of fetal anoxia or fetal or neonatal cerebrovascular hemorrhage

Addiction to narcotics, such as heroin, morphine, or codeine, can create another problem: fetal addiction. Withdrawing the drug from the addicted woman before delivery causes the fetus to experience withdrawal distress as a result of visceral vasoconstriction and reduced circulation to the uterus. Intrauterine death may occur. However, when addiction continues, the infant is born with drug addiction. The addicted newborn is twice as likely to die soon after birth as the non-addicted baby. If the newborn does not die, it will experience withdrawal in two to four days. This is the *acute* period. The baby may require up to 40 days of treatment during the *withdrawal* period. The limited ability of the newborn to

Neonatal Narcotic Abstinence Syndrome: Manifestations of Narcotic Withdrawal

Central Nervous System
(signs appear within first 24 hours)

- Hyperirritability
- Hyperactivity: hard to hold; failure to mould to mother's body
- Restlessness
- Incessant shrill cry
- Inability to sleep, disturbed REM sleep
- Hypertonia of muscles
- Hyperactive reflexes
- Stretching
- Tremors
- Poor temperature regulation; fever
- Possible generalized convulsions

Respiratory System

- Rapid irregular breathing
- Yawning
- Sneezing
- Nasal stuffiness, congestion
- Excessive secretions
- Intermittent cyanosis
- Respiratory alkalosis
- Periods of apnea

Cardiovascular System

- Tachycardia

Gastrointestinal System

- Frantic sucking of hands; disorganized sucking behaviour
- Difficulty sucking and feeding; poor closure of lips around nipple
- Appearance of being very hungry
- Sensitive gag reflex
- Regurgitation
- Vomiting
- Diarrhea
- Progressive weight loss

Skin

- Pallor
- Sweating
- Excoriation

Musculoskeletal System

- Small head size
- Short length

metabolize and eliminate these fat-soluble drugs may be responsible for postponement of withdrawal symptoms. However, the withdrawal does not end the problems. Babies born addicted to opiates may suffer effects of addiction until at least age six.[360,361]

The Brazelton Neonatal Behavioural Assessment Scale can be used to evaluate normality of responses to environmental stimuli.[362,363] Finnegan's Neonatal Narcotic Abstinence Syndrome (NSA) is useful for assessing neonatal withdrawal.[364] The specific pattern of symptoms is dependent on (1) the type, amount, and combination of drugs used by the mother, (2) the length of time between drug exposure and delivery, and (3) the fetal ability to metabolize the drug. See the box entitled "Neonatal Narcotic Abstinence Syndrome" for a list of the symptoms and signs that are typically observed in the neonate who has been addicted during pregnancy to cocaine, heroin, or another narcotic.[365–369]

The effect of addictive drugs on the child extends beyond the neonatal and infancy periods. In early childhood babies who were addicted may weigh less and be shorter than the norm, and overall be less well adjusted. These children score lower on perceptual and learning ability tests, are more anxious, and do not perform as well in school.[370–374]

Clinical assessment for substance abuse should include evaluation of physical appearance, since demeanour and hygiene may give clues; a thorough history and physical examination; and a substance abuse interview: a history may reveal multiple drug use or exposure to more than one teratogen. Urine samples of mothers are effective to screen for ingestion of illicit drugs.

Effects of drug use on the fetus, neonate, and child depend on the type of drug ingested, dose, duration of drug use before and during pregnancy, and state of maternal nutrition. There are fewer infant symptoms when the pregnant woman stops drug use in the first trimester of pregnancy than if drug use continues. Thus it is imperative to prevent drug use and to support the mother's efforts to stop drug use and to encourage adequate prenatal care and nutrition.[375,376]

Prenatal care must include increased surveillance for drug-related complications in coordinated, comprehensive, family-oriented drug treatment programs. Rehabilitation and support efforts should continue after delivery and address issues that lead to and maintain patterns of abuse.[377]

Alcohol. *Alcohol* ingested before or during pregnancy *serves as another* common cause of abnormal changes in the fetus and may increase perinatal mortality.[378]

Alcohol circulates to every tissue and through the placenta. The blood alcohol concentration (BAC) in the woman is influenced by the amount ingested, duration of drinking, body size, health, when food was last eaten, body metabolism, and genetic makeup. *The BAC is the same in the fetus as in the pregnant woman.* Alcohol is cleared from the woman's body in one to one-and-a-half hours; it takes about eight to 12 hours to be eliminated from the fetus. Both the first and third trimesters are critical periods, increasing the possibility of birth defects, fetal alcohol syndrome (FAS), premature labour, and obstetric complications.[379]

The *combination of alcohol and smoking may reduce birth weight to a substantial degree.*[380] New research finds that caffeine (found in coffee, cola, tea, chocolate) has no detrimental effect on birth weight, except in pregnant women who consume large amounts of alcohol (21 to 43 drinks per week). Cultural habits regarding smoking and the intake of alcohol and caffeinated beverages can explain the differences between levels of consumption reported for different countries.[381]

For women who are (or may become) pregnant, the smart choice is to totally abstain from alcohol.[382] In a study of 11 698 Danish women, alcohol consumption of more than 120 g per week was associated with a five times greater reduction in average birth weight in babies of smokers versus babies of nonsmokers.[383] Alcoholism in the father may inhibit spermatogenesis and also act as a teratogen that contributes to chromosomal breaks or damaged genes, resulting in spontaneous abortion or birth defects.[384] Even abstinence during the gestational period seems to be "too little, too late" for infants born to mothers who have had a history of heavy alcoholic intake before conception.

Prior to the introduction of the identification of fetal alcohol spectrum disorder (FASD), the conditions fetal alcohol syndrome (FAS) and fetal alcohol effects (FAE) were used solely to describe birth defects caused by maternal ingestion of alcohol.[385,386] It has been recorded that the rate of FAS/FAE in some First Nations and Inuit communities is much higher than the national average due to the history of colonization and the devaluation of culture.

FAS manifests itself through the following characteristics:[387–390]

- Low birth weight
- Small head
- Flat facial profile or deformity
- Ear and eye abnormalities
- Poor motor coordination
- Disturbed sleep patterns
- Extra digits
- Heart defects

FAE refers to the cognitive and behavioural problems of children exposed to alcohol while in utero but who lack the typical diagnostic characteristics of full-blown FAS.[391] Investigations of children with FAE have demonstrated that they will have better cognitive abilities than those with FAS, but their behavioural functions, such as poor social skills, have been termed secondary disabilities.[392] A number of ongoing health and developmental problems in the child are associated with alcohol consumption in the mother during pregnancy. Several of these include sluggish and weaker sucking in infancy, impaired gross and fine motor development, and lower overall school performance.[393–396]

Continued, regular use of alcohol by the mother who breastfeeds further impedes motor development of the infant.[397–399] Alcohol-induced damage to the developing brain encompasses a long developmental time frame, affects more cell populations, occurs at lower levels of exposure, produces greater numbers of permanent effects, and is modulated by more factors than were initially suspected in earlier studies.[400,401] Community education, treatment for the alcohol-abusing mother, parenting education, and early identification and intervention with the alcohol-affected child are essential.[402,403]

One of the recommendations to reduce the number of infants with FAS is to conduct further research into (1) discovering why some women drink alcohol so heavily during pregnancy, (2) assessing drinking patterns more effectively, and (3) assisting women to avoid the consumption of alcohol during pregnancy.[404]

The Canadian government has been highly instrumental in focusing on substance abuse. For example, the 1999 federal budget included special funding earmarked specifically to address the FAS/FAE issues.[405]

A recent Health Canada document entitled "Fetal Alcohol Spectrum Disorder: A Framework for Action" was produced in collaboration with many organizations and individuals nationwide.[406] **Fetal alcohol spectrum disorder (FASD)** is an umbrella term used increasingly to describe the spectrum of disabilities (and diagnoses) associated with prenatal exposure to alcohol. The diagnoses grouped under the FASD umbrella include fetal alcohol syndrome (FAS), partial FAS (pFAS), alcohol-related neurodevelopmental disorder, and alcohol-related birth defects. The FASD document not only encourages people to understand FASD, but includes the basic building blocks required for concerted action within communities, provinces, and territories, as well as within the federal government.[407] The document reflects the ideas and advice for the prevention of FASD and the treatment of those with the disability (see Figure 6–3); its five broad goals for action are as follows:

1. Increase public and professional awareness and understanding of FASD as well as the impact of alcohol use during pregnancy.
2. Develop and increase the capacity to identify and meet the needs of children, youth, adults, and families affected by FASD.
3. Create effective national screening, diagnostic, and data-reporting tools and approaches.
4. Expand the knowledge base and facilitate information exchange between people and professionals in all types of settings.
5. Increase commitment and support for action on FASD.

The Addictions Foundation of Manitoba, through the efforts of Zenon Lisakowski, Pat Hayward, and members of the Adult Education Service Team, has developed a *Participant Manual for Alcohol Related Birth Defects*. The manual's diagnostic criteria have been developed through the work of Dr. Ann Streissguth and her colleagues from the University of Washington and the University of Victoria. For more information regarding FASD, visit the Addictions Foundation of Manitoba's site at http://www.afm.mb.ca or call 1-866-877-0050.

CRITICAL THINKING

What types of questions (linear, convergent, divergent, and circular) can a health professional ask the family for the purpose of circumventing denial regarding prenatal alcohol exposure?

Maternal Infections: Hazardous Influence on the Fetus

The pregnant woman is more susceptible to infections. The placenta cannot screen out all infectious organisms; therefore, infectious diseases in the vaginal region can travel up to the

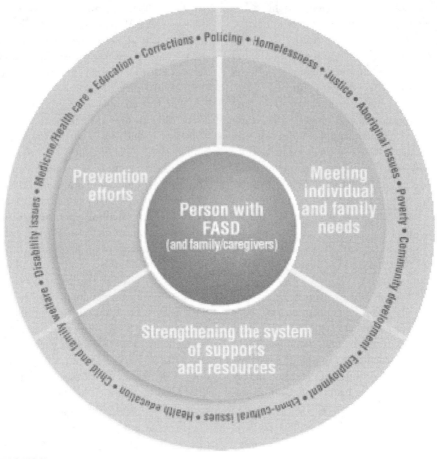

FIGURE 6–3

Setting the stage for future action on FASD. Individual and collaborative action is required in all sectors, at all levels—federal/national, provincial/territorial and community. Future effort needs to build on the excellent work done to date, focusing on prevention, meeting current needs of people with FASD, and strengthening and expanding the system of supports, services, and resources.

CONTROVERSY DEBATE

What Do You Do Now?

You have been invited to teach a preventative program on alcohol abuse to a classroom of 13- and 14-year-olds. After the presentation, a student approaches you. She informs you that her mother, a lone parent, became pregnant "accidentally." Her mother, the girl reports, is depressed and drinks a lot of alcohol. The girl pleads with you to come home with her right now to make her mother stop drinking.

1. With what decisions will you be faced in the next five minutes?

2. What are your professional and personal options?

3. How do you help this child?

---

amniotic sac and penetrate its walls and infect the amniotic fluid. Viral, bacterial, and parasitic diseases that have a mild effect on the mother may have a profound effect on the development of the fetus, depending on gestational age.[408]

Rubella (German measles) can manifest as a maternal infection that may occur during the first trimester with harmful effects. At the preconception visit, women at risk for rubella should be identified and, if not actively trying to become pregnant, should be immunized.[409] Rubella may go unnoticed by the mother, but it can cause severe effects and even death.[410–413] Screening by serology at the first prenatal visit is indicated. In fact, screening of serologic-negative women should be performed after exposure or if the women have a possible rubella infection. Women who have negative serology should be immunized postpartum.[414]

New cases of congenital rubella are fewer compared with years past; however, surviving victims of the epidemic continue to deal with its effects.[415] Amniocentesis can be used to detect the presence of rubella in utero.[416] The fetus suffers an abnormal decrease in the absolute number of cells in most organs because of the viral interference with cell multiplication. The virus also causes adverse changes in the small blood vessels of the developing fetus and does profuse damage to the placental vascular system as well, thus interfering with fetal blood flow and oxygenation.[417–419]

Rubeola ("red measles") is also associated with congenital defects. If a pregnant woman has been exposed to measles, and her immunity status is in doubt, she should be tested for measles antibodies. Immune globulin (0.25ml/kg for a healthy adult; 0.5 ml/kg if immuno-compromised) is recommended within six days of the last exposure to measles for several reasons: (1) if the client is immuno-compromised, (2) if measles immune status in unknown or questionable, and (3) if measles IgG serology is either negative or cannot be obtained before six days from the last exposure.[420] Immune globulin is not recommended if the woman was born before 1957, if she has had documented natural measles, or if she has had two doses of vaccine in a minimum of one month apart.[421]

HIV and **AIDS** in men and women is a worldwide concern because of transmission between sexual partners as well as in nonpartnered sexual relationships. The number of HIV-infected women of childbearing age is rising worldwide. Because of the long incubation period (at least five years), the pregnant woman may be unaware that she has the virus. Transmission appears more likely when the mother has full-blown AIDS than when she is HIV-positive but not yet experiencing AIDS symptoms. Infection may depend on the strain of virus to which the fetus is exposed.

Three concepts support the idea of offering HIV testing to every pregnant woman during pregnancy: (1) the increasing rates of HIV infection in women, (2) the devastating effect on the baby of vertical transmission from the mother, and (3) the proven efficacy of AZT in reducing vertical transmission.[422] Therefore, it is recommended that HIV testing be offered to all pregnant women. Women should be provided with basic information about HIV testing, which includes learning of the risks and benefits of discovering a positive result, and stressing the success of treatment in reducing vertical transmission.[423]

Katz states that the care for the pregnant woman who has HIV is highly complex.[424] It is important for health professionals to become aware of certain issues in caring for the woman. One such issue, due to the major focus on treatment, has been the reduction of the risk of perinatal transmission. Therefore, the decision to initiate drug therapy is important. Nurses must be aware of the dosage levels and adverse effects, and must help the woman deal with adherence issues.[425]

6-2 BONUS SECTION IN CD-ROM
Effects of Maternal Infection and Disease

An informative table cites the disease, the critical period for transmission, its effects on the embryo/fetus, and preventive measures. Eight different diseases are featured.

CRITICAL THINKING

What are some of the social aspects of HIV infection among pregnant women?

Screening of **syphilis** by serology at either the preconception or early pregnancy visit is indicated according to provincial and territorial regulations. For women at risk, a repeat test in the third trimester is indicated.[426] It is important that maternal syphilis be identified before or early in pregnancy to prevent devastating consequences for the neonate.[427] Poor prenatal care and lack of maternal treatment for syphilis contribute to these consequences.[428] Although necrosis of the umbilical cord (vein) is a clear indication that the newborn is infected, other symptoms may not appear until the 14th

week of life. Or the child may appear healthy at birth, with symptoms appearing in two to six weeks. Occasionally, symptoms may not appear for two years.[429,430] Treatment of the mother also ensures treatment of the ill fetus because penicillin or erythromycin readily crosses the placenta.

Chlamydia trachomatis and **gonorrhea** are two genital infections that are easily transmitted and can produce pelvic inflammatory disease (PID). For example, tubal adhesions resulting from PID are an important factor in the occurrence of ectopic pregnancies.[431] Both diseases affect the fetus and neonate. For chlamydia, health care professionals should offer screening to women who are believed to be at increased risk, such as women younger than 20, those with multiple sex partners (or who have partners with multiple sexual partners), and women with a history of sexually transmitted diseases.[432] Evidence exists to support routine screening of pregnant women with chlamydia.[433] For gonorrhea, on the other hand, screening of high-risk populations (as for chlamydia) by cervical culture is recommended at the first visit—especially if the woman is symptomatic (e.g., has cervicitis).[434]

CRITICAL THINKING

What is your priority in caring for a pregnant woman with chlamydia?

The incidence of **herpes simplex virus (HSV)** *infection of the genital area* is increasing. The routine prenatal screening by culture is not indicated for those with a positive history. However, what is indicated is a single culture to confirm diagnosis when lesions are present.[435] Caesarean section is indicated in women with clinically apparent HSV infection at delivery to protect the newborn against infection. The primary source is maternal in nature in that genital herpes infections are sexually transmitted; consequently, affected women are mainly in the childbearing age group. The majority of genital infections are asymptomatic and difficult to recognize on clinical examination, thus making the identification of a mother whose fetus is in jeopardy very difficult.[436–440]

Congenital and neonatal herpes simplex viral infections often prove lethal.[441] A mortality rate of 60% and serious central nervous system and eye damage have been identified in half the survivors. Neonates may be asymptomatic. Drug therapeutic measures taken thus far to cure the mother and newborn have been ineffective; thus research in prevention and treatment of the infectious disease continues.[442,443]

For **cytomegalovirus (CMV),** no pregnancy screening is indicated.[444] The potential public health effect of preconception screening remains to be determined because of the possibility of recurrent infections.[445]

Toxoplasmosis is an infection that was first discovered in 1909 in a rodent in Africa. The parasite is harboured in the bodies of cattle, sheep, and pigs, and the intestinal tracts of cats. It is contracted by eating infected meat or eggs that are raw or undercooked or through contact with the feces of an infected cat. An educational program at the preconception and/or first pregnancy visit is appropriate. Screening by serology at the first pregnancy visit may be appropriate, but only for a woman known to be at risk (e.g., one who has a new or outside cat or eats raw meat), with a repeat test at 16 to 20 weeks. Converters may be referred to a tertiary centre for percutaneous fetal blood sampling and culturing and, if possible, treatment or termination. Due to the high prevalence and seriousness of maternal infection and prenatal transmission, a potential health benefit to routine preconception exists.[446] For example, should the mother become infected during pregnancy, there is a good possibility that the parasite will cross the placental barrier. The presence of antibodies provides reassurance about immunity. The absence of antibodies underscores the need for education and vigilance.[447] Health education on how to avoid contact with the parasite should be emphasized by the nurse. Chronic maternal alcohol use acts as a predisposition to infection. Alcoholics are more susceptible to pulmonary infections; alcohol has adverse effects on all components of the immune system.[448–451]

Fetal Infection

Intrauterine fetal infection caused by group B *Streptococcus* species probably occurs with greater frequency than is clinically diagnosed. In the most serious cases, the clinical signs—apnea, respiratory distress, and shock—emerge at birth or within 48 hours.[452] Immediate treatment is mandatory for survival. The death rate may be particularly high in preterm infants who show early signs and symptoms. Evidence points to the passage of this infectious agent during the birthing process via the maternal genital tract. Only penicillin is indicated for use as an antibiotic because with this drug no severe allergic reaction to the fetus or newborn has been reported.[453]

In Canada, regarding group B Streptococcus (GBS), the Society of Obstetricians and Gynaecologists of Canada (SOGC) states that an urgent need exists for research in this area. They recommend that the process of identification and management of women whose newborns might be at increased risk of GBS disease is initiated by one of the following methods: (1) universal screening of all pregnant women at 35 to 37 weeks gestation with a single combined vaginal-anorectal swab and the offer of intrapartum chemoprophylaxis to all GBS-colonized women,[454] or (2) no universal screening but intrapartum chemoprophylaxis for all women with identified risk factors. This strategy should also be used in cases where universal screening is the policy, but either the screening was not done, or the test results are not available.[455]

CRITICAL THINKING

What is a research question that a health professional can develop regarding group B Streptococcus affecting the neonate?

Immunologic Factors

The fetus is immunologically foreign to the mother's immune system, yet the fetus is sustained. Selected antibodies of measles, chickenpox, hepatitis, poliomyelitis, whooping cough, and diphtheria are transferred to the fetus. The resulting immunity lasts for several months after birth. Antibodies to dust, pollen, and common allergens do not transfer across the placenta.[456] *Incompatibility between maternal and infant blood factors* is the most commonly

encountered interference with fetal development resulting in various degrees of circulatory difficulty for the baby. When a fetus's blood contains a protein substance, the Rh factor (Rh-positive blood), but the mother's blood does not (Rh-negative blood), antibodies in the mother's blood may attack the fetus and possibly cause spontaneous abortion, stillbirth, jaundice anemia, heart defects, mental retardation, or death. Usually the first Rh-positive baby is not affected adversely, but with each succeeding pregnancy the risk becomes greater. A vaccine can be given to the Rh-negative mother within three days of childbirth or abortion that will prevent her body from making Rh antibodies. Babies affected by the Rh syndrome can be treated with repeated blood transfusions.[457] In-depth information can be attained from a physiology or obstetrics text.[458,459]

Maternal Emotions

The physical–psychological interdependence between mother and fetus still is being studied; effects of the mother's elation, fear, and anxiety on the behaviour and other developmental aspects of the baby are poorly understood. Anxiety and fear, resulting from physical abuse, worries about the current living situation or finances, or violence in the neighbourhood or community produce a variety of physiologic changes in the person. These changes occur because of activation of the hypothalamus and the sympathetic division response of the autonomic nervous system, which stimulates the adrenal medulla to produce adrenaline. Adrenaline, in turn, stimulates the anterior lobe of the pituitary to produce adrenocorticotropic hormone (ACTH), which activates the adrenal cortex to release cortisone. The results are increased heart rate, constriction of peripheral vessels, dilation of coronary vessels, decrease in gastrointestinal motility, and changed carbohydrate and protein metabolism, which also affects many body functions and changes in the adrenocortical hormonal system.[460,461] These changes occurring in the pregnant woman contribute to hyperactivity of the fetus because increased maternal cortisone is secreted and enters the blood circulation, crossing the placenta to the fetus.[462–464] Further, fetal circulatory and nutritional processes may be affected, interfering with intrauterine development. Because the fetus experiences only the consequences and not the cause of the emotion itself, the experience may mean nothing to the fetus; however, some studies indicate that maternal fear and anxiety induce the same sensations in the fetus.[465] *Maternal stress, therefore, may be considered a teratogen, resulting in physical and psychological alterations of the developing person before and following birth.*

The effects of job stress on pregnant women have not been adequately researched and study results are contradictory. One study of 15 000 women on perinatal outcome of broken marriages (separated, divorced, widowed) found that these women are at higher risk for low-birth-weight infants than married mothers (odds ratio, 5:1) or single mothers. The low birth weight was attributed to reduced growth rather than to prematurity and was associated with substance abuse.[466] Other studies that compared the outcomes of pregnancies of female medical residents with those of wives of male medical residents showed no significant difference despite long work hours, lack of sleep, and high occupational stress of the former group of women.[467,468]

Other studies showed no direct relationship between work-related psychosocial stress during pregnancy and preterm or low-birth-weight delivery.[469,470] However, personal motivation toward work, as well as physical effect of work, should be considered in evaluating the impact of a job's psychological effects on pregnancy outcome. Women who did not want to remain in the workforce were more likely to experience work-related stress and preterm, low-birth-weight delivery.[471]

Domestic violence is a severe and common stressor for the pregnant woman. Physical abuse during pregnancy has been associated with unemployment, substance abuse and addiction, poverty, and family dysfunction that may be both past and current. Thus, it is difficult to determine the relative contribution of each of these risks.[472,473] The results of a Canadian study found that 95% of women who were abused in the first trimester of their pregnancies were also abused in the three-month period after delivery. The study also indicated that the abuse increased after the baby was born.[474] Battering a pregnant woman may represent an extreme response of jealousy toward the unborn baby and anger at being displaced from the centre of the woman's attention. Men also may fear and envy women's reproductive power. Such men deal with fear and envy by asserting physical power over women, often forcing themselves sexually on women to the extent of manifesting sexual addiction or rape.[475]

Maternal anxiety reactions are also related to physiologic responses of pregnancy, such as nausea and vomiting, backaches, and headaches, which, in turn, affect the fetus. The woman who begins pregnancy with fewer psychic reserves is especially vulnerable to the stresses and conflicting moods that accompany pregnancy.[476]

Do not assume harmony between the partners or happiness about the coming baby. The mother-to-be may have many feelings to resolve during pregnancy, as might the father-to-be. However, maternal emotionality during pregnancy has not been correlated with specific mother–child behavioural interaction.

CRITICAL THINKING

What questions would you ask a pregnant women who has been abused?

Birth Defects Transmitted by the Father

Genes of both mother and father and the prenatal maternal environment may cause birth defects. Genetic mutations or abnormalities in sperm are being formed in an increasingly greater percentage of the population. It is interesting to note

Causes of Paternal Contributions to Birth Defects in the Child

Direct (occur at conception)

- Damage to spermatozoa caused by chemicals such as fumigants, solvents, vinyl chloride, methyl mercury, hypothermia, radiation, pesticides, diethylstilbestrol (DES), alcohol, or lack of vitamin C
- Alterations in seminal fluid.
- Factor or agent affects chromosomes or cytogenic apparatus in sperm cells or their precursors.
- Drugs and chemicals cross into testes and male accessory reproductive organs for secretion in semen.

Indirect (occur before conception)

- Genetic constitution contributed by father to fetus may make fetus more susceptible to environmental factors to which it is later exposed. (Responses to teratogens may in part depend on genotype of exposed individual.)
- Transmission of chemicals to the pregnant woman through the man's skin, hair, or contaminated clothing.

Examples of Paternal Contributions to Causes of Fetal Defects

- Down syndrome (trisomy 21): paternal nondisjunction and extra chromosome; 20% to 30% of cases occur when father is 55 years or older at time of conception.
- Sex chromosome disorders in child.
- Adverse outcomes such as spontaneous abortion and perinatal death (stillbirth) due to methadone and morphine dependency and chemicals such as fumigants, solvents, and vinyl chloride.
- Infertility in the couple due to drugs or other chemicals.
- Hemophilia: coagulation disorder in child; deficiency of factor VIII.
- Marfan syndrome: connective tissue disorder with elongated extremities, hands.
- Progeria: premature aging, growth deficiency.
- Decreased neonatal survival due to methadone and morphine dependency.
- Birth defects if father is epileptic (especially if taking phenytoin) or if father is exposed to lead, waste, anaesthetic gases, Agent Orange, or dioxin.
- Tumours of nervous system if father is miner, printer, pulp or paper mill worker, electrical worker, or auto mechanic

that more male than female cells undergo genetic mutation. Mutations may be caused by exposure to irradiation, infection, drugs, and chemicals. These mutations occur more frequently as a man ages and may be responsible for various inborn disorders and congenital anomalies (see the box entitled "Causes of Paternal Contributions to Birth Defects in the Child").[477–480] For males, this "cut-off" is 45 years of age; risks for chromosomal abnormalities may double when the male is 55 years or older.[481,482] The male may affect the unborn child in other ways as well.

VARIABLES RELATED TO CHILDBIRTH THAT AFFECT THE BABY

Use the following information in assessment of and intervention with mother and baby.

Medications

Analgesics and general anaesthetics given during childbirth cross the placental barrier, affecting the newborn for days after delivery. Respiration after birth is negatively affected; artificial resuscitation may be needed for severe respiratory depression. Motor skills are also less developed and more crying irritability is seen after birth.

Thus, **analgesics,** or *drugs to reduce pain,* and sedatives, or mild tranquilizers to reduce anxiety, are given in early labour. Epidural block, one form of local anaesthesia, is being used increasingly rather than general anaesthesia. However, all drugs and local anaesthetics also indirectly affect the fetus by reducing blood flow to the uterus, thus affecting the fetal heart rate. The APGAR score may be low (see Chapter 7). Drugs given during labour remain in the infant's bloodstream for a few days.[483–485]

Childbirth without drugs was first introduced in 1914 by Grantly Dick Read. He was followed by Dr. Fernand Lamaze. The natural childbirth method has become popular with both mothers and fathers because they can both actively participate in the birth of their child. During natural childbirth classes, the mother and father (or partner) learn about the physiology of pregnancy and childbirth, exercises that strengthen the mother's abdominal and perineal muscles, and techniques of breathing and relaxation during labour and delivery. The father or partner acts as encourager and coach throughout the prenatal classes and during labour and delivery so that the birth experience is shared between the couple. Equally of benefit is the child who comes into the world without any ill effects from medication. Refer to literature from the American Society for Psychoprophylaxis in Obstetrics and obstetric nursing texts for more information on prepared childbirth.

Method and Place of Delivery

Birth can be difficult, even dangerous. Forceps may be needed to withdraw the baby, because of maternal or fetal reasons, and are safe if the cervix is completely dilated and the head is

within 5 cm of the mouth of the vagina. Abdominal surgery, or caesarean section, is done when the baby, for a number of reasons, cannot be born vaginally. This major surgery should not be done unless absolutely necessary. No evidence exists to indicate that the site at which the baby is born has any effect on long-term development.[486] Adequate prenatal care and safety for mother and baby are the important factors.

CRITICAL THINKING

What are some special features of home delivery that may be available to the mother and newborn that may not be available in a family birthing centre?

Inadequate Oxygenation

Anoxia, *decreased oxygen supply,* and increased carbon dioxide levels may result during delivery. Some degree almost routinely occurs from compression of the umbilical cord, reduced blood flow to the uterus, or placental separation. Fortunately, newborn babies are better able to withstand periods of low oxygenation than are adults. Other causes of asphyxia, however, such as drug-induced respiratory depression or apnea, kinks in the umbilical cord, wrapping of the cord around the neck, very long labour, and malpresentation of the fetus during birth, have more serious effects. Longitudinal studies of anoxic newborns revealed lower performance scores on tests of sensorimotor and cognitive-intellectual skills and personality measures than for children with minimal anoxia at birth. Anoxia is also the principal cause of perinatal death and a common cause of mental retardation and cerebral palsy.[487–489]

Premature or Preterm Birth and Low Birth Weight

Prematurity may have long-term consequences for the child. **Preterm** birth is defined as *birth before 38 weeks of gestation.*

Prematurity is defined as *the birth at a gestational age of 37 weeks or earlier, combined with birth weight of less than 2500 g (5.5 pounds).* Risk of death is greater for premature or low-birth-weight babies. Causes have been discussed earlier in this chapter.

Later developmental and behavioural problems such as physical and mental retardation and hyperactivity may also be correlated with prematurity.[490,491] Treatment of the premature neonate in sterile, precisely controlled incubators causes an absence of environmental and sensory stimuli, which also contributes to retardation. Research shows that gentle rubbing hourly throughout the 24-hour day promotes positive effects immediately and later for infants in isolettes—they are more active and gain weight faster, and later they perform better on tests of motor development, while appearing healthier and more active than premature children who suffer tactile and sensory deprivation.

The small-for-gestation age or **low-birth-weight infants** (*less than 2500 g or 5.5 pounds*) may not be premature; some are small for gestational age. The baby may have completed the 38th week in utero.[492] The **very-low-birth-weight (VLBW)** *baby weighs less than 1500 grams (3.3 pounds).* The **extremely low birth weight (ELBW)** *baby weighs less than 1000 grams (a little over 2 pounds).* Both the VLBW and ELBW baby will be of low gestational age or premature.[493] The **small-for-date** *(growth-retarded)* baby may be born after nine months' gestation but be too small because of a slow-down in prenatal growth[494] (see Chapter 7).

The following *maternal factors contribute to a higher risk of low-birth-weight babies:*[495–501]

- Underweight before pregnancy
- Less than 21 pounds gained during pregnancy
- Inadequate prenatal care
- Age of 16 years or younger or 35 years or older
- Low socioeconomic level
- Poor nutrition during pregnancy
- Smoking cigarettes during pregnancy
- Use of addictive drugs or alcohol during pregnancy
- History of abortion
- Complications during pregnancy, poor health status, exposure to infections
- High stress levels, including physical or emotional abuse

Risk of low birth weight is associated with financial problems or living in high-crime areas, irrespective of the variables of race, poor health habits, and complications during pregnancy.[502] A study of low-birth-weight children born

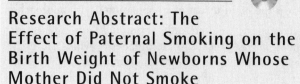

6-3 BONUS SECTION IN CD-ROM

Research Abstract: The Effect of Paternal Smoking on the Birth Weight of Newborns Whose Mother Did Not Smoke

This research abstract describes a study of 1219 newborns in a large health maintenance organization in Arizona. The study focused on the effect of passive exposure of the mother to paternal smoking, and lower birth weight. Strong health care implications resulted from this study.

to disadvantaged families showed that those who had received sensory stimulation in the nursery and additional sensorimotor stimulation from their mothers throughout the first year of life performed better on tests of intellectual and sensorimotor development at the end of the year than the children who had not received extra stimulation.

Heaman states that at the Canadian Consensus Conference on Preterm Birth Prevention, held in 1998, consensus was reached on the facts regarding preterm birth prevention. Suggestions were made for research and community and clinical action. Recommendations for action emphasized the adoption of a population health approach to prevent preterm birth.[503]

EVIDENCE-BASED PRACTICE

Risk Factors for Spontaneous Preterm Birth (SPB)

In Manitoba, the incidence of preterm birth has been increasing and the rate is higher among Aboriginal than non-Aboriginal women. The purpose of this study was to identify risk factors for spontaneous preterm birth in Manitoba women, and to compare risk factors among Aboriginal and non-Aboriginal women. In this case-control study, cases delivered a live singleton infant at less than 37 weeks gestation (n = 226; 36% Aboriginal), while controls delivered between 37 and 42 weeks gestation (n = 458; 38% Aboriginal). An interview was conducted with each subject on the postpartum unit, and information was collected from the health record. Using stratified analyses to control for race/ethnicity, several risk factors for preterm birth had a uniform effect measure across strata, while others demonstrated heterogeneity. After adjusting for other maternal characteristics in a multivariate logistic regression model, significant risk factors emerged.

Significant risk factors for all women included:

1. previous preterm birth
2. two or more previous spontaneous abortions
3. vaginal bleeding after 12 weeks gestation
4. gestational hypertension

5. antenatal hospitalization, and
6. prelabour rupture of membranes

Potentially modifiable risk factors included:

1. low weight gain during pregnancy for all women
2. inadequate prenatal care for all women
3. high levels of perceived stress for Aboriginal women

Practice Implications

1. Strategies to increase women's access to, and utilization of, prenatal care should be implemented. There should be more use of outreach into the community by a multidisciplinary team for the provision of prenatal care to Aboriginal women.
2. Prenatal care providers should consider women with low pregnancy weight gain at increased risk for preterm delivery.
3. Women need to be counselled about appropriate rates of weight gain in pregnancy based on national guidelines.
4. The need exists to develop culturally appropriate stress reduction strategies.

Source: Heaman, M.I. Risk Factors for Spontaneous Preterm Birth among Aboriginal and Non-Aboriginal Women in Manitoba. Ph.D. dissertation, University of Manitoba, 2001. Used with permission.

CRITICAL THINKING

What is the main thrust of a population health approach?

Premature children differ from full-term infants in a number of ways, including sleep patterns, which are poorly organized with poorly differentiated sleep states. Shorter and less regular periods of each sleep state are exhibited and may persist beyond infancy. Because more growth hormone is released during sleep, disturbed sleep patterns in the premature infant may affect physical growth and size generally.[504–506]

EARLY CHILDHOOD VARIABLES THAT AFFECT THE PERSON

Use the following information in assessment of and health promotion interventions with the child and adults in the childbearing years.

Nutrition

Nutrition can exert an important influence on growth and development, especially if nutritional deficiency diseases occur. Too many children under the age of 12 go to bed hungry every night, despite available nutrition programs. Unfortunately, minimum, optimum, and toxic levels of nutrients are not well researched to date; however, inadequate nutrition may slow normal growth and apparently causes a permanent effect of low intellectual ability. The possibility of as many as 30% of the brain's neurons may never be formed if protein intake is inadequate during the second trimester of pregnancy or the first six months of life. Children who suffer starvation do not catch up with growth norms for their group, although later in life adequate nutrition and socioemotional support help to offset the differences.[507,508]

If the child is fed a **vegetarian or macrobiotic diet,** the diet must be nutrient- and calorie-dense, and not high in fibre. Because an infant's stomach capacity is less than an adult's, the volume of food that can be consumed is limited. Growth retardation is the major visible marker for an inadequate diet. *In your nutritional counselling, emphasize that there must be enough calories to support adequate growth, so that protein that is consumed is not used primarily for energy, instead of growth and repair.*[509–511]

Too much fibre will be hard to digest, with the result that the child loses energy and weight. The diet may be low in fat because it lacks animal products. Plant foods must be combined in such a way to supply essential amino acids in the proportions needed for growth. Legumes, cereals, nuts, seeds, avocados, and olives are nutrient dense, but they must be prepared and cooked so they can be eaten by the infant and young child. Infant cereal can be given to the age of 18 months, since it is fortified with iron. Fortified soy milk and mineral supplementation can be given through the childhood years to ensure adequate calcium intake if dairy products are not eaten. Tofu, green leafy vegetables, legumes, almonds, and sesame seeds help supply calcium. To prevent rickets, which have been seen in children on macrobiotic diets, vitamin D supplementation, sunlight, and cod-liver oil should be supplied. Vitamin B_{12} has no practical plant food source; without supplementation there is likely to be a deficiency after one year of age and even in breastfed infants. Vitamin B_{12} deficiency causes fretfulness, apathy, decreased responsiveness, and loss of motor control. Neurological damage may be permanent. Iron deficiency is common in vegetarian children because the usual meat sources are not eaten. A good source of ascorbic acid at each meal will improve absorption of whatever iron is ingested. Zinc deficiency may occur unless sufficient legumes, nuts, seeds, tofu, hard cheese, and eggs are eaten. Some vegetarians refuse supplementation. They must select a diet carefully for themselves and their children.[512–514]

Obesity in childhood more likely is related to eating patterns than to genetics, according to a study of weight differences between infants of obese and nonobese foster mothers. The babies weighed 2 kg (4.5 pounds) at birth and entered the foster homes at 3.5 weeks of age. Children cared for by obese foster parents also became obese. The mean weight of all children of obese mothers was greater at all ages than for children of nonobese mothers. Children with excess cell mass from excessive caloric intake develop adult adipose cells early in life. Adipose stores continue to increase because of the increased number of adipose cells.[515–518]

Breast milk is considered the food of choice for the newborn and infant for at least six months.[519] Yet, breastfeeding is not completely safe. Many substances and drugs ingested by the mother are excreted in human milk. The newborn is susceptible to foreign substances because the body's principal detoxifying mechanisms are not functional, the enzyme system is immature, and kidney function is incompletely developed.[520–522] Media reports indicate that pesticides in food and other environmental pollutants unknowingly ingested by the mother are excreted in human milk.

Stress

Stress comes in various forms to young children as well as to individuals of any age; there may be illness and hospitalization; day-to-day frustrations; neglect, abuse, or abandonment by parents; emotional and sensory deprivation; natural disasters; and wars. The environment up to age three is especially critical. Adverse and harsh or stressful living environments or life experiences cause a heightened sympathetic system activity and can alter the structure of the brain. The young child is especially vulnerable. Brain neurotransmitters also appear to be affected long term. In turn, reduced functioning of the neurotransmitter serotonin can increase risks for ill health. Animal studies reveal that insufficient maternal care reduces serotonin function, causing increased aggression and reduced ability to respond to or give affection. A steady flood of stress chemicals in the brain alters the brain's system of response, causing depression, a shutting down emotionally, unresponsiveness to stimuli, withdrawal, and intermittent impulsiveness and acting out.[523–527]

Neurobiological discoveries add to the emotional, social, and spiritual reasons for giving children adequate nurturing, attention, love, support, and guidance in emotional and cognitive skills. Only then can they develop, learn, cope, and be healthy.

Effects of Practice on Neuromuscular Development

Effects of exercise or practice on developing early motor skills remain contradictory in reports. Apparently certain motor behaviour appears when the body has the neuromuscular maturity for that behaviour; practice of the behaviour before its natural appearance does little to speed up long-term development, although it may appear that the child can do an activity earlier. Unpractised children catch up, often doing the same activity only a few days later.[528]

Endocrine Function

Mediation of hormones is crucial to the child and person throughout life. A **hormone** is a *chemical substance produced by an endocrine gland and carried by the bloodstream to another part of the body (the target organ) where it controls some function of the target organ.* The major functions of hormones include integrative action, regulation, and morphogenesis. **Integration,** *permitting the body to act as a whole unit in response to stimuli, results from hormones travelling throughout the body and reaching all cells of the body.* For example, the response of the body to epinephrine during fright is generalized. Estrogen, which is more specific in its action, affects overall body function. **Regulation,** *maintaining a constant internal environment or homeostasis, results from all the hormones.* The regulation of salt and water balance, metabolism, and growth are examples. In **morphogenesis,** the *rate and type of growth of the organism,* some hormones play an important part.[529]

Growth hormone (GH) or *somatotropic hormone (STH),* secreted by the anterior pituitary gland and regulated by a substance called *growth hormone–releasing factor (GHF),* produced in the hypothalamus, affects morphogenesis by promoting the development and enlargement of all body tissues that are capable of growing. Growth hormone has three basic effects on the metabolic processes of the body: (1) protein synthesis is increased; (2) carbohydrate conservation is increased; and (3) use of fat stores for energy is increased.[530]

Growth hormone is secreted in spurts instead of at a relatively constant rate. The lowest concentrations of plasma GH are found in the morning after arising; the highest concentrations occur between 60 and 90 minutes after falling asleep at night. The peak of GH is clearly related to sleep; thus, the folk belief that sleep is necessary for growth and healing has been supported.[531]

Environmental Pollution

Children are especially affected by environmental pollution. Children are exposed to more toxic chemicals because they ingest more food, water, and air than their parents, pound for pound. The life of a child is exploration: on hands and knees they encounter pesticides, lead, and other poisons lurking in soil, house dust, and carpets, which they swallow while sucking on their hand or thumb. Further, these contaminants are more toxic to children than adults and are more likely to cause permanent damage. The child is not fully developed at birth; the brain and the neurological, immune, endocrine, and reproductive systems pass through numerous critical periods when they are especially vulnerable. Damage from even minor exposure can last a lifetime.[532]

The incidence of childhood asthma and cancer has increased sharply. Asthma is the leading chronic illness in children; cancer is second only to accidents as a cause of childhood death. Increases in both diseases are attributed in part to environmental hazards, as are increasing numbers of hypospadias and precocious development in girls.[533,534] A pilot study was conducted to determine the prevalence of impaired lung function in school-aged First Nations children. Results indicated that many children in the study had already established airflow obstruction and may be at risk for asthma or chronic obstructive pulmonary disease (COPD). Somewhat surprisingly, exposure to mould appeared to be protective. The researchers claim that further research is needed to evaluate the lung health concerns of this population.[535]

CRITICAL THINKING

Why might mould be a protective factor in the pilot study conducted with school-aged First Nations children? (See Williams, 1999.[536])

Asthma is caused in part, and attacks are prolonged, by air pollution. However, the main causative factors are allergens that are inhaled because today's children spend more time in tightly sealed buildings, where they have greater exposure to mould, dust mites, animal dander, and cockroach droppings. A child who has asthma has an underlying immune system dysfunction, making him or her overreactive to substances in the environment. The child's early experience can change the relative proportion of T-cells and development of the immune system; contaminant exposure before birth has been linked to altered T-cells; the higher the mother's level of PCBs and dioxin, the greater the change in the T-cells. The result can be immune suppression, allergy, or autoimmunity.[537,538]

SOCIOCULTURAL FACTORS THAT INFLUENCE THE DEVELOPING PERSON

Use the following information with the information in Chapter 1 for assessment and health promotion.

Cultural and Demographic Variables

Culture, social class, race, and ethnicity of the parents; foods eaten by the pregnant woman; prenatal care and childbirth practices; childrearing methods; expected patterns of behaviour; language development and thought processes during childhood and adulthood; and health practices—all affect the person from the moment of conception. The person, however, will demonstrate some behaviours outside the cultural norm. If the child's parents are from a different ethnic or social background from most citizens of the area, the child may learn to talk, act, and think differently from most people. Conflict results between the person and the representatives (people and institutions) of the main culture, which, in turn, affects the child's ongoing development and care. Refer to Chapter 1 for in-depth discussion.

The health care given to the child by the parents is related to sociocultural status. For example, in urban areas parents of children who are adequately immunized are likely to have the following characteristics: (1) they perceive childhood diseases as serious; (2) they know about the effectiveness of vaccination; (3) they are older in age; (4) they are better educated; (5) they have smaller family size (number of children); and (6) they read newspapers, listen to radio or television promotions of immunizations, and respond to these community educational efforts. Inadequately immunized children in urban areas are found in families in which the parents are young, poor, and minimally educated, and have a large number of children. The parents do not perceive childhood diseases as serious, do not know about the effectiveness of vaccines, or do not pay attention to health education in the mass media.[539–541] All the advantages of inheriting a good brain can be lost if the child does not have the right environment in which to develop it.

Child–caregiver interaction; lifestyle factors such as adequate rest, smoking, and drug and alcohol use; use of health promotion measures; poor food habits that result in either malnutrition or obesity; along with toxic factors in the environment and infections all together are major determinants of how closely the genetic potential can be reached. All of these factors affect the child's growth and development, learning ability, functional capacity, and health, and eventually affect the health and longevity of adults.

Socialization Processes

Socialization is the *process by which the child is transformed into a member of a particular society and learns the values, standards, habits, skills, and roles appropriate to sex, social class, and ethnic group or subculture to become a responsible, productive member of society.*

All humans experience socialization, the shaping of the person into a socially acceptable form, especially during the early years of life. Thus heritage and culture are perpetuated. The newborn is a biological organism with physical needs and inherited characteristics, which will be socialized or shaped along a number of dimensions: emotional, social, cognitive, intellectual, perceptual, behavioural, and expressive. During the period of socialization, various skills, knowledge, attitudes, values, motives, habits, beliefs, needs, interests, and ideals are learned, demonstrated, and reinforced. Various people are key agents in the socialization process: parents, siblings, relatives, peers, teachers, and other adults. Certain forces will impinge on the person and interact with all the individual is and learns; these forces include culture, social class, religion, race or ethnicity, the community, the educational system, mass media, and various organizations. Certain

factors may limit or enhance the socialization process: age, sex, rate and stage of development, general constitution, and innate intelligence. Integration of all the various individual and socializing forces will form the adult character, personality traits, role preferences, goals, and behavioural mode.

Socialization is a lifelong process of social learning or training through which the person acquires knowledge, skills, attitudes, values, needs, motivations, and cognitive and affective patterns that relate to the sociocultural setting. The success of the socialization process is measured by the person's ability to perform in the roles he or she attempts and respond to rapid social change and a succession of life tasks. The person learns to think and behave in ways consonant with the roles to be played; performance in a succession of roles leads to predictable personality configurations.[542]

Community Support System

Community relationships influence primarily the parents, but they also influence the child. An emotional support system for the parents, physical and health care resources in the community, and social and learning opportunities that exist outside the home promote the child's development and prepare him or her for later independence and citizenry roles. If the parents are unable to meet the child's needs adequately, other people or organizations in the community may make the difference between bare survival and eventual physical and emotional normalcy and well-being.

Cultures vary in the degree to which the new mother is given help. Prenatal classes can bring together women and families who are often isolated in Western society.[543]

Physical health of the baby and emotional health of the mother in the months following delivery depend in part on whether or not she had assistance with infant care and a support system during the first month after delivery. Ongoing support is essential for healthy development and life.[544–546]

Family Factors

The family structure, developmental level and roles of family members, their health and financial status, their perception of the baby, and community resources for the family influence the child's development and well-being, before birth and afterwards. Social and environmental factors that produce low birth weight, for instance, are likely to continue to operate on the infant and child as well. The child learns to behave differently and, as an adult, will have different values and expectations if he or she is reared in a single-parent, nuclear, extended, matrifocal, or patriarchal family or in a poor or wealthy family. The number of siblings, their sexes, and birth order influence how the child is treated and perceives him- or herself. The family's presence or absence of work, leisure, travel, material comforts, habits of daily living, and the façade put on for society will affect the child's self-concept, learning, physical well-being, and eventual lifestyle. Refer to Chapter 4 for more information.

A study was conducted by Ford-Gilboe to determine which variables would predict *choice of health promotion options in single-parent and two-parent families.* The convenience sample in a mid-size city in southern Ontario consisted of 138 families (68 single-parent families, 70 two-parent families) with at least one preadolescent child. The majority of subjects were Caucasian, identifying with the Canadian culture, but from a variety of ethnic backgrounds. Mothers and children closest to age 12 completed questionnaires. Mother's education was the only demographic variable significantly related to choice of health options. Family pride, family cohesion, mother's nontraditional sex role orientation, general self-reliance, network support, and community support were significantly related to choice of health options. Single-parent families and two-parent family types were similar on all demographic variables, but two-parent families were found to have more community support, higher income, and more resources.[547]

Vulnerable and Resilient Children

Both vulnerable and resilient children develop within the same family system. Siblings brought up under chaotic situations, with alcoholic or drug-using parents, or in impoverished circumstances do not all develop the same personality traits. One becomes physically or emotionally ill, whereas the sibling thrives. No single set of qualities or circumstances characterizes such resilient children, but they are different from their vulnerable siblings from birth. Children who are exposed to more than one adverse factor or long-term crisis or who do not have a consistent caring adult are less able to offset the negative effects of stress and maintain resiliency.[548–550]

Resilient children appear to be *endowed with innate characteristics that insulate them from the pain of their families, allow them to reach out to some adult who provides crucial emotional support, and to bounce back from circumstances.* Characteristics of these children include the ability to:[551–553]

- Use some talent or personality traits to draw some adult to them as a substitute parent; have compensating experiences
- Recover quickly from stressors; be adaptable, resourceful, and creative
- Be more alert to their surroundings from birth
- Establish trust with the mother or with mothering person
- Have warm and secure relationships with the mother or mother surrogate, regardless of other circumstances
- Be more independent, easygoing, friendly, enthusiastic for activities, and able to tolerate frustration by age two
- Be more cheerful, flexible, and persistent in the face of failure and seek help from adults by age three-and-a half
- Be sensitive to others
- Feel that they can exert some control over life
- Demonstrate good school performances and good problem-solving skills

Vulnerable children *are closest emotionally to the distressed parent and are most likely to show signs of distress.* These children are more likely to be self-derogatory, anxious, depressed, and physically ill; however, hardships can leave even the resilient children with psychological scars, although they tend not to become emotionally disabled. Even apparently well-adjusted, successful, resilient children may pay a subtle psychological cost. In adolescence they are more likely to cling to a moralistic outlook. In intimate relationships they are apt to be disagreeable and judgmental. They tend to be constricted and overcontrolled. If the disturbed parent is of the opposite sex, the resilient person is often emotionally distant in intimate relationships, breaking off relationships as they become more intimate. Some seek partners with problems, with the idea of rescuing or curing them.[554,555]

Child Maltreatment

Child abuse is a negative influence on the developing person. It is currently an epidemic, and children are suffering more serious and brutal injuries. Parents who abuse their children may be from any race, creed, ethnic origin, or economic level.[556,557] You are crucial in preventing child abuse through your assistance to parents. **Child maltreatment** is *physical abuse, neglect, sexual abuse and emotional maltreatment of children.*[558] Abused children range in age from neonate through adolescence.[559]

You may be the first health worker to encounter such a child in the community. Be alert for signs of child abuse as you assess the injured or ill child. Nonaccidental physical injury includes multiple bruises or fractures from severe beatings; poisonings or overmedication; burns from immersion in hot water or from lighted cigarettes; excessive use of laxatives or enemas; and human bites. The trauma to the child is often great enough to cause permanent blindness, scars on the skin, neurological damage, subdural hematoma, and permanent brain damage or death. **Sexual abuse,** *exploitation of the child for the adult's sexual gratification,* includes rape, incest, exhibitionism to the child, or fondling of the child's genitals. **Emotional maltreatment** includes *excessively aggressive or unreasonable parental behaviour to the child,* placing unreasonable demands on the child to perform above his or her capacities, verbally attacking or constantly belittling or teasing the child, or withdrawing love, support, or guidance. **Neglect** includes *failure to provide the child with basic necessities of life* (food, shelter, clothing, hygiene, or medical care), *adequate mothering, or emotional, moral, or social care.*[560–565] The parents' lack of concern is usually obvious. Abandonment may occur. In all forms of abuse, the child frequently acts fearful of the parents or adults in general. The child is usually too fearful to tell how he or she was injured.

There are a number of characteristics of the potentially or actually abusive parent. Typically the abuser:

- Is young
- Is emotionally unstable, unable to cope with the stress of life or even usual personal problems
- Was insufficiently mothered, rejected, or abused as a child
- Is lonely, has few social contacts, and is isolated from people
- Is unable to ask for help; lacks friends or family who can help with child care
- Does not understand the development or care needs of children
- Is living through a very stressful time such as unemployment, spousal abuse, or poverty

- Has personal emotional needs previously unmet; has difficulty in trusting others
- Is angered easily; has negative self-image and low self-esteem
- Has no one from whom to receive emotional support, including partner
- Expects the child to be perfect and to cause no inconvenience
- May perceive the child as different, too active, or too passive, even if the child is normal or only mildly different

Sometimes the child has mild neurological dysfunction and is irritable, tense, and difficult to hold or cuddle. The child may have been the result of an unwanted pregnancy or be premature or have a birth defect. Usually only one child in a family becomes the scapegoat for parental anger, tension, rejection, and hate. The child who does not react in a way to make the parent feel good about his or her parenting behaviour will be the abused one.[566–572]

Additional information about child and adolescent abuse is found in Chapters 7 through 11.

Prolonged Separation

Early separation for more than three months from a mothering person leads to serious consequences, because from approximately three to 15 months of age, the presence of a consistently loving caretaker is essential. Physical and intellectual growth is impaired, and the baby will not learn to form and maintain trust or a significant relationship. He or she will either withdraw or seek precociously to adapt by getting attention from as many people as possible. Death may result even with the best possible physical care.[573,574]

Maternal Deprivation and Failure to Thrive

Maternal deprivation and **failure to thrive** are the terms used to describe *infants who have insufficient contact with a mothering one and who do not grow as expected in the absence of an organic defect.* These infants may be institutionalized or have a parent who does not exhibit affectionate maternal behaviour. Deprivation during the second six months occurs when a previously warm relationship with the mother is interrupted. This deprivation is more detrimental to the child than the lack of a consistent relationship during the first six months. Another cause for failure to thrive is **perceptual deprivation,** *lack of tactile, vestibular, visual, or auditory stimuli,* resulting from either organic factors or the lack of mothering.[575,576] Touch and cuddling are essential for the infant; the skin is the primary way in which baby comes to know self and the environment.

Although damage to the child from maternal deprivation may be severe, not every deprived child becomes delinquent or a problem adult. Some infants who have lacked their mother's love appear to suffer little permanent damage. The age of the child when deprived or abused, the length of separation or duration of abuse, the parent–child relationship before separation or in later childhood, care of the child by other adults during separation from the parents, and the stress produced by the separation or abuse all affect the long-range outcome.

Spiritual Factors

Religious, philosophic, and moral insights and practices of the parents (and of the overall society) influence how the child is perceived, cared for, and taught. These early underpinnings— or their lack—will continue to affect the person's self-concept, behaviour, and health as an adult, even when he or she purposefully tries to disregard these early teachings. Refer to Chapter 3 for more information.

Macroenvironmental Factors That Influence the Developing Person

The overall environment of the region in which the person lives and in the home affects development and health. The climate the person learns to tolerate, water and food availability, emphasis on cleanliness, demands for physical and motor competency, social relationships, opportunities for leisure, and inherent hazards depend on whether the child lives on a farm or in the city, on the seacoast or inland, in a mining town or a mountain resort area. Added to these effects are the hazards from environmental pollution that affect all societies, whether it is excrement from freely roaming cattle or particles from industrial smokestacks. No part of the world is any longer uncontaminated by pesticides; all parts have disease related to problems of waste control. On a more immediate level, the size, space, noise, cleanliness, and safety within the home will affect the person's behaviour and health and the home environment he or she will eventually build.

The *media and national and international sports* also constitute the microenvironment. The media has informed the public in recent years of the various forms of drug abuse practised by professional and Olympic athletes who wish to excel in competition. These drugs build muscles, stamina, and strength, and prevent fatigue. It is widely acknowledged that *taking* these *nonregulation and nonmedicinal drugs* (**doping**) causes serious health problems and even death. Increasingly children in community school sports are being pushed to excel in competition, and when famous athletes, their role models, use drugs, so will school children and adolescents. Examples have already been reported in the media.

HEALTH CARE AND NURSING APPLICATIONS

Your support, assistance, and teaching with the pregnant woman and her significant support system will contribute to more nurturing parenting. Ways to prevent or overcome deterrents to development or teratogen agents are discussed throughout this chapter. Refer to texts on obstetric and maternal–child nursing for additional information about nursing care of the woman during pregnancy, labour, delivery, and after delivery. Information is also given in Chapters 2 and 7 through 11 that can be shared with the pregnant woman and parents for health promotion.

The following health promotion strategies are useful:

- Consider the principles of growth and development as you assess people in different developmental eras.

- Carefully assess pregnant women to determine whether they are at risk because of any of the negative influencing factors.
- Consider also the sociocultural and religious background and the lifestyle of the person you are caring for so that you do not overlook or misinterpret factors that are significant to the pregnant woman and her family.
- Help those who are at risk to get the care necessary to prevent fetal damage and maternal illness.
- Teach potential parents about the many factors discussed in this and following chapters that can influence the welfare of their offspring.
- Be aware of community services such as genetic screening and counselling, family planning, nutritional programs, prenatal classes, counselling for prevention of child abuse, and medical services.
- Join with other citizens in attempts to reverse environmental and child abuse hazards.

Your role with the child-abusing parent and the maltreated child is a significant one. To help parents and child, you must first cope with your own feelings as you give necessary physical care to the child or assist parents in getting proper care for the baby. Often parents who feel unable to cope with the stresses of childrearing will repeatedly bring the child to the emergency room for a variety of complaints of minor, vague illnesses or injuries.

CRITICAL THINKING

What other health promotion strategies would you develop to use with a culturally diverse population?

Certain health promotion strategies are useful:

- Be alert to the subtle message; talk with the parent(s) about himself or herself, the management of the child, feelings about parenting and the child, and who helps in times of stress.
- Establish rapport; act like a helpful friend; convey a feeling of respect for them as people (which may be difficult if you feel that the child abuser is a monster).
- Avoid asking probing questions too quickly.
- Do not lecture or scold the parent about his or her childrearing methods.
- Help parents to feel confident and competent in any way possible.
- Form a cool, mothering relationship with the parent(s). Make yourself consistently available but do not push too close emotionally. Often the mother responds well to having a grandmotherly person (usually a volunteer) spend time with her. This person could go to the home, where she could mother the mother, assist with a variety of household chores, and give the mother time to spend with her baby while unharried by demands of other children or household tasks.
- Be a model on how to approach, cuddle, and discipline the child; the parent may expect the six-month-old baby to obey commands.

- Convey that consistency of care is important. Realize that the parent will need long-term help in overcoming the abusive pattern.
- Use the principles of therapeutic communication and crisis intervention discussed in Chapters 4 and 5 to avoid driving the parent away from potential help or becoming more abusive to the child.
- Intervene sensibly with the parents and the child to avoid further harm and to avoid disrupting any positive feelings that might exist between parents and child. Foster home care is not necessarily the answer; foster parents are sometimes abusive, too. Rapid court action may antagonize parents to the point of murdering the child or moving to a different geographic location where they cannot receive help.

Further, cooperate with legal, medical, and social agencies to help the parent(s) and to prevent further child abuse—and possible death or permanent impairment of the child. Child maltreatment is against the law in every province and territory. Any citizen or health worker can anonymously report a case of child maltreatment to authorities without fear of recrimination from the abuser. An investigation by designated authorities of the danger to the child is carried out shortly after reporting; the child may be placed in a foster home or institution by court order if the child's life is threatened. The goal of legal intervention is to help the parents and child, not to punish.

INTERESTING WEBSITES

FOLIC ACID

http://www.hc-sc.gc.ca/; Site navigation at Health Canada home page: select A-Z index, folic acid
Folic acid, or folate, is one of the B vitamins important for healthy growth of an unborn baby. It is essential to the normal development of the baby's spine, brain, and skull, especially during the first four weeks of pregnancy. This site provides information and several related links.

CANADA PRENATAL NUTRITION PROGRAM

http://www.hc-sc.gc.ca; search: "Buns in the Oven"
If you're young and pregnant in Ottawa, feel overwhelmed and lonely and aren't always able to eat nutritiously, then one place to go is **Buns in the Oven.** This program offers food ideas, peer support, and prenatal and parenting education. It is sponsored by a coalition of four Ottawa agencies. Through a community development approach, the CPNP aims to reduce the incidence of unhealthy birth weights, improve the health of both infant and mother, and encourage breastfeeding.

CANADA'S FOOD GUIDE TO HEALTHY LIVING

http://www.hc-sc.gc.ca/; Site navigation at Health Canada home page: select A-Z index, Food and Nutrition, Canada Food Guide to Healthy Eating
The Nutrition Resource Centre presents the *Cultural Adaptations of Canada's Food Guide to Healthy Eating.* The

adaptations are available for use with the Chinese, Portuguese, Punjabi, Spanish, Tamil, Urdu, and Vietnamese-speaking communities. These guides feature culturally specific foods and full-colour illustrations. Each adaptation has been produced in three languages: the language of the cultural group (e.g., Chinese), English, and French.

FETAL ALCOHOL SYNDROME/FETAL ALCOHOL EFFECTS

http://www.healthcanada.ca/fas

Fetal alcohol syndrome (FAS) is the medical term used to describe certain birth defects that result from drinking alcohol during pregnancy. Fetal alcohol effects (FAE) is a similar condition that has some, but not all, of the characteristics of FAS. It estimated that every day in Canada, at least one child is born with FAS, which can lead to a variety of life-long disabilities. Both FAS and FAE are preventable. The smart choice for women who are, or may become, pregnant is to abstain totally from alcohol. Explore this site and learn much more.

FIRST NATIONS AND INUIT HEALTH BRANCH

http://www.hc-sc.gc.ca/fnihb

The Primary Health Care and Public Health (PHCPH) Directorate is responsible for primary health care delivered in partnership with First Nations and Inuit health authorities. All PHCPH activities have as their goals the support of knowledge and the building of capacity, among First Nations and Inuit, to facilitate First Nations and Inuit control of health programs and resources. This site provides current news, links, and general information.

CANADIAN CENTRE ON SUBSTANCE ABUSE

http://www.ccsa.ca

The Canadian Centre on Substance Abuse (CCSA) is an arm's length, national agency that promotes informed debate on substance abuse issues; encourages public participation in reducing the harm associated with drug abuse; disseminates information on the nature, extent, and consequences of substance abuse; and supports and assists organizations involved in substance abuse treatment, prevention, and educational programming.

MOTHERISK

http://www.motherisk.org

This site is a source of evidence-based information about the safety or risk of drugs, chemicals, and disease during pregnancy and lactation.

FETAL ALCOHOL SPECTRUM DISORDER

http://www.faspartnership.ca

The Canada Northwest Fetal Alcohol Spectrum Disorder Partnership is an alliance for the development and promotion of an interprovincial/territorial approach on the prevention, intervention, care, and support of people affected by fetal alcohol spectrum disorders. This new site offers "single-window" access to related sites around the country.

SUMMARY

1. Childhood is the foundation period of life, and development follows a definable, predictable, sequential pattern.
2. The person is unique, yet similar to other people in patterns of development, characterized by wholism (physical, emotional, cognitive, social, and spiritual/moral dimensions).
3. Development, developmental tasks, maturation, and learning are key terms to understanding the developing person throughout the life span.
4. Several principles of growth explain the pattern of development.
5. Prenatal influences on development include heredity, various physiologic processes, and age, health, and nutritional status of the mother and father.
6. Environmental hazards, drugs, alcohol, infections, and other conditions are teratogens that may adversely affect the developing organism, especially during the critical period of the first trimester.
7. Certain variables, such as medication in the mother, may negatively affect the fetus during labour and delivery.
8. Early childhood variables that affect the developing person include nurturance from the parents, nutrition, stressors, physiologic functions in the infant, and various sociocultural and family characteristics.

ENDNOTES

1. Papalia, D., S. Olds, and R. Feldman, *Human Development* (9th ed.). Boston: McGraw-Hill, 2004.
2. *Ibid.*
3. *Ibid.*
4. *Ibid.*
5. *Ibid.*
6. Bee, H., *Lifespan Development* (2nd ed.). New York: Longman, 1998.
7. Gormly, A., *Lifespan Human Development* (6th ed.). Fort Worth TX: Harcourt Brace, 1997.
8. Papalia et al., *op. cit.*
9. Seifert, K., R. Hoffnung, and M. Hoffnung, *Lifespan Development.* Boston: Houghton Mifflin, 1997.
10. Gormly, *op. cit.*
11. Guyton, A. *A Textbook of Medical Physiology* (9th ed.). Philadelphia: W.B. Saunders, 1996.
12. *Ibid.*
13. *Ibid.*
14. Seifert, *op. cit.*
15. Hakansson, A., Equality in Health and Health Care During Pregnancy: A Prospective Population-Based Study From Southern Sweden, *Acta Obstetricia et Gynecologica Scandinavica,* 73, no. 9 (1994), 674–679.
16. Papalia et al., *op. cit.*
17. Gormly, *op. cit.*
18. Erikson, E., *Childhood and Society* (2nd ed.). New York: W.W. Norton, 1963.
19. *Ibid.*
20. Cunningham, F., P. MacDonald, and N. Gant, *Williams Obstetrics* (18th ed.). Norwalk, CT: Appleton & Lange, 1989.
21. Papalia et al., *op. cit.*
22. Guyton, *op. cit.*
23. Wong, D., *Whaley and Wong's Nursing Care of Infants and Children* (6th ed.). St. Louis: C.V. Mosby, 1999.

24. Erikson, *op. cit.*
25. Sherwen, L., M. Scoleveno, and C. Weingarten, *Nursing Care of the Childbearing Family* (3rd ed.). Norwalk, CT: Appleton & Lange, 1999.
26. Wong, *op. cit.*
27. Sherwen et al., *op. cit.*
28. Wong, *op. cit.*
29. Maslow, A., *Motivation and Personality* (2nd ed.). New York: Harper and Row, 1970.
30. Gormly, *op. cit.*
31. Maslow, *op. cit.*
32. Wong, *op. cit.*
33. Gormly, *op. cit.*
34. Guyton, *op. cit.*
35. *Ibid.*
36. *Ibid.*
37. Sherwen et al., *op. cit.*
38. Wong, *op. cit.*
39. Sherwen et al., *op. cit.*
40. Wong, *op. cit.*
41. Sherwen et al., *op. cit.*
42. Wong, *op. cit.*
43. Guyton, *op. cit.*
44. Sherwen et al., *op. cit.*
45. Wong, *op. cit.*
46. Sherwen et al., *op. cit.*
47. Wong, *op. cit.*
48. Baltes, P.B., U.M. Staudinger, and U. Lindenberger. Lifespan Psychology: Theory and Application to Intellectual Functioning. *Annual Review of Psychology,* 50 (1999), 471–507.
49. Lindenberger, U., and P.B. Baltes. Life Span Psychology Theory. *American Psychological Association: Encyclopedia of Psychology,* Volume 5 (2000), 52–57.
50. Lindenberger, U. Lifespan Theories of Cognitive Development. *International Encyclopedia of the Social and Behavioral Sciences,* 13 (2001), 884–885.
51. Lindenberger and Baltes, *op. cit.*
52. Guyton, *op. cit.*
53. Papalia et al., *op. cit.*
54. Sherwen et al., *op. cit.*
55. Wong, *op. cit.*
56. Guyton, *op. cit.*
57. Papalia et al., *op. cit.*
58. Sherwen et al., *op. cit.*
59. Wong, *op. cit.*
60. Guyton, *op. cit.*
61. Papalia et al., *op. cit.*
62. Guyton, *op. cit.*
63. Papalia et al., *op. cit.*
64. Guyton, *op. cit.*
65. Papalia et al., *op. cit.*
66. Guyton, *op. cit.*
67. Papalia et al., *op. cit.*
68. Guyton, *op. cit.*
69. Papalia et al., *op. cit.*
70. Cunningham et al., *op. cit.*
71. Mariano, C., and R. Hickey. Multiple Pregnancy, Multiple Needs. *The Canadian Nurse,* 94, no. 9 (1998), 26–30.
72. Blondel, B., and M. Kaminski. Trends in the Occurrence, Determinants, and Consequences of Multiple Births, *Seminars in Perinatology,* 26 (2002), 239–249.
73. Mariano and Hickey, *op. cit.*
74. Health Canada, *Assisted Human Reproduction Legislation Becomes Law,* News Release, Website: http://www.hc-sc.gc.ca/, June 2004.
75. Cunningham et al., *op. cit.*
76. *Ibid.*
77. Guyton, *op. cit.*
78. Cunningham et al., *op. cit.*
79. Guyton, *op. cit.*
80. Seifert, *op. cit.*
81. Sherwen et al., *op. cit.*
82. Wong, *op. cit.*
83. Cunningham et al., *op. cit.*
84. Papalia et al., *op. cit.*
85. Seifert, *op. cit.*
86. Sherwen et al., *op. cit.*
87. Wong, *op. cit.*
88. Cunningham et al., *op. cit.*
89. Guyton, *op. cit.*
90. Papalia et al., *op. cit.*
91. Cunningham et al., *op. cit.*
92. Guyton, *op. cit.*
93. Papalia et al., *op. cit.*
94. Dykens, E., R. Hodapp, and J. Leckmann, *Behavior and Development in Fragile X Syndrome.* Thousand Oaks, CA: Sage, 1994.
95. Wong, *op. cit.*
96. Cunningham et al., *op. cit.*
97. Papalia et al., *op. cit.*
98. Bee, *op. cit.*
99. Papalia et al., *op. cit.*
100. Cunningham et al., *op. cit.*
101. Seifert, *op. cit.*
102. Sherwen et al., *op. cit.*
103. Wong, *op. cit.*
104. Dryburgh, H. Teenage Pregnancy. *Health Reports,* 12, no. 1 (2002), 9–19.
105. Health Canada, *Canadian Perinatal Health Report.* Ottawa: Minister of Public Works and Government Services Canada, 2003.
106. Singh, S., and J. E. Darroch, Adolescent Pregnancy and Childbearing: Levels and Trends in Developing Countries, *Family Planning Perspectives,* 32, no. 1 (2000), 14–23.
107. Bee, *op. cit.*
108. Papalia et al., *op. cit.*
109. Seifert, *op. cit.*
110. Sherwen et al., *op. cit.*
111. Wong, *op. cit.*
112. Sherwen et al., *op. cit.*
113. Wong, *op. cit.*
114. Health Canada, *Canadian Perinatal Health Report.*
115. Health Canada, *Congenital Anomalies in Canada—A Perinatal Health Report.* Ottawa: Minister of Public Works and Government Services Canada, 2002. Catalogue No. H39-641/2002E.
116. Berkowitz, G.S., M.L. Skovron, R.H. Lapinski, and R.L. Berkowitz. Delayed Childbearing and the Outcome of Pregnancy. *New England Journal of Medicine,* 322 (1990), 659–664.
117. *Ibid.*
118. Prysak, M., R.P. Lorenz, and A. Kisly. Pregnancy Outcome in Nulliparous Women 35 Years and Older. *Obstetrics and Gynecology,* 85 (1995), 65–70.
119. Cunningham et al., *op. cit.*
120. Sherwen et al., *op. cit.*
121. Wong, *op. cit.*
122. Bee, *op. cit.*
123. Papalia et al., *op. cit.*
124. Seifert, *op. cit.*
125. Cunningham et al., *op. cit.*
126. Guyton, *op. cit.*
127. Papalia et al., *op. cit.*
128. Sherwen et al., *op. cit.*
129. Wong, *op. cit.*

130. Cunningham et al., *op. cit.*
131. Sherwen et al., *op. cit.*
132. Wong, *op. cit.*
133. Cunningham et al., *op. cit.*
134. Guyton, *op. cit.*
135. Cunningham et al., *op. cit.*
136. Guyton, *op. cit.*
137. Cunningham et al., *op. cit.*
138. Menton, R.K., et al., Transplacental Passage of Insulin in Pregnant Women with Insulin-Dependent Diabetic Macrosomia, *New England Journal of Medicine,* 323, no. 5 (1990), 309–315.
139. Uphold, C., and M. Graham, *Clinical Guidelines in Family Practice* (3rd ed.), Gainesville, FL: Barmarrae Books, 1999.
140. Goto, M.P., and A.S. Goldman, Diabetic-Embryopathy: Current Opinion, *Pediatrics,* 6, no. 4 (1994), 486–491.
141. Cunningham et al., *op. cit.*
142. Menton et al., op cit.
143. Uphold and Graham, *op. cit.*
144. Cunningham et al., *op. cit.*
145. Sherwen et al., *op. cit.*
146. Wong, *op. cit.*
147. Sherwen et al., *op. cit.*
148. Health Canada, *Nutrition for a Healthy Pregnancy: National Guidelines for the Childbearing Years.* Ottawa: Minister of Public Works and Government Services Canada, 1999.
149. *Ibid.*
150. Health Canada, *Review of Canada's Food Guide to Healthy Eating, Interpretation of Findings and Next Steps.* Her Majesty The Queen in Right of Canada, 2004. Catalogue No. H44-63/2004E-PDF.
151. National Academy of Sciences. *Dietary Reference Intakes: Applications in Dietary Planning,* Web Search Engine: EBrooks@Bracken Health Science Library, June 2004.
152. *Ibid.*
153. Health Canada, *Canadian Guidelines for Body Weight Classification in Adults,* Website: http://www.healthcanada.ca/nutrition/, June 2004.
154. Health Canada, *Nutrition for a Healthy Pregnancy: National Guidelines for the Childbearing Years.*
155. *Ibid.*
156. Human Resource Development Canada and Health Canada, *The Well-Being of Canada's Young Children.* Government of Canada Report, 2003. SP-545-11-03E. Cat. No. RH64-20/2003.
157. Health Canada, *Nutrition for a Healthy Pregnancy: National Guidelines for the Childbearing Years.*
158. *Ibid.*
159. Duyff, R., *The American Dietetic Association's Complete Food and Nutrition Guide.* Minneapolis: Chronomed Publishing, 1998.
160. Williams, S., *Nutrition and Diet Therapy* (10th ed.). St. Louis: C.V. Mosby, 1995.
161. Papalia et al., *op. cit.*
162. Seifert, *op. cit.*
163. Williams, *op. cit.*
164. Duyff, *op. cit.*
165. Cunningham et al., *op. cit.*
166. Luke, V., Nutritional Influences on Fetal Growth, *Clinical Obstetrics and Gynecology,* 37, no. 3 (1994), 538–549.
167. Health Canada. *Nutrition for a Healthy Pregnancy: National Guidelines for the Childbearing Years.*
168. Health Canada, *Preconception Health and Folic Acid, Primary Prevention of Neural Tube Defects with Folic Acid,* Web Search Engine: Health Canada Folic Acid, Backgrounder, June 2004.
169. Duyff, *op. cit.*
170. Williams, *op. cit.*
171. Health Canada, *Nutrition for a Healthy Pregnancy: National Guidelines for the Childbearing Years.*
172. *Ibid.*
173. *Ibid.*
174. *Ibid.*
175. *Ibid.*
176. Community Health Services, *Preconceptual Health Series,* Website: http://www.lambtonhealth.on.ca/pregnancy/preconception/nutritio.asp, June 2004.
177. Williams, *op. cit.*
178. Duyff, *op. cit.*
179. Williams, *op. cit.*
180. Rodwell Williams, S., and E.D. Schlenker, *Essentials of Nutrition and Diet Therapy* (8th ed.). St Louis: Mosby, 2003.
181. National Institute of Nutrition, *Nutrition for a Healthy Pregnancy—National Guidelines, 2001,* Website: http://www.nin.ca/public_html/Publications/Rapport/rapp4_99.html#weight_gain, June 2004.
182. Cunningham et al., *op. cit.*
183. Sherwen et al., *op. cit.*
184. Williams, *op. cit.*
185. National Institute of Nutrition, *op. cit.*
186. Duyff, *op. cit.*
187. Sherwen et al., *op. cit.*
188. Williams, *op. cit.*
189. Health Canada, *Preconception Health and Folic Acid, Primary Prevention of Neural Tube Defects with Folic Acid.*
190. Cunningham et al., *op. cit.*
191. Health Canada, *Preconception Health and Folic Acid, Primary Prevention of Neural Tube Defects with Folic Acid.*
192. Cunningham et al., *op. cit.*
193. Duyff, *op. cit.*
194. *Ibid.*
195. Cunningham et al., *op. cit.*
196. Luke, *op. cit.*
197. Sherwen et al., *op. cit.*
198. Williams, *op. cit.*
199. Wong, *op. cit.*
200. Harrington, K., and S. Campbell, Fetal Size and Growth, *Current Opinion in Obstetrics & Gynecology of North America,* 18, no. 4 (1991), 907–931.
201. Otto, C., and L.D. Platt, Fetal Growth and Development, *Obstetrics and Gynecology Clinics of North America,* 18, no. 4 (1991), 907–931.
202. National Institute of Nutrition, *op. cit.*
203. Health Canada, *First Nations and Inuit Health Branch, Clinical Practice Guidelines for Nurses in Primary Care.* Minister of Public Works and Government Services Canada, 2000. Cat. No. H34-109/2000E.
204. Uphold and Graham, *op. cit.*
205. Williams, *op. cit.*
206. Cunningham et al., *op. cit.*
207. Willows, N.D., J. Morel, and K. Gray-Donald, Prevalence of Anemia Among James Bay Cree Infants of Northern Quebec, *Canadian Medical Association Journal,* 162, no. 3 (2000), 323–326.
208. Willows, N.D., E. Dewally, and K. Gray-Donald, Anemia and Iron Status in Inuit Infants from Northern Quebec, *Canadian Journal of Public Health,* 91, no. 6 (2000), 407–410.
209. Cunningham et al., *op. cit.*
210. Sherwen et al., *op. cit.*
211. Uphold and Graham, *op. cit.*
212. Williams, *op. cit.*
213. Wong, *op. cit.*
214. Duyff, *op. cit.*
215. Sherwen et al., *op. cit.*
216. Williams, *op. cit.*
217. Health Canada, *Nutrition for a Healthy Pregnancy: National Guidelines for the Childbearing Years.*

218. Duyff, *op. cit.*
219. Sherwen et al., *op. cit.*
220. Uphold and Graham, *op. cit.*
221. Williams, *op. cit.*
222. Wong, *op. cit.*
223. Health Canada, *Nutrition for a Healthy Pregnancy: National Guidelines for the Childbearing Years.*
224. Gormly, *op. cit.*
225. Papalia et al., *op. cit.*
226. Cunningham et al., *op. cit.*
227. *Ibid.*
228. Guyton, *op. cit.*
229. Papalia et al., *op. cit.*
230. Sherwen et al., *op. cit.*
231. Wong, *op. cit.*
232. Chasnoff, I.J., Prenatal Cocaine Exposure Is Associated with Respiratory Pattern Abnormalities, *American Journal of Disabled Children,* 144, no. 2 (1990), 583–587.
233. Chasnoff, I.J., and D. Griffith, Cocaine: Clinical Studies of Pregnancy and the Newborn. *Annals of the New York Academy of Sciences,* 562 (1989), 260–266.
234. Chasnoff, I.J. et al., Temporal Patterns of Cocaine Use in Pregnancy: Perinatal Outcomes, Journal of the *American Medical Association,* 261, no. 12 (1989), 1741–1749.
235. Papalia et al., *op. cit.*
236. Cunningham et al., *op. cit.*
237. *Ibid.*
238. Papalia et al., *op. cit.*
239. Sherwen et al., *op. cit.*
240. Wong, *op. cit.*
241. Cunningham et al., *op. cit.*
242. Sherwen et al., *op. cit.*
243. Wong, *op. cit.*
244. Bee, *op. cit.*
245. Cunningham et al., *op. cit.*
246. Del Gandio, D., and D. Menonna-Quinn, Chemotherapy: Potential Occupational Hazards, *American Journal of Nursing,* 98, no. 11 (1998), 59–65.
247. Dumanoski, D., Child's Plague, *Sierra,* November/December 1997, 47–51, 80.
248. Gormly, *op. cit.*
249. Luke, B., et al., The Association Between Occupational Factors and Preterm Birth: A United States Nurses' Study, *American Journal of Obstetrics and Gynecology,* 173 (1995), 849–862.
250. Papalia et al., *op. cit.*
251. Seifert, *op. cit.*
252. Worthington, K., Workplace Hazards: The Effect on Nurses As Women, *The American Nurse,* February 1998, 15.
253. Van Dongen, C., Environmental Health Risks, *American Journal of Nursing,* 98, no. 9 (1998), 16B–16E.
254. Community Health Services, *Preconceptual Health Series, Male Issues,* Website: http://www.lambtonhealth.on.ca/pregnancy/pre-conception/male.asp, June 2004.
255. Papalia et al., *op. cit.*
256. Van Dongen, *op. cit.*
257. Community Health Services, *Preconceptual Health Series, Male Issues.*
258. Hakansson, *op. cit.*
259. Luke et al., *op. cit.*
260. Henriksen, T.B., D.A. Savitz, M. Hedegaard, and N.J. Secher, Employment During Pregnancy in Relation to Risk Factors and Pregnancy Outcomes, *British Journal of Obstetrics and Gynaecology,* 101, no. 10 (1994), 858–865.
261. Homer, C., S. James, and E. Siegel, Work-Related Psychosocial Stress and Risk of Preterm, Low Birthweight Delivery, *American Journal of Public Health,* 80 (1990), 173–177.
262. Peoples-Sheps, M., E. Siegel, C. Suchindran, H. Origisa, A. Ware, and A. Barakat, Characteristics of Maternal Employment During Pregnancy: Effects on Low Birthweight, *American Journal of Public Health,* 81 (1991), 1007–1012.
263. Simpson, J.L., Are Physical Activity and Employment Related to Preterm Birth and Low Birth Weight? *American Journal of Obstetrics and Gynecology,* 168, no. 4 (1993), 1231–1238.
264. Dumanoski, op. cit.
265. *Ibid.*
266. *Ibid.*
267. *Ibid.*
268. Van Dongen, *op. cit.*
269. Ayotte, P., G. Muckle, J.L. Jacobson, S.W. Jacobson, and E. Dewailly, Assessment of Pre- and Postnatal Exposure to Polychlorinated Biphenyls: Lessons from the Inuit Cohort Study. *Environmental Health Perspectives,* 111, no. 9 (2003), 1253–1258.
270. Van Dongen, *op. cit.*
271. Health Canada, *Tobacco Control Program,* Website: http://www.hc-sc.gc.ca/ hecs-sesc/tobacco/index.html, June 2004.
272. *Ibid.*
273. Adatsi, G., Health Going Up in Smoke: How Can You Prevent It? *American Journal of Nursing,* 99, no. 3 (1999), 63–66.
274. Bee, *op. cit.*
275. Cunningham et al., *op. cit.*
276. Adatsi, *op. cit.*
277. Bee, *op. cit.*
278. Cunningham et al., *op. cit.*
279. Chomitz, V., L. Cheung, and E. Lieberman, The Role of Lifestyle in Preventing Low Birth Weight, *The Future of Children,* 5, no. 1 (1995), 121–138.
280. Cunningham et al., *op. cit.*
281. Papalia et al., *op. cit.*
282. Cunningham et al., *op. cit.*
283. Wong, *op. cit.*
284. Adatsi, *op. cit.*
285. Cunningham et al., *op. cit.*
286. Chomitz et al., *op. cit.*
287. Cunningham et al., *op. cit.*
288. Kallen, K., Maternal Smoking during Pregnancy and Limb Reduction Formations in Sweden, *American Journal of Public Health,* 87, no. 1 (1997), 29–32.
289. Wilcos, A.J., Birth Weight and Perinatal Mortality: The Effect of Maternal Smoking, *American Journal of Epidemiology,* 137, no. 20 (1993), 1098–1104.
290. Wong, *op. cit.*
291. Kallen, *op. cit.*
292. Adatsi, *op. cit.*
293. Chomitz et al., *op. cit.*
294. Kallen, *op. cit.*
295. Papalia et al., *op. cit.*
296. Wilcos, *op. cit.*
297. Kallen, *op. cit.*
298. Wilcos, *op. cit.*
299. Adatsi, *op. cit.*
300. Little, R. E., and D.R. Petersen, Sudden Infant Death Syndrome Epidemiology: A Review and Update, *Epidemiology Review,* 12 (1990), 241–246.
301. Papalia et al., *op. cit.*
302. Sherwen et al., *op. cit.*
303. Papalia et al., *op. cit.*
304. Wakefield, M.A., and W.R. Jones, Cognitive and Social Influences on Smoking Behavior During Pregnancy, *New Zealand Journal of Obstetrics and Gynecology,* 31, no. 3 (1991) 235–239.
305. Community Health Services, *Preconceptual Health Series.*
306. Wong, *op. cit.*
307. Sherwen et al., *op. cit.*

308. Wong, *op. cit.*

309. Papalia et al., *op. cit.*

310. Sherwen et al., *op. cit.*

311. Wong, *op. cit.*

312. Dykens, E., R. Hodapp, and J. Leckmann, *Behavior and Development in Fragile X Syndrome.* Thousand Oaks, CA: Sage, 1994.

313. Cunningham et al., *op. cit.*

314. Health Canada, *Preconception Health and Folic Acid, Primary Prevention of Neural Tube Defects with Folic Acid.*

315. Milberger, S., J. Biederman, S. Farame, et al., Is Maternal Smoking During Pregnancy a Risk Factor for Attention Hyperactivity Disorder in Children? *American Journal of Psychiatry,* 153, no. 9 (1996), 1138–1142.

316. Olds, D., C. Henderson, and R. Talelbaum, Intellectual Impairment in Children of Women Who Smoke Cigarettes During Pregnancy, *Pediatrics,* 93 (1994), 221–227.

317. Papalia et al., *op. cit.*

318. Sherwen et al., *op. cit.*

319. Wong, *op. cit.*

320. Condon, J.T., and C.A. Hilton, A Comparison of Smoking and Drinking Behaviors in Pregnant Women: Who Abstains and Why, *Medical Journal of Australia,* 148 (1988), 381–385.

321. Society of Obstetricians and Gynaecologists of Canada, Healthy Beginnings: Guidelines for Care During Pregnancy and Childbirth, *Journal of SOGC,* Policy Statement No. 71 (1998).

322. Johnson, J.L., P.A. Ratner, J.L. Bottorff, W. Hall, and S. Dahinten, Qualitative Study: Preventing Smoking Relapse in Postpartum Women, *Nursing Research,* 49, no. 1 (2000), 44–52.

323. *Ibid.*

324. Canadian Nurses Association, *Position Statement, Tobacco: The Role of Health Professionals in Smoking Cessation, Joint Statement,* Website: http://www.cna-nurses.ca, June 2004.

325. *Ibid.*

326. Windsor, R., J. Lowe, L. Perkins, D. Smith-Yoder, L. Artz, M. Crawford, K. Amburgy, and N. Boyd, Health Education for Pregnant Smokers: Its Behavioral Impact and Cost Benefit, *American Journal of Public Health,* 83 (1993), 201–206.

327. Olds et al., *op. cit.*

328. Zhang, J., and J. Ratcliffe, Paternal Smoking and Birthweight in Shanghai, *American Journal of Public Health,* 83, no. 2 (1993), 207–210.

329. Olds et al., *op. cit.*

330. Papalia et al., *op. cit.*

331. *Drugs in Pregnancy,* Website: http://www.theberries.ns.ca/ Archives/drugs_pregnancy.html, July 2004.

332. Society of Obstetricians and Gynaecologists of Canada, *op. cit.*

333. Motherisk, Website: http://www.motherisk.org, July 2004.

334. Wong, *op. cit.*

335. Bee, *op. cit.*

336. Cunningham et al., *op. cit.*

337. Papalia et al., *op. cit.*

338. Sherwen et al., *op. cit.*

339. Cunningham et al., *op. cit.*

340. *Ibid.*

341. *Ibid.*

342. Sherwen et al., *op. cit.*

343. Robinson, L., J. Buckley, A. Daigle, et al., Maternal Drug Use and Risk of Childhood Nonlymphoblastic Leukemia Among Offspring, *Cancer,* 63 (1989), 1904–1911.

344. Chasnoff, I.J., Prenatal Cocaine Exposure Is Associated With Respiratory Pattern Abnormalities.

345. Chasnoff, I. J., and D. Griffith, Cocaine: Clinical Studies of Pregnancy and the Newborn.

346. Chasnoff, et al., Temporal Patterns of Cocaine Use in Pregnancy: Perinatal Outcomes, *Journal of the American Medical Association,* 261, no. 12 (1989), 1741–1749.

347. Cocaine Before Birth, *The Harvard Mental Health Letter,* 15, no. 6 (1998), 1–4.

348. Williams, *op. cit.*

349. Windsor et al., *op. cit.*

350. Zuckerman, B., et al., Effect of Maternal Marijuana and Cocaine Use on Fetal Growth, *New England Journal of Medicine,* 320 (1989), 762–768.

351. Chasnoff, Prenatal Cocaine Exposure Is Associated With Respiratory Pattern Abnormalities.

352. Chasnoff and Griffith, Cocaine: Clinical Studies of Pregnancy and the Newborn.

353. Chasnoff, et al., Temporal Patterns of Cocaine Use in Pregnancy: Perinatal Outcomes.

354. Cocaine Before Birth, *The Harvard Mental Health Letter,* 15, no. 6 (1998), 1–4.

355. Williams, *op. cit.*

356. Windsor et al., *op cit.*

357. Wong, *op. cit.*

358. Zuckerman et al., *op. cit.*

359. Motherisk, Cocaine Use by Pregnant Women in Toronto, Website: http://www.motherisk.org/updates/index.php?id=106, July 2004.

360. Papalia et al., *op. cit.*

361. Wong, *op. cit.*

362. Sherwen et al., *op. cit.*

363. Wong, *op. cit.*

364. Strachan-Lindenberg et al., *op. cit.*

365. Chasnoff, I.J., Prenatal Cocaine Exposure Is Associated With Respiratory Pattern Abnormalities.

366. Chasnoff, I. J., and D. Griffith, Cocaine: Clinical Studies of Pregnancy and the Newborn.

367. Chasnoff et al., Temporal Patterns of Cocaine Use in Pregnancy: Perinatal Outcomes.

368. Strachan-Lindenberg et al., *op. cit.*

369. Zuckerman et al., *op. cit.*

370. Cocaine Before Birth.

371. Mott, L., *Children at Risk.* San Francisco: Natural Resources Defense Council, 1997.

372. Papalia et al., *op. cit.*

373. Robinson et al., *op. cit.*

374. Seifert, *op. cit.*

375. Wong, *op. cit.*

376. Zuckerman et al., *op. cit.*

377. Wheeler, S.F., Substance Abuse During Pregnancy, *Primary Care in Office Practice,* 20, no. 1 (1993), 191–207.

378. Little, R. E., and J.K. Wendt, The Effects of Maternal Drinking in the Reproductive Period: An Epidemiologic Review, *Journal of Substance Abuse,* 3, no. 2 (1991), 187–204.

379. Blackman, J., *Medical Aspects of Developmental Disabilities in Children From Birth to Three* (2nd ed.). Rockville, MD: Aspen Publishers, 1990.

380. Isen, J., A. de Costa Pereira, and S.F. Olsen, Does Maternal Tobacco Smoking Modify the Effect of Alcohol on Fetal Growth? *American Journal of Public Health,* 81, no. 1 (1991), 69–73.

381. Larroque, B., M. Kaminski, N. Lelong, D. Subtil, and P. Dehaene, Effects on Birth Weight of Alcohol and Caffeine Consumption During Pregnancy, *American Journal of Epidemiology,* 137, no. 9 (1993), 941–950.

382. Health Canada, *Healthy Living, Fetal Alcohol Syndrome/Fetal Alcohol Effects,* Website: http://www.hc-sc.gc.ca/english/lifestyles/fas.html, June 2004.

383. Wong, *op. cit.*

384. Spagnolo, A., Teratogenesis of Alcohol, *Annali dell' Instituto Suyperidi Sanit[[lang]]*, 29, no. 1 (1993), 89–96.

385. Larroque et al., *op. cit.*

386. Health Canada, *First Nations and Inuit Health Branch, Community Programs: FAS/FAE*, Website: http://www.hc-sc.gc.ca/fnibh/ep/fas_fae/introduction.html, June 2004.

387. Cunningham et al., *op. cit.*

388. Day, N.L., and G.A. Richardsen, Prenatal Alcohol Exposure: A Continuum of Effects, *Seminars in Perinatology*, 15, no. 4 (1991), 271–279.

389. Little and Wendt, *op. cit.*

390. Streissguth, A., F. Bookstein, P. Sampson, and H. Barr, Attention: Prenatal Alcohol and Continuities of Vigilance and Attentional Problems From 4 Through 14 Years, *Development and Psychopathology*, 7 (1995), 419–446.

391. Motherisk, *Fetal Alcohol Syndrome: Role of the Family Physician*, Website: http://www.motherisk.org/updates/index.php?id=299, July 2004.

392. Koren, G. *The Children of Neverland. The Silent Human Disaster.* Toronto: The Kids in Us Ltd., 1997.

393. Little and Petersen, *op. cit.*

394. Papalia et al., *op. cit.*

395. Sherwen et al., *op. cit.*

396. Dykens et al., op. cit.

397. Health Canada, First Nations and Inuit Health Branch, Community Programs, *op. cit.*

398. Duyff, *op. cit.*

399. Williams, *op. cit.*

400. Duyff, *op. cit.*

401. Williams, *op. cit.*

402. Smith, I.E., and C.D. Coles, Multilevel Intervention for Prevention of Fetal Alcohol Syndrome and Effects of Prenatal Alcohol Exposure, *Recent Developments in Alcoholism*, 9 (1991), 165–180.

403. Day and Richardsen, *op. cit.*

404. Koren, *op. cit.*

405. Health Canada, *It Takes a Community: Framework for the First Nations and Inuit Fetal Alcohol Syndrome and Fetal alcohol Effects Initiative*, Website: http://www.hc-sc.gc.ca/fnihb/cp/fas_fae/publications/it_takes_community.pdf, July 2004.

406. Health Canada, *Fetal Alcohol Spectrum Disorder (FASD)*, Website: http://www.hc-sc.gc.ca/dca-dea/publications/pdf/fasd-etcaf_e.pdf, July 2004.

407. Health Canada, *The Framework for Action on FASD*, Website: http://www.hc-sc.gc.ca/dca-dea/publications/fasd-etcaf/framework_e.html, July 2004.

408. Cunningham et al., *op. cit.*

409. Society of Obstetricians and Gynaecologists of Canada, *op. cit.*

410. Givens, K.T., D. A. Lee, T. Jones, and D.M. Ilstrup, Congenital Rubella Syndrome: Ophthalmic Manifestations and Associated Systematic Disorders, *British Journal of Ophthalmology*, 77, no. 6 (1993), 358–383.

411. Seifert, *op. cit.*

412. Sherwen et al., *op. cit.*

413. Wong, *op. cit.*

414. Society of Obstetricians and Gynaecologists of Canada, *op. cit.*

415. Health Canada, *The Framework for Action on FASD*.

416. Skovorc-Ranko, R., H. Lavola, P. St. Denis, M. Gagnou, R. Chicoine, M. Boucher, J. Gulmond, and Y. Dontigny, Intrauterine Diagnosis of Cytomegalovirus and Rubella Infections by Amniocentesis, *Canadian Medical Association Journal*, 145 (1991), 649–664.

417. Cunningham et al., *op. cit.*

418. Sherwen et al., *op. cit.*

419. Wong, *op. cit.*

420. Society of Obstetricians and Gynaecologists of Canada, *op. cit.*

421. *Ibid.*

422. Health Canada, *Division of Childhood and Adolescence*, Website: http://www.hc-sc.gc.ca/dca-dea/prenatal/fcmcl_e.html, June 2004.

423. Society of Obstetricians and Gynaecologists of Canada, *op. cit.*

424. Katz, A., The Evolving Art of Caring For Pregnant Women with HIV Infection. *Journal of Obstetrics, Gynecologic, and Neonatal Nursing*, 32, no.1 (2003), 102–108.

425. Health Canada, *Division of Childhood and Adolescence*.

426. Society of Obstetricians and Gynaecologists of Canada, *op. cit.*

427. McFarlin, S., S.F. Bottoms, B.S. Dock, and N.B. Isada, Epidemic Syphilis: Maternal Factors Associated with Congenital Infection, *American Journal of Obstetrics and Gynecology*, 170 (1994), 535–540.

428. Rawstron, S.A., S. Jenkins, P.W. LiBlanchard, and K. Bromberg, Maternal and Congenital Syphilis in Brooklyn, N.Y.: Epidemiology, Transmission, and Diagnosis, *American Journal of Diseases of Children*, 147 (1993), 7727–7731.

429. Sherwen et al., *op. cit.*

430. Wong, *op. cit.*

431. Sheffield, P.A., D.E. Moore, L.F. Boigt, D. Scholes, S.P. Wang, J.T. Grayston, and J.R. Darling, The Associations Between *Chlamydia Trachomatis* Serology and Pelvic Damage in Women with Tubal Ectopic Gestations, *Fertility and Sterility*, 60 (1993), 870–876.

432. Society of Obstetricians and Gynaecologists of Canada, *op. cit.*

433. *Ibid.*

434. *Ibid.*

435. *Ibid.*

436. Corcoran, G.D., and G.L. Ridgway, Antibiotic Chemotherapy of Bacterial Sexually Transmitted Diseases in Adults: A Review, *International Journal of SID and AIDS*, 5, no. 3 (1994), 165–171.

437. Cunningham et al., *op. cit.*

438. Sherwen et al., *op. cit.*

439. Lindenberger, *op. cit.*

440. Wong, *op. cit.*

441. *Ibid.*

442. Cunningham et al., *op. cit.*

443. Wong, *op. cit.*

444. Society of Obstetricians and Gynaecologists of Canada, *op. cit.*

445. *Ibid.*

446. *Ibid.*

447. *Ibid.*

448. Ausman, L.F., Toxoplasmosis and Pregnancy, *Canadian Nurse*, 89, no. 4 (1993), 31–32.

449. Sheffield et al., *op. cit.*

450. Cunningham et al., *op. cit.*

451. Seifert, *op. cit.*

452. Cunningham et al., *op. cit.*

453. *Ibid.*

454. Society of Obstetricians and Gynaecologists of Canada, *op. cit.*

455. The Society of Obstetricians and Gynaecologists of Canada and Canadian Paediatric Society, National Consensus Statement on the Prevention of Early-Onset Group B Streptococcal Infections in the Newborn. *Journal of the SOGC*, 19, no.7 (1997), 751–758.

456. Cunningham et al., *op. cit.*

457. *Ibid.*

458. *Ibid.*

459. Guyton, *op. cit.*

460. Cunningham et al., *op. cit.*

461. Guyton, *op. cit.*

462. Cunningham et al., *op. cit.*

463. Sherwen et al., *op. cit.*

464. Wong, *op. cit.*

465. *Ibid.*

466. McIntosh, L.J., N.E. Roumayah, and S.F. Bottoms, Perinatal Outcome of Broken Marriage in the Inner City, *Obstetrics and Gynecology*, 85, (1995), 233–236.
467. Henriksen et al., *op. cit.*
468. Osborn, L.M., D.C. Harris, M.C. Reading, and M.B. Prather, Outcome of Pregnancies Experienced During Residency, *Journal of Family Practice*, 31, no. 6 (1990), 618–622.
469. Homer et al., *op. cit.*
470. Hoff, L., *Battered Women as Survivors*, New York: Routledge, 1990.
471. Homer et al., *op. cit.*
472. Stewart, D.E., Incidence of Postpartum Abuse In Women With A History Of Abuse During Pregnancy. *Canadian Medical Association Journal*, 151, no. 11 (1994), 1601–1604.
473. Seifert, *op. cit.*
474. Stewart, *op. cit.*
475. Hoff, *op. cit.*
476. Stewart, *op. cit.*
477. Crow, J., How Much Do We Know About Spontaneous Human Mutation Rates? *Environmental and Molecular Mutagenesis*, 21 (1993), 122–129.
478. Cunningham et al., *op. cit.*
479. Papalia et al., *op. cit.*
480. Zhang and Ratcliffe, *op. cit.*
481. Hoff, *op. cit.*
482. Papalia et al., *op. cit.*
483. Cunningham et al., *op. cit.*
484. Sherwen et al., *op. cit.*
485. Wong, *op. cit.*
486. Papalia et al., *op. cit.*
487. Cunningham et al., *op. cit.*
488. Sherwen et al., *op. cit.*
489. Wong, *op. cit.*
490. Sherwen et al., *op. cit.*
491. Wong, *op. cit.*
492. *Ibid.*
493. Bee, *op. cit.*
494. Gormly, *op. cit.*
495. Health Canada, *Nutrition for a Healthy Pregnancy: National Guidelines for the Childbearing Years.*
496. Gormly, *op. cit.*
497. Nesbitt, T., E. Larson, R. Rosenblatt, and L. Hart, Access to Maternity Care in Rural Washington: Its Effect on Neonatal Outcomes and Resource Use, *American Journal of Public Health*, 87, no. 1 (1997), 85–88.
498. Sherwen et al., *op. cit.*
499. Lindenberger, *op. cit.*
500. Williams, *op. cit.*
501. Wong, *op. cit.*
502. Papalia et al., *op. cit.*
503. Heaman, M.I., A.E. Sprague, and P.J. Stewart, Reducing the Preterm Birth Rate: A Population Health Strategy. *Journal of Obstetric, Gynecologic, and Neonatal Nursing*, 30, no. 1 (2001), 20–29.
504. Cunningham et al., *op. cit.*
505. Papalia et al., *op. cit.*
506. Seifert, *op. cit.*
507. Duyff, *op. cit.*
508. Williams, *op. cit.*
509. Duyff, *op. cit.*
510. Johnston, P., Getting Enough to Grow On, *American Journal of Nursing*, 84, no. 3 (1984), 336–339.
511. Williams, *op. cit.*
512. Duyff, *op. cit.*
513. Heaman et al., *op. cit.*
514. Williams, *op. cit.*
515. Cunningham et al., *op. cit.*
516. Sherwen et al., *op. cit.*
517. Williams, *op. cit.*
518. Wong, *op. cit.*
519. Society of Obstetricians and Gynaecologists of Canada, *op. cit.*
520. Cunningham et al., *op. cit.*
521. Sherwen et al., *op. cit.*
522. Wong, *op. cit.*
523. Beck, C., The Effects of Postpartum Depression on Maternal-Infant Interaction: A Meta-analysis, *Nursing Research*, 44 (1995), 298–303.
524. Bustan, M., and A. Coker, Maternal Attitude Toward Pregnancy and the Risk of Neonatal Death, *American Journal of Public Health*, 84 (3), 1994, 411–414.
525. Garbarino, J., N. Dubrow, K. Kosteling, and C. Pardo, *Children in Danger: Coping with Consequences of Community Violence.* San Francisco: Jossey-Bass, 1992
526. Rogers, A., P. Wingert, and T. Hayden, Why the Young Kill, *Newsweek*, May 3, 1999, 32–35.
527. Williams, R., Social Ties and Health, *The Harvard Mental Health Letter*, 15, no. 19 (1999), 4–5.
528. Papalia et al., *op. cit.*
529. Guyton, *op. cit.*
530. *Ibid.*
531. *Ibid.*
532. Dumanoski, *op. cit.*
533. *Ibid.*
534. Van Dongen, *op. cit.*
535. Sin, D.D., H.M. Sharpe, R.L. Cowie, S.F. Man, Spirometric Findings Among School-Aged First Nations Children on a Reserve: A Pilot Study, *Canadian Respiratory Journal*, 11, no. 1 (2004), 45–48.
536. Williams, R., Social Ties and Health.
537. Dumanoski, *op. cit.*
538. Van Dongen, *op. cit.*
539. Montgomery, L., J. Kiely, and G. Pappas, The Effects of Poverty, Race, and Family Structure on U.S. Children's Health: Data from the NHIS, 1978 Through 1980 and 1989 Through 1991, *American Journal of Public Health*, 86, no. 10 (1996), 1401–1405.
540. Parish, N., Lack of Good Housing Hurts Children's Health, Study Says, *St. Louis Post-Dispatch*, April 8, 1999, B1, B3.
541. Wong, *op. cit.*
542. Buhler, C., The Developmental Structure of Goal Setting in Group and Individual Studies, in C. Buhler, and F. Massarik, eds., *The Course of Human Life*, New York: Springer-Verlag, 1968.
543. Society of Obstetricians and Gynaecologists of Canada, *op. cit.*
544. Johnston, *op. cit.*
545. Sherwen et al., *op. cit.*
546. Wong, *op. cit.*
547. Ford-Gilboe, M., Family Strengths, Motivation and Resources as Predictors of Health Promotion Behavior in Single-Parent and Two-Parent Families, *Research in Nursing and Health*, 20, no. 3 (1997), 205–217.
548. Bee, *op. cit.*
549. Papalia et al., *op. cit.*
550. Werner, E., Risk and Resilience in Individuals with Learning Disabilities: Lessons Learned from the Kauai Longitudinal Study, *Learning Disabilities: Research and Practice*, 8, 28–34.
551. Bee, *op. cit.*
552. Papalia et al., *op. cit.*
553. Ford-Gilboe, *op. cit.*
554. Papalia et al., *op. cit.*
555. Ford-Gilboe, *op. cit.*
556. Sherwen et al., *op. cit.*
557. Wong, *op. cit.*

558. Health Canada, *Canadian Incidence Study of Reported Child Abuse and Neglect*, Website: http://www.hc-sc.gc.ca/pphb-dgsp-sp/publicat/chirpp-schirpt/20se01/, July 2004.
559. Bustan and Coker, *op. cit.*
560. *Ibid.*
561. Stewart, *op. cit.*
562. Sin et al., *op. cit.*
563. Sherwen et al., *op. cit.*
564. Wong, *op. cit.*
565. Werner et al., *op. cit.*
566. Bee, *op. cit.*
567. Gormly, *op. cit.*
568. Papalia et al., *op. cit.*
569. Sachs, B., L. Hall, M. Lulenbacker, and M. Rayens, Potential for Abusive Parenting by Rural Mothers with Low-Birth-Weight Children, *IMAGE: Journal of Nursing Scholarship,* 31, no. 1 (1995), 21–25.
570. Seifert, *op. cit.*
571. Sherwen et al., *op. cit.*
572. Wong, *op. cit.*
573. Sherwen et al., *op. cit.*
574. Wong, *op. cit.*
575. Sherwen et al., *op. cit.*
576. Wong, *op. cit.*

Part 3

THE DEVELOPING PERSON AND FAMILY: INFANCY THROUGH ADOLESCENCE

CHAPTER 7

ASSESSMENT AND HEALTH PROMOTION FOR THE INFANT

CHAPTER 8

ASSESSMENT AND HEALTH PROMOTION FOR THE TODDLER

CHAPTER 9

ASSESSMENT AND HEALTH PROMOTION FOR THE PRESCHOOLER

CHAPTER 10

ASSESSMENT AND HEALTH PROMOTION FOR THE SCHOOLCHILD

CHAPTER 11

ASSESSMENT AND HEALTH PROMOTION FOR THE ADOLESCENT AND YOUTH

Chapter 7

ASSESSMENT AND HEALTH PROMOTION FOR THE INFANT

THE GREAT SPIRIT GAVE US CHILDREN. . . .
That is why we must love them.

Elder, Awasis Training Institute of Northern Manitoba (1994)

OBJECTIVES

STUDY OF THIS CHAPTER WILL ENABLE YOU TO:

1. Define terms and give examples of basic developmental principles pertinent to the neonate and the infant.

2. Comprehend the issue of birth as a crisis for the family. Identify factors that influence parental attachment for the neonate and infant. Ascertain details of your role in assisting the family to adapt to the challenges and joys of the birth crisis.

3. Identify and describe the adaptive physiological changes that occur at birth for the mother and for the child.

4. Assess the neonate's physical characteristics and the manner in which psychosocial needs begin to be filled.

5. Determine the normal or expected characteristics of a neonate and infant regarding physiology, motor activity, cognitive abilities, emotional responses, and social characteristics including adaptive mechanisms.

6. Determine the normal range of sleep, movement, and play patterns of an infant.

7. Interpret an immunization schedule, and discuss safety and health promotion measures with a parent.

8. Discuss in a health care team setting your role in assisting parents: to foster the development of trust with each other and to develop positive self-concepts regarding the new baby.

9. State the developmental tasks of the infant. Describe the behaviours that indicate these tasks are being achieved.

10. Compare thriving parent–infant behaviours to faltering parent–infant behaviours.

11. Discuss your role in promoting parental attachment.

12. Begin to implement health-promoting strategies with parents and baby after delivery and during the first year of life.

This chapter discusses the normal growth and development of the baby during the first year of life, baby's effect on the family, and the family's influence on baby. *Measures to promote the infant's well-being that are useful in health promotion and nursing practice and that can be taught to parents are described throughout the chapter.*

In this chapter the terms **neonate** and **newborn** refer to the *first four weeks of life;* **infant** refers to the *first 12 months* (or in some texts, 15 months). Practices vary from culture to culture. In most Asian cultures, the child is considered one year old at birth. Traditional Chinese custom adds one year to an infant's age on January 1, regardless of the birthday.[1] **Mother** or **parent(s)** is the term used to denote *the person(s) responsible for the child's care and long-term well-being.*

You can refer to an embryology and obstetric nursing textbook for detailed information on fetal development, prenatal changes, and the process of labour and delivery. This chapter builds on information presented in Chapters 4 and 6 and focuses on the developmental tasks of the infant and family after birth. The authors are aware that some characteristics and developmental tasks of the infant and family described here may vary among cultures. The infant will certainly be slower to develop some characteristics if he or she is born where there is famine, economic deprivation, political unrest or war, or devastation from natural disaster.

FAMILY DEVELOPMENT AND RELATIONSHIPS

The coming of the child is a **crisis**, a *turning point in the couple's life in which old patterns of living must be changed for new ways of living and new values.*[2] The crisis will be less severe if the baby is wanted than if the couple had planned not to have children. Many couples look forward to starting a family, and they initially make plans to accommodate a pregnancy. But having a baby is always a crisis—a change. The woman may first feel the crisis as she recognizes body changes and new emotional responses. For example, Sally, age 28, who has just become pregnant, may wonder about losing her slim figure, question how long she can work, and worry about balancing work and childrearing. Further, Sally may be concerned about making spatial changes in the home or moving to a new home to accommodate the new baby. She might be anxious, too, about balancing the budget to meet additional expenses.

The crisis is greater when the baby is not planned, or not wanted. Such may be the case with Jane who was devastated when she found out she was pregnant. Although she did not deliberately seek an abortion, she began to skip meals and to exercise vigorously in an effort to maintain a slim figure. Jane did not have anyone to talk to about her feelings and felt very much alone. She was frightened and eventually became ill at work. Jane's co-workers helped her to find medical attention.

At times, even though the pregnancy may have been planned, the man becomes fearful of fatherhood because of the consequent responsibility and loss of freedom due to the birth of the baby. When John learned that his wife, Nancy, was pregnant, he withdrew emotionally, was apathetic about the baby, and spent more time with his male friends and work associates. Nancy, in turn, spent much time alone and felt increasingly rejected, abandoned, depressed, and angry. These behaviours may bring John and Nancy to separate unless they find help, admit to their problem, work through their feelings, and recommit their love for one another.

7-1 BONUS SECTION IN CD-ROM
Baby Crisis

What happens when a couple learns they are going to have a baby? This question and the lifestyle changes that accompany the event are considered.

Whether perceived as positive or negative, change always involves a sense of loss of the familiar, for the way it used to be. The vacuum created by the loss is a painful one and one for which parents are usually ill-prepared. The couple's life will never again be "normal" as they once knew it, but together the family now needs to find a "new normal."

If pregnancy and parenting create a crisis for a couple who may want a baby, these events are even more stressful for the adolescent or for the single woman—either unmarried, or, if married, left by her husband to face pregnancy, birth, and childrearing alone. This adolescent or woman needs the support of and help from at least one other person during this period. A parent, relative, or friend can be a resource. Often the support and help of a number of people are needed. You may be the primary source of support. Your empathetic listening, acceptance, practical hints for better self-care and baby care, and general availability can make a real difference in the outcome of the pregnancy and in the mother's and father's ability to parent and to handle future crises.

In Canada, the *Family-Centred Maternity and Newborn Care: National Guidelines*, developed through a collaborative process involving health care providers and consumers, is a multidimensional, dynamic, and complex process that responds to the physical, emotional, and psychosocial needs of women and families. These guidelines not only view pregnancy and birth as normal, healthy events (a celebration), but consider pregnancy and birth to be unique for each woman. One of the guiding principles stresses that health care providers form a trusting relationship between women and their families based on respect in order for the woman to give birth safely and with dignity.[3] Referral to other resources and self-help groups (such as Parents Without Partners, which is found both in Canada and United States) as well as to a counsellor may also be of great help to the mother. Another Canadian prenatal resource is Motherisk, which has a useful website.[4]

CRITICAL THINKING

Assume you were working in a remote community in northern Canada. How would you access resources for a pregnant woman and her family?

Growth and Development of Parents

Parenting is an inexact science. An increasing number of people are not prepared either intellectually or emotionally for family life because of the lack of nurturing or because of the difficult family life they experienced in childhood. Every parent hopes that their child will grow to be an independent and happy adult. However, creating and maintaining a family unit is difficult in today's society. Therein lies the challenge for every parent. Many occupations demand travel, frequent change of residence, and working on Sundays and holidays, the traditional family days. The rapid pace of life and available opportunities interfere with family functions. For example, Gloria and Don, who both work, seem always to be on the go with their three young school-age children. At times they take turns driving them to either dancing or piano lessons, or to various sports activities. They find that their dinner schedule varies from day to day.

For Aboriginal people, the term **family** denotes the *biological unit of both parents and children residing together in a household*.[5] However, Aboriginal children receive nurturing not only from their family of origin, but also from the elders, extended family, and the community. Because children are valued and hold a special place in the Aboriginal community, the task of fostering child development in a healthy way becomes very important.[6] Even though Aboriginal communities are evolving and are in the process of demographic change in Canada, the centrality of the family remains important.[7] In fact, health care providers need to promote and reinforce Aboriginal parenting skills and traditional teachings.[8] Brenda and Fred, who reside in a northern community, maintain their traditional beliefs and cultural practices. Brenda, who is pregnant with their first child, views her pregnancy as a natural event. She is somewhat anxious and shy about attending a prenatal clinic, but she soon realizes that the health professionals are approachable and display culturally sensitive and caring practices that are meaningful to her. Following are some general guidelines for health professionals who might interact with Aboriginal families:

1. Demonstrate friendliness during the visit with the family and show a genuine interest in topics that come up for discussion.

2. Demonstrate a nonjudgmental attitude.

3. Respect the child and family as they are.

4. Listen, listen, and listen again, as Aboriginal people have a strong oral tradition and stress the value of observing.

5. Learn to recognize the rights of the family and extended family who might be caring for the child.

6. Give everyone an opportunity to speak regarding the well-being of the child, and mainly, learn to recognize that "the child must be understood as a whole being in the total context of his or her family, culture, community and physical environment."[9]

Pregnancy is preparation for the birth event, whereas parenting is a process that continues for many years. Becoming a parent involves grieving the loss of one's own childhood and former lifestyle. The person must be in touch with and be able to express and work through feelings of loss before he or she can adapt and move on to a higher level of maturation. Being aware of the tremendous influence of parents on their children's development, parents may feel challenged to become the best persons they are capable of being. New parents may need to develop a confidence that they do not feel, an integrity that has been easy to let slide, and values that can tolerate being scrutinized. To grow and develop as a parent, the person needs to make peace with his or her past so that unresolved conflicts are not inflicted on the child.

After a baby joins the family, a number of problems must be worked through. The mother must deal with the separation from a symbiotic relationship with the baby. The reality of child care and managing a household may be a disillusionment after exposure to the ideals inculcated by the mass media and advertising. Even though many parents exhibit strengths, problems always exist. It is important for you, as a health professional, to validate the couple's strengths to promote their health and well-being.

One of the potential problem areas that you can explore with parents is that of re-establishing a mutually satisfying sexual relationship, which is not a simple process but has intricate psychological overtones for man and woman. You may also need to address the couple's desire for family planning. (See Table 11-5 for information on contraceptive measures.) Sexual relationships usually decrease during pregnancy, childbirth, and the postpartum period. However, couples can resume sexual intercourse once the episiotomy has healed and the lochia flow has stopped. This usually occurs by the end of the third week. Prior to the six-week check-up, it is important that the woman and her partner be informed about what to expect regarding sexual activity. For example, the couple should be informed that since the vaginal vault is dry (hormone poor), some form of lubrication might be necessary during intercourse.[10] By six weeks after birth, the woman's pelvis is back to normal, lochia has ceased, and involution is complete. Whether or not she is ready physically for an active sex life depends upon the person and the situation. But the mother may be so absorbed in and fatigued by the challenges and responsibilities of motherhood that the father is pushed into the background. He may feel in competition with the baby, resenting both the baby and his wife.

Either parent may take initiative in renewing the role of lover, in being sexually attractive to the other. The woman may choose to do this by getting a new hairdo or stylish clothes for her now slimmer outward figure. Inwardly, she can strengthen flabby perineal muscles through prescribed exercise. Patience on the part of the man is necessary, for if an episiotomy was done before delivery, healing continues for some time, and the memory of pain in the area may cause the woman involuntarily to tense the perineal muscles and wish to forgo intercourse. Happy couples who have a sound philosophy and communication system soon work out such problems, including the fact that the needs of the baby will sometimes interrupt intimacy. For couples whose earlier sex life was unsatisfactory and who do not work together as a team, such problems may be hard to surmount. Your support, suggestions, and assistance in helping the couple seek and accept help from family and friends will foster their ability to manage.

Given the whole realm of stresses and life changes associated with a baby's birth, it is understandable that, at least initially, parenting is at best a bittersweet experience. Parents may have strongly ambivalent thoughts and feelings toward this child whom they have together created.

The following stress indicators may be used in your assessment to predict the likelihood of postpartum difficulties:[11,12]

- Woman is having her first baby (primipara).
- No relatives are available to help with baby care.
- Complications occurred during pregnancy.
- Woman's mother is dead.
- Woman is ill apart from pregnancy.
- Woman was ill on bed rest during pregnancy.
- Woman has distant relationship or conflict with own mother.
- Male partner is often away from home or not involved with pregnancy or childrearing.
- Woman has no previous experience with babies.

Postpartum difficulties are also more likely if the parent is an adolescent or has suffered child abuse, especially sexual abuse or incest. Strass claims that the assessment and treatment of postpartum depression is overlooked, and that all geographical health regions in Canada should offer appropriate assessment and health promoting strategies to such families.[13]

Parenting is a risky process. It involves facing the unknown with faith because no one can predict the outcome when the intricacies of human relationships are involved. Parents grow and develop by taking themselves and their child one day at a time and by realizing the joy that can be part of those crazy, hectic early weeks and months. The feelings of joy and involvement increase as the parent–child attachment is cemented.

Because establishing this attachment is crucial to the long-term nurturing of the child and parental interest in the child, the process is explored in depth to assist you in assessment and intervention.

CRITICAL THINKING

Differentiate between the type of health care information on pregnancy and delivery you would provide for a couple living in an urban area, compared to that which you would provide to a couple living in Nunavut.

Infant–Parent Attachment

Attachment *is an emotional tie between two persons.* Thus, it is *a human phenomenon characterized by certain behaviours.* It is described as a *close, reciprocal relationship between two people that involves contact with and proximity to another that endures over time.* It is only when these behaviours are directed to one or a few persons rather than to many persons that the behaviours indicate attachment (Figure 7–1). Health care professionals often use the term *attachment* to describe behaviours between caregivers and their infants. Authors and investigators have devoted considerable attention to and interest in the formation of early maternal–infant and, more recently, paternal–infant ties of affection. Authors often use the term *attachment* interchangeably with the term *bonding*. The term **bonding** first appeared in behavioural research and referred to the *sensitive period for the establishment of a tie between animal mothers and their offspring.* The term now *refers to the initial maternal feeling and attachment behaviour immediately following delivery.* **Engrossment** is the term authors use to describe the *father's initial paternal response to the baby.* Interest in the concept of bonding went beyond the maternal–infant dyad to consider the father–infant dyad. This concept developed along with the concept of maternal–infant bonding.[14–18]

When considering infant behaviour, **temperament** is a concept frequently linked with attachment. **Temperament** is described as *a behavioural style* and is defined as *a characteristic way of thinking, behaving, or reacting in a given situation.* While it is believed that from birth children are predisposed to respond to the environment in different ways, these differences influence the way others respond to them and their needs. Temperament is believed to have a major impact on behaviour and development as it influences the dynamic interactions, including attachment behaviours, between children and other people in their environment.[19]

Rubin describes the beginning of the mother–child relationship as similar to the beginning of any new relationship. She writes that "identification of the partner in the relationship is a universal prerequisite. Even before any interaction occurs, there are certain relevant pieces of information to be obtained about the newcomer—sex, condition, and size. Each member must obtain introductory information before any interaction can occur."[20] Table 7-1 outlines some behaviours of the infant, mother, and father in the typical order of progression in establishing this initial relationship.[21–31]

Recent investigations and review articles conclude that there is no firm scientific evidence supportive of immediate parent–infant bonding.[32–34] But Palkovitz found that media presentations, anecdotal reports, and survey data indicate that a majority of lay respondents expressed a strong belief not only in the phenomenon of bonding, but also in the existence of scientific evidence to support this concept.[35–38] In the view of the general public's beliefs concerning bonding, health care workers, especially childbirth educators, must present scientific information in an objective manner to decrease the possibility that parents will experience guilt or disappointment concerning their role in the intrapartum or postpartum period. It is important that childbirth educators inform parents that early contact with the infant in the postpartum period can be a fulfilling, but neither necessary nor sufficient, experience. The media and other authors continue to present information about the importance of parental nurturing and attachment over time.[39–44]

Some research shows that all mothers do not initially follow the sequence of handling that is described in most of the literature and in Table 7-1. Some mothers initially use palms or arms to handle the infant and then their fingers to explore the infant. Often mothers simultaneously use fingers and palms and then arms and trunk to explore and hold the baby. Some mothers may be initially hesitant or awkward in touching or holding the baby, or hold the baby differently from most mothers, and yet feel very maternal. These differences should be considered in assessment of maternal bonding and attachment.[45] Realize also that there are cultural differences in expression of attachment. In some cultures, the parents of the woman or the man take care of the newborn and mother for a designated time. Further, out of respect for the elderly, the new parents will comply with their parents' wishes, regardless of what professionals tell the young parents.

The state of the infant is a strong predictor of the relative frequency with which fathers display interactive, affectionate, and comforting behaviour toward the infant. Very young crying infants are comforted or shown affectionate behaviour. One study found that fathers are most likely to stimulate by touch those infants who are awake but not crying. Fathers are as likely to talk in a stimulating manner to infants who are either crying or not crying and, similarly, to infants who are sleeping or awake. Perhaps fathers perceive talking as less soothing to crying infants than touch and talking as less disturbing than touch to sleeping infants. Recently, a study found that fathers are less consistent than mothers are at responding to infant cues. Sometimes fathers respond and at other times they don't.[46]

Studies in bonding and attachment have included primarily middle-class, reasonably well-educated Caucasians.

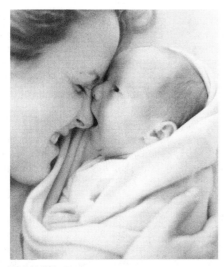

FIGURE 7–1

Mother–infant attachment develops mutually over the first year of life.

Bonding and attachment behaviours, especially for the male, could be different in other racial and cultural groups. Some cultures emphasize the mother as caretaker of the infant; the bond or attachment between father and child is less overt and may be emphasized later in childhood. For Aboriginal people, "the family is the recognized cornerstone of First Nations cultures, and a distinctive feature of that cornerstone is the central position of the child."[47] In the culture a close relationship with the child is important, and the display of affection and kindness to the child is paramount. For example, the time period during the construction of cradleboards provides opportunities for bonding to occur between the mother and the child. Designing and decorating the cradleboard give special attention to welcome the child and keep his or her spirit happy. Although cradleboards are not as common in current generations of Aboriginal peoples, the significance of time taken during the cradleboard construction exemplifies the continuing importance of teaching nurturing behaviour and recognizing the importance of child development.[48]

Some investigators have found a positive relationship between the first holding of the infant and the development of attachment feelings, but indicated that attachment began when the infant was first held, regardless of how long after delivery the holding occurred.[49]

Some authors believe that in addition to causing increased alertness in the baby, effective maternal–infant bonding can promote the baby's physical health in the following ways: (1) transference of maternal nasal and respiratory flora to baby may prevent the baby from acquiring hospital strains of infectious organisms; (2) maternal body heat is a reliable source of heat for the newborn; and (3) regular breastfeedings can pass on the antibodies IgA and T- and B-lymphocytes to the baby to protect against enteric pathogens.

Development of attachment between parent and baby continues through infancy. It involves emotional, cognitive, and socialization processes: loving through cuddling, touching, stroking, kissing, cooing and talking to, laughing, playing with, and reinforcing and teaching baby. Such contact should be consistent and done while caring physically for baby. The touching, cooing, talking, and laughing can also be focused on baby while the mother (or father) is preparing a meal, doing a household task, or waiting in a grocery line. The parent's voice across the room can also soothe and promote attachment. Further, just as the parent may need to learn to respond to the infant, sometimes the child needs prompting to be responsive to the parent and to signal needs and not just wait for every need to be automatically met.

TABLE 7-1
Infant–Parent Attachment Behaviours

Infant	Mother	Father
Reflexively looks into mother's face, *establishes eye-to-eye contact* or "*face tie*"; moulds body to mother's body when held	*Reaches* for baby; *holds high against breast-chest-shoulder area;* handles baby smoothly	Has great *interest in baby's face and notes eyes*
Vocalizes, cries, and *stretches out arms* in response to mother's voice; responds to mother's voice with "*dance*" or *rhythmic movements*	Talks softly in *high-pitched voice* and with intense interest to baby; puts baby face-to-face with her (*en face position*); eye contact gives baby sense of identity to mother	*Desires to touch, pick up, and hold baby;* cradles baby securely; shows fingertip touching and smiling to male baby; has more eye contact with infant delivered by forceps or caesarean section
Roots, licks, then *sucks* mother's nipple if in contact with mother's breast, cries, smiles	*Touches* baby's extremities; examines, strokes, massages, and kisses baby shortly after delivery; puts baby to breast if permitted; oxytocin and prolactin released	*Looks for distinct features;* thinks newborn resembles self; perceives baby as beautiful in spite of newborn characteristics
Reflexively embraces, clambers, clings, using hands, feet, head, and mouth to maintain body contact	*Calls baby by name;* notes desirable traits; *expresses pleasure* toward baby; *attentive* to reflex actions of grunts and sneezes	*Feels elated,* bigger, proud after birth; has strong *desire to protect and care for child*
Odour of mother distinguished by breastfeeding baby by fifth day	*Recognizes odour* of own child by third or fourth day	

NOTE: Similar behaviours are seen with a premature baby but the timing will vary.

EVIDENCE-BASED PRACTICE

Mother–Infant Interaction: Achieving Synchrony

Twenty-nine first-time mothers were randomly assigned to either an intervention or a control group. Extra education, received by the intervention group about two weeks prior to their expected due date, consisted of a 45-minute videotape based on the *Keys to Caregiving* program about infant behaviour. The videotape contained information on infant states, communication cues, and ways to increase social and cognitive growth-fostering behaviours. The control group attended routine teaching sessions only, consisting of information on cord care, infant bath, and risk factors with early discharge. The purpose of the research was to study differences in mother–infant interaction within the first 24 hours following birth. The Nursing Child Assessment Teaching Scale was the questionnaire used to test the mother's sensitivity to, and understanding of, the infant's behaviour. In addition, the mother was videotaped when teaching her child to look at a rattle. The scores between groups were compared to determine the effect of education on the interaction that occurred between the dyads.

The results showed that:

1. In the treatment group there was a high correlation between the infant's clarity of cues and responsiveness to the care given.
2. There was a moderate correlation between the infant's responsiveness to the caregiver and caregiver total scores in both treatment and control group.
3. Based on t-test analysis, the education provided in the prenatal period did affect the quality of interaction that occurred between mother and infant.

Practice Implications

Prenatal classes need to include information about how the baby communicates, cues to respond to, and ways to respond to different infant states. Doing so, coupled with the reinforcement of such behaviour postnatally in community health clinics and well baby clinics, would facilitate mother–infant synchrony.

Source: Leitch, D., Mother–Infant Interaction: Achieving Synchrony, Nursing Research, 48, no. 1 (1999), 55–57. Used with the permission of Lippincott, Williams & Wilkins.

Observe for maternal–child attachment. Research indicates that educating the mother prenatally via videotape about infant behaviours, developmental norms, and communication cues facilitates a more positive mother–infant interaction in the postpartum period. The infant develops effective reciprocal interactions with the caregiver when the caregiver is responsive to the infant.[50]

An article by Byrd[51] gives suggestions on how to approach maternal–child home visits and ask questions about the quality of caregiving during the home visit.

Factors Influencing Maternal Attachment

Motherly feelings do not necessarily accompany biological motherhood. Various factors affect the mother's attachment and caretaking. Variables that are difficult or impossible to change include the woman's level of emotional maturity, how she was reared, what her culture encourages her to do, relationships with her family and partner, experience with previous pregnancies, and planning for and experiencing events during the course of this pregnancy.[52–55]

Deterrents to adequate mothering include the mother's own immaturity or lack of mothering, stress situations, fear of rejection from significant people, loss of a loved one, financial worries, lack of a supportive partner, and even the sex and appearance of the child. Separating mother and infant the first few days of life, depersonalized care by professionals, rigid hospital routines, and the current practice of early discharge from the hospital without adequate help also interfere with establishing attachment and maternal behaviours.[56–59] Assess

for these deterrents. Your nurturing of the mother and helping her seek additional help may offset the negative impact of these factors.

Nurturing will be essential for the mother who returns home within the 24-hour period after delivery. She will be exhausted, sore, and possibly overwhelmed with emotion and responsibility. The community health nurse is one support system; relatives or friends will also be needed for help. The nurse's assessment regarding mother's physical and emotional status and need for information about child care is critical and is also essential to determine status of the newborn. The first 72 hours of the baby's life is a significant period of transition and stabilization and also a time when malformations or cardiorespiratory or feeding problems are evidenced. Infection in both mother and baby may occur in this initial period.

Parenting skills can be manifested in various ways. Although eye contact, touch, and cuddling are important, love can be shown by a tender, soft voice and loving gazes. *Observe for other indications of warm parenting feelings:*

- Calls the baby by name
- Expresses enjoyment of the baby and indicates that the baby is attractive or has other positive characteristics
- Looks at the baby and into baby's eyes
- Talks to the baby in a loving voice
- Takes safety precautions for the baby
- Responds to the baby's cues for attention or physical care

Factors Influencing Paternal Attachment

Fatherly feelings do not necessarily accompany fatherhood. Bonding and attachment feelings in the father appear related to various factors: general level of education, participation in prenatal classes, sex of infant, role concept, attendance at delivery, type of delivery, early contact, and feeding method for the baby.[60]

Support from the mother is most effective in reducing stress levels in expectant fathers; support from others is critical only if the expectant woman cannot be supportive. This may be because intimacy and self-disclosure for men are maintained primarily in the partner relationship. For the expectant woman, support from both the partner and others is critical in coping with stress, perhaps because women are socialized to value and depend on social relations to a greater extent than men.[61]

The father is increasingly recognized as an important person to the infant and young child, not only as a breadwinner but also as a nurturer. Lack of a father figure can cause developmental difficulties for the child. Just as the mother is not necessarily endowed with nurturing feelings, the father is not necessarily lacking nurturing feelings. Some fathers seem to respond better to this role than the mothers do.[62–66] Lorne, for example, is assuming the basic childrearing responsibilities, while his wife, Gwen, pursues the major family career. Both parents are content in carrying out their individual family responsibilities. Today, such undertakings by couples are generally accepted.

Behaviour Characteristic of Parental Difficulty in Establishing Attachment

Realize that parents tend to project their own feelings onto their child, turning the child into a figure from their own past. Negative feelings in the parent can create a dysfunctional relationship with the child.

Note the methods of relating to and holding the infant that would indicate the parent's *difficulty in establishing attachment*:[67–70]

- Maintains little or no eye contact with baby
- Does not touch baby, or picks up baby at times to meet own needs
- Does not support baby's head
- Holds baby at a distance, at arm's length after initial visits, loosely, or not at all
- Appears disinterested in baby, is preoccupied with something else when baby is present, and has a flat, fixed facial expression or unconvincing smile in response to your enthusiasm about baby
- Perceives baby as unattractive or looking like someone who is disliked
- Talks or coos to baby little or not at all
- Has passive response to baby; allows baby to be placed in arms rather than reaching out to baby
- Calls baby "it" rather than saying "my baby" or calling baby by name
- Notes defects or undesirable traits in baby, even if baby is normal, or is convinced baby is abnormal
- Avoids talking about baby, even when someone else initiates the topic
- Expresses dissatisfaction with or revulsion about care of baby
- Ignores baby's communications of cries, grunts, sneezes, and yawns
- Gets upset when baby's secretions, feces, or urine touch body or clothes; perceives care of baby as revolting
- Readily gives baby to someone else
- Does not take adequate safety precautions with baby (e.g., in relation to diapering, feeding, covering baby, or baby's movements)
- Handles the baby roughly, even after the baby has eaten or vomited
- Gives inappropriate responses to baby's needs such as overfeeding or underfeeding, or underhandling
- Thinks baby does not love him or her

NARRATIVE VIGNETTE

You are a nurse in a northern community. A month ago you managed, after completing a generous maternity leave, to regain your full-time appointment at the local hospital, and, as before, you are frequently called in for overtime work. You and your spouse, an RCMP officer at the local detachment, have a 10-month-old infant, Sarah, your first. For the times when you and your spouse are working at the same time, you have hired a local grandmother, Clara, to look after Sarah in her home. All seems well for your family, except when disruptions occur—which can happen at any time. For example, you are called to the hospital frequently on weekend evenings when the emergency ward is very busy. Weekends are especially demanding for the police force and overnight flights into the interior are routine for all RCMP members. Clara has not been too enthusiastic recently about having Sarah overnight two or three times per week. And it seems that Sarah is becoming less regular at sleeping through the night and is fussing more.

1. What issues will you take into consideration?

2. What plans will you make to facilitate your own, and your spouse's, attachment with Sarah?

- Expresses dislike of self, finds attribute in baby that is disliked in self
- Complains of being too tired to take care of baby
- Expresses fears that baby might die of a minor illness

You may not observe all these behaviours in the mother initially, or in the mother or father later, but a combination of several should alert you to actual or potential difficulty with being a parent.

CRITICAL THINKING

On repeated occasions, you experience that an older mother readily hands her baby to you as you begin a home visit. What possible reasons might the mother have for doing this?

Personalizing Nursing Care to Promote Attachment

Certain interventions directed to the parents will help them to develop attachment with the infant:

- Call the child, mother, and father by their names during your care.
- Inquire about the mother's well-being; too often all the focus is on the baby. She is in a receptive state and must be emotionally and physically cared for.
- The father also needs nurturance before he can show caring and be helpful to the mother and baby.
- Make favourable comments about the infant's progress.
- Compliment the mother on her intentions or ability to comfort, feed, or identify her baby's needs. Speak of the pleasure baby shows in response to the parent's ministrations.
- Reassure parents that positive changes in baby are a result of their care, and avoid judgmental attitudes or guilt statements.

Interventions that support, teach, and counsel parents about how to promote attachment and optimum infant stimulation are:

- Encourage both parents to cuddle, look at, and talk to the baby; if necessary, demonstrate how to stroke, caress, and rock baby.
- Encourage parents to be prompt and consistent in answering the infant's cry.
- Assist parents in gaining confidence in responding effectively to baby's cry through recognizing the meaning of the cry, meeting the child's needs, and using soothing measures, such as rocking, redundant sounds, and swaddling.
- Explain the infant's interactive abilities and help the parents develop awareness of their own initial effective responses to the newborn's behaviour.
- Explain the basis of early infant learning as the discovery of associations, connections, and relationships between self and repeated occurrences. Explore how to provide variety; a gradually increasing level of stimulus

complexity, sights, sounds, smells, movements, positions, temperatures, and pressure all provide learning opportunities and opportunities for emotional, perceptual, social, and physical development.

- Call attention to baby and those behaviours that indicate developmental responsiveness, such as reflex movements, visual following, smiling, raising chin off bed, rolling over, and sitting alone. Pupil dilation in the presence of the parent begins at approximately four weeks of age. During the first few weeks of life baby prefers the human face to other visual images.
- Differentiate between contact stimulation and representative behaviours present in fetal life. Pressure and touch sensation is present a few months before birth; thus the newborn responds well to touch and gentle pressure. Rooting and hand–mouth activity occur in fetal life and are major adaptive activities after birth.
- Emphasize the importance of visual and auditory skills for developing social behaviours during the first two months of life.
- Encourage mutual eye contact between parent and baby; all infant's efforts to vocalize should be reinforced. Eye contact between the parent and baby increases during the first three months of life and is soon accompanied by other social responses—smiling and vocalization.
- Encourage regular periods of affectionate play when the infant is alert and responsive. Mother and father may pick up and hold the baby close, encourage visual following and smiling, and talk to the infant, repeating sounds. Rhythm and repetition are enjoyed. Often baby is most alert after a daytime feeding.
- Promote awareness in other family members of baby's competencies so that they can also respond to and reinforce the infant.

Incorporate the parents' cultural beliefs, values, and attitudes into your nursing care and modern health care practices whenever possible.[71] Maintaining important cultural traditions is one way to individualize care. Satz[72] gives specific examples of how she incorporated the values of the Navajo in promoting attachment. Specific traditions may extend to naming or bathing the baby, prenatal and postnatal care of mother, how to hold or dress baby, inclusion or exclusion of father from the delivery, and roles of various family members. Be sensitive to the preferences of clients who represent a culture different from your own. Listen to and observe carefully their requests. Listen to what is said and implied. Suggest rather than advise or direct when you teach.

Listen attentively for information and signs that give you clues to the parents' feelings about themselves, where they are in their own developmental growth, whom they rely on for strength, their ideas about child discipline, and their expectations of the new child. As you see weaknesses or gaps in necessary information, you can instruct. If your approach is right, the parents will recognize you as a helpful friend. Mothers are receptive to your information and to your reinforcement of mothering skills.

Help parents realize that soon the complete focus on mother–father–new baby will be gone. Other roles will be re-established: husband, wife, employer or employee, student, daughter, son, friend. The new parents will have to allow for all aspects of their personalities to function again. Baby will have to fit in.

While you are caring for the baby, you will no doubt feel great satisfaction. Remember, however, that the child belongs to the parents; this is *not your* baby. Do not become so involved that through your actions you push aside the parents and cause them to feel ineffective.

Baby's Influence on Parents

Some babies have a high activity level and warm up easily to the parent; some are quiet, withdrawn, with a low activity level; and various other mixtures of activity level and temperament exist. The infant's dominant reaction pattern to new situations manifests an innate temperament, and the temperament affects the reactions of others, especially the parents. They, in turn, will mould baby's reaction pattern.[73]

It is easy to love a lovable baby, but parents have to work harder with babies who are not highly responsive. Assess the reactions between baby and parents, as the style of child care that will develop has its basis here. A highly active mother who expects an intense reaction may have a hard time mothering a low-activity, quiet baby because she may misinterpret the baby's behaviour, feel rejected, and in turn reject the child. The baby will be denied the stimulation necessary for development. If the mother is withdrawn, quiet, and inexpressive and has a high-activity baby, she may punish the baby for normal energetic or assertive behaviour and ignore the bids for affection and stimulation. The child needs to feel his or her behaviour will produce an effect or he or she will stop contacting the parents.[74] Extreme parental rejection or lack of reaction causes the syndrome of neglect and deprivation, emotional illness, and **autistic behaviour,** characterized by *self-absorption, isolation from the world, and obsession with sameness, repetitive behaviour, and lack of language communication with others.*[75] An assertive child may become controlling with an indecisive mother and not learn that others also have needs and rights. If the baby is controlled by the mother, he or she cannot develop trust, independence, or ability to cope with persons on equal terms. If the mother overanticipates the child's needs, the child becomes passive and dependent.

Help parents understand the *mutual response* between the baby and themselves, and help them learn to read the baby's signals and to give consistent signals to the baby. All parents feel incompetent and despairing at times when they are unable to understand the child's cues and meet needs, but if self-confidence is consistently lacking, the parent's despair may turn to anger, rejection, and abuse.

Expansion of Intrafamily Relationships

Grandparents-to-be and other relatives frequently become more involved with the parents-to-be (bringing gifts and advice) than is necessarily desired. Yet their gifts and supportive presence can be a real help if the grandparents respect the independence of the couple, if the couple has resolved their earlier adolescent rebellion and dependency conflicts, and if the grandparents' advice does not conflict with the couple's philosophy or the doctor's advice. The couple and grandparents should collaborate rather than compete. Grandparents should be reminded not to take over the situation, and the couple's autonomy should be encouraged in that they can listen to the various pieces of advice, evaluate the statements, and then as a unit make their own decision. In addition, parents should refrain from expecting the grandparents to be built-in baby-sitters and to rescue them from every problem. Grandparents usually enjoy brief rather than prolonged contact with baby care. For the single parent, the grandparents or other relatives can be a major source of emotional and financial help and can provide help with child care.

You may assist the parent(s) in working with grandparents, resolving feelings of either being controlled or not adequately helped, understanding grandparents' feelings, accepting help, and avoiding excessive demands.

In some cultures, the maternal grandmother has a major role in care of the pregnant and postpartum daughter and in care of the infant. The grandmother may give advice about nutrition, self-care, or baby care to the daughter; however, the advice may be contrary to scientific and medical knowledge and practices. Establish rapport with both the grandmother and the mother or mother-to-be. Respect the role of the grandmother. Often the advice she gives is culturally based—the practices have maintained the group for centuries. The practices may be carried out along with modern-day health and medical practices. If the advice is truly harmful to the mother or baby, your rapport, nonjudgmental approach, and well-timed, low-key teaching of the grandmother may help her to accept the teaching you direct to the mother. Indeed, if either or both grandparents are considered the head of the household, direct your attention initially to them and direct your teaching to them. Initial or exclusive focus on their daughter is likely to alienate them, so that they discontinue coming for care or become resistant and do not allow their daughter to carry out your teaching.

CRITICAL THINKING

What would you say to a grandfather who insists his only daughter remain in the maternity unit with the healthy baby for a week?

Child Maltreatment

A common area of concern for the nurse who cares for infants and their families is **child maltreatment** *(physical abuse, neglect,* *sexual abuse, and emotional maltreatment).* Brief descriptions of these four categories of child maltreatment are provided below:

- **Physical abuse** is the *application of force to any part of the child's body. This may involve shaking, choking, biting, burning or poisoning a child or any other dangerous use of force.*[76]

- **Sexual abuse** is the *use of a child for sexual gratification such as touching and fondling the genitals, including exposure to pornographic material.*[77]

- **Neglect** *occurs when the caregiver does not give appropriate attention to the child's needs, such as physical neglect, abandonment, and educational and medical neglect.*[78]

- **Emotional maltreatment** *involves threatening, intimidating, terrorizing, and socially isolating a child.*

The Canadian Incidence Study of Reported Child Abuse and Neglect (CIS)) was the first Canada-wide study to examine incidence of child maltreatment based on 7672 investigations from 51 sites in all provinces and territories.[79,80] The results of substantiated cases indicated the following: inappropriate punishment (69%) and shaken baby syndrome (1%) were related to physical abuse; touching and fondling of the genitals (68%) were related to sexual abuse; exposure to family violence (58%) was related to emotional maltreatment; and failure to supervise leading to physical harm (48%) was related to neglect. The primary category of abuse was physical in nature. In Canada, an estimated 21.52 cases of child abuse and neglect per 1000 children occurred. Of these, 9.71 cases per 1000 were confirmed or verified.[81] Data collection for the second cycle of the study (CIS-2) commenced in the fall of 2003.[82]

In Canada, all individuals in jurisdictions with reporting statutes are obliged to report suspected child abuse to the appropriate child protection authorities. For health professionals, the reporting statute overrides statutory rules regarding confidentiality.[83]

Child maltreatment is not a simple phenomenon. It is a complex sequence of events that lead to children being hurt. Theorists have proposed numerous models to explain child maltreatment. No single theoretical framework has been recognized as the definitive explanation of child abuse and neglect, but rather models include a complex interaction of personal, social, and environmental factors.

Whenever the developing person and family and influences on development and behaviour are considered, the microsystem, exosystem, and macrosystem are all contributors. Each of these components is discussed in relation to child abuse, maltreatment, and neglect.

The **microsystem** *consists of the family.* Maltreating parents are angry and anxious, have poor impulse control and low self-esteem, are under great stress, and are lonely and depressed. In general, they cannot cope with the demands of childrearing. They do not understand normal child development; they become enraged because the child does not meet their expectations for behaviour to not cry or to stay clean. Many of the parents, especially the mother, are young and hold a lone-parent status. They are highly stressed, for example, by behaviour most parents take in stride. Some of these

parents are emotionally ill or have antisocial personalities or have experienced a history of child abuse. At times the pregnancy has been unplanned, or a negative attitude is exhibited toward the pregnancy. They are less effective in resolving problems with their children or with the spouse or other family members. Often these parents are cut off from any support system; they are lonely and isolated. Then, too, the child may need more care because of a disability or a demanding nature. As children are *abused,* some become more aggressive, which causes even more abuse from the parent. In contrast, *neglectful* parents tend to be apathetic, incompetent in relationships, irresponsible, and emotionally withdrawn.[84] Children who are sexually abused generally reside in a family without a natural parent; usually a stepfather. These children tend to relate poorly with their parents.[85]

The **exosystem**—*the outside world*—can be a contributor. Poverty, unemployment, job dissatisfaction, social isolation, and lack of assistance from others all contribute to stress, rage, and withdrawal. The low-income neighbourhood with no sense of community, criminal activity, lack of facilities or resources, inadequate safety overall, and poor political leadership also affects families and their ability to cope and care for themselves. A neighbourhood may be poor, but if there are strong social support networks and a sense of community, there is less child abuse.[86] However, the social support system may also be an obstacle. For example, individuals within a social support system may protect the abuser instead of the abused.[87]

The **macrosystem**—*cultural values and patterns of punishment*—is key. In Canada and the United States, high rates of violence exist in various forms: child abuse rates are especially high. In one-third of physical abuse cases, the victims are under one year of age. The most common offender is the baby's father or the mother's boyfriend, who is typically young, in his 20s.[88] In countries where violent crime is less frequent, such as Japan, China, and Tahiti, child abuse is rare.[89] The Hollow Water First Nation Holistic Healing Circle (CHCH) is a mature healing process that is widely acclaimed in Canada. The goal is that the community takes responsibility of their own offender and the offending actions. CHCH has facilitated a strong relationship between the community and the justice system.[90] For a summary of the theoretical models of abuse and neglect of children, see Baker.[91]

Professionals must be aware of the parent who has difficulty with attachment where maltreatment can result. Chapter 4 describes characteristics and behaviours of parents who have difficulty with parenting skills. Further information about maltreatment is presented in Chapters 6, 8, 9, and 10.

MacMillan describes the Preventive Interventions for Child Maltreatment:

1. Perinatal and early childhood programs aimed primarily at prevention of child physical abuse or neglect:
    a. Home visitation by nurses during perinatal period through infancy for the first-time mothers of low socioeconomic status, single parents, or teenage parents
    b. Comprehensive health care program and parent education or support program

c. Combination of services including case management, education, and psychotherapy
d. Intensive pediatric contact with home visits
e. Extended parent–child contact
f. Free access to health care centre

Note: Of the strategies listed, only home visitation to first-time disadvantaged mothers has been shown effective in preventing physical abuse and neglect.

2. Educational programs aimed primarily at prevention of sexual abuse:
   a. sexual abuse and abduction prevention programs for children

Note: Improved knowledge of sexual abuse, and enhanced awareness of safety skills; no studies have determined effectiveness of programs in reducing incidence of sexual abuse or abduction.[92]

Other preventative approaches include the Kids Help Line (1-800-668-6868), which is a national, toll-free confidential hotline for children and adolescents in need of help and support.[93] The Population Health Perspective (PHP), which takes into account the determinants of health, may be used as a framework in studying child maltreatment. Child maltreatment is a serious population health problem because its consequences early and later in life are widespread and detrimental to health.[94] The significant contribution of PHP is its holistic approach—taking into consideration both societal and personal factors.[95]

Shaken baby syndrome (SBS) *is a form of child abuse that is caused by vigorous shaking of the child, with or without impact. It produces acceleration and deceleration forces in the head and consequent damage, with little or no evidence of external cranial trauma.* Because of the nature of the situation, there are no accurate statistics regarding the incidence of SBS in Canada or the United States. There is consensus that head trauma is the leading cause of death of abused children and that shaking is involved in many of these cases. The majority of perpetrators are males. Infants who have been shaken display symptoms ranging from irritability or lethargy and vomiting, to seizures or unconsciousness with interrupted breathing or death.[96] Many survivors of SBS suffer brain damage, resulting in lifelong impairments. The victims of SBS are usually less than one year of age, with the majority under the age of six months.[97–100]

However, children as old as age five are vulnerable to SBS, but children two to four months old are especially at risk.[101] SBS is a crime punishable by imprisonment.[102] Risk factors, manifestations, and prevention strategies are provided by Monteleone, Monteleone, and Brodeur.[103,104] Prevention efforts should be built on a population health basis. Strategies should be provided to the general public regarding the adverse effects of shaking a baby along with guidance for coping with a baby.[105] Health professionals also need to be provided with guidelines to ensure appropriate and consistent care to SBS victims. These guidelines must ensure that health-promoting strategies are provided for families regarding the care of an infant. Susan, a nurse unit manager on a pediatric unit, always makes certain the staff handbook on the unit is up to date on shaken baby syndrome.

CONTROVERSY DEBATE

You have recently graduated with your baccalaureate degree in nursing, and you are pleased to have obtained a position 10 months ago in the pediatric respiratory unit of a large children's hospital in a major city in Saskatchewan.

During the past week, you have been caring for Ricki, an infant in the hospital with asthma. When Ricki's mother comes in each day, with Ricki's five-year-old brother Shawn, you notice that the mother is very caring and attentive to Ricki, while Shawn spends most of his time talking quietly to himself and exploring the room near Ricki's bed, by touching and manipulating things. Strangely, Shawn does not seem to be very interested in Ricki.

Two days ago, you happened to see his mother grab Shawn rather roughly by the arm. Mother shook Shawn two or three times quickly, telling him harshly to leave the tissue box alone. Shawn struggled, cried out in apparent pain, and sobbed for a few minutes while sitting on the floor. Soon, he pulled a small ball from his pocket and held it as he slowly cruised about the room looking at, but not approaching, any of the other children. Mother had immediately turned her attention back to Ricki.

Today, a few minutes ago, when Shawn and his mother came to visit, you noticed a fresh bruise on Shawn's cheek. When you cheerfully asked about it, Shawn cowered and his mother quickly mentioned a fall from his tricycle and moved on. You are concerned that Shawn might be a victim of physical abuse. The unit chart shows that Shawn's mother is professionally employed and lives with her husband.

1. What are your options now, as a health care professional, while the mother and Shawn are still in Ricki's room, and you must attend to other children on the ward?
2. Your nurse unit manager is unavailable to you for at least two hours. What is your plan of action?

Teach parents, both mother and father (or stepparent if involved), to better understand normal infant behaviour and how to manage their frustrations to avoid abusive behaviour. If the parent feels angry, he or she should avoid touching the baby, step back, and leave the room to calm down. Consider causes for crying: the child may be hungry, soiled, teething, tired, ill, injured, or frightened. The need behind the crying needs to be addressed.

PHYSIOLOGIC CONCEPTS

The following information will assist you in assessment and intervention with the neonate and in parental education.

Neonate: Physical Characteristics

The neonatal period of infancy includes the critical transition from parasitic fetal existence to physiologic independence. The normal newborn is described in the following pages.[106–109] Transition begins at birth with the first cry. Air is sucked in to inflate the lungs. Complex chemical changes are initiated in the cardiopulmonary system so that the baby's heart and lungs can assume the burden of oxygenating the body. The foramen ovale closes during the first 24 hours; the ductus arteriosus closes after several days. For the first time, the baby experiences light, gravity, cold, and firm touch.

The newborn is relatively resistant to the stress of anoxia and can survive longer in an oxygen-free atmosphere than an adult. The reason is unknown, as are the long-term effects of *mild* oxygen deprivation.

General Appearance

The newborn does not match the baby ads and may be a shock to new parents. The misshapen head, flat nose, puffy eyelids and often undistinguished eye colour, discoloured skin, large tongue and undersized lower jaw, short neck and small sloping shoulders, short limbs and large rounded abdomen with protruding umbilical stump that remains for three weeks, and bowed skinny legs may prove very disappointing if the parents are unprepared for the sight of a newborn. The head, which accounts for one-fourth of the total body size, appears large in relation to the body.

The **anterior fontanel,** a *diamond-shaped area at the top of the front of the head,* and the **posterior fontanel,** a *triangular-shaped area at the centre back of the head,* are often called **soft spots.** These unossified areas of the skull bones, along with the suture lines of the bones, allow the bones to overlap during delivery and also allow for expansion of the brain as they gradually fill in with bone cells. The posterior fontanel closes by two or three months; the anterior fontanel closes between eight and 18 months. These soft spots may add to the parents' impression that the newborn is too fragile to handle.

Reassure the parents that the newborn, although in need of tender, gentle care, is also resilient and adaptable. The head and fontanels can be gently touched without harm, although strong pressure or direct injury should be avoided. Reassure them also that the baby will soon take on the features of the family members and look more as they expected.

Apgar Scoring System

The physical status of the newborn is determined with the Apgar tool one minute after birth and again five minutes later. The newborn's respirations, heart rate, muscle tone, reflex activities, and colour are observed. A maximum score of 2 is given to each sign, so that the Apgar score could range from 0 to 10, as indicated in Table 7-2. A score of less than 7 means that the newborn is having difficulty adapting, needs even closer observation than usual, and may need life-saving intervention.

Gestational Age Assessment

In addition to using the Apgar score, assessment includes estimating gestational age to use parameters other than weight to assess an infant's level of maturity. By considering *both birth weight* and *gestational age,* you can categorize infants into one of several groupings. Problems can then be anticipated and, if present, be identified and treated early. Assessment can be done as early as the first day of life and should be done no later than the fifth day of life because external criteria such as hip abduction, square window, dorsiflexion of foot, and size of breast nodules change after five to six days of life. If the neonate is examined on the first day of life, he or she should be examined again before the fifth day to detect neurological changes. The score can be affected by asphyxia or maternal anaesthesia.

To assess gestational age, several scales can be used. From *Wong's Nursing Care of Infants and Children,* the *Classification of Newborns by Intrauterine Growth and Gestational Age* scale uses weight, length, and head circumference to determine normal values for gestational age.[110] The *Dubowitz Guide to Gestational Age Assessment* examines 10 neurological and 11 external signs.[111] Ballard et al. modified the Dubowitz scale. The "new" Ballard *Gestational Age Assessment,* which is a revision of the original scale, determines neuromuscular and physical maturity in relation to gestational age. This tool includes scores that reflect signs of extremely premature infants (Figure 7–2). To ensure accuracy, it is recommended that the initial examination be done within the first 48 hours of life.[112]

TABLE 7–2 Assessment of the Newborn: Apgar Scoring System			
Sign	0	1	2
Heart rate	Absent	Less than 100 beats/min	More than 100 beats/min
Respirations	Absent	Slow, irregular	Cry; regular rate
Muscle tone	Flaccid	Some flexion of extremities	Active movements
Reflex irritability	None	Grimace	Cry
Colour	Body cyanotic or pale	Body pink; extremities cyanotic	Body completely pink

Sources: Sherwen, L., M. Scoloveno, and C. Weingarten, Maternity Nursing: Care of the Childbearing Family *(3rd Ed.). Norwalk, CT: Appleton & Lange, 1999; and Wong, D.,* Wong's Nursing Care of Infants and Children *(7th ed.). St. Louis: Mosby, 2003.*

NEUROMUSCULAR MATURITY

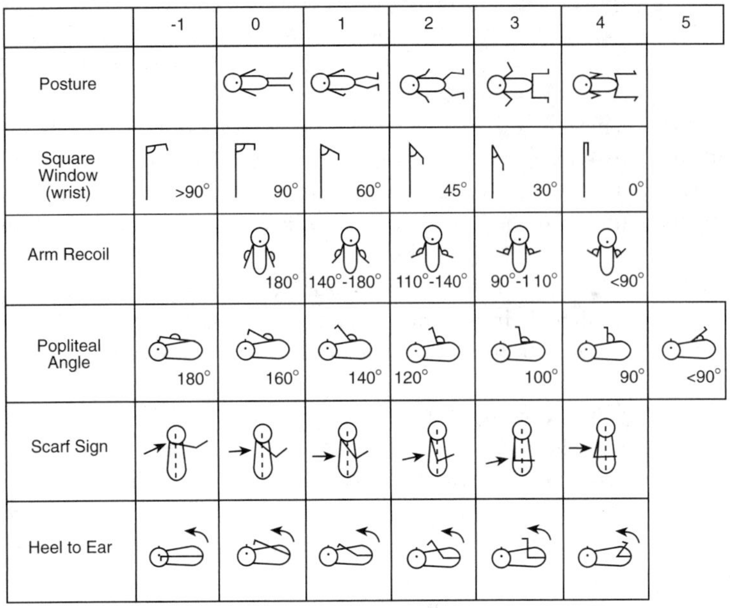

	-1	0	1	2	3	4	5
Posture							
Square Window (wrist)	>90°	90°	60°	45°	30°	0°	
Arm Recoil		180°	140°-180°	110°-140°	90°-110°	<90°	
Popliteal Angle	180°	160°	140°	120°	100°	90°	<90°
Scarf Sign							
Heel to Ear							

MATURITY RATING

score	weeks
-10	20
-5	22
0	24
5	26
10	28
15	30
20	32
25	34
30	36
35	38
40	40
45	42
50	44

PHYSICAL MATURITY

Skin	sticky; friable; transparent	gelatinous; red; translucent	smooth; pink; visible veins	superficial peeling &/or rash; few veins	cracking; pale areas; rare veins	parchment; deep cracking; no vessels	leathery; cracked; wrinkled
Lanugo	none	sparse	abundant	thinning	bald areas	mostly bald	
Plantar Surface	heel-toe 40-50 mm: -1 <40 mm: -2	>50 mm; no crease	faint red marks	anterior transverse crease only	creases ant. 2/3	creases over entire sole	
Breast	imperceptible	barely perceptible	flat areola; no bud	stippled areola; 1-2 mm bud	raised areola; 3-4 mm bud	full areola; 5-10 mm bud	
Eye/Ear	lids fused loosely: -1 tightly: -2	lids open; pinna flat; stays folded	sl. curved pinna; soft; slow recoil	well-curved pinna; soft but ready recoil	formed & firm; instant recoil	thick cartilage; ear stiff	
Genitals male	scrotum flat; smooth	scrotum empty; faint rugae	testes in upper canal; rare rugae	testes descending; few rugae	testes down; good rugae	testes pendulous; deep rugae	
Genitals female	clitoris prominent; labia flat	prominent clitoris; small labia minora	prominent clitoris; enlarging minora	majora & minora equally prominent	majora large; minora small	majora cover clitoris & minora	

SCORING SECTION

	1st Exam=X	2nd Exam=O
Estimating Gest Age by Maturity Rating	_____Weeks	_____Weeks
Time of Exam	Date _____ Hour _____ am pm	Date _____ Hour _____ am pm
Age at Exam	_____Hours	_____Hours
Signature of Examiner	_____ M.D./R.N.	_____ M.D./R.N.

FIGURE 7–2
Ballard scale for newborn maturity rating.

Source: Ballard, J., et al., New Ballard Score Expanded to Include Extremely Premature Infants, Journal of Pediatrics, 119 (1991), p. 417.

Skin

The skin is thin, delicate, and usually mottled, varies from pink to reddish, and becomes very ruddy when the baby cries. **Acrocyanosis,** *bluish colour of the hands and feet,* is the result of the sluggish peripheral circulation that occurs normally only for a few days after birth. **Lanugo,** *downy hair of fetal life,* most evident on shoulders, back extremities, forehead, and temples, is lost after a few months and is replaced by other hair growth. The *cheesy skin covering,* **vernix caseosa,** is left on for protective reasons; it rubs off in a few days. **Milia,** *tiny white spots that are small collections of sebaceous secretions,* are sprinkled on the nose and forehead and should not be squeezed or picked; they will disappear. **Hemangioma,** *pink spots* on the upper eyelids, between eyebrows, on the nose, upper lip, or back may or may not be permanent. **Mongolian spots** are *slate-coloured areas* on buttocks, lower back, thighs, ankles, and arms of children of colour, especially black (90%), Asian, and Aboriginal (80%). In contrast, only about 9% of Caucasian children have Mongolian spots. The dark areas usually disappear by the end of the first year.

If a birthmark is present, parents should be assured it is not their fault. **Jaundice,** *yellowish discolouration of skin,* should be noted. If it occurs during the first 24 hours of life, it is usually caused by blood incompatibility between mother and baby and requires medical investigation and possibly treatment. **Physiologic jaundice** normally appears on the third or fourth day of life *because the excess number of red blood cells present in fetal life that are no longer needed are undergoing hemolysis, which in turn causes high levels of bilirubin (a bile pigment) in the bloodstream.* The jaundice usually disappears in approximately one week when the baby's liver has developed the ability to metabolize the bilirubin. If bilirubin levels are excessively high, the neonate is placed under full-spectrum lights (phototherapy) to promote bilirubin breakdown. The baby's eyes must be covered during phototherapy.

Parents should be reassured about these and other conditions of the skin that normally occur. Foot or hand prints are made for identification, as these lines remain permanently. **Desquamation,** *peeling of skin,* occurs in two to four weeks.

Umbilical Cord

The *bluish-white, gelatinous structure that transports maternal blood from placenta to fetus* is the **umbilical cord.** It is cut 3.8 to 7.5 cm (1.5 to 3 inches) from the baby's abdominal wall. Because of the high water content, the stump of the cord dries and shrinks rapidly, losing its flexibility by 24 hours after birth. By the second day, it is a very hard yellow or black (blood) tab on the skin. Slight oozing where the cord joins the abdominal wall is common and offers an excellent medium for bacterial growth.

The area should be cleaned with cotton balls and alcohol several times daily until the cord has dropped off (six to 14 days) and for two or three days after the cord falls off when the area is completely healed. Parents should be taught this procedure.

Circumcision

In Canada, you may inform the parents that the Canadian Paediatric Society does not recommend circumcision as a routine procedure for newborns because the benefits and harms of circumcision are so evenly balanced.[113] Parents are advised to seek advice on the current state of medical knowledge regarding the benefits and harms of circumcision. Often, the parents' decision will reflect their personal, religious, or cultural beliefs.

Weight, Length, and Head Circumference

In newborns these circumferences provide an index to the normality of development, and measurements should be accurate. The **average birth weight** of Caucasian infants in North America is 3400 g (7.5 pounds) for boys and 3100 g (7 pounds) for girls. In Canada, most babies weigh between 2500 and 4499 g at birth.[114] Healthy birth weight indicates probable healthy development in utero, and subsequently, in the first year of life.[115] Newborn infants of African, Aboriginal, and Asian population groups are smaller, on the average, at birth. On average, babies of African descent weigh 240 grams less, are 2 cm shorter, and 0.7 cm less in circumference at birth than Caucasian babies, even when variables of income, maternal age, smoking, and marital status are the same.[116]

There is a difference in risk for low birth weight among ethnic groups in general and among major Asian groups in particular. The risk of low birth weight was greatest for blacks and Filipinos.[117] Maternal age, parity, lifestyle, and the woman's previous state of nutrition and prenatal care also influence birth weight. In all instances, female babies are somewhat smaller than males. Shortly after birth the newborn loses weight, up to 10% of birth weight, because of water loss, and parents should be told that this is normal before a steady weight gain, which begins in one or two weeks. Tissue turgor shows a sense of fullness because of hydrated subcutaneous tissue.[118,119]

In Canada, the rate of low birth weight is defined as the number of live births under 2500 grams per 100 live births.[120] Infants less than 1500 grams are considered to be of very low birth weight.[121] According to the Manitoba Population-Based Study (2001), compiled in the Manitoba provincial health database, low-birth-weight infants may be at greater risk for developmental problems, and are a high cost to health services due to neonatal care services.[122] Low birth weight outcomes in Canada focus on very young and older mothers. *The First Nations and Inuit Regional Health Survey* claims that the rate of low birth weight among Aboriginal people in 1996–97 did not differ significantly from national norms in 1994–1995. However, the rate of high birth weight associated with neonatal mortality was significantly higher.[123] One explanation proposed is that Aboriginal people have a genetic predisposition to heavier babies. More research is needed to understand this pattern of heavy birth weight and to explore the role of nutrition.[124] The prevention of low birth weight is a public health challenge because no clearly defined medical-at-risk group exists. However, there are multiple risk factors such as smoking, drinking, drug use, physical or emotional abuse, and other stresses that contribute to low birth weight.[125] Health promotion strategies in the community hold great promise for all families. Resources must be made available in all communities, stressing the importance of support for the mother and family.

In developing countries a large percentage of babies are born at home. Babies are not weighed at birth because scales are not available; however, measurements within 24 hours of birth of chest circumference (at nipple line) and midarm circumference (midway between acromium process and bend of elbow), when combined, were predictors of birth weight in one study. Based on accurate (92% to 97%) studies of 402 newborns in Thailand, the *Chulalongkorn University Birth Weight Estimation Device,* a circular nomographic chart, has been developed. Estimation, if not precise measurement, of birth weight is important because low birth weight is the major factor associated with death of infants within the first four weeks of life.[126]

Length is measured by having the child supine on a hard surface, extending the knees, placing the soles upright, and measuring from the soles of the feet to the vertex (tip) of the head. The **average length** of American infants at birth is just less than 50.8 cm (20 inches). Boys range from 48.2 to 53.3 cm (19 to 21 inches); girls average slightly less. In Canada, the average length at birth is between 50 and 52 cm (19.7 to 20.5 inches).[127] The bones are soft, consisting chiefly of cartilage. The back is straight and curves with sitting. The muscles feel hard and are slightly resistant to pressure.[128,129]

Measurement of **head circumference** is important in assessing the speed of head growth to determine if any abnormalities, such as too rapid or too slow growth, are present. The measurement is taken over the brow just above the eyes and across the posterior occipital protuberance. This standard measure of head size averages approximately 31 to 37 cm (12.4 to 14.8 in.) at birth, but variations of 1.3 cm (one-half inch) are common. In Canada, the average head circumference is 33 to 35 cm.[130] Chest circumference is usually approximately 2.5 cm (one inch) less than head size.[131,132] Parents should be prepared for moulding of the skull during vaginal delivery; **caput succedaneum,** *irregular edema of the scalp,* which disappears approximately the third day; or for **cephalohematoma,** *a collection of blood beneath the fibrous covering of the skull bones,* usually the parietal bones.

The baby's characteristic *position* during this period is one of flexion, closely imitating the fetal position, with fists tightly closed and arms and legs drawn up against the body. The baby is aware of disturbances in equilibrium and will change position, reacting with the Moro reflex.

It is recommended that the physical assessment of the newborn be conducted with the parents present.[133] Their presence provides the health professionals with the opportunity to reassure the parents of their newborn's normalcy, and to answer any questions that the parents might have. At the same time, health-promoting strategies for the parents and newborn can be discussed. For example, one strategy would be to ensure that the mother and family know how to obtain emergency help and parent information.

CRITICAL THINKING

What would be the role of the health professional, such as the nurse, in genetic diagnostic testing and counselling?

Neonate—Other Characteristics

Several other characteristics are also normal and resolve themselves shortly after birth: swollen breasts that contain liquid in boys and girls; swollen genitalia with undescended testicles in the boy; and vaginal secretions in the girl, caused by maternal hormones. Genital size varies for boys and girls. Urine is present in the bladder, and the baby voids at birth. Obstruction of the nasolacrimal duct is also common, and the excessive tearing and pus accumulation usually clear up when the duct opens spontaneously in a few months.

Vital Signs

In the newborn, vital signs are not stable.

Respiratory Efforts. Respiratory efforts at birth are critical and immediate adaptations must occur to counter the decreasing oxygen level and increasing carbon dioxide level in the blood. Causes of respiratory initiations include cutting of the umbilical cord, which causes hypoxia, resulting in carbon dioxide accumulation; physical stimulation of the birth process; the sudden change in baby's environment at birth; the exposure to firm touch; and the cool air. If the mother was medicated during labour or if the baby is premature, the respiratory centre of the brain is less operative, and the baby will have more difficulty with breathing. Respirations range from 50 to 80 per minute during the first hour after birth and then decrease to 30 to 60 per minute. Respirations are irregular, quiet, and shallow and may be followed by an intermittent five- to ten-second pause in breathing.

Body Temperature. Body temperature ranges from 36.1°C to 37.7°C (97°F to 100°F) because:

- The heat-regulating mechanism in the hypothalamus is not fully developed.
- Shivering to produce heat does not occur.
- There is less subcutaneous fat.
- Heat is lost to the environment by evaporation, conduction, convection, and radiation.

At birth amniotic fluid increases temperature loss by evaporation from the skin; thus, diligent efforts to dry the skin are necessary. The wet newborn can lose heat about four times as fast as adults, up to 200 calories of heat per kilogram per minute (90 calories per minute is the maximum the adult can lose). If the room is cool and the baby is placed in contact with cold objects, heat loss occurs by convection, radiation, and conduction. Excessive heat loss or cold stress may lead to apnea, respiratory depression, and hypoglycemia.[134,135]

Thus, baby should be placed next to mother's abdominal skin or breast initially and then wrapped well in blankets before being placed in a warm crib. Several mechanisms occur to help the newborn conserve heat:

- Vasoconstriction, by which constricted blood vessels maintain heat in the inner body
- Flexion of the body to reduce total amount of exposed skin (the premature baby does not assume flexion of the extremities onto the body)
- Increased metabolic rate, which causes increased heat production

■ Metabolism of adipose tissue that has been stored during the eighth month of gestation

This *adipose tissue* is called **brown fat** because it is *brown in colour from a rich supply of blood vessels and nerves,* and it is unique in that it *aids adaptation to the stress of cooling.* Brown fat, located between the scapulae around the neck, behind the sternum, and around the kidneys and adrenal glands, accounts for 2% to 6% of the neonate's body weight and is metabolized quickly.[136,137]

Body temperature of the baby normally drops approximately 1°C (1°F to 2°F) immediately after birth, but in a warm environment, begins to rise slowly after eight hours. It is critical to maintain the birth area at 23 to 25°C, with a draft-free environment.[138] Thus, prevention of heat loss, especially during the first 15 minutes, is crucial to adaptation to extrauterine life.[139,140] Also, babies who have lost excessive amounts of heat cannot produce surfactant. **Surfactant** is a *thin lipoprotein film produced by the alveoli that reduces surface tension of the alveoli, allows them to expand, and allows some air to remain in alveoli at end of expiration.* Thus it takes less effort to re-expand the lungs.[141,142]

The temperature should be taken at the axillary site for five minutes. Rectal thermometers may cause infection, raise blood pressure, lower arterial blood oxygen, and unnecessarily stimulate defecation, causing loss of fluid and calories.[143] A tympanic thermometer probe may be inserted into the auditory canal.

Heart Rate. Heart rate ranges at birth from 100 to 160 beats per minute because of the immature cardiac regulatory mechanism in the medulla. The heart rate may increase to 170 to 180 beats per minute when the newborn cries and drop to 90 beats per minute during sleep. The pulse rate gradually decreases during the first and subsequent years.[144,145]

Blood Pressure. Systolic blood pressure may range from 40 to 50 mm Hg depending on cuff size or the instrument used for measurement. By the end of the first month, blood pressure averages 80/40 mm Hg, increases slowly the first year, and remains under 90/60 mm Hg.[146,147]

Meconium

Meconium, the *first fecal material,* is sticky, odourless, and tarry, and is passed from eight to 24 hours after birth. Transitional stools, which last for a week, are loose, contain mucus, are greenish-yellow and pasty, and have a sour odour. There will be two to four stools daily. If the neonate takes cow's milk, the stools will become yellow and harder and average one to two daily. Once feeding begins the stools change colour.[148]

Reflex Activity

Reflex activity is innate or built in through the process of evolution and develops while the baby is in utero. **Reflex** is an *involuntary, unlearned response elicited by certain stimuli,* and it indicates neurological status or function. Individual differences in the newborn's responses to stimulation are apparent at birth. Some respond vigorously to the slightest stimulation; others respond slowly, and some are in between. Several types of reflexes exist in the neonate and young infant: consummatory, avoidant, exploratory, social, and attentional. **Consummatory**

reflexes, *such as rooting and sucking, promote survival through feeding.* **Avoidant reflexes** are *elicited by potentially harmful stimuli* and include the Moro, withdrawing, knee jerk, sneezing, blinking, and coughing reflexes. **Exploratory reflexes** *occur when infants are wide awake and are held upright so that their arms move without restraint.* The visual object at eye level elicits both reaching and grasping reflexes. **Social reflexes,** such as smiling, *promote affectionate interactions between parents and infants* and thus have a survival value. Crying in response to painful stimuli, loud noise, food deprivation, or loss of support; quieting in response to touch, low soft tones, or food; and smiling in response to changes in brightness, comforting stimuli, or escape from uncomfortable stimuli are examples of innate reflexes that can be modified by experience and that persist throughout life. **Attentional reflexes,** including orienting and attending, *determine the nature of the baby's response to stimuli* and have continuing importance through development.[149,150]

The nervous system of the newborn is both anatomically and physiologically immature, and reflexes should be observed for their presence and symmetry. These reflexes are described in Table 7-3.[151–155]

Sensory Abilities

The newborn has more highly developed sensory abilities than was once supposed. Apparently a moderately enriched environment, one without stimulus bombardment or deprivation, is best suited for sensory motor development. Even premature babies placed in a stimulus-rich environment until discharged from the hospital learn more quickly and are healthier at four months than premature babies who lived in the traditional environment.[156–158]

The infant's use of the senses, innate abilities, and environment lay the ground work for intellectual development. Studies show that 20 minutes of extra handling a day will result in earlier exploring and grasping behaviour by the infant. He or she is very sensitive to touch and vestibular (rocking, holding upright) stimulation; cutaneous and postural stimulation is necessary for development of the nervous system, skin sensitivity, and emotional health.[159,160] Moderate, gentle kinesthetic stimulation daily results in a baby who is quieter, gains weight faster, and shows improved socioemotional function.

The first impressions of life, security, warmth, love, pleasure, or lack of them come to the infant through touch. Knowledge of the people around him or her, initially of mother, is gradually built from the manner in which the baby is handled. He or she soon learns to sense mother's self-confidence and pleasure as well as her anxiety, lack of confidence, anger, or rejection. These early touch experiences and the infant's feelings through them apparently lay the foundation for feelings about people throughout life.

Sensitivity to Pain, Pressure, and Temperature. Sensitivity to pain, pressure, and temperature extremes is present at birth; pain is shown by a distinct cry.[161–163] The baby is especially sensitive to touch around the mouth and on the palms and soles. Females are more responsive to touch and pain than males. The newborn reacts diffusely to pain, as he or she has little ability to localize the discomfort because of incomplete myelinization of the spinal tracts and cerebral cortex; however,

TABLE 7-3
Assessment of Infant Reflexes

Reflex	Description	Appearance/Disappearance
Rooting	Touching baby's cheek causes head to turn toward the side touched.	Present in utero at 24 weeks; disappears 3–4 months; may persist in sleep 9–12 months
Sucking	Touching lips or placing something in baby's mouth causes baby to draw liquid into mouth by creating vacuum with lips, cheeks, and tongue.	Present in utero at 28 weeks; persists through early childhood, especially during sleep
Bite	Touching gums, teeth, or tongue causes baby to open and close mouth.	Disappears at 3–5 months when biting is voluntary, but seen throughout adult years in comatose person
Babkin	Pressure applied to palm causes baby to open mouth, close eyes.	Present at birth; disappears in 2 or 4 months
Pupillary response	Flashing light across baby's eyes or face causes constriction of pupils.	Present at 32 weeks of gestation; persists throughout life
Blink	Baby closes both eyes.	Remains throughout life
Moro or startle	Making a loud noise or changing baby's position causes baby to extend both arms outward with fingers spread, then bring them together in a tense, quivery embrace	Present at 28 weeks of gestation; disappears at 4–7 months
Withdrawing	Baby removes hand or foot from painful stimuli.	Present at birth; persists throughout life
Colliding	Baby moves arms up and face to side when object is in collision course with face.	Present at birth or shortly after; persists in modified form throughout life
Palmer grasp	Placing object or finger in baby's palm causes his or her fingers to close tightly around object.	Present at 32 weeks of gestation; disappears at 3–4 months, replaced by voluntary grasp at 4–5 months
Plantar grasp	Placing object or finger beneath toes causes curling of toes around object.	Present at 32 weeks of gestation; disappears at 9–12 months
Tonic neck or fencing (TNR)	Postural reflex is seen when infant lies on back with head turned to one side; arm and leg on the side toward which he or she is looking are extended while opposite limbs are flexed.	Present at birth; disappears at approximately 4 months
Stepping, walking, dancing	Holding baby upright with feet touching flat surface causes legs to prance up and down as if baby were walking or dancing.	Present at birth; disappears at approximately 2–4 months; with daily practice of reflex, infant may walk alone at 10 months
Reaching	Hand closes as it reaches toward and grasps at object at eye level.	Present shortly after birth if baby is upright; comes under voluntary control in several months
Orienting	Head and eyes turn toward stimulus of noise, accompanied by cessation of other activity, heartbeat change, and vascular constriction.	Present at birth; comes under voluntary control later; persists throughout life

(continued)

TABLE 7-3 *(continued)*
Assessment of Infant Reflexes

Reflex	Description	Appearance/Disappearance
Attending	Eyes fix on a stimulus that changes brightness, movement, or shape.	Present shortly after birth; comes under voluntary control later; persists throughout life
Swimming	Placing baby horizontally, supporting him under abdomen, causes baby to make crawling motions with his or her arms and legs while lifting head from surface as if he or she were swimming.	Present after 3 or 4 days; disappears at approximately 4 months; may persist with practice
Trunk incurvation	Stroking one side of spinal column while baby is on his or her abdomen causes crawling motions with legs, lifting head from surface, and incurvature of trunk on the side stroked.	Present in utero; then seen at approximately third or fourth day; persists 2–3 months
Babinski	Stroking bottom of foot causes big toe to rise while other toes fan out and curl downward.	Present at birth; disappears at approximately 9 or 10 months; presence of reflex later may indicate disease
Landau	Suspending infant in horizontal, prone position and flexing head against trunk cause legs to flex against trunk.	Appears at approximately 3 months; disappears at approximately 12–24 months
Parachute	Sudden thrusting of infant downward from horizontal position causes hands and fingers to extend forward and spread as if to protect self from a fall.	Appears at approximately 7–9 months; persists indefinitely
Biceps	Tap on tendon of biceps causes biceps to contract quickly.	Brisk in first few days, then slightly diminished; permanent
Knee jerk	Tap on tendon below patella or on patella causes leg to extend quickly.	More pronounced first 2 days; permanent

Sources: Sherwen, L., M. Scoloveno, and C. Weingarten, Maternity Nursing: Care of the Childbearing Family *(3rd Ed.). Norwalk, CT: Appleton & Lange, 1999; and Wong, D.,* Wong's Nursing Care of Infants and Children *(7th ed.). St. Louis: Mosby, 2003.*

the baby's response to pain increases each day in the neonatal period. Visceral sensations of discomfort, such as hunger, overdistension of the stomach, passage of gas and stool, and extremes of temperature, apparently account for much of the newborn's crying. At first the cry is simply a primitive discharge mechanism that calls for help. He or she wails with equal force regardless of stimulus. In a few weeks baby acquires subtle modifications in the sound of the cry that provide clues to the attentive parent about the nature of the discomfort so that response can be adjusted to the baby's need.[164,165]

Vision. Vision is the least well-developed sense at birth. The eyes of the newborn are smaller than those of the adult; retinal structures are incomplete; the optic nerve is underdeveloped. The visual abilities change from birth to four months of age.[166]

The following are *characteristics of newborn vision*:[167]

- *Initial state:* Vision is blurred.

- *Acuity:* Clarity of vision at a specific distance begins within the first day; 20 to 50 cm distance is necessary for focus.
- *Fixation:* The newborn is able to direct his or her eyes at the same point in space for a specific time (four to ten seconds).
- *Tracking:* The newborn visually follows large moving objects, beginning a day after birth.
- *Discrimination:* The newborn demonstrates a preference for particular sizes, shapes, colours, or patterns; discriminates large from small and intensity of colour; and prefers less complex stimuli and large pictures or objects.
- *Conjugation:* The newborn is able to move the eyes together; refixation is more frequent.
- *Sensitivity to light:* The newborn's sensitivity to light is equal to that of adults.
- *Scanning:* The newborn is able to move her or his eyes over the visual field and focus on a satisfying image.

■ *Accommodation:* The newborn is able to adjust the eyes for distance. The preferred distance is 20 cm for infants up to one month in age.

■ *Visual preference:* Amount of time spent looking at different sights in the environment.

The infant maintains contact with the environment through visual fixation, scanning, and tracking and pays more attention to stimuli from the face than to other stimuli (Figure 7–3). The newborn looks at mother's face while feeding and while sitting upright follows the path of an object, crying or pulling backward if it comes too close to his or her face.

The *newborn has the following visual abilities*:[168,169]

1. Can see objects from 20 to 50 centimetres away[170]

2. Can look at face of mother while feeding or sitting upright

3. Prefers human face to mobile toy

4. Pulls back if object comes too close to face

5. Has pupillary reflex at four weeks of age; can differentiate between brightness and darkness; bright lights cause discomfort

6. Prefers black and white to bright colours; prefers strong contrasts

7. Can focus attention on patterned object, such as geometric, symmetrical, and complex shapes; large circles, dots, and squares

8. Prefers to scan edges and contours of complex shapes; peripheral vision is narrow

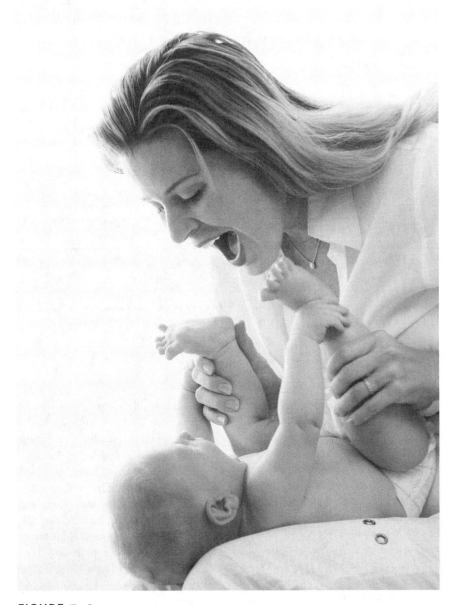

FIGURE 7–3

Infant has the ability to fix on the mother's face beginning one day after birth and finds geometric objects interesting.

By the age of one month, baby can distinguish between face of mother and stranger.

Teach parents that baby needs eye contact and the opportunity to see the human face and a variety of changing scenes and colours. Providing a mirror or chrome plate that reflects light and objects and rotating the bed help the baby use both eyes, avoiding one-sided vision. Hang cardboard black-and-white mobiles, especially those that make sound, and have them within reach of baby's kicking feet. Later the infant enjoys other colours and designs that are within grasp. By age two months, baby can see the ceiling and decorations on it. As baby grows older, the crib should be low enough for baby to see beyond the crib.

Parents should be reassured that the antibiotic ointment correctly placed in baby's eyes at birth will not damage vision but prevents blindness if the mother should have an undetected gonorrheal infection.[171]

Hearing. Hearing is developed in utero when the fetus is exposed to internal sounds of mother's body, such as the heartbeat and abdominal rumbles (heard at five months), and external sounds, such as voices, music, and a cymbal clap (heard at seven months). Hearing is blurred the first few days of life because fluid is retained in the middle ear, but hearing loss can be tested as early as the first day.[172] The neonate cannot hear whispers but can respond to voice pitch changes. A low pitch quiets and a high pitch increases alertness. Baby responds to sound direction—left or right—but responds best to mother's voice, to sounds directly in front of his or her face, and to sounds experienced during gestation.[173–175] Baby often sleeps better with background songs or a tape recording of mother's heartbeat. By three days of age, the newborn discriminates between the voice of mother and another female.[176] Differentiation of sounds and perception of their source take time to develop, but there are startle reactions. The baby withdraws from loud noise.[177]

In Canada, hearing loss is estimated to occur in 1.5 to 6.0 cases per 1000 live births.[178] It is advocated that babies who are at increased risk for hearing loss may have screening completed in their place of birth. However, other appropriate arrangements should be made within three months of birth.[179] Some factors associated with increased hearing loss are birth weight less than 1500 g, congenital infections such as rubella, herpes, syphilis, and a family history of childhood sensory hearing loss.[180] It is important that health care professionals assist the parents to locate appropriate resources. One such resource is the Parenting Helpline (888-603-9100), a toll-free line that provides support and information on parenting concerns.

CRITICAL THINKING

What steps would you take to assist parents of a child with hearing loss to learn about resources available to them in their province or territory?

Taste and Smell. Taste is not highly developed at birth, but acid, bitter, salt, and sweet substances evoke a response. Taste buds for sweet are more abundant in early than late life. Breathing rhythm is altered in response to fragrance, showing some ability to smell. The sense of smell is well developed in the newborn; infants can discriminate the smell of mother's

body from other bodies or objects and can sense the odours that adults sense.

Neonates differ in their appearance, size, function, and response. Girls are more developmentally advanced than boys and blacks more than Caucasians. The most accurate assessment is made by comparing the neonate against norms for the same sex and race.[181–183]

Checklist to Detect Presence of Hearing in Infancy

From Birth to 2 Weeks Does Baby:

- Jump or blink when there is a sudden loud sound
- Stop crying when you start to talk
- Seem aware of your voice
- Stir in sleep when there is continuous noise close by
- Jump or blink when there is a sudden soft click such as a light switch or a camera click when the noise is otherwise quiet
- Stop sucking momentarily when there is a noise or when you start to talk
- Look up from sucking or try to open eyes when there is a sudden noise

From 2 to 10 Weeks Does Baby:

- Stop crying when you talk to him or her
- Stop movements when you enter the room
- Seem aware of your voice
- Sleep regardless of noises
- Waken when the crib or bassinet is touched
- Respond to comforting only when held against mother or familiar caretaker
- Cry at sudden loud noises
- Blink or jerk at sudden loud noises

From 2½ to 6 Months Does Baby:

- Always coo with pleasure when you start to talk
- Turn eyes to the speaker
- Know when father comes home and wriggle in welcome (if awake)
- Startle when you bend over the crib after awakening
- Seem to enjoy a soft musical toy (e.g., a crib musical toy)
- Cry when exposed to sudden, loud unexpected noise
- Stop movements when a new sound is introduced
- Try to turn in the direction of a new sound or a person who starts to talk
- Make many different babbling sounds when alone
- Try to "talk back" when you talk
- Start wriggling in anticipation of a bottle when you start preparing it (if the baby is awake and the preparation is out of sight, as the refrigerator door opening, and so on)
- Know own name (smiles, turns, or otherwise gives an indication)

Note: The Hearing Foundation of Canada supports a broad range of services for deaf and hard of hearing children and adults across Canada.

Special Considerations in Physical Assessment of the Neonate

When a newborn is examined, the primary concerns are neurological status, congenital deformities, and metabolic disturbances. Any history of hereditary diseases and pregnancy and delivery information is essential. Reflex status indicates neurological development and some congenital deformities. The following are particular aspects to check when physically assessing the neonate.[184,185]

A *small chin*, called **micrografthia,** means that the neonate may experience breathing difficulties, because the tongue can fall back and obstruct the nasopharynx.

Ear position is important because there is a strong association between low-set ears and renal malformation or a chromosomal aberration such as Down syndrome. The top of the ear should be in alignment with the inner and outer canthi of the eyes. The eustachian tube is shorter and wider than in the adult. To examine the neonate with an otoscope, the head should be stabilized and the pinna of the ear pulled back and up.

Discharges from the eye may result from chemical irritation or ophthalmic neonatorum from gonorrhea in the mother. A mongoloid slant in a Caucasian infant may suggest a chromosome abnormality.

Ptosis (*drooping*) of the eyelids should be a cause for concern. Drooping eyelids reduce the amount of light entering the retina and can decrease development of sight.

Conjunctival hemorrhage is usually of no significance. An infant lid retractor may be used to view the fundus if the muscles of the newborn keep the eyelids closed.

The **nose** should be patent. Flaring of the nostrils usually represents respiratory distress. A thick bloody discharge from the nose suggests congenital syphilis.

The **mouth** should be inspected for cleft lip and cleft palate. Although spitting up is common in the newborn, projectile vomiting is not. The newborn should have very little saliva, and tonsillar tissue should not be present at birth.

The **chest** and **abdomen** are considered a unit in the newborn. The anteroposterior diameter is usually equal to the transverse diameter. Wide-set nipples may indicate Turner syndrome, a genetic disorder. Smaller breasts that contain liquid are not uncommon in both males and females. The breath sounds in the infant are bronchovesicular. If heart murmurs exist, they are usually best heard over the base of the heart rather than at the apex.

The **umbilical** cord should have two arteries and one vein. Auscultation of bowel sounds should precede palpation for masses, an extremely important procedure in the newborn.

The **genitalia** are examined for deformities. Only the external genitalia are examined in children. In uncircumcised males up to three months of age, the foreskin should not be retracted to avoid tearing the membrane. The testes should be palpated in the scrotum, although sometimes they are still undescended. A **hydrocele,** *a collection of watery fluid in the scrotum or along the spermatic cord,* and **hernia,** *a protrusion of part of the intestine through the abdominal muscles,* are common findings in males.

A bloody or mucous vaginal discharge may be present in girls. Fused labia are a serious anomaly, but simple adhesion may be due to inflammation.

Taking temperatures rectally can rule out **imperforate anus** (*lacking normal anal opening*).

The spine should be palpated for **spina bifida,** *a congenital neural tube defect characterized by anomaly in posterior vertebral arch.* Observation for symmetric bilateral muscle movements of the hips and knees is essential. The **hips** should be examined for dislocation by rotating the thighs with the knees flexed.

Extremities should be noted for the right number of fingers and toes and bilateral movements, and position of hands and feet should be checked.

Signs of prematurity include low birth weight and small size, thick lanugo, excess vernix, slow or absent reflexes, undescended testicles in the male, and nipples not visible.[186]

Infant—Physical Characteristics

General Appearance

The growing infant changes in appearance as he or she changes size and proportion.[187–192] The face grows rapidly; trunk and limbs lengthen; back and limb muscles develop; and coordination improves. By one month the baby can lift the head slightly when prone and hold the head up briefly when the back is supported. By two months the head is held erect, but it bobs when he or she is sitting unsupported.

Skull enlargement occurs almost as rapidly as total body growth during the first year and is determined mainly by the rate of brain expansion. From birth to four weeks, the head size increases to 37.5 cm (14.75 inches); at three months to 39.5 cm (15.75 inches); at 20 weeks to 41 cm (16.5 inches); and at 30 weeks to 43 cm (17 inches). By the end of the first year, the head will be two-thirds of adult size.

Physical Growth and Emotional, Social, and Neuromuscular Learning

Physical growth and these areas of learning are concurrent, interrelated, and rapid in the first year. The first year of life is one of the two periods of rapid physical growth after birth. (The other period is prepuberty and postpuberty.) Baby gains about 20 g per day in the first five months and 14 g per day for the next seven months. Birth weight doubles by five to six months and triples by 12 months. Baby grows approximately 30.5 cm (12 inches) in the first year. The skeletal system should be assessed for any orthopedic problems.

Physical and motor abilities are heavily influenced by genetic, biological, and cultural factors; nutrition, maturation of the central nervous system; skeletal formation; overall physical health status; environmental conditions; stimulation; and consistent loving care.[193–197] Do you have any photographs of yourself as an infant? If you do, examine the photographs carefully. Note, if you can, the physical growth characteristics that you have attained in each one of them.

Table 7-4 divides further developmental sequence into three-month periods for specific assessment.[198–204] *It is only a guide,* not an absolute standard. Great individual differences occur among infants, depending on their physical growth and

TABLE 7-4
Assessment of Physical Characteristics of the Infant

1–3 Months	3–6 Months	6–9 Months	9–12 Months
Many characteristics of newborn, but more stable physiologically	Most neonatal reflexes gone Temperature stabilizes at 37.5°C (99.4°F)		Temperature averages 37.7°C (99.7°F)
Heartbeat steadies at about 120–130 beats/min		Pulse about 115/min	Pulse about 100–110/min
Blood pressure about 80/40; gradually increases		Blood pressure about 90/60	Blood pressure 96/66
Respirations more regular at 30–40/min; gradually decrease		Respirations about 32/min	Respirations 20–30/min
Appearance of salivation and tears			
Weight gain of 141.75–198.45 g (5–7 oz.) per week	Weight gain of 85–141 g (3–5 oz.) per week		Weight gain of 85–141.75 g (3–5 oz.) per week
Weight at 3625–5900 g (8–13 lb.)	Weight at 7–7.3 kg (15–16 lb.) by 6 months	Birth weight doubled by 6 months	Birth weight tripled; average 10 kg (22 lb.)
Head circumference increases up to 40 cm (16 in.)	Head size increases 2.5 cm (1 in.)	Head size 43.2 cm (17.8 in.)	Head size increases slightly more, to 45–46 cm (18.3 in)
Chest circumference 40 cm (16 in.)	Chest size increases more than 2.5 cm (up to 43–44 cm or 17.3 in.)	Chest circumference increases by 1.25 cm (to 44–45 cm or 17.8 in.)	Chest circumference increases to 45–46 cm (18.3 in.)
Body length: Growth of 2.5 cm (1 in.) monthly	Growth of 1.25 cm (½ in.) monthly	Growth of 1.25 cm (½ in.) monthly	Growth of about 1.25 cm monthly; height 72.5–75 cm (29–30 in.), increased by 50% since birth
Tonic neck and Moro reflexes rapidly diminishing	Most neonatal reflexes gone Palmar reflex diminishing		
Arms and legs found in bilaterally symmetrical position			
Limbs used simultaneously, but not separately	Movements more symmetric		
Hands and fingers played with			
Clenched fists giving way to open hands that bat at objects			

(continued)

TABLE 7-4 *(continued)*
Assessment of Physical Characteristics of the Infant

1–3 Months	3–6 Months	6–9 Months	9–12 Months
Reaches for objects	Reaches for objects with accurate aim and flexed fingers	Palmar grasp developed Picks up objects with both hands; bangs toys	Throws objects
Plays with hands	Objects transferred from one hand to another by 6 months Bangs with objects held in one hand Scoops objects with hands Begins to use fingers separately	Holds bottle with hands; holds own cookie Preference for use of one hand Probes with index finger Thumb opposition to finger (prehension) by 7 months	Puts toys in and out of container Points with finger Brings hands and thumb and index finger together at will to pick up small objects Releases objects at will
Can follow moving objects with eyes when supine; begins to use both eyes together at about 2 months	Binocular depth perception by about 5 months Looks for objects when they are dropped Improving eye–hand coordination Eruption of one or two lower incisors	Explores, feels, pulls, inspects, tastes, and tests objects Hand–mouth coordination Feeds self cracker and other finger foods Begins weaning process	Makes mark on paper Eats with fingers; holds cup, spoon Has 6 teeth, central and lateral incisors; eruption of first molars at about 12 months
Attends to voices	Binaural hearing present		
Raises chin while lying on stomach at 1 month	Turns head to sound	Turns to sounds behind self	
Raises chest while lying on stomach at 2 months; raises head and chest 45° to 50° off bed, supporting weight on arms			
Holds head in alignment when prone at 2 months; holds head erect in prone position at 3 months			
Supports self on forearms when on stomach at 3 months	Rolls over completely by 6 months		Rolls over easily from back to stomach

(continued)

TABLE 7-4 *(continued)*
Assessment of Physical Characteristics of the Infant

1–3 Months	3–6 Months	6–9 Months	9–12 Months
Sits if supported	Sits with support at 4 months Holds head steady while sitting Pulls self to sitting position Begins to sit alone for short periods Plays with feet Kicks vigorously Begins to hitch (scoot) backward while sitting Bears portion of own weight when held in standing position Pushes feet against hard surface to move by 3 or 4 months	Sits erect unsupported by 7 months Creeps or crawls by 8 or 9 months Pulls self to stand by holding onto support Cruises (walking sideways while holding onto object with both hands) by 10 months Begins to walk with help	Sits alone steadily Pivots when seated Puts feet in mouth Hitches with backward locomotion while sitting Sits from standing position without help Stands alone for a minute Walks when led by 11 months Walks with help by 12–14 months Lumber and dorsal curves developed while learning to walk Turning of feet and bowing of legs normal Beginning to show regular bladder and bowel patterns; has one or two stools per day; interval of dry diaper does not exceed 1 to 2 hours Not ready for toilet training
Smiles reflexively at comforting person	Smiles at person deliberately during interaction Displays joy, frustration, rage	Experiences separation anxiety about 7–9 months Engages in social play; elicits response from others	Attachment to caregiver Sociable increasingly with others
Coos, chuckles, laughs	Babbles; plays with sounds		Begins to cooperate in dressing; puts arm through sleeve; takes off socks Improves previously acquired skills throughout this period

emotional, social, and neuromuscular responses. Girls usually develop more rapidly than boys, although the activity level is generally higher for boys. Even with these cautions, the table can be a useful tool if you observe overall behaviour patterns rather than isolated characteristics.

Neurological System

The neurological system is immature, but it continues the fetal pattern of developing a functional capacity at a rapid rate. Consistent stimulation of the nervous system is necessary to maintain growth and development, or function is lost and cannot be regained.[205–208]

Vision. *By two months of age,* the infant can:[209]

1. Focus both eyes on object steadily
2. Look longer at colours of medium intensity (yellow, green, pink) than at bright (red, orange, blue) or dim (grey, beige) colours
3. Distinguish red from green
4. Accommodate better, lenses have become more flexible
5. Use broader peripheral vision, which has doubled since birth
6. Follow path of an object

By four months of age, the infant can:[210]

1. Distinguish between red, green, blue, and yellow, and prefers red and blue
2. Use binocular vision (both eyes focus), which allows perception of depth and distance and ability to distinguish stripes and edges
3. Accommodate on an adult level

Under four months of age, baby does not look for an object hidden after seeing it, and when the same object reappears, it is as if the object were a new object. The infant has no knowledge that objects have a continuous existence: the object ceases to exist when it is not seen.[211,212] The baby coordinates both eyes and attends to and prefers novel stimuli. *At four months,* he or she can focus for any distance and perceive shape constancy when the object is rotated at different angles. Infants look longer at patterned stimuli of less complexity than at stimuli that have more complex designs or no lines or contours and can detect change of pattern. The infant prefers faces but is attracted by checkerboard designs, geometric shapes, and large pictures (circles, dots, and squares at least 7.5 cm high and with angles rather than contours). Full depth perception develops at approximately nine months when the images received in the central nervous system from the macula of each eye are integrated.

Visual stimulation of both eyes simultaneously is necessary for the baby to develop binocular vision. Otherwise **amblyopia** (*lazy eye*), *which is a gradual loss of the ability to see in one eye because of lack of stimulation of visual nerve pathways,* develops without damage to the retina or other eye structures. If visual stimulation is not lacking for too many weeks, the condition reverses itself. If one eye continues to do all the work for several months, blindness results in the other eye.

Vital Signs. During infancy vital signs (temperature, pulse, respirations, and blood pressure) stabilize, as shown in Table 7-4.

Intersensory Integration. At birth, perceptual skills are greater than previously believed. In infancy, information from two sense modalities is interrelated. Four-month-old infants respond to relationships between visual and auditory stimuli that carry information about an object. Six-month-old infants look longer at television when both picture and sound are on than when only the picture is on. They look longer at patterns on television than other types of stimuli.

Touch. The haptic system is that body system pertaining to tactile stimulation. There are different neural receptors for heat, warmth, cold, dull pain, sharp pain, deep pressure, vibration, and light touch. At birth all humans possess central nervous system ability to register and associate sensory impressions received through receptor organs in the skin and from kinesthetic stimuli that originate with neuromuscular stimulation from their contact with other humans. Sensory pathways subserving kinesthetic and tactile activities are the first to complete myelinization in infancy, followed by auditory and visual pathways.[213–215]

Touching the infant from birth on provides the basis for higher-order operations in the neurological, perceptual, muscular, skeletal, and cognitive systems. Each tactile act carries a physiologic impact with psychological and sociocultural meaning. Much information is gained through discriminating one physical stimulus from another, with the form or quality of touch changing the perception of the tactile experience. Tactile stimulation is essential for both beginning body image development and other learning.[216] Encourage parents to stroke, massage, and cuddle baby; to talk and sing to baby; and to provide toys that have primary colours, different textures, and movement.

Endocrine System

The endocrine system begins to develop primarily in infancy and childhood; it is limited in fetal life. Thus the child is very susceptible to stress, including fluid and electrolyte imbalance, during the first 18 months because the pituitary gland and adrenal cortex do not function well together and the adrenal gland is immature. The pituitary gland continues to secrete growth hormone and thyroid-stimulating hormone (begun in fetal life), which influence growth and metabolism.[217]

Respiratory System

The structures of the upper respiratory tract remain small and relatively delicate and provide inadequate protection against infectious agents. Close proximity of the middle ear, wide horizontal eustachian tube, throat, short and narrow trachea, and bronchi result in rapid spread of infection from one structure to the other. Mucous membranes are less able to produce mucus, causing less air humidification and warming, which also increases susceptibility to infection. The rounded thorax, the limited alveolar surface for gas exchange, and the amount of anatomic dead air space in the lungs or portion of the tracheobronchial tree, where inspired air does not participate in gas exchange, means that more air must be moved in and out per minute than later in childhood. This causes increased respiratory rate. By one year of age, the lining of the airway resembles that of the adult. The respiratory rate at rest decreases gradually during the first year.[218]

Gastrointestinal System

The gastrointestinal system matures somewhat after two to three months, when the baby can voluntarily chew, hold, or spit out food. Saliva secretion increases and composition becomes more adult-like. The Canadian Medical Association recommends that from the age of four to six months, the baby will be ready to sample solid food.[219] The stomach's emptying time changes from two-and-a-half to three hours to three to six hours. Gastric hydrochloric acid is low; pepsinogen secretion nears adult levels at three months. Tooth eruption begins at approximately six months and stimulates saliva flow and chewing.[220]

The small intestine is proportionally longer than it is in an adult; the large intestine is proportionally shorter. Peristaltic waves mature by slowing down and reversing less after approximately eight months; then stools are more formed and baby spits up or vomits less. **Colic,** a term that indicates *daily periods of distress,* usually occurs between two to three weeks and two to three months and seems to have no remedy. X-ray films taken of such infants show unusually rapid and violent peristaltic waves throughout the intestinal tract. These movements are normally set off by a few sucking movements. Gas pressure in the rectum is also three times greater than in the average infant.[221,222] Some physicians believe colic is caused by a deficiency of vitamin K, A, or E. Some mothers find that changing formula and giving plain, low-fat yogurt helps reduce the pains. When small yogurt feedings do not help, vitamin A and E supplements have been found effective. Apparently colic disappears as digestive enzymes become more complex, and normal bacterial flora accumulates as the baby ingests a larger variety of food. It is important that health professionals assist the mother and family to cope with colic. It is also important that mothers do not resort to medications, but that they try to soothe the baby by cuddling, keeping the baby in motion, or rubbing the stomach in a rhythmic motion. It may be especially helpful for the mother to have an occasional evening out, and leave her partner or a competent caregiver in charge of the baby.[223,224]

CRITICAL THINKING

What other health promoting activities can you suggest for a mother who is having a difficult time coping with her baby who is experiencing colic?

By two months, baby usually has two **stools** (*bowel movements*) daily. By four months there is a predictable interval of time between feeding and bowel movements. Breastfed babies usually have soft, semi-liquid stools that are light yellow. Breastfed babies may vary more in the bowel movement pattern: the baby may have three or four watery stools a day or may go several days without a bowel movement. The stools of the formula-fed baby are more brown and formed.

The liver occupies a larger part of the abdominal cavity than an adult's liver does and remains functionally immature until age one year. Glycogen and vitamin storage is less effective than it is later in life.

As the autonomic nervous system and gastrointestinal tract mature, interconnections form between higher mental functions and the autonomic nervous system; the infant's gastrointestinal tract responds to emotional states in self or someone close to him or her.[225,226]

Muscular Tissue. At birth muscular tissue is almost completely formed; growth results from increasing size of the already existing fibres under the influence of growth hormone, thyroxin, and insulin. As muscle size increases, strength increases in childhood. Muscle fibres need continual stimulation to develop to full function and strength.[227,228]

Skin

Structures typical of adult skin are present, but they are functionally immature; thus baby is more prone to skin disorders. The epidermal layers are very permeable, causing greater loss of fluid from the body. Dry, intact skin is the greatest deterrent to bacterial invasion. Sebaceous glands, which produce sebum, are very active in late fetal life and early infancy, causing milia and cradle cap, which go away at approximately six weeks. Production of sebum decreases during infancy and remains minimal during childhood until puberty.

Eccrine (sweat) glands are not functional in response to heat and emotional stimuli until a few months after birth, and function remains minimal through childhood. The inability of the skin to contract and shiver in response to cold or perspire in response to heat causes ineffective thermal regulation.[229,230]

Urinary System

Renal structural components are present at birth; by five months tubules have adult-like proportions in size and shape. The ureters are relatively short, and the bladder lies close to the abdominal wall. Renal function, however, is not mature until approximately one year; therefore, the child is unable to handle increased intake of proteins, which are ingested if cow's milk is given too early.[231]

Immune System

Components of the immune system are present or show beginning development. The phagocytosis process is mature, but the inflammatory response is inefficient and unable to localize infections. The ability to produce antibodies is limited; much of the antibody protection is acquired from the mother during fetal life. Development of immunologic function depends on the infant's gradual exposure to foreign bodies and infectious agents.[232,233]

Red Blood Cell and Hemoglobin Levels

High at birth, red blood cell and hemoglobin levels drop after two or three months and then gradually increase when erythropoiesis begins. Iron deficiency anemia becomes apparent around six months of age if the physiologic system does not function adequately to sustain red blood cell and hemoglobin levels. By the end of infancy, the level of white blood cells, high at birth, declines to reach adult levels. Red blood cell and hemoglobin levels reach adult norms in late childhood.[234,235]

Increasingly, studies show that the health of the adult is influenced considerably by the person's health status in early life. Obesity, discussed in Chapters 10, 11, and 12, is an example. Blood pressure in the adult years is apparently set by age one; the mix of genetic and environmental influences such as diet, stress, and infections is unknown.

Nutritional Needs

The feeding time is a crucial time for baby and mother: a time to strengthen attachment, for baby to feel love and security, a time for mother and baby to learn about self and each other, and a time for baby to learn about the environment. See Table 7-5 for a stage-by-stage guide to infant feeding.

Breastfeeding

Breastfeeding is a learning process for mother and baby as well as the family. The American Academy of Pediatrics *recommends breastfeeding for the first 10 to 14 months of life;* however, a large percentage of infants are bottle-fed. Only about 15% of North American mothers nurse their baby for a year, a rate lower than in most other parts of the world. Children as old as two years can benefit from the antibodies and folic acid in mother's milk.[236] The *Joint Statement on Nutrition for Healthy Term Infants* from the Canadian Paediatric Society,

TABLE 7-5
A Stage-by-Stage Guide to Infant Feeding

Stage/Age	What to Do	Drinks	Meals and Feedings				
			EARLY AM	BREAK-FAST	LUNCH	DINNER	BED-TIME
Weeks 1 and 2 Age 6 months (ages are guidelines only)	Give small tastes of baby cereal or fruit or vegetable puree at lunchtime, halfway through the breast- or bottle-feeding. Give the same food for three days to accustom your baby to it.	If you are bottle-feeding, offer your baby occasional drinks of cooled boiled water.	□	□	□■□	□	□
Weeks 3 and 4 Age 6¹/² months	Introduce solid food at breakfast, halfway through the feeding; baby cereal or other single-grain cereal is ideal. Increase the amount of solid food at lunchtime to 3-4 teaspoonfuls.	Offer cooled boiled water or diluted fruit juice in a bottle. Don't worry if she doesn't want any	□	□■□	□■□	□	□
Weeks 5 and 6 Age 7 months	Introduce solid food at dinner, halfway through the feeding. A week later, offer two courses at lunch; follow a vegetable puree with a fruit one, giving 2-3 teaspoonfuls of each.	Introduce a trainer cup, but don't expect her to be able to drink from it yet—it's just a toy.	·	□■□	□■■□	□■□	□
Weeks 7 and 8 Age 7¹/² months	Offer solid food as the first part of lunch then give breast or bottle to top up. She can have two courses at dinner now, a vegetable and a piece of banana, for example. At breakfast and dinner, continue giving the feeding first. She may eat 5-6 teaspoonfuls of solid food at each meal now.	You can start to give your baby drinks in her cup, but hold it for her as she drinks from it.	·	□■□	■■□	□■■□	□

(continued)

TABLE 7–5 *(continued)*
A Stage-by-Stage Guide to Infant Feeding

Stage/Age	What to Do	Drinks	Meals and Feedings				
			EARLY AM	BREAK-FAST	LUNCH	DINNER	BED-TIME
Weeks 9 and 10 Age 8 months	After lunch solids, offer a drink of formula or breast milk from a cup. After a few days with no lunchtime breast or bottle, offer solid food as the first part of dinner.	Offer formula or breast milk in a cup at each meal and water or diluted juice at other times.	·	□■□	■■	■■□	□
Weeks 11 and 12 Age 8¹/² months	Offer your baby a drink of breast or formula milk in a cup instead of a full feeding after her dinner. You may find she often refuses her breast or bottle feeding after her breakfast solids now.	As before.	·	□■	■■	■■	□
Week 13 onwards Age 9 months	Offer a drink in a cup instead of the feeding before breakfast; now your baby is having solids at three meals a day. Breast or formula milk should be the main milk drink until one year. She can have cow's milk from 12 months.	As before. Your baby may possibly be able to manage her own trainer cup now.	·	■	■■	■■	□
			Key	□ feeding		■ solid food	

Source: Canadian Medical Association, Complete Book of Mother and Baby Care: Parents Practical Handbook from Conception to 3 Years *(3rd ed.). Toronto, Tourmaline Eds. Inc., 2001, p. 113. Copyright Dorling Kindersley Limited.*

Dieticians of Canada, and Health Canada, recommends exclusive breastfeeding for at least the first four months of life and to continue breastfeeding for up to two years.[237]

Breastfeeding is not recommended in Canada and the United States for babies whose mothers are HIV-positive or who have AIDS. If the mother is taking antidepressant medication, in general, breastfeeding is not recommended for the first 10 to 12 weeks. In Canada, infants who have galactosemia should not be breastfed. In addition, mothers who have untreated active tuberculosis or who are receiving long-term chemotherapy should not breastfeed.[238] However, decisions must be made with each individual mother, depending on the benefit to mother and risk to infant.[239,240] Alcohol, nicotine, many medications, including laxatives and barbiturates, and drugs and foreign substances, such as chemical pollutants and pesticides, *pass into the milk and to the infant.* The mother should be informed of these hazards to her baby if she breastfeeds so that she can avoid harmful substances if possible. Organic food without preservatives or dyes can be purchased; some food can be home-grown by families if they wish to exert the effort and have the space. The trend toward shorter postnatal stays carries important implications for breastfeeding outcomes. For example, stimulants such as caffeine, found in coffee and tea, can affect breastfeeding. Women who choose to breastfeed should be provided with the appropriate resource contacts, should any such issues or concerns arise. One of the main health promoting strategies for the mother is encouraging healthy lifestyle choices. Strategies include following a healthy eating pattern according to *Canada's Food Guide to Healthy Eating*, and being involved in an active lifestyle by following *Canada's Physical Guide*.[241] The *Northern Food Guide* is available from the North West Company in Winnipeg, Manitoba.

Human milk is considered ideal because it is sterile, digestible, available, and economical; and it contains the necessary nutrients, except for vitamins C and D and iron. Further, even in undernourished women, the composition of breast milk is adequate, although vitamin content depends on the mother's diet. Breast milk is sufficient for all that baby needs during the first four months of life. It contains higher levels of lactose, vitamin E, and cholesterol and less protein than cow's milk. The additional cholesterol may induce production of hormones required for cholesterol breakdown in adulthood. Breast milk has a more efficient nutritional balance of iron, zinc, vitamin E, and unsaturated fatty acids.[242,243]

Because of the host-resistant factors in human milk, breast milk offers many advantages to the infant, including the premature infant. Immunoglobulins and antibodies and many types of microorganisms—especially those found in the intestinal tract—and enzymes that destroy bacteria are obtained from human milk. Living milk leukocytes, which further promote disease resistance, are also present in breast milk. Respiratory and gastrointestinal diseases, infantile obesity, and meningitis occur two to three times less frequently in breastfed babies than in those who are bottle-fed. Breastfed babies are also less prone to allergies. Human milk kept refrigerated in a sterile container (not pasteurized and not frozen) can be given to premature infants to prevent necrotizing enterocolitis, an often fatal bacterial invasion of the colon wall. *Even a brief period of breastfeeding gives immunologic and other benefits.*[244,245] Breastfeeding also promotes maternal–infant attachment and may provide some protection against sudden infant death syndrome (SIDS).[246]

The mother's decision either to breastfeed or to bottle-feed can be influenced by the obstetrician, pediatrician, nurse, hospital staff, husband, friends, and how her own mother fed her children, or there may be no decision making at all. It may be assumed from the start that the mother will feed either one way or the other. Health professionals can influence the mother in a positive manner regarding her attitude toward breastfeeding. The need for health professionals not only to promote but to support breastfeeding as the healthiest choice for both infant and mother is well recognized.[247]

Critical Thinking
How would you explain to a group of mothers how cultural forces and geography influence breastfeeding?

The woman who works can be encouraged to breastfeed when at home; although in some work sites women can bring their babies so that breastfeeding can be continued. Teach the mother the benefits of breastfeeding to the baby, how to express milk to be used by the caregiver, and suggestions given by community resources such as La Leche League.

Any woman is physiologically able to nurse her baby, with very rare exceptions.[248] But childbirth, breastfeeding, and childrearing are sexual experiences for the woman. The woman's success in breastfeeding is related to other aspects of her psychosexual identity. She may choose not to breastfeed or to limit the lactation period because of personal preference, illness, or employment in a place where she cannot take baby with her. It is important to note that women who have been sexually or physically abused may not wish to breastfeed.[249] It becomes imperative that psychosocial and spiritual assessment become an integral part of prenatal care.

A positive social support system is essential for the woman who breastfeeds because fear of failure, embarrassment, anxiety, exhaustion, frustration, humiliation, anger, fear, or any stress-producing situation can prevent the effect of oxytocin and can block the flow of milk. The pregnant woman's level of information and motivation for achievement are positively related to successful breastfeeding.

Preparation for breastfeeding begins during pregnancy. An adequate diet during pregnancy is an initial step toward successful lactation and breastfeeding. Through the National Academy of Sciences (NAS), Canada and the United States are currently reviewing the scientific data on nutrient requirements. Special attention must be given to folate, calcium, vitamin D, iron, and essential fatty acids, because inadequate intakes exist for some groups of women.[250,251] When inadequate nutrient intake is suspected, vitamin or mineral supplementation may be considered with modification of the diet. Women also may be informed to consult their physician about appropriate supplementation well before pregnancy. The woman may consult La Leche League literature for help.

The baby should be put to breast immediately after delivery and fed within eight hours of birth to reduce hypoglycemia and hyperbilirubinemia.[252] In fact, it would be beneficial to breastfeed during the first half-hour after birth as the baby is most alert at that time.[253] The first nourishment the baby receives after delivery from breastfeeding is **colostrum,** a *thin yellow secretion* for two to four days after delivery. Colostrum has higher levels of antibodies than the later milk; is rich in carbohydrates, which the newborn needs; and serves as a laxative in cleaning out the gastrointestinal tract. Colostrum fed immediately after birth prevents against infection because it triggers antibody production. Depending on how soon and how often the mother nurses, true milk comes in the first few days.[254–256]

If a mother nurses after delivery, the pituitary gland secretes prolactin. The high levels of estrogen from the placenta that inhibited milk secretion during pregnancy are gone. As the baby sucks, the nipple is in the back of the mouth, and the jaws and tongue compress the milk sinuses. These tactile sensations trigger the release of the hormone oxytocin from the pituitary gland, which, in turn, causes the "let-down" response. The sinuses refill immediately, and milk flows with very little effort to the baby. This is the crucial time to learn breastfeeding. Oxytocin also causes a powerful contraction of the uterus, lessening the danger of hemorrhage.[257,258]

Every effort should be directed toward making breastfeeding a comfortable, uninterrupted time. Effective techniques for mother getting into a comfortable position, holding the baby, and putting the baby to nipple are described in La Leche League literature, obstetric nursing and other child care books, and some booklets prepared by formula companies. Some babies take time to orient to the breast, others may latch and suckle well. Mother needs an encouraging partner or family member, knowledgeable and supportive nursing and medical personnel to assist, acquaintance with other successful nursing mothers, to be with her for feeding when the baby is hungry and her breasts are full. The mother whose milk does not let-down may need oxytocin, a period of relaxation, or perhaps a soothing liquid before feeding. She should, in any case, be encouraged to increase her fluid intake and meet the increased recommended dietary allowances for lactating women.[259–263]

The baby may nurse every hour or two at first or on demand, perhaps 15 to 30 minutes each time, but graduate to three- to four-hour intervals, by four months, obtaining more milk in shorter feeding sessions. If anxieties, excessive stimuli, and fatigue are dealt with appropriately, the mother's milk supply will increase or decrease to meet the demand. Alternating breasts with each feeding and emptying the breasts will prevent caking. The infant should grasp the areola completely to avoid excess pressure on the nipples. Generally breastfeeding babies get enough to eat; the child whose growth and weight are within the norm is being breastfed adequately. The large or active infant may need supplemental feeding in addition to breast milk, even when mother's supply is not compromised; however, usually extra formula or baby food is not necessary before the fourth to fifth month. Food in addition to breast milk (or formula) should be introduced from age four to six months.[264] If the mother received ample amounts of iron during pregnancy, her baby's iron stores should last four to 12 months, even on an iron-poor diet.[265,266]

Premature infants can breastfeed earlier and with less effort than they can bottle-feed, but they need time to learn to suck. Physiologically, breastfeeding is an advantage; premature infants suck for approximately 25 minutes at one time, but the longer feeding fills the stomach more slowly. The infant controls the pace of breastfeeding and also avoids gastric distension, in contrast to bottle feeding, and the caregiver's controlling feeding pace, amount, and time.[267,268]

Breastfeeding the premature infant is possible and desirable and can be a rewarding option for the mother and nutritionally and emotionally beneficial to the baby. Breast milk is more digestible, and milk from mothers with preterm babies has adequate protein, sodium, potassium, and chloride. It is not at that point adequate in calcium, phosphorus, iron, zinc, and copper. These substances can be provided in supplementary feedings designed for premature infants.[269] Several investigators describe (1) the specific procedure for pumping the breasts; (2) how the mother can maintain a milk supply; (3) ways to enhance the experience for the mother, baby, and intensive care nursery staff; and (4) continuation of breastfeeding after discharge.[270,271]

Commercial Formulas

In Canada, it is important for all health care facilities to be "breastfeeding friendly." Health care facilities should not be centres for marketing infant formulas, for they then become in conflict with the baby-friendly initiative.[272] The amount of fluoride in formula (ready to use, concentrated, and powdered) is regulated by Health Canada to help ensure that infants receive the appropriate amount of fluoride.[273]

Teach parents that care must be taken if the bottle is heated; it is not essential to heat it. Instruct the parents why baby bottles should preferably not be heated in the microwave. The bottle, nipple, and milk all become too hot and will cause oropharyngeal and esophageal burns. Further, the formula-filled disposable plastic liner of a commercial nurser may explode after removal of the heated bottle from the microwave, causing body burns.

Cow's Milk

The Canadian Paediatric Society states that babies under 9 to 12 months of age should not be given cow's milk.[274] Cow's milk contains from two to three times as much protein as does human milk, and a much greater percentage of the protein is casein, which produces a large, difficult-to-digest curd. It is higher in saturated fats and lower in cholesterol than is human milk, but the total fat contents are comparable; however, the butterfat is poorly absorbed. Cow's milk contains half as much total lactose as human milk and also has galactose and glucose. Although it contains more sodium, potassium, magnesium, sulphur, and phosphorus than human milk, like human milk, it is a relatively poor source of vitamins C and D and iron. One striking difference between cow's milk and human milk is the calcium content. Cow's milk contains over four times the calcium of human milk; and babies who are fed cow's milk have larger and heavier skeletons. Whether or not this is normal or better is debatable. Low fat (2% milk fat) or skim milk should not be fed to infants because they will not gain weight and they need the fat content.[275–277]

Before parents make the switch from breast milk or formula to cow's milk, they need to check with their baby's doctor. If a mother in Canada is unable to provide her own breast milk for her baby, then she should contact a breastfeeding support clinic (contact the local hospital or health clinic for referral). If the mother feels unable to breastfeed, one option, particularly for an ill or a high-risk infant, is to receive pasteurized human milk from Canada's human milk bank located in Vancouver. The mother is required to pay a processing fee and the cost of transportation for the milk. (The milk bank's address is: B.C. Women's Milk Bank, Children's and Women's Lactation Services, 4480 Oak St., Vancouver, BC, V6H 3V1.) Whole cow's milk is the main milk drink from 10 to 12 months.[278]

Water

Normally, healthy term breastfeeding babies should receive only breast milk, without other foods and fluids, unless a medical situation exists. Supplementation interferes with milk production.[279] In fact, supplemental foods intended to minimize dehydration are not routinely required. Failure of the baby to void (at least three times daily during the first two days, and six times per day subsequently) may indicate dehydration. Dehydration may be confirmed by identification of weight loss and examination of the anterior fontanel, skin turgor, and skin perfusion.[280] Infants become dehydrated more quickly than adults because they have a smaller total fluid volume in the body compared with body size.[281] Health teaching should be implemented to the parents regarding the *signs of dehydration*.

Fluoridated drinking water does not harm the fetus and is beneficial to the mother's teeth during pregnancy when hormonal changes may lead to possible dental problems. Breast milk is relatively low in fluoride but the fluoride still benefits the infant's teeth.[282] In Canada, some individuals may assume that bottled water is safer than municipal tap water, but no evidence exists to support this. Pre-packaged water (bottled water) is considered to be food and is regulated under the Food and Drug Regulation.[283]

Nutrient Requirements

After the initial period of adjustment (seven to ten days after birth), the baby needs a daily average of 2.2 g of protein and 117 calories per kilogram (or 53 per pound) of body weight to grow and gain weight satisfactorily. Moderate protein intake is apparently well used and increases growth. No specific fat requirement is set, but some fats are necessary because they contain essential fat-soluble vitamins, furnish more energy per unit than carbohydrates and protein, promote development of the nervous system, and contribute to diet palatability. Adequate intake of vitamins and minerals, especially iron and fluoride is essential.[284] Recommendations for various ages can be found in a nutrition text.[285,286] By two to three weeks of age, babies return to birth weight and 14 g to 28 g per day for the first few months.[287]

Feeding Comfort

Mothers frequently need instruction about times and methods of **burping** (*bubbling, or gently patting baby's back*) the baby to reduce gaseous content of the stomach during feeding, because the cardiac sphincter is not well developed. Young babies must be bubbled after every ounce and at the end of a feeding. Later they can be bubbled halfway through and again at the end. The infant should be moved from a semi-reclining to an upright position while the feeder gently pats the back. Because a new infant's gastrointestinal tract is unstable, milk may be eructated with gas bubbles. Adequate bubbling should occur before the infant is placed into the crib to prevent milk regurgitation and aspiration. The infant should be positioned on back or on side.

Solid Foods

There is no rigid sequence in adding solid foods to the infant's diet. The case situation also presents an effective approach. Whatever solid food is offered first or at what time is largely a matter of individual preference of the mother or of the pediatrician. Ideally the infant's needs and developmental achievements such as eye–hand–mouth coordination and fine pincer grasp should be considered when introducing solids. A large, active baby who is bottle-fed may need cereal added to the diet at two months to satisfy hunger. A smaller, more lethargic baby may find it awkward to accept such supplements before three or four months.

The mother or nurse introducing the baby to solid foods should make it a pleasant experience. The foods offered should be smooth and well-diluted with milk or formula. The infant should not be hurried, coaxed, or allowed to linger more than 30 minutes. New foods should be offered one at a time and early in the feeding while he or she is still hungry. Emphasize *not to add* salt or sugar to feedings to please the feeder's taste buds. Honey should *not* be added to feedings the first year because of the possibility of infant botulism.[288,289]

Teach parents that when the baby is first fed puréed foods with a spoon, he or she expects and wants to suck. The protrusion of the tongue, which is needed in sucking, makes it appear as if baby is pushing food out of the mouth. Parents misinterpret this as a dislike for the food, but it really is the result of immature muscle coordination and possibly surprise at the taste and feel of the new items in the diet. This reflex gradually disappears by seven to eight months.

Infant nutritional status can be assessed by measuring head circumference, height, and weight. Small stature may indicate undernutrition unless there is a genetic influence from small-sized parents. Signs of nutritional deprivation include smaller-than-normal head size, pale skin colour, poor skin turgor, and low hemoglobin levels and hematocrit.[290,291]

Teach parents to avoid overfeeding—either milk or foods. Theories hold that babies who are fed more calories than they use daily develop additional fat cells to store unused energy sources. These fat cells proliferate in infancy and continue to replace themselves during childhood. Adults who were fat infants will have excess fat cells to fill through life and may have difficulty with weight control or may be obese. Another theory about the effect of infant feeding on adult weight is that eating patterns are difficult to change, especially if food symbolizes love, attention, or approval.

In addition to discussing the food quantities, quality, and nutrients needed by the baby, teach parents that food and mealtime are learning experiences. The baby gains motor control and coordination in self-feeding; he or she learns to recognize colour, shape, and texture. Use of mouth muscles stimulates the ability to make movements necessary for speech development. He or she continues to develop trust with the consistent, loving atmosphere of mealtime. Food should not be used as reward or punishment (by withholding food). The child should learn moderation in feeding quantity, and between-feeding snacks should be avoided or, if used, should be healthful, small in quantity, and given because the child is hungry despite eating at mealtime.[292]

Unless you are an experienced mother, you may feel uncomfortable in teaching about feeding or other child care. Yet, you can share information gleaned from the literature, experiences of other mothers you have helped, and your own experiences if you have worked in the newborn nursery or helped a family member with a new baby. Do not tell the mother what method is best; give her the available information and then support her in *her* decision. Because feeding is one of the first tasks as a mother, she will need your guidance, assistance, and emotional support. You can offer suggestions such as the posture that will ensure a comfortable position for her as she cradles the baby in her arms close to her body. Whether breast- or bottle-fed, the baby needs the emotional warmth and body contact. The bottle should never be propped because choking may result. Further, nursing-bottle mouth may develop: tooth decay is much higher in children when mothers use the bottle of milk, juice, or sugar water as a pacifier. The upper front teeth are most affected because liquids pool around these teeth when the baby is drowsy or sleeping.[293]

Mother–child contacts after birth are a continuation of the symbiotic prenatal relationship. The dependence of the baby on the mother and the reciprocal need of the mother for satisfaction from the child, proving her dependability and giving her confidence, are necessary to develop and continue the relationship. A successful feeding situation sets the foundation for the infant's personality and social development. It is the main means of establishing a relationship with another person and consequently the most basic opportunity to establish trust. Thus, feeding is much more than a mechanical task. Your teaching attitude can convey its importance. If a father will be a primary nurturer, teach him the same way you would teach the mother.

Weaning

The *gradual elimination of breastfeeding or bottle-feeding in favour of cup and table feeding* (**weaning**) is usually completed by the end of the first year. The ideal time to wean is when mother and baby are both ready. Baby shows signs of making this transition: muscle coordination increases, teeth erupt, and he or she resists being held close while feeding. The two methods should overlap and allow baby to take some initiative and allow mother to guide the new method. Mother's consistency in meeting the new feeding schedule is important to development of a sense of trust.

The most difficult feeding to give up is usually the bedtime feeding because baby is tired and is more likely to want the "old method." After the maxillary central incisory teeth erupt, a night bottle should contain no carbohydrate, to reduce decay in the deciduous teeth. During periods of stress the baby will often regress. Baby is also learning to wait longer for food and may object vigorously to this new condition.

The need to suck varies with different children. Some children, even after weaning, will suck a thumb or use a pacifier (if provided). The baby should not be shamed for either of these habits because they are not likely to cause problems with the teeth or mouth during the first two years.

CRITICAL THINKING

How would you explain the process of weaning to a woman with limited understanding of English?

Cultural Influences on Infant Nutrition

In both Canada and the United States middle- and upper-socioeconomic-level Caucasian women are more likely to breastfeed than other groups. Members of subcultures vary to the extent to which they engage in breastfeeding. Cultural values influence (1) women's perceptions about breastfeeding in terms of nutritional importance, (2) the father's beliefs and preferences, (3) acceptance of breast exposure, (4) sexuality issues, and (5) considerations related to convenience. For immigrant groups, bottle-feeding may be viewed as more modern and prestigious. In Canada, breastfeeding rates are positively related to maternal education.[294] Breastfeeding trends vary across Canada. For example, the First Nations and Inuit Regional Health Survey (FNIRHS) report that mothers were less likely to initiate breastfeeding than the National Longitudinal Survey on Children and Youth (NLSCY) mothers.[295] This suggests that we need to encourage Aboriginal women to increase the initiation rate of breastfeeding.

7-2 BONUS SECTION IN CD-ROM

Breastfeeding Variations in Asian and Latino Cultures

Cultural variation is often interesting—especially if some of your clients are members of the culturally "different" group. Asian and Latino practices regarding breastfeeding are compared; and the *Yin-Yang Theory* is considered.

7-3 BONUS SECTION IN CD-ROM

Breastfeeding and Weaning: First Year

Come and meet Sue! Sue gives a first-hand account of her breastfeeding and weaning experience. Her account will provide helpful information for health care practice. Be cautious, however, the costs quoted are in U.S. funds.

Sleep Patterns

One of the most frequent concerns of a new mother is when, where, and how much baby sleeps. Awake, alert periods are altered by different types of feeding schedules. Sleep patterns are unique to each infant, but some generalizations can be made.

The infant exhibits at least six states or levels of arousal:[296,297]

■ Regular or quiet sleep: Eyes are closed, breathing is regular, and the only movements are sudden, generalized startle motions. Baby makes little sound. This is the low point of arousal; infant cannot be awakened with mild stimuli.

■ Irregular, active rapid eye movement (REM) sleep: Baby's eyes are closed, breathing is irregular, muscles twitch slightly from time to time, and there are facial responses of smiles or pouts in response to sounds or lights. Baby may groan, make faces, or cry briefly.

■ Quiet wakefulness: Eyes are open, the body is more active, breathing is irregular, and there is varying spontaneous response to external stimuli.

■ Active wakefulness: Eyes are open; there is visual following of interesting sights and sounds, body movements, and vocalizations that elicit attention.

■ Crying.

■ Indeterminate state: Transition from one state of alertness to another.

Newborn and young infants spend twice as much time in REM sleep than adults. In this state baby shows continual slow rolling eye movements on which are superimposed rapid eye movements. Additionally, respirations increase and are irregular, and small muscle twitching movements are seen.[298,299]

As the infant's nervous system develops, baby will have longer periods of sleep and wakefulness that gradually become more regular. By six weeks, baby's biological rhythms usually

EVIDENCE-BASED PRACTICE

Impressions of Breastfeeding Information and Support among First-Time Mothers within a Multi-Ethnic Community

A telephone survey was conducted to a sample of 108 immigrant and Canadian-born mothers (average age 29.4 years) in an ethnically diverse local community service centre in Quebec. All participants were primiparous, breastfeeding mothers at three weeks postpartum. The purpose of the study was to examine mothers' perceptions of breastfeeding information and support received from health professionals within a multi-ethnic community.

Overall, mothers' evaluations of professional breastfeeding support were found to be positive, despite their reports of what breastfeeding experts would consider less than optimal standards of hospital and community-care practice concerning breastfeeding.

Additional findings from the survey revealed the following:

1. Immigrant and Canadian-born mothers differ in their perceptions of breastfeeding support:
   a. Immigrant mothers were more likely to experience practices detrimental to breastfeeding success (e.g., in-hospital formula supplementation).
   b. Immigrant mothers' evaluations of in-hospital breastfeeding support were more positive than those of Canadian-born mothers.
   c. Immigrant mothers were more likely than Canadian-born mothers to receive breastfeeding support from community health services.
   d. Immigrant mothers were less positive than Canadian-born mothers about the follow-up care that was provided.
2. Overall, the breastfeeding information that was provided tended to focus more on the successful initiation of breastfeeding rather than on strategies to incorporate breastfeeding into the lifestyle of the mother.
3. Despite evidence in the literature claiming that "perceived inadequate milk supply" is the most common reason for early termination of breastfeeding, mothers were provided with minimal information on ensuring adequate milk production.
4. As good sources of information, both books and nurses (hospital and community-based), were identified by both types of mother as valuable; nurses in particular were identified as significant by the immigrant mothers.
5. Canadian-born mothers were more likely to use fee-for-service lactation consultants.

Practice Implication

Nurses must continue to provide to mothers support and complete information on breastfeeding.

Source: Loiselle, C., S. Semenic, B. Cote, M. Lapointe, and R. Gendron. *Impressions of Breastfeeding Information and Support among First-Time Mothers within a Multiethnic Community,* Canadian Journal of Nursing Research, 33, no. 3 (2001), 31–46. Used with permission.

coincide with daytime and night-time hours, and he or she may be sleeping through the night. Babies sleep an average of 16 to 20 hours a day for the first week. By 12 to 16 weeks these hours will be reduced to 14 or 15 a day. Usually this pattern will continue through the first year, with nap times getting shorter until the morning nap is eliminated. By seven or eight months, baby may sleep through the night without awakening.

Help parents understand that when a baby goes through the stage of separation anxiety at about eight months of age, bedtime becomes more difficult because he or she does not want to leave mother or other people. Because the baby needs sleep, the parent should be firm about getting the child ready for bed. Prolonging bedtime adds to fatigue. By the end of the first year, the baby may sleep 12 to 14 hours at night and nap one to four hours during the day.[300]

The infant should at least have a consistent place for sleeping (be it box, drawer, or crib) and a clean area for supplies. A baby can sleep comfortably in an infant crib or bassinet during the first few weeks, but as soon as active arms and legs begin to hit the sides, he or she should be moved to a full-sized crib. Note that cribs manufactured only after September 1986 are considered safe. Cribs made before this date do not meet current standards and put children at risk.[301] No pillows should be used. The crib should have a crib border placed at the bottom of the slats to prevent catching the head between the bars. It should be fitted with a firm, waterproof, easy-to-clean mattress and with warm light covers loosely tucked in. The sides of the crib should fit closely to the mattress so that the infant will not get caught and crushed if he or she should roll to the edge. Thin plastic sheeting can cause suffocation and should never be used on or around the baby's crib. Teach these safety measures to the parents.

Caressing or singing softly while holding baby in a sleeping position in bed is calming. If the mother is available when the baby first awakes, he or she anticipates this pleasure, and sleep is associated with return of mother. If the baby awakes and cries during the night, the parent should wait briefly. Many times the crying will subside with the baby's growing ability to control personal anxiety feelings. Persistent crying indicates unmet needs and should be attended.

Frequently a mother becomes concerned if baby sleeps too long during the day, perhaps six or seven hours without a feeding. If this happens frequently, it may help to awaken the baby during the day for regular feedings and attempt to establish a better routine with longer sleeping periods at night. Occasional oversleeping is little cause for concern.

Co-sleep, when *baby sleeps in the bed with the parent(s),* is sometimes frowned upon. However, this is considered normal in some cultures. Co-sleep can help the baby regulate respiration, heart rate, and body temperature in cold climates and is convenient for breastfeeding. Because of the baby's movements, it may be difficult for the parents to sleep, and baby between parents decreases their intimacy. Further, it can be difficult to get the child to break this habit. The Canadian Child Care Federation claims that bed sharing is a common practice for many families. Further, no evidence exists that a baby who shares the bed with a parent or sibling has a reduced risk of sudden infant death syndrome (SIDS). The risk of SIDS increases if the individual who shares the bed is a smoker or has taken alcohol or other drugs that may alter responsiveness.[302]

Rates of SIDS are lower because parents are following recommendations for positioning the infant during sleep. However, in Canada three children die per week from SIDS.[303] Health Canada recommends placing the child on the back, and on a firm (not soft and fluffy) mattress. SIDS probably has other causes; the occurrence is higher in infants whose mothers smoke tobacco or use cocaine.[304] Other health promoting strategies include keeping the baby warm, not hot, and promoting breastfeeding strategies.

Play Activity

The infant engages in play with self: with the hands or feet, by rolling, getting into various positions and with the sounds he or she produces. Baby needs playful activity from both mother and father to stimulate development in all spheres. Share the following information with parents. You may need to teach the parents how to touch, cuddle, talk to, and play with the baby.

Certain toys are usually enjoyed at certain ages because of changing needs and developing skills. The box entitled "Guide to Play Activities" lists age, characteristics that influence play interest and activities, and suggested activities, toys, and equipment.[305–307]

Guide to Play Activities

Age	Characteristics Development	Suggested Activities and Equipment
4 weeks	Tonic neck reflex postion Rolls partway to side Disregards ring in midplane Eyes follow ring in midplane Hand clutches on contact Drops rattle immediately Attends bell Activity diminishes Marked head lag when pulled to sitting position Head sags forward; back evenly rounded Head rotation; in prone position Startles easily to sudden sounds or movements	Much tender loving care Mobiles and other hanging objects which can be followed by eyes but which can't be grasped—bright in colour Musical mobiles
16 weeks	Head position in midplane Plays with hands at midplane Regards ring immediately, arms activate Holds rattle in fist Head fairly steady in sitting position On verge of rolling Laughs aloud; coos; carries on "conversation" Spontaneous social smile Knows mother; stares at strangers Smiles at strangers who are friendly	Enjoys cuddling and motion Cradle gym for brief periods (20–30 minutes) Rattles Soft, stuffed, small toys to touch and squeeze Soothing music (humming, singing, CDs) Rattles, bells, musical toys Crinkling paper, clap, or snap of fingers Large wooden or nonsplintering plastic toys, beads, spools
28 weeks	Transfers small toys (blocks, bells, etc.) from one hand to the other Mouths objects Lifts head in supine position Reaches with one hand Sits momentarily by self leaning on hands Feet to mouth Regards image in mirror	Small toys Soothing music Cradle gym (30–40 minutes) Peek-a-boo Pat-a-cake Noise makers (bells, squeak toys) Moderately active bouncing on lap Use of mirror to see self and others

(continued)

Guide to Play Activities *(continued)*

Age	Characteristics Development	Suggested Activities & Equipment
	Polysyllabic vowel sounds	Outdoor excursions—walks
	Bounces actively	Reading to child, letting child touch and pat books
	Prompt grasp	Splashing in water, water toys
	Pivots in prone position	
	Plays contentedly alone	
40 weeks	Knocks blocks together in hands	Small (2.5 cm) square blocks
	Approaches objects with index finger	Soft, small toys
	Prehends pellet, inferior pincer grasp	Assorted objects of varying colour having interesting texture
	Grasps bell by handle and waves it	Peek-a-boo
	Sits with good control	Pat-a-cake
	Goes from sitting to prone position	Rides in buggy or stroller
	Creeps	Parallel play
	Pulls to standing position	Nesting, stock, or climbing boxes and blocks
	Waves bye-bye	Kitchen utensils
	Increasing imitation	Bath toys
	Adjusts to simple commands	Cups and boxes to pour (water, sand) and fill
	Is fascinated with words and other sounds	
12 months	Walks with help	Open and close simple boxes
	Throws and rolls ball	Empty and fill toys
	Offers objects, but frequently does not release them	Push-pull toys
	Vocabulary of 3–10 words	Strongly strung large beads
	Vigorous imitative scribble	Small, brightly colored blocks
		Rag and oil cloth books
		Balls, bells, floating bath toys
		Cuddle toys
		Nursery rhymes
		Music and singing to child

The baby can remain satisfied playing with self for increasing amounts of time but prefers to have people around. Baby enjoys being held briefly in various positions, being rocked, swinging for short periods, being taken for walks.

Because much of baby's play involves putting objects into the mouth, a clean environment with lead-free paint is important. A small object that baby swallows, such as a coin, is passed through the digestive tract; however, small batteries used in cameras, calculators, and other electronic equipment may be hazardous if swallowed because they can rupture and release poisonous chemicals. Surgical removal may be necessary. Children gradually build immunity to the germs encountered daily on various objects; however, health may be threatened by that which goes unnoticed. Sitting and playing in dirt or sand contaminated by dioxin, other pesticides or herbicides, or radiation is dangerous to the developing physiologic systems. Children's or parents' reading material, which can become play objects, may also be hazardous.

Toys need not be expensive, but they should be colourful (and without leaded paint), safe, sturdy, and easily handled and cleaned. They should be large enough to prevent aspiration or ingestion; they should be without rough or sharp edges or points, detachable parts, or loops to get around the neck, and some should make sounds and have moving parts.

Baby needs an unrestricted play area, such as the floor, that is clean and safe, although use of a playpen may be necessary for short periods. Excess restriction or lack of stimulation inhibits curiosity, learning about self and the environment, and development of trust. Therefore baby should not wear clothing that is restraining, and he or she should not be kept constantly in a playpen or crib.

Stationary play stations, an exersaucer play gym that turns, rocks, and bounces, should be used no more than 20 minutes a day. If overused, the baby is likely to have poor posture and weak back and stomach muscles and delay walking. Children learn through activity; they need supervised "tummy time" and "scoot time" and a clean, safe floor to develop back, neck, abdominal, and buttock muscles.[308] Baby needs play objects and a loving parent who provides stimulating surroundings.

Verzemnieks discusses ways to stimulate sensory development of the hospitalized child during routine care measures and common items in the hospital that can be used as toys, such as medicine cups, soufflé cups, empty tape cylinders, and various boxes. She also lists common household items that can be used in the home for toys that can provide fun and stimulate creativity, more so than some of the expensive toys on the market.[309] The best educational toys are likely to be in household cupboards and closets.[310]

Parents should know the dangers of overstimulation and rough handling. Fatigue, inattention, and injury may result. The playful, vigorous activities that well-intentioned parents engage in, such as tossing the baby forcefully into the air or jerking the baby in a whiplash manner, may cause bone injuries or subdural hematomas and cerebrovascular lesions that later could cause mental retardation. Premature infants and male babies are twice as vulnerable as full-term girls, because of the relative immaturity of their brains.

For Aboriginal people, toys and playthings are important tools through which the child can become better acquainted with the world around him or her. Any parent buying a toy should look for those that will enhance positive social-emotional development, help to build pride in identity, provide fun and enrich the child's growth, and help to encourage creative and dramatic play.[311] Hammersmith and Sawatsky state that ways for socializing the child toward his or her identity may include the use of cultural events, puppets, music, dance, and body movement.[312]

Health Promotion and Health Protection

In addition to measures already discussed, including the safety measures in the previous section on play activity, the following measures also promote health.

At birth the neonate should have an antibiotic ointment instilled in the eyes to prevent gonococcal or chlamydia ophthalmia neonatorum. The possibility of blindness in the infant, along with the low cost and effectiveness of the treatment, makes this procedure mandatory.[313]

Injecting 1 mg of vitamin K is effective in preventing hemorrhagic disease, which is caused in one of 2000 to one of 3000 live births by a transient deficiency of factor VIII production. Sickle cell screening can be obtained from in-cord blood.

During the first week of life the infant should be screened for **phenylketonuria (PKU),** *an inborn metabolic disorder characterized by abnormal presence of phenylketonuria and other metabolites of phenylalanine in the urine.* Screening for thyroid function and hemoglobin abnormalities is also recommended for all newborns.

Immunizations

Immunizations, *promoting disease resistance through injection of attenuated, weakened organisms or products produced by organisms,* are essential to every infant as a preventive measure. Before birth, baby is protected from certain organisms by the placental barrier and mother's physical defence mechanisms. Birth propels baby into an environment filled with many microorganisms. Baby has protection against common pathogens for a time, but as he or she is gradually exposed to the outside world and the people in it, further protection is needed through routine immunizations. Immunizations have been considered the most effective health promotion intervention; and they have had a positive impact on health in Canada. See Chapter 10 regarding parental concerns about immunization and ways of approaching these concerns. In 1995, the National Advisory Committee on Immunization initiated a process to develop guidelines for childhood immunization practices. These guidelines have been officially endorsed by many professional bodies.[314] A harmonized routine infant immunization schedule does not exist in Canada. It is important that health professionals encourage parents to check with their local health departments concerning provincial and territorial variations.[315] Table 7–6 outlines the routine immunization schedule for infants and older children.

Teach parents about the importance of immunizations. Parents should keep a continuing record of the child's immunizations. Your teaching, encouragement, community efforts, and follow-up are vital.

A mailed reminder about the date for immunization of the infant increases the chances that baby will receive the scheduled immunization, especially in families that have a record of not keeping clinic appointments. A telephone reminder may help in getting mothers to return for well-baby immunizations.

As a result of worldwide efforts, worldwide immunization of children is now increasing, according to the World Health Organization. Currently 80% of the world's children are immunized against six diseases: diphtheria, measles, pertussis, poliomyelitis, tetanus, and tuberculosis. About 25% of children's deaths in the developed world could be prevented by immunization. In the province of Manitoba, registered First Nations children, both "on-reserve" and "off-reserve," have far lower complete immunization rates than all other Manitoba children at ages one (62% versus 89%) and two (45% versus 77%).[316]

CRITICAL THINKING

Regarding immunization, what would you tell a mother who has an infant born prematurely?

Safety Promotion and Injury Control

Safety promotion and injury control are based on the understanding of infant behaviour. Accidents are a major cause of death in individuals less than 26 years of age. Risk factors that influence the occurrence of fatal childhood accidents include (1) host factors, such as age and sex; (2) environmental factors, such as hazardous play equipment, flammable clothing, and accessible poisons; and (3) parental characteristics, such as socioeconomic status.[317] Although infant mortality rates have been decreasing in the past four decades, in 1996 the United States ranked 24th (9.22) and Canada ranked 6th (6.82) in the number of infant deaths per 100 000 live births.[318] Differences in infant mortality are noted in terms of socioeconomic and educational variables. Substantial differences in infant mortality between the various ethnic and racial groups have been documented.[319]

Epidemiologic studies report that the main causes of death for the infant are drowning; suffocation by inhalation or ingestion of food or by mechanical means (in bed or cradle, by plastic bag, or by polystyrene-filled pillows); transport accidents; and falls.[320] Contrary to common belief, the baby is not immobile: he or she will not necessarily stay where placed. Baby rolls, crawls, creeps, walks, reaches, and explores.

TABLE 7-6
Routine Immunization Schedule for Infants and Children

Age at Vaccination	DTaP[1]	IPV	Hib[2]	MMR	Td[3] or dTap[10]	Hep B[4] (3 doses)	V	PC	MC
Birth									
2 months	X	X	X					X[8]	X[9]
4 months	X	X	X			Infancy		X	X
6 months	X	(X)[5]	X			or		X	X
12 months				X		preadolescence	X[7]	X	
18 months	X	X	X	(X)[6] or		(9-13 yrs)			or
4-6 years	X	X		(X)[6]					
14-16 years					X[10]				X[9]

DTaP[1] Diphtheria, tetanus, pertussis (acellular) vaccine

IPV Inactivated poliovirus vaccine

Hib *Haemophilus influenzae* type b conjugate vaccine

MMR Measles, mumps and rubella vaccine

Td Tetanus and diphtheria toxoid, adult type with reduced diphtheria toxoid

dTap[10] Tetanus and diphtheria toxoid, acellular pertussis, adolescent/adult type with reduced diphtheria and pertussis components

Hep B Hepatitis B vaccine

V Varicella

PC Pneumococcal conjugate vaccine

MCM eningococcal C conjugate vaccine

Notes:

1. DTaP (diphtheria, tetanus, acellular or component pertussis) vaccine is the preferred vaccine for all doses in the vaccination series, including completion of the series in children who have received ≥ 1 dose of DPT (whole cell) vaccine.

2. Hib schedule shown is for PRP-T or HbOC vaccine. If PRP-OMP is used, give at 2, 4 and 12 months of age.

3. Td (tetanus and diphtheria toxoid), a combined adsorbed "adult type" preparation for use in people ≥ 7 years of age, contains less diphtheria toxoid than preparations given to younger children and is less likely to cause reactions in older people.

4. Hepatitis B vaccine can be routinely given to infants or preadolescents, depending on the provincial/territorial policy; three doses at 0, 1 and 6 month intervals are preferred. The second dose should be administered at least 1 month after the first dose, and the third at least 2 months after the second dose. A two-dose schedule for adolescents is also possible.

5. This dose is not needed routinely, but can be included for convenience.

6. A second dose of MMR is recommended, at least 1 month after the first dose for the purpose of better measles protection. For convenience, options include giving it with the next scheduled vaccination at 18 months of age or with school entry (4-6 years) vaccinations (depending on the provincial/territorial policy), or at any intervening age that is practicable. The need for a second dose of mumps and rubella vaccine is not established but may benefit (given for convenience as MMR). The second dose of MMR should be given at the same visit as DTaP IPV (± Hib) to ensure high uptake rates.

7. Children aged 12 months to 12 years should receive one dose of varicella vaccine. Individuals ≥ 13 years of age should receive two doses at least 28 days apart.

8. Recommended schedule, number of doses and subsequent use of 23 valent polysaccharide pneumococcal vaccine depend on the age of the child when vaccination is begun.

9. Recommended schedule and number of doses of meningococcal vaccine depends on the age of the child.

10. dTap adult formulation with reduced diphtheria toxoid and pertussis component.

Source: Health Canada, Canadian Immunization Guide (6th ed.). Ottawa: Minister of Public Works and Government Services, 2002, p. 56. Reproduced with the permission of the Minister of Public Works and Government Services Canada, 2003.

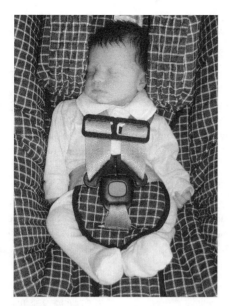

FIGURE 7-4

Infants should be transported in an approved automobile infant seat or harness.

As he or she is helpless in water, the baby should never be left alone or with an irresponsible person while in water. The home and car have many often-unnoticed hazards; thus, the baby should never be left alone in either and should never roam freely in the car while it is in motion. Parents should use an approved car infant seat or harness (Figure 7–4).

Falls can be avoided if the parents or nurse are responsible for doing the following:

- Keep crib rails up and securely fastened.
- Maintain a firm grasp of the baby while carrying or caring for him or her and support the head during the first few months.
- Use a sturdy highchair and government-approved car infant seat.
- Strap child securely in grocery cart, if used.
- Lock windows if infant can climb onto windowsills.
- Have a gate at the top of the stairs or in front of windows or doors that are above the first story.
- Keep room free of loose rugs or trailing cables or cords to avoid child falling over them as he or she becomes mobile.
- Keep furniture, lamps, and heavy or breakable objects secure so child does not pull them on self when becoming mobile.
- Clean up spills immediately from floor.

Suffocation at home and in the health care setting can be avoided:

- Remove any small objects from floor or accessible surroundings that could be inhaled or ingested (safety pins, small bead, coins, toys, paper clips, nuts, raisins, popcorn, chips, parts of broken toys, balloons).
- Keep plastic bags, Venetian blind cords, or other cords out of reach.
- Avoid the use of pillows in the crib or excessively tight clothing or bedcovers.

- Choose stair gate with opening too small for head; avoid accordion or expandable gates.

Burns can also be avoided:

- Place the crib away from radiators or fireplaces.
- Use warm-air vaporizers with caution.
- Disconnect unused appliances; cover electric outlets.
- Avoid tablecloths that hang over the table's edge.
- Place crib, play materials, and highchair away from heater and fans.
- Turn pot handles inward on the stove.
- Avoid excessive sun exposures; use sunscreen.
- Avoid smoking around the baby.
- Use sturdy screens in front of fireplace; keep child away from stoves.

Encourage parents to take a first-aid course (one directed toward cardiopulmonary resuscitation, preventing airway obstruction, and other home and family concerns) that enables them to recognize hazards and take appropriate measures to avoid injury to loved ones. Teaching parents about the child's normal developmental pattern will also enable them to foresee potential accidents and take precautions. Because some infants are quite mobile by 10 or 12 months, the safety precautions discussed in Chapter 8 may also apply.

Parents must also consider another threat to the safety of the child and to the integrity of their family unit: stealing, kidnapping, or abduction of their infant. Burgess et al. describe characteristics of the abductor and legal ramifications of the crime.[321]

Common Health Problems: Prevention and Treatment

Various conditions are common in the infant. Table 7-7 summarizes the problems, their signs or symptoms, and methods to prevent or treat them.[322,323] Refer also to Chapters 2 and 6 for illnesses that can result from various teratogens or infectious diseases in the mother (see Figures 6-1 and 6-2).

Because of the contact with a variety of microorganisms, infants who are in daycare centres have about twice as many respiratory infections as those who are reared entirely at home. Infants in small group care fall somewhere in between. Counsel parents about careful selection of daycare services in relation to hygiene measures that are followed, the number of children being served, and policies related to whether or not sick children are kept for the day. However, when children raised entirely at home go to school, their illness rates are higher because of exposure to new germs.[324]

Advise parents against the harmful effects of smoking. Discuss both active and passive effects of smoking. The incidence of *acute respiratory disease, bronchitis,* and *pneumonia* increases with the increasing number of cigarettes smoked by the mother or other family members, particularly in infants aged six to nine months. Infants of smoking mothers have significantly more admissions for bronchitis or pneumonia

TABLE 7-7
Common Health Problems in Infancy

Problem	Definition	Symptoms/Signs	Prevention/Treatment
Atopic dermatitis	Chronic inflammatory disease of skin, characterized by itching	Family history of allergic disease, especially asthma Onset usually after 2 months Rough, red, papular scaling areas, mainly on scalp, behind ears, on forearms and legs	Use warm water for baths. Apply lotions. Use soft cotton clothing. Keep fingernails short.
Diaper dermatitis	Inflammation of skin covered by diaper	Itching, irritability Redness on buttocks, genitalia; papules, vesicles, and pustules	Keep area clean and dry. Allow air to circulate. Apply bland ointment or Burrow's solution.
Seborrheic dermatitis ("cradle cap")	Oily, scaly condition occurring in areas with large numbers of sebaceous glands	Scaly eruptions spreading to eyebrows, eyelids, nasolabial folds	Shampoo and massage scalp. More severe cases may require a selenium sulphide (e.g., Selsun) shampoo.
Oral candidiasis ("thrush")	Fungal infection found in mouth of infants	White, irregular plaques found in mouth	Administer oral medication (e.g., nystatin [Mycostatin]).
Constipation	Difficulty in passing stool; excessive firmness of stool; decreased frequency of defecation	Straining on defecation, lack of stool passage Sometimes anal or perianal abscess	Give warm sitz bath. Apply petroleum jelly to anus. Give additional water to drink.
Iron deficiency anemia	Anemia associated with inadequate supply of iron for synthesis of hemoglobin	Hematocrit value less than 30 Pallor, lethargy Anorexia Poor weight gain Splenomegaly	Discontinue whole cow's milk and substitute commercial formula. Increase intake of foods high in iron content. Give ferrous sulphate.
Roseola infantum	Acute benign febrile illness; fever stops as rash appears	High sudden fever lasting 3–4 days with few other symptoms Rash lasts 24–48 hours	Use antipyretic therapy.
Colic	Periods of unexplained irritability, usually in first 3 months; apparently associated with abdominal pain	Intense crying, legs drawn up to abdomen, hands clenched, passes flatus	Reassure parents. Consider formula change. If breastfeeding, review mother's intake. Review feeding and feeding technique. Apply warmth to abdomen. Put to sleep in prone position. Hold with rhythmic movement. Feed warm water during attack. Try Mylicon drops.
Umbilical cord granuloma	Small pink lesion that forms at the base, believed to be result of mild infection	Pink granulation tissue on umbilicus, seropurulent discharge	Keep area clean and dry. Parents may clean with alcohol.

Sources: Boynton, R.W., E.S. Dunn, and G.R. Stephens, Manual of Ambulatory Pediatrics *(3rd Ed.). Philadelphia: J. B. Lippincott, 1994; Sherwen, L., M. Scoloveno, and C. Weingarten,* Maternity Nursing: Care of the Childbearing Family *(3rd Ed.). Norwalk, CT: Appleton & Lange, 1999; Wong, D.,* Wong's Nursing Care of Infants and Children *(7th Ed.). St. Louis: Mosby, 2003.*

and more injuries. In households in which the mother smokes, the infant's urine cotinine levels are higher, especially in breastfed babies during nonsummer months; however, infants in a family in which any member smokes will suffer the effects of passive smoking from absorption of environmental tobacco smoke.[325,326]

Breastfeeding for at least six months helps to prevent diseases such as otitis media, lower respiratory tract illness, allergies, diarrhea, and meningitis. Additionally, normal cognitive development is promoted through breastfeeding.[327]

PSYCHOSOCIAL CONCEPTS

The following information will facilitate assessment and intervention with the infant and parents.

The *intellectual, emotional, social, and moral components can be combined into what is often referred to as* **psychosocial development.** The separation of these facets of growth is artificial for they are closely interrelated. Similarly, psychosocial, physical, and motor developments greatly influence each other. Babies are born cognitively flexible rather than with preset instinctual behaviour. A level of physiologic maturation of the nervous system must be present before environmental stimulation and learning opportunities can be effective in promoting emotional and cognitive development. In turn, without love and tactile, kinesthetic, verbal, and other environmental stimuli, some nervous system structures do not develop. Babies adapt and react to the environment with which they are confronted. Low-birth-weight and premature infants have neurological deficits that predispose to an increased risk for developmental delays, and they are apt to have behavioural styles that are more difficult to handle, which reduces maternal involvement and the stimulation needed for development.[328,329]

Cognitive Development

Intelligence is the *ability to learn or understand from experience, to acquire and retain knowledge, to respond to a new situation, and to solve problems.* It is a system of living and acting developed in a sequential pattern through relating to the environment. Each stage of operations serves as a foundation for the next.[330] **Cognitive behaviour** includes *thinking, perceiving, remembering, forming concepts, making judgments, generalizing, and abstracting.* Cognitive development is learning and depends on innate capacity, maturation, nutrition, gross and fine motor stimulation, touch, appropriate stimulation of all senses through various activities, language, and social interaction.[331]

Sequence in Intellectual Development

The sequence described by Piaget corresponds rather roughly in time span to those described for emotional development. The infant is in the *sensorimotor period of cognitive development.*[332–334]

The infant arrives in the world with great potential for intellectual development, but at birth intellectual capacities are completely undifferentiated.

Stage 1: The Reflex Stage. This stage covers the neonatal period when behaviour is entirely reflexive. Yet all stimuli are being assimilated into beginning mental images through reflexive behaviour and from human contact.

Stage 2: Primary Circular Reactions. Primary circular reactions are response patterns, where a stimulus creates a response and gratifying behaviour is repeated. At one to four months, life is still a series of random events, but hand–mouth and ear–eye condition is developing. The infant's eyes follow moving objects; eyes and ears follow sounds and novel stimuli. Responses to different objects vary. Baby does not look for objects removed from sight. He or she spends much time looking at objects in the environment and begins to separate self from them. Beginning intention of behaviour is seen; he or she reproduces behaviour previously done. For example, the eight-week-old infant can purposefully apply pressure to a pillow to make a mobile rotate, smile at familiar faces, and anticipate a routine such as diapering.

Stage 3: Secondary Circular Reactions. Stage 3 covers four to eight months. Baby learns to initiate and recognize new experiences and repeat pleasurable ones. Intentional behaviour is seen. Increasing mobility and hand control help him or her become more oriented to the environment. Reaching, grasping, listening, and laughing become better coordinated. Memory traces are apparently being established: baby anticipates familiar events or a moving object's position. The child repeats or prolongs interesting events. Activities that accidentally brought a new experience are repeated. Behaviour becomes increasingly intentional. Habits developed in previous stages are incorporated with new actions. Baby will imitate another's behaviour if it is familiar and not too complex.

Stage 4: Coordination of Secondary Schemata. In this stage, from eight to 12 months, baby's behaviour is showing clear acts of intelligence and experimentation. Baby uses certain activities to attain basic goals. He or she realizes for the first time that someone other than self can cause activity, and activity of self is separate from movement of objects. He or she searches for and retrieves a toy that has disappeared from view. Shapes and sizes of familiar objects are recognized, regardless of the perspective from which they are viewed. Because of the baby's ability to differentiate objects and people from self and the increased sense of separateness, he or she experiences separation (eighth month) anxiety when the mothering figure leaves. Baby is more mobile; sitting, creeping, standing, or walking gives a new perception of the environment. Baby understands words that are said. Thus coordination of schema involves using one idea or mental image to attain a goal and a second idea or image to deal with the end result. Baby systematically imitates another while observing another's behaviour.[335–338]

Reaffirm with parents that they can greatly influence the child's later intellectual abilities by the stimulation they provide for baby, the loving attention they give, and the freedom they allow for baby to explore and use his or her body in the environment.[339] Many educational toys are on the market, but common household items can be made into educational toys. For example, a mobile of ribbons and colourful cut-outs will attract as much attention as an expensive mobile from the store. Unbreakable salt and pepper shakers or small cardboard boxes partly filled with rice, sand, or pebbles and then taped securely

Examples of Educational Toys for the Infant

1–3 Months—Mobiles, unbreakable mirrors, and large colourful rings attached over crib; rattles of various sizes and geometric shapes; stuffed animals with black and white patterns; music boxes or tapes of music—need to change the tune and words from time to time.

4–6 Months—Plastic or paper streamers attached over crib, so child sees but cannot chew or choke on them; squeaky toys; colourful stuffed animals that are not too large; small beach ball or soft plastic ball; chunky bracelets; books made of cloth or vinyl; small barriers that encourage playing peek-a-boo.

7–9 Months—Larger stuffed animals, without buttons or small parts that can be detached and cause choking; nesting cylinders of various size, unbreakable cartons; pop-up toys; cloth blocks; large dolls and puppets; bath toys; mirror available so child can see self during adult play of "so big" and pat-a-cake.

10–12 Months—Push-pull toys; household objects like empty egg cartons or large spoons; stacked rings on a spindle; balls—soft, of various sizes and colours.

Note: Toys or items like a music box or audiotape that were enjoyed in the prior months continue to be enjoyed throughout infancy, especially if they are not continuously available.

shut make good rattles. Various sizes of pots, pans, lids, and unbreakable plastic wastebaskets or smooth blocks are effective play objects.[340] Use the box entitled "Examples of Educational Toys for the Infant" as a guide for teaching parents.

Piaget's views have been challenged by some researchers, who suggest that very young babies have more understanding of object permanence than Piaget has indicated.[341]

CRITICAL THINKING

How do you differentiate between a good learning toy and a poor learning toy?

Communication, Speech, and Language Development

Communication between people involves facial expressions, body movements, other nonverbal behaviour, vocalizations, speech, and use of language. A newborn is ready to communicate if parents and caretakers know how to read the messages. The first communications are through eye contact, crying, and body movements.

Several lay references give an understandable explanation about processes involved in and influences on language development.[342–344] Refer parents to the variety of readable literature available to help them realize the importance of their verbal and nonverbal interaction with the infant from birth on.

Speech awareness *begins before birth. In utero the fetus hears a melody of language,* equivalent to overhearing two people talk through the walls of a motel room. *This creates a*

CASE SITUATION
Infant Development

Michael, eight months old, is sitting on the lap of his babysitter, Aunt Jennifer, who is reading a story to him. As she reads to Michael, Aunt Jennifer smiles and chuckles. Michael responds by mimicking her mouth movements. She says, "Ooooohh" with a widened O-shaped mouth, and Michael imitates the O-shape of her mouth while she speaks. Michael makes a long, loud "Ooooohh" sound. Aunt Jennifer responds with smiles and exclamations of enthusiasm, recognizing his achievement. Michael smiles and continues to repeat "Ooooohh."

Michael then attempts to imitate Aunt Jennifer's actions in reading the book. He reaches toward the book and makes babbling sounds as he swats at the book. Michael's coordination of vision, hearing, and tactile senses as he repeatedly imitates his aunt's facial expressions, reaches for the book, and engages in prespeech babbling demonstrates a common behaviour of children in this age group. These behaviours demonstrate Piaget's Stage 3, secondary circular reactions of the sensorimotor stage of cognitive development.

QUESTIONS

1. Suppose that you have been asked to observe this episode with Michael and Aunt Jennifer. Using your knowledge of Piaget's Stage 3, secondary circular reactions, what information about Michael's intellectual development would you be able to relate to his mother?

2. In what ways would you reinforce Aunt Jennifer's behaviour regarding Michael's intellectual development, especially regarding secondary circular reactions? Can you think of any suggestions or insights you might provide to Aunt Jennifer on Michael's behalf?

3. What new sensorimotor behaviours would you expect Michael to exhibit in the next two or three weeks? In the next two or three months?

4. What challenges or criticisms of Piaget's sensorimotor stages theory have you found?

sensitivity that after birth provides the child with clues about sounds that accompany each other. If babies have been read to in utero, after birth they appear to prefer the sound of the stories they had heard in utero.[345,346]

Speech is the *ability to utter sounds;* **language** refers to *the mother tongue of a group of people,* or the *combination of sounds into a meaningful whole to communicate thoughts and feelings.* Speech development begins with the cry at birth, and the cry remains the basic form of communication for the infant. The newborn cries an average of one to four hours a day. *Baby's cry is undifferentiated for the first month;* the *adult listener cannot distinguish between cries of hunger, pain, fear, and general unhappiness.* Parents learn to distinguish the meanings of different cries and grunts the baby makes in the first two or three months. Baby responds, with similar sounds at first, to both soothing and distressing stimuli. Then *other prespeech sounds heard are as follows:*

- **Cooing,** *the soft murmur or hum of contentment,* beginning at two to three months
- **Babbling,** *incoherent sounds made by playing with sounds,* beginning at two to three months; the number of sounds produced by babbling gradually increases, reaches a peak at eight months, and gives way for true speech and language development
- *Squealing* and *grunting*
- **Lalling,** *the movement of the tongue with crying and vocalization,* such as "m-m-m"
- *Sucking sounds*
- Gestures

Smiles, frowns, and other facial expressions often accompany the baby's vocalizations as do gestures of reaching or withdrawing to convey feelings.[347,348]

There is a biological basis for speech; the brain has amazing ability to process and interpret verbal expressions over an infinite range; however, parent–child interaction is essential for the child to learn language and conversation. Further, there is a critical period during which young children need environmental stimuli, or they will not learn to speak even when the sensory stimulation is exchanged for sensory deprivation.[349,350]

At first vocalizations are reflexive: no difference exists between the vocalizations of hearing babies and deaf babies before six months of age. Later, vocalizations are self-reinforcing; that is, the baby finds pleasure in making and hearing his or her own sounds, and responses from others provide further reinforcement. Reinforcement when desired sounds are made and when certain sounds are omitted is necessary for the infant to progress to language development. The child must also hear others speak to reinforce further the use of the sounds and language of the culture. Effective mothers speak to their children frequently, even while they are doing their housework.[351,352]

By nine months baby will have made every sound basic to any human language. The sounds made in infancy are universal, but when he or she learns the native language, the potential to say all universal sounds is lost.[353,354]

At every age the child comprehends the meaning of what others say more readily than he or she can put thoughts and feelings into words. In speech comprehension, the child first associates certain words with visual, tactile, and other sensations aroused by objects in the environment. Between nine and 12 months, baby learns to recognize his or her name and the names of several familiar objects, responds to "no," echoes and imitates sounds, repeats syllables, and may occasionally obey the parent.[355,356]

Baby tries to articulate words from sounds heard. Words are invented such as "didi" to mean a toy or food. Language is **autistic;** *he or she associates meanings with sounds made by the self, but the sounds are not meaningful to others,* often even to the parents. By trial and error, by imitation and as a result of reinforcement from others, the baby makes the first recognizable words, such as "mama," "dada," "no," and "bye-bye" between 10 and 18 months. (If the correct sound is directed

to the appropriate parent, the sound is reinforced, and the baby continues speech.) Words such as "mama" and "nana" are universal to babies in every culture because they result from the sounds the infant normally makes in babbling. By age one, the baby has a vocabulary of approximately six words. Nouns typically are learned first. He or she learns to associate meaning with an object, such as its name, size, shape, use, and sound; then a word becomes a symbol or label for the object. Learning to speak involves pronouncing words, building a vocabulary, distinguishing between sounds such as "p*e*t" and "p*a*t" or "*h*ear" and "*n*ear" and then making a sentence. The baby's first sentence usually consists of one word and a gesture.[357,358]

Teach parents that many factors influence speech and language development: innate intelligence, ability to hear, modification of the anatomic structures of the mouth and throat, sense of curiosity, parental verbal stimulation and interest, and encouragement to imitate others.[359]

Emotional Development

Eight psychological stages in the human life cycle are described by Erikson.[360,361] He elaborates on the core problems or crisis with which each person struggles at each of these levels of development. In addition to these problems, the child has other tasks to accomplish that relate to the psychosocial crisis, such as learning to walk. Emotional or personality development is a continuous process.

It is estimated about 50% of the child's personality is determined by genes. However, DNA is *not* destiny. Experience plays a powerful role. The infant must have a caring, nurturing adult to develop normally, including developing trust and other emotional expressions.[362] No person succeeds or fails completely in attainment of the goal to reach at a particular point in personality development.

Developmental Crisis
According to Erikson,[363] the psychosexual crisis for infancy is trust versus mistrust. **Basic trust** involves *confidence, optimism, acceptance of and reliance on self and others, faith that the world can satisfy needs, and a sense of hope or a belief in the attainability of wishes is spite of problems and without overestimation of results.* A sense of trust forms the basis for a sense of hope and for later identity formation, social responsiveness to others, and ability to care about and love others. The person accepts self, develops reachable goals, assumes life will be manageable, and expects people and situations to be positive. A sense of trust may be demonstrated in the newborn and infant by the ease of feeding, the depth of sleep, the relaxation of the bowels, and the overall appearance of contentment. **Mistrust** is a *sense of not feeling satisfied emotionally or physically, an inability to believe in or rely on others or self.* See the box entitled "Consequences of Mistrust."

Security and trust are fostered by the prompt, loving, and consistent response to the infant's distress and needs and by the positive response to happy, contented behaviour. You can teach parents that they do not "spoil" a baby by promptly answering the distress signal—his or her cry. Rather, they are

Consequences of Mistrust

Infant

- Is lethargic
- Fails to gain weight
- Eats poorly
- Sleeps poorly
- Experiences excessive, persistent colic
- Fails to thrive

Child and Adult

- Is pessimistic, hopeless
- Lacks self-confidence
- Is gullible, easily hurt
- Is suspicious, unsure of self or others
- Is dependent on others, clings to others
- Is antagonistic toward others
- Is bitter to others
- Is withdrawn, asocial
- Avoids new relationships or new experiences, *or*
- Bullies others; is aggressive, sarcastic, controlling
- Is pathologically optimistic (takes risks, gambles on everything, sure nothing can go wrong)
- Is unable to delay gratification

teaching trust by relieving tension. Parents should understand the meaning they convey through such care as changing diapers. Even if the techniques are not the best, baby will sense the positive attitude if it exists. If the parents repeatedly fail to meet primary needs, fear, anger, insecurity, and eventual mistrust result. If the most important people fail him or her, there is little foundation on which to build faith in others or self and little desire to be socialized into the culture. The world cannot be trusted. If the baby is abused, neglected, or deprived, he or she may suffer irreversible effects, as discussed in Chapter 6.

The infant who is in a nurturing, loving environment and who has developed trust is a happy baby most of the time. He or she is sociable and responsive to others. Attachment to the parent has been formed so that separation or stranger anxiety is experienced at approximately seven to nine months of age and may extend to ten to 12 months. After a time the infant will again respond to strangers. Sociable babies have sociable mothers, and sociable, friendly babies score higher on cognitive tests than less sociable or mistrusting infants.[364–367]

The working mother may discuss her situation with you. Emotional development of the infant is not compromised by the working mother if she has time and energy to maintain consistent, loving, and stimulating responses when she is with baby. Quality of care rather than quantity of time is the essence of parenting and promoting emotional development. When work is not stressful and is a source of personal satisfaction for the mother, she is a more contented mother and gives the baby better care. The father's nurturance is also important, and often he is more involved in caring for the child when the

mother works, which contributes to quality care. The lowest scores of adequate mothering are found in unsatisfied homemakers. Further, the effective mother does not devote the bulk of her day in the home to childrearing. Instead she designs a loving environment that is adequately stimulating, and helpful to the child in gaining competency.[368,369]

Because so many mothers work outside the home today, an important subject to discuss is child-care arrangements or baby-sitting services. Even if the parent does not work, some time away from the baby is rejuvenating and enhances the quality of parenting. Each parent has different ideas about how often, if at all, to leave the baby with a sitter. Discuss characteristics to consider in a sitter. Point out that parents will probably be most satisfied with a sitter whose childrearing philosophy and guidance techniques coincide with theirs; and who has had some child-care training or experience.

The *sitter,* or nanny, should be physically and emotionally healthy, be acquainted with the baby and the home, and like the baby. If possible, parents should keep the baby with the same person consistently, especially around seven or eight months, when baby recognizes mother and familiar people and is experiencing separation anxiety. The sitter or nanny should have exact instructions about where the parents can be reached; special aspects of care; telephone numbers of doctor, police, and fire department; name and telephone number of another family member; and telephone number of a poison control centre. As more mothers return to the workforce shortly after childbirth, there has been an increasing trend toward infant daycare centres. Factors to consider in choosing daycare services are discussed in Chapter 9.

CRITICAL THINKING

What do you think are the factors needed for building trust in an infant within a family unit?

Development of Self-Concept and Body Image

Body image, the *mental picture of one's body,* includes the external, internal, and postural picture of the body, although the mental image is not necessarily consistent with the actual body structure. Included also are attitudes, emotions, and personality reactions of the individual in relation to his or her body as an object in space, with a distinct boundary and apart from all others and the environment. The body image, gradually formulated over a period of years, is included in the **self-concept** (*awareness of self or me*) and *derives from reactions of others to his or her body, perceptions of how others react, experiences with his or her own and other bodies, constitutional factors, and physiologic and sensory stimuli.*[370]

At birth the infant has diffuse feelings of hunger, pain, rage, and comfort but no body image. For the first month, the main goal is fulfillment of needs for survival and comfort. Pleasurable sensations come mainly from the lower face, the mouth and nose area, which has considerable enervation. At first all the baby knows is self. Baby has the same attitude toward his or her body as toward other objects in the environment; the external world is an extension of self. Gradually, baby distinguishes his or her body from other animate and inanimate objects in the environment as he or she bites a hand, bangs the head, grasps and mouths a toy, and experiences visceral, visual, auditory, kinesthetic, and motor sensations.[371,372]

A primitive ego or self-development begins at approximately three months. Weaning, contact from others, and more exploration of the environment also heighten self-awareness. As the child approaches the first birthday, there is some coordination of these sensory experiences that are being internalized into the motor body image. There is increased locomotor function and ability to explore the environment, and a sense of separateness of self. He or she is aware that some body parts give greater pleasure than other parts and that there are differences in sensation when his or her body or another object is touched.[373]

Without adequate somatosensory stimulation, body image and ego development are impaired as shown by studies of premature incubator infants who lacked rocking, stroking, and cuddling.[374] The infant's initial experiences with his or her body, determined largely by maternal care and attitudes, are the basis for a developing body image and how he or she later likes and handles the body and reacts to others.

Adaptive Mechanisms

Adaptive mechanisms are *learned behavioural responses that aid adjustment and emotional development.* At first the baby cries spontaneously. Soon baby learns that crying brings attention. Consequently he or she cries when uncomfortable, hungry, or bored. Other tools besides crying used in adaptation are experimentation, exploration, and manipulation. Baby uses the body in various ways to gain stimulation. He or she grabs and plays with whatever is within reach, whether it is father's nose or a toy. By the end of infancy, emotions of anger, fear, delight, and affection are expressed through vocalization, facial expression, and gestures.

The young infant does not understand waiting. But a baby meets with security and feels a sense of tenderness from caretakers; he or she begins to wait a short time between feeling hunger pains and demanding food. Instead of immediately screaming when a toy cannot be reached, baby will persist in repeating the action that will get him or her to the object. The baby is beginning to respond to the expectations of others and adapt to the family's cultural patterns.

If, however, care does not foster trust, the infant constantly feels threatened. At first he or she cries and shows increased motor activity, perhaps expressing rage, but may eventually feel powerless and become apathetic.

Adaptive mechanisms in infancy are called **primary processes.** Some of these rudimentary methods of handling anxiety are symbolization, condensation, incorporation, and displacement. **Symbolization** *occurs when an object or idea comes to stand for something else because of associated characteristics.* For example, taking milk from mother's breast satisfies hunger. Soon the act also means pleasurable body contact, emotional response, and security. **Condensation** is the *reverse process. Several objects are fused into a single symbol.* The word *toy,* for example, comes to represent a variety of objects. **Incorporation** occurs when the *representation of mother or other objects is taken into the self and becomes a part of the*

understanding and is the basis for the child's separation anxiety or attachment to parents. **Displacement** occurs when *emotions are transferred from an original object to another,* such as from the mother to other family members or the babysitter.[375,376]

Adaptive behaviour is developed through structuring of the baby's potential. He or she needs both freedom to explore and exercise and consistent, pleasant restraints for personal safety, which together enable learning of self-restraint. Constantly saying "No" or confining the child to a walker or playpen does not help the learning of adaptive behaviour.

The infant may be temporarily deflected off course by premature birth, prolonged hospitalization, and illness around the time of birth, but once he or she is exposed to an even minimally appropriate environment, natural self-righting mechanisms have the potential to bring him or her back into the maturational trajectory characteristic of the species. Further, the infant is changing and growing within the context of a transactional, organic milieu. Negative past events become less important as the child, the parents, and the environment influence one another. The child elicits and reinforces parental responses, and parental behaviours and characteristics support developmental gains. The quality of the home environment and the passage of time significantly affect the outcome.[377,378]

Research indicates that education of the mother about infant behaviours, emotional states, and communication cues facilitates mother–infant interaction, which has a positive effect on attachment, nurturing, and the child's development and adaptation.[379]

Recent media publicity that peers have more effect than parents on their children is questionable.[380,381] While peers are important at a later age, the nurturing that occurs in infancy and the first years of life is critical, as described by Begley,[382,383] Cole,[384] and other writers.[385–393] You can foster the nurturing that will get the next generation off to a good start.

Sexuality Development

Sexuality may be defined as a *deep, pervasive aspect of the total person and the sum total of one's feelings and behaviour as a male or female, the expression of which goes beyond genital response.* Sexuality includes the attitudes that are necessary to maintain a stable and intimate relationship with another person. Sexuality culminates in adulthood, but it begins to develop in infancy.[394]

Gender or sex assignment occurs at birth. The parents' first question is usually "Is it a boy or a girl?" The answer to this question often stimulates a set of adjectives to describe the newborn: soft, fine-featured, little, passive, weak girl; robust, big, strong, active boy, regardless of size or weight. The name given to baby also reflects the parents' attitudes toward the baby's sex and may reflect their ideas about the child's eventual role in life. Mothers, however, engage in less sex-typing stereotypes than fathers.[395]

Occasionally external genitalia are ambiguous in appearance, neither distinctly male nor distinctly female. When this occurs, parents should be given as much support and information as possible to cope with the crisis; sex assignment based on chromosomal studies or appearance should be made as soon as possible.[396]

The stereotypes about sex do have some basis in fact, because at birth males usually are larger and have more muscle mass, are more active, and are more irritable than girls. Females are more sensitive to auditory, tactile, and painful stimuli. At three weeks of age males are still more irritable and are sleeping less than females.[397]

Initially, mothers seem to respond more to male infants than to female infants (perhaps because male infants have traditionally been more highly valued). But by three months this trend reverses, and mothers are thought to have more touch and conversational contact with female infants, even when they are irritable. This reverse may occur because mothers are generally more successful in calming irritable daughters than irritable sons.[398]

By five months baby responds differently to male and female voices, and by six months he or she distinguishes mother from father and as distinct people. At six months the female infant has a longer attention span for visual stimuli and better fixation on a human face, is more responsive to social stimuli, and prefers complex stimuli. The male infant has a better fixation response to a helix of light and is more attentive to an intermittent tone.[399]

Also, when the babies are six months old, mothers imitate the verbal sounds of their daughters more than their sons, and mothers continue to touch, talk to, and handle their daughters more than their sons. Throughout infancy and childhood, female children talk to and touch their mothers more, whereas boys are encouraged to be more independent, exploratory, and vigorous in gross motor activity.[400]

Fathers tend to treat the baby girl more softly and the baby boy more roughly during the last six months of infancy. At nine months, a baby girl behaves differently with her mother than with her father. She will be rougher and more attention seeking with her father.[401]

By nine to 12 months, baby responds to his or her name, an important link to sex and role. Research indicates that girl babies are more dependent and less exploratory by one year than boys because of different parental expectations. Parents appear to reinforce sex-coded behaviour in infancy so that sex role behaviour is learned on the basis of parental cues.[402]

Infants receive stimulation of their erogenous zones during maternal care. The mouth and lower face are the main erogenous zones initially, providing pleasure, warmth, and satisfaction through sucking. Both sexes explore their genitalia during infancy. Erection in the male and lubrication in the female occur.

Explore sexuality development with parents. Help them be aware of the importance for sexuality development of their tone of voice, touch, behaviour, and feelings toward the boy or girl. Help them develop ways to relate optimally to and promote trust and well-being in the child.

Developmental Tasks

Infancy is far from what some have assumed—a time for rigidly and mechanically handling the baby because he or she seems to have so little capability as an adapting human being. The following developmental tasks are to be accomplished in infancy:[403]

- Achieve equilibrium of physiologic organ systems after birth

- Establish self as a dependent person but separate from others
- Become aware of the alive versus inanimate and familiar versus unfamiliar and develop rudimentary social interaction
- Develop a feeling of and desire for affection and response from others
- Adjust somewhat to the expectations of others
- Begin to manage the changing body and learn new motor skills, develop equilibrium, begin eye–hand coordination, and establish rest–activity rhythm
- Begin to understand and master the immediate environment through exploration
- Develop a beginning symbol or language system, conceptual abilities, and preverbal communication
- Direct emotional expression to indicate needs and wishes

Explore these tasks with parents. Help them realize specific ways in which they can enable their baby to achieve these tasks.

HEALTH CARE AND NURSING APPLICATIONS

Your role with the infant and family has been discussed with each section throughout this chapter. You can also be instrumental in establishing or working with community agencies that assist parents and infants. You may be called on to work with families who have adopted a child or with the single parent or with the stepfamily who then has their own child (see also Chapter 4). You may work with a family whose child is not healthy or is born prematurely (see also Chapter 4), or you may work with a family who experiences the sudden death of the infant. For more information, see the box entitled "Selected Nursing Diagnoses Related to the Infant."

Establishment and Use of Community Resources for Continuity of Care

Some sources of help that may be found in your community are summarized in the box entitled "Community Resources for Parents."

In one large city two maternity nurses identified a need for a local organization that would offer courses in parenting. In addition to course offerings, the organization now hosts discussion groups for expectant and new mothers and for parents of toddlers. Recently a "postpartum hotline" was started. The despair of couples who experience postpartum problems is pointed out repeatedly. For example, "This is Julie… We had our baby on the fourteenth. But (*tears*) you must have to be a pediatrician to be a mother. The baby is crying all the time; I don't know if I can continue to nurse her.… Everything is horrible!" (A home visit and a series of follow-up phone calls played a part in this mother's nursing her baby happily for eight months.)

Instead of using referral to a community agency, a hospital may provide its own postpartum home care services, especially for mothers and babies who are discharged from the hospital 12 to 24 hours after delivery. Early discharge can have the

Pattern I: Exchanging

Altered Nutrition: More than Body Requirements
Altered Nutrition: Less than Body Requirements
Constipation
Diarrhea
Ineffective Breathing Pattern
Risk for Injury
Risk for Suffocation
Risk for Poisoning
Risk for Trauma
Risk for Aspiration
Altered Protection
Risk for Impaired Skin Integrity

Pattern 6: Moving

Impaired Physical Mobility
Sleep Pattern Disturbance
Ineffective Breastfeeding
Ineffective Infant Feeding Pattern
Altered Growth and Development
Disorganized Infant Behaviour

Pattern 7: Perceiving

Sensory/Perceptual Alterations
Unilateral Neglect

Pattern 9: Feeling

Pain
Anxiety

Other of the NANDA diagnoses are applicable to the ill infant.

Source: North American Nursing Diagnosis Association, *NANDA Nursing Diagnoses Definitions & Classification 1999–2000*. Philadelphia: North American Nursing Diagnosis Association, 1999.

Community Resources for Parents

Classes on Parenting, Prenatal or Postnatal Care, Lamaze or Psychoprophylaxis Method of Childbirth

- Canadian Parents Online (http://www.canadianparents.com)
- Hospitals
- Community health nursing services

Breastfeeding Information

- La Leche League

Parent Support

- Canadian Association of Midwives
- Perinatal bereavement services
- Support groups for children who are challenged
- SIDS Canada Bereavement Support
- Health Canada Shaken Baby Syndrome
- Parents of Multiple Birth

Crisis Attendance or Counselling

- Crisis hotlines
- Clergy or other counsellors

advantages of treating mother and baby as well, not ill, reducing family separation time, and more directly involving the father in care. Every woman or family, however, is not a candidate for early discharge. Prenatal preparation is necessary. Mother and baby must show no potential complications, which often occur in the third or fourth day after delivery. Medical backup care must be quickly available. Further, at times mother may get more rest and emotional support in the hospital than at home, depending on home and family conditions. In fact, visits by a nurse one hour daily for two or three days may *not* provide sufficient care.

Whenever visits are made in the home, assessment tools that can be used, if administered by a qualified person, are the *Denver II—Revision and Restandardization of the Denver Developmental Screening Test (DDST)* (see Figure 9–2), a general scale that measures personal and social skills, language, and gross and fine motor abilities,[404] and the *Home Observation for Measurement of the Environment (HOME),* in which the home-rearing situation is assessed.

Although nurses work with many ill infants in hospitals, they have many opportunities to care for well infants in the communities. Even when caring for hospitalized infants, nurses should emphasize attainment of developmental tasks regardless of the illness.[405] Examples of wellness diagnosis include:

- Progressive development of motor skills
- Beginning sense of trust
- Beginning recognition of object permanence
- Progressive interaction with family members.[406]

In addition, examples of wellness diagnoses related to the caregiver include providing a safe environment, providing adequate nutrition, and creating learning opportunities for the child.[407]

Care of the Premature Baby and the Baby with Congenital Anomalies

The principal threats to infant health are low birth weight and its major antecedent, preterm delivery, and birth defects. The infant mortality rate in Canada has declined dramatically in the last 35 years.[408] In 1996, it dropped below the level of six infant deaths per 1000 live births for the first time. Although the U.S. has relatively high infant mortality rates in international comparisons, infant mortality rates have been declining in the U.S. and many other countries. This decline results primarily from advances in neonatal care systems. More than three-quarters of infant deaths are caused by babies being born too small or too early.[409,410] While the mortality rate of preterm infants has dramatically improved as a result of education of care providers, regionalization of care providers and care, and improved technology, paradoxically, there has not been a corresponding improvement in neonatal morbidity in the U.S.

Babies born of adolescent mothers, particularly young adolescent mothers, are at higher risk of low birth weight and infant mortality than babies born of older mothers. Also, poverty is strongly and consistently associated with low birth weight, but the precise social and environmental conditions that produce preterm delivery are not understood.[411–413]

There are several individual factors, such as cigarette smoking, the use of drugs, and diet, that influence fetal growth. Cessation of smoking during pregnancy is the single largest modifiable factor affecting low birth weight and infant mortality. Other behaviours such as diet and the abuse of alcohol and other drugs, while important in reducing the rates of low birth weight and preterm birth, do not have nearly the impact that cigarette smoking has. Thus, a woman can adopt healthful lifestyle changes that will increase her chances of having a healthy, normal-weight child. Refer also to Chapter 6 for more information on the negative effects of cigarette smoking, alcohol and drug use and abuse, and inadequate diet on prenatal and infant development.

While low-birth-weight infants are at a higher risk of death or long-term illness and disability than are infants born at normal weight, the majority of low-birth-weight infants have normal outcomes. The sequelae associated with prematurity include higher rates of subnormal growth, illnesses, and neurodevelopment problems. Further, problems with cognition, attention, and neuromotor problems may occur and may still be apparent in adolescence.[414,415]

Birth defects are a leading cause of infant death in Canada and the United States. The most common defects are heart problems, central nervous system disorders, and defects of the respiratory system. Another leading cause of death is a combination of low birth weight, prematurity, and respiratory distress syndrome. These children also receive neonatal intensive care unit (NICU) treatment.[416–418]

In 2000, Health Canada brought together participants from every province and territory to discuss **congenital anomalies** (*defects in physical structure or function*).[419] Of the 350 000 children born in Canada each year 2% to 3% will be born with a serious congenital anomaly.[420,421] Infant mortality due to congenital anomalies has decreased significantly in Canada. In spite of the frequency of occurrences of congenital anomalies, the underlying causes for most remain obscure.

The prevalence of maternal substance abuse has escalated over the last quarter century. Infants exposed to drugs may exhibit many physical and psychological effects, including those discussed in Chapter 6, related to effects of medications, effects of addictive drugs, the narcotic abstinence (withdrawal) syndrome in the neonate, effects of alcohol use and abuse, and FASD (a set of birth defects associated with the maternal consumption of alcohol during pregnancy).

A generation of babies has already been affected and will present major problems to our society because of their developmental disabilities, uncontrollable behaviour and rage, learning deficits, and lack of superego and remorse. There are

not enough treatment centres and foster homes. Mothers or grandmothers are likely to bear the brunt of this crisis. For many parents and their families, birth of a baby will not bring joy but fear, grief, and depression—for a long time.[422]

There are times, however, when the baby is preterm or premature or has a lasting problem for no known reason. Further, there are families who reach out to these babies with love and caring; as a result, the baby develops to the maximum potential. Supportive nursing care is a key factor for these families.[423]

Cultures vary in the care of the premature. Premature babies in some countries are placed with their mothers two to three hours after birth and are sent home soon after birth because of economic status of the parents, problems with cross-infections, and deep respect for natural processes. In some countries the premature child has no chance of survival.

Parents of the baby with congenital anomalies will need the same considerations as parents of the premature infant. They should be encouraged to see their infant as soon as possible to avoid fantasies that are often worse than the anomaly. The manner in which the nurse presents the infant to the parents may well set the tone for the early parent–child relationship.

Show them the normal parts and emphasize the baby's positive features. Above all, show your acceptance of the infant: hold, cuddle, and look at the infant as you talk to him or her. Give information about the anomaly and the possible prognosis. This is a difficult time for parents, and they will need ample time to express their grief, guilt, and worries. Your patience and support will be most helpful. Various references provide more in-depth information to share with parents pertinent to the specific disability.[424,425] Refer to Chapter 4 for additional information on nursing practice with the family.

Numerous *ethical issues* arise in the context of care of the infant born with a congenital anomaly and the preterm or low-birth-weight infant. This is especially true if the infant has a severe congenital anomaly, is born extremely early, or weighs very little. The values of individuals (health care professionals and parents) involved in caring for infants influence their clinical decision making. In this group of infants, these values include preserving life, decreasing morbidity, and relieving pain and suffering.[426,427]

Parents and members of the health care and judicial systems continue to debate hotly the anticipated length and quality of many infants' lives. Some infants who are saved will continue as a financial and care burden on their parents for the rest of the parents' lives.

The ethical, personal, and economic dilemmas posted by the use of life-sustaining technologies are considerable and have caused policymakers to consider withholding treatment from selected infants. Using high-technology treatment methods may be experimentation and research shrouded in the guise of treatment. The pivotal case of Baby Doe has come to exemplify just such an event. The case is discussed at length by Wakefield-Fisher.[428]

The advanced technology to maintain life has posed a major ethical dilemma for parents and professionals: Should life be continued with machines, or when and how should the critically ill infant or child be allowed to die? Schloman and Fister describe the perspectives of parents in their study.[429]

Nurses increasingly must have understanding of both the questions and legal and ethical responses related to withholding life-sustaining treatment from infants. Nurses must participate in the decision making, based on adequate knowledge of the issue.

Care of the Family Experiencing Adoption and Infant Death

Mothers Who Give Their Newborns for Adoption

These mothers are confronted with a crisis that involves bereavement. Ambivalence prevails during the prenatal period: love for baby, guilt about abandonment, and concern for his or her future. Therapeutic intervention begins prenatally by exploring with the mother the anticipatory grief, anger, depression, decisions about seeing the baby, and choice of post delivery care. To promote bonding would be cruel, but the mother should have the opportunity—the reality—of holding and inspecting. Not to recognize the infant is to deny the pregnancy; seeing the infant gives concrete focus to the mother's grief. A maternity nurse-specialist should consult the relinquishing mother on a scheduled basis to promote the woman's personal growth, self-respect, and dignity. Refer also to Chapter 4 for more information on the adoptive process and family.

Parents Whose Infant Dies

If the newborn dies, there are no magic words. Certain actions are helpful: (1) give parents mementos, such as a footprint sheet, identification band, or photograph; (2) be patient and compassionate; and (3) help the family say goodbye. Parents must work through the affection-symbiotic bond developed in anticipation of the baby as perfect. Full expression of the grief, guilt, and anger is necessary.

Parents should, if they desire, be permitted to view, touch, and hold their dead infant. Within the beliefs of the parents, some traditional bereavement service should be arranged to promote grieving and making the death real. The spirituality of the parents influences their emotional, mental, and physical responses to bereavement.[430] Meeting with the parents after the death of the infant or attending the funeral can assist them through mourning. Contact or meet with the parents within the next two to three weeks and in three to six months. During these visits you can effectively listen, encourage expression of feelings, and assist the parents in working through their feelings and reactions.[431,432]

The thrust for the nurse is in helping the parents or caretakers deal with their guilt, grief, and future psychological balance. The health care professional must recognize that the normal grieving process is fluid in nature with much fluctuation between phases.[433] You should be able to direct these people to national or local help. In some health departments there are nurses who are designated to make visits for as long as needed. Self-help groups have been formed to assist parents with mourning and feelings of guilt, failure, and isolation after their infant's death.

No matter what birth takes place—normal or abnormal—the family is going through a type of *rebirth* in that their lives are forever changed by the event. Your guidance in this process may be felt for years.

CRITICAL THINKING

If the parents approached you wondering whether or not to take their dying child home from the hospital, how would you counsel them?

INTERESTING WEBSITES

CANADIAN CHILD CARE FOUNDATION

http://www.cccf-fcsge.ca/affiliates_en.html

The CCCF was founded in 1987 as a national nonprofit organization whose mission is to improve the quality of child care services for Canadian children and families. Among its associations are Child and Family Canada, Children's Health, Early Learning Canada, and Working Family Tips. All are linked to the CCCF site.

CANADIAN INCIDENCE STUDY OF CHILD ABUSE

http://www.cecw-cepb.ca/Pubs/PubsCIS.shtml

This is the first nationwide study to examine the incidence of child maltreatment in Canada.

FIRST NATIONS AND INUIT HEALTH BRANCH

http://www.hc-sc.gc.ca/fnihb-dgspni/fnihb/

Detailed information is available at this site about FNIHB, its organization, mandate and priorities, and the branch organization.

FAMILY-CENTRED MATERNITY AND NEWBORN CARE: NATIONAL GUIDELINES

http://www.hc-sc.gc.ca/english/media/ releases/2000/2000_48ebk.htm

Head here for a complete copy of the guidelines, which were facilitated in 2000 by Health Canada, the Canadian Institute of Child Health, and 70 Canadian professionals and consumers.

SHAKEN BABY SYNDROME

http://www.cps.ca/english/statements/IP/cps01-01.htm

This site provides a *Joint Statement on Shaken Baby Syndrome*. The 11-page document contains the statement of purpose, what can be done, recommendations, and an extensive bibliography.

SUMMARY

1. Childbirth is a crisis to the parents. Life is changed with birth of a baby.
2. Development of infant–parent attachment is essential for the child's total development.

3. Infant and parent behaviours are reciprocal.

4. Maltreatment of the infant by parents or others must be reported. Intervention is essential.

5. The neonatal period, the first 30 days of life, and infancy, the first year of life, constitute an era that is a critical period for the child.

6. Physiological adaptations are necessary to survive after birth.

7. The first year is a period of rapid physical growth and cognitive development.

8. Adequate nutrition, play, safety, health promotion, and illness prevention and treatment are essential for the infant's growth and development.

9. Culture influences all areas of the child's growth and development.

10. The first year is emotionally critical in order to thrive, to learn to trust, and to achieve developmental tasks. The infant must be consistently loved and cared for as a whole person.

11. The box entitled "Considerations for the Infant and Family in Health Care" summarizes what you should consider in assessment and health promotion with the infant.

Considerations for the Infant and Family in Health Care

- Cultural background and experiences of the family of the infant
- Reaction of the mother and father to the crisis resulting from the baby's birth
- Attachment behaviours and the binding-in process of the mother, attachment of father and other family members
- Parental behaviours that indicate difficulty in establishing attachment or potential/actual abuse of the infant
- Physical characteristics and patterns, such as eating, sleeping, elimination, and activity in the neonate/infant, that indicate health and are within the age norms for growth
- Cognitive characteristics and behavioural patterns in the neonate/infant that indicate age-appropriate norms for intellectual development
- Communication characteristics and behavioural patterns in the neonate/infant that indicate intact neurological and sensory status, speech awareness, and ability to respond with age-appropriate sounds (prespeech)
- Overall appearance and behavioural and play patterns in the neonate/infant that indicate development of trust, rather than mistrust, and continuing age-appropriate emotional development
- Behavioural patterns and characteristics that indicate the infant has achieved developmental tasks
- Parental behaviours that indicate knowledge about how to care physically and emotionally for the neonate/infant
- Parental behaviours that indicate they are promoting positive self-concept and sexuality development in the infant
- Evidence that the parents provide a safe and healthful environment and the necessary resources for the neonate/infant
- Parental behaviours that indicate they are achieving their developmental tasks for this era

ENDNOTES

1. Andrews, M., and J. Boyle, *Transcultural Concepts in Nursing Care* (3rd ed.). Philadelphia: Lippincott, 1999.

2. Hoff, L., *People in Crisis: Understanding and Helping* (4th ed.). Stamford, CT: Appleton-Lange, 1995.

3. Health Canada, *Family Centred Maternity and Newborn Care: National Guidelines,* Website: www.hc-sc.gc.ca/dca-dea/publications/fenc11_e.html, July 2004.

4. Motherisk, Website: www.motherisk.org, July 2004.

5. Canada, Royal Commission on Aboriginal Peoples. *Report. Vol 3.* Ottawa, 1996, p 11.

6. Health Canada, *A Handbook for First Nations & Inuit Communities: Brighter Futures Initiative.* Ottawa: Health Canada, 1994, pp. 76–77.

7. Kioke, S.J., "Revisiting the Past: Discovering Traditional Care and the Cultural Meaning of Pregnancy and Birth in a Cree Community" (master's thesis). Kingston: Queen's University, 1999, p. 92.

8. Health Canada, *A Handbook for First Nations & Inuit Communities.*

9. Hammersmith, B., and L. Sawatsky, *The Beat of a Different Drum: An Aboriginal Cross-Cultural Handbook for Child-Care Workers,* Saanichton, BC: Association of Aboriginal Friendship Centres, 2000.

10. London, M.L., P.W. Ladewig, J.W. Ball, and R.C. Bindler, *Maternal-Newborn & Child Nursing: Family-Centered Care,* Upper Saddle River: Pearson Education, Inc., 2003.

11. Hoff, *op. cit.*

12. Maloni, J., and M. Ponder, Father's Experience of Their Partner's Antepartum Bed Rest, *IMAGE: Journal of Nursing Scholarship,* 29, no. 2 (1997), 183–187.

13. Strass, P., Postpartum Depression Support, *Canadian Nurse,* 98, no 3 (2002), 25–28.

14. Ainsworth, M.D., The Development of Infant-Mother Attachment, in Caldwell, B., and Ricciuti, H., eds., *Child Development Research.* Chicago: University of Chicago Press, 1973, pp. 1–94.

15. Bowlby, J., *Attachment and Loss, Vol. 1.* New York: Basic Books, 1969.

16. Cole, E., Set Your Course for Maximized Fatherhood, *Believer's Voice of Victory,* 26, no. 6 (1998), 12–14.

17. Becker, P., et al., Outcomes of Developmentally Supportive Nursing Care for Very Low Birth Weight Infants, *Nursing Research,* 40, no. 3 (1991), 150–155.

18. Pressler, J., Promoting Attachment, in Craft, M., and J., Denehy, eds., *Nursing Interventions for Infants & Children.* Philadelphia: W.B. Saunders, 1990, pp. 4–17.

19. Chess, S., and A. Thomas, Infant Bonding: Mystique and Reality, *American Journal of Orthopsychiatry,* 52, (1982), 421–425.

20. Rubin, R., The Family–Child Relationship and Nursing Care, *Nursing Outlook,* 8 (1964), 36–39.

21. Ainsworth, *op. cit.*

22. Bowlby, *Attachment and Loss, Vol. 1.*

23. Bowlby, J., Disruption of Affectional Bonds and Its Effect on Behaviour, *Canada's Mental Health Supplement,* no. 59 (January–February, 1969), 2–12.

24. Robson, K., The Role of Eye-to-Eye Contact in Maternal–Infant Attachment, *Journal of Child Psychology and Psychiatry,* 8 (1976), 13–25.

25. Rubin, *op. cit.*

26. Attainment of the Maternal Role—Part I, *Nursing Research,* 16, no. 3 (1967), 237–245.

27. Attainment of the Maternal Role—Part II, *Nursing Research,* 16, no. 4 (1967), 342–346.

28. Cognitive Style in Pregnancy, *American Journal of Nursing,* 70, no. 3 (1970), 502–508.

29. Binding-in in the Postpartum Period, *Maternal-Child Nursing Journal*, 6 (1977), 67–75.

30. Rubin, R. *Maternal Identity and the Maternal Experience.* New York: Springer, 1984.

31. Toney, L., The Effects of Holding the Newborn at Delivery on Paternal Bonding, *Nursing Research*, 32, no. 1 (1983), 16–19.

32. Eyer, D.E. *Mother-Infant Bonding: A Scientific Fiction.* New Haven, CT: Yale University Press, 1992.

33. Goldberg, S., *Parent-Infant Bonding: Another Look.* Child Development, 54 (1983), 1355–1382.

34. Palkovitz, R., Fathers: Birth Attendance, Early Contact and Extended Contact With Their Newborns: A Critical Review, *Child Development*, 56, no. 2 (1985), 392–406.

35. Eyer, *op. cit.*

36. Goldberg, *op. cit.*

37. Palkovitz, R., Laypersons: Beliefs about the "Critical" Nature of Father-Infant Bonding: Implications for Childbirth Educators, *Maternal-Child Nursing Journal*, 15, no. 1 (Spring 1986), 39–46.

38. Palkovitz, R., Sources of Father-Infant Bonding Beliefs: Implication for Childbirth Educators, *Maternal-Child Nursing Journal*, 17, no. 2 (Summer 1988), 101–113.

39. Begley, S., How to Build a Baby's Brain, *Newsweek (Special Issue)*, Spring/Summer (1997), 28–32.

40. Chess, S., and A. Thomas, Infant Bonding: Mystique and Reality, *American Journal of Orthopsychiatry*, 52, (1982), 421–425.

41. Bettelheim, B., and A. Freedgood, *A Good Enough Parent: A Book on Child-rearing.* New York: Random, 1988.

42. Greenberg, S., The Loving Ties that Bond, *Newsweek (Special Issue)*, Spring/Summer (1997), 68–69, 70.

43. Stearns, P.N., Fatherhood in Historical Perspective: The Role of Social Change, in Bosett, F.W., and S.M.H. Hanson, eds., *Fatherhood and Families in Cultural Context.* New York: Springer, 1991, pp. 28–52.

44. Van Boven, S., Giving Infants a Helping Hand, *Newsweek (Special Issue)*, Spring/Summer (1997), 45.

45. Tulman, L., Mothers and Unrelated Persons' Handling of Newborn Infants, *Nursing Research*, 34, no. 4 (1985), 205–210.

46. Harrison, M., J. Magill-Evans, and K. Benzies, Fathers' Scores on the Nursing Child Assessment Teaching Scale: Are they Different than Those of the Mothers? *Journal of Paediatric Nursing*, 14, (1999), 1–8.

47. Hammersmith and Sawatsky, *op. cit.*

48. *Ibid.*

49. Mercer, R.T., and S.L. Ferketich, Predictors of Parental Attachment during Early Parenthood, *Journal of Advanced Nursing*, 15 (1990) 268–280.

50. Letch, D., Mother-Infant Interaction: Achieving Synchrony, *Nursing Research*, 48, no. 1 (1999), 55–57.

51. Byrd, M., Questioning the Quality of Maternal Caregiving during Home Visiting, *IMAGE: Journal of Nursing Scholarship*, 31, no. 1 (1999), 27–32.

52. Brazelton, T., and B. Cramer, *The Earliest Relationship.* Reading, MA: Addison-Wesley, 1990.

53. Klaus, M., and J, Kennell, *Parent-Infant Bonding* (2nd ed.). St. Louis: C.V. Mosby, 1982.

54. Attainment of the Maternal Role—Part I.

55. Cognitive Style in Pregnancy.

56. Ainsworth, *op. cit.*

57. Beck, C., The Effects of Postpartum Depression on Maternal-Infant Interaction: A Meta Analysis, *Nursing Research*, 44 (1995), 296–302.

58. Palkovitz, Fathers: Birth Attendance, Early Contact and Extended Contact With Their Newborns: A Critical Review.

59. Gelfand, D., and D. Teti, How Does Maternal Depression Affect Children? *The Harvard Mental Health Letter*, 12, no. 5 (1995), 8.

60. Toney, *op. cit.*

61. Brown, M., Social Support, Stress, and Health: A Comparison of Expectant Mothers and Fathers, *Nursing Research*, 36, no. 2 (1986), 74–76.

62. Cole, *op. cit.*

63. Ferketich, S., and R. Mercer, Predictors of Role Competence for Experienced and Inexperienced Fathers, *Nursing Research*, 44 (1995), 89–95.

64. LaRossa, R., Fatherhood and Social Change, *Family Relations*, 37 (1988) 451–457.

65. Mercer and Ferketich, *op. cit.*

66. Rustia, J.G., and D.A. Abbott, Father Involvement in Infant Care: Two Longitudinal Studies, *International Journal of Nursing Studies*, 30, no. 6 (1993), 467–476.

67. Becker et al., *op. cit.*

68. Attainment of the Maternal Role—Part I.

69. Cognitive Style in Pregnancy.

70. Sherwen, L., M. Scoloveno, and C. Weingarten, *Maternity Nursing: Care of the Childbearing Family* (3rd ed.). Norwalk, CT: Appleton & Lange, 1999.

71. *Ibid.*

72. Satz, K., Integrating Navajo Tradition into Maternal-Child Nursing, *IMAGE, Journal of Nursing Scholarship*, 14, no. 3 (1982), 89–91.

73. Peyser, M., and A. Underwood, Emotions: Shyness, Sadness, Curiosity, Joy: Is It Nature or Nurture? *Newsweek (Special Issue)*, Spring/Summer (1997), 60–63.

74. *Ibid.*

75. Bettelheim and Freedgood, *op. cit.*

76. Health Canada, *Canadian Incidence Study of Reported Child Abuse and Neglect*, Website: www.hc-sc.gc.ca/pphb-dgspsp/cm-vee/cish101/index.html, June 2004.

77. *Ibid.*

78. *Ibid.*

79. *Ibid.*

80. Trocmé, N., B. MacLaurin, B. Fallon, J. Daciuk, M. Tourny, and D. Billingsley, Canadian Incidence Study of Reported Neglect: Methodology, *Canadian Journal of Public Health*, 92, no. 4 (2001), 259–263.

81. Health Canada, *Canadian Incidence Study of Reported Child Abuse and Neglect.*

82. *Ibid.*

83. Loo, S., N. Bala, M. Clarke, and J. Hornick, *Child Abuse: Reporting and Classification in Health Care Settings.* Ottawa: National Clearinghouse on Family Violence, Family Violence Prevention Division, Health Canada, 1998.

84. Papalia, D., S. Olds, and R. Feldman, *Human Development* (7th ed.). Boston: McGraw-Hill, 1998.

85. MacMillan, H., Child Maltreatment: What We Know in the Year 2000, *Canadian Journal of Psychiatry*, 45, no. 8 (2000), 702–709.

86. Papalia et al., *op. cit.*

87. Tonmyr, L., H. MacMillan, E. Jamieson, and K. Kelly, The Population Health Perspective as a Framework for Studying Child Maltreatment Outcomes, *Chronic Diseases in Canada*, 23, no. 4 (2002), 123–129.

88. Poussaint, A., and S. Linn, Fragile: Handle with Care, *Newsweek (Special Issue)*, Spring/Summer (1997), 33.

89. Papalia et al., *op. cit.*

90. Aboriginal Peoples Collection, Solicitor General of Canada, *A Cost-Benefit Analysis of Hollow Water's Community Holistic Circle Healing Process*, Ottawa: Solicitor General of Canada, 2001.

91. Baker, M., *Changing Trends in Canada* (4th ed.). Toronto: McGraw-Hill Ryerson, 2001.

92. MacMillan, *op. cit.* Reprinted in part with the permission of Dr. H. MacMillan.

93. Baker, *op. cit.*

94. Tonmyr et al., *op. cit.*
95. *Ibid.*
96. Canadian Paediatric Society, *Joint Statement on Shaken Baby Syndrome,* Website: www.cps.ca/english/statements/IP/cps01-01.htm, June 2004.
97. Showers, J., *Never, Never, Never Shake a Baby: The Challenges of Shaken Baby Syndrome.* Washington, D.C: National Association of Children's Hospitals and Related Institutions, 1999.
98. U.S. Advisory Board on Child Abuse and Neglect. *A Nation's Shame: Fatal Child Abuse and Neglect in the United States,* Washington, DC: U.S. Government Printing Office, 1995.
99. Wiehe V.R., *Understanding Family Violence: Treating and Preventing Partner, Child, Sibling, and Elder Abuse.* Thousand Oaks, CA: Sage, 1998.
100. Canadian Paediatric Society, Joint Statement on Shaken Baby Syndrome.
101. Poussaint and Linn, *op. cit.*
102. *Ibid.*
103. Wiehe, *op. cit.*
104. Bee, H., *Lifespan Development* (2nd ed.). New York: Longman, 1998.
105. Canadian Paediatric Society, Joint Statement on Shaken Baby Syndrome.
106. Bee, *op. cit.*
107. Papalia et al., *op. cit.*
108. Seifert, K., R. Hoffnung, and M. Hoffnung, *Lifespan Development.* Boston: Houghton Mifflin, 1997.
109. Sherwen et al., *op. cit.*
110. Wong, D., *Wong's Nursing Care of Infants and Children* (7th ed.). St. Louis, Mosby, 2003, 249
111. Dubowitz, L., and V. Dubowitz, *A Clinical Manual: Gestational Age of the Newborn.* New York: Addison-Wesley, 1977.
112. Ballard, J. et al., A Simplified score for Assessment of Fetal Maturation in Newly Born Infants, *Journal of Pediatrics, 95* (1979), 769–774.
113. Health Canada, *Family Centred Maternity and Newborn Care,* Chapter 6: Early Postpartum Care of the Mother and Infant and Transition to the Community, Website: www.hc-sc.gc.ca/dca-dea/publications/femc06_e.html, June 2004.
114. Canadian Institute of Child Health, *The Health of Canada's Children* (3rd ed.). Ottawa: Canadian Institute of Child Health, 2000.
115. MacMillan, *op. cit.*
116. Health Canada, *Pediatric Clinical Practice Guidelines for Nurses in Primary Care,* Website: www.hc-sc.gc.ca/fnihb/ons/nursing/resources/pediatric_guidelines/chapter_1.htm, July 2004.
117. Singh, G., and S. Yu, Birth Weight Differentials among Asian Americans, *American Journal of Public Health, 84* (1994), 1444–1449.
118. Sherwen et al., *op. cit.*
119. Ballard, et al., *op. cit.*
120. MacMillan, *op. cit.*
121. *Ibid.*
122. Manitoba Centre for Health Policy and Evaluation, *Assessing the Health of Children in Manitoba: A Population-Based Study,* Winnipeg: Manitoba Centre for Health Policy and Evaluation, 2001.
123. Health Canada, *Population Health Approach, Toward a Healthy Future: Second Report on the Health of Canadians,* Website: www.hc-sc.gc.ca/hppb/phdd/report/toward/back/how.html, June 2004.
124. MacMillan, *op. cit.*
125. *Ibid.*
126. Dusitin, N., et al., Development and Validation of a Simple Device to Estimate Birth Weight and Screen for Low Birth Weight in Developing Countries, *American Journal of Public Health, 81,* no. 9 (1991), 1201–1205.
127. Baker, *op. cit.*
128. Sherwen et al., *op. cit.*
129. Ballard et al., *op. cit.*
130. Baker, *op. cit.*
131. Sherwen et al., *op. cit.*
132. Ballard et al., *op. cit.*
133. Papalia et al., *op. cit.*
134. Sherwen et al., *op. cit.*
135. Ballard et al., *op. cit.*
136. Sherwen et al., *op. cit.*
137. Ballard et al., *op. cit.*
138. Papalia et al., *op. cit.*
139. Sherwen et al., *op. cit.*
140. Ballard et al., *op. cit.*
141. Sherwen et al., *op. cit.*
142. Ballard et al., *op. cit.*
143. Temperature Recording in Infants and Children, *Pediatric Nursing, 19* (1992).
144. Sherwen et al., *op. cit.*
145. Ballard et al., *op. cit.*
146. Sherwen et al., *op. cit.*
147. Ballard et al., *op. cit.*
148. Canadian Medical Association, *Complete Book of Mother and Baby Care: A Parent's Practical Handbook from Conception to Three Years* (3rd ed.). Toronto: Tourmaline Editions Inc, 2001.
149. Sherwen et al., *op. cit.*
150. Ballard et al., *op. cit.*
151. Health Canada, *Canadian Incidence Study of Reported Child Abuse and Neglect.*
152. Papalia et al., *op. cit.*
153. Trocmé et al., *op cit.*
154. Sherwen et al., *op. cit.*
155. Ballard et al., *op. cit.*
156. Kramer, M., et al., Extra Tactile Stimulation of the Premature Infant, *Nursing Research, 24,* no. 5 (September–October 1975), 324–334.
157. Sherwen et al., *op. cit.*
158. Ballard et al., *op. cit.*
159. Brazelton and Cramer, *op. cit.*
160. Wiehe, *op. cit.*
161. Fuller, B., Acoustic Discrimination of Three Types of Infant Cries, *Nursing Research, 40,* no. 3 (1991), 156–160.
162. Sherwen et al., *op. cit.*
163. Ballard et al., *op. cit.*
164. Gesell, A, et al., *The First Five Years of Life.* New York: Harper Brothers, 1940.
165. Troy, N., Early Contact and Maternal Attachment Among Women Using Public Health Care Facilities, *Applied Nursing Research, 6,* no. 4 (1993), 161–166.
166. Papalia et al., *op. cit.*
167. Lack, J., Turning on the Motor, *Newsweek (Special Issue),* Spring/Summer (1997), 26–27.
168. Sherwen et al., *op. cit.*
169. Ballard et al., *op. cit.*
170. U.S. Advisory Board on Child Abuse and Neglect, *op. cit.*
171. Ballard et al., *op. cit.*
172. *Ibid.*
173. Trocmé et al., *op. cit.*
174. Sherwen et al., *op. cit.*
175. Ballard et al., *op. cit.*
176. *Ibid.*
177. Sherwen et al., *op. cit.*
178. Papalia et al., *op. cit.*
179. *Ibid.*
180. *Ibid.*
181. Andrews and Boyle, *op. cit.*
182. Sherwen et al., *op. cit.*

183. Ballard et al., *op. cit.*
184. Sherwen et al., *op. cit.*
185. Ballard et al., *op. cit.*
186. *Ibid.*
187. Health Canada, *Canadian Incidence Study of Reported Child Abuse and Neglect.*
188. Edelman, C., and C. Mandle, *Health Promotion Throughout The Life Span* (4th ed.). St. Louis: Mosby, 1998.
189. Papalia et al., *op. cit.*
190. Trocmé et al., *op. cit.*
191. Sherwen et al., *op. cit.*
192. Ballard et al., *op. cit.*
193. Begley, *op. cit.*
194. Bettelheim and Freedgood, *op. cit.*
195. Papalia et al., *op. cit.*
196. Peyser and Underwood, *op. cit.*
197. Wingert, P., and A. Underwood, First Steps, *Newsweek (Special Issue),* Spring/Summer (1997), 12–15.
198. Andrews and Boyle, *op. cit.*
199. Seifert et al., *op. cit.*
200. Horn, B., Cultural Concepts and Postpartal Care, *Journal of Transcultural Nursing,* 2, no. 1 (1990), 48–51.
201. Papalia et al., *op. cit.*
202. Trocmé et al., *op. cit.*
203. Sherwen et al., *op. cit.*
204. Ballard et al., *op. cit.*
205. Papalia et al., *op. cit.*
206. Trocmé et al., *op. cit.*
207. Sherwen et al., *op. cit.*
208. Ballard et al., *op. cit.*
209. Papalia et al., *op. cit.*
210. *Ibid.*
211. Piaget, J., *The Construction of Reality in the Child* (M. Cook, Transl.). New York: Basic Books, 1954.
212. Piaget, J., *The Origins of Intelligence in Children.* New York: International University Press, 1952.
213. Papalia et al., *op. cit.*
214. Sherwen et al., *op. cit.*
215. Ballard et al., *op. cit.*
216. Montagu, A., *Touching: The Human Significance of the Skin* (3rd ed.). New York: Columbia University Press, 1986.
217. Sherwen et al., *op. cit.*
218. Ballard et al., *op. cit.*
219. U.S. Advisory Board on Child Abuse and Neglect, *op. cit.*
220. Ballard et al., *op. cit.*
221. Sherwen et al., *op. cit.*
222. Ballard et al., *op. cit.*
223. U.S. Advisory Board on Child Abuse and Neglect, *op. cit.*
224. Toronto Public Health, *Growing Healthy Together: Birth to Two Years,* Toronto, 1998.
225. Sherwen et al., *op. cit.*
226. Ballard et al., *op. cit.*
227. Sherwen et al., *op. cit.*
228. Ballard et al., *op. cit.*
229. Sherwen et al., *op. cit.*
230. Ballard et al., *op. cit.*
231. *Ibid.*
232. Sherwen et al., *op. cit.*
233. Ballard et al., *op. cit.*
234. Sherwen et al., *op. cit.*
235. Ballard et al., *op. cit.*
236. Duyff, R., *The American Dietetic Association's Complete Food & Nutrition Guide.* Minneapolis: Chronimed Publishing, 1998.
237. Health Canada, *Nutrition for a Healthy Pregnancy: National Guidelines for the Childbearing Years,* Ottawa, 2000.
238. Kramer et al., *op. cit.*
239. *Ibid.*
240. *Ibid.*
241. *Ibid.*
242. *Ibid.*
243. Williams, S.R., *Nutrition and Diet Therapy* (11th ed.). St. Louis: Times Mirror/Mosby, 2001.
244. Kramer et al., *op. cit.*
245. Fuller, *op. cit.*
246. MacMillan, *op. cit.*
247. Papalia et al., *op. cit.*
248. Fuller, *op. cit.*
249. Papalia et al., *op. cit.*
250. Kramer et al., *op. cit.*
251. Health Canada, Medical Services Branch, *Native Foods and Nutrition: An Illustrated Reference Manual,* Ottawa, 1994.
252. Fuller, *op. cit.*
253. Papalia et al., *op. cit.*
254. Kramer et al., *op. cit.*
255. Sherwen et al., *op. cit.*
256. Fuller, *op. cit.*
257. Sherwen et al., *op. cit.*
258. Ballard et al., *op. cit.*
259. Kramer et al., *op. cit.*
260. Sherwen et al., *op. cit.*
261. Fuller, *op. cit.*
262. Ballard et al., *op. cit.*
263. Canadian Medical Association, *Complete Book of Mother and Baby Care: A Parent's Practical Handbook from Conception to Three Years.*
264. U.S. Advisory Board on Child Abuse and Neglect, *op. cit.*
265. Kramer et al., *op. cit.*
266. Fuller, *op. cit.*
267. Sherwen et al., *op. cit.*
268. Ballard et al., *op. cit.*
269. Kramer et al., *op. cit.*
270. *Ibid.*
271. Fuller, *op. cit.*
272. Papalia et al., *op. cit.*
273. Calgary Health Region, *Fluoridation: Prenatal and Breastfeeding,* Website: www.crha-health.ab.ca./pophlth/hp/fluoride/default.htm, July 2004.
274. Caring for Kids, *Cow's Milk,* Website: www.caringforkids.cps.ca/babies/CowMilk.htm, August 2004.
275. Kramer et al., *op. cit.*
276. Fuller, *op. cit.*
277. Ballard et al., *op. cit.*
278. U.S. Advisory Board on Child Abuse and Neglect, *op. cit.*
279. Health Canada, *Family Centred Maternity and Newborn Care: National Guidelines.*
280. *Ibid.*
281. Fuller, *op. cit.*
282. Troy, *op. cit.*
283. Health Canada, *Food Program 2000,* Website: www.hc-sc.gc.ca/food-aliment/mh-dm/mhe-dme/e_faqs_bottle_eng.html, July 2004.
284. Fuller, *op. cit.*
285. Kramer et al., *op. cit.*
286. Fuller, *op. cit.*
287. Papalia et al., *op. cit.*
288. Kramer et al., *op. cit.*
289. Fuller, *op. cit.*
290. *Ibid.*
291. Ballard et al., *op. cit.*
292. Fuller, *op. cit.*
293. Kramer et al., *op. cit.*
294. MacMillan, *op. cit.*
295. *Ibid.*
296. Sherwen et al., *op. cit.*
297. Ballard et al., *op. cit.*

298. Sherwen et al., *op. cit.*

299. Ballard et al., *op. cit.*

300. Sherwen et al., *op. cit.*

301. Health Canada, *Crib Safety*, Website: http://www.hc-sc.gc.ca/hecs-sesc/cps/pdf/cribguide.pdf, August 2004.

302. Canadian Child Care Foundation, *Health Watch, Back to Sleep*, Website: http://www.cccf-fcsge.ca/practice/health520watch/sleep_en.html, June 2004.

303. Health Canada, *SIDS*, Website: http://www.hc-sc.gc.ca/dca-dea/prenatal/sids_e.html, July 2004.

304. Piaget, *The Construction of Reality in the Child*.

305. Gelfand and Teti, *op. cit.*

306. Verzemnicks, I., Developmental Stimulation for Infants and Toddlers. *American Journal of Nursing*, 84, no. 6 (1984), 749–752.

307. Wadsworth, B., *Piaget's Theory of Cognitive and Affective Development Foundations of Constructivism* (5th ed.). New York: Longman, 1996.

308. Wingert, P., and A. Underwood, First Steps, *Newsweek (Special Issue)*, Spring/Summer (1997), 12–15.

309. Piaget, *The Origins of Intelligence in Children*.

310. Rosenberg, D., and L. Reibstein, Pots, Blocks, and Socks, *Newsweek (Special Issue)*, Spring/Summer (1997), 34–35.

311. Hammersmith and Sawatsky, *op. cit.*

312. *Ibid.*

313. Rubin, *op. cit.*

314. Health Canada, *Canadian Immunization Guide* (6th ed.). Ottawa: Minister of Public Works and Governmental Services, 2002.

315. Canadian Paediatric Society, Vaccine Schedules, *Paediatric Child Health*, 8, no. 1 (2003).

316. Manitoba Centre for Health Policy, *The Health and Health Care Use of Registered First Nations People Living in Manitoba: A Population-Based Study*, Winnipeg, 2002.

317. Ballard et al., *op. cit.*

318. Andrews and Boyle, *op. cit.*

319. *Ibid.*

320. Ballard et al., *op. cit.*

321. Burgess, A., E. Dowdell, C. Hartman, C. Nakemy, and J. Rabun, Infant Abductors, *Journal of Psychosocial Nursing*, 33, no. 9 (1995), 30–37.

322. Kalb, C., The Top 10 Health Worries, *Newsweek (Special Issue)*, Spring/Summer (1997), 42–43.

323. Riccitiello, R., and J. Adler, "Your Baby Has a Problem," *Newsweek (Special Issue)*, Spring/Summer (1997), 46– 47, 48.

324. Health Canada, *Canadian Incidence Study of Reported Child Abuse and Neglect*.

325. Chilmonczyk, B., et al., Environmental Tobacco Smoke Exposure during Infancy, *American Journal of Public Health*, 80, no. 10 (1990), 1205–1208.

326. Calgary Health Region, *op. cit.*

327. Kramer et al., *op. cit.*

328. Sherwen et al., *op. cit.*

329. Ballard et al., *op. cit.*

330. Health Canada, *Population Health Approach, Toward a Healthy Future: Second Report on the Health of Canadians*.

331. Papalia et al., *op cit.*

332. Manitoba Centre for Health Policy and Evaluation, *op. cit.*

333. Health Canada, *Population Health Approach, Toward a Healthy Future: Second Report on the Health of Canadians*.

334. Papalia et al., *op cit.*

335. Seifert et al., *op. cit.*

336. Manitoba Centre for Health Policy and Evaluation, *op. cit.*

337. Health Canada, *Population Health Approach, Toward a Healthy Future: Second Report on the Health of Canadians*.

338. Papalia et al., *op cit.*

339. Dusitin, *op. cit.*

340. Duyff, *op. cit.*

341. Bee, H., D. Boyd, and P. Johnson, *Lifespan Development* (Canadian ed.). Toronto: Pearson Education Canada, Inc., 2003.

342. Begley, *op. cit.*

343. Greenberg, *op. cit.*

344. Van Boven, *op. cit.*

345. Begley, *op. cit.*

346. Dusitin, *op. cit.*

347. Begley, *op. cit.*

348. Trocmé et al., *op. cit.*

349. Sherwen et al., *op. cit.*

350. Ballard et al., *op. cit.*

351. Bettelheim and Freedgood, *op. cit.*

352. Papalia et al., *op. cit.*

353. Health Canada, *Canadian Incidence Study of Reported Child Abuse and Neglect*.

354. Bettelheim and Freedgood, *op. cit.*

355. *Ibid.*

356. Papalia et al., *op. cit.*

357. Bettelheim and Freedgood, *op. cit.*

358. Papalia et al., *op. cit.*

359. Bettelheim and Freedgood, *op. cit.*

360. Erikson, E., *Childhood and Society* (2nd ed.). New York: W.W. Norton, 1963.

361. Erikson, E., *Toys and Reasons*. New York: W.W. Norton, 1977.

362. Peyser and Underwood, *op. cit.*

363. Health Canada, *SIDS*.

364. Adler, I., It's a Wise Father Who Knows, *Newsweek (Special Issue)*, Spring/Summer (1997), 23.

365. Bettelheim and Freedgood, *op. cit.*

366. Peyser and Underwood, *op. cit.*

367. Van Boven, *op. cit.*

368. Chess and Thomas, *op. cit.*

369. Bettelheim and Freedgood, *op. cit.*

370. Schilder, P., *The Image and Appearance of the Human Body*. New York: International University Press, 1951.

371. Bettelheim and Freedgood, *op. cit.*

372. Wingert and Underwood, *op. cit.*

373. *Ibid.*

374. Wiehe, *op. cit.*

375. Bettelheim and Freedgood, *op. cit.*

376. Wingert and Underwood, *op. cit.*

377. Becker, P., et al., Outcomes of Developmentally Supportive Nursing Care for Very Low Birth Weight Infants, *Nursing Research*, 40, no. 3 (1991), 150–155.

378. Low-Birth-Weight Infants Catch Up in Adolescence, *American Journal of Nursing*, 98, no. 10 (1998), 9.

379. Letch, D., Mother–Infant Interaction: Achieving Synchrony, *Nursing Research*, 48, no. 1 (1999), 55–57.

380. Chess and Thomas, *op. cit.*

381. Harris, J., *The Nurture Assumption*. New York: Free Press, 1998.

382. Begley, *op. cit.*

383. Chess and Thomas, *op. cit.*

384. Cole, *op. cit.*

385. Bettelheim and Freedgood, *op. cit.*

386. Greenberg, *op. cit.*

387. Pressler, J., Promoting Attachment, in *Nursing Interventions for Infants & Children*, 1990, pp. 4, 13. Craft, M., and J. Denehy, eds.

388. Koniak-Griffin, D., Maternal Role Attainment, *IMAGE: Journal of Nursing Scholarship*, 25, no. 3 (1993), 257–262.

389. Health Canada, *Family Centred Maternity and Newborn Care, Chapter 6: Early Postpartum Care of the Mother and Infant and Transition to the Community*.

390. Peyser and Underwood, *op. cit.*

391. Van Boven, *op. cit.*

392. Walker, L., and E. Montgomery, Maternal Identity and Role Attainment's Long-Term Relations to Children's Development, *Nursing Research,* 43, no. 2 (1998) 105–110.
393. Montagu, op. cit.
394. Dusitin, *op. cit.*
395. *Ibid.*
396. Ballard et al., *op. cit.*
397. Dusitin, *op. cit.*
398. *Ibid.*
399. *Ibid.*
400. *Ibid.*
401. Bettelheim and Freedgood, *op. cit.*
402. Papalia et al., *op. cit.*
403. Duvall, E., and B. Miller, *Marriage and Family Development* (6th ed.). New York: Harper & Row, 1984.
404. Frankenburg, W.K., and J.B. Dodd, The Denver Developmental Screening Test, *Journal of Pediatrics,* 71 (1967), 181–191.
405. Stolte, K.M., *Wellness: Nursing Diagnosis for Health Promotion,* Lippincott, 1996.
406. Bee et al., *Lifespan Development* (Canadian ed.).
407. Ibid.
408. Baker, *op. cit.*
409. Federal Interagency Forum on Child and Family Statistics, America's Children: Key National Indicators of Well-Being, *Federal Interagency Forum on Child and Family Statistics,* Washington, DC: U.S. Government Printing Office, 1998.
410. Shiono, P., and R. Behrman, Low Birth Weight: Analysis and Recommendations. In *The Future of Children: Low Birth Weight,* 5, no. 1 (Spring, 1995), Los Altos State: The David and Lucile Packard Foundation, Center for the Future of Children.
411. Erikson, *Childhood and Society.*
412. Gardner, S., K. Garland, S. Merenstein, and L. Lubchenco, The Neonate and the Environment: Impact on Development, in G. Merenstein, and S. Gardner, eds., *Handbook of Neonatal Intensive Care* (3rd ed.). St. Louis: Mosby, 1993.
413. Paneth, N., The Problem of Low Birth Weight, *The Future of Children: Low Birth Weight,* 5, no. 1 (Spring 1995), Los Altos,
CA: The David and Lucile Packard Foundation, Center for the Future of Children.
414. Erikson, *Childhood and Society.*
415. Burgess et al., *op. cit.*
416. Calgary Health Region, *op. cit.*
417. Caring for Kids, *op. cit.*
418. Sandling, J., B. Carter, C. Moore, and J. Sparks, Ethics in Neonatal Intensive Care, in G. Merenstein and S. Gardner, eds., *Handbook of Neonatal Intensive Care* (3rd ed.). St. Louis: Mosby, 1993.
419. Health Canada, Canadian Perinatal Surveillance System, *Congenital Anomalies in Canada: A Perinatal Health Report,* Ottawa: Minister of Public Works and Government Services Canada, 2002.
420. Low-Birth-Weight Infants Catch Up in Adolescence.
421. Health Canada, Canadian Perinatal Surveillance System, *Perinatal Health Indicators for Canada: A Resource Manual.* Ottawa: Minister of Public Works and Government Services Canada, 2000.
422. Dorris, M., *The Broken Cord.* New York: HarperCollins, 1991.
423. Becker, P., et al., Outcomes of Developmentally Supportive Nursing Care for Very Low Birth Weight Infants, *Nursing Research,* 40, no. 3 (1991), 150–155.
424. Sherwen et al., *op. cit.*
425. Ballard et al., *op. cit.*
426. Becker et al., *op. cit.*
427. Tyson, J., Evidence-Based Ethics and the Care of Premature Infants, *The Future of Children: Low Birth Weight,* 5, no. 1 (1995). Los Altos, CA: The David and Lucile Packard Foundation, Center for the Future of Children.
428. Wakefield-Fisher, M., Balancing Wishes with Wisdom: Sustaining Infant Life, *Nursing and Health Care,* no. 11 (1987), 517–520.
429. Schloman, P., and S. Fister, Parental Perspectives Related to Decision-making and Neonatal Death, *Pediatric Nursing,* 21 (1995), 243–248.
430. Canadian Paediatric Society, *Guidelines for Health Care Professionals Supporting Families Experiencing a Perinatal Loss,* Website: www.cps.ca/english/statements/FN/fn01-02.htm, July 2004.
431. Cole, *op. cit.*
432. Ballard et al., *op. cit.*
433. Frankenburg and Dodd, *op. cit.*

Chapter 8

ASSESSMENT AND HEALTH PROMOTION FOR THE TODDLER

Train up a child in the way he should go, and
when he is old, he will not depart from it.

Proverbs 22:6

OBJECTIVES

STUDY OF THIS CHAPTER WILL ENABLE YOU TO:

1. Explore the reciprocal effects of family and toddler within a family system.

2. Describe the significance of attachment behaviour and parenting practices.

3. Examine with parents ways to meet their toddler's developmental tasks.

4. Assess a toddler's physical and motor characteristics and related needs, including nutrition, rest, exercise, play, safety, and health protection measures.

5. Assess a toddler's cognitive, language, emotional, and sexuality development.

6. Evaluate specific methods of guidance and discipline for the toddler; and consider the significance of the family's philosophy about guidance and discipline.

7. Discuss with parents their role in contributing to the toddler's cognitive, language, emotional, self-concept, and moral development.

8. Describe the commonly used adaptive mechanisms that promote autonomy of the toddler; and analyze your role in assisting parents to foster the development of the child's autonomy.

9. State the toddler's developmental tasks, and identify ways to help him or her to achieve these tasks.

10. Work effectively with a toddler and the family in the health care and nursing situation, either in a hospital or a community setting.

In this chapter development of the toddler and the family relationships are discussed. *Nursing and health care responsibilities for the promotion of health for the child and family in any setting are discussed throughout the chapter.*

Within the first year of life children make remarkable adaptation internally and externally to their environment. They sit, walk, remember, recognize others and begin to socialize, communicate more purposefully with speech, and show more specific emotional responses.

The **toddler stage** *begins when the child takes the first steps alone at 12 to 15 months and continues until approximately three years of age.* The family is very important during this short span of the child's life as he or she acquires language skills, increases cognitive achievement, improves physical coordination, and achieves control over bladder and bowel sphincters. These factors lead to new and different perceptions of self and the environment, new incentives, and new ways of behaving.

CRITICAL THINKING

What family experiences can you recall from when your siblings or cousins were toddlers?

FAMILY DEVELOPMENT AND RELATIONSHIPS

Behaviourally, the toddler changes considerably between 12 months and three years, a change that in turn affects family relationships. Because of new skills, the child begins to develop a sense of independence, establishes physical boundaries between self and mother, and gains the sense of a separate, self-controlled being who can do things on his or her own. From the age of two years the child moves toward independence—from the protracted dependency of childhood toward adulthood independence, self-reliance, and object relations. The child attempts self-education through mastery and engaging parents and others in help when necessary. Without the myriad attempts to do things for himself or herself, the child would obtain no degree of autonomy in skills. The periods of practice that ensure reliable performance and skills are often periods of independent action; however, dependence on others and gratification of dependency needs are essential for optimum ego development. Dependency does not mean passivity, for the child is quite active in obtaining help by crying, screaming, taking an adult by the hand and pulling him or her to another area, or asking how to solve a problem. The toddler should neither be kept too dependent nor forced too quickly into independence.

The family of a toddler can be quiet and serene one minute and in total upheaval the next, resulting from the imbalance between the child's motor skills, lack of experience, and mental capacities. One quick look away from the toddler can result in a broken object, spilled glass of milk, or an overturned dish. Teach parents that this behaviour is normal and necessary for maturation. Expecting, planning for, and trying to handle patiently each situation will reduce parent frustration.

Having a new baby arrive in the toddler's world is a crisis. Prepare the child for the arrival by explaining why mother's shape is becoming larger or changing, and prepare the toddler to sleep in a different bed if the crib is needed for the baby. Emphasis on the positive features of becoming a "big girl" or "big boy" is helpful. When baby arrives, the toddler will need more attention, especially while giving baby care.

The toddler is frequently jealous of younger siblings because of having to vie for the centre of attention that was once his or her own; older siblings are resented because they are permitted to do things he or she cannot. Power struggles focusing on feeding and toilet training occur between parent and child. Family problems may also arise when the toddler's activities are limited because of parental anxieties concerning physical harm or because of their intolerance of the child's energetic behaviour.

Inform parents that their social teaching likely will centre on cleanliness and establishing reasonable controls over anger, impulsiveness, and unsafe exploration.

INFLUENCE OF THE FAMILY

The chief moulder of personality is the family unit, and home is the centre of the toddler's world. Family life nurtures in the child a strong affectional bond, a social and biological identity, intellectual development, attitudes, goals, and ways of coping and responding to situations of daily life. The family life process also imparts tools such as language and an ethical system, in which the child learns to respect the needs and rights of others and which provide a testing ground before he or she emerges from home. A loving, attentive, healthy, responsible family is essential for maximum physical, mental, emotional, social, and spiritual development in childhood. The importance of the father's role with the child and the mother is being affirmed.[1–3] In fact, fathers are more involved with their children now, and they are no longer merely providers. The greater number of women in the job market, higher divorce rate, and the more egalitarian division of roles and responsibilities are all factors that explain why men now play a more active role as fathers.[4]

CRITICAL THINKING

What character strengths and personality qualities have you seen fathers display while interacting with a toddler?

Parents with high self-esteem provide the necessary conditions for the toddler to achieve trust, self-esteem, and autonomy (self-control) through allowing age-appropriate behaviour. Parents with low self-esteem provoke feelings of shame, guilt, defensiveness, decreased self-worth, and "being bad" in the child by overestimating the child's ability to conform, inappropriately or forcefully punishing or restraining the child, denying him or her necessities, and withdrawing love.[5]

Help parents work out their feelings about self in relation to the child. Changing parental attitudes are often evident. If the parent is delighted with a dependent baby and is a competent parent to an infant, the parent may be threatened by the independence of the toddler and become less competent. Some parents have difficulty caring for the dependent infant but are creative and loving with the older child. But if the parent's development was smooth and successful, and if he or she understands self, parental behaviour can change to fit the maturing child.

Attachment Behaviours

Attachment behaviour is very evident during the toddler years. The symbiotic mother–child relationship is slowly being replaced by more interaction with father[6] and the larger family unit, but the toddler still needs mother close.[7] Children need to be touched, cuddled, hugged, and rocked. All young mammals need physical contact for normal brain tissue development and for the brain to develop receptors that inhibit secretion of adrenal hormones (glucocorticoids)—the stress hormones. Thus, both the immune and neurological systems are affected positively by touch and by emotional attachment.[8]

The toddler shows attachment behaviour by maintaining proximity to the parent. Even when out walking, the child frequently returns part or all the way to the parent for reassurance of the parent's presence, to receive a smile, to establish visual, and sometimes touch, contact, and to speak before again moving away.[9]

Although attachment is directed to several close people such as father, siblings, babysitter, and grandparents, it is usually greatest toward one person, mother. Attachment patterns do not differ significantly between children who stay home all day versus those who go to daycare centres, because attachment is related to the intensity of emotional and social experience between child and adult rather than to physical care and more superficial contact. Attachment is as great or greater if the mother shows warm affection less frequently than if she is present all day but not affectionate. Schneider, Atkinson and Tardif, a group of Canadian researchers, found that for children early attachment seems to affect later social functioning. The researchers state that the child–mother attachment literature lends itself to rich speculation, but presently there is insufficient literature regarding implications of child–father attachment on children's peer relations.[10] Further, Pederson and Moran, researchers from the University of Western Ontario, claim that for the study of attachment behaviours, the home setting is more natural to measure such behaviours than using the "Strange Situation," which measures mother–infant interactions in a laboratory setting. They developed this new, more natural setting claiming that the richer fabric of a home environment may reveal differences in the relationships that are not found in the Strange Situation. By using both methods to compare expressions of attachment relationships between the infant and the mother, the researchers determined that in a secure type of a relationship, mothers were more sensitive to the needs of their infants; and infants displayed less fussy behaviour and enjoyed physical contact with the mother.[11,12]

Separation anxiety, the *response to separation, from mother,* intensifies at approximately 18 and 24 months. Anxiety can be as intense for the toddler as for the infant if the child has had a continuous warm attachment to a mother figure because he or she thinks an object ceases to exist when it is out of sight. The child who is more accustomed to strangers will suffer less from a brief separation. When separated, the child experiences feelings of anger, fear, grief, and revenge. An apathetic, resigned reaction at this age is a sign of abnormal development. The child who is separated from the parent for a period, as with hospitalization, goes through three phases of *grief and mourning*—protest, despair, and denial, which may merge somewhat—as a result of separation anxiety.[13]

During **protest,** *lasting a few hours or days and seen for short or long separations, the need for mother is conscious, persistent, and grief laden. The child cries continually, tries to find her, is terrified, fears he or she has been deserted, feels helpless and angry that mother left him or her, and clings to her on her return.* If he or she is also ill, additional uncomfortable body sensations assault the toddler.[14] The child needs mother at this time.

Despair *is a quiet stage, characterized by hopelessness, moaning, sadness, and less activity. The child does not cry continuously but is in deep mourning. He or she does not understand why mother has deserted him or her. The child makes no demands on the environment nor responds to overtures from others, including at times the mother. Yet the child clings to her if permitted.* Mother may feel guilty and want to leave to relieve her distress, as she may feel her visits are disturbing to the child, especially when the child does not respond to her.[15]

Parents need help in understanding that the child's and their reactions are normal and that the child desperately needs parental presence.[16] If she can be present, you can promote family-centred care through your explanations to the mother and child, by not being rigid about visiting hours, by attending to the comfort and needs of mother (or father), and by letting the parent help care for the child. Protests, in the form of toddlers' screams and crying, will thus be less intense. Be accepting if a parent cannot stay with the child. Parents may live great distances from the hospital or have occupational or family responsibilities that indeed prevent them from visiting the child as often as they desire. The parent may also be ill or injured. Be as nurturing to the toddler as possible while the parent is away. Tell the toddler how much Mommy and Daddy love him or her and want to be present but cannot. If possible, have the parent leave an article with the child that is a familiar representation of the parent.

Denial, *which occurs after prolonged separation, defends against anxiety by repressing the image of and feelings for mother and may be misinterpreted for recovery.* The child now begins to take more interest in the environment, eats, plays, and accepts other adults. Anger and disappointment at mother are so deep that the child acts as if he or she does not need her and shows revenge by rejecting her, sometimes even rejecting gifts she brings. To prevent further estrangement, mother should understand that the child's need for her is more intense than ever.[17]

Continue the above interventions that promote family-centred care. Give the mother, or father, and child time together undisturbed by nursing or medical care procedures. Provide toys that help the child to act out the fears, anxiety, anger, and mistrust experienced during the hospitalization and separation. Encourage the parent to talk about and work through feelings related to the child's illness and absence from the family.

With prolonged hospitalization, the child may fail to discover a person to whom he or she can attach for any length of time. If the child finds a mother figure and then loses her, the pain of the original separation is re-experienced. If this happens repeatedly, the child will eventually avoid involvement with anyone but invest love in self and later value material possessions more highly than any exchange of affection with people.

Teach parents that immediate aftereffects of separation include changes in the child's behaviour—regression, clinging, and seeking out extra attention and reassurance. If extra affection is given to the child, trust is gradually restored. If the separation has been prolonged, the child's behaviour can be very changed and disturbed for months after return to the parents. The parent needs support in accepting the child's expressions of hostility and in meeting his or her demands. Counteraggression or withdrawal from the child will cause further loss in trust and regression. Parenting can be hard work. You may inform the parents if they need to talk to someone they may call the Parent Help Line toll-free at 1-888-603-9100. There is someone available 24 hours a day.[18]

Child maltreatment may begin or continue at this age. Even when parents seem concerned and loving, a child is not immune from abuse. Further, children today are exposed to a variety of potential abusers—babysitters, daycare workers, the parent's live-in lover or occasional friend, stepparents, extended family members, and neighbours. The results of one study, conducted by Onyskiw, indicated that children exposed to domestic violence had lower health status and more conditions or health problems. Theses factors, in turn, limited the child's participation in normal age-related activities compared to children in nonviolent families. In addition, more child witnesses of violence regularly used prescription medication than children who were not exposed to violence at home.[19] *Be alert to signs and symptoms of child maltreatment,* discussed in Chapters 4, 6, and 7.

You often must be very patient and observant to detect child maltreatment because the child does not have the language skills to tell you what has happened. The child's nonverbal behaviour, play, and artwork may provide clues. Observation of the latter takes time and patience as well as the parent's presence.[20,21] The boxes entitled "Parental Behaviour Characteristic of Psychological Maltreatment of the Toddler," "Physical Signs of Abuse of a Child," and "Interaction Signs of Parental Abuse of a Child" present assessment data to aid you in recognizing signs of abuse.

CRITICAL THINKING

Kari, a toddler, has multiple bruises on her body. There is evidence that she has been beaten by her mother. What health promoting strategies can you employ with this family?

Parental Behaviour Characteristic of Psychological Maltreatment of the Toddler

Rejecting

- Excludes actively from family activities
- Refuses to take child on family outings
- Refuses to hug or come close to child
- Places the child away from the family

Isolating

- Teaches the child to avoid social contact beyond the parent–child relationship
- Punishes social overtures to children and adults
- Rewards child for withdrawing from opportunities for social contact

Terrorizing

- Uses extreme gestures and verbal statements to threaten, intimidate, or punish the child
- Threatens extreme or mysterious harm (from monsters or ghosts or bad people)
- Gives alternately superficial warmth with ranting and raging at the child

Ignoring

- Is cool and apathetic with child
- Fails to engage child in daily activities or play
- Refuses to talk to child at mealtimes or other times
- Leaves child unsupervised for extended periods

Corrupting

- Gives inappropriate reinforcement for aggressive or sexually precocious behaviour
- Rewards child for assaulting other children
- Involves the child sexually with adolescents or adults

Source: Garbonino, J. E. Guttmao, and J. Seeley, *The Psychologically Battered Child: Strategies for Identification, Assessment, and Intervention.* San Francisco: Jossey-Bass, 1987. Copyright 1986. Adapted by permission of Jossey-Bass, Inc., a subsidiary of John Wiley & Sons, Inc.

Physical Signs of Abuse of a Child

- An injury for which there is no explanation or an implausible explanation is present.
- Injury is not consistent with the type of accident described (e.g., child would not suffer both feet burned by stepping into hot tub of water, he or she would step in with one foot at a time, a child who tips a pot of hot coffee on his or her hand has a splash-effect burn, not a mitten appearance.)
- Inconsistencies exist in the parents' stories about the reason for child's injuries.
- Parents quickly blame a babysitter or neighbour for an accidental injury.
- Child does not have total appearance of an accident—dirty clothes, face smudged, hair tousled.
- Large number of healed or partially healed injuries is observed.
- Large bone fracture, multiple fractures, or tearing of periosteum caused by having limb forcibly twisted are evident.
- Child flinches when your fingers move over an area not obviously injured, but it is tender due to abusive handling.
- Human bite marks are evident.
- Fingernail indentations or scratches are noted.
- Old or new cigarette burns are evident.
- Loop marks from belt beating are present.
- Soft tissue swelling and hematomas are noted.
- Clustered or multiple bruises are observed on trunk or buttocks, in body hollows, on back of neck, or resembling hand prints or pinch marks.
- Bald spots are observed.
- Retinal haemorrhage from being shaken or cuffed about the head is assessed.
- History of unusual number of accidents exists.

Sources: Papalia, D., S. Olds, and R. Feldman, *Human Development* (7th ed.). Boston: McGraw-Hill, 1998; Seifert, K., R. Hoffnung, and M. Hoffnung, *Lifespan Development.* Boston: Houghton Mifflin, 1997; Wong, D., *Whaley and Wong's Nursing Care of Infants and Children* (6th ed.). St. Louis: C. V. Mosby, 1999.

- Determining whether or not they will have any more children
- Rededicating themselves, among many dilemmas, to their decision to be a childbearing family[22]

Help parents to be cognizant of these tasks. Encourage them to talk through concerns, feelings, and practical aspects related to fulfilling these tasks. Refer them to a counsellor or community agency if help is desired.

PHYSIOLOGIC CONCEPTS

Physical Characteristics

Information in this section will assist you in assessment of the toddler and teaching the parents about normal development and health promotion measures.

Family Developmental Tasks

The family with a toddler faces many new developmental tasks:

- Meeting the spiralling costs of family living
- Providing a home that is safe and comfortable and has adequate space
- Maintaining a sexual involvement that meets both partners' needs
- Developing a satisfactory division of labour
- Promoting understanding between the toddler and the family

Interaction Signs of Parental Abuse of a Child

- Child flinches or glances about nervously when you touch him or her.
- Child seems afraid of parents or caregivers and is reluctant to return home.
- Parent issues threat to crying child such as "Just wait 'till I get you home."
- Parent remains indifferent to child's distress.
- Parent(s) blames child for his or her own injuries (e.g., "He's always getting hurt" or "He's always causing trouble").
- Parental behaviour suggests role reversal; parent solicits help or protection from child by acting helpless (when child cannot meet parent's needs, abuse results).
- Parent repeatedly brings healthy child to emergency room and insists child is ill (parent feeling overwhelmed by parental responsibilities and may become abusive).
- Child has had numerous admissions to an emergency room, often at hospitals some distance from the child's home.

Sources: Papalia, D., S. Olds, and R. Feldman, *Human Development* (7th ed.). Boston: McGraw-Hill, 1998; Seifert, K., R. Hoffnung, and M. Hoffnung, *Lifespan Development*. Boston: Houghton Mifflin, 1997; Wong, D., *Whaley and Wong's Nursing Care of Infants and Children* (6th ed.). St. Louis: C. V. Mosby, 1999.

General Appearance

The appearance of the toddler has matured from infancy. He or she has lost the roly-poly look of infancy with abdomen protruding, torso tilting forward, legs at stiff angles, and flat feet spaced apart, by 12 to 15 months. Limbs are growing faster than torso, giving a different proportion to the body. By 12 to 15 months, chest circumference is larger than head circumference. The child increasingly looks like a family member as face contours fill out with the set of deciduous teeth. By age two, he or she has 16 teeth. Gradually the chubby appearance typical of the infant is lost; muscle tone becomes firmer as the fat-storing mechanisms change. Less weight is gained as fat; more weight is gained from muscle and bone.[23–26]

Rate of Growth

During toddlerhood, *growth is slower than in infancy; but it is even, and development follows the cephalocaudal, proximodistal, and general-to-specific principles discussed in Chapter 6.* Although the rate of growth slows, bone growth continues rapidly with the development of approximately 25 new ossification centres during the second year.[27]

Between the first and second years the average height increase is 10 to 12 cm (4 to 5 inches) Average height increase the next year is 6 to 8 cm ($2^1/_2$ to $3^1/_2$ inches). Weight gain averages 2.25 to 2.75 kg (5 to 6 pounds) between the first and second years. *Birth weight is quadrupled by age two.* The two-year-old child stands 81 to 84 cm (32 to 33 inches) and weighs 11 to 13 kg (26 to 28 pounds) At 30 months average height is 91.5 cm (36 in) and weight is approximately 13.6 kg (30 pounds). *By age two, the girl has grown to 50% of final adult height; by age two-and-a-half, the boy to 50% of adult height.*[28–31]

The Indian and Inuit Health Committee of the Canadian Paediatric Society believes that no single growth chart for all Native children should be produced due to regional variation. They make the following recommendations:

- The growth charts prepared from the U.S. National Ambulatory Health and Nutrition Survey are suitable for use in Native communities.
- Throughout childhood, measurements of height and weight and of head circumference for the first three years should be taken at all well-child contacts and plotted.
- The Medical Services Branch should catalogue areas where head circumference tends to be larger than in Caucasian children.
- Health care workers must first comprehend how to use growth charts, and second they must be made aware of local variations in weight or head circumference as part of their orientation.[32]

CRITICAL THINKING

What other factors besides the child's environment and family history should be taken into account in assessing growth abnormalities?

8–1 BONUS SECTION IN CD-ROM

Research Abstract: The Effects of Maternal Psychosocial Factors on Parenting Attitudes of Low-Income Single Mothers with Young Children

Neuromuscular Maturation

Neuromuscular maturation and repetition of movements help the child further develop skills. **Myelinization,** *covering of the neurons with the fatty sheath called myelin,* is almost complete by two years. This enables the child to support most movement and increasing physical activity and to begin toilet training. Additional growth also occurs as a greater number of connections form among neurons, and the complexity of these connections increases. Lateralization or specialization of the two hemispheres of the brain has been occurring; evidence of signs of dominance of one hemisphere over the other can be seen. The left hemisphere matures more rapidly in girls than in boys; the right hemisphere develops more rapidly in boys. These differences may account for language ability in girls and spatial ability in boys. Handedness is demonstrated, and spatial perception is improving.[33–37] (Spatial ability will be complete at approximately age ten.) The limbic system is mature; sleep, wakefulness, and emotional responses become better regulated. The toddler responds to a wider range of stimuli, responds voluntarily to sounds, and has greater control over behaviour. The brain reaches 80% of adult size by age two.[38] The growth of the glial cells accounts for most of the change.[39,40]

Motor Coordination

Increasing gross motor coordination is shown by leg movement patterns and by hand–arm movements. Table 8-1 summarizes the increasing motor coordination skills manifested during the toddler years.[41–45]

TABLE 8-1
Motor Coordination During the Toddler Years

Age (months)	Characteristics
12–15	Walks alone; legs appear bowed
	Climbs steps with help; slides down stairs backward
	Stacks two blocks; scribbles spontaneously
	Grasps but rotates spoon; holds cup with both hands
	Takes off shoes and socks
15–18	Runs but still falls
	Walks backward and sideways (17 months)
	Climbs to get to objects
	Falls from riding toys or in bathtub
	Hammers on pegboard
	Grasps with both hands
	Picks up small items off floor; investigates electric outlets; grabs cords and table cloths (15 months)
	Clumsily throws ball
	Unzips large zipper
	Takes off easily removed garments
	Stacks three to four blocks (18 months)
18–24	Falls from outdoor play equipment
	Walks stairs with help (20 months)
	Walks up and down stair steps alone, holding rail, both feet on step before ascending to next step
	Can reach farther than expected, including for hazardous objects
	Fingers food
	Brushes paint; finger-paints
	Takes apart toys; puts together large puzzle pieces
24–30	Runs quickly; falls less
	Walks downstairs holding to rail; does not alternate feet
	Jumps off floor with both feet (28 months)
	Throws ball overhand
	Puts on simple garments
	Stacks six blocks
	Turns door handles
	Plays with utensils and dishes at mealtimes; pours and stacks
	Turns book pages
	Uses spoon with little spilling; feeds self
	Brushes teeth with help
30–36	Walks with balance; runs well
	Balances on one foot; walks on tiptoes (30 months)
	Jumps from chair (32 months)
	Pedals tricycle (32 months)
	Jumps 25–30 cm off floor (36 months)
	Climbs and descends stairs, alternating feet (36 months)
	Rides tricycle
	Sits in booster seat rather than highchair
	Stacks 8–10 blocks; builds with blocks
	Pours from pitcher
	Dresses self completely except tying shoes; does not know back from front
	Turns on faucet
	Assembles puzzles
	Draws; paints

Sources: Bee, H., Lifespan Development (2nd ed.). New York: Longman, 1998; Gormly, A., Lifespan Human Development (6th Ed.). Fort Worth: Harcourt Brace College Publishers, 1997; Papalia, D., S. Olds, and R. Feldman, Human Development (7th ed.). Boston: McGraw-Hill, 1998; Seifert, K., R. Hoffnung, and M. Hoffnung, Lifespan Development. Boston: Houghton Mifflin, 1997; Wong, D., Whaley and Wong's Nursing Care of Infants and Children (6th ed.). St. Louis: C.V. Mosby, 1999.

Vision

Visual acuity and the ability to **accommodate,** *to make adjustments to objects at varying distances from the eyes,* are slowly developing. Vision is **hyperopic,** *farsighted,* testing approximately 20/10 at two years. Visual perceptions are frequently similar to an adult's, even though the child is too young to have acquired the richness of symbolic associations. The child's eye–hand coordination also improves. At 15 months he or she reaches for attractive objects without superfluous movements. Between 12 and 18 months, the toddler looks at pictures with interest and identifies forms.[46,47]

Endocrine System

Endocrine function is not fully known. Production of glucagons and insulin is labile and limited, causing variations in blood sugar. Adrenocortical secretions are limited, but they are greater than they were in infancy. Growth hormone, thyroxin, and insulin remain important secretions for regulating growth.[48]

Respiratory System

Respirations average 20 to 30 per minute. Lung volume is increased, and susceptibility to respiratory infections decreases as respiratory tract structures increase in size.[49]

Cardiovascular System

The pulse decreases, averaging 105 beats per minute. Blood pressure increases, averaging 80 to 100 systolic and 64 diastolic. The size of the vascular bed increases, thus reducing resistance to flow. The capillary bed has increased ability to respond to hot and cold environmental temperatures, thus aiding thermoregulation. The body temperature averages 37.2°C (99°F).[50]

Gastrointestinal System

Foods move through the gastrointestinal tract less rapidly, and digestive glands approach adult maturity. Acidity of gastric secretion increases gradually. Liver and pancreatic secretions are functionally mature. Stomach capacity is 500 mL.[51]

Skin

The skin becomes more protective against outer invasion from microorganisms, and it becomes tougher, with more resilient epithelium and less water content. Less fluid is lost through the skin as a result. The skin remains dry because sebum secretion is limited. Eccrine sweat gland function remains limited. At this age eczema improves and the frequency of rashes declines.[52]

Urinary System

By age three, the bladder has descended into the pelvis, assuming adult position. Renal function is mature; except under stress, water is conserved, and urine is concentrated on an adult level.[53]

Immune System

Specific antibodies have been established to most commonly encountered organisms, although the toddler is prone to gastrointestinal and respiratory infections when he or she encounters new microorganisms. Lymphatic tissues of adenoids, tonsils, and peripheral lymph nodes undergo enlargement, partly because of infections and partly from growth. By age three years, the adenoid tissue reaches maximum size and then declines, whereas tonsils reach peak size around seven years.[54]

Blood Cell Components

Blood cell counts are approaching adult levels, although the hemoglobin and erythrocyte (red blood cell) counts are lower. Sufficient iron intake is necessary to maintain an adequate erythrocyte level. Erythrocytes are formed in the bone marrow of the ribs, sternum, and vertebrae as in adulthood. During stress, the liver and spleen also form erythrocytes and granulocytes.[55]

Overall Development

Development does not proceed equally or simultaneously in body parts and maturational skills. Sometimes a child concentrates so intently on one aspect of development (e.g., motor skills) that other abilities (e.g., toilet training) falter or regress. Illness or malnutrition may slow growth, but a catch-up growth period occurs later so that the person reaches the developmental norms. The brain is more vulnerable to permanent injury because destroyed cells are not replaced, although some brain cells may take over some functions of missing cells. Most children also show seasonal spurts in growth. Caucasians, for example, show more height increase in spring and more weight increase in fall. There are also cultural differences in growth and development. Teach parents about physical characteristics of the toddler to help them adjust to his or her changing competencies.

Physical Assessment of the Young Child

The approach to the physical examination depends on the age of the individual. Adequate time should be spent in becoming acquainted with the child and the accompanying parent. A friendly manner, quiet voice, and relaxed approach help make the examination more fruitful. Hands should always be warmed before giving an examination, but especially so in the case of the child.

No assessment is complete without knowing the antenatal, natal, and neonatal history. When the child is old enough, let him or her tell what conditions surround the visit even if the message is only "stomach hurt."

CRITICAL THINKING

Which details should a pediatric history include as compared to an adult history?

Many times you will be learning about the young child from the mother and will be learning about the mother's attitude. If other siblings are present, observe the interaction among the family members.

What are the mother's facial expressions? In what tone of voice does she talk? Does she look away or comfort the child if the child seems disturbed with a procedure?

What are the other siblings' reactions toward the toddler, the mother, and the health care worker? What are the siblings' reactions in general?

Although the child may not talk much, general appearance can reveal a considerable amount of information. Does the child look ill or well? What is the activity level? How do you describe his or her co-ordination? Gait, if walking? What are the child's reactions to parents, siblings, and examiner? What is the nature of the child's cry, if present? What do you learn from the child's facial expressions?

Before six months of age the infant usually tolerates the examining table. Between six months and three to five years, most of the examination can be done from the mother's or caretaker's lap. After age four, much depends on the relationship established with the child.

The sequence of the examination with the young child should be from least discomfort to most discomfort. Undressing can be a gradual procedure as children are often shy about this process. Some examiners prefer to go from toe to head or at least to start with auscultation, which is painless and sometimes fascinating to the child. Measurement of length and height should be part of every health maintenance visit (along with the measurement of head circumference in the first two years of life). It is necessary to record these parameters on gender-appropriate growth curves, so measurements may be compared to the appropriate norm. These measurements should form part of the child's health record.[56]

It is best to leave the ears, nose, and mouth to the end because examination of these areas often initiates a negative response. Generally the temperature should be taken rectally during the first years of life. Blood pressure should be taken with the cuff that will snugly fit the arm. The first reading is recommended at age three. The inflatable bladder should completely encircle the arm but not overlap. Artificially high blood pressure results if the cuff is too narrow or too short.[57] Because this procedure causes some discomfort and it is important to get readings in a low-anxiety state, sensitive timing is needed to get desired results. It sometimes helps to make a game out of the procedure by allowing the toddler to help pump up the bulb or read the numbers on the gauge.

The skin can be examined for turgor by feeling the calf of the leg, which should be firm. **Spider nevi,** *pinhead-sized red dots from which blood vessels radiate,* are commonly found, as are **Mongolian spots,** *large, flat black or blue-and-black spots.* One or two *patches of light brown, nonelevated stains,* called **café au lait spots,** are within normal findings, but more may be indicative of fibromas or neurofibromas. **Bruises** (*ecchymoses*) are not abnormal in healthy active children, but their location is important. Bruises not on the extremities or on areas easily hit when falling may

indicate child abuse, or excessive bruising may indicate blood dyscrasias.[58]

Lymph nodes are palpable in almost all healthy young children. Small, mobile, nontender nodes often point to previous infection.[59]

When examining the head region, consider the following:

- The auricles of the ears should be pulled back and down in young children and back and up in older children.
- A complete hearing test with an audiometer should be done before a child enters school. Before that, the whisper technique or the use of a tuning fork is adequate.
- A Snellen E-chart can be used for testing visual acuity before the child knows the alphabet. Visual acuity at three years is 20/40, and at four to five years is 20/30.
- Other aspects of the visual examination depend on the child's age and the suspected problem (e.g., after surgery for congenital cataracts).
- Teeth should be examined for their sequence of eruption, number, character, and position.[60]

When examining the thorax and lungs, remember that breath sounds of young children are usually more intense and more bronchial and expiration is more pronounced than in adults. The heart should be examined with the child erect, recumbent, and turned to the left. Sinus arrhythmia and extrasystoles can be benign and are not uncommon.[61]

When standing, a child's abdomen may be protuberant; when lying down, it should disappear. The skilled examiner should be able to palpate both the liver and the spleen.[62]

When examining the male genitalia, the testicles should be examined while the male is warm and in a sitting position, holding his knees with heels on the seat of the chair or examining table. Without warmth and abdominal pressure, the testes may not be in the scrotum.[63]

Examination of the female genitalia is basically visual unless a specific problem in the area has developed.

When examining the extremities, the examiner may note bowlegs, which are common until 18 months. Knock-knees are common until approximately age 12. The toddler may appear flat-footed when first walking. All these characteristics are usually short term.[64]

The neurological examination is conducted throughout and is not much different from the sequence in the adult examination; however, the appropriate maturation level must be kept in mind.

NARRATIVE VIGNETTE
Toddler Check-up

You are working in a nursing station in rural Nova Scotia. A mother has brought her three-year-old son for his yearly check-up. He has been sitting quietly on the floor playing, but looks up wide-eyed and appears somewhat anxious as you approach.

1. How will you begin your assessment?

2. What information will you seek from the mother?
3. Which of the child's behaviours might be noteworthy? For what reason(s)?
4. What significant health issues will you ensure that the mother comprehends?

Nutritional Needs

Toddlerhood is an exciting time for change. Attitudes are forming. Bodies are growing and maturing. Skills are being mastered. Youngsters get to know their world by utilizing their senses such as smelling and tasting.[65] Most two- and three-year-olds take pleasure in experimenting with new food. Two- and three-year-olds are striving for greater autonomy. They practise controlling their environment by deciding whether or not to eat something. For example, one day they may really like a particular food, and the next day they may reject it. It is important to understand that these whims are normal. Many toddlers insist on having their milk in a certain cup or their food arranged or cut up in certain shapes. Most prefer meals and snacks on a regular schedule because they seek a sense of security.[66] New foods may be refused with a common phrase like "I don't like it," or an even more common phrase—"No!"

Canada's Food Guide has been adapted for children by taking into account the smaller portions of food they eat. Consequently, the guide has become a useful tool for everyone in the family over two years of age.[67]

The *Food Guide* gives a lower and higher number of servings for each food group. The range of these servings allows the *Food Guide* to be sufficiently flexible to use with family members with different energy and nutrient needs.[68] The following general guidelines apply when choosing a number of servings for toddlers and preschoolers:

- A wide range of grain products (5–12), and vegetables and fruit (5–10). The toddler or preschool child will usually choose child-size servings from the lower end of the range for these food groups each day.

- The *Food Guide* recommends two to three servings per day of milk products. Toddlers and preschoolers should drink 500 mL (2 cups) of milk every day because it is their main dietary source of vitamin D. This amount can be counted as two servings. In addition, they may choose to include a child-size serving of other milk products such as cheese and yogurt.

- They can choose two or three child-size servings of meat and alternatives each day. See the box entitled "Examples of One Child-Size Serving."

Some *suggestions to teach parents to avoid having mealtime be a battleground* are:[69]

1. Serve food in small portions.

2. Serve finger foods or cut food so that it can be eaten with the fingers.

3. Let the child choose (it is not necessary for the toddler to sample every food served).

4. Avoid high-fat, high-salt, or carbohydrate foods such as soda, candy, and cake or empty nutrition snack foods in the choice.

5. Offer a food again if it has been rejected one time, without fussing about it.

6. Avoid insisting that the child eat everything on the plate.

The toddler is a great imitator; he or she eats the kind of foods eaten by the parents. Parental pressure or reprimands when the child does not eat a particular food convey anxiety or anger

Examples of One Child-Size Serving

Grain Products	1/2–1 slice of bread 15–30 g cold cereal 75–175 mL (1/3–3/4 cup) hot cereal 1/4–1/2 bagel, pita or bun 1/2–1 muffin 50–125 mL (1/4–1/2 cup) pasta or rice 4–8 soda crackers
Vegetables and Fruit	1/2–1 medium-size vegetable or fruit 50–125 mL (1/4–1/2 cup) fresh, frozen or canned vegetables or fruit 125–250 mL (1/2–1 cup) salad 150–125 mL (1/4–1/2 cup) juice
Milk Products	25–50 g cheese 75–175 g (1/3–3/4 cup) yogourt Preschoolers should consume a total of 500 mL (2 cups) of milk every day.
Meat and Alternatives	25–50 g meat, fish or poultry 1 egg 50–125 mL (1/4–1/2 cup) beans 50–100g (1/4–1/3 cup) tofu 1 5–30 mL (1–2 Tbsp) peanut butter

Source: Health Canada, Office of Nutrition Policy and Promotion, *Canada's Food Guide to Health Eating Focus on Preschoolers— Background for Educators and Communicators*, 2002, Website: http://www.hc-sc.gc.ca/hpfb-dgpsa/onpp-bppn/food_guide_ preschoolers_e.html, page 7. Reproduced with the permission of Public Works and Government Service Canada, 2004.

and reinforce not eating, because of either the negative attention received or the stress response felt by the child. Toddlers can be fussy eaters or go on "food jags," preferring only a certain food. Advise parents to give the requested food for a few days until the child gets bored with it, while continuing to offer alternative foods. Or the toddler may overeat if parents overeat. If there is a high caloric intake, obesity may result. Excessive weight gain interferes with the physical mobility that is a part of being a normal toddler. *Teach parents to maintain caloric balance by substituting fibre foods* because they give a sense of fullness.

Teach parents about the nutritional needs and eating patterns of the toddler. Avoid serving too large a portion, which can be the beginning of overeating or cause refusal to eat all the food, with resultant conflict between parent and toddler.

Malnutrition may lead to slower growth, tooth decay, lowered resistance to disease, and even death. Signs of malnutrition include abdominal swelling, lethargy, lack of attention to stimuli, lack of energy, diminished muscle strength and coordination, changes in skin colour, and hair loss. Females apparently are buffered better against effects of malnutrition or illness than males. Malnutrition delays growth, but children have great recuperative powers if malnutrition does not continue too long. When nutrition improves, growth takes place unusually fast until norms for weight, height, and skeletal development are reached. For example, children who suffered early malnutrition but were provided good nutrition later performed as well on intellectual tests as their peers.[70–72]

A hospitalized toddler frequently regresses; refusing to feed self is one manifestation. The child needs a lot of emotional support and to feel some kind of control over his or her destiny and that he or she is not totally helpless and powerless. A way of ensuring some area of control is by permitting the child to choose foods and encouraging him or her to feed self.[73]

Play, Exercise, and Rest

Play and Exercise

Play is the business of the toddler. During play he or she exercises, learns to manage the body, improves muscular coordination and manual dexterity, increases awareness and organizes the surrounding world by scrutinizing objects, and develops beginning spatial and sensory perception. The child learns language and to pay attention and releases emotional tensions as he or she channels unacceptable urges such as aggression into acceptable activities; translates feelings, drives, and fantasies into action; and learns about self as a person. Through play the toddler becomes socialized and begins to learn right from wrong. The child learns to have fun and to master. For more information on activities to try with children, visit http://www.healthcanada.ca/paguide or call 1-888 334-9769.

The child has little interest in other children except as a curious explorer. **Play** is solitary and **parallel;** *he or she plays next to but not with other children.* There is little overt exchange, but there is satisfaction in being close to other children. The toddler is unable to share toys and is distressed by demands of sharing as he or she has a poorly defined sense of ownership. The toddler will play cooperatively with guidance, however.

Play time and positive relationships with the parents, siblings, and other family members help the toddler learn how to interact and to be sociable, and over time, how to make friends. By the end of two years, most children imitate adults in dramatic play by doing such things as setting the table and cooking. When selecting play materials for the toddler, remember likes and dislikes and choose a variety of activities because the attention span is short. (Safety and durability aspects of toys, as discussed in Chapter 7, must be considered.)

Father is likely to continue the same kind of play pattern with the toddler as with the infant. Fathers tend to jostle the young child more and devote more time to play than do mothers. Fathers are more likely than mothers to use their own body as a portable, interactive monkey bar or rocking horse. From infancy on, father helps the child to individuate by being willing to let the child move out of sight and will let a child crawl or move twice as far than mother allows before retrieving the child. When a child confronts a novel situation, a new toy, a stranger, or a dog, mothers move closer to support the child and offer reassurance with their presence, while fathers stay back and let the child explore by him- or herself. The child needs to be exposed to both the comforting and the challenge.[74]

However, when the father is the primary caregiver, he interacts with the young child in much the same way as has the mother, traditionally, by smiling frequently and imitating

the child's facial expressions and vocalizations. The father still remains quite physical with the child in interaction. As fathers assume greater responsibility for young child care due to changing social and cultural conditions and expectations, mothers and fathers are likely to interact more similarly with their young children.[75]

Table 8-2 presents suggested play activities and equipment for the child 18 months or two years of age.

TABLE 8-2
Suggested Play Activities and Equipment for Toddlers

Age (months)	Toy, Equipment, or Activity
18	Push-pull toys (cars, trucks, farm tools)
	Boxes and toys for climbing
	Empty and fill toys (plastic food containers, kitchen utensils, small boxes, and open-close toys)
	Big picture books—thick-paged, colourful, sturdy (child will turn two or three pages at a time, tear at thin pages, can identify one picture at a time)
	Stuffed animals with no detachable parts
	Baby dolls, large enough to hug, carry, cuddle, dress, and feed
	Big pieces of plain paper or newspaper layers and crayons for scribbling
	Small blocks—builds a tower of two or three at a time
	Shape-sorting blocks or cubes
	Small chair; small furniture to play "house"
	Toy farm animals or equipment
	Rubber or soft ball; throws overhand
	Phonograph record, preferably sturdy plastic that child can manipulate by self; musical and sound toys; musical instruments simple to use
	Rocking horse; rocking chair
24	All of the above are enjoyed; child now turns book or magazine pages singly—still tears; builds tower of seven blocks and aligns cubes
	Makes circular strokes with crayon, enjoys finger-paints
	Puppets
	Pedal toys; dumping toys (dump trucks)
	Sandbox toys
	Play dough and clay; mud
	Jungle gym for climbing; sand box; small water pool for waterplay
	Pounding toys—hammer and pegs, drums, small boards
	Picture puzzles—two to four pieces (wooden or thick cardboard)
	Large, coloured wooden beads to string
	Simple trains, cars, boats, planes to push-pull or sit on and pedal
	Kicks ball
	Likes to run

Teach parents the importance of play and safety. A relation exists between the quality of attachment between mother and baby and the quality of play and problem-solving behaviour at two years of age. Toddlers who are securely attached at 18 months of age are more enthusiastic, persistent, cooperative, and able to share than if secure attachment has not developed. There is also more frequent and sophisticated interaction with peers at three years when secure attachment has formed in infancy.[76] Discuss play patterns and toys with the parents.

Help parents realize the importance of offering playthings that can transform into any number of toys, depending on the child's mood and imagination at the time. The adult can be available or initially start a play activity with the child; however, the child should be encouraged to play independently, developing mastery, autonomy, and self-esteem in the process.

CRITICAL THINKING

What role does gender play today in parental choice of play activities for toddlers?

Verzemnieks[77] describes developmental stimulation, play activities, and toys for the hospitalized child. See the box entitled "Techniques for Using Play While Caring for the Child" for a summary of how play can be used effectively with the ill child.

Rest

Rest is as essential as exercise and play, and although a child may be tired after a day full of exploration and exerting boundless energy, bedtime is often a difficult experience. Bedtime means loneliness and separation from fun, family, and, most important, the mother figure. The toddler needs an

Techniques for Using Play While Caring for the Child

Physical Assessment

- Talk soothingly and calmly. Explain what you are doing as you do it.
- Blow on the stethoscope. Ask child to imitate.
- Have child listen to own heartbeat with stethoscope.
- Name body parts and touch them. "Foot. Here is my foot." "Where are your eyes?" "There are your eyes!" "Where is your nose?" Guide the child's hands to touch.
- Use diversions—another toy, tickles (especially abdomen).
- Play peek-a-boo: cover your eyes, then child's. Hide your head with blanket, then child's head. When child covers own head, say "Where's [name?]" Then delight in discovery.
- Use body movement, exercising child's arms and legs rhythmically while doing assessment.
- Sing a nonsense tune or talk animatedly.
- Talk about sensations: warm or cold, soft or rough as sensations are presented.
- Name body position: up or down, over.
- Encourage child to do examination of doll, teddy bear, or toy animal.

Bathing

- Experiment with the properties of water in a small tub. Use items that float and sink—washcloth, plastic soap dish, paper cup, plastic lid, empty plastic cylinders, or toys at child's crib side. Talk about what happens.

- Identify body parts as you wash them. Give simple directions: "Close your eyes." "Raise your arms." "Wash your hair." Be sure to praise all help.
- Encourage child to "bathe" a doll, teddy bear, or toy animal.

Feeding

- Place the child in highchair or walker when he or she can sit unsupported. Tie toy or utensil to high chair to facilitate retrieval.
- Discuss the food: hot or cold, colours, textures, which utensils to use.
- Use an extra spoon and cup: one for you, one for baby.
- Experiment with food: finger-paint with food on tray, make lines.

Diagnostic Procedures

- Explain to the child what you plan to do and are doing. Be honest but gentle.
- Tell the child it is all right to cry; comfort if child cries.
- Set up situation so child can do procedure on doll or toy animal. While child is imitating, talk about how much it hurts. Cuddle and comfort the child, cooing, singing softly, and rocking after the procedure.
- Distract the child with empty dressing packages, encouraging crushing and listening to sounds.
- Make the sounds and touch different parts of child's body.
- Vocalize sounds related to procedure. Have child imitate you.

---

average of 10 to 12 hours of sleep nightly plus a daytime nap. The sleep schedule may be as follows:

15 months	Morning nap is shorter; needs afternoon nap.
17–24 months	Will have trouble falling asleep.
18 months	Brings stuffed toy or pillow.
19 months	Sleeps fairly well, tries to climb out of bed.
20 months	May awaken with nightmares.
21 months	May rest quietly and sleep less time in afternoon nap at times.
24 months	Total sleep time reduced, tries to delay bedtime; continues to need afternoon nap or rest.
2–3 years	Can be changed from crib to bed; needs rails on side to not tumble out.

Teach the following guidelines to parents for establishing a bedtime routine for the toddler:

- Set a definite bedtime routine and adhere to it. If the child is overly tired, he or she becomes agitated and difficult to put to sleep.
- Establish a bedtime ritual, including bath, a story, soft music (some young children prefer classical), quiet talking and holding, and a tucking-in routine. Reduce noise

and stimuli in the house. Avoid television, movies, or videos that show aggressive scenes and are too loud. Begin approximately 30 minutes before bedtime. The tucking-in should be caring and brief.

- If the child cries, which most children do, briefly go back in a few minutes to provide reassurance. Do not pick up the child or stay more than 30 seconds. If the crying continues, return in five minutes and repeat the procedure. Thus the parent can determine whether there is any real problem, and the child feels secure.
- If extended crying continues, lengthen the time to return to the child to ten minutes. Eventually fatigue will occur, the cry will turn to whimpers, and the child will fall asleep.
- The child should remain in his or her bed rather than sleep for all or part of the night with parents. Bedtime routine becomes a precedent for other separations; however, if the parents make an occasional exception such as during a family crisis of major loss, trauma, or transition or if the child is ill, neither the marriage relationship nor the child's development will be hindered. It is important that the exception not become the routine.
- As the child grows older, limit the number of times the child can get up, for any reason, after going to bed.

Sleep problems during hospitalization may show up through restlessness, insomnia, and nightmares. Increasingly, hospitals are permitting parents to spend the night in the child's room to lessen fears and separation anxiety. Cuddling is still important to a toddler, especially if hospitalized. If a parent cannot remain with a frightened child, you can hold and rock him or her while he or she holds a favourite object.

CRITICAL THINKING

What other strategies might you pursue with a frightened child who is unable to sleep?

Health Promotion and Health Protection

Routine Immunizations

Immunizations remain a vital part of health care. The toddler needs to continue the immunization process that was begun in infancy. (See Table 7–6 on page 328 for an immunization schedule, or visit http://www.caringforkids.cps.ca/immunization/Schedule.htm.)

Safety Promotion and Injury Control

Common health threats at the toddler stage are accidents. The main causes of accidents include motor vehicles, burns, suffocation, drowning, poisoning, and falls. Accidents are a major cause of death.

Because children delight in exploring the world around them, 80% of injuries to young children happen at home.[78] Thus it is necessary to childproof the home. *Teach parents they can prevent injury from furniture by:*

- Selecting furniture with rounded corners and a sturdy base
- Packing away breakable objects
- Putting safety catches on doors to prevent the child opening furniture doors or pulling furniture on self
- Disconnecting unused appliances; wrapping cords; securing cords in use

    They can prevent falls by:

- Avoiding hazardous waxing
- Discarding throw rugs
- Keeping traffic lanes clear
- Placing gates at tops of stairways (Figure 8–1) and screens on the windows
- Placing toys and favourite objects on a low shelf
- Using appropriate child safety seats in the car and grocery cart

Burns are prevented by blocking access to electric outlets, heating equipment, matches, lighters, hot water or hot food, and stoves, fireplaces, and appliances that heat. Handles of pans should be turned to the back of the stove. Electric cords attached to appliances that heat should not drape over the top edge of a work or counter surface. Fireworks should never be used when a young child is nearby. Placing tools and knives high on the wall or in a locked cabinet can *prevent lacerations or more serious injury*. Any surface that is sharp may cut the child and should be covered, if possible, or kept out of the way of the child. It is important to note that areas outside the home—the yard, the street, the grocery cart—have greater hazard because today there is more contact with them.

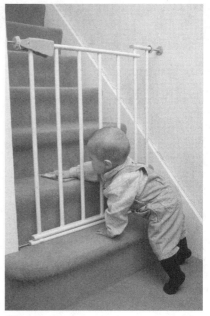

Figure 8–1

Toddlers should be prevented from climbing stairs, for example, by a portable gate.

Due to the numerous accidentally caused fires occurring in homes, it is important to make certain that the home is well equipped with working smoke alarms. Further, it is highly recommended that families develop and practise a fire escape plan together.

CRITICAL THINKING

How would you go about teaching a family home fire safety in a rural area?

Parents may call you to help when their child has been injured or is ill. *Know emergency care.* Many cities have poison-control centres to treat and give information to parents and professionals. Suggest that parents visit http://www.safekid.org/pcc.htm, or call Safe Kids Canada (1-888-SAFE-TIPS) or the Infant and Toddler Safety Association (519-570-0181). The local Canadian Red Cross is also a source of first-aid information, as is the St. John Ambulance. To find the contact information for the St. John Ambulance branch nearest you, visit http://www.sja.ca.

Explore thoroughly safety promotion with the parents, as the following normal developmental characteristics make the toddler prone to accidents. He or she:

- Moves quickly and is impulsive
- Is inquisitive and assertive
- Enjoys learning by touch, taste, and sight
- Enjoys playing with small objects
- Likes to attract attention
- Has a short attention span and unreliable memory
- Lacks judgment
- Has incomplete self-awareness
- Imitates the actions of others

Educate parents to teach the toddler to swim and always stay with the child when he or she is near water; not to allow boisterous play or sharp objects near a swimming pool, jungle gym, or sandbox; and to provide safety equipment and supervision. Regarding product safety, urge adults to keep cleaners and other poisons away from toddlers. It is important to keep all cleaners in their original containers and to show children the hazard symbols.[79] See the box entitled "Parent Teaching to Prevent Poisoning."

Common Health Problems: Prevention and Treatment

The child must be carefully assessed for infections and other disease conditions because he or she lacks the cognitive, verbal, and self-awareness capacities to describe discomforts. Table 8-3 summarizes common conditions.[80–83]

Parent Teaching to Prevent Poisoning

- Teach the child that medication and vitamins are not candy; keep them locked. Discard old medicine.
- Keep medicines, polishes, insecticides, drain cleaners, bleaches, household chemicals, garage products, and other potentially toxic substances in a locked cabinet out of the child's reach. Do not store them in containers previously used for food.
- Store nonfood substances in original containers with labels attached, not in food or beverage containers.
- If you are interrupted while pouring or using a product that is potentially harmful, take it with you. The toddler is curious and impulsive and moves quickly.
- Keep telephone numbers of the physician, poison control centre, local hospital, and police and fire departments by the telephone.
- Teach the child not to eat berries, flowers, or plants; some are poisonous.

CONTROVERSY DEBATE

Safety with Cleansers

You are conducting a home visit with a young lone parent, Susan, who has a three-year-old toddler and an infant. Susan proudly shows you that she has placed each of her cleaning agents in its own container, which is identical to all the others. She states that it took her a lot of time to label each container with felt marker and to cut out the hazard labels from the original containers and attach them to the new container.

1. How should you respond to Susan?
2. What health promoting strategies will you teach to Susan?

TABLE 8-3
Common Health Problems of Toddlers

Problem	Definition	Signs/Symptoms	Prevention/Treatment
Myopia	Nearsightedness	Squinting, not seeing far away	Prescribed glasses, use Allen cards to check vision; 30 ft (9 m) represents maximum distance at which child should identify object; if identified at 15 ft (4.5 m), vision is 15/30
Astigmatism	Unequal curvature in the refractive surfaces of the eyes	Cannot clearly focus	Prescribed glasses, use Allen cards to check vision; 30 ft (9 m) represents the maximum distance at which child should identify object; if identified at 15 ft (4.5 m), vision is 15/30
Strabismus	Eyes are not straight or properly aligned	One or both eyes may turn in, turn out, turn up or down; may be consistent or come and go	Prescribed treatment to bring the deviating eye back into binocular vision before age 6 by wearing a patch over the better aligned eye

(continued)

TABLE 8-3 *(continued)*
Common Health Problems of Toddlers

Problem	Definition	Signs/Symptoms	Prevention/Treatment
Hearing impairment	Hearing less than normal for age group	Inability to speak by age 2; failure to respond to out-of-sight noise; tilting the head while listening	Observe child carefully for appropriate hearing; check with practitioner to see if ear or upper respiratory problem is to blame; teach lip reading and sign language if appropriate
Otitis media	Infection of middle ear with accumulation of seropurulent fluid in middle ear cavity	Earache; fever; upper respiratory infection; decreased hearing; bulging tympanic membrane; disappearance of landmarks	Medication (antibiotic), sometimes decongestant; follow-up examination
Dental caries	Tooth decay often related to excess concentrated sweets or bottle mouth syndrome	Obvious dark places or breakdown of teeth; pain	Supplemental fluoride; avoidance of sweets; directions to parents for cleaning teeth (hydrogen peroxide on gauze before 18 months; then a soft toothbrush) Prepare for first dental visit with explanation, role play, and positive image If problem with discoloured teeth, infection, chipping, see dentist immediately
Malabsorption syndrome	Lactose intolerance	Chronic vomiting; diarrhea; abdominal discomfort; flatulence, irritability; poor sleep pattern	Try other products besides milk (e.g., soybean formula)
Impetigo	Lesions caused by microorganism (usually *Streptococcus Species*), often a complication of insect bites, abrasions, or dermatitis	Upper layers of skin have honey-coloured, fluid-filled vesicles that eventually crust, surrounded by a red base	Identification of lesions significant because acute glomerulonephritis can follow if not properly treated; trim fingernails to avoid scratching; wash and scrub lesions gently three times daily; wash towels used on infected areas separately; oral or topical antibiotics
Pharyngitis	Inflammation of pharynx or tonsils, or both, caused by virus or group A *Streptococcus Species* and rarely *Mycoplasma pneumonia* and *Corynebacterium diphtheria*	Red throat, exudates, enlarged lymph nodes; fever; other upper respiratory infectious symptoms	Get specific diagnosis with throat culture; treat with antibiotic if bacterial cause to avoid further disease complications; antipyretic medicine if fever present. Do not give salicylates to children because of possible Reye's syndrome, a rare but sometimes fatal disease. Warm saline gargle if able; increased fluid intake

(continued)

TABLE 8-3 *(continued)*
Common Health Problems of Toddlers

Problem	Definition	Signs/Symptoms	Prevention/Treatment
Acute nonspecific gastroenteritis (simple *diarrhea*)	Inflammation of the gastrointestinal tract during which stools are more liquid and frequent than usual	May cause dehydration with signs of sunken eyes, dry mucous membranes, decreased skin turgor, and weight loss	Discontinue milk; give small amounts of clear liquids such as flat soda (at room temperature) alternating with an electrolyte solution; add simple foods slowly
Varicella (*chickenpox*)	Acute, highly contagious disease caused by varicella zoster virus	Rash consisting of lesions that appear in crops and that go from flat macules to fluid-filled vesicles that crust in 6–8 hours; spread is from trunk to periphery and sometimes into the mouth; itching; fever; headache; general malaise; loss of appetite	Give vaccine when available; keep fingernails short; use lotions or prescription drug if itching intense; antipyretic drug if fever; isolate until lesions are all crusted
Rubella (*3-day measles*)	Viral disease characterized by rash and lymph node enlargement	Rash on face or neck, spreading to trunk and extremities; rash usually gone in 3 days	Prevention: immunization—a very serious disease during pregnancy, associated with high degree of congenital malformation; mild disease treated symptomatically for the toddler, but to be avoided by all
Pinworms (*Enterobius vermicularis*)	Most common parasite infestation in North America; cycle begins with oral infection of pinworm eggs which pass through intestinal tract in 15–28 days, hatch into larva and then into adult worms	Possibly asymptomatic; itching around anus; 2.5 cm (1-inch) white thread-like worms visible on perineum, especially when child at rest	Medication (treat all family members); personal hygiene; washing all laundry and bedclothes in hot water; clean favourite stuffed animals, chairs, and rugs, which may harbour eggs
Miliaria rubra ("*heat rash*" or "*prickly heat*")	Erythematous papular rash distributed in area of sweat glands	Fine red, raised rash; itching, pustules in neck and axillary region	Keep environment cool and dry; use air conditioner/fan; tepid baths; light clothing; use Caldesene powder; use sparingly 1% hydrocortisone cream
Viral croup (*laryngotracheo-bronchitis*; usually caused by Para influenza virus in late fall or early winter)	Inflammation of the respiratory mucosa of all airways; edema of the larynx and subglottic area	Gradual onset of upper respiratory infection; inspiratory stridor; low-grade fever; barking cough; wheezing; hoarseness; high-pitched sound on inspiration	Keep child well hydrated; use cool mist vaporizer; force liquids; take child in bathroom and turn on hot water; take child outside; if airway obstruction present, seek help immediately

Consult pediatric nursing texts for additional information on childhood illnesses and their assessment, care, and prevention.[84]

PSYCHOSOCIAL CONCEPTS

The following information will assist you to understand the toddler's behaviour; plan and give developmentally based care, promote health, and teach parents about the child.

Cognitive Development

The intellectual capacity of the toddler is limited. The child has all the body equipment that allows for an assimilation of the environment, but he or she is just beginning intellectual maturity.

Learning occurs through several general modes:[85–87]

- Natural unfolding of the innate physiologic capacity
- Imitation of others
- Reinforcement from others as the child engages in acceptable behaviour
- Insight, gaining understanding in increasing depth as he or she plays, experiments, or explores
- Identification, taking into self values and attitudes like those with whom he or she is closely associated through use of the other modes

The toddler's attention span lengthens. He or she likes songs, nursery rhymes, and stories, even though he or she does not fully understand simple explanations of them. He or she can name pictures on repeated exposure, plays alone sometimes but prefers being near people, and is aware of self and others in a new way.

Part of the toddler's learning is through imitation of the parents, helping them with simple tasks such as bringing an object, trying new activities on his or her own, ritualistic repetition of activity, experimenting with language, and expressing self emotionally. According to Piaget, the toddler finishes the fifth and sixth stages of the sensorimotor period and begins the preoperational period at approximately age two.[88]

In the **fifth stage of the sensorimotor period** (12–18 months) the child consolidates previous activities involving body actions into *experiments* to discover new properties of objects and events and achieve new goals instead of applying habitual behaviour. He or she no longer keeps repeating the same behaviour to achieve a goal and performs familiar acts without random manoeuvres. The child differentiates self from objects in the environment. Understanding of *object permanence, space perception,* and *time perception* can be observed in new ways. The child is aware that objects continue to exist even though they cannot be seen; he or she accounts for sequential displacements and searches for objects where they were *last* seen. Toddler manipulates objects in new and various ways to learn what they will do. For the first time, objects outside the self are understood as causes of action. Activities are now linked to internal representations or symbolic meaning of events or objects (memories, ideas, and feelings about past events).[89]

The **sixth stage of the sensorimotor period** (18–24 months) seems primarily a transitional phase to the preoperative period. Now the child does less trial-and-error thinking but uses memory of past experience and imitation to act as if he or she arrived at an answer. He or she imitates another who is out of sight. Toddler begins to solve problems, to foresee manoeuvres that will succeed or fail, and to remember an object that is absent and search for it until it is found.[90]

In the **preoperational period** (two to seven years) thought is more symbolic; memory continues to form; and the child internalizes mental pictures of people, the environment, and ideas about rules and relationships. The child begins to arrive at answers mentally instead of through physical activity, exploration, and manipulation. Symbolic representation is seen in:

1. Use of language to describe (symbolize) objects, events, and feelings.
2. Beginning of symbolic play (crossing two sticks to represent a plane).
3. Delayed imitation (repeating a parent's behaviour hours later).[91]

The toddler can understand simple abstractions, but thinking is basically concrete (related to tangible events) and literal. He or she is **egocentric** (*unable to take the viewpoint of another*); the ability to differentiate between subject and object, the real object and the word symbol, is not developed. He or she knows only one word for any object and cannot understand how the one word *chair* can refer to many different styles of chairs. If the flower is called *flower* and *plant,* the child will not understand that more than one word can refer to the same object. Concept of time is *now* and concept of distance is whatever can be seen. The child imitates the thinking and behaviour observed in another but lacks the past experience and broader knowledge that is essential for logical thought. This level of learning will continue through the preschool era.[92,93]

Over the past decade a considerable body of research has been generated toward understanding cognitive development in infancy. Piaget's views on infancy have dominated the field for many years. Recent research suggests, however, that infants have the ability to conceptualize earlier than believed.[94] In fact, Aguiar and Baillargeon conducted a study to examine whether 8.5-month-old infants take into account the width and compressibility of an object when determining whether or not it can be inserted into a container. Their results indicated that by 8.5 months of age, infants are already capable of sophisticated reasoning about containment events.[95]

Pushing children to read and write at an early age has not been shown to produce long-lasting positive effects. It may cause the child to lose initiative, curiosity, desire to use ingenuity, and ability to cope with ordinary life stresses. The child knows inside what he or she can do. If the parents whom the child looks to for support and guidance are manipulating him or her to meet their needs, the child may come to mistrust parents and self. Before parents put the child in a preschool that emphasizes formal academics, they should consider what the child is not learning from missed playtime. Play that is parallel to and cooperative with peers helps the child develop language, motor, cognitive, nonverbal, and social skills; positive self-esteem; a sense of worth as an individual; and unique problem-solving skills in the face of stress.[96,97]

Teach parents about this aspect of development. See the box entitled "Examples of Educational Toys and Play for the Toddler." This period can be trying and should be tempered by supportive guidance and discipline: parents' saying what is meant, providing environmental stimulation, showing interest in the child's activities and talking and working with the child, reinforcing intellectual attempts, and showing a willingness to teach with simple explanations. Much of the intellectual development now depends on the achievements of infancy, how parents used the baby's potential, and the *quality of parent–child interaction rather than the amount of time, per se, that is spent with the child*.[98] This interactive system between the mother and the child is important. It depends upon the mother's development of an emotional synchronization with her child. That is, the mother's ability to be in tune with the infant's states and to respond accordingly is significant. This process enables the mother and infant to engage in meaningful teaching/learning interaction.[99] Lipari[100] provides a particularly insightful explanation of emotional synchrony.

CRITICAL THINKING

On a biological level, what may be the effects of emotional synchronization?

Language Development

Learning to communicate in an understandable manner begins during this era. Through speech the toddler will gradually learn to control unacceptable behaviour, exchange physical activity for words, and share the view of reality held by society. The child is capable of considerable learning, including more than one language and words of simple songs and prayers.[101,102] That is, long before they can speak, children are initiated into their culture and speech by the language and words of their parents and significant caregivers.[103]

Examples of Educational Toys and Play for the Toddler

13–15 months

Toy telephone
Toy horse for rocking, rocking chair
Carriage or other toys for pushing and pulling
Household objects, such as pots or pans and unbreakable cups, or food cartons of various sizes for nesting and stacking
Pot lids for banging together
Wooden blocks of various sizes and shapes for stacking
Large plastic clothespins
Larger balls or stuffed animals
Toys that encourage acrobatic movement

16–18 months

Sandbox and toys that can be pushed through sand
Simple musical instruments, such as tambourine or drum
Large coloured beads
Jack-in-the-box
Equipment for blowing bubbles, with adult help

19–21 months

Rocking horse
Kiddie cars
Toys to take apart and fit together
Small rubber balls
Digging toys
Large crayons, large sheets of paper
Easy puzzles, with large and few pieces, colourful, pictures of animals, foods, and other objects in the environment, made of sturdy material or wood
Dirt for making mud pies
Big cardboard boxes to play hide and seek (self and others)

22–24 months

Kiddie lawn mower
Kitchen sets for make believe play, including toy utensils
Modelling clay
Construction blocks or sets
Action toys (e.g., toy trains, dump trucks, cars, and fire engines)
Old magazines that can be used to point out pictures and also torn up
Baskets, boxes, and tubes of various sizes have multiple uses in action and fantasy play
Containers (e.g., pots, pans) with lids

2–3 years

Dolls, male *and* female, various ethnicities, with accessories like clothing, strollers, baby bottle, feeding utensils
Beginner tricycle
Kiddie swimming pool
Mini-trampoline
Age-appropriate roller skates
Swing set, mini-basketball hoop
Dress-up clothes (parents' and older siblings' clothing no longer used) for male *and* female
Crayons, markers, finger paints, large sheets of paper
Colouring books, not too detailed in design
Easel or chalkboard and chalk
Kiddie cassette player and tapes
Kiddie woodworking bench

Note: Toys played with at an earlier age continue to be enjoyed, especially if they can be used in different ways or with different actions. Puppets and age-appropriate musical tapes and cloth or vinyl books should be available throughout toddlerhood.

The ability to speak words and sentences is not governed by the same higher centre that controls understanding. The child understands words before they are used with meaning, and some children develop adequate comprehension but cannot speak.[104]

Various theories explain language acquisition. Although behavioural or learning theory explains some language learning through receiving reinforcement for imitation of language sounds, the number of specific stimulus-response connections that would be necessary to speak even one language could not be acquired in a lifetime. Nor do behaviourists explain the sequence of language development, regardless of culture; however, learning principles can be used to modify acquired language deficits.[105]

Interactionist theory is used by most theorists to explain language development. Language develops through interaction between heredity, maturation, encounters with people and environmental stimuli, and life experiences. Humans are biologically prepared for language learning, but experience with the spoken word and with loving people who facilitate language acquisition is equally essential. Further, the child has an active role in learning language rather than a passive one. Adults modify their speech when talking to a child and the child is more attentive to simplified speech. Mothers and fathers use different conversational techniques to talk with the child, which in turn, teaches the child language in a broader way.[106] At York University in Toronto, researchers related mothers' scaffolding to their toddlers' vocabulary at 15 months. They concluded that the more scaffolding was associated with the toddler having a larger vocabulary.[107] Scaffolding refers to the structuring of a child's learning experience.[108]

Speech and language are major adaptive behaviours being developed during the second year. Speech enables the child to become more independent and to better make needs known. Speech is the mediation for thought processes. The greater the comprehension and vocabulary a child has, the further a child can go in cognitive processes. As the child and parents respond verbally and nonverbally to each other, the child learns attitudes and values and behaviours and ideas. The child first responds to patterns of sounds rather than to specific word sounds; if others speak indistinctly to the child, he or she will also speak indistinctly. The normal child will begin to speak by 14 months, although some children may make little effort to speak until after two years. By age three, children may still mispronounce more than half the sounds.

The toddler speaks in the present tense initially, using **syncretic speech,** in which *one word stands for a certain object, and has a limited range of sounds.* Single words represent entire sentences; for example, "go" means "I want to go." By 18 to 20 months he or she uses telegraphic speech, *two- to four-word expressions that contain a noun and verb and maintain word order,* such as "go play" and "go night-night." Variety on intonation also increases. A two-year-old will introduce additional words and say "I go play" or "I go night-night." Conversation with parents involves contraction and expansion. The *child shortens into fewer words what the parent says but states the main message* (**contraction**); the *parent elaborates on, uses a full sentence, and interprets what the child says* (**expansion**). Expansion helps the child's language development.[109] The toddler frequently says "no,"

perhaps in imitation of the parents and their discipline techniques, but may often do what is asked even while saying "no." Stuttering is common because ideas come faster than the ability to use vocabulary.

Recognizable language develops sequentially. See Table 8-4 for a summary of language and speech development.[110-114]

The toddler's speech is **autistic** because *vocalizations have specific meaning only to the child.* He or she plays with sounds and incorrectly produces the majority of consonant sounds.

Apparently the child learns to speak in a highly methodical way, breaking down language into its simplest parts and developing rules to put the parts together. Children proceed from babbling to one-word and two-word sentences, use of word order and plurals, use of negative sentences, and the importance of phonetics or a sound system. To communicate effectively, the child must learn not only the language and its rules, but also the use of social speech, which takes into account the knowledge and perspective of another person.[115] This begins in toddlerhood and continues to develop through childhood as the child gains interpersonal and social experiences.

CRITICAL THINKING

What are a few strategies to help the child use more words?

Teach parents that this is facilitated when they teach social language strategies to the child as they introduce him or her to life experiences. Through conversation with the family at mealtime and in other activities, vocabulary is enlarged, and the child learns family expressions that aid socialization. Mealtime provides a miniature society in which the toddler can feel secure in attempting to imitate speech. He or she gets positive reinforcement for speech efforts, especially for words that are selected, repeated frequently, and reinforced by eager parents. In addition, *being talked with, using adult words rather than baby talk frequently throughout the day, being read to, and having an opportunity to explore the environment increases the child's comprehension of words and rules of grammar as well as organization and size of vocabulary and use of word inflections.*[116] Researchers from Carleton University in Ottawa claim that shared book reading provides a rich source of linguistic stimulation for young children.[117] The findings from their two experiments suggest that storybook experiences during the preschool years (ages three to six) may be an important influence on the development of language skills for children.[118]

Language development requires a sense of security and verbal and nonverbal stimulation. For a child to speak, he or she must have a loving, consistent relationship with a parent or caretaker. Unless the toddler feels that this person will respond to his or her words, the toddler will not be motivated to speak. The toddler may not talk when separated from mother, such as during hospitalization or the first day at daycare. When being prepared for hospital procedures, the toddler needs simple and succinct explanations, with gestures pointing to the areas of the body being cared for, and verbal and physical displays of affection.

If a child is *delayed in speech,* carefully assess the child and family. Causes may include deafness or the inability to listen,

TABLE 8-4
Assessment of Language and Speech Development

Characteristics	1 Year	1¹/₂ Years	2 Years	2¹/₂ Years
		Age		
Language understanding and basic communication	Understands "no-no" inhibition; knows "bye-bye" and pat-a-cake; says "mama," "dada," or some similar term for caretakers	Understands very simple verbal instructions accompanied by gesture and intonation; identifies 3 body parts; points to 5 simple pictures; points for wants	Identifies 5 body parts; finds 10 pictures; obeys simple commands	Points to 15 pictures; obeys 2 or 3 simple commands
Appearance of individual sounds	10 vowels, 9 consonants in babbling and echoing	*p, b, m, h, w* in babbling		*t, d, n, k, g, ng* in words
Auditory memory imitation and repetition	Lalls; imitates sound; echoes or repeats syllables or some words (may not have meaning)		Meanings increasingly becoming associated with words	Repeats 2 digits; remembers 1 or 2 objects
Numerical size of vocabulary	1 or 2 words	Adds 10–20 words a week	50–300 words if consistently spoken to	400–500 words
Word type	Nouns	Nouns, action verbs, some adjectives	Nouns, verbs, adjectives, adverbs	Pronouns, "I"
Sentence length	Single word	Single words expanding to 3 or 4 words, noun and verb	2–5 words; elemental sentence	Basic sentence
Description of vocalization and communication	Babbling, lalling, echolalia (repeating sounds)	Leading, pointing, jargon, some words, intonations, gestures	Words, phrases, simple sentences	Developmental language problems first seen
Purpose of vocalization and communication	Pleasure	Attention getting	Meaningful social control; wish requesting	Interaction; express needs; convey yearnings
Speech content and style			Possessive "mine"; pronouns last grammar form learned; grammar depends on what is heard	
Percent intelligibility		20–25% for person unfamiliar with child	60–75%; poor articulation of some words	Vowel production—90%

Sources: Gormly, A., Lifespan Human Development (6th ed.). Fort Worth: Harcourt Brace College Publishers, 1997; Papalia, D., S. Olds, and R. Feldman, Human Development (7th ed.). Boston: McGraw-Hill, 1998; Seifert, K., R. Hoffnung, and M. Hoffnung, Lifespan Development. Boston: Houghton Mifflin, 1997; Wong, D., Whaley and Wong's Nursing Care of Infants and Children (6th ed.). St. Louis: C.V. Mosby, 1999.

mental retardation, emotional disturbance, maternal deprivation or separation from the parents, lack of verbal communication within the family and to the child, inconsistent or tangential responses to the child's speech, presence of multiple siblings, or parents anticipating the needs of the child before he or she has a chance to communicate them.[119,120]

Verbal interaction, an environment with a variety of objects and stimuli, and freedom to explore are crucial to help the young child use his or her senses and emerging motor skills and thereby are necessary to learn during the sensorimotor and pre-operational stages.

In Canada, the majority of Aboriginal peoples are adamant that language be promoted, protected, preserved, and practised, even at an early age.[121] Kirkness firmly states that language is the principal means by which culture is transmitted from one generation to another. That is, language is culture and culture is language.[122]

CRITICAL THINKING

In health care settings, how can you help to preserve Aboriginal language?

Emotional Development

The toddler is a self-loving, uninhibited, dominating, energetic little person absorbed in self-importance, always seeking attention, approval, and personal goals. Sometimes the toddler is cuddly and loving. At other times, he or she bites or pinches and looks almost happy, feeling no sense of guilt or shame. There is little self-control over exploratory or sadistic impulses. The toddler only slowly realizes that he or she cannot have everything desired and that some behaviour annoys others. He or she experiments with abandon in the quest for independence, yet becomes easily frightened and runs to the parent for protection, security, reassurance, and approval.

Because the toddler still relies so much on the parents and wants their approval, he or she learns to curb the negativism without losing independent drives, to cooperate increasingly, and to develop socially approved behaviour. Need for attention and approval is one of the main motivating forces in ego development and socialization.

The toddler often repeats performances and behaviour that are given attention and laughed at; he or she likes to perform for adults and pleases self as much as the audience. He or she has a primitive sense of humour, laughs frequently, especially at surprise sounds and startling incongruities, and laughs with others who are laughing and at his or her own antics. Parents should give sufficient attention but not make the child show off for an audience, verbally or physically, and they should not overstimulate with laughter or games. Further, adults must realize the child fears separation, strangers, darkness, sudden or loud noises, large objects and machines, and hurtful events such as traumatic procedures.

Developmental Crisis

According to Erikson, the psychosexual crisis for the toddler is autonomy versus shame and doubt.[123] **Autonomy** is *shown in the ability to gain self-control* over motor abilities and sphincters; to make and carry out decisions; to feel able to cope adequately with problems or get the necessary help; to wait with patience; to give generously or to hold on, as indicated; to distinguish between possessions or wishes of self and of others; and to have a feeling of good will and pride. Autonomy is characterized by the oft-heard statement, "Me do it." Mastery accomplished in infancy sets the basis for autonomy.

The toddler is demonstrating developing autonomy and maintaining a sense of security and control through the following behaviours:

1. Using negativism.
2. Displaying temper.
3. Dawdling.
4. Using rituals.
5. Exploring even when parents object.
6. Developing language skills; saying "no" although he or she may do as asked.
7. Increasing control over his or her body or situations.

Ritualistic behaviour is normal and peaks at about two-and-a-half years, especially at bedtime and during illness. Although autonomy is developing, emotions are still contagious. The toddler reflects others' behaviour and feelings. For example, if someone laughs or cries, he or she will imitate for no apparent reason.

Teach parents that reasonable limits help the toddler gain positive experiences and responses from others and build a sense of self and autonomy. Accepting the toddler's behaviours and allowing some self-depression and choice fosters autonomy.

CRITICAL THINKING

What type of ritualistic behaviours can the parents initiate when the toddler is ill?

Shame and doubt are felt if autonomy and a positive self-concept are not achieved.[124] **Shame** is *the feeling of being fooled, embarrassed, exposed, small, impotent, dirty, wanting to hide, and rage against self.* **Doubt** is *fear, uncertainty, mistrust, lack of self-confidence, and feeling that nothing done is any good and that one is controlled by others rather than being in control of self.*[125]

There is a limit to how exposed, dirty, mean, and vulnerable one can feel. If the child is pushed past the limit, disciplined or toilet trained too harshly, or abused, he or she can no longer discriminate about self, what he or she should be and can do. If everything is planned and done *for* and *to* the child, he or she cannot develop autonomy. The toddler's self-concept and behaviour will try to measure up to the expectations of parents and others, but there is no close attachment to an adult. The box entitled "Consequences of Shame and Doubt" outlines traits and behaviours of a child who develops stronger feelings of shame and doubt than of autonomy. Too much shaming does not develop a sense of propriety but rather a secret determination to get away with things.

Children in Crashes: Mechanisms of Injury and Restraint Systems

Motor vehicle crashes (MVCs) are the leading cause of injury, disability, and death in Canadian children. The objective of this study was to explore the levels of protection offered to children involved in motor vehicle collisions. This joint study by Children's Hospital of Eastern Ontario (CHEO) in Ottawa and Transport Canada was conducted in two phases. The retrospective phase from 1990 to 1997 involved analysis, in a series of 45 children after MVCs, by location of spinal injury versus seatbelt type. The second phase was a prospective study of 22 children injured in 15 MVCs. Interventions included a biomechanical assessment of the vehicle and its influence on the injuries sustained. The main outcome measurements were the nature and extent of injuries sustained, the vehicle dynamics, and associated occupant kinematics.

Results

The odds ratio of sustaining a spinal injury while wearing a two-point belt versus a three-point belt was 24, indicating a much higher incidence with a lap belt than a shoulder strap.

Conclusions

Proper seatbelt restraint reduces the morbidity in children involved in MVCs. Children under the age of 12 years should not be front seat passengers until the sensitivity of air bags is improved. Three-point pediatric seatbelts should be available for family automobiles to reduce childhood trauma in MVCs.

Practice Implications

1. Because all chance fractures in this study were associated with a poorly fitting lap belt, the ideal position for the belt is on the anterior inferior iliac spines.
2. Proper belt fit with a lap belt is sometimes impossible to achieve. This occurs when seat depth is greater than femur length, forcing the child into a slouched position. A booster seat allows better fit of the belt across the bony pelvis, using either two-point or three-point devices, preventing a slouched position.
3. The addition of a crotch strap would prevent submarining and maintain the belt on the pelvis in the younger child.
4. Airbags used as supplemental restraints have worked to prevent injury; they have also been implicated in its cause. For example, children have suffered injuries both directly from airbag inflation and indirectly by contact with the gear shift after being pushed into it. Therefore, children under 12 years should not be seated in the front passenger seat until airbags are rendered more sensitive to smaller occupants.

Source: Lapner, P.C., M. McKay, A. Howard, B. Gardner, A. German, and M. Letts, Children in Crashes: Mechanisms of Injury and Restraint Systems, Canadian Journal of Surgery, 44, no. 6 (2001), 445–449. Used with permission. © 2001 Canadian Medical Association.

8-2 BONUS SECTION IN CD-ROM

Research Abstract: Parental Sensitivity to Infants and Toddlers in Dual-Earner and Single-Earner Families

Consequences of Shame and Doubt

- Has difficulty with eating, digestion, elimination, sleep
- Has low self-esteem
- Has low frustration tolerance, gives up easily
- Is apathetic, withdrawn
- Is passive, too compliant, easily controlled or manipulated
- Is excessively negative, defiant
- Is impulsive
- Is physically overactive, aggressive
- Is angry about being controlled or manipulated by others
- Is stubbornly assertive, obstinate
- Has little sense of responsibility
- Is sneaky, wanting to get away with things
- Is compulsive
- Hoards
- Is overmeticulous or excessively messy

Discourage parents from creating an emotional climate of excessive expectations, criticism, blame, punishment, and over-restriction for the toddler because within the child's consciousness a sense of shame and doubt may develop that will be extremely harmful to further development. The child should not be given too much autonomy, or he or she will feel all-powerful. When a toddler fails to accomplish what he or she has been falsely led to believe could be achieved, the self-doubt and shame that result can be devastating. Aggressive behaviour results if the child is severely punished or if parents are aggressive. With the proper balance of guidance and discipline, the toddler gains a sense of personal abilities and thus has the potential to deal with the next set of social adjustments.

Toilet Training

Toilet training is a major developmental accomplishment and relates directly to the crisis of autonomy versus shame and doubt or to what Freudian theorists call the **anal stage.** Independence and autonomy (self-control), not cleanliness, are the critical issues in teaching the child to use the toilet. For the process to work, the parents must do little more than arrange for the child to use the toilet easily. The parent supports rather than acts as a trainer and is interested in the child, not just the act. The toddler is interested in the products he or she excretes. Toilet learning readiness should not be dictated by a child's chronological age. The child-oriented approach advocates that a child must be physiologically and psychologically ready to begin the process.[126] By the time the child reaches 18 months of age, reflex sphincter control has matured and the myelinization of extrapyramidal tracts has occurred; both processes are necessary for bowel and bladder control.[127]

In some cultures, the mother begins toilet training before the child is one year, and the child is expected to achieve dryness by 18 months. In other cultures, the child is not expected to be toilet trained until about five years of age.[128] The Canadian Paediatric Society recommends a child-oriented approach, where the timing and method of toilet training is individualized as much as possible.[129]

Parents and all caregivers should be prepared to begin toilet training by ensuring that time is set aside for the process and that the arrangements are suitable for the entire family. The process should not be initiated at a stressful time in the child's life (e.g., after a traumatic event or after the birth of a new sibling). Parents should be prepared emotionally for the unavoidable accidents that will occur before the process is completed.

A few signs of the child's toilet readiness include:

- Able to walk to the potty chair
- Able to remain dry for several hours in a row
- Able to follow one or two simple instructions
- Able to use expressive language skills to communicate the need to use the potty
- Desire for independence and control of bladder and bowel function[130]

Parents can facilitate a child's toilet training by:

- Deciding on what vocabulary to use
- Encouraging the child to inform the parent when he or she needs to void
- Praising the child and avoiding negative reinforcement and punishment
- Ensuring a consistent approach to toilet training from all caregivers[131]

If toilet training does not work, it is usually because the child is not ready. Further, if the child refuses to use the potty, a break from potty training should be taken for about one to three months. For a child with special needs, a consultation with a physician is warranted.[132]

CRITICAL THINKING

What other strategies can you teach parents to use if toilet training with their toddler does not work?

Body Image and Self-Concept Development

Body Image

Body image development gradually evolves as a component of self-concept. The toddler has a dim self-awareness, but with a developing sense of autonomy, he or she becomes more correctly aware of the body as a physical entity and one with emotional capabilities. The toddler is increasingly aware of pleasurable sensations in the genital area and on the skin and mouth and is learning control of the body through locomotion, toilet training, speech, and socialization.

Self-Concept

Self-concept is also made up of the *feelings about self, adaptive and defensive mechanisms, reactions from others, and one's perceptions of these reactions, attitudes, values, and many of life's experiences.*

The sense of self as a separate being continues to develop; the individuation process is complete between 24 and 36 months. When the child is able to sustain a mental image of the loved person who is out of sight, separation anxiety is resolved.[133]

As the child incorporates approval and disapproval, praise and punishment, gestures that are kind and forbidding, he or she forms an opinion about self as a person. Experiences of discomfort are first with mother and then are generalized to other people, and much behaviour becomes organized to avoid or minimize discomfort around others. Thus, he or she gradually evolves adaptive and defensive behaviours and learns what to do to get along with others. The **self-system** gradually develops as an *organization of experiences that exists to defend against anxiety and to secure satisfaction.*[134]

Self-awareness is demonstrated as the child says "mine" and "me" more often, beginning at about 18 to 24 months. The possessiveness with toys and inability to share that is typical of the two-year-old may be a reflection of greater awareness of self, not just selfishness. The action may actually be an attempt to be sociable with another child.[135]

The child is fully aware of reactions that convey approval, love, and security, and because these make him or her feel good, a concept of **good-me** forms. *He or she likes self because others do—the basis of a positive self-concept.* Reactions of disapproval or punishment from significant adults increase the child's anxiety, and if this cycle continues, **bad-me,** a *negative self-concept,* results. If negative reaction is never-ending, the child may evolve defensive behaviours such as denial that prevent noticing the negative evaluations. Some appraisals from others evoke severe discomfort or panic; these *feelings and awareness of the situation are repressed and dissociated from the rest of the personality,* forming the **not-me** part of the self. These are the *ideas, feelings, or body parts that later seem foreign to the person.* For example, severe toilet training or punishing the child for masturbating or touching the genitals may be so traumatic and panic producing that he or she becomes almost unaware of the genital area. Later the person does not include the lower half of the body or the genital area in self-drawings or does not speak of sexual matters; he or she may be very inhibited about toileting; and a disturbed sex identity may be evident through behaviour. The more feelings or life experiences that are dissociated, the more rigid the personality and the less aware of self he or she is in later life. Each person attempts to find ways to keep feelings of *good-me* and reduce the uncomfortable feelings elicited by the *bad-me.*[136]

The child's major caretaker should have a positive self-concept and feel good about being a mother (or father). If others in the family or if society debases the mothering one, there is injury to the child's self-esteem. Be mindful of body image and self-concept formation as you care for toddlers, for it determines their reaction. Only through repetitious positive input can you change a negative self-concept to one that is positive. By stimulating a positive self-image, you are promoting emotional health. Teach parents to provide an environment in which the child can successfully exercise skills such as running, walking, and playing and feel acceptance of his or her body and behaviour. Help them realize that as the child's autonomy develops so too will a more appropriate mental picture of his or her body and emotions.

Adaptive Mechanisms

Before the child is two years old, he or she is learning the basic response patterns appropriate for the family and culture; a degree of trust and confidence, or lack of it, in the parents; how to express annoyance and impatience and love and joy; and how to communicate needs.

The toddler begins to adapt to the culture because of **primary identification.** He or she *imitates the parents* and responds to their encouragement and discouragement. With successful adaptation, the child moves toward independence. Other major adaptive mechanisms of this era include repression, suppression, denial, reaction formation, projection, and sublimation.[137]

Repression *unconsciously removes from awareness the thoughts, impulses, fantasies, and memories of behaviour that are unacceptable to the self.* The *not-me* discussed earlier is an example and may result from child abuse. **Suppression** *differs from repression in that it is a conscious act.* For example, the child forgets that he or she has been told not to handle certain articles. **Denial** is *not admitting, even when warned, that certain factors exist,* for example, that the stove is hot and will cause a burn. **Reaction formation** is *replacing the original idea and behaviour with the opposite behaviour characteristics.* For example, the child flushes the toilet and describes feces as dirty instead of playing in them, thus becoming appropriately tidy. **Projection** occurs when *he or she attributes personal feelings or behaviours to someone else.* For example, if the babysitter disciplines toddler, he or she projects dislike for her by saying, "You don't like me." **Sublimation** is *channelling impulses into socially acceptable behaviour rather than expressing the original impulse.* For example, he or she plays with mud, finger paints, or shaving cream, which is socially acceptable, instead of playing with feces.

Teach parents that the child's adaptive behaviour is strengthened when he or she is taught to do something for self and permitted to make a decision *if that decision is truly his or hers to make.* If the decision is one that must be carried out regardless of the toddler's wish, it can best be accomplished by giving direction rather than by asking the child if he or she wants to do something.

Sexuality Development

Traditionally parents have handled sons and daughters differently during infancy, and the results became evident in toddlerhood.

Because parents encourage independent behaviour in boys and more dependency in girls, by 13 months the boy ventures farther from mother, stays away longer, and looks at or talks to his mother less than does the girl. The girl at this age is encouraged to spend more time touching and staying near mother than is the boy; however, the separation process later seems less severe for girls. Perhaps boys should be touched and cuddled longer.[138]

Boys play more vigorously with toys than do girls, and they play more with nontoys such as doorknobs and light switches. Yet basically there is no sexual preference for toys, although parents may enforce a preference. A boy responds with more overt aggression to a barrier placed between him and his mother at 13 months of age than a girl does. Boys show more exploratory and aggressive behaviour than girls, and this behaviour is encouraged by the father. The female remains attentive to a wide variety of stimuli and complex visual and auditory stimuli. The female demonstrates earlier language development and seems more aware of contextual relationships, perhaps because of the more constant stimulation from the mother.[139]

Primary identification, *imitation, and observation of the same-sexed parent,* contributes to sex identity. The child by 15 months is interested in his or her own and others' body parts. Both boys and girls achieve sexual pleasure through self-stimulation, although girls masturbate less than boys (possibly because of anatomic differences).

By 21 months the child can refer to self by name, an important factor in the development of identity. By two years of age, the child can categorize people into boy and girl and has some awareness of anatomic differences if he or she has had an opportunity to view them.[140]

By the end of toddlerhood, the child is more aware of his or her body, the body's excretions, and his or her actions, and he or she can be more independent in the first steps of self-care. Ability to communicate verbally expands to the point that he or she can ask questions and talk about sexual topics with parents and peers.

Help parents to understand the developing sexuality of their child and to be comfortable with their own sex identification and sexuality so that they can cuddle the child and answer questions. Help them understand that a wide variety of play experiences will prepare the child for adult behaviour and competence. They may talk through their concerns about a son's becoming a sissy if he plays with dolls or wears mother's high heels in dramatic play. Help parents realize that a daughter's playing with trucks does not mean she will become a truck driver.

CRITICAL THINKING

What types of play experiences may help the child to be comfortable with his or her own sexuality later in life?

Guidance and Discipline

Discipline is *guidance that helps the child learn to understand and care for self and to get along with others.* It is not just punishing, correcting, or controlling behaviour, as is commonly assumed.

Everything in the toddler's world is new and exciting and meant to be explored, touched, eaten, or sat on, including porcelain figurines from Spain or boiling water. In moving away from complete dependency, the toddler demonstrates energy and drive and requires sufficient restrictions to ensure physical and psychological protection and at the same time enough freedom to permit exploration and autonomy. Because mother must now set limits, a new dimension is added to the relationship established between mother and toddler. Before, mother met his or her basic needs immediately. With the toddler's increasing ability, freedom, and demands, the parent sometimes makes him or her wait or denies a wish if it will cause harm. The transition should be made in a loving, consistent, yet flexible manner so that the child maintains trust and moves in the quest for independence. Excessive limitations, overwhelming steady pressure, or hostile bullying behaviour might cause an overly rebellious, negativistic, or passive child. Complete lack of limitations can cause accidents, poor health, and insecurity.

Through guidance and the parent's reaction, the child is being socialized, learning what is right and wrong. Because the child cannot adequately reason, he or she must depend on and trust the parents as a guide for all activities. He or she can obey simple commands. Later, the child will be capable of internalizing rules and mores and will become self-disciplined as a result of having been patiently disciplined. Setting limits is not easy. Parents should not thwart the toddler's curiosity and enthusiasm, but they must protect him or her from harm. Parents who oppose the toddler's desire of the moment are likely to meet with anything from a simple "no" to a temper tantrum.

Teach parents the importance of constructive guidance and discipline. Temper tantrums result because the toddler hates being thwarted and feeling helpless. Once the feelings are discharged, the child regains composure quickly and without revenge. If temper tantrums, a form of negativism, occur, the best advice is to ignore the outburst; it will soon disappear. The parent's calm voice, expressing understanding of feelings and introduction of an activity to restore self-esteem are important to teaching self-control.

Because parents are sometimes confused about handling the toddler's behaviour, you can assist them by teaching some *simple rules for guiding the toddler*:[141]

- Provide an environment in which the child feels respected.
- Decide what is important and what is not worth a battle of will. For example, the child may not be wearing matched clothing but resists parental attempts to change. Avoid negativism and an angry scene by deciding that today it is all right for the child to wear an unmatched outfit.
- Changing the mind, pursuing an alternate activity, or letting the child have his or her way is not giving in, losing face, being a poor parent, or letting the child be manipulative. When limits are consistent, changing a direction of behaviour can be a positive learning experience for the child. The child is becoming aware of being a separate person, able to assert self and influence others.
- Remove or avoid temptations such as breakable objects within reach or candy that should not be eaten to avoid having to repeatedly say "no."
- Try not to ask open-ended questions for the child to decide about an activity when the decision is not really one the child can make.
- Consider limits as more than restrictions but also as a distraction *from* one prohibited activity to another in which

the child can freely participate. Distraction with alternatives or a substitute is effective with the toddler because attention span is short.
- Reinforce appropriate behaviour through approval and attention. The child will continue behaviour that gains attention, even if the attention is punitive, because negative attention is better than none to the child.
- Set limits consistently so that the child can rely on the parent's judgment rather than testing the adult's endurance in each situation.
- State limits clearly, concisely, simply, positively, and in a calm voice. For example, if the child cannot play with a treasured object, he or she should not be allowed to handle it. Say "Look with your hands behind your back" or "Look with your eyes, not your hands" rather than "Don't touch."
- Set limits only when necessary. Some rules promote a sense of security, but too many confuse the child.
- Provide a safe area where the child is free to do whatever he or she wants to do.
- Do not overprotect the child; he or she should learn that some things have a price such as a bruise or a scratch.
- Do not terminate the child's activity too quickly; tell him or her that the activity is ending.

Each situation will determine the extent of firmness or leniency needed. The toddler needs gradations of independence.

Moral-Spiritual Development

Birth through the toddler era might be termed the *pre-religious stage*. This label does not deny religious influences but simply points out that the toddler is absorbing basic intellectual and emotional patterns regardless of the religious conviction of the caretakers. The toddler may repeat some phrases from prayers while imitating a certain voice tone or body posture that accompanies those prayers. The child only knows that when he or she imitates or conforms to certain rituals, affection and approval come that add to the sense of identification and security. The "good" and "bad" are defined in terms of physical consequences to self.

Teach parents that the toddler can benefit from a nursery-school type of church program in which emphasis is on positive self-image and appropriate play and rest rather than on a lesson to learn. The toddler also needs to have others to imitate who follow the rules of society, and he or she needs rewards and reinforcement for good or desirable behaviour.

Developmental Tasks

Developmental tasks for the toddler may be summarized as follows:[142]

- Settling into healthy daily routines
- Mastering good eating habits
- Mastering the basics of toilet training
- Developing the physical skills appropriate to the stage of motor development
- Becoming a family member
- Learning to communicate efficiently with an increasing number of others

The constantly sensitive situation of the toddler, gaining autonomy and independence—at times overreaching and needing mother's help, at times needing the freedom from mother's protection—is one you can help parents understand. The child's future personality and health will depend partially on how these many opportunities are handled now. *Your role in teaching and support is critical.*

CRITICAL THINKING

What may be some consequences for the child who is unable to meet a few developmental tasks?

HEALTH CARE AND NURSING APPLICATIONS

Your role with the toddler and family has been discussed with each section throughout this chapter. The box entitled "Selected Nursing Diagnoses Related to the Toddler" lists some *nursing diagnoses* based on assessments that would be accomplished from knowledge presented in this chapter. Interventions include

your role modelling of caring behaviour to the toddler and family; parent and family education, support, and counselling; or direct care to meet the toddler's physical, emotional, cognitive, and social needs.

Although health professionals work with ill children in various settings, they also work with healthy children who receive care in daycare centres and preschools. It is important that the health professional recognizes the strengths in these children. Fostering the strengths assists the child to progress through the appropriate developmental tasks (see the box entitled "Wellness Nursing Diagnoses").[143]

SELECTED NURSING DIAGNOSES RELATED TO THE TODDLER*

Pattern 1: Exchanging
Altered Nutrition: More than Body Requirements
Risk for Infection
Risk for Injury
Risk for Suffocation
Risk for Poisoning
Risk for Trauma
Risk for Aspiration

Pattern 2: Communicating
Impaired Verbal Communication

Pattern 3: Relating
Impaired Social Interaction
Risk for Altered Parent/Child Attachment

Pattern 6: Moving
Impaired Physical Mobility

Pattern 7: Perceiving
Self-Esteem Disturbance
Sensory/Perceptual Alterations

Pattern 9: Feeling
Pain
Anxiety
Fear

---

* Other of the NANDA diagnoses are applicable to the ill toddler.

Source: North American Nursing Diagnosis Association, NANDA Nursing Diagnosis Definitions & Classification 1999–2000. *Philadelphia: North American Nursing Diagnosis Association, 1999.*

Wellness Nursing Diagnoses

- Progressive refining of motor skills
- Initiating a sense of autonomy
- Increase in language skills
- Increase in social interaction through imitation
- Increase in self-expression in play activities

Source: Stolte, K.M., *Wellness: Nursing Diagnosis for Health Promotion* (Chapter 6), Philadelphia: Lippincott-Raven, 1996.

INTERESTING WEBSITES

FIRST NATIONS CHILD & FAMILY CARING SOCIETY OF CANADA

http://www.fncfcs.com
The purpose of the Caring Society is to promote the well-being of all First Nations children, youth, families, and communities, with a particular focus on the prevention of, and response to, child maltreatment.

FIRST NATIONS RESEARCH SITE ONLINE JOURNAL

http://www.fncfcs.com/pubs/onlineJournal.html
The *First Peoples Child & Family Review* is a new, online journal, published jointly by the First Nations Research Site, Centre of Excellence for Child Welfare, and the First Nations Child and Family Caring Society of Canada. The purpose of the journal, to be published twice yearly from Summer 2004, is to "reach beyond the walls of academia" to promote child welfare research, practice, policy, and education from a First Nations/Aboriginal perspective.

CANADIAN PAEDIATRIC SOCIETY

www.cps.ca
This site has information on programs and issues related to children's health, including immunization, street smarts, healthy eating, childhood infections, choosing car seats, and injury prevention.

CANADIAN COALITION FOR IMMUNIZATION AWARENESS AND PROMOTION

http://www.immunize.cpha.ca

This site has information on types of immunization, schedules, and Canadian statistics on rates of immunization, as well as discussions of facts and myths related to the subject.

CHILDREN'S SAFETY ASSOCIATION OF CANADA

http://www.safekid.org/welcome.htm

Visit this site for information on a wide variety of safety topics.

SUMMARY

1. The toddler grows at a slower pace physically than the infant; but physical growth is steady and there is considerable gain in neuromuscular skills.

2. Emotionally, socially, and behaviourally, the toddler makes great strides in development during these two years.

3. The child gains control over basic physiologic processes, such as toileting; and gains competency in behaviour patterns.

Considerations for the Toddler and Family in Health Care

- Family cultural background and support systems for the family of the toddler
- Attachment behaviours of the parents; separation reactions of the toddler
- Parental behaviours that indicate difficulty with attachment or potential/actual abuse of the toddler
- Physical characteristics or patterns, such as eating, toilet training, sleep/rest, and play, that indicate health and are within age norms for growth
- Cognitive characteristics and behavioural or play patterns in the toddler that indicate age-appropriate norms for intellectual development
- Communication patterns and language development that indicate age-appropriate norms for the toddler
- Overall appearance and behavioural or play patterns in the toddler that indicate development of autonomy rather than shame and doubt, positive self-concept, sense of sexuality, and continuing age-appropriate emotional development
- Behavioural patterns that indicate the toddler is beginning moral-spiritual development
- Behavioural patterns and characteristics that indicate the toddler has achieved developmental tasks
- Parental behaviours that indicate knowledge about how to physically and emotionally care for the toddler
- Parental behaviours and communication approaches that indicate effective guidance of the toddler
- Evidence that the parents provide a safe and healthful environment and the necessary resources for the toddler
- Parental behaviours that indicate they are achieving their developmental tasks for this era

4. Developmental or autonomy tasks are achieved in his or her own unique way as parents and family members provide consistent love and guidance and adequate resources to foster physical, cognitive, emotional, social, and moral development.

5. The box entitled "Considerations for the Toddler and Family in Health Care" summarizes what you should consider in assessment and health promotion with the toddler.

6. The unique toddler characteristics of curiosity, impulsivity, advancement of motor skills beyond verbal and cognitive development, and assertion of will must be considered by parents and health care professionals in relation to safety and health promotion measures.

ENDNOTES

1. Begley, S., Your Child's Brain, *Newsweek,* February 19 (1996), 55–61.
2. LaRossa, R., Fatherhood and Social Change, *Family Relations,* 37 (1988), 451–457.
3. Papalia, D., S. Olds, and R. Feldman, *Human Development* (7th ed.). Boston: McGraw-Hill, 1998.
4. Dubeau, D., The Involved Father. *Transition Magazine,* 32, no. 2 (2002), 8–14.
5. Wong, D., *Whaley and Wong's Nursing Care of Infants and Children* (6th ed.). St. Louis: C.V. Mosby, 1999.
6. LaRossa, *op. cit.*
7. Gottlieb, L., and J. Bailles, Firstborn's Behaviors During a Mother's Second Pregnancy, *Nursing Research,* 44 (1995), 356–362.
8. Why Children Need Their Parents' Time, *AFA Journal,* April (1991), 17–18.
9. Bowlby, J., *Attachment and Loss, Vol. I: Attachment.* New York: Basic Books, 1969.
10. Schneider, B.H., L. Atkinson, and C. Tardif, Child-Parent Attachment and Children's Peer Relations: A Quantitative Review. *Developmental Psychology,* 37, no. 1 (2001), 86–100.
11. Pederson, D.R., and G. Moran, Expressions of the Attachment Relationship Outside of the Strange Situation. *Child Development,* 67 (1996), 915–927.
12. Pederson, D.R., K.E. Gleason, G. Moran, and S. Bento, Maternal Attachment Representations, Maternal Sensitivity, and the Infant–Mother Attachment Relationship. *Developmental Psychology,* 34, no. 5 (1998), 925–933.
13. Bowlby, *op. cit.*
14. *Ibid.*
15. *Ibid.*
16. *Ibid.*
17. *Ibid.*
18. Health Canada, *Mental Health Promotion, First Connections,* Website: http://www.hc-sc.gc.ca/hppb/mentalhealth/mhp/pub/fc/par_needtoknow.html, May 2004.
19. Onyskiw, J.E., Health and the Use of Health Services of Children Exposed to Violence in Their Families, *Canadian Journal of Public Health,* 93, no. 6 (2002), 416–420.
20. Kalk, C., and T. Namuth, When a Child's Silence Isn't Golden, *Newsweek (Special Issue),* Spring/Summer (1997), 23.
21. Seifert, K., R. Hoffnung, and M. Hoffnung, *Lifespan Development.* Boston: Houghton Mifflin, 1997.
22. Duvall, E., and B. Miller, *Marriage and Family Development* (6th ed.). New York: Harper & Row, 1986.
23. Bee, H., *Lifespan Development* (2nd ed.). New York: Longman, 1998.
24. Papalia et al., *op. cit.*

25. Seifert, *op. cit.*
26. Wong, *op. cit.*
27. *Ibid.*
28. Bee, *op. cit.*
29. Gormly, A., *Lifespan Human Development* (6th ed.). Fort Worth: Harcourt Brace College Publishers, 1997.
30. Papalia et al., *op. cit.*
31. Seifert, *op. cit.*
32. Indian and Inuit Health Committee, Canadian Paediatric Society, Growth Charts for Indian and Inuit Children. *Canadian Medical Association Journal,* 136, no. 1 (1987), 118–119.
33. Bee, *op. cit.*
34. Gormly, *op. cit.*
35. Lack, J., Turning on the Motor, *Newsweek (Special Issue),* Spring/Summer (1997), 26–27.
36. Papalia et al., *op. cit.*
37. Seifert, *op. cit.*
38. Wong, *op. cit.*
39. Papalia et al., *op. cit.*
40. Wong, *op. cit.*
41. Bee, *op. cit.*
42. Boynton, R., E. Dunn, and G. Stephens, *Manual of Ambulatory Pediatrics* (3rd ed.). Philadelphia: J.B. Lippincott, 1994.
43. Gormly, *op. cit.*
44. Papalia et al., *op. cit.*
45. Seifert, *op. cit.*
46. Papalia et al., *op. cit.*
47. Wong, *op. cit.*
48. *Ibid.*
49. *Ibid.*
50. *Ibid.*
51. *Ibid.*
52. *Ibid.*
53. *Ibid.*
54. *Ibid.*
55. *Ibid.*
56. Health Canada, First Nations and Inuit Health Branch, *Pediatric Clinical Practice Guidelines for Nurses in Primary Care,* Website: http://www.hc-sc.gc.ca/msb/fnihb, July 2004.
57. Hoole, A., C. Pickard, R. Ouimette, J. Lohr, and W. Powell. *Patient Care Guidelines for Nurse Practitioner* (5th ed.). Philadelphia: J.B. Lippincott, 1999.
58. *Ibid.*
59. *Ibid.*
60. *Ibid.*
61. *Ibid.*
62. *Ibid.*
63. *Ibid.*
64. *Ibid.*
65. Health Canada, *Office of Nutrition Policy and Promotion,* Website: http://www.hc-sc.gc.ca/hpfb-dgpsa/onpp-bppn/food_guide_preschoolers_e.html, June 2004.
66. *Ibid.*
67. *Ibid.*
68. Health Canada, *Using the Food Guide.* Ottawa: Minister of Health, 1997.
69. Williams, S., *Nutrition and Diet Therapy* (10th ed.). St. Louis: C.V. Mosby, 1995
70. Duyff, R., *The American Dietetic Association's Complete Food and Nutrition Guide.* Minneapolis: Chronimed Publishing, 1998.
71. Williams, *op. cit.*
72. Wong, *op. cit.*
73. Ibid.
74. Papalia et al., *op. cit.*
75. Seifert, *op. cit.*
76. *Ibid.*
77. Verzemnieks, I., Developmental Stimulation for Infants and Toddlers, *American Journal of Nursing,* 84, no. 6 (1984), 749–752.
78. Parents Canada, *Keeping Your Child Safe: Common Household Hazards,* Website: http://www.parentscanada.com/301/Keeping_Your_Child_Safe:_Common_Household_Hazards_.htm, July 2004.
79. Health Canada, Division of Childhood and Adolescence, *Home: Is Your Child Safe?* Website: http://www.hc-sc.gc.ca/dca-dea/allchildren_touslesenfants/she_security_e.html, May 2004.
80. Bee, *op. cit.*
81. Boynton et al., *op. cit.*
82. Hoole et al., *op. cit.*
83. Wong, *op. cit.*
84. Hockenberry, M.J., D. Wilson, M.L. Winkelstein, and N.E. Kline, *Wong's Nursing Care of Infants and Children, Seventh Edition.* St Louis: Mosby, 2003.
85. Onyskiw, *op. cit.*
86. Papalia et al., *op. cit.*
87. Seifert, *op. cit.*
88. Wadsworth, B., *Piaget's Theory of Cognitive and Affective Development: Foundations of Constructivism* (5th ed.). New York: Longman, 1996.
89. *Ibid.*
90. *Ibid.*
91. *Ibid.*
92. Papalia et al., *op. cit.*
93. Wadsworth, *op. cit.*
94. Mandler, J.M., A New Perspective on Cognitive Development in Infancy, *American Scientist,* 78 (1990), 236–243.
95. Aguiar, A., and R. Baillargeon, Eight-and-a-Half-Month-Old Infants' Reasoning About Containment Events, *Child Development,* 69, no. 3 (1998), 636–653.
96. Begley, *op. cit.*
97. Papalia et al., *op. cit.*
98. Begley, *op. cit.*
99. Lipari, J. Four Things You Need to Know about Raising Baby, in K.L. Freiberg, ed., *Annual Editions: Human Development* (31st ed., pp. 34–35). Guilford, CN, McGraw-Hill/Dushkin, 2003/2004.
100. *Ibid.*
101. Begley, *op. cit.*
102. Cowley, G., The Language Explosion, *Newsweek (Special Issue),* Spring/Summer (1997), 16–17, 22.
103. Craig, G.J., M.D. Kermis, and N.L. Digdon, *Children Today* (2nd Canadian ed.). Toronto: Prentice Hall. 2001.
104. Papalia et al., *op. cit.*
105. *Ibid.*
106. Papalia et al., *op. cit.*
107. Stevens, E., J. Blake, G. Vitale, and S. MacDonald, Mother-Infant Object Involvement at 9 and 15 Months: Relation to Infant Cognition and Early Vocabulary, *First Language,* 18 (1998), 203–222.
108. Bee, H., D. Boyd, and P. Johnson, *Lifespan Development* (Canadian Study ed.). Toronto: Pearson Education Canada, 2005.
109. Papalia et al., *op. cit.*
110. Cowley, *op. cit.*
111. Gormly, *op. cit.*
112. Kalk and Namuth, *op. cit.*
113. Papalia et al., *op. cit.*
114. Seifert, *op. cit.*
115. Papalia et al., *op. cit.*
116. Bossard, J.H.S., and E.S. Boll, *The Sociology of Child Development* (4th ed.). New York: Harper & Row, 1966.
117. Senechal, M., J-A. LeFevre, E. Hudson, and E. P. Lawson, Knowledge of Storybooks as a Predictor of Young Children's Vocabulary, *Journal of Educational Psychology,* 88, no. 3 (1996), 520–536.

118. *Ibid.*

119. Kalk and Namuth, *op. cit.*

120. Wong, *op. cit.*

121. Kirkness, V.J., The Critical State of Aboriginal Languages in Canada, *Canadian Journal of Native Education,* 22, no. 1 (1998), 93–107.

122. *Ibid.*

123. Erikson, E.H., *Childhood and Society* (2nd ed.). New York: W.W. Norton, 1963.

124. *Ibid.*

125. *Ibid.*

126. Community Paediatrics Committee, Canadian Paediatric Society, Toilet Learning: Anticipatory Guidance with a Child-Oriented Approach, *Paediatrics and Child Health,* 5, no. 6 (2000), 333–335.

127. *Ibid.*

128. Andrews, M., and J. Boyle, *Transcultural Concepts in Nursing Care* (3rd ed.). Philadelphia: Lippincott, 1999.

129. Community Paediatrics Committee, Canadian Paediatric Society, *op. cit.*

130. Canadian Child Care Federation, *Flexible Toilet Learning: A Child-Oriented Approach,* Website: http://www.cccf-fcsge.ca/practice/health%20watch/toiletlearning_en.htm, May 2004.

131. *Ibid.*

132. *Ibid.*

133. Gormly, *op. cit.*

134. Sullivan, H.S., *Interpersonal Theory of Psychiatry.* New York: W.W. Norton, 1953.

135. Gormly, *op. cit.*

136. Sullivan, *op. cit.*

137. Papalia et al., *op. cit.*

138. *Ibid.*

139. *Ibid.*

140. Papalia et al., *op. cit.*

141. *Ibid.*

142. Duvall and Miller, *op. cit.*

143. Stolte, K.M. *Wellness: Nursing Diagnosis for Health Promotion.* Philadelphia: Lippincott-Raven, 1996.

Chapter 9

ASSESSMENT AND HEALTH PROMOTION FOR THE PRESCHOOLER

If the child is safe, the people are safe.

Marian Wright Edelman

OBJECTIVES

STUDY OF THIS CHAPTER WILL ENABLE YOU TO:

1. Compare and contrast the family relationships between the preschool and previous developmental eras.

2. Differentiate among the types of influence exerted upon the preschooler by parents, siblings, and non–family members.

3. Explore, with the family, the expected developmental tasks for the child, and consider the best ways to help the child meet them.

4. Evaluate the values and services available to parents and the child from several daycare centres and nursery schools.

5. Discuss the necessary adaptations required by the preschooler in each daycare and nursery school setting.

6. Assess physical, motor, mental, language, play, and emotional characteristics of a three-, four-, and five-year-old.

7. Describe (1) the health needs of the preschooler, including nutrition, exercise, rest, safety, and immunization, and (2) measures to meet these needs.

8. Examine with parents their role in contributing to the preschooler's cognitive, language, self-concept, sexuality, moral-spiritual, emotional development, and physical health.

9. Analyze measures to diminish the trauma of hospitalization for this age group.

10. Explore with parents effective ways to enhance the development of the preschooler through communication, guidance, and discipline.

11. Describe (1) the developmental crisis of initiative versus guilt, (2) the adaptive mechanisms commonly used to promote a sense of initiative, and (3) the implications of this crisis for later maturity.

12. Examine the developmental tasks and your role in promoting the achievement of them.

13. Demonstrate the process of working effectively with a preschooler in a nursing situation.

In this chapter development of the preschool child and the family relationships are discussed. *Nursing and health care responsibilities for health promotion for the child and family are discussed throughout the chapter. The information regarding normal development and needs serves as a basis for assessment. Your role is to use information on assessment and health promotion in health education counselling of families, and care of the preschooler in communities and various other health settings.*

The **preschool years,** *ages three through five,* along with infancy and the toddler years, form a crucial part of the person's life. The preschool child is emerging as a social being. He or she participates more fully as a family member but begins to grow slowly out of the family, spending more time in association with **peers,** who are *children of the same age.* Physical growth is slowing, but the body is well proportioned and control and coordination are increasing. Emotional and intellectual growth is progressively apparent in the ability to form mental images; and the expression of self occurs in a range of emotions. The child can identify with the play group and follow rules; control primitive *(id)* impulses; and begin to be self-critical with references to a standard set by others *(superego formation).*

Explore with parents ways to separate themselves from their growing child and how to revise decisions about how much free expression and initiative to permit the child while setting certain limits. Thus gradually promoting more independence during the preschool years allows both the child and parents to be more comfortable about the separation that occurs when he or she goes to school.

FAMILY DEVELOPMENT AND RELATIONSHIPS

The family unit, regardless of the specific form, is important to the preschooler, and in turn, the preschooler affects relationships within the family by his or her behaviour. The close relationship of the baby to the mother and father gradually expands to include other significant adults living in the home, siblings, and other relatives, and they will have some effect on the child's personality.

There are several *dominant parenting styles:*[1–4]

- **Authoritarian:** *Demanding, impose many rules, expect instant obedience, and do not give reasons for rules.* No consideration given to the child's view. Rely on physical punishment to gain compliance.

- **Authoritative:** *Exert control, demanding but responsive to and accepting of child.* Give reasons for rules. Expect mature behaviour. Encourage independence and child meeting own potential. Maintain balance between control, socialization, and individualization.

■ **Permissive:** *Accepting of and responsive to child. Rarely make demands or exert control. Indulgent.* Encourage child to express feelings and impulses.

■ **Neglectful:** *Low in demand and control but also low in acceptance and responsiveness. Uninvolved* in child's upbringing. May be rejecting to child. So involved in own needs and problems that they have no energy to set and enforce rules.

■ **Intimidated:** *Lack ability to be firm with child. No control over child,* but frustrated or angry with self and child's behaviour.

■ **Secure:** *Confident in own childrearing. Accept self and child.* Realize they will make mistakes and are willing to change. Assume they and child will cope successfully.

CRITICAL THINKING

What effects do you think that the parenting styles of your own parents had on your development?

Parenting behaviours vary with the culture. In addition, the child's temperament affects the parent's behaviour.[5,6] A cross-cultural study was conducted regarding child-rearing attitudes and behavioural inhibition in Chinese and Canadian toddlers. The Chinese toddlers were significantly more inhibited than were their Canadian counterparts. In the Canadian sample, inhibition was associated positively with mothers' punishment orientation and negatively with mothers' acceptance and encouragement of achievement. In the Chinese sample, however, the directions of the relations were opposite. Child inhibition was associated positively with mothers' warm and accepting attitudes and negatively with rejection and punishment orientation. In summary, the researchers claim that the results indicate the existence of different adaptation meanings of behavioural inhibition across cultures.[7]

Research has indicated that maternal interaction patterns differ on the basis of the child's medical history. Mothers had developed a pattern of higher involvement with the child if the child had been preterm or at high-risk, medically, at birth, than with the child who was normal and healthy at birth. Mothers of very ill preterm babies demonstrated high-quality and appropriate involvement that did not contribute to the child's developmental delay. Generally speaking, all of the children who were most competent in cognition, linguistics, and problem solving had mothers with higher interaction scores, who were more responsive, and who used appropriate control styles. The qualities of maternal interaction patterns appear to diminish adverse effects of medical morbidity or maternal education deficits.[8] Canadian researchers Magill-Evans and Harrison concluded that early parent–child interactions contributed to the child's development in both healthy preterm and full-term infants.[9]

Mothers' and fathers' interactions with their child are similar in many aspects. For example, Harrison, Magill-Evans, and Benzies concluded that mothers and fathers of infants aged two to 12 months were equally sensitive to their infant's cues. However, fathers were less contingent in interaction with their

infants.[10] In another study, Broom used three subscales of the Nursing Child Assessment Scale (NCATS) with first-time parents. The results did not show differences between white, well-educated, middle-class mothers and fathers when their child was three months old.[11] Meanwhile, Harrison, Magill-Evans, and Sadoway observed fathers of 49 Canadian children (ages 13 to 24 months) interacting with their child at home using the NCATS. They concluded that when compared with the NCATS reference data for 164 mothers of similar ethnicity and marital status with similar–aged children, mothers were more responsive than fathers in the interactions.[12] It appears that to reach confident generalizations further research is warranted regarding fathers' interaction with their children. The possibility of comparing maternal and paternal traits seems to have led to a somewhat negative image of fathers. Dubeau states that (1) future research must focus on fathers' strengths and motivations and (2) we must interpret these traits in a different cultural and historical context than we do for mothers.[13]

CRITICAL THINKING

What is one research question you might pose regarding fathers and their interaction with their young child?

Effect of parenting styles on preschoolers and their parents can be divided into several categories of behaviour as depicted in the box entitled "Effect of Parenting Style on Child's Behaviour."[14–16]

Relationships with Parents

The preschooler's early emotional and physical closeness or attachment to the parents now leads to a different kind of relationship with them. This is the stage of the **family triangle,** or what Freud called the **Oedipal** or **Electra complex.**[17]

During this stage, *positive, possessive, or love feelings are directed mainly toward the parent of the opposite sex, and the parent of the same sex may receive competitive, aggressive, or hostile feelings.* Help parents recognize these feelings as developmentally normal. During this phase the child is establishing a basis for his or her own eventual adult relationship; the parents' positive response is crucial.[18]

Help the parents feel comfortable with the sexuality of the child and with their own sexuality so that they are neither threatened by nor ignore or punish the child's remarks and behaviour.

In the preschool years, **secondary identification** *occurs through introjection or internalization of attitudes, feelings, values, and actions about sexual, moral, social, and occupational roles and behaviour.*[19–21]

The child watches and listens to the parents and demonstrates what they do and say in his or her own unique way, depending on the child's perceptions. Through this process of internalization and behaving, the child develops an inner parent, which is the core of the *superego* or *conscience.* Through identification, the child also gains a sexual or gender identity.

Attachment continues to develop in the preschool years. The attachment that began with parents in infancy was extended to others in toddlerhood. Parallel and then cooperative play

Effect of Parenting Style on Child's Behaviour

Parent's Behaviour	Child's Behaviour
Controlling, detached, rather than loving and warm	Discontented, withdrawn, moody, unhappy, easily annoyed, aimless, lacks self-reliance, lacks confidence in own decision-making abilities
More controlling, demanding, loving overtly than most parents	Friendly, self-controlled, self-reliant, cheerful, socially responsible, cooperative with adults and peers
Highly permissive, warm and friendly	Low levels of self-reliance and self-control, rebellious, low levels of independence and achievement orientation
Relatively demanding, loving	Self-reliant, more independent, better adjusted
Warm, loving, expect a great deal of child at early age, demanding of child, show interest in child's activities	Highly creative, high need for achievement, independent, highly competent, works toward set goals

with other children is a continuation of the attachment learned in infancy. By age three, the child realizes that others may not think like him or her, but the child wants to interact. Thus the child learns to share or play, even when there are differences. The four- or five-year-old has a best friend, likes to participate in many social activities, and plays with other peers because of the earlier experiences with attachment and parental guidance with socialization. In the process, a child learns to like and accept self, and then others. Moss and her associates examined a sample of 121 French-Canadian school-age children. The contributions of attachment, maternal reported stress, and mother–child interaction to the prediction of teacher-reported behaviour problems were examined. The researchers' results support the importance of attachment in explaining school-age adaptation and validity of attachment coding for children of this age.[22]

It seems reasonable to conclude that a nonresponsive, neglectful, or abusive environment produces angry, depressed, or hopeless children by age two, three, or four years.

CRITICAL THINKING

What events in a preschooler's life might be associated with insecure attachments?

Parental nurturing cannot be overemphasized. If the child has been neglected in infancy, brain scans show that the brain region responsible for emotional attachments has never fully developed. *Without early close relationships, there may be biological, as well as learned, reasons for the child to be unable later to form relationships and caring social behaviour.*

Relationships in One-Parent or Stepparent Families

In the *one-parent or stepparent family* (or in the abusive home), achieving identification may be more difficult. In the *one-parent home,* the little girl raised by a male may not fit in with other girls at school or may not feel comfortable and relate to women later in life. The boy raised by a woman may relate better to women than to men. The 2001 Census collected information for the first time on the numbers of same-sex couples across Canada.[23] Today, gay and lesbian parents are becoming more visible in society, and they are being seen at child-care centres, soccer fields, and school concerts. Research has made it clear that fears about the negative outcomes for children raised in gay and lesbian families have been refuted.[24] However, despite these findings, gay and lesbian couples and their children continue to be confronted by public and private homophobia.

CRITICAL THINKING

How can homophobia be considered in the health care system? What health promoting strategies might be implemented to address homophobia?

Let us shift our consideration from children of gay and lesbian families to children of divorced parents. Children of divorced parents manifest higher levels of depression and lower levels of self-esteem compared to samples of children from intact parents. Interestingly, children who hold irrational beliefs and feelings about divorce are most likely to develop behavioural and psychological problems.[25] Recently, the study of the impact of divorce on young children has expanded to consider the longer-term consequences of divorce through longitudinal studies of young adult children. Another recent investigation has looked at studies of intergenerational ties between young adult children and their divorced parents.[26,27] In one example, Connidis, from the University of Western Ontario, conducted a qualitative study involving 86 adults from ten three-generation families to illustrate the extensive reach of divorce across time and generations. She concluded that multiple voices from three generations demonstrate (1) the complexity of family relationships over time and (2) the reverberation of life course transitions of individuals throughout family networks.[28]

Sexual or Gender Identity through Parental Relationships

Teach parents that sexual or gender identity is reinforced through name, clothing, colour of clothing and room, behaviour toward, and expectations of the child. The innumerable contacts between the child and significant adults contribute to sexual and gender identification and should occur in this developmental period.[29–31]

The sex of the child is a great determinant in personality development because each sex has different tasks and roles in every culture. However, you cannot predict the child's personality traits by knowing only the sex. Achieving a firm identity as a man or woman is basic to emotional stability and ego development, and cultural expectations and influences are important. These are expressed by the family socialization.[32]

Explain parental reactions to and expectations of the child. Help them clarify their feelings and behaviour and convey their respect to the child, regardless of sex. The sex assigned to the child by significant adults may be physically realistic or unrealistic. The feelings and needs of the parents strongly influence their reactions to the child so that sex assignment within the family can override biological factors.

This phase brings the development of sexuality to the foreground. The child is interested in the appearance and function of his or her own body, in variations of clothing and hairstyles (the child at first assigns sex on this basis), and in the bodies of others, especially in their sex organs.[33] Children at this age feel a sense of excitement—first, in seeing and feeling their own and others' nude bodies and, second, in exposing themselves to other children or adults.

Teaching Sexuality

Teaching sexuality to the child is enmeshed in the acquisition of sex identity and positive feelings about the self. The basis for sex education begins prenatally with the parents' attitudes about the coming child. Parents and other caretakers, including health care providers, continue daily thereafter to form attitudes in the child and impart factual knowledge in response to questions.

Because of the child's consuming curiosity, he or she asks many questions: Will the man in the television come out? How do I tie my shoes? Why is that lady's tummy so big? What is lightning? These questions are originally asked with equal curiosity. The adult's response will determine into what special category the child places questions about sex.

For example, you can teach parents that it may be beneficial to reward the question when the child asks "Where did I come from?" by stating, "That is a good question, I am glad you asked me." It is critical for parents to comprehend that the child's ability to think and understand is influenced by the level of his or her development. Parents need not explain everything at once. Timing is important.[34] Although talking about sexuality with children can cause some anxiety for parents, it is usually well worth the effort. Such discussions tend to bring the child closer to the parents; and hopefully they will show the child that they are able to come to the parent when they need to talk.[35]

Although sex education must be tailored to the individual child's needs and interests and to the cultural, religious, and family values, the following suggestions are also applicable to all children and can be shared with parents:

- Recognize that education about the self as a sexual person is best given by example in family life through parents' showing respect and love for the self, mate, and the child.
- Understand that the child who learns to trust others and to give and receive love has begun preparation for satisfactory adulthood, marriage, and parenthood.
- Observe the child at play; listen carefully to statements of ideas, feelings, and questions and ask questions to understand better his or her needs.
- Respond to the child's questions by giving information honestly, in a relaxed, accepting manner, and on the child's level of understanding. Avoid isolated facts, myths, or animal analogies. The question, "Where does baby come from?" could be answered, "Mommy carried you inside her body in a special place," rather than saying "The stork brought baby," "Baby was picked up at the hospital after a special order," or "God makes babies." Religious beliefs can be worked into the explanation while acknowledging human realities.
- Teach the child anatomic names rather than other words for body parts and processes. Parents may hesitate to do this because they do not want the child to blurt out *penis* or *vagina* in public. Parents can teach the child that certain topics such as sexual and financial matters are discussed in the home, just as certain activities such as urinating are done in private.
- Grabbing the genitals and some masturbation are normal. Children explore their bodies, especially body parts not easily seen and that give pleasurable sensations when touched. Masturbation is acceptable to many families if it occurs in the home. The child should be taught that this is not normal behaviour in public.

- Playing doctor or examining each other's body parts is normal for preschool children. Parents should not overreact and should calmly affirm that they want the children to keep their clothes on while they play. Diversion from "playing doctor" is useful. If children seem to be using each other in a sexual way, they should be instructed that this is not acceptable.

- Realize that sex education continues throughout the early years. The child's changing self motivates the same or different questions again and again. Remain open to his or her ongoing questions. Explanation about reproduction may begin with a simple statement, for example: "A man and a woman are required to be baby's father and mother. Baby is made from the sperm in the daddy's body and an egg in the mother's body." A simple explanation of sperm and egg would be needed. Later the child can be given more detail.

CRITICAL THINKING

How can you respond to the question, "How does the baby get started?"

Relationships with Siblings

An attachment for the child that began with the parents extends to siblings in late infancy and continues to deepen during the toddler and preschool years. Often parents are emotionally warmer to subsequent children after the firstborn. Possibly they feel more experienced and relaxed after the first birth. In the following discussion, you should realize that the relationships described could occur at other developmental eras in childhood, but in the preschool years siblings begin to make a very definite impact.[36–39]

The preschool child often has **siblings,** *brothers or sisters,* either younger or older, so that family interaction is complex with many **dyads,** *groups of two people.* Siblings become increasingly important in directing the child's early development, partly because of their proximity but also because the parents change in their role with each additional child. Downey and Condron analyzed a sample of kindergartners. They endeavoured to replicate the often-noted negative relationship between the number of siblings and cognitive outcomes. They then demonstrated that this pattern does not extend to social skills. These researchers concluded that the findings were consistent with the view that children negotiate peer relationships better when they grow up with at least one sibling.[40] On the other hand, Mendelson, Aboud, and Lanthier, from McGill University in Montreal, found that popular kindergartners tended to feel positively about, and to identify with, a sibling; and if they had an older sibling, the sibling tended to report high companionship. In contrast, kindergartners who rated a same-sex friendship, or who were observed to be friendly with a same-sex friend, tended not to feel positively about a same-sex sibling. Interestingly, if they had an older sibling, the sibling tended to report low companionship.[41] A question that arises is what are the reasons for positive and negative links between the preschooler and the sibling?

The sibling may be part of a multiple birth: twins, triplets, or more. Identical twins share traits, emotional bonds, and pain and communicate with each other in their own language in uncanny or mysterious ways, often when they are great distances apart. Studies of identical twins who are reared separately in different environments can help to sort out the relative influence of heredity and environment. Twins seem to think about each other more than other siblings, so some of the ESP-like communication or experiences may be coincidence. Yet the extreme intimacy can be pathologic; there may be jealousy of each other or a symbiotic interdependence that interferes with identity formation of each individual. For the parents, raising twins creates a delicate balance. Refer to Chapter 4 for more information on multiple births.

Preschooler and New Baby

The arrival of a new baby changes life: the preschooler is no longer the centre of attention but is expected by the parents to delight in the baby. It is important for parents to prepare the young child (toddler or preschooler) for a new arrival (Figure 9–1). Although a space of three to four years is ideal, such ideal spacing does not always occur.

When pregnancy is apparent, there are some ways for parents to prepare the older child:

- Share the anticipation in discussions and planning. Let the child feel fetal movements. Show the child a picture of when he or she was a newborn. Talk about what he or she needed as a baby and the necessary responsibilities. Read books that explain reproduction and birth on his or her level.

- Include the child as much as possible in activities such as shopping for furniture for the baby or decorating baby's

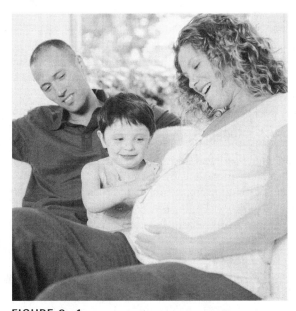

FIGURE 9–1

As birth approaches, parents can help prepare the preschooler for the arrival of the new sibling.

room. The preschool child likes to feel important, and being a helper enhances this feeling.

■ Accept that the child may act out, regress, or express dependency or separation anxiety during the pregnancy as well as after the new baby arrives.

■ Have the child attend sibling preparation classes, if available. Encourage relatives and friends to bring a small surprise gift for the older child when they visit and bring a gift for the baby. Have them spend time with the older child also, rather than concentrating only on the baby.

■ Prepare child to be with mother during birth, if family considers this appropriate and if permitted by birthing centre. Have the child visit mother and baby at the hospital, if rules permit, after delivery, or the older child can talk to mother by phone.

Accepting the family's affection toward the baby is difficult for the firstborn, and jealousy is likely to occur if more attention is focused on the baby than on him or her. The following behaviour may result:

1. The preschooler may regress, overtly displaying a need to be babied. He or she may ask for the bottle, soil self, have enuresis, lie in the baby's crib, or demand extra attention.
2. The child may harm the baby, directly or indirectly, through play or handling baby roughly.
3. He or she may appear to love the baby excessively, more than is normal.
4. The child may show hostility toward the mother in different ways: direct physical or verbal attacks, ignoring or rejecting her, or displacing anger onto the daycare, nursery, or Sunday school teacher.

Teach parents that these outward behaviours and the underlying feelings should be accepted, for they are better handled with overt loving behaviour than repressed through punishment. *Jealousy can be handled by the parents in a variety of ways:*

1. Tell the child about the pregnancy but not too far in advance, because a young child has a poor concept of time.
2. Involve him or her in preparing for the new baby. Although the preschooler may have to give up a crib, getting him or her a new big bed can seem like a promotion rather than a loss.
3. Convey that the child is loved as much as before, provide a time for him or her only, and give as much attention as possible.
4. Emphasize pleasure in having the child share in loving the new arrival and give increasing responsibility and status without overburdening him or her.
5. Encourage the child to talk about the new situation or express hostility in play.
6. Reading stories about feelings of children with new siblings can help the child express personal feelings.

There is other effective advice you can give about ways to handle jealous behaviour:

1. Do not leave the preschooler alone with the baby.
2. Give him or her a pet or doll to care for as mother cares for the baby.

3. Encourage the child to identify with the parents in helping to protect the baby because he or she is more grown up.
4. Avoid overemphasis of affection for the baby.

Older Sibling and Preschooler

The older sibling in the family who is given much attention for accomplishments may cause feelings of envy and frustration as the preschooler tries to engage in activity beyond his or her ability to get attention also. If the younger child can identify with the older sibling and take pride in the accomplishments while simultaneously getting recognition for his or her own self and abilities, the child will feel positive about self. If the younger child feels defeated and is not given realistic recognition, he or she may stop emulating the older sibling and regress instead. In turn, the older sibling can be helpful to the younger child if he or she does not feel deprived or is not reprimanded too much because of the preschooler.

Explore sibling relationships with parents and present suggestions for preventing conflicts. Often positive feelings exist between siblings. Quarrels are quickly forgotten if parents do not get overly involved. Because siblings have had a similar upbringing, they have considerable empathy for each other, similar values, similar superego development, and related perceptions about situations. Sibling values may be as important as the parents' values in the development of the child. *Often recognition and other feelings of the sibling are of such importance to the child that he or she may conceal ability rather than move into an area in which the sibling has gained recognition, or may engage in activity to keep the sibling from being unhappy.* Children tend to learn to develop roles, such as "the boss" or "the angry monster," or they regulate space among themselves to avoid conflicts. Other problems can arise if conflictual behaviour is given undue attention, or if the children are manipulated against each other by the significant adults.

A warm sibling relationship and play promotes a definition of self, helps the child learn to take others' perspectives, and enhances the child's ability to form relationships later because he or she learned to cooperate, compete, negotiate, and be sociable.[42]

CRITICAL THINKING

What interpersonal skills can the preschooler gain from the presence of older brothers and sisters?

Relationship with Grandparents

According to Rosenthal and Gladstone, grandparenting is a complex social process, which carries different types of meanings for grandparents.[43] This process is reflected both in the feelings that grandparents have toward their grandchildren and in the ways they interact with their grandchildren. Sometimes the relationship with the grandparent is deeper than with either parent, especially if the parents (1) are abusive or neglectful, (2) are busily employed professionals, (3) travel a great deal as part of a job, or (4) have separated or divorced.

Grandparents participate in different types of activities with their grandchildren and are resources to them in both instrumental and symbolic ways.[44] They serve as babysitters and pass down traditions whereby the child learns about "olden days," family history, the meaning of old pictures and objects, and the child's own roots. Grandparents are ideal mentors if they take the time and trouble: the child can learn to fix, to build, and to create. Grandparents provide spiritual sustenance to children of indifferent parents and answer questions about God.[45] Interesting books and courses are available to help grandparents to develop a sense of competency in their role.[46] An example is that grandparents may be taught the importance of boundary issues regarding "parenting" limits.

Nurses practise in many settings, such as pediatric units in hospitals or community health clinics, where they may encounter grandparents who are raising grandchildren. It is important to be aware of the issues that the grandparents face and to conduct appropriate assessments of the needs of the grandparents, the children, and the home.[47]

A growing number of grandparents are losing contact with their grandchildren as a result of parental divorce, conflict between parents, death of an adult child, or adoption of a grandchild after remarriage. After divorce, the grandparent may wish to be the child's legal custodian but may not be permitted by his or her own child or the courts. Increasingly, in cases of divorce, grandparents are seeking legal means to ensure visitation rights and sometimes to gain custody.[48] Further, recent trends in fertility among today's young adults may possibly result in slightly lower percentages of individuals experiencing grandparenthood in the future. It does seem apparent, however, that most people will still have grandchildren.[49]

CRITICAL THINKING

How do grandchildren benefit their grandparents?

CONTROVERSY DEBATE

Grandmother as Parent

Jody is a preschooler who started care with you yesterday on the pediatric unit. At that time you met Jody's grandmother, Mrs. Jones, who informed you that because of her daughter's recent separation from her husband, she will be taking full parenting responsibilities for the next few months. During your interaction with Mrs. Jones, you learned that she has recently had a mastectomy. She also informed you that Jody loves to be picked up and cuddled often. It is clear to you that Mrs. Jones enjoys a deep and emotional closeness with Jody.

You wonder whether or not Mrs. Jones has received discharge teaching regarding lifting activities.

1. Design the plan of action you will take with Mrs. Jones regarding her recent surgery.

2. Because of Mrs. Jones's emotional closeness with Jody, how will you address the matter of "taking full parental responsibilities"?

Influence of Other Adults and Non-Family Members

Help parents realize that other people may be significant to the child, depending on frequency and duration of contact, warmth of the relationship, and how well the parents meet the child's needs.[50]

Other significant adults may include relatives, especially grandparents, aunts, uncles, and cousins who are peers; the teacher at the daycare centre or nursery school; the babysitter; or neighbours. Relatives and friends also contribute to the development of a child's identity, if contact is frequent. *Guests* in the child's home introduce the child to new facets of family life and to their parents' behaviour. Visits to others' homes helps the child to become socialized through the comparison of households, the ability to separate from home, and interactions with people in new places. *Domestic pets* can be particularly useful in meeting certain needs: loving and being loved; companionship; learning a sense of responsibility; and learning about sex in a natural way.

If the family uses daycare, nursery school, or other early schooling for the child, the adults in the agency may exert a strong influence on the child. The child learns a variety of skills often not available in home life that can in turn form a foundation for extracurricular activities in the school years, or even for a later vocation.[51] The advantage of the year-round program is that the child retains and adds to learning; children who are not in a structured program in summer lose some of what was learned unless they have parents who continue to engage them in new experiences and with new resources.[52]

In Canada, child care is a significant component in the lives of more than two million Canadian children and their families.[53] In fact, many children enter child care before they are one year old, and many of them spend more waking hours in the child-care setting than in their own home. The child's environment is very important to him or her. According to the Canadian Child Care Federation (CCCF), the environment must not only protect a child's health and safety but it must promote optimal child development.[54] The CCCF is a national charitable organization committed to improving the quality of child care services for families in Canada. It does so by strengthening the infrastructure of the child-care community at the national and grassroots level. In addition, it provides a national focus for commentary, information, and dialogue on current issues relating to child care.[55]

There are three main types of child care available in Canada:

- Care provided in one's own home, called *own-home care*
- Care provided in the caregiver's home, called *other-home care*
- Care provided in a centre, or *centre care*[56]

It is important to note that no single type of child care is considered to be the right type for all infants or toddlers. All three types of child care may be good if they provide the warmth, supervision, individual attention, and activity that each child needs.

In Canada, child care may be licensed or unlicensed. The provincial or territorial government must license all centres, as well as some other-home facilities.[57] Each province and territory sets its own licensing standards. These standards vary from province to province, but usually the standards specify the number and ages of children. Included in the standards are health, safety, and nutritional requirements, group size, and staff–child ratios. The requirements also include a program of child-focused activities.[58] A licence is not a guarantee of quality care. It is only an indicator that minimum standards that can be enforced by law are being met. A licence means that the program can be inspected at any time. However, in some parts of Canada inspection may be minimal or infrequent.[59] For specific information about licensing regulations call your provincial/territory licensing authority.

The Canadian Child Care Federation (CCCF) and its affiliate organizations recognize their responsibility to promote ethical practices and attitudes on the part of the child care practitioners.[60] The CCCF Code of Ethics is intended to guide child care practitioners to protect the children and families with whom they work. The eight ethical principles are as follows:

1. Promote the health and well-being of all children.
2. Enable children to engage to their full potential in carefully planned environments and to facilitate the child's progress in a holistic way.
3. Demonstrate a caring attitude to all children.
4. Work in a collaborative way with parents in meeting their responsibilities to their children.
5. Work in partnerships with colleagues and other service providers.
6. Work in ways that enhance human dignity in trusting, caring, and cooperative relationships that respect the worth and uniqueness of the individual.
7. Pursue the knowledge and skills that are needed to be professionally competent.
8. Demonstrate integrity in all professional relationships.

Ethical practice must reflect these eight principles. In situations where ethical dilemmas occur the practitioner must carefully think through the likely consequences of giving priority to particular principles.[61]

CRITICAL THINKING

What are some ethical dilemmas with which a child care practitioner may be confronted?

Parents may ask you about each agency: the differences between them, their significance for the child, and the criteria for selection. Share the following information to the best of your ability. You may also assist with primary prevention and health consulting to teachers, children, and parents in agencies.

Generally speaking, **daycare** is *a licensed, structured program that provides care daily for some portion of the day, for 13 or more children away from home, five days a week year round, for compensation. The age of the children can range from infancy to 13 years;* most children will be of preschool age. *Daycare is child-oriented in program and in the physical structure of the facilities.*

Family daycare *is the arrangement by a caregiver to provide care for a small group of mixed-age children in his or her home*

while the parent works. In some jurisdictions, if there are more than four children, the family daycare must meet licensing requirements, and many caregivers choose to avoid undergoing the regulations, procedures, and remodelling that would be involved in licensing.[62]

Home daycare *is provision of child care in the child's home by someone (father or mother, other relative, nonrelative) during the parent's working hours. The number of children tends to be small* (one to four); thus, there is not much opportunity for diverse peer interaction and limited adult contact. *There is usually no structured program.*[63]

Nursery school is usually a *half-day program that emphasizes an educational, socialization experience for the children to supplement home experiences.*

Early school experiences may include a *Montessori program, a compensatory program, or kindergarten,* which has now become the first step before school entry for most children. **Montessori programs** evolved from the Italian educator Maria Montessori, who developed preschool education in Europe. They *emphasize (1) self-discipline of the child; (2) intellectual developmental through training of the senses; (3) freedom for the child within a structure and schedule; and (4) meaningful individual cognitive experiences that are provided in a quiet, pleasant, educational environment.* **Compensatory programs** *focus on making up for deprived conditions in the child's life, and include (1) giving physical care (good nutrition, dental care, immunizations); (2) fostering curiosity, exploring creativity, and learning about the self and environment; (3) promoting emotional health through nurturing, positive self-concept, self-confidence, and self-discipline; and (4) teaching social skills and behaviours, how to interact with peers, teachers, and parents.*[64]

Kindergarten is a *half- or whole-day educational program* for the five-year-old child that may be an extension of either a nursery school or a part of the public elementary school system. The social behaviours that are learned prepare the child to be better disciplined in the school setting and to interact appropriately with teacher and peers. The half-day program helps the child and parents to separate from each other for a period, if that has not been done through nursery school or day care.

More corporations are recognizing the need to address employees' child care needs to reduce parental anxiety and missed workdays, and enhance productivity.[65] You can be an advocate for such programs.

Criteria for selection of the daycare centre or nursery school may be discussed with parents as they seek assistance with child care and education. Some of the same criteria are useful in selecting family daycare, Montessori, or compensatory programs (Table 9-1).

The criteria in Table 9-1 also are applicable to home daycare, although they would be applied to one adult in a home setting. The following questions should be asked:

- Is there backup help available to the adult if it is needed (e.g., in case the daycare provider is ill or if his or her child or another child was injured or became ill)?
- Does the adult take the children for trips in a vehicle? If so, are there child safety seats or belts appropriate to the child's age?
- Is care provided on weekends, holidays, or in the evening?

TABLE 9-1
Criteria for Selection of Day Care Facility

1. Operated by reputable person, agency, or industry. Either profit or nonprofit programs can offer quality care.
2. Licensed or certified by local and provincial regulatory bodies. However, this only ensures meeting minimum standards.
3. Located convenient to home or workplace, open at the hours needed by the parent(s).
4. Committed to a philosophy of and beliefs about childrearing and discipline that are similar to those of the parents.
5. Staffed with certified teachers and other workers in appropriate staff–child ratio. Teacher and staff have a low turnover rate in employment.
6. Provision of an environment in which children and staff are happy and interacting. Children are having fun and learning.
7. Provision for grouping children according to age and developmental level so that children are safe and can learn from each other.
8. Provision of adequate space that is safe with well-controlled temperature; attractive; clean (but not sterile in appearance) and appropriate for age of child; psychomotor and sensory stimulation (height of windows, level floor); colourful but simple decor.
9. Provision of safe space and a variety of equipment, materials, and supplies for different types of play, such as:
   - Creative: art, music, reading, water play
   - Quiet: games, puzzles
   - Active: pedal toys, blocks
   - Outdoor: jungle gym, balls
   - Dramatic: Playhouse, farm, fire station
10. Provision of place for child to keep personal belongings.
11. Provision for snacks and mealtime. Kitchen facilities meet health department standards. Tables and chairs are available for children and staff to sit and eat together.
12. Provision for child to be alone for short period, if desired, and for midday rest (floor mats provided).
13. Provision of age-appropriate toilet facilities and sinks.
14. Provision of separate room supplied to give emergency health services to an impaired or ill child until parents, or their designate, or emergency medical services can arrive.
15. Provision for occasional extra event, or short trip, such as a visit by a firefighter or trip to the local fire station.
16. Operated at a cost comparable to other similar facilities or programs or on a sliding scale basis.
17. Willingness by staff for anyone to visit unannounced.
18. Daily interaction of teachers with parents and talk with parents about child's behaviour, progress, or health, as indicated.
19. Discussion between teachers and administrator(s) and parents about the contract for services, policies and procedures and their rationale, and explanation of planned changes well in advance.
20. Satisfaction of parents, child, teachers, administrator(s), and staff with decision to have child attend program.

The nursery school operated by a reputable person or organization provides the aforementioned, except for a full noon meal. Usually only a mid-session snack is served. In either centre the parent should observe the program to learn about the philosophy of the staff regarding childrearing, care, and discipline; administrative policies; the use of professional consultants for educational, social, or medical concerns; and the educational qualifications of the staff. They should note the warmth, emotional characteristics, and competence of the staff as they and children work and play together. Cost of the program, when services are available, and the parents' obligations to the agency are other aspects to consider.

In either program, *the child, under guidance of qualified staff, will have many experiences and will develop a variety of skills such as the following:*

- Following rules
- Socializing with others; being cooperative in peer play
- Investigating the environment
- Doing imaginative experimentation with a variety of toys
- Developing creative abilities
- Doing basic problem solving
- Becoming more independent, secure, and self-confident in a variety of situations
- Handling emotions, broadening self-expression
- Learning basic hygiene patterns
- Learning about the surrounding community

Whether or not parents feel well-informed, parents are the ones who ultimately decide which child care arrangements they will trust and support.[66]

In a paper entitled "Developing Cross-Cultural Partnerships: Implication for Child Care Quality Research and Practice,"[67] Pence and McCallum claim that working across cultural and institutional differences is a significant challenge. However, they provide an example of the partnership experience with Meadow Lake Tribal Council in Saskatchewan and the School of Child and Youth Care at the University of Victoria. They conclude that caring was an especially important element in the dynamic process inherent in the partnership.[68]

There are no accurate predictors of later academic success for preschool children. Some studies show that when infants and young children from poor families were given a planned educational experience aimed at preventing retardation and promoting parental interaction, environmental stimulation, and experiential opportunity, the experimental group showed superior cognitive abilities at age five-and-a-half, compared with children in a control group raised in the usual way. Other studies showed that three-year-old children who were given special educational opportunities showed better intellectual performance at the end of second grade than did children in a control group.[69] Other authors say that pushing the child to develop reading and mathematics skills too early will create problems: fatigue, stress-related illnesses, disciplinary problems, and parental burnout.[70-72]

If parents use a daycare centre, family daycare, nursery school, or early school program, help them understand that they remain the most important people to the child and that their love and involvement with the child are crucial for later learning and adjustment to life. Help the working mother realize that her working does not necessarily deprive the child. Many career women tend to do better parenting than full-time homemakers. They do not see the child as an end in itself; they allow the child to develop autonomy and initiative in creative ways because they have a sense of self-fulfillment in their own lives.

You can help the parents and child prepare for the separation if the child will be enrolled in a nursery school or daycare centre. Help the parents realize, too, that the child's emotional and social adjustment and overall learning depend on many factors. Because each child interprets entrance into the agency on the basis of his or her own past experience, each differs in adjustment. Being with a number of children can be an upsetting experience. The child needs adequate preparation to avoid feeling abandoned or rejected.

The parents must have confidence in the agency so that she can convey a feeling of pleasurable expectation to the child. The child should accompany the mother and/or father to see the building, observe the program, and meet the teachers and other children before enrolment. Ideally the child should begin attending when parents and child feel secure about the ensuing separation, and the mother or father should be encouraged to stay with the child the whole first day or for a shorter period for several days until he or she feels secure without mother. If possible, the parent, rather than a neighbour or stranger, should take the child each day, assuring the child of the parent's return at the end of the day.

CRITICAL THINKING

As a parent, what other criteria would you include in choosing a child care centre?

Developmental Tasks of the Family

While the preschool child and siblings are achieving their developmental tasks, the parents are struggling with childrearing and their own personal developmental tasks. A discussion of parental developmental tasks, while raising a preschooler, should include the following:

- Encourage and accept the child's evolving skills rather than elevating the parent's self-esteem by pushing the child beyond his or her capacity. Satisfaction is found through reducing assistance with physical care and giving more guidance in other respects.
- Supply adequate housing, facilities, space, equipment, and other materials needed for life, comfort, health, and recreation.
- Plan for predicted and unexpected costs of family life such as insurance, education, babysitter fees, food, clothing, and recreation.
- Maintain some personal privacy and an outlet for tension of family members, while including the child as a participant in the family.
- Share household and child-care responsibility with other family members, including the child.
- Strengthen the partnership with the mate and express affection in ways that keep the relationship from becoming humdrum.
- Learn to accept failures, mistakes, and blunders without piling up feelings of guilt, blame, and recrimination.
- Nourish common interests and friendships to strengthen self-respect and self-confidence and to remain interesting to the spouse.
- Maintain a mutually satisfactory sexual relationship and plan whether or not to have more children.
- Create and maintain effective communication within the family.
- Cultivate relationships with the extended family.
- Tap resources and serve others outside the family to prevent preoccupation with self and family.
- Face life's dilemmas and rework moral codes, spiritual values, and a philosophy of life.

Explore with parent the challenges and practical ways of meeting these tasks within the specific family unit.

PHYSIOLOGIC CONCEPTS

The following information will be useful in assessment of the child and teaching of parents.

Physical Characteristics

Growth

Growth during the preschool years is *relatively slow*, but changes occur that transform the chubby toddler into a sturdy child who appears taller and thinner. Limb growth is greater in proportion to trunk growth. Although development does not proceed at a uniform rate in all areas or for all children, *development follows a logical, precise pattern or sequence*.[73-76] The preschool child grows approximately 6 to 7.5 cm (2-1/2 to 3 inches) and gains less than 2.2 kg (5 pounds) *per year*. The child appears tall and thin because he or she grows proportionately more in height than in weight. The average height of the three-year-old is 94 cm (37 inches); of the four-year-old, 104 cm (41 inches, *or double the birth length*); and of the five-year-old, 110 to 130 cm (43 to 52 inches). At three the child weighs approximately 15 kg (33 pounds); at 4 years, 17 kg (38 pounds); and at 5 years, approximately 18 to 23 kg (40 to 50 pounds).

Vital Signs

The *body temperature* is 36.7° to 37.2°C (98° to 99°F). The *pulse rate* is normally 80 to 110 and the *respiratory rate* approximately 30 per minute. *Blood pressure* is approximately 90/60 mm Hg.

Other Characteristics

Vision in the preschooler is farsighted; the five-year-old has 20/40 to 20/30 vision and is visually discriminative. *Eye–hand coordination* improves. By age four-and-a-half, the *motor nerves are fully myelinated* and the *cerebral cortex* is fully connected to the cerebellum, permitting better coordination and control of bowel and bladder and fine muscle movements, such as tying shoelaces, cutting with scissors, or holding a pencil or crayon. *Internal organs* are larger; at five years, the *brain* is at 90% of the weight of the adult brain, the child has 20 *teeth,* and by the end of the preschool period, the child begins to lose deciduous teeth.[77–80] Physical characteristics to assess in this child are listed in Table 9-2. Because each child is unique, the normative listings indicate only where most children of a given age are in the development of various characteristics. Characteristics are listed by age in all following tables for reasons of understanding sequence and giving comparison. Consideration of only the chronologic age is misleading as a basis for assessment and care. For example, opportunity for muscle movement and exercise and nutritional status, rather than gender, influences strength. Still, by using the norms for the child at a given age, you can assess how far the child deviates from the norm. With more parental guidance, the child may reach norms ahead of age. Certain situations, such as prenatal alcohol or drug exposure, are likely to cause the child to be below the norms.[81]

Developmental Assessment

The Denver II—Revision and Restandardization of the Denver Developmental Screening Test (DDST) evaluates four major categories of development: gross motor, fine motor–adaptive, language, and personal–social (Figure 9–2 on pages 388–389). It is used to determine whether a child is within normal range for various behaviours or is developmentally delayed. Like the original DDST, the Denver II is applicable to children from birth through six years of age. The age divisions are monthly until 24 months and then every six months until six years of age.[82,83]

Although it is not the purpose of this discussion to describe the administration and interpretation of the Denver II, the following points should be noted. First, to avoid errors in administration and interpretation, and hence invalid screening results, the examiner should carefully follow the protocol outlined by the test's authors. A manual and workbook, videotape, and proficiency test have been developed to ensure accurate administration and interpretation by examiners. Second, before administering the test, explanations should be given to both the child and parent(s). Parents should be advised that the Denver II is

not an intelligence test but rather a means of assessing what the child can do at a particular age.[84,85]

Because the Denver II is nonthreatening, requires no painful or unfamiliar procedures, and relies on the child's natural activity of play, it is an excellent way to begin the health assessment. It provides a general assessment tool that can help guide treatment and teaching. The Denver II form and instruction manual can be obtained from Denver Developmental Materials, Inc., P.O. Box 371079, Denver, CO 8037-5075; (303) 355–4729.

It is important to consider genetics, family factors, nutrition, and social environment when you assess and care for children who are *developmentally delayed.*[86–89] Occasionally a child does not attain height within the norms for his or her age, although torso to leg proportions are normal, because the pituitary gland does not produce enough growth hormone.[90] **Growth hormone deficiency,** *which causes dwarfism in a preschool child,* can now be treated with a synthetic growth hormone. The person still remains short in stature but is within a normal height range. The treatment is important because children who lag behind peers in growth are often teased, are kept from participating in certain play activities, and may have difficulty finding clothes or play equipment, such as a bicycle, that is of correct size. The child may be regarded by others as retarded intellectually. He or she may feel inferior, suffer a negative self-concept, lack initiative, and become withdrawn, depressed, or antisocial in later childhood or adult years.[91,92]

Nutritional Needs

As stated in Chapter 8, *Canada's Food Guide* has been adapted for children by taking into account the smaller portions of food they eat. As a result, the guide has become a useful tool for everyone in the family over two years of age.[93] The dietary requirements of preschoolers are similar to those of toddlers. Preschooler children consume slightly more than toddlers, and nutrient density is more important than quantity.[94]

Slower growth rate and heightened interest in exploring the environment may lessen interest in eating. Because preschoolers have relatively high needs for energy, in addition to small stomachs, they may need to eat small amounts of food frequently throughout the day. This need is best achieved by three meals with a nutritious snack between meals. The amount of food a preschooler needs depends on age, body size, activity level, growth rate, and appetite.[95] See the box entitled "Examples of One Child-Size Serving" in Chapter 8.

Children who are reared in *vegetarian families* may be shorter and weigh less, but by the end of the preschool era, the child's growth velocity approaches the norm. However, children who follow a vegetarian diet are especially at risk for protein and vitamin deficiencies, such as vitamin B.[96]

Eating assumes increasing social significance for the preschooler and is still an emotional and physiologic experience. The child needs the right foods physically and a warm, happy atmosphere in which he or she is included in mealtime conversation. The family mealtime promotes socialization in relation to meal preparation, behaviour during mealtimes, language skills, and understanding of family rituals and situations. The training

TABLE 9-2
Assessment of Physical Characteristics: Motor Control

Age 3 Years	Age 4 Years	Age 5 Years
Occasional accident in toileting when busy at play; responds to routine times; tells when going to bathroom	Independent toilet habits; manages clothes without difficulty Insists on having door shut for self but wants to be in bathroom with others	Takes complete charge of self; does not tell when going to bathroom
Verbalizes difference between how male and female urinate Needs help with back buttons and drying self Night time control of bowel and bladder most of time	Asks many questions about defecation function	Self-conscious about exposing self Boys and girls go to separate bathrooms Voids four to six times during waking hours; occasional nighttime accident
Runs more smoothly than before, turns sharp corners, suddenly stops; trunk rotates with run	Runs easily with coordination Skips clumsily Hops on one leg Legs, trunk, shoulder, arms move in unison Aggressive physical activity	Runs with skill, speed, agility, and plays games simultaneously Starts and stops abruptly when running Increases strength and coordination in limbs
Walks backward Climbs stairs with alternate feet Jumps from low step	Heel-toe walk Walks a plank Climbs stairs without holding onto rail Climbs and jumps without difficulty	May still be knock-kneed Jumps from three to four steps
Tries to dance but has inadequate balance, although sense of balance improving	Enjoys motor stunts and gross gesturing	Balances self on toes and on one leg; dances with some rhythm Balances on one foot approximately 10 sec.
Pedals tricycle Swings	Enjoys new activities rather than repeating same ones	Jumps rope Roller skates Hops and skips on alternate feet Enjoys jungle gym
Sitting equilibrium maintained but combined awkwardly with reaching activity	Sitting balance well maintained; leans forward with greater mobility and ease Exaggerated use of arm extension and trunk twisting; touches end of nose with forefinger on direction	Maintains balance easily Combines reaching and placing object in one continuous movement Arm extension and trunk twisting coordinated Tummy protrudes, but some adult curve to spine
Undresses self; helps dress self Undoes buttons on side or front of clothing Goes to toilet alone if clothes simple Washes hands, feeds self May brush own teeth	Dresses and undresses self except tying bows, closing zipper, putting on boots and snowsuit Does buttons Distinguishes front and back of self and clothes Brushes teeth alone	Dresses self without assistance; ties shoelaces Requires less supervision of personal duties Washes self without wetting clothes

(continued)

TABLE 9-2 *(continued)*
Assessment of Physical Characteristics: Motor Control

Age 3 Years	Age 4 Years	Age 5 Years
Catches ball with arms fully extended one out of two to three times	Greater flexion of elbow	Uses hands more than arms in catching ball
Hand movement becoming better coordinated	Catches ball thrown at 1.5 m two to three times	Pours fluid from one container to another with few spills; bilateral coordination
Increasing coordination in vertical direction	Throws ball overhand	
Pours fluid from pitcher, occasional spills	Judges where a ball will land	Uses hammer to hit nail on head
Hits large pegs on board with hammer	Helps dust objects	Interest and competence in dusting
	Likes water play	Likes water play
Builds tower of 9 to 10 blocks; builds three-block gate from model	Builds complicated structure extending vertically and laterally; builds five-block gate from model	Builds things out of large boxes
		Builds complicated three-dimensional structure and may build several separate units
Imitates a bridge	Notices missing parts or broken objects; requests parents to fix	Able to disassemble and reassemble small object
Copies circle or cross; begins to use scissors; strings large beads	Copies a square or simple figure	Copies triangle or diamond from model
	Uses scissors without difficulty	Folds paper diagonally
Shows hand preference	Enjoys finer manipulation of play materials	Definite hand preference
Trial-and-error method with puzzle	Surveys puzzle before placing pieces	Does simple puzzles quickly and smoothly
	Matches simple geometric forms	
	Prefers symmetry	Prints some letters correctly; prints first name
	Poor space perception	
Scribbles	Less scribbling	Draws clearly recognized lifelike representatives; differentiates parts of drawing
Tries to draw a picture and name it	Form and meaning in drawing apparent to adults	

Sources: Frankenburg, W., and J.B. Dobbs, Denver II—Revision and Restandardization of the Denver Developmental Screening Test. Denver: Denver Developmental Materials, 1990; Gormly, A., Lifespan Human Development (6th ed.). Fort Worth: Harcourt Brace College Publishers, 1997; Papalia, D., S. Olds, and R. Feldman, Human Development (7th ed.). Boston: McGraw-Hill, 1998; Seifert, K., R. Hoffnung, and M. Hoffnung, Lifespan Development. Boston: Houghton Mifflin, 1997; Wong, D., Whaley and Wong's Nursing Care of Infants and Children (6th ed.). St. Louis: C. V. Mosby, 1999.

is positive or negative, depending on the parents' example. Such learning is missed if there are no family mealtimes. Table manners need not be rigidly emphasized; accidents will happen, and parental example is the best teacher.

The preschooler likes to eat one thing at a time. Of all food groups, vegetables are least liked, whereas fruits are a favourite. The child usually prefers vegetables and fruits crisp, raw, and cut into finger-sized pieces. New foods can be gradually introduced; if a food is refused once, offer it again after several days. It is important not to pressure the child to eat. By trusting their hunger cues, preschoolers can learn to choose an amount they can expect to eat.[97]

A child may be eating insufficiently, for the following reasons:

- Eating too much between meals
- Experiencing unhappy mealtime atmosphere
- Seeking attention
- Mimicking parental eating habits
- Responding to excessive parental expectations
- Having inadequate variety and quantity
- Suffering tooth decay, which may cause nausea or toothache with chewing
- Feeling sibling rivalry
- Experiencing overfatigue or physical illness
- Experiencing emotional disturbance

Eating a variety of foods is one of the best ways to ensure an adequate intake of nutrients. If a child is eating according to the Food Guide, is growing well, and is healthy, vitamin-mineral supplements are rarely necessary. However, vitamin D supplements may be indicated for special situations such as for children who do not consume enough vitamin D–fortified milk.[98]

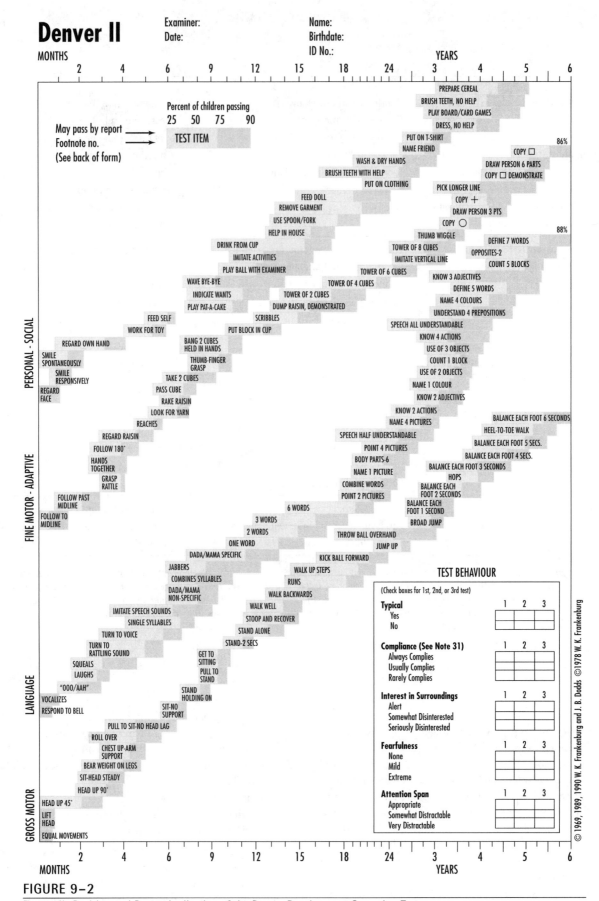

FIGURE 9–2

Denver II—Revision and Restandardization of the Denver Development Screening Test

Source: Frankenberg, W.K., and J.B. Dobbs, Denver II—Revision and Standardization of the Denver Developmental Screening Test. Denver Developmental Materials, *1990.*

DIRECTIONS FOR ADMINISTRATION

1. Try to get child to smile by smiling, talking or waving. Do not touch him/her.
2. Child must stare at hand several seconds.
3. Parent may help guide toothbrush and put toothpaste on brush.
4. Child does not have to be able to tie shoes or button/zip in the back.
5. Move yarn slowly in an arc from one side to the other, about 8" (20 cm) above child's face.
6. Pass if child grasps rattle when it is touched to the backs or tips of fingers.
7. Pass if child tries to see where yarn went. Yarn should be dropped quickly from sight from tester's hand without arm movement.
8. Child must transfer cube from hand to hand without help of body, mouth, or table.
9. Pass if child picks up raisin with any part of thumb and finger.
10. Line can vary only 30 degrees or less from tester's line. $\lor$
11. Make a fist with thumb pointing upward and wiggle only the thumb. Pass if child imitates and does not move any fingers other than the thumb.

| 12. Pass any enclosed form. Fail continuous round motions. | 13. Which line is longer? (Not bigger.) Turn paper upside down and repeat. (pass 3 of 3 or 5 of 6) | 14. Pass any lines crossing near midpoint. | 15. Have child copy first. If failed, demonstrate. |

When giving items 12, 14, and 15, do not name the forms. Do not demonstrate 12 and 14.

16. When scoring, each pair (2 arms, 2 legs, etc.) counts as one part.
17. Place one cube in cup and shake gently near child's ear, but out of sight. Repeat for other ear.
18. Point to picture and have child name it. (No credit is given for sounds only.)
    If less than 4 pictures are named correctly, have child point to picture as each is named by tester.

   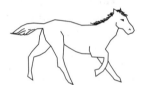   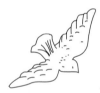   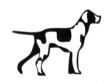   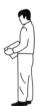

19. Using doll, tell child: Show me the nose, eyes, ears, mouth, hands, feet, tummy, hair. Pass 6 of 8.
20. Using pictures, ask child: Which one flies?...says meow?...talks?...barks?...gallops? Pass 2 of 5, 4 of 5.
21. Ask child: What do you do when you are cold?...tired?...hungry? Pass 2 of 3, 3 of 3.
22. Ask child: What do you do with a cup? What is a chair used for? What is a pencil used for?
    Action words must be included in answers.
23. Pass if child correctly places *and* says how many blocks are on paper. (1, 5).
24. Tell child: Put block **on** table; **under** table; **in front of** me, **behind** me. Pass 4 of 4.
    (Do not help child by pointing, moving head or eyes.)
25. Ask child: What is a ball?...lake?...desk?...house?...banana?...curtain?...fence?...ceiling? Pass if defined in terms of use, shape, what it is made of, or general category (such as banana is fruit, not just yellow). Pass 5 of 8, 7 of 8.
26. Ask child: If a horse is big, a mouse is _____ ? If fire is hot, ice is _____ ? If the sun shines during the day, the moon shines during the _____ ? Pass 2 of 3.
27. Child may use wall or rail only, not person. May not crawl.
28. Child must throw ball overhand 3 feet (approx 1 metre) to within arm's reach of tester.
29. Child must perform standing broad jump over width of test sheet (8 1/2 inches or 22 cm).
30. Tell child to walk forward ⬭⬭⬭⬭⬭ → heel within 1 inch (2.5 cm) of toe. Tester may demonstrate.
    Child must walk 4 consecutive steps.
31. In the second year, half of normal children are noncompliant.

OBSERVATIONS:

FIGURE 9-2

(continued)

CRITICAL THINKING

What criteria should be taken into account for an accurate nutritional assessment of a preschooler?

Exercise, Rest, and Sleep

This is the period when the child seems to have a surplus of energy and is on the move. The child needs time and space for physical exercise through play. Clothing and shoes should be comfortable and allow for easy movement. Shoes should provide flexibility, yet be stable, and conform to the plantar arch contours.[99] Children of all ages can, and should, be involved in a variety of different activities. Of course, the kinds of activities in which they participate depend on their age and stage of development. Although children follow a basic developmental pattern, they grow and develop at different rates.[100] The following three types of physical activities should be combined when planning activities for preschoolers:

- Endurance activities that strengthen the vital organs such as the heart and lungs, such as running, jumping, and swimming
- Flexibility activities that encourage a child to bend, stretch, and reach, such as gymnastics and dancing
- Strength-building activities that build strong muscles and bones, such as climbing[101]

For more information, visit Canada's Physical Activity Guide for Children at http://www.healthcanada.ca/paguide.

CRITICAL THINKING

What are some suitable physical activities for the preschooler?

The preschooler may still take a favourite toy to bed; he or she likes to postpone bedtime and is ritualistic about bedtime routines, such as prayers, a story, or music. Sleeping time decreases from ten to 12 hours for the younger preschooler to nine to 11 hours for the older preschooler. Dreams and nightmares may awaken the three- or four-year-old, causing fear and a move into bed with parents or older siblings. The five-year-old sleeps quietly through the night without having to get up to urinate and has fewer nightmares.

If the parent responds with special attention to the child who awakens during the night, the sleep disturbance becomes worse. Parents should not become a sleep adjunct to the child (e.g., holding child in lap until he or she falls asleep again, picking up child as soon as he or she cries) because the child will not learn to fall asleep alone. The parent reinforces the waking behaviour. Instead, help the restless child develop sleep strategies, such as cuddling a teddy bear or blanket or babbling to an imaginary friend. Parents should provide reassurance, and set and stick to limits.

Dreams and nightmares occur during the light stages of sleep as a way to resolve emotional conflicts. In night terrors the child screams or cries, may thrash and squirm, is confused, does not respond to parents, behaves abnormally, and has tachycardia and tachypnea, dilated pupils, and sometimes facial contortions and diaphoresis.

Help the parents understand that calm reassurance is needed with night terrors. Wait out the attack without trying either to comfort or to arouse the child. Further stimulation intensifies agitation. After 15 minutes or so, the child usually collapses back into sleep without memory of what happened. Sleep problems usually subside spontaneously, but the child and parents may need therapy if the problem persists several times weekly or over a period.

Health Promotion and Health Protection

Immunization Schedules
For immunization schedules for children of this age group, refer to Table 7-6 on page 328, or visit http://www.immunize.cpha.ca/English/schedule.htm.

Dental Care
Because caries frequently begin at this age and spread rapidly, dental care is important. Deciduous teeth guide in the permanent ones; they should be kept in good repair. If deciduous teeth are lost too early, permanent teeth grow in abnormally. Teeth should be brushed after eating, using a method recommended by the dentist, and intake of refined sugars limited to help prevent tooth decay. The Canadian Dental Association advises against fluoride supplements in young children before permanent teeth erupt.[102]

Before entering school the child is usually required to have a physical examination (including urinalysis) and a dental examination.

Safety Promotion and Injury Control
The preschooler has more freedom, independence, initiative, and desire to imitate adults than the toddler but still has an immature understanding of danger and illness. This combination is likely to get him or her into hazardous situations.

A major responsibility of caretaking adults is safety promotion and injury control: the child needs watchfulness and a safe play area. The adult serves as a bodyguard while slowly teaching caution and keeping the environment as safe as possible. Other siblings can also take some, but not total, responsibility for the preschooler. Protecting the firstborn is simple as you can put dangerous objects away and there is likely to be more time and energy for supervision. When there are a number of children in a family, the activities of the older children may provide objects or situations that are dangerous to the younger ones. As the child learns to protect self, he or she should be allowed to take added responsibility for personal safety and should be given appropriate verbal recognition and praise that reinforce safe behaviour. Also, if the parent voices fear constantly, natural curiosity and the will to learn will be dulled; the child may fear every new situation.

Explore information in this section with parents so that they and you can use these safety suggestions:

- Begin safety teaching early. Teaching done in the toddler years, for example, pays off later.
- Avoid constant threats and frequent physical punishment. Incessant "don'ts" should be avoided because the child will

learn to ignore them, feel angry or resentful, and purposefully rebel or defy adults, thus failing to learn about real danger.

- When you must forbid, use simple command words in a firm voice without anger to convey the impression that you expect the child to obey—for example, "stop," "no."
- Phrase safety rules and their reasons in positive rather than negative terms when possible. For example, say: "Play in the yard, not the street, or you'll get hurt by cars"; "Sit quietly in the car to avoid hurt"; "Put tiny things (coins, beads) that you find in here (jar, bowl, box)."
- Teach the child his or her full name, address including postal code, and telephone number, and teach the child how to use police or adults in service roles for help (e.g., 911, emergency services, fire department).
- Teach the child not to give information over the phone about him- or herself or the family.
- Encourage the child to share "secrets"; emphasize that he or she does not need to fear saying anything.
- Tell the child not to leave home alone or with a stranger. He or she should use a "buddy" system when going somewhere.
- Never leave the child alone in public or unattended in a car.
- Teach the child escape techniques, for example, how to unlock home doors or car doors.
- Never leave the child home alone. Make sure that the babysitter is reliable.
- Never allow play in or near a busy driveway or garage. Forbid street play if other play areas are available. Teach children to look carefully for, and to get away from, cars. Drivers must take all possible precautions. A fenced yard or playground is ideal, although not always available.
- Teach the child how to cross the street safely.
- Teach the child to refuse gifts or rides from strangers, to avoid walking or playing alone on a deserted street, road, or similar area, and about the possibility of child molesters or abductors.
- Keep matches in containers and out of reach.
- Dispose of, or store out of reach and in a locked cabinet, all of the poisons you have in the house: rat and roach killer, insecticides, weed killer, kerosene, cleaning agents, furniture polish, medicines. Suntan lotion, shampoo, deodorants, nail polish, and cosmetics remain potential hazards; the child should be taught their *correct* use. The child is less likely to pull them out of cabinets or swallow them than when he or she was a toddler, but brightly coloured containers or pills, powders, or liquids raise curiosity and experimentation. Keep medications out of the child's reach. Bright-coloured pills can be mistaken for candy. Keep the Poison Control Centre telephone number readily seen.
- Observe your child closely while he or she plays near water. Cover wells and cisterns. Be sure to fence ponds and swimming pools.
- Keep stairways and nighttime play areas well lit.
- Equip upstairs windows with sturdy screens and guards. Have handrails for stairways.
- Store knives, saws, and other sharp objects or lawn or power tools out of reach.

- Remove doors from abandoned appliances and cars; campaign for legislation for appropriate disposal of them and for mandatory door removal.
- Discourage playing with or in the area of appliances or power tools while they are in operation: a washing machine with a wringer, a lawn mower, a saw, or clothes dryer.
- Use safety glass in glass doors or shower stalls; place decals on sliding doors at child's eye level (and adult's eye level, too) to prevent walking or running through them.
- Use adhesive strips in the bathtub.
- Avoid scatter rugs, debris, or toys cluttered on the floor in areas of traffic.
- Use seatbelts in the car that are appropriate for the weight of the child.
- Teach the child sun safety rules: cover up, find shade, and use sun-safe products and sunscreens.

If the child continually fails to listen or obey, ask the following questions: Is the child able to hear? Is he or she intellectually able to understand? Are demands too numerous, or expectations too great? Are statements too lengthy or abstract? Is anger expressed with teaching and discipline to the point that it interferes emotionally with the child's perception and judgment? Perhaps most important, do the parents demonstrate safety-conscious behaviour with equipment, movements, or use of sun safety rules? Although imitation is a major way to learn, let us pay a brief visit to one recent, and relevant, Canadian research study.

Bruce and her colleagues examined the relationship between two groups of Canadian preschoolers (injured and noninjured) and their parents' risk perceptions, safety behaviours, parenting stress, and children's risk behaviours. They found significantly higher numbers of injury behaviour in the group of injured children. Contrary to the researchers' hypothesis, parents' perception of risk and hazard were not found to be significantly less among those parents of injured children. However, the parents of injured children had a higher score for perceived dangers for their children and less parent stress.[103] The researchers conclude that injury behaviour screening may provide a useful tool for health care professionals in practical environments to target injury prevention counselling for those children and families most at risk.[104]

CRITICAL THINKING

What elements should be included in an injury behaviour screening tool?

Accidents

Accidents are the most common cause of death of children. *Teach parents about prevention and emergency treatment of these conditions.* Approximately one-third of accidental deaths are caused by motor vehicles; the next most common causes are drowning, burns from fire or hot water, and poisonings. Running through sliding glass doors in homes, locking self in an abandoned refrigerator or freezer, and electric shocks from electrical equipment also frequently cause severe injury or death. Falls can cause minor bumps, bruises, and lacerations. Animal bites are common.[105]

Minor head injury *is any trauma to the head that does not alter normal cerebral functioning.* What appears to be a very minor head injury can result in a subdural or epidural hematoma—the preschooler bears very close monitoring. Parents or caretakers should be taught to check the preschooler every two hours in the first 24 hours after injury. If the preschooler cannot be awakened; is mentally confused; is unusually restless, disturbed, or agitated; starts vomiting; has a severe headache; has unequally sized pupils (unless previously that way); has weakness of arms or legs; has drainage from ears or nose; or has some sort of fit or convulsion, medical help must be sought.[106–109]

Minor lacerations and *cuts* should be examined for dirt and foreign objects even after they have been cleaned with warm water and soap. The laceration should be covered with a loose bandage that will keep out dirt and protect the wound from additional trauma. The parent or caretaker should watch for signs of infection: redness, heat, swelling, and drainage. The child should have tetanus prophylaxis updated.[110,111]

Burns *are thermal injuries to the skin.* A **first-degree burn** *usually shows redness only;* a **second-degree burn** causes *blister formation,* sometimes with peeling and weeping. Scalds often produce this type of burn. A **third-degree burn** *chars the skin, causing a whitish appearance, and involves tissue under the skin.* It may cause anaesthesia. Flame and hot metal often cause third-degree burns.[112–114]

For a first-degree burn the affected area should be plunged into cold water for a few minutes. Gentle washing with soap and water should be sufficient. A second-degree burn should have the same initial treatment. Blisters that form should be left intact, and the burned area should be covered with a nonadherent gauze and a bulky, dry, sterile dressing. Tetanus immunization should be up to date. A third-degree burn, any second-degree burn that covers an area greater than an adult's hand size, any facial burns, and any burn in which child maltreatment is suspected should be seen by the health care provider and physician.[115–117]

Accidental ingestions and poisonings may occur in children under the age of five, sometimes even when preventive measures as discussed in Chapter 8 are used. These ingestions can cause a great variety of symptoms and signs. *The following guidelines should be taught to parents:*

1. Look for an empty container nearby if sudden unusual symptoms or abnormal odour to breath or clothes is observed.
2. Try to determine what and how much was ingested and when.
3. Call the poison control centre for help.
4. If there are no contraindications to vomiting (either from reading the side of the container or from getting directions at the poison control centre), induce vomiting with syrup of ipecac. Mechanical stimulation of the posterior pharynx can be used to induce vomiting *except* with ingestion of corrosive agents, such as lye, gasoline, and kerosene.
5. Take the child to the nearest clinic that is set up to deal with these problems.[118–121]

The *bite of any animal* will probably have few symptoms other than pain at the site of puncture wounds or small lacerations. Dog bites are most common, although the child may have contact with other animals that bite or scratch. Bites from other children can also occur. The chief concern is the possibility of rabies. It is essential to establish the vaccination status of the biting animal, if possible, for if the animal is properly vaccinated, there is little chance of acquiring and transmitting the disease to humans. Rabies prophylaxis will be determined by the physician. The wound should be washed with copious amounts of soap and water. Tetanus prophylaxis should be up to date.[122]

Lead poisoning, especially in preschoolers, will produce **encephalopathy,** or *brain dysfunction.* The onset is insidious, with weakness, irritability, weight loss, and vomiting, followed by personality changes and developmental regression. Convulsions and coma are late signs. Often history will reveal pica, involving cracking paint in old homes, lead toys, old yellow and orange crayons, artist's paints, leaded gasoline, or fruit tree sprays.[123,124]

Prevention lies in keeping the preschooler in a lead-free environment as much as possible. You may call the housing inspector, with the family's permission, to test paint for lead. In many cities landlords are required to repaint the house interior when lead paint is found. Treatment for severe cases of lead poisoning involves hospitalization.

Common Health Problems: Prevention and Treatment

Teach parents that scheduled health maintenance visits to the doctor or nurse practitioner are important for early detection of problems. Table 9-3 summarizes some common health problems.[125–128]

Child Maltreatment

In Canada, child maltreatment is classified as physical abuse, sexual abuse, neglect, and emotional maltreatment.[129,130] The selection of best practices for the prevention and treatment of child maltreatment is critical. Canadian child abuse programs have been delineated into three levels: tertiary, secondary, and primary.[131] Tertiary programs are implemented in families where child abuse has occurred. Secondary prevention programs of child maltreatment consist of the early identification of parents who are at risk for abusing their children. A parenting program called First Nations Parenting is available to First Nations communities served by the Awasis Agency of Northern Manitoba. Primary prevention programs are focused at the general population to address underlying causes and to decrease the incidence of maltreatment.[132] The purpose of these programs is to reduce the risk for families under stress and to promote wellness in families that are functioning adequately.[133] The main intent of prevention and health promotion programs regarding child abuse should address the aspect of quality living with emphasis on wellness and primary prevention. Some children who are frequently or severely maltreated develop post-traumatic stress disorder (PTSD), which involves extreme levels of anxiety. Other symptoms include nightmares, feelings of isolation, flashback memories of episodes of abuse, guilt feelings, and other sleep disturbances.[134] Also see the section entitled "Child Maltreatment" in Chapter 7.

TABLE 9-3
Common Health Problems of Preschooler

Problem	Definition	Signs/Symptoms	Prevention/Treatment
Strabismus	Eyes not straight or properly aligned	Double vision (diplopia), followed by irreversible loss of vision in suppressed eye (amblyopia)	Appropriate vision testing E chart or Allen cards Use toy to go through visual field testing Test for colour blindness Functional amblyopia remedied through corrective lens, contact lens, and prisms
Conjunctivitis	Inflammation of the eyelids or conjunctivae or both; caused by bacteria or virus	Redness of conjunctivae; mild irritation; excessive lacrimation; normal vision	Cool compresses Appropriate eye drops
Hearing loss	Hearing less than normal for age group	Inability to speak by age 2; failure to respond to out-of-sight noise; tilting the head while listening	Use play technique to evaluate hearing Use earphones to transmit sounds and have child put peg in board when hearing sound
Otitis media	Infection of middle ear with accumulation of serop-urulent fluid in middle ear cavity	Earache, fever, upper respiratory infection; decreased hearing; bulging tympanic membrane; disappearance of landmarks	Lymphatic tissue, tonsils, and adenoids more abundant now than later and, therefore, are often involved in the infectious process
Acute cervical adenitis	Inflammation of one or more cervical nodes in response to an infection in the ear, nose or throat; group A streptococcal often the cause	Painful swelling of neck; possibly high fever; usually unilateral cervical nodes enlarged and tender	Appropriate antibiotic Antipyretic Warm compresses
Urinary tract infection	Bacterial infection of part or all of urinary tract, collect-ing system of kidneys, and bladder	May be asymptomatic; urgency and frequency of urination; dysuria; flank and suprapubic pain; foul-smelling urine; fever	Appropriate antibiotic Increased water intake Personal hygiene
Enuresis	Involuntary passage of urine; occurs at night in 10–15% of 5-year-olds	Bedwetting	Reduction of liquid intake in the evening Maintaining appropriate attitude Signal device sometimes helpful Getting child up at specified times to urinate
Nonspecific vulvovaginitis	Inflammation of vulva and vagina; usually nonspecific organism responsible	Discharge; pruritus; erythema,	Personal hygiene Wearing cotton underwear Avoidance of bubble baths and perfumed soaps Cold compresses to vulva

(continued)

TABLE 9-3 *(continued)*
Common Health Problems of Preschooler

Problem	Definition	Signs/Symptoms	Prevention/Treatment
Measles	Highly contagious viral disease with severe complications	Rash (beginning at face and descending down body); 3C's—coryza, cough, conjunctivitis; Koplik's spots (red) on buccal mucosa; fever	Prevention: immunization *If disease: isolation* No specific therapy Symptomatic treatment
Diarrhea	Inflammation of gastrointestinal tract caused at this age by *Giardia lambdia* and *Salmonella*	Stools more frequent and liquid than usual; abdominal cramps; foul-smelling stool; weight loss	Sometimes antibiotics Personal hygiene; safe drinking water Staying out of wading pools
Postural problems	Deviation of normal posture and normal spinal curves	Deviation seen as child bends anteriorly, laterally, posteriorly	Exercises prescribed by knowledgeable health care practitioner
Juvenile hypertension	Child more than age 3 who has diastolic pressure greater than 90 mm Hg	Probably none other than blood pressure elevation	Referral for overall cardiovascular investigation
Hypochromic anemia	Prevalent nutritional problem in childhood, caused by inadequate intake of absorbable iron	Associated with poor hygiene, chronic disease; major part of diet is milk or milk products	Encourage parents to feed child eggs, meat, fish, fruits, cereals, and dark green leafy vegetables Normal, not excessive, amounts of milk

Sources: Gesell, A., and F. Ilg, The Child From Five to Ten (rev. ed.). New York: Harper & Collins, 1977; Sherman, J., Jr., and S. Fields, Guide to Patient Evaluation (5th ed.). Garden City, NY: Medical Examination Publishing, 1989; Uphold, C., and M. Graham, Clinical Guidelines in Family Practice (2nd ed.). Gainesville, FL: Barmarrae Books, 1994; Wong, D., Whaley and Wong's Nursing Care of Infants and Children (6th ed.). St. Louis: C.V. Mosby, 1999.

CRITICAL THINKING

What steps are involved in designing a primary prevention program on child maltreatment in the community?

9–1 BONUS SECTION IN CD-ROM

Abuse

A comprehensive overview of abuse from the U.S. legal perspective is provided. With the Canadian treatment of abuse in the text, comparisons can be made by the reader on child maltreatment in the two countries.

Reactions to Illness and Hospitalization

During this stage, when the child has heightened feelings of sexuality, fears of dependency and separation, fantasies, feelings of narcissism, and rivalry with parents, he or she is particularly vulnerable to fears about body damage. The child perceives and fears dental, medical, and surgical procedures as mutilating, intrusive, punishing, or abandoning. The resulting conflicts, fears, guilt, anger, or excessive concern about the body can persist and influence personality development into adulthood.

Teach parents that many of these negative reactions can be averted by introducing the child to medical facilities and health workers when he or she is well. The best teaching is positive example. If the parent takes the child with him or her to the physician and dentist and if the child observes courteous professionals, a procedure that does not hurt (or an explanation of why it will hurt), and a positive response from the parent, a great deal of teaching is accomplished. These visits can be reinforced with honest answers to the many questions the preschooler will have. Research also indicates that being away from mother on a daily basis, in some kind of alternative daycare experience, moderates the separation anxiety and negative reaction to hospitalization.[135]

Hospitalization should be avoided if possible. Preparation for hospitalization is important to reduce the separation anxiety and grief and mourning response described in Chapter 8. Most families have had some experience with a hospital and can give some explanation to the child.

Although children are forbidden in certain areas of a hospital, parents may arrange for a tour of the pediatric ward. The child should be told that special caring people work there and that if he or she is ever hospitalized, the parents will stay close by. The child can be further prepared through play, books, and appropriate films. Emphasize the importance of continued, ample contact with the child whenever either parent or child is hospitalized. You should advise parents to:

1. Trust their intuition (they know the child best).
2. Shop for a doctor and hospital.
3. Prepare themselves so that they can prepare the child.
4. Prepare the child a few days before hospitalization.
5. Be present at important times.

You will be in a position to offset the negative effects of hospitalization through planning individualized care, use of play or art therapy, and involvement in decision and policy making. The hospital personnel must make the ward as homelike as possible through cheerful decor and furnishings and provision for toys, a playroom, and central dining area. The staff members usually wear pastel uniforms or smocks and provide for the child to remain in his or her own clothes, keep a favourite toy, eat uninterrupted by procedures, and follow normal living routines when possible. Flexible visiting hours are essential, as the presence of the mother can dramatically revive a child's interest in getting well and improve eating, sleeping, and general behaviour. The family should be seen as collaborators in care. Answer questions and ask questions related to parents' questions to clarify further and inform or reinforce their ideas. Ideally, if the parent wishes, he or she should be allowed to stay with the child during care, procedures, tests, or treatments. If not feasible, one nurse should consistently care for the child while involving the parent as much as possible.

The parent needs to see the child receiving competent care and to feel that he or she is important to the child and capable as a parent, even if staying with the child is not possible. Encourage the parent to talk about feelings of fear, anxiety, guilt, shame, or sadness that may be present and related to the child's illness or hospitalization or children left at home. Help parents to talk about the unique aspects of their child's or family life so that care can be truly individualized. For example, the child may prefer to wear his shorts instead of pyjamas in bed. Obtain a developmental history from the mother on admission and use it to plan care to follow the child's usual living routine. Help the child displace aggression onto toys or staff rather than onto parents. Allow the child to be angry. Objective involvement is also important to avoid showing favouritism to only certain children. Several authors describe practical ways to help the child prepare for and cope with painful procedures.[136,137] Be aware of cultural differences in the family. For example, the Filipino family provides primary support during illness; and many members of the extended family become involved in the care.[138]

CRITICAL THINKING

What constitutes a developmental history of a child?

Psychosocial Concepts

Use the following information in assessment, teaching, and health promotion with the child and parent(s).

Cognitive Development

The child in this stage is perceptually bound, unable to reason logically about concepts that are discrepant from visual cues. The child learns by interacting with more knowledgeable people, being confronted with others' opinions, and being actively involved with objects and processes.[139] More important than the facts learned are the attitudes the child forms toward knowledge, learning, people, and the environment. Cognition and learning, at least partly a result of language learning and perceptual ability, can be studied through the child's handling of the physical environment and in connection with the concepts of number, causality, and time, abstractions highly developed in Western civilization.[140]

By helping parents understand the cognitive development of their child, including concept formation, you will help them stimulate intellectual growth realistically, without expecting too much. **Concepts** *come about by giving precepts (events, things, and experiences) a meaningful label; the name or label implies similarity to some other things having the same name and difference from things having a different name.* **Concept formation** *develops with perception progressing from diffuse to roughly differentiated and finally to sharply differentiated* awareness of stable and coordinated objects. The first concept is formed when a word comes to designate a crudely defined area of experience. As the late toddler and early preschooler acquire a number of words, each presenting a loosely defined notion or thing, the global meaning becomes a simple concrete concept. As perceived characteristics of things and events become distinguished from each other, the child becomes aware of differences among words, objects, and experiences, such as dog and cat, baby and doll, men and daddy, approval and disapproval; however, the preschooler cannot yet define attributes and cannot make explicit comparisons of the objects. The attributes are an absolute part of the object, such as bark and dog; hence the child is said to *think concretely.* What he or she sees or hears can be named, which is different from conceptual or abstract thinking about the object.[141,142]

Concrete concepts become true concepts when the late preschooler can compare, combine, and describe them and think and talk about their attributes. At this point the child can deal with differences between concepts, such as "dogs bark, people talk," but not until after age six or seven will he or she be able to deal with opposites and similarities together.[143–147] For further information, see the box entitled "Categories of Concepts that Develop in the Preschool Years."

Some of the influences on concept development include the following:

- The child's inability to distinguish between his or her own feelings and outside events
- The ability to be impressed by the external, obvious features of a situation or thing rather than its essential features
- Awareness of gaps in a situation
- Emotional or contextual significance of words

Categories of Concepts that Develop in the Preschool Years

- **Life:** ascribes living qualities to inanimate objects
- **Death:** associates death with separation, lack of movement; thinks dead people capable of doing what living people do
- **Body functions:** has inaccurate understanding about body functions and birth process
- **Space:** judges short distances accurately; aware of direction and distance in relation to body
- **Weight:** estimates weight in terms of size; by age five can determine which of two objects feels heavier, notion of quantity—more than one, big, small
- **Numbers:** understands up to five
- **Time:** has gradually increasing sense of time; present-oriented; knows day of week, month, and year
- **Self:** knows sex, full name, names of outer body parts by age three; when begins to play with other children, self-concept begins to include facts about his or her abilities and race but not socioeconomic class
- **Sex roles:** has general concept of sex, identity, and appropriate sex roles developed at age five or six
- **Social awareness:** is egocentric but forms definite opinions about others' behaviour as "nice" or "mean"; intuitive; concept of causality is magical, illogical
- **Beauty:** names major colours; prefers music with definite tune and rhythm
- **Comedy:** considers as comic funny faces made by self or others, socially inappropriate behaviour, and antics of pets

The concreteness typical of a preschooler's concepts is found in the rambling, loosely jointed circumstantial descriptions. Everything is equally important and must be included. One must listen closely to get the central theme as young children learn things in bunches and not in a systematic, organized way. They can memorize and recite many things, but they cannot paraphrase or summarize their learning.[148–150]

Concepts of Relationships
These *concepts involve time, space, number, and causation, are more abstract than those based on the immediately observable properties of things, and are greatly determined by culture.*[151] See Table 9-4 for the pattern of mental development.

Time Concept
For the preschooler, time is beginning to move; the past is measured in hours, and the future is a myth. At first formal time concepts have nothing to do with personal time. Adults are seen as changeless, and the child believes that he or she can mature in a hurry; thus the preschooler thinks he or she can grow up fast and marry his or her parent. Time concepts are further described in Table 9-4.[152–155]

Spatial Concepts
These concepts differ markedly in children and adults. There are five major stages in the development of spatial concepts. First, there is **action space,** *consisting of the location or regions* to which the child moves. Second, **body space** *refers to the child's own awareness of directions and distances in relation to his or her own body.* Third, there is **object space,** *in which objects are located relative to* each other and without reference to the child's body. The fourth and fifth stages, **map space** and **abstract space,** *are interrelated and depend on knowing directions of east, west, south, and north; allocating space in visual images to nations, regions, towns, rooms; and the ability to deal with maps, geographic or astronomic ideas, and three-dimensional space* that use symbolic (verbal or mathematical) relationships.[156,157]

The preschool child has action space and moves along familiar locations and explores new terrain. He or she is beginning to orient self to body space and object space through play and exploration of his or her own body, up and down, front and back, sideways, next to, near and far, and later left and right. The child is not able until approximately age six to understand object space as a unified whole; he or she will first see a number of unrelated routes or spaces. He or she is generally aware of specific objects and habitual routes. The child does not see self and objects as part of a larger integrated space with multiple possibilities for movement. *Map space and abstract space are not understood until later.*

Quantitative Concepts
Notions of quantity such as one and more than one, bigger, and smaller are developed in the early preschool years. Understanding of the quantity or amount represented by a number is not related to the child's ability to count to 10, 20, or higher, nor can he or she transfer numbers to notions of value of money, although he or she may imitate adults and play store, passing money back and forth. Ordinal numbers, indicating successions rather than totals, develop crudely in "me first" or "me last"; the concept of second or third develops later. The preschooler cannot simultaneously take account of different dimensions such as 1 quart equals 2 pints and equal volume in different-shaped containers (see Table 9-4).[158,159]

Klein and Bisanz of the University of Alberta presented a nonverbal form of arithmetic problems to facilitate performance by helping children create an appropriate mental model of the tasks. They used poker chips in lieu of numbers for counting. They concluded that for two-term problems (e.g., $a + b$), the maximum number of units that must be held in working memory at the same time during problem solution is a major constraint on preschoolers' success in solving addition and subtraction problems when a nonverbal format is used. Some children, in a three-term problem (e.g., $a + b - b$) indicated the spontaneous use of procedures based on the arithmetic principle of inversion. This principle arises from give and take (subtraction and addition), and it occurs in play with other children and adults when solving such a problem. These findings could help teachers to optimize the instructional process so that children can learn to link the knowledge they have gained prior to formal schooling with the instruction offered in school.[160]

Concepts of Causality
The way of perceiving cause and effect is marginal. Things simply are. The child may be pleased or displeased with events but does not understand what brought them about. He or she

TABLE 9–4
Assessment of Mental Development

Age 3 Years	Age 4 Years	Age 5 Years
Knows he or she is a person separate from another Knows own sex and some sex differences	Senses self one among many	Aware of cultural and other differences between people and the two sexes Mature enough to fit into simple type of culture Can tell full name and address Remains calm if lost away from home
Resists commands but distractible and responsive to suggestions Can ask for help Desire to please Friendly Sense of humour	States alibis because more aware of attitude and opinions of others Self-critical; appraises good and bad of self Does not like to admit inabilities; excuses own behaviour Praises self; bosses or criticizes others Likes recognition for achievement Heeds others' thoughts and feelings; expresses own	Dependable Increasing independence Can direct own behaviour; but fatigue, excessive demands, fantasy, and guilt interfere with assuming self-responsibility Admits when needs help Moves from direct to internalized action, from counting what he or she can touch to counting in thought; uses more clues
Use language rather than physical activity to communicate	Active use of language Active learning Likes to make rhymes, to hear stories with exaggeration and humour, dramatic songs Knows nursery rhymes Tells action implied in picture books	Improves use of symbol system, concept formation Repeats long sentences accurately Can carry plot in story Defines objects in terms of use States relationship between two events
Imaginative Better able to organize thoughts Can be bargained with Sacrifices immediate pleasure for promise of future gain	Highly imaginative yet literal, concrete thinking Can organize his or her experience Increasing reasoning power and critical thinking capacity Makes crude comparisons	Less imaginative Asks details Can be reasoned with logically More accurate, relevant, practical, sensible than 4-year-old Asks to have words defined Seeks reality
Understands simple directions; follows normal routines of family life and does minor errands	Concept of 1, 2, 3; counts to 5; does some home chores Generalizes	Begins to understand money Does more home chores with increasing competence Can determine which of two weights heavier Idea in head precedes drawing on paper or physical activity Interested in meaning of relatives
Know age Meagre comprehension of past and future Knows mostly today	Realizes birthday is one in a series and that birthday is measure of growth Knows when next birthday is	Understands week as a unit of time Knows day of week Sense of time and duration increasing

(continued)

TABLE 9-4 *(continued)*
Assessment of Mental Development

Age 3 Years	Age 4 Years	Age 5 Years
	Knows age	Know how old will be on next birthday
	Birthdays and holidays significant because aware of units of time	Knows month and year
		Adults seen as changeless
	Loves parties related to holiday	Memory surprisingly accurate
	Conception of time	
	Knows day of week	
Has attention span of 10–15 minutes	Has attention span of 20 minutes	Has attention span of 30 minutes

does pre-causal thinking, confusing physical and mechanical causation or natural phenomena with psychological, moral, or sequential causes. He or she frequently says "n' then," indicating causal sequence. When the child asks "why?" he or she is probably looking for justification rather than causation. Most things are taken for granted; the child assumes that people, including self, or some motivated inanimate being is the cause of events. Perception of the environment is **animistic,** *endowing all things with the qualities of life Westerners reserve for human beings.* There is little notion of accident or coincidence. It takes some time to learn that there are impersonal forces at work in the world. Thinking is also **egocentric:** *things and events are seen from a personal and narrow perspective and are happening because of self.*[161,162]

CRITICAL THINKING

What is an example of an egocentric verbalization from a preschooler?

The late preschooler fluctuates between reality and fantasy and a materialistic and animistic view of the world; most adults never completely leave behind the magical thinking typical of the preschooler. The child plays with the idea of a tree growing out of the head, what holes feel like to the ground, and growing up starting as an adult. The adult finds no meaning in music, art, literature, love, and possibly even science and mathematics without fantasy or magic.

Preoperational Stage

According to Piaget the preschooler is in the preoperational stage of cognitive development. The preoperational stage is divided into the preconceptual and intuitive phases.[163] During the **preconceptual phase,** *from two to four years of age, the child gathers facts as they are encountered but can neither separate reality from fantasy nor classify or define events in a systematic manner.* Ability to define properties of an object or denote hierarchies or relationships among elements in a class is lacking. He or she is beginning to develop mental strategies from concept formation; concepts are constructed in a global way. He or she is capable of perceiving gross outward appearances but sees only one aspect of an object or situation at a time. For example, if you say, "Take the yellow pill," he or she will focus on

either yellow or pill but cannot focus on both aspects at once. The child is unable to use time, space, equivalence, and class inclusion in concept formation. During the **intuitive phase,** *lasting from approximately four to seven years,* the child gains increasing, but still limited, ability to develop concepts. He or she defines one property at a time, has difficulty stating the definition, but knows how to use the object. The child uses **transductive logic,** *going from general to specific in explanation,* rather than deductive or inductive logic. He or she begins to label, classify in ascending or descending order, do seriation, and note cause–effect relationships, even though true cause–effect understanding does not occur.[164–166]

In addition to the previously described characteristics of concept development, the preoperational stage is characterized by the following:[167–169]

- Egocentric thought
- Literal thinking with absence of reference system
- Intermingling of fantasy, intuition, and reality
- **Absolute thought,** *seeing all or nothing without shades of grey or any relativity*
- **Centring,** *focusing on a single aspect of an object,* causing distorted reasoning
- Lack of concept of **reversibility,** *for every action, there is one that cancels it*
- Static thinking
- Difficulty remembering what he or she started talking about so that when the sentence is finished he or she is talking about something else
- Inability to state cause–effect relationships, categories, or abstractions, believing that events that occur together belong together

Sociocultural Perspective

Another approach to understanding how people learn is Vygotsky's sociocultural theory, which was not fully described because of his death at the age of 38. Lev Vygotsky formulated the sociocultural perspective to cognitive and language development. His main theme was that cognitive growth occurs in a sociocultural context and evolves out of the child's social interactions. He believed that what people knew, thought, and said was shaped by the culture and historical time in which they lived. Each culture has certain "tools of the mind," as well as knowledge that it passes on to its members: languages, problem-solving tactics, and memory strategies. Thereby cognitive development differs between cultures; some do not have formal operational thinking, for example. The child, with an adult's help at a new task, expands the zone of cognitive development as the adult questions, demonstrates, explains, and encourages independent thinking or praises a decision or outcome.[170]

From a sociocultural view, language is the primary vehicle through which adults teach culturally valued ways of thinking and problem solving, as well as what is to be learned. Piaget believed cognitive development influenced language development. Vygotsky believed just the opposite.[171] Refer to Table 9-5 for a summary of Piaget's and Vygotsky's theories.[172]

In general, the preschooler has a consuming curiosity. Learning is vigorous, aggressive, and intrusive. The imagination creates many situations he or she wishes to explore. Judgment is overshadowed by curiosity and excitement. The preschooler has begun to develop such concepts as friend, aunt, uncle; accepting responsibility; independence; passage of time and spatial relationships; use of abstract words, numbers, and colours; and the meaning of cold, tired, and hungry. Attention span is lengthening.

The child's ability to grasp reality varies with individual intelligence and potential intelligence, the social milieu, and opportunities to explore the world, solve problems independently, ask questions, and get answers. Table 9-4 summarizes major characteristics of mental development to help you in assessment.[173–177]

The Family's Role in Teaching the Preschooler

Parents can enhance the child's growth by realizing the importance of the following approaches and their work with the child. Share this information with them.

The single most critical factor in the child's learning is a loving caretaker, because that is who the child imitates. How the mothering person speaks to, touches, and plays with the child governs the potential for socialization and cognitive development. This is true even for the child who had a low birth weight and was at risk for developmental lag or disability.[178,179] A child's problem-solving abilities are shaped by the parents' method for coping with problems and by opportunities for problem solving. In families in which everyone gets a chance to speak out and jointly explore a problem, the child learns to express him- or herself logically. Automatic obedience or acceptance of parental commands or decisions will interfere with reasoning.[180] Also important are the opportunities provided for the child to learn, explore, ask questions, and play a variety of games. Teaching involves demonstration, listening, and talking about the situation in direct and understandable terms and giving reasons. Cognitive development includes more than fluency with words, a good verbal memory, and information. It includes ability to use imagination, form mental pictures, and engage in fantasy appropriately, along with art, music, and other creative activities. It includes expanding skills in logical thinking. Most important, it involves increasing integration of many kinds of brain functions. Much integrated learning comes from the child's engaging in motor activity, play, and language games; talking with adults and peers; and paying attention to both trivial and important aspects of the environment.[181]

CRITICAL THINKING

What specific examples of play activities can stimulate cognitive development?

The amount of prosocial behaviour displayed by children varies from one child to another. One type of prosocial behaviour is altruism. Eisenberg and her associates found that a prosocial personality disposition emerges early in childhood and is somewhat consistent over time.[182] A group of Canadian researchers have been studying relations among emotional expressiveness, empathy, and prosocial behaviour in children.

TABLE 9-5
Comparison of Piaget's and Vygotsky's Theories of Cognitive Development

Piaget's Cognitive Theory	Vygotsky's Sociocultural Theory
1. Cognitive development is mostly the same universally.	1. Cognitive development differs from culture to culture and in different historical eras.
2. Cognitive development results from the child's independent exploration of the world.	2. Cognitive development results from guided participation or social interactions.
3. Each child constructs knowledge on his or her own.	3. Children and adults or more knowledgeable persons or peers co-construct knowledge.
4. Individual egocentric processes and language become more social.	4. Social processes or interactions with others become individual psychological processes.
5. Peers are important because children must learn to take peer's perspectives.	5. Adults are important because they know the culture's way and tools of thinking.
6. Development precedes learning; children cannot master certain things until they have the requisite cognitive structures.	6. Learning precedes development; tools learned with adult help are internalized.

They conclude that boys' level of empathy is a strong predictor of prosocial behaviour compared to girls. Girls' level of empathy, as related to prosocial behaviour, was modest. This finding may possibly be due to social norms which require girls to be prosocial whether they feel empathetic or not.[183] Other Canadian researchers claim that as children grow they eventually find themselves in situations which offer to them opportunities to consider their own future well-being (prudent behaviour) and the well-being of others (altruistic behaviour). The results of the children's considerations may conflict, however, with what is desirable for them at the present moment. Thompson and her colleagues at Dalhousie University concluded that between three and four years of age children acquire the ability to deal with future-oriented situations through the development of some common mechanism that affects both future-oriented prudence and altruism.[184] They state that the findings of similar, age-related changes in performance provide support for the claim that four-year-olds, but not three-year-olds, have the ability to imagine various mental states that conflict with the child's own current states and involve a noncurrent situation. This ability has been described as double imagination and appears only in four-year-olds. In addition, the resolution of conflicts between current and future desires may involve other processes as well.[185] Further research is needed to examine more closely the processes involved in dealing with these kinds of conflicts during age-four transition.

Canada has a stellar reputation in the area of children's television programming.[186] Canadian networks are required to air a certain amount of domestic programming mainly to make certain that Canadian children have a sense of their own culture. Children's television in Canada has a long history of providing a gentler alternative to a few of the over-the-top programs being shown elsewhere. Classic programs such as *Mr. Dressup* and *The Friendly Giant* allow children to engage in a more interactive experience with the program hosts.[187] Treehouse TV is unique in that it is the only national speciality network in North America solely dedicated to children age six years and under. It offers a variety of high-quality programming from Canada and around the world. Treehouse TV has launched three original series: *Ants in Your Pants*, a music show featuring Canadian performers; *Crazy Quilt*, a program that features storytelling and easy craft-making; and *Wee 3*, a show about three tiny monsters who analyze their fears and feelings through signing and playing out scenarios. For kids from preschool age to teenagers, *Teletoon*, Canada's speciality channel which is totally dedicated to animation, offers 24-hour programming, 12 hours of which is guaranteed to be suitable for unsupervised viewing (violence free), while the preschool block is commercial free.[188]

Another option for kids is YTV, Canada's leading youth network, which is seen in more than 8 million homes. YTV Jr. broadcasts 40 hours of commercial-free programming per week for preschoolers. The network has Canada's number-one afterschool block with programs such as the messy game show *Hugo*. It is helpful to know that Canadian children will always have the option of watching quality television programming.[189]

A conservative estimate is that preschoolers spend more than a third of their waking time watching television.[190] In fact, many young children spend more time watching television than they spend in conversation with adults or siblings. In today's world, if children watch prime-time television, what may be the effects of television violence on children?

Television has many roles. It can teach children about stereotypes and provide them with violent models of aggression. On the other hand, television can teach the child that it is better to behave in positive prosocial ways than in negative, antisocial ways.[191] However, it is essential that professionals concerned with the health and well-being of children include TV violence in their work with families in both rural and urban communities.[192]

CRITICAL THINKING

Develop a series of critical guidelines that you could provide to parents to assist them in making television a more positive influence in their children's lives.

Communication Patterns

People have three types of communication at their disposal: (1) somatic or physical symptoms such as flushed skin colour and increased respirations; (2) action such as play or movement; and (3) verbal expression. The preschool child uses all of them.

Learning to use verbal expression—language—to communicate is an ongoing developmental process that is affected directly by the child's interaction with others.

Vygotsky's sociocultural approach to language development helps us understand the preschooler as he or she learns. Preschoolers often talk to themselves as they play or go about daily activities. Two preschoolers together may be in a collective monologue rather than truly conversing. Instead of the egocentric speech of preoperational thought, such speech can be considered **private speech,** *speech that guides one's thoughts and behaviour.* Private speech is heavily used when the child is struggling to solve difficult problems.[193] It is a step toward mature thought and a forerunner of the silent thinking-in-words that adults use daily. Private speech gets expanded by **social speech,** or *conversations with others.* Then the child develops **inner speech,** or *mutterings, lip movements, and silent verbal thoughts.* The use of private speech increases during preschool years; and then it decreases during early elementary school years. **Guided participation,** or *learning in collaboration with more knowledgeable adults or companions who are more knowledgeable,* helps the child incorporate the learned problem-solving strategies into his or her own thinking.[194]

The *child uses language for many reasons:*

- To maintain social rapport
- To gain attention
- To get information
- To seek meaning about his or her experience
- To note how others' answers fit personal thoughts
- To play with words
- To gain relief from anxiety
- To learn how to think and solve problems

He or she asks why, what, when, where, how, repeatedly.

A child learns language from hearing it and using it. Words are at first empty shells until he or she has experiences to match. Parents should provide age-appropriate experiences so the child learns that words and actions go together. Equally important, parents should avoid saying one thing and doing another. Attaining trust in the utility and validity of verbal communication and learning that talking helps rather than hinders life are crucial to transition from infancy to school years. If talking does not gain a response from others or help the child solve problems and relate to those he or she needs, or if the world is too troublesome, the child is likely to find refuge in fantasy and neglect social, communicative meanings of language.

Directing his or her life depends on language and an understanding of the meaning of words and the logic with which they are used. When the child acquires language, he or she gradually becomes freed from tangible, concrete experiences and can internalize visual symbols, develop memory and recall, fragment the past, project the future, and differentiate fantasy from reality.

Language is also learned from being read to and having printed material available. Share the following suggestions with

parents for choosing books for the preschooler. The book should be durable, have large print that does not fill the entire page, and be colourfully illustrated. The concepts should be expressed concretely in simple sentences and should tell a tale that fits the child's fantasy conception of the world, such as a story with animals and objects who can talk and think like people. Or the story should tell about the situations he or she ordinarily faces, such as problems with playmates, discovery of the preschooler's world, nightmares, and the arrival of a new baby.

Use and share with the significant adults in the child's life these effective ways of talking with the preschooler (Table 9-6).

Table 9-7 is a guide for assessing language skills of the preschooler. During assessment keep in mind that the ways in which the child's parents and other family members speak, and the language opportunities the child encounters, all considerably influence his or her language skills.

Gaines states that good interaction skills have been related to lifelong success in academic, social and vocational spheres of life.[195] However, many children with communication and language disorders are usually not identified until three years of

TABLE 9-6
Guidelines for Communication with a Preschooler

1. Be respectful as you talk with the child.
2. Do not discourage talking, questions, or the make-believe in the child's language; verbal explorations are essential to learn language. Answers to questions should meet needs and give him or her awareness of adult attitudes and feelings about the topics discussed.
3. Tell the truth to the best of your ability and on the child's level of understanding. Do not say an injection "won't hurt." Say, "It's like a pin prick that will hurt a short time." Admit if the answer is unknown, and seek the answer with the child. A lie is eventually found out and causes a loss of trust in that adult and in others.
4. Do not make a promise unless you can keep it.
5. The child takes every word literally. Do not say, "She nearly died laughing," or "I laughed my head off." Do not describe surgery as "putting you to sleep."
6. Respond to the relationship or feelings in the child's experience rather than the actual object or event. Talk about the child's feelings instead of agreeing or disagreeing with what he or she says. Help the child understand what he or she feels rather than why he or she feels it.
7. Precede statements of advice and instruction with a statement of understanding of the child's feelings. When the child is feeling upset emotionally, he or she cannot listen to instructions, advice, consolation, or constructive criticism.
8. Do not give undue attention to slang or curse words, and do not punish the child for using them. The child is demonstrating initiative and uses these words for shock value, and attention or punishment emphasizes the importance of the words. Remain relaxed and give the child a more difficult or different word to say. If he or she persists in using the unacceptable word, the adult may say, "I'm tired of hearing that word, say _____"; ask him or her not to say the word again since it may hurt others, or use distraction. Children learn unacceptable words as they learn all others, and parents would be wise to listen to their own vocabulary.
9. Sit down if possible when participating or talking with children. You are more approachable when at their physical and eye level.
10. Seek to have a warm, friendly relationship without thrusting yourself on the child. How you feel about the child is more important than what you say or do.
11. Through attentive listening and interested facial expression, convey a tell-me-more-about-it attitude to encourage the child to communicate.
12. Regard some speech difficulties as normal. Ignore stuttering or broken fluency that does not persist. Do not correct each speech error and do not punish. Often the child thinks faster than he or she can articulate speech. Give the child time when he or she speaks.
13. Talk in a relaxed manner. Do not bombard the child with verbal information.

TABLE 9-7
Assessment of Language Development

Age 3 Years	Age 4 Years	Age 5 Years
Appearance of individual sounds *y, f,* and *v* in words	Appearance of individual sounds *s, z, th, r, ch, j* in words	Appearance of individual sounds *sh, zh, th* in words
Vocabulary of at least 900, up to 2000, words	Vocabulary of at least 1500, up to 3000, words	Vocabulary of at least 2100, up to 5000, words
Uses language understandably; uses same sounds experimentally	Uses language confidently	Uses language efficiently, correctly
Understands simple reasons	Concrete speech	No difficulty understanding other's spoken words
Uses some adjectives and adverbs	Increasing attention span	Meaningful sentences; uses future tense
	Uses "I" and other pronouns	Increasing skill with grammar
	Imitates and plays with words	Knows common opposites
	Defines a few simple words	
	Talks in sentences; uses past tense	
	Uses plurals frequently	
	Comprehends prepositions	
Talks in simple sentences about things	Talks incessantly while doing other activities	Talks constantly
Repeats sentence of six syllables	Asks many questions	No infantile articulation
Uses plurals in speech	Demands detailed explanations with "why"	Repeats sentences of 12 or more syllables
Collective monologue; does not appear to care whether another is listening	Carries on long involved conversation	Asks searching questions, meaning of words, how things work
Some random, inappropriate answers	Exaggerates; boasts; tattles; may use profanity for attention	Can tell a long story accurately, but may keep adding to reality to make story more fantastic
Intelligibility is 70–90%	Frequently uses "everything"	Intelligibility good; some distortion in articulation of *t, s*
Sings simple songs	Tells family faults outside of home without restraint	Sings relatively well
	Tells story combining reality and fantasy; appears to be lying	
	Intelligibility is 90%; articulation errors with *l, r, s, z, sh, ch, j, th*	
	Variations in volume from a yell to a whisper	
	Likes to sing	
Knows first and family name	Calls people names	Counts to 10 or further without help
Names figures in a picture	Names three objects he or she knows in succession	Repeats five digits
Repeats three digits	Counts to 5 without help	Names four colours, usually red, green, blue, yellow
Likes to name things	Repeats four digits	
	Knows which line is long	
	Names one or more colours	
Talks to self or imaginary playmate	Talks with imaginary playmate of same sex and age	Sense of social standards and limits seen in language use
Expresses own desires and limits frequently	Seeks reassurance	
	Interested in things being funny	
	Likes puns	

age or later. Early identification, including hearing testing, may prevent many difficulties related to and resulting from speech, language, and communication disorders. In fact, the earlier intervention begins, the better the outcome. In 1997, the Ontario Ministry of Health provided funding to initiate First Words, the Preschool Speech and Language Program in the Ottawa region.[196] This program was the result of a provincial initiative to give enhanced dollars to serve the preschool population. A system of services, including a screening clinic, was developed to prevent and identify early speech and language disabilities in children. Now a system of services, including the screening clinic, is accessible to the general public.

Community care nurses can play a vital role in efforts to improve early detection of speech-language difficulties in children.[197] In a special health promotion endeavour, nurses can provide assistance to families concerned about a child's communication skills.

CRITICAL THINKING

What limitation in, or absence of, communication behaviours indicates that a child might have difficulties in talking and/or understanding?

Play Patterns

Play is the work of the child. Play occupies most of the child's waking hours and serves to consolidate and enlarge his or her previous learning and promote adaptation. Play has elements of reality, and there is earnestness about it. Piaget described play as assimilation; play behaviour involves taking in, moulding, and using objects for pleasure and learning.[198]

The preschooler is intrusive in play, bombarding others by purposeful or accidental physical attack. He or she is into people's ears and minds by loud, assertive talking; into space by vigorous gross motor activities; into objects through exploration; and into the unknown by consuming curiosity.[199]

The preschool years are the pre-gang stage, in which the child progresses from solitary and parallel play to cooperating for a longer time in a larger group. He or she identifies somewhat with a play group; follows rules; is aware of the status of self compared with others; develops perception of social relationships; begins the capacity for self-criticism; and states traits and characteristics of others that he or she likes or dislikes. At first the child spends brief, incidental periods of separation from the parents. The time away from them increases in length and frequency, and eventually the orientation shifts from family to peer group.[200]

A **peer** is a *person with approximately equal status, a companion, often of the same sex and age,* and with whom one can share mutual concerns. The **peer group** is a *relatively informal association of equals who share common play experiences with emphasis on common rules and understanding the limits that the group places on the individual.* The preschool play group differs from later ones in that it is loosely organized. The activity of the group may be continuous; but membership changes as the child joins or leaves the group at will, and the choice of playmates is relatively restricted in kind and number. This is

the first introduction to a group that assesses him or her as a child from a child's point of view. The preschooler is learning about entering a new, different, very powerful world when he or she joins the group. Although social play is enjoyed, the child feels a need for solitary play at times.[201,202]

The number and sex of siblings and the parents' handling of the child's play seem to influence behaviour with the play group. If the family rejects the child, he or she may feel rejected by peers, even when the child is not rejected, causing self-isolation, inability to form close friendships, and ultimately real rejection.

Purposes of Play

The natural mode of expression for the child is play. *Purposes of play include the following:*

- Develop and improve muscular strength, coordination, and balance; define body boundaries
- Work off excess physical energy; provide exercise
- Communicate with others, establish friendships, learn about interpersonal relations, and develop concern for others
- Learn cooperation, sharing, and healthy competition
- Express imagination, creativity, and initiative
- Imitate and learn about social activity, adult roles, and cultural norms
- Test and deal with reality, gain mastery over unpleasant experiences
- Explore, investigate, and manipulate features of the adult world; sharpen the senses and concentration
- Learn about rules of chance and probability and rules of conduct and that at times one loses, but it is all right
- Build self-esteem
- Feel a sense of power, make things happen, explore and experiment
- Provide for intellectual, sensory, and language development and dealing with concrete experiences in symbolic terms
- Assemble novel aspects of the environment
- Organize life's discrepancies privately and with others
- Learn about self and how others see him or her
- Practise leader and follower roles
- Have fun, express joy, and feel the pleasure of mastery
- Act out and symbolically work through a painful physical or emotional state by repetition in play so that it is more bearable and assimilated into the child's self-concept; master overwhelming stimuli
- Develop the capacity to gratify self and to delay gratification
- Formulate a bridge between concrete experiences and abstract thought

The boxes entitled "Types of Play Related to Social Characteristics" and "Common Themes in Children's Play" give more insight into children's play.[203–208]

CRITICAL THINKING

A farm family has one preschool child. The child's parents are wondering how frequently they should take their child to town to play with a cousin. What advice would you give the parents?

Types of Play Related to Social Characteristics

- **Unoccupied play:** Child stands by, aimlessly engaged in activity, such as pace, run, hit.
- **Onlooker play:** Child watches others with no interactions or movement toward participation (e.g., use of television).
- **Parallel play:** Child plays independently but next to other children; displays no group association.
- **Associative play:** Children play together in similar or identical play without organization, division of labour, leadership, or mutual goals.
- **Cooperative play:** Play is organized in group with others. Planning and cooperation begin before play starts to form goals, division of labour, and leadership.
- **Solitary play:** Child, either by choice or because of lack of peers, entertains self in play. Play is often imaginative or studious in nature.
- **Supplementary play:** Play shifts from large group activities or games to focus on smaller group or board games.

Sources: Papalia, D., S. Olds, and R. Feldman, Human Development (7th ed.). Boston: McGraw-Hill, 1998; Seifert, K., R. Hoffnung, and M. Hoffnung, Lifespan Development. Boston: Houghton Mifflin, 1997; Sigelman, C., Life-Span Human Development (3rd ed.). Pacific Grove, CA: Brooks/Cole, 1999; Wong, D., Whaley and Wong's Nursing Care of Infants and Children (6th ed.). St. Louis: C. V. Mosby, 1999.

Common Themes in Children's Play

Various issues in the child's life will be repeated four to five times in each play session. These issues are shown in different styles of play, but the theme is the thread that ties all the different styles together, as the pieces of a quilt unite to form the pattern of the whole.

- Power/control
- Anger/sadness
- Trust/relationships/abandonment
- Nurturing/rejection/security
- Boundaries/intrusion
- Violation/protection
- Self-esteem
- Fears/anxiety (separation, monsters, ghosts, animals, the dark, noises, bad people, injury, death)
- Confusion
- Identity
- Loyalty/betrayal
- Loss/death
- Loneliness
- Adjustment/change

Play Materials

These materials should be simple, sturdy, durable, and free from unnecessary hazards. They need not be expensive. The child should have adequate space and equipment that is unstructured enough to allow for creativity and imagination to work unfettered. He or she will enjoy trips to parks and playgrounds. Often, creative, stimulating toys can be made from ordinary household articles: plastic pot cleaners, empty thread spools, a bell, yarn, or empty boxes covered with washable adhesive paper. The child may like the box more than the toy.

Increasing emphasis is being placed on high-technology, interactive, and weaponry toys. These toys actually stifle imagination and discovery, and weaponry toys may cause fears, heighten aggressive fantasies, and cause injury and sometimes death. Weaponry toys should be avoided as much as possible. Young children need to direct their games to be in control of their play and their fantasies. They use play to work out problems, to practise skills, and to act out roles in preparation for later real-life experiences

The play materials that are available will determine the play activities. Play materials are enjoyed for different reasons. For example, **physical activity,** *which facilitates development of motor skills,* is provided through play with musical instruments and records for marching and rhythm, balls, shovel, broom, ladder, swing, trapeze, slide, boxes, climbing apparatus, boards, sled, wagon, tricycle, bicycle with training wheels, wheelbarrow, and blocks. Swimming, ice-skating, roller-skating, and skiing are being learned. **Dramatic play,** *which is related to the ability to classify objects correctly, take another's perspective, and do problem solving,* is afforded through large building blocks, sandbox and sand toys, dolls, housekeeping toys, nurse and doctor kits, farm or other occupational toys, cars and other vehicles, and worn-out adult clothes for dress-up. This is a predominant form of play in childhood and also can include aspects of physical play. **Creative playthings,** *which promote constructive, nonsocial, cognitive, and emotional development,* include blank sheets of paper, crayons, finger or water paints, chalk, various art supplies, clay, plasticine, or other manipulative material; blunt scissors, paste, cartons, scraps of cloth, water-play equipment, and musical toys. **Symbolic play** *is play that enables the child to create new images or symbols to represent objects, people, and events.* It results from opportunities to do dramatic and creative play. **Quiet play,** *which promotes cognitive development and rest from physical exertion,* is achieved through books, puzzles, records, and table games. Children's songs, nursery rhymes, and fairy tales can absorb anxiety, entertain, soothe, reassure that life's problems can be solved, and support the child's superego.[209,210]

The *role of the adult in child's play* is to provide opportunity, equipment, and safety and to avoid interference or structuring of play. Mothers and fathers tend to play differently with the child. How fathers play with their children appears to be determined not just by biology but also by cultural influences. Studies of fathers in Sweden, Germany, Africa, and New Delhi showed that they do not play with children in a highly physical way, as in North America. Rather, they play more quietly; and New Delhi fathers were notably gentle.[211] Dubeau states that because immigrants make up 17% of Canada's population, we need research on the impact of various cultural models on fatherhood.[212] Becoming and being a father is a significant step in one's life, and for the child having a father is stimulating and enriching because each parent interacts with the child in different ways.

Parents should be taught the following:

1. Allow the child to try things and enjoy personal activities.
2. Assist only if he or she is in need of help.
3. The child is not natural in play when he or she thinks adults are watching; avoid showing amusement or ridicule of play behaviour or conversation.
4. Allow playmates to work out their own differences.
5. Distract, redirect, or substitute a different activity if the children cannot share and work out their problems.
6. There are times to play with the child, but avoid over-stimulation, teasing, hurry, or talking about the child as if he or she were not present.
7. Avoid doing the activity for the child. Let him or her take the lead.
8. Try to enter the child's world. If he or she wants you to attend the teddy bear's 100th birthday party, go.

Even when free time, space, and toys are limited, most children find a way to play. They use household objects such as pots, pans, and furniture, and outdoor items such as trees, sticks, rocks, sand, empty cans, and discarded equipment—all for dramatic and fantasy play.

Table 9-8 summarizes play characteristics as a further aid in assessment and teaching.[213–216]

Share the above information with parents and explore their feelings about child's play and their role with the child.

TABLE 9-8
Assessment of Play Characteristics

Age 3 Years	Age 4 Years	Age 5 Years
Enjoys active and sedentary play	Increasing physical and social play	More varied activity More graceful in play
Likes toys in orderly form Puts away toys with supervision	Puts away toys when reminded	Puts away toys by self
Fantasy not yielding too much to reality Likes fairy tales, books	Much imaginative and dramatic play Has complex ideas but unable to carry out because of lack of skill and time	More realistic in play Less interested in fairy tales More serious and ready to know reality Restrained but creative
Likes solitary and parallel play with increasing social play in shifting groups of two or three	Plays in groups of two or three, often companions of own sex Imaginary playmates Projects feelings and deeds onto peers or imaginary playmates May run away from home	Plays in groups of five or six Friendships stronger and continue over longer time Chooses friends of like interests Spurred on in activity by rivalry
Cooperates briefly Willing to wait turn and share with suggestion	Suggests and accepts turns but often bossy in directing others Acts out feelings spontaneously, especially with music and arts	Generous with toys Sympathetic, cooperative, but quarrels and threatens by word or gesture Acts out feelings Wants rules to do things right; but beginning to realize peers cheat, so develops mild deceptions and fabrications
Some dramatic play-house or family games Frequently changes activity Likes to arrange, combine, transfer, sort, and spread objects and toys	Dramatic and creative play at a peak Likes to dress up and help with household tasks; plays with dolls, trucks Does not sustain role in dramatic play; moves from one role to another incongruous role No carry over in play from day to day Silly in play	Dramatic play about most life events, but more realistic Play continues from day to day Interested in finishing what started, even if it takes several days More awareness of yesterday and tomorrow

(continued)

TABLE 9-8 *(continued)*
Assessment of Play Characteristics

Age 3 Years	Age 4 Years	Age 5 Years
Able to listen longer to nursery rhymes Dramatizes nursery rhymes and stories Can match simple forms Identifies primary colours Enjoys cutting, pasting, block building	Concentration span longer Sometimes so busy at play forgets to go to toilet Re-enacts stories and trips Enjoys simple puzzles and models with trial-and-error method Poor space perception	Perceptive to order, form, and detail Better eye–hand coordination Rhythmic motion to music; enjoys musical instruments Likes excursions Interested in world outside immediate environment; enjoys books
Enjoys simple puzzles, hand puppets, large ball Enjoys sand and water play	Uses constructive and manipulative play material increasingly Enjoys sand and water play; cups, containers, and buckets for carrying and pouring	Interested in the many hues and shades of colours Enjoys cutting out pictures, pasting, working on special projects, puzzles
Enjoys dumping and hauling toys Rides tricycle	Identifies commonly seen colours Enjoys crayons and paints, books Enjoys swing, jungle gym, toy hammer or other tools, pegboards	Likes to run and jump, play with bicycle, wagon, and sled Enjoys sand and water play; dramatic and elaborative in play Enjoys using tools and equipment of adults

Guidance and Discipline

The child learns how to behave by imitating adults and by using the opportunities to develop self-control. The child needs consistent, fair, and kind limits to feel secure, to know that the parents care for and love him or her enough to provide protection—a security he or she does not have when allowed to do anything, regardless of ability. Limits should be set in a way that preserves the self-respect of the child and parent. Only when the child can predict the behaviour of others can he or she accept the need to inhibit or change some of his or her behaviour and work toward predictable and rational behaviour. The parent should be an ally to the child as he or she struggles for control over inner impulses and convey to the child that he or she need not fear impulses.

"Bad behaviour" springs from wanting to get attention, exert independence or control, or frustration and anger. Children learn to strike out or hit others from other children or by imitating parents. It is important to stop immediately behaviour that hurts another by holding the child's arm gently and quietly saying, "No." Explain the reason. Spanking should be avoided; it only teaches the child it is all right to hit.[217]

Some children are more difficult to discipline even though the parents appear to be using the right strategies. Some people are born with a larger variety of dopamine-4 receptor genes and are biologically predisposed to be thrill-seekers. The gene makes them less sensitive to pain and physical sensation. Such children are more likely to crash their tricycles into a wall, to jump from high places, to ignore cautious directions, to pound the fist on hard objects, to break objects, and to be a daredevil.

Attention deficit hyperactivity disorder (ADHD) may be associated with this neurotransmitter difference. It is noteworthy to mention that Washbusch and his colleagues reviewed three cases in the assessment and treatment of ADHD. These case studies highlighted the importance of the need for systematic, comprehensive, and individualized treatments for children with ADHD. In fact, pharmacological intervention is the most common form of treatment for children with ADHD, along with behavioural interventions.[218]

CRITICAL THINKING

What types of support can you, as a health professional, provide to parents who have a child with ADHD?

A behaviour modification technique that can be used to discipline an aggressively acting out child is *time-out*. Time-out involves immediately placing the child after a mean act in a quiet, uninteresting place (hall, small room, or corner of a room) for five to 15 minutes to remove the child from positive reinforcement. Time-out stops the misbehaviour and is unpleasant enough to increase the possibility that the child will not repeat the undesirable act. *The child should be helped to realize that time-out means that his or her behaviour—not the child—is rejected; thus, the use of rewards to reinforce desired behaviour is necessary* in conjunction with this time-out method.

Emotional Development

If the child has developed reasonably well and if he or she has mastered earlier developmental tasks, the preschooler is a source

Kalisha is an active, 38-month-old girl, who weighs 15.45 kg (34 pounds) and is 95 cm (38 inches) tall. She is playing on the sidewalk in front of her parents' home with her brother Marvin, four years old, and her next-door neighbour Lori, aged five years.

Kalisha is riding her small, two-wheeled bicycle, which has training wheels. Marvin and Lori are riding their small bicycles or scooters. Kalisha rides for a while, and then stops to watch the others. Although involved in the same activity, she plays next to rather than with the older children. Several times Kalisha rides her bicycle into the path of her brother's approaching bicycle. The preschooler is typically intrusive in play, bombarding others by purposeful or accidental attack. Kalisha continues to ride and stop, always staying within her mother's view as she moves farther away and then nearer on her bicycle. She demonstrates the attachment behaviour typical of this age by maintaining proximity to her mother.

When Marvin and Lori ride down the street, leaving Kalisha, Kalisha asks her mother to go with her to join them. She pulls her mother's hand insistently several times, and they walk together down the street. When she approaches the other children, Kalisha runs to them, laughing, and then gives Lori a hug. Lori chases Kalisha up the street, and Kalisha laughs and runs to her mother, seeking protection, security, assurance, and approval. Through this behaviour she affirms that her mother is still the most important person in her life.

As the older children ride their bicycles on the sidewalk toward Kalisha, she laughs and shouts, then waves her arms, telling them, "I am the stop sign." She tells Lori to stop, but Lori rides by, laughing and saying, "You'll have to give me a ticket." On the return trip, Lori stops at Kalisha's command. Kalisha and Lori repeat this pattern several times, and each time Kalisha becomes more animated. She demonstrates autonomy and beginning initiative in these interactions, displaying the egocentrism typical of the preschooler as she commands events for her own needs and purposes and gains a sense of power through symbolic play.

1. What may be some other images or symbols, other than "I am the stop sign," which Kalisha might use to demonstrate symbolic play?

2. How do you interpret Kalisha's behaviour of riding her bicycle into the pathway of her brother? How should her mother react to this behaviour?

3. Project yourself, if you can, into the mind and body of Kalisha to respond to this question. What is your interpretation of the "sense of power" Kalisha experiences as she plays out the part of the stop sign?

status and development. Tolerance of frustration is still limited, but flares of temper and frustrations over failure pass quickly. As the child is learning to master things and handle independence and dependence, so is he or she increasing mastery of self and others and learning to get along with more people, both children and adults. The preschooler attempts to behave like an adult in realistic activity and play and is beginning to learn social roles, moral responsibility, and cooperation, although he or she still grabs, hits, and quarrels for short bursts of time.

If the child has the opportunity to establish a sense of gender and to identify with mature adults, if the attitude about self is sound and positive, and if he or she has learned to trust and have some self-control, he or she is ready to take on the culture. The preschooler begins to decide what kind of person he or she is, and self-concept, ego strength, and superego will continue to mature. Self is still very important, but he or she does not feel omnipotent.

Developmental Crisis

The psychosexual crisis for this era is initiative versus guilt, and all the aforementioned behaviours are part of achieving initiative.[219] **Initiative** is *enjoyment of energy displayed in action, assertiveness, learning, increasing dependability, and ability to plan.* Natural initiative is desirable; however, it is important for parents not to expect too much or to push the child excessively. If the child does not achieve the developmental task of initiative, there is an overriding sense of guilt from the tension between the demands of the superego, or expectations, and actual performance.

Guilt is a *sense of defeatism, anger, feeling responsible for things that he or she is not really responsible for, feeling easily frightened from what he or she wants to do, feeling bad, shameful, and deserving of punishment.* A sense of guilt can develop from sibling rivalry, lack of opportunity to try things, or restriction on or lack of guidance in response to fantasy or when parents interfere with the child's activity. If the guilt feelings are too strong, the child is affected in a negative way. Excessive guilt does not enhance moral or superego development, although the child must experience realistic guilt for wrong behaviour.[220–222]

Help parents understand that if the child is to develop a sense of initiative and a healthy personality, they and other significant adults must encourage use of imagination, creativity, activity, and plans. Parents should encourage the child's efforts to cooperate and share in the decisions and responsibilities of family life. The child develops best when he or she is commended and recognized for accomplishments. Appropriate behaviour should be reinforced so that it will continue. Affirming a child's emotional experience is as important as affirming his or her physical development. The preschooler needs to learn what feelings of love, hate, joy, and antagonism are and how to cope with and express them in ways other than physically. He or she needs guidance toward mature behaviour.

of pleasure to adults. He or she is more a companion than someone to care for. The various behaviours discussed under development of physical, mental, language, play, body image, and moral-spiritual aspects contribute to his or her emotional

CRITICAL THINKING

How can a child who has a chronic illness develop a sense of initiative?

Self-Concept: Body Image and Sexuality Development

Self-concept, including body image and sex role behaviour, are gradually developing in these years.[223–225] Positive self-concept develops from parental love, effective relations with peers and others, success in play and other activities, and gaining skills and self-control in activities of daily living. Body boundaries and sense of self become more definite to the preschooler because of developing sexual curiosity and awareness of how he or she differs from others, increased motor skills with precision of movement and maturing sense of balance, improved spatial orientation, maturing cognitive and language abilities, ongoing play activities, and relationship identification with his or her parents.

Learning about the body—where it begins and ends, what it looks like, and what it can do—is basic to the child's identity formation. Included in the growing self-awareness is discovery of feelings and learning names for them. The child is beginning to learn how he or she affects others and others' responses, and he or she is learning the rudiments of control over feelings and behaviour. The concept of body is reflected in the way the child talks, draws pictures, and plays. The child with no frame of reference in relation to self has increased anxiety and misperception of self and others.

The artistic productions of the preschooler tell us about self-perceptions. The three-year-old draws a man consisting of one circle, sometimes with an appendage, a crude representation of the face, and no differentiation of parts. The four-year-old draws a man consisting of a circle for a face and head, facial features of two eyes and perhaps a mouth, two appendages, and occasionally wisps of hair or feet. Often the four-year-old has not really formulated a mental representation of the lower part of the body. The five-year-old draws an unmistakable person. There is a circle face with nose, mouth, eyes, and hair; there is a body with arms and legs. Articles of clothing, fingers, and feet may be added. The width of the person is usually approximately one-half the length.[226] The child may think of the body as a house.[227] For example, while eating, he or she may name the various bites as fantasy characters that will go down and play in his or her house. The child may create an elaborate play area for them. (You can take advantage of this fantasy if eating problems arise.)

When the three-year-old is asked his or her sex, the child is likely to give his or her name; the four-year-old can state sex, thus showing a differentiation of self.

Discuss with the parents the concept of body image and how they can help the child's formulation of self. The child needs opportunities to learn the correct names and basic functions of body parts and to discover his or her body with joy and pride. Mirrors, photographs of the child, drawings of self and others such as parents and siblings, weighing, and measuring height enhance the formation of his or her mental picture. The child needs physical and mental activity to learn body mastery and self-protection and to express feelings of helplessness, doubt, or pain when the body does not accomplish what he or she would like or during illness. The preschooler needs to manipulate the tools of his or her culture to learn the difference between self and machines, equipment, or tools. The child needs to be encouraged to "listen" to the body—the aches of stretched muscles, tummy rumblings, stubbed toes—and to understand what he or she feels. To deny, misinterpret, misname, or push aside physical or emotional activities and feelings promotes an unrealistic self-understanding and eventually a negative self-concept and unwholesome body image. Specific nursing measures after illness or injury help the child reintegrate body image.[228]

Adaptive Mechanisms

Development proceeds toward increasing differentiation, articulation, and integration. **Differentiation** involves a *progressive separation of feeling, thinking, and acting and an increased polarity between self and others.* Differentiation is seen in the child's ability to **articulate** or *talk about the perceived experience of the world and the experience of self as a being.* **Integration** is seen in the *development of structured controls and adaptive or defensive mechanisms.*[229]

The preschooler has gained both language and conceptual ability, greater experience, and a greater imagination. Now he or she can talk about and play out the fears of being alone, ghosts, masks, the dark, strange noises, strangers, dogs, tigers, spiders, bears, and snakes, closed places, thunderstorms, and separation from loved ones. These fears decline by age five but may persist until age seven or eight.

The child encounters a variety of frustrations as he or she engages in new activities, expects more of self, and others expect more of the child. Disappointments arise. The *child must learn to cope with frustrations just as he or she learns to handle and overcome fears. Teach parents that they can help by:*

1. Showing concern and acceptance of the child's feelings.
2. Helping the child talk about the feelings.
3. Exploring with the child possible causes for the feelings.
4. Helping the child realize that emotions have reasons and that they can discover causes for personal feelings.
5. Emphasizing that the child is neither expected to be perfect nor should expect that everything will always go as desired.
6. Helping the child make a decision about handling the frustrating situation, thus learning problem-solving strategies.

How the parent handles frustrations and problems sets an example for the child.

Sibling conflict is one of the most frequently reported child management problems that occur in families, and parents face complex issues in deciding how to manage such conflict.[230] Perlman and Ross examined the impact of parental intervention on the quality of children's conflict behaviour. The data used was from 40 English-speaking Canadian families with two- and four-year-old children. The researchers concluded that parental interventions in sibling conflict have beneficial effects in terms of the quality of children's fighting.[231] Parental intervention seemed to both decrease the level of intensity of conflict and allow the children to behave in ways that are more sophisticated than what they were capable of on their own.

CRITICAL THINKING

What are your thoughts about parental interventions in sibling conflict?

Moral-Spiritual Development

Great influences on the child during these early years are the parents' attitude toward moral codes (the human as creative being, spirituality, religion, nature, love of country, the economic system, and education) and their behaviour in the presence of the child. They convey to the child what is considered good and bad, worthy of respect or unworthy. With the developing superego and imitation of and identification with adults, the child is absorbing a great deal of others' attitudes and will retain many of them throughout life. He or she is also beginning to consider how his or her actions affect others.

There are some general considerations you may find helpful pertaining to moral and religious education. *The child cannot be kept spiritually neutral. He or she hears about morals and religion from other people and will raise detailed questions about the basic issues of life:* Where did I come from? Why am I here? Why did the bird (or Grandpa) die? Why is it wrong to do . . .? Why can't I play with Joey? How come Billy goes to church on Saturday and we go to church on Sunday? What is God? What is heaven? Mommy, who do you like best: Santa Claus, the Easter Bunny, the tooth fairy, or Jesus? These questions, often considered inappropriate from the adult viewpoint, should not be lightly brushed aside, for how they are answered is more important than the information given.

The first religious responses are social in nature; bowing the head and saying a simple prayer is imitated but is like brushing teeth to the young preschooler. The child likes prayers before meals and bedtime, and the three-year-old may repeat them like nursery rhymes. The four-year-old elaborates on prayer forms, and the five-year-old makes up prayers.

Encourage parents to discuss religion and related practices with the child. The preschool child is old enough to go to Sunday school, vacation Bible school, or classes in religious education that are on an appropriate level for the child. Religious holidays raise questions, and the spirit of the holiday and ceremonies surrounding it should be explained.

Conscience, or Superego, Development

This development is related to moral-spiritual training, discipline, conditioning of behaviour (smiles, loving words), modelling of parents and others for correct behaviour, being given reasons for behaviour, and other areas of learning. The **superego,** *that part of the psyche that is critical to the self and enforces moral standards,* forms as a result of identification with parents and an introjection of their standards and values, which at first are questioned.[232] At this point the child is in the preconventional period (Stage 2) of moral development.[233]

The preschooler usually behaves even if there is no external authority standing around, to avoid disapproval, although he or she will slip at times. The child continues use of **social referencing,** or *turning to mother or father for guidance in unfamiliar situations to seek tacit permission, or to determine disapproval,* that was begun as a toddler. Thus, the child learns to feel proud or a realistic guilt about what is done. Preschoolers retain the sense of a parent guiding them and imitate socially acceptable behaviours, even when the parent is not nearby.

Superego development will continue through contact with teachers and other significant adults. If the superego remains too strict, self-righteous, or intolerant of others, the person in adulthood will develop a reaction formation of moralistic behaviour so that prohibition rather than initiative will be a dominant pattern of behaviour. If the superego does not develop, and if no or few social values are internalized, the child will increasingly be regarded as mischievous or bad in his or her behaviour.

The child continues the moral development previously begun, learning a greater sense of responsibility, empathy, mercy, compassion, and fairness. The parents are the major teachers as they relate to the child fairly with compassion and gentleness. They teach also by being reliable and responsive. Further, they teach when they point out to the child the consequences of his or her behaviour to others. If the child hurts another child physically or emotionally, the child needs to know that. Then the child learns an appropriate sense of guilt. Discuss with parents the importance of superego development and beginning moral development during this period.

Developmental Tasks

In summary, the developmental tasks for the preschooler are the following:

- Settle into a healthful daily routine of adequately eating, exercising, and resting.
- Master physical skills of large- and small-muscle coordination and movement.
- Become a participating member in the family.
- Conform to others' expectations.
- Express emotions healthfully and for a wide variety of experiences.
- Learn to communicate effectively with an increasing number of others.
- Learn to use initiative tempered by a conscience.
- Develop ability to handle potentially dangerous situations.
- Lay foundations for understanding the meaning of life, self, the world, and ethical, religious, and philosophical ideas.

Discuss with parents how these tasks may be achieved and encourage them to talk about their concerns or problems as they help the child mature in these skills.

If maladaptive behaviour such as failure in language development, destructiveness, or excessive bedwetting persists, the parents and child need special guidance. You can obtain information on causes, associated behaviour, and care for these and other special problems from a pediatric nursing book or from resources in the community.

HEALTH CARE AND NURSING APPLICATIONS

Your role with the preschooler and family has been discussed in each section throughout this chapter. The box entitled "Selected Nursing Diagnoses Related to the Preschooler" lists some *nursing diagnoses* that may apply to the preschooler based on assessments that would result from knowledge presented in this chapter. *Interventions* include your role modelling of caring behaviour to the preschooler and family; child, parent, and family education, support, and counselling; and direct care to meet the preschooler's physical, emotional, cognitive, social, or spiritual and moral needs.

As a general conclusive statement, it can be said that the nurse must develop wellness diagnoses for health promotion in the preschooler and the family. General assessment areas may include psychosocial development, cognitive development, role learning, and play activity. Stolte states that assessment of each of these areas provides data for the formation of a wellness diagnosis.[234]

CRITICAL THINKING

Develop at least one wellness diagnosis in each of the different domains (motor development, psychosocial development, and cognitive development).

Because child maltreatment and abuse, especially sexual abuse, is of great concern, some detail about the nurse's role is described. It is critical that the nurse and other health team members intervene to protect the child and work with the family to improve parenting.

Assessment

Assessment must be done carefully. The TRIADS checklist assesses the dimensions of child abuse. This acronym represents the following assessment areas:[235]

Type of abuse (physical, neglect, emotional maltreatment, sexual)
Role relationship of victim to offender (intrafamilial or extrafamilial)
Intensity of abuse (way abuse began and ended, number of times abuse occurred, and number of offenders involved)
Autonomic response of the child
Duration of abuse (length of time over which abuse occurred, ranging from days to years)
Style of offender or abuse

Style of abuse relates to the offender's techniques and access to the child:[236] (1) whether it occurs spontaneously and explosively and without anticipation on the part of the child; (2) if there are antecedent cues that alert the child to a series of acts;

Selected Nursing Diagnoses Related to the Preschooler

Pattern 1: Exchanging

Altered Nutrition: More than Body Requirements
Altered Nutrition: Less than Body Requirements
Altered Nutrition: Risk for More than Body Requirements
Risk for Infection
Risk for Injury
Risk for Poisoning
Risk for Trauma
Risk for Impaired Skin Integrity
Altered Dentition

Pattern 2: Communicating

Impaired Verbal Communication

Pattern 3: Relating

Impaired Social Interaction
Risk for Altered Parenting
Altered Family Process

Pattern 5: Choosing

Impaired Adjustment

Pattern 6: Moving

Impaired Physical Mobility
Fatigue

Sleep Pattern Disturbance
Feeding Self-Care Deficit
Bathing/Hygiene Self-Care Deficit
Dressing/Grooming Self-Care Deficit
Toileting Self-Care Deficit
Altered Growth and Development

Pattern 7: Perceiving

Body Image Disturbance
Self-Esteem Disturbance
Unilateral Neglect
Hopelessness

Pattern 8: Knowing

Knowledge Deficit
Altered Thought Processes

Pattern 9: Feeling

Pain
Anxiety
Fear

Other NANDA diagnoses are applicable to the ill preschooler.
Source: North American Nursing Diagnosis Association, NANDA Nursing Diagnoses Definitions & Classification 1999–2000. *Philadelphia: North American Nursing Diagnosis Association, 1999.*

EVIDENCE-BASED PRACTICE

Mother's Resilience, Family Health Work, and Mother's Health-Promoting Lifestyle Practices in Families with Preschool Children

Hypotheses derived from the developmental model of health and nursing (DMHN) were tested by examining relationships among mother's resilience (health potential), family health-promoting activity (health work), and mother's health-promoting lifestyle practices (competence in health behaviour) in 67 southern Ontario families with at least one preschool child, three to five years of age. Mothers completed a mailed survey containing self-report measures of the study variables and a demographic form.

Health work, the central concept in the DMHN, reflects the process through which families develop healthy ways of living by learning how to cope with life events and by promoting healthy development of the family unit and its members. *Coping* is viewed as a function of problem solving—a process of attempting to deal with or solve challenging health situations. *Development* relates to growth-seeking behaviour seen in the family's ability to mobilize strengths and resources to achieve health goals.

Results

As hypothesized, both mother's resilience and family health work were positively related to mother's health-promoting lifestyle practices. Mother's resilience was also associated with health work.

Practice Implications

1. According to the DMHN, nurses must identify and support factors that contribute to family health promotion efforts to assist families in developing healthy ways of living. Both mother's resilience and health work were positively related to mother's health-promoting lifestyle practices, suggesting that attention to the development and support of each of these qualities is a potentially important nursing role.

2. Personal and family efforts to promote health may be quite intertwined, suggesting that attention be paid to developing programs and services aimed at both mothers and groups of family members.

3. Supportive learning environments should also be established that provide mothers and their families with opportunities to develop and use coping and goal attainment processes and to further identify and develop their health potential, particularly internal resources or strengths.

4. Mothers, fathers, children who are developmentally ready to participate, and other people who are considered to be family could be involved in such activities.

5. Viewing the family as a system that is influenced by a multitude of internal and external factors should direct nurses to be open to identifying and supporting a range of factors that influence both health work and healthy lifestyle practices. The combination of many different aspects of health potential may have the most persuasive influence on health work.

6. Nurses may be able to foster the development of resilient qualities such as optimism, perseverance, and confidence in mothers as a means of supporting family health promotion processes and mother's lifestyle choices.

7. Nurses can help mothers positively reframe difficult situations by pointing out successes, and by providing positive feedback for their efforts. Such efforts can contribute to a sense of confidence and optimism.

8. There is sufficient evidence to justify nurses' lobbying government bodies to promote adequate education and a level of income for all families that is sufficient to sustain, if not promote, health.

Source: Monteith, B., and M. Ford-Gilboe, The Relationships among Mother's Resilience, Family Health Work, and Mother's Health-Promoting Lifestyle Practices in Families with Preschool Children, Journal of Family Nursing, 8, no. 4 (2002), 383–407. Reprinted by permission of Sage Publications, Inc.

or (3) if acts are repetitively patterned, ritualistic, or ceremonial to control how the child can act.

If you suspect abuse, establish rapport and talk with the child alone; however, do not pry. If the child finds it difficult to talk, gently offer to draw some pictures or play with the child to *gain information as follows:*

1. *What* has happened to you?
   a. Has anyone ever told you to take off your panties?
   b. Has anyone ever put his or her finger (or another object) between your legs?
   c. Does anyone ever get in bed with you at night?
2. *Who* did this to you? Explain.
3. *How* did it happen? Tell me what happened just before that.
4. *Where* did this happen?
5. *When* did this happen?

6. *Who* saw this happen to you?
7. *Who* else have you told?
   a. What did they say?
   b. What did they do?

The child may not answer because he or she (1) thinks abuse is normal, (2) is terrified that parents will be more abusive if they know he or she told, (3) feels loyalty to the parents and fears desertion, or (4) believes abuse is deserved.

When you talk with the parents about the subject of child abuse, do not give the impression that you are criticizing them, trying to impart your own values, or acting as their judge. Putting them on the defensive will not make them cooperate, and it may keep them from accepting help from other health care professionals. Do your best to be tolerant and understanding. Try to determine how realistically they perceive the child, how they cope with the stresses of parenting, and to whom they turn for support. As you talk, *attempt to get the parents' answers to the following questions:*[237,238]

- What do you do when he or she cries too much? If that does not work, what do you do?
- Does the child sleep well? What do you do when he or she does not sleep?
- How do you discipline him or her?
- How do you feel after you have disciplined the child?
- Are you ever angry because the child takes up so much of your time?
- Does he or she take up more time than your other children, or require more disciplining? If yes, why is this so?
- Do you think he or she misbehaves on purpose?
- Whom do you usually talk to when your child upsets you? Is that person available now?
- Does the child remind you of a relative or former spouse that is disliked? (Explore this possibility with gentle questions: "It must be really upsetting for you when he acts like his father. What goes through your mind then?" "In what ways is she like your mother? Do those characteristics irritate you?")

As you discuss things, try to determine what the situation is at home. Does one or both of the parents seem unduly distressed? Perhaps they are facing other stresses with which they cannot cope such as a job loss, loneliness, illness, or alcoholism.

If you suspect **sexual abuse,** *find out the following from the parents:*

- What words or names does the child use to describe various body parts?
- What are the names of family members and frequent visitors?
- Who babysits for the child?
- What are the family's sleeping arrangements?
- Does the child have behavioural problems such as excessive masturbation?
- Does the child have any phobias or excessive fears of any person or place? Does he or she have any nightmares?

Parents may not be involved in the sexual abuse and may be unaware of its occurrence. Work up gradually to the subject of their child's being abused. Inform them of your suspicions in private and without judgment. Do not bombard the parents with questions they will interpret as accusatory. Offer your support, telling them of your concern for the child. Suggest counsellors who would be helpful for the child and parents. Give them ideas on how to help the child work through feelings about the trauma. Advise parents not to punish or scold the child when he or she works through emotions through masturbation or by playing with dolls.[239–245]

A pelvic examination is necessary if the child has been sexually abused; however, this procedure should be done carefully after explanation is given to the child, questions are answered, rapport is established, and the child feels some sense of security. A visual examination of the whole body, including the genital and rectal regions, should be done before a pelvic examination.

Allow plenty of time for every step of the examination. The prepubescent vagina is extremely sensitive, and the doctor may want to sedate or anaesthetise the child before the examination. A sterile plastic medicine dropper lubricated with sterile water should be used to obtain specimens. A nasal speculum or infant-sized vaginoscope, lubricated with water and warmed, can be used with the young child. Test the child for venereal disease (girls who are past menarche should be tested for pregnancy).[246]

Intervention

You are a key factor in intervention; however, do not engage in rescue fantasies. You are limited in what you can do, although reporting to the appropriate professionals is necessary action for intervention.

Interventions for the abused child include the following:[247–253]

1. Relaxation techniques and psychopharmacology to reduce hyperactivity, nightmares, enuresis, and startle responses— sensory disruption
2. Thought stopping, clarification, and reframing of beliefs and linking distress directly to the trauma experience to reduce perceptual-cognitive disruptions
3. Desensitizing the child to fearful involvement with others, focused role-playing to discriminate threatening exploitative behaviour from safe behaviour, and empathy training to reduce interpersonal disruption

Treatment objectives for the sexually abused child, using play therapy, include the following:

1. Child will express feelings about being sexually abused.
2. Child will re-enact incidents of sexual trauma; anatomic dolls will be used for the child to show where she or he has been touched by the adult and to allow the child to vent anger felt for the adult.
3. In an appropriate but satisfying way, child will diffuse anger, shame, humiliation, tension from secrecy, fear, and guilt and work through feelings of being damaged.
4. Child will learn to respect her or his body and the right to have physical and psychological boundaries.
5. Child will learn to improve judgment process with adults and strangers and to handle sexual confrontations.
6. Child will demonstrate less acting out at school or home.
7. Child will discuss bad dreams and nightmares to be reassured of safety.

Crayons, paints, chalkboards, punching bags, bean bags, and dolls may be used in treatment. Simple teaching tools, basic vocabulary, and keen observation are essential. Repetition of stories, recreation of telephone conversations with the perpetrator, and drawing and painting are essential for beginning resolution.[254,255]

If you are in a health care facility and suspect child abuse, report it to the doctor and appropriate health team members. Also report your suspicions to the proper agency—the police, the district attorney's office, a child-protective service, or a social service group. *Carefully document all evidence of abuse,* your interview of and actions with parents and child, any agencies or persons contacted about the abuse, and any agencies to which the parents were referred. List the names of children who are repeatedly brought to the hospital with injuries. Make sure the notes on the chart include what the parents said, how they reacted, and how they explained the accident. Provide other hospitals in the area with the names on file. Urge them to do the same with their files. Take the time to check with other hospitals when you have a case you question.[256]

A **neglected child** needs help as much as one who has been abused. Careful assessment and interviewing of child and parents are essential. Notify your community's child protection service and thoroughly document your findings and interventions. Many of the guidelines described above are applicable.

INTERESTING WEBSITES

CHILD AND INFANT HEALTH

http://www.ottawa.ca/city_services/yourhealth/children_en.shtml

Keeping your child healthy requires a combination of knowledge, planning, and nurturing. Sometimes, being able to get the right information quickly is the best support. Click the links to get up-to-date information about important health issues relevant to young children.

CANADIAN CHILD CARE FEDERATION AND FAMILY CHILD CARE

http://www.cfc-efc.ca/menu/childcare_en.htm

This site is a place to share news, information, and ideas; access resources; and connect with the family child care community across Canada and elsewhere.

HEALTHY START FOR LIFE

http://www.dieticians.ca/healthystart/index.asp

Healthy Start for Life is a collaboration between Dieticians of Canada and nine organizations whose shared goal is to promote healthy eating and physical activity among toddlers and preschool age children. The program aims to help parents and child care providers learn more about the nutrition and physical activity needs of preschoolers; suggest activities that promote positive attitudes toward healthy eating and active living; provide strategies to help tackle common preschool feeding issues, plan meals, and keep preschoolers active; and help prevent childhood obesity, diabetes, and other health problems in later life.

SUMMARY

1. The preschooler grows at a steady pace; motor coordination is increasing.
2. The preschooler makes considerable gains in neuromuscular, cognitive, emotional, and social and moral and spiritual behaviours.
3. Parents' provision of consistent love, guidance, and new experiences is essential for holistic development.

4. The child develops the ability to carry out basic hygiene and routine activities.
5. The child begins to participate within the family, and to communicate and relate more effectively with adults and significant others in the community.
6. The child slowly reaches out from the family, establishes beginning peer relationships, and learns to follow rules of the play group.
7. The box entitled "Considerations for the Preschool Child and Family in Health Care" summarizes what you should consider in assessment and health promotion with the preschooler.

Considerations for the Preschool Child and Family in Health Care

- Family, cultural background and values, support systems, and community resources for the family
- Parents as identification figures for the child, secondary identification of the preschool child with the parents
- Behaviours that indicate gender identity and sense of sexuality in the preschool child
- Behaviours that indicate ability of the preschool child to relate to siblings, adults in the extended family, and other adults and authority figures in the environment
- Parental behaviours that indicate difficulty with parenting or potential of actual abuse of the preschool child
- Physical characteristics and patterns, such as neuromuscular development, nutrition, exercise, and rest or sleep, which indicate health and are within age norms for growth for the preschool child
- Cognitive characteristics and behavioural patterns in the preschool child that demonstrate curiosity, increasingly realistic thought, expanding concept formation, and continuing mental development
- Communication patterns—verbal, nonverbal, and action—and language development that demonstrate continuing learning and age-appropriate norms for the preschool child
- Behaviours that indicate that the child can participate in and enjoys early childhood education experiences
- Overall appearance, behaviour, and play patterns in the preschool child that indicate development of initiative rather than excessive guilt, positive self-concept, body image formation, and a sense of sexuality
- Use of adaptive mechanisms by the preschool child that promote a sense of security, control of anxiety, and age-appropriate emotional responses
- Behavioural patterns that indicate that the preschool child is forming a superego, or conscience, and is continuing moral and spiritual development
- Behavioural patterns and characteristics that indicate that the preschool child has achieved developmental tasks
- Parental behaviours that indicate knowledge about and how to guide and discipline the child, and how to assist the child in becoming more independent
- Parental behaviours that indicate the child is achieving his or her developmental tasks for this era

ENDNOTES

1. Bee, H., *Lifespan Development* (2nd ed.). New York: Longman, 1998.

2. Maccoby, E., and J. Martin, Socialization in the Context of Family: Parent-Child Interaction. In E. Hetherington, (ed.), *Handbook of Child Psychology, Vol. 4: Socialization, Personality, and Social Development,* (4th ed.). New York: Wiley,

3. Seifert, K., R. Hoffnung, and M. Hoffnung, *Lifespan Development.* Boston: Houghton Mifflin, 1997.

4. Sigelman, C., *Life-Span Human Development* (3rd ed.). Pacific Grove, CA: Brooks/Cole, 1999.

5. Bee, *op. cit.*

6. Seifert et al., *op cit.*

7. Chen, X., P.D. Hastings, K.H. Rubim, H. Chen, G. Cen, and S.L. Stewart, Child-Rearing Attitudes and Behavioural Inhibition in Chinese and Canadian Toddlers: A Cross-Cultural Study, *Developmental Psychology,* 34, no. 4 (1998), 677–686.

8. McGrath, M., M. Sullivan, and R. Seifer, Maternal Interaction Patterns and Preschool Competence in High Risk Children, *Nursing Research,* 47, no. 6 (1998), 309–316.

9. Magill-Evans, J., and M.J. Harrison, Parent-Child Interactions and Development of Toddlers Born Preterm, *Western Journal of Nursing Research,* 21, no. 3 (1999), 292–307.

10. Harrison, M.J., J. Magill-Evans, and K. Menzies, Fathers' Scores on the Nursing Child Assessment Teaching Scale: Are They Different from Those of Mothers? *Journal of Pediatric Nursing,* 14, no. 4 (1999), 248–254.

11. Broom, B.L., Parental Differences and Changes in Marital Quality, Psychological Well-Being, and Sensitivity with First-Born Children, *Journal of Family Nursing,* 4 (1998), 87–112.

12. Harrison, M.J., J. Magill-Evans, and D. Sadoway, Scores on the Nurses Child Assessment Teaching Scale for Father-Toddler Dyads, *Public Health Nursing,* 18, no. 2 (2001), 94–100.

13. Dubeau, D. The Involved Father, *Transition Magazine,* 32, no. 2 (2002), 8–14.

14. Bee, *op. cit.*

15. Maccoby and Martin, *op. cit.*

16. Sigelman, *op. cit.*

17. Lidz, T., *The Person: His and Her Development Throughout the Life Cycle* (2nd ed.). New York: Basic Books, 1983.

18. *Ibid.*

19. Kornhaber, A., and K. Woodward, *Grandparent Power.* New York: Random House, 1995.

20. Lidz, *op. cit.*

21. Sigelman, *op. cit.*

22. Moss, E., D. Rousseau, S. Parent, D. St-Laurent, and J. Saintonge, Correlates of Attachment at School Age: Maternal Reported Stress, Mother-Child Interaction, and Behaviour Problems, *Child Development,* 69, no. 5 (1998), 1390–1405.

23. Arnup, K. Lesbian and Gay Parents, in N. Mandell and A. Duffy (eds.), *Canadian Families* (3rd ed., pp. 176–177). Toronto: Thomson Nelson, 2005.

24. *Ibid.*

25. Skitka, L., and M. Frazier, Ameliorating the Effects Of Parental Divorce: Do Small Group Interventions Work? *Journal of Divorce and Marriage,* 24 (1995), 3–4.

26. Finch, J., and J. Mason, Divorce, Remarriage, and Family Obligations, *The Sociological Review,* 38 (1990), 219–246.

27. Ross, C.E., and J. Mirowsky, Parental Divorce, Life-Course Disruption, and Adult Depression, *Journal of Marriage and the Family,* 61 (1999), 1034–1045.

28. Connidis, I.A., Divorce and Union Dissolution: Reverberations over Three Generations, *Canadian Journal of Aging,* 22, no. 4 (2003), 353–368.

29. Gormly, A., *Lifespan Human Development* (6th ed.). Fort Worth: Harcourt Brace College Publishers, 1997.

30. Newman, B., and P. Newman, *Development Through Life: A Psychosocial Approach* (7th ed.). Belmont, CA: Wadworth, 1999.

31. Sigelman, *op. cit.*

32. Papalia, D., S. Olds, and R. Feldman, *Human Development* (7th ed.). Boston: McGraw-Hill, 1998.

33. Lidz, *op. cit.*

34. Child and Infant Health, *Talking with Preschool and School Aged Children about Sexuality,* Website: http://www.hc-sc.gc.ca/hppb/mentalhealth/mhp/pdf/booklet.pdf, August 2004.

35. *Ibid.*

36. Burgess, A., Intra-familial Sexual Abuse, in J. Campbell and I. Humphreys, eds., *Nursing Care of Victims of Family Violence.* Reston, VA: Reston, 1984.

37. Duyff, R., *The American Dietetic Association's Complete Food and Nutrition Guide.* Minneapolis: Chronimed Publishing, 1998.

38. Papalia et al., *op. cit.*

39. Seifert et al., *op. cit.*

40. Downey, D.B., and D.J. Condron, Playing Well with Others in Kindergarten: The Benefit of Siblings at Home, *Journal of Marriage and Family,* 66, no. 2 (2004), 333–350.

41. Mendelson, M.J., F.F. Aboud, and R.P. Lanthier, Kindergartners' Relationships with Siblings, Peers, and Friends, *Merrill-Palmer Quarterly,* 40, no. 3 (1994), 416–435.

42. Burgess, *op. cit.*

43. Vanier Institute of the Family, *Contemporary Family Trends—Grandparenthood in Canada,* Website: http://www.vifamily.ca/library/cft/grandparenthood.html, August 2004.

44. *Ibid.*

45. Kornhaber and Woodward, *op. cit.*

46. Strom, R., and S. Strom, Building a Theory of Grandparent Development, *International Journal of Aging and Human Development,* 45, no. 4 (1997), 255–286.

47. Inwood, S., Grandparents Raising Grandchildren, *Canadian Nurse,* 98, no. 4 (2002), 21–25.

48. Newman and Newman, *op. cit.*

49. Vanier Institute of the Family, *Contemporary Family Trends—Grandparenthood in Canada.*

50. Lidz, *op. cit.*

51. Gormly, *op. cit.*

52. Newman and Newman, *op. cit.*

53. Child and Family Canada, *Bibliography on Quality Child Care,* Website: http://www.cfc-efc.ca/docs/cccf/00000066.htm, August 2004.

54. *Ibid.*

55. Child and Family Canada, *National Statement on Quality Child Care,* Website: http://www.cfc-efc.ca/docs/cccf/00000111.htm, August 2004.

56. Child and Family Canada, *Choosing a Child Care, Types of Child Care* (Chapter 2), Website: http://www.cfc-efc.ca/docs/cccf/00000278.htm, August 2004.

57. *Ibid.*

58. *Ibid.*

59. *Ibid.*

60. Canadian Child Federation, *Code of Ethics,* Website: http://www.cccf-fcsge.ca/practice/ethical%20dilemmas/codeofethics_en.htm, August 2004.

61. *Ibid.*

62. Bee, *op. cit.*

63. Gormly, *op. cit.*

64. Papalia et al., *op. cit.*

65. Newman and Newman, *op. cit.*

66. Larner, M., and D. Phillips, Defining and Valuing Quality as a Parent, in P. Moss and A. Pence, eds., *Valuing Quality in Early*

Childhood Services: New Approaches to Defining Quality (pp. 43–51). New York: Teachers College Press, Teachers College, Columbia University, 1994,

67. Pence, A., and M. McCallum, Developing Cross-Cultural Partnerships: Implications for Child Care Quality Research and Practice, in P. Moss and A. Pence, eds., *Valuing Quality in Early Childhood Services: New Approaches to Defining Quality* (pp. 108–116). New York: Teachers College Press, Teachers College, Columbia University, 1994.

68. Pence and McCallum, *op. cit.*

69. Papalia et al., *op. cit.*

70. Bee, *op. cit.*

71. Newman and Newman, *op. cit.*

72. Papalia et al., *op. cit.*

73. Bee, *op. cit.*

74. Newman and Newman, *op. cit.*

75. Papalia et al., *op. cit.*

76. Seifert et al., *op. cit.*

77. Gormly, *op. cit.*

78. Papalia et al., *op. cit.*

79. Seifert et al., *op. cit.*

80. Wong, D., *Whaley and Wong's Nursing Care of Infants and Children* (6th ed.). St. Louis: C.V. Mosby, 1999.

81. *Ibid.*

82. Cadman, D., et al., The Usefulness of the Denver Developmental Screening Test to Predict Kindergarten Problems in a General Community Population, *American Journal of Public Health,* 74, no. 110 (1984), 1093–1097.

83. Frankenburg, W., and J.B. Dobbs, *Denver II—Revision and Restandardization of the Denver Developmental Screening Test.* Denver: Denver Developmental Materials, 1990.

84. Cadman et al., *op. cit.*

85. Frankenburg and Dobbs, *op. cit.*

86. Gormly, *op. cit.*

87. Papalia et al., *op. cit.*

88. Seifert et al., *op. cit.*

89. Sigelman, *op. cit.*

90. Wong, *op. cit.*

91. Uphold, C., and M. Graham, *Clinical Guidelines in Family Practice* (2nd ed.). Gainesville, FL: Barmarrae Books, 1994.

92. Wong, *op. cit.*

93. Health Canada, Office of Nutrition Policy and Promotion, Website: http://www.hc-sc.gc.ca/hpfb-dgpsa/onpp-bppn/food_guide_preschoolers_e.html, June 2004.

94. Potter, P.A., A. Griffin Perry, J.C. Ross-Kerr, and M.J. Wood, *Canadian Fundamentals of Nursing* (2nd ed.). Toronto: Mosby, 2001.

95. Health Canada, Office of Nutrition Policy and Promotion.

96. Potter et al., *op. cit.*

97. Health Canada, Office of Nutrition Policy and Promotion.

98. *Ibid.*

99. Schuster, R., Footgear Modifications for Children in the Preschool to Pre-Teen Ages, *Proceedings National Academies of Practice Fourth National Health Policy Forum,* April 24–25 (1992), 81–85.

100. Potter et al., *op. cit.*

101. Health Canada, *Physical Activity Guide to Healthy Active Living,* Ottawa: Minister of Public Works and Government Service Canada, 2002. Cat. H39-611/2002-2E.

102. Canadian Dental Association, *Canadian Dental Association Advises AGAINST Fluoride Supplements in Young Children,* Website: http://www.mercola.com/2000/aug/13/fluoride_supplements.htm, August 2004.

103. Bruce, B.S., J.P. Lake, V.A. Eden, and J.C. Denny, Children at Risk of Injury, *Journal of Pediatric Nursing,* 19, no. 2 (2004), 121–127.

104. *Ibid.*

105. Wong, *op. cit.*

106. Gesell, A., and F. Ilg, *The Child From Five to Ten* (rev. ed.). New York: Harper & Collins, 1977.

107. Sherman, J., Jr., and S. Fields, *Guide to Patient Evaluation* (5th ed.). Garden City, NY: Medical Examination Publishing, 1989.

108. Uphold and Graham, *op. cit.*

109. Wong, *op. cit.*

110. Uphold and Graham, *op. cit.*

111. Wong, *op. cit.*

112. Gesell and Ilg, *op. cit.*

113. Uphold and Graham, *op. cit.*

114. Wong, *op. cit.*

115. Gesell and Ilg, *op. cit.*

116. Uphold and Graham, *op. cit.*

117. Wong, *op. cit.*

118. Gesell and Ilg, *op. cit.*

119. Sherman and Fields, *op. cit.*

120. Uphold and Graham, *op. cit.*

121. Wong, *op. cit.*

122. *Ibid.*

123. Sherman and Fields, *op. cit.*

124. Wong, *op. cit.*

125. Gesell and Ilg, *op. cit.*

126. Sherman and Fields, *op. cit.*

127. Uphold and Graham, *op. cit.*

128. Wong, *op. cit.*

129. Health Canada, *Canadian Incidence Study of Reported Child Abuse and Neglect,* Website: http://www.hc-sc.gc.ca/pphb-dgspsp/cm-vee/cish101/index.html, July 2004.

130. Trocmé, N., B. MacLaurin, B. Fallon, J. Daciuk, M. Tourigny, and D. Billingsley, Canadian Incidence Study of Reported Neglect: Methodology, *Canadian Journal of Public Health,* 92, no. 4 (2001), 259–263.

131. Ateah, C., A., J.E. Durrant, and J. Mirwaldt, Physical Punishment and Physical Abuse of Children: Strategies for Prevention, in C. Ateah and J. Mirwaldt, eds., *Within our Reach: Preventative Abuse across the Lifespan* (pp. 11–25). Winnipeg: Fernwood, 2004.

132. *Ibid.*

133. *Ibid.*

134. Barnett, O., C.L. Miller-Perrin, and R.D. Perrin, *Family Violence Across the Lifespan: An Introduction, Second Edition.* Thousand Oaks, CA: Sage, 2005.

135. Youngblut, J., and D. Brooten, Alternate Child Care, History of Hospitalization, and Preschool Behavior, *Nursing Research,* 48, no. 1 (1999), 29–34.

136. Heiney, S., Helping Children through Painful Procedures, *American Journal of Nursing,* 91, no. 11 (1991), 20–24.

137. Wong, *op. cit.*

138. Pacquiao, D.F. People of Filipino Heritage, in L.D. Purnell and B.J. Paulanka, eds., *Transcultural Health Care: A Culturally Competent Approach* (2nd ed., pp. 138, 145). Philadelphia: F.A. Davis, 2003.

139. Webb, P., Piaget: Implications for Teaching, *Theory Into Practice,* 19, no. 2 (1980), 93–97.

140. Wadsworth, B., *Piaget's Theory of Cognitive and Affective Development: Foundations of Constructivism* (5th ed.). New York: Longman, 1996.

141. Papalia et al., *op. cit.*

142. Wadsworth, *op. cit.*

143. Gormly, *op. cit.*

144. Papalia et al., *op. cit.*

145. Piaget, J., *The Equilibration of Cognitive Structures: The Central Problem of Intellectual Development* (Transl. by T. Brown and K.J. Thampy). Chicago: University of Chicago Press, 1985.

146. Sigelman, *op. cit.*

147. Wadsworth, *op. cit.*
148. Gormly, *op. cit.*
149. Lidz, *op. cit.*
150. Wadsworth, *op. cit.*
151. *Ibid.*
152. Gormly, *op. cit.*
153. Papalia et al., *op. cit.*
154. Wadsworth, *op. cit.*
155. Webb, *op. cit.*
156. Piaget, *op. cit.*
157. Wadsworth, *op. cit.*
158. *Ibid.*
159. Webb, *op. cit.*
160. Klein, J.S., and J. Bisanz, Preschoolers Doing Arithmetic: The Concepts Are Willing but the Working Memory Is Weak, *Canadian Journal of Experimental Psychology,* 54, no.1 (2000), 105–115.
161. Lidz, *op. cit.*
162. Wadsworth, *op. cit.*
163. *Ibid.*
164. Lidz, *op. cit.*
165. Wadsworth, *op. cit.*
166. Webb, *op. cit.*
167. Lidz, *op. cit.*
168. Wadsworth, *op. cit.*
169. Webb, *op. cit.*
170. Bodrova, E., and D. Leong, *Tools of the Mind: The Vygotskian Approach to Early Childhood Education.* Englewood Cliffs, N.J.: Prentice-Hall, 1996.
171. *Ibid.*
172. Sigelman, *op. cit.*
173. Lidz, *op. cit.*
174. Child and Infant Health, *Talking with Preschool and School Aged Children about Sexuality.*
175. Seifert et al., *op. cit.*
176. Wadsworth, *op. cit.*
177. Webb, *op. cit.*
178. Bodrova and Leong, *op. cit.*
179. Wong, *op. cit.*
180. Bodrova and Leong, *op. cit.*
181. Lidz, *op. cit.*
182. Eisenberg, N., I.K. Guthrie, B.C. Murphy, S.A. Shepard, A. Cumberland, and G. Carlo, Consistency and Development of Prosocial Dispositions: A Longitudinal Study, *Child Development,* 70, no. 6 (1999), 1360–1372.
183. Roberts, W., and J. Strayer, Empathy, Emotional Expressiveness, and Prosocial Behavior, *Child Development,* 67 (1996), 449–470.
184. Thompson, C., J. Barresi, and C. Moore, The Development of Future-Oriented Prudence and Altruism in Preschoolers, *Cognitive Development,* 12 (1997), 199–212.
185. *Ibid.*
186. iParenting Canada, *Top-Notch TV, Canadian Children's Television,* Website: http://iparentingcanada.com/resources/articles/tv.htm, August 2004.
187. *Ibid.*
188. *Ibid.*
189. *Ibid.*
190. LeFrançois, G.R, *Of Children: An Introduction to Child and Adolescent Development* (9th ed.). Toronto: Wadsworth/Thomson Learning, 2001.
191. Santrock, John W., Anne Mackenzie-Rivers, Kwan Ho Leung, and Thomas Malcomson, *Life-Span Development* (1st Canadian ed.). Toronto: McGraw-Hill Ryerson, 2003.
192. Johnson, M.O., Television Violence and Its Effect on Children, *Journal of Pediatric Nursing,* 11, no. 2 (1996), 94–99.
193. Bodrova and Leong, *op. cit.*
194. *Ibid.*

195. Gaines, B.R, Screening for Childhood Speech-Language Problems, *Canadian Nurse,* 98, no. 5 (2002), 15–16.
196. *Ibid.*
197. *Ibid.*
198. Piaget, *op. cit.*
199. Erikson, E.H., *Childhood and Society* (2nd ed.). New York: W.W. Norton, 1963.
200. Lidz, *op. cit.*
201. Gormly, *op. cit.*
202. Papalia et al., *op. cit.*
203. Le Vieux-Anglin, L., and E. Sawyer, Incorporating Play Interventions into Nursing Care, *Pediatric Nursing,* 19 (1993), 459–462.
204. Lidz, *op. cit.*
205. Newman and Newman, *op. cit.*
206. Papalia et al., *op. cit.*
207. Seifert et al., *op. cit.*
208. Wong, *op. cit.*
209. Lidz, *op. cit.*
210. Warren, S., D. Oppenheim, and R. Emde, Can Emotions and Themes in Child's Play Predict Behavior Problems? *Journal of the American Academy of Child and Adolescent Psychiatry,* 35, no. 10 (1996), 1331–1337.
211. Papalia et al., *op. cit.*
212. Dubeau, *op. cit.*
213. Heiney, *op. cit.*
214. Lidz, *op. cit.*
215. Papalia et al., *op. cit.*
216. Seifert et al., *op. cit.*
217. Miller, S., and L. Reibstein, Good Kid, Bad Kid, *Newsweek (Special Issue),* Spring/Summer (1997), 64–65, 68.
218. Waschbusch, D.A., H.L. Kipp, and W.E. Pelham Jr., Generalization of Behavioural and Psychostimulant Treatment of Attention-Deficit/Hyperactivity Disorder (ADHD): Discussion and Examples, *Behaviour Research and Therapy,* 36, nos. 7–8 (1998), 675–694.
219. Erikson, *op. cit.*
220. *Ibid.*
221. Lidz, *op. cit.*
222. Schulman, M., *Moral Development Training: Strategies for Parents, Teachers, and Clinicians.* Menlo Park, CA: Addison-Wesley, 1985.
223. Gormly, *op. cit.*
224. Lidz, *op. cit.*
225. Wong, *op. cit.*
226. Newman and Newman, *op. cit.*
227. Lidz, *op. cit.*
228. Wong, *op. cit.*
229. Lidz, *op. cit.*
230. Perlman, M., and H.S. Ross, The Benefits of Parent Intervention in Children's Disputes: An Examination of Current Changes in Children's Fighting Styles, *Child Development,* 64, no. 4 (1997), 690–700.
231. *Ibid.*
232. Lidz, *op. cit.*
233. Kohlberg, L., *Recent Research in Moral Development.* New York: Holt, Rinehart, Winston, 1977.
234. Stolte, K.M. *Wellness: Nursing Diagnosis for Health Promotion.* Philadelphia: Lippincott, 1996.
235. Burgess, A. C. Hartman, and S. Kelley, Assessing Child Abuse: The TRIADS Checklist, *Journal of Psychosocial Nursing and Mental Health Services,* 28, no. 4 (1990), 6–14.
236. *Ibid.*
237. Critchley, D., Therapeutic Group Work with Abused Preschool Children, *Perspectives in Psychiatric Care,* 20, no. 2 (1982), 79–85.
238. Wong, *op. cit.*
239. Burgess, A., Intra-familial Sexual Abuse.

240. Burgess et al., Assessing Child Abuse: The TRIADS Checklist.
241. Burgess, A., C. Hartman, and T. Baker, Memory Presentations of Childhood Sexual Abuse, *Journal of Psychosocial Nursing*, 33, no. 9 (1995), 9–16.
242. Burgess, A., M. McCausland, and W. Wolbert, Children's Drawings as Indicators of Sexual Trauma, *Perspectives in Psychiatric Care*, 19, no. 2 (1981), 50–58.
243. Burgess, A., et al., Child Molestation: Assessing Impact in Multiple Victims (Part I), *Archives of Psychiatric Nursing*, 1, no. 1 (1987), 33–39.
244. Mendelson et al., *op. cit.*
245. Thompson et al., *op. cit.*
246. Wong, *op. cit.*

247. Burgess, A., Intra-familial Sexual Abuse.
248. Burgess et al., Assessing Child Abuse: The TRIADS Checklist.
249. Burgess et al., Memory Presentations of Childhood Sexual Abuse.
250. Burgess et al., Children's Drawings as Indicators of Sexual Trauma.
251. Burgess et al., Child Molestation: Assessing Impact in Multiple Victims (Part I).
252. Stolte, *op. cit.*
253. Wong, *op. cit.*
254. Federation, S., Sexual Abuse: Treatment Modalities for the Younger Child, *Journal of Psychosocial Nursing*, 24, no. 7 (1986), 21–24.
255. Wong, *op. cit.*
256. *Ibid.*

Chapter 10

ASSESSMENT AND HEALTH PROMOTION FOR THE SCHOOLCHILD

If you are concerned about yourself, plant rice. If you are concerned about your family, plant trees. If you are concerned about your nation, educate your children.

Chinese Proverb

OBJECTIVES

STUDY OF THIS CHAPTER WILL ENABLE YOU TO:

1. Discuss the family relationships of the schoolchild.

2. Examine the influence of the child's peers and of adults, other than parents, on the schoolchild.

3. Explore developmental tasks with the family members and determine the most effective ways to achieve them.

4. Compare and assess the physical changes and needs, including nutrition, rest, exercise, safety, and health protection, for the juvenile and preadolescent.

5. Assess intellectual, communication, play, emotional, self-concept, sexuality, and moral–spiritual development in the juvenile and preadolescent and influences on these areas of development.

6. Discuss the crisis of school entry and determine ways to help the child adapt to the experience of formal education, including latch key care.

7. Analyze the physical and emotional adaptive mechanisms of the schoolchild.

8. Discuss the significance of peers and the chum relationship to the psychosocial development of the child.

9. Explore with parents their role in communication with, and guidance of, the child to foster healthy development in a holistic way.

10. Describe the influence that the media can exert upon behaviour.

11. State the developmental tasks of the schoolchild and discuss your role in helping him or her to achieve these tasks.

12. Work effectively with the schoolchild in the nursing setting.

As growth and development continue and the child leaves the confines of the home, he or she emerges into a world of new experiences and responsibilities. If previous developmental tasks have been met and the child has developed a healthy personality,

he or she will continue to acquire new knowledge and skills steadily. If previous developmental tasks have not been met and the child's personality development is immature, the child may experience difficulties mastering the developmental tasks of the school-age child. Peers, parents, and other adults can have a positive, maturing influence if the child is adequately prepared for leaving home, if individual needs are considered, and if he or she has some successful experiences.

The **school-age** years can be divided into **middle childhood** (*six to eight years of age*) and **late childhood** (*eight to 12 years of age*). The school-age years can also be divided into the juvenile and preadolescent periods. *At approximately age six, the **juvenile period** begins, marked by a need for peer associations.* **Preadolescence** *usually begins at nine or ten years of age and is marked by a new capacity to love, when the satisfaction and security of another person of the same sex is as important to the child as personal satisfaction and security.* Preadolescence ends at approximately 12 years with the onset of puberty. Preadolescence is also called **prepubescence** *and is characterized by an increase in hormone production in both sexes,* which is preparatory to eventual physiologic maturity. Psychological and social changes also occur as the child slowly moves away from the family. *This chapter discusses characteristics to assess and intervention measures for you to use in relation to promote health care for the child and family.*

In today's world many conditions influence the development of a child. One of them is poverty. In Canada, approximately one in four children under the age of seven years lives in poverty. The absolute number of children living in poverty grew by over 700 000 between 1981 and 1996, despite a House of Commons all-party resolution in 1989 to eliminate child poverty by the year 2000.[1] Given the importance of the early years to the long-term healthy growth and development of children, the high rate of poverty of families with young children is a cause of serious concern.[2] Although children in families living in poverty (i.e., those with family incomes below the Statistics Canada low income cut-offs) are at significant risk for many physical and mental health problems, it is important to note that the majority of children with these problems do not come from poor families. The fact is that the majority of families with children do not live in poverty. Note, however, that the "low-income cut-offs" of Statistics Canada defines people who live in poverty as those who spend more than 58.5% percent of their total income on food, clothing, and shelter.[3] Nevertheless, children from families with the lowest incomes are more likely to exhibit manifestations of conduct disorder, emotional problems, and hyperactivity; and they are more prone to engage in delinquent behaviours.[4] Poverty does mean hunger, and many Canadian families resort to food banks.

A group of Canadian researchers claim that few data exist to establish whether or not low income alone affects infant morbidity.[5] Few studies have involved Canadian children specifically, and almost all of the available information comes from American research. It is difficult to generalize the results of U.S. studies to the Canadian situation partly because of the different health care systems in the two countries.[6]

Health care professionals can endeavour to combat the effects of poverty and violence on the health of children and families. Regardless, money, effort, and time are necessary to do the following:

■ Help children who are at risk of dropping out of school with special tutoring so that academic performance and self-esteem can be strengthened.

■ Counsel parents and children in homes where child maltreatment, abuse, and violence are present.

■ Assist parents with child care; support efforts of parents who are trying to improve their incomes and life.

■ Provide daycare or after-school care for children when parents cannot be in the home because of job demands.

■ Advocate at federal, provincial, territorial, and local governmental levels for policies and programs that will assist children (such as healthy school lunches) as well as eliminate causes of poverty (such as employment conditions) for families.

■ Work at the community level to reduce violence in the neighbourhoods, community, school, and nation.

■ Support families in their efforts to protect their children from violence through church, community, and school programs.

CRITICAL THINKING

What steps would you take in developing a health promotion program in a community to address the need for a food bank?

FAMILY DEVELOPMENT AND RELATIONSHIPS

Share the following information with parents to promote health.

Relationships with Parents

Although parents remain a vital part of the schoolchild's life, the child's position within the family is altered with his or her entry into school. Parents play a major role in socializing the child to the adult world. They contribute to the socialization process in at least five ways:

1. By assuming the role of love providers and caretakers
2. By serving as identification figures
3. By acting as active socialization agent
4. By determining the sort of experiences the child will have
5. By participating in the development of the child's self-concept[7-9]

The schoolchild now channels energy into intellectual pursuits, widens social horizons, and becomes familiar with the adult world. He or she has identified with the parent of the same sex and, through imitation and education, continues to learn social roles and the tasks and routines expected by the culture or social group. The family atmosphere has much impact on the child's emotional development and future response within the family when he or she becomes an adolescent. Research indicates that children can become positive in their behaviour whether they are reared in authoritarian or permissive homes, if parents are consistent in their approach.

Although parental support is needed, the schoolchild pulls away from overt signs of parental affection. Yet during illness or when threatened by his or her new status, the child turns to parents for affection and protection. Parents get frustrated with behavioural changes, antics, and infractions of household rules.

The child changes ideas about and behaviour toward parents and adults as he or she grows. See the box entitled "The School Child's View of Parents and Adults."[10-13]

The School Child's View of Parents and Adults

Ages 6–8
■ Is still primarily family-oriented
■ Sees parents as good, powerful, and wise
■ Seeks parental approval
■ Becomes emotionally steadier and freer from parents

Ages 9–12
■ Begins to question parental authority
■ Tends to feel smarter than parents, teachers, and adults in general
■ Sees same-sex parent as more harsh disciplinarian

As you work with families and children, realize that there is no "typical family" for school-age children. In fact, Cloutier and Alain from Laval University state that the contemporary family is undergoing transformation, with the emergence of a greater variety of profiles and trajectories.[14] This development in family mobility has been observed for several decades and the trend it represents can be regarded as a lasting one. The population must accept the changing families and adapt to the family's process of transition. As well as a series of transitions, that are part of the normal cycle of a family, including growth and the development of children (known as developmental transitions), a family may also be significantly affected by nondevelopmental transitions, such as placement of a child in substitute care, a death in the family, and parental separation.[15]

CRITICAL THINKING

What resources are available in your community to help a family with school-age children in transition?

According to the 2001 Canadian Census, the proportion of "traditional" families continues to decline. Children are living with common-law parents and more young adults are living with their parents. The size of the Canadian household is declining; and living alone is on the rise. Regarding same-sex couples, male couples outnumber female couples. In addition, more seniors are living with a spouse, more are living alone, and fewer are living in health care institutions.[16] The Aboriginal population is much younger than the Canadian average, and Aboriginal children represent 5.6% of all children in Canada.[17]

However, whatever the family structure, a child's adjustment is associated with the quality of parenting and not the structure of the family. For example, with at least one positive, warm, and authoritative parent, children of divorce are likely to be competent and well adjusted.[18] The responsibility for family life and for looking after children must be shared by parents, caregivers, employers, and the community. Because of the time pressures that parents face nowadays, many children need caring adults in their lives. These significant adults can be drawn from grandparents, aunts and uncles, neighbours, teachers, coaches, and child care providers.[19] For more information regarding Canada's children and their families, see http://www.cfc-efc.ca/docs/vanif/00000899.htm.

The structural level of child poverty in Canada has hardly changed in almost 30 years. In 1973, the child poverty rate stood at 16.4%, it improved to 15.7% in 1980, and decreased further to 14.9% in 1989.[20] However, by 2001, the child poverty rate was 15.6%. Child poverty increased to a record high in the early 1990s as Canada experienced a deep recession and high unemployment. Although the rate began to decline at the end of the 1990s, the decline did not happen as quickly as economic growth might suggest. Generally speaking, children, women, certain minorities (especially Aboriginals), and those who live in rural areas are all at a higher risk of experiencing poverty.[21] To achieve a sustained reduction and end to child poverty, governments need to adopt a comprehensive multi-pronged social investment strategy, which might include the following:

■ Income security to protect families
■ Significant steps to improve the availability of good jobs with decent living wages and working conditions
■ A well-designed system of early childhood education and care
■ Affordable housing that meets the needs of all families[22]

CRITICAL THINKING

How can you, as a health professional, lobby the government for a decrease in child poverty?

Refer to Chapter 4 for more information about trends in family life. More and more, studies are being reported about how the parent(s) can better focus quality time on the child, effects of both parents being employed, effects of being in a single-parent home or stepparent home, and how much the child needs the love and support of parents. Studies also focus on feelings of parents as they try to juggle the demands of child care and work.

Health Canada's publication *Because Life Goes on...Helping Children and Youth Live with Separation and Divorce* is intended to reach out to Canadian families in need of information and resources to help their children to live through the process of separation and divorce.[23] Many factors are important as the separation or divorce is initiated. However, keep in mind that however an adult understands or experiences the situation, the children see it and experience it differently. Younger children typically view divorce as the enemy; preteens and teenagers tend to hold their parents accountable for the divorce.[24] It is critical to remember that the emotional experience of anger is common to all children, but they express it differently. Talking to the children about separation and divorce is often the most difficult step parents must take in the process; yet how parents handle this crucial step can set the patterns for future discussions and influence the level of trust children feel in the future.[25]

Review with families the tasks summarized in Table 10-1 that must be resolved by children after divorce.[26]

Although the poor child frequently shares the helplessness of an unemployed parent, the higher-income child often feels the relentless pressure on the parent who is a high-powered corporate executive, lawyer, professor, or government official preoccupied with his or her own survival. Too often the demands of the workplace encroach on the needs and happiness of the family.

You will care for families in which abuse, neglect, or maltreatment occur. Refer to Chapters 4, 6, 7, and 9 for background information about precipitating factors, characteristics of abusing parents, and signs, symptoms, and treatment of abuse. Table 10-2 summarizes risk factors for sexual abuse.

The research of Garbarino, Guttmann, and Seeley[27] shows the physiological abuse or maltreatment of the schoolchild is demonstrated by the behaviour described in the box entitled "Parental Behaviour Characteristic of Psychological Maltreatment of the Schoolchild."[28-34]

The **latch key child,** the *child who has the door key because no one is home when the child returns from school,* is seen increasingly as more women with children under 18 work outside of the home. Children voice different feelings about the working mother and having no one home to meet them after school. Some like it. They enjoy the solitude, privacy, responsibility, and closeness of each other at day's end. Some hate it for the same reasons. Some tolerate it out of necessity, disliking the separation and lack of time together. Some are afraid for themselves and their mothers. Some are proud of mother and how they are managing together. Some become discipline problems. All understand the financial reasons and sometimes the career and emotional reasons that are usually the basis for mother working. Hunt states that children stay home alone because their working parents cannot find, or cannot afford, a regulated child care space, or cannot establish a stable informal care arrangement.[35] Clearly, children who care for themselves at home are at an increased risk for injury, missing meals, and other health and well-being problems.[36]

Canada Safety Council's advice to the parents includes:

■ Set firm rules, with dos and don'ts
■ Prepare the child to deal with events that may arise
■ Specify how his or her time is to be spent

TABLE 10-1
Psychological Tasks for Children After Divorce

Task I: Understanding the Divorce

Schoolchildren

1. Understand the immediate changes.
2. Differentiate fantasy from reality.
3. Manage concerns regarding abandonment, placement in foster care, not seeing departed parent again.

Adolescents and Young Adults

1. Understand what led to marital failure.
2. Evaluate parents' actions.
3. Draw useful conclusions for their own lives.

Task II: Strategic Withdrawal

1. Acknowledge concern and provide appropriate help to parents and siblings.
2. Avoid divorce as the total focus and get back to their own interests, pleasures, activities, peer relationships.
3. Children allowed to remain children.

Task III: Dealing with Loss

1. Deal with loss of intact family and loss of presence of one parent, usually the father.
2. Deal with feelings of rejection and blame for making one parent leave.
3. Task is easier if child has good relationship with both parents; this may be most difficult task.

Task IV: Dealing with Anger

1. Manage anger at parents for deciding to divorce.
2. Be aware of parents' needs, anxiety, and loneliness.
3. Diminish anger and forgive.

Task V: Working Out Guilt

1. Deal with sense of guilt for causing marital difficulties and driving wedge between parents.
2. Separate guilty ties and get on with their lives.

Task VI: Accepting Permanence of Divorce

1. Overcome early denial and fantasies of parents getting back together.
2. Task may not be completed until parent remarries or child mourns loss.

Task VII: Taking a Chance on Love

1. Remain open to love, commitment, marriage, fidelity.
2. Able to turn away from parents' model.
3. Most important task for growing children, adolescents, and young adults.

- Keep in touch—a cell phone or pager may be an asset
- Make certain the home is safe and secure
- Limit the time in leaving the child alone[37]

TABLE 10-2
Sexual Abuse of the Schoolchild

Risk Factors

- Having a stepfather
- Poor relationship between child and parent
- Mothers who work outside the home or are emotionally distant
- Having a parent who does not live with the child
- Sex: 25% of all females and 10% of all males by age 18

Family Characteristics

- An emotionally dependent adult male in the home
- Sexual estrangement between the parents or parental figures
- Mother deserted the family (literally or figuratively)
- Sexual offender suffers a crisis, such as loss of job
- Daughter begins to mature sexually
- Parent has poor impulse control
- Problems such as substance abuse, personality disorders, psychoses, and mental retardation in parent(s)

CRITICAL THINKING

If you were asked by the Canada Safety Council to add more pointers for parents, what would you add to the list?

In Canada, the age at which children can legally be left home alone for short periods varies from province to province, but ranges from 10 to 12 years. Therien, the president of the Canada Safety Council, urges parents not to consider letting a child stay at home alone before age 10—and then only if the child is mature enough. The maximum time to be spent alone is an hour or two—and only if there is a responsible adult nearby to help out if needed.[38]

To prepare children for the responsibilities of self care, the Canada Safety Council prepared the booklet *At Home On My Own*, which focuses on how to prevent problems, handle real-life situations, and keep children safely and constructively occupied.[39]

As a health care professional, you care for the family and the individual child. As a community nurse, your assessment may be the key to a child's receiving necessary care. You can conduct many of the health promotion activities that are described throughout this chapter. You can counsel and teach both parents and children. Be aware of cultural beliefs and practices as you work with children and families. A family who has lived in this country for several generations may follow the same cultural patterns as the newly emigrated family.

Relationships with Siblings

Although parental influence is of primary importance, the child's relationship with siblings affects personality formation. The influence of siblings on the development of the school-age child depends on a number of factors, including age and sex of the siblings, number of children in the family, proximity of their ages, and type of parent–child interaction.

Parental Behaviour Characteristic of Psychological Maltreatment of the Schoolchild

Rejecting

- Communicates negative definitions of self to the child
- Creates a sense of "bad-me" or negative self-concept by consistently calling child negative names such as stupid, dummy, monster
- Belittles child's accomplishments regularly
- Scapegoats child in the family system

Isolating

- Removes child from normal social relations with peers
- Prohibits child from playing with or inviting children into the home
- Withdraws child from school

Terrorizing

- Places child in double bind
- Demands opposite or conflicting behaviour or emotions simultaneously from the child
- Forces child to choose one of the two parents
- Changes rules of the house or of relationships with parents frequently
- Criticizes constantly so that child has no prospect of meeting expectations

Ignoring

- Fails to protect child from threats or intervene on behalf of the child
- Does not protect child from assault from siblings or other family members
- Does not respond to child's request for help or feedback

Corrupting

- Rewards child for stealing, substance abuse, assaulting other children, and sexual precocity
- Goads child into attacking other children
- Exposes child to pornography
- Encourages drug use
- Reinforces sexually aggressive behaviour
- Involves child sexually with adolescents or adults

Source: Garbarino J., E. Guttman, and J. Seeley, The Psychologically Battered Child: Strategies for Identification, Assessment and Intervention. San Francisco: Jossey-Bass, 1987. Copyright 1986. Adapted by permission of Jossey-Bass, Inc., a subsidiary of John Wiley & Sons, Inc.

CONTROVERSY DEBATE

Home Alone

Your neighbours routinely allow their seven-year-old child to be alone in their home for several hours each day after school until they arrive home from work. You have seen the child come home from school, sometimes alone, and at others with a small group of age mates. One day, after seeing the child with eight other children go into the house, you decide to phone the home to see how they are doing. The telephone does not get answered—even after you check the number and redial.

1. What is your immediate responsibility as a neighbour?
2. How will you approach the parents?

Relationships between the school-age child and siblings vary from jealousy, rivalry, and competition to protectiveness and deep affection. Siblings tend to get along more harmoniously when they are the same sex, but boys usually are more physically aggressive at all ages. Although sibling jealousy is less acute in school-age children than in preschool children, it still exists. An older child may be jealous of the attention given to younger siblings and may resent having to help with their care. The younger school-age child may feel jealous of the freedom given to older siblings. School-age children may feel the need to compete for parental attention and academic excellence. Parental comparisons of siblings' scholastic and artistic abilities or behaviour should be avoided as they add to jealousy and resentment.

Sibling relationships are likely to influence social interactions in later life. Siblings teach each other how to negotiate, cooperate, compete, support, and reward one another and how to work and play with others. Siblings of chronically ill children may work hard at being helpful to parents and the ill child, or even be overprotective, to receive attention and approval as well as to convey love, depending on how the family approaches care of the ill child. The siblings may also become depressed, withdraw, or act out in various ways to receive attention. In part, how the siblings react depends on the psychological health of parents and their marital adjustment, and on the parents' ability to allow siblings to express anger, guilt, exclusion, deprivation, jealousy, fears of family break-up, or other feelings related to how their life differs from the life patterns of their friends (e.g., fewer outings, increased chores, less money for desired items). Siblings should have an opportunity to talk with health care professionals about the illness and their feelings.

Family Development Tasks

Family activities with the school-age child revolve around expanding the child's world. Tasks include the following:[40]

- Take on parenting roles.
- Adjust the marital system and the lifestyle to allow physical, emotional, and social space for the child or children.
- Keep lines of communication open among family members.
- Work together to achieve common goals.
- Plan a lifestyle within economic means.
- Find creative ways to continue a mutually satisfactory married life or satisfactory single parenthood.
- Maintain close ties with relatives.

- Realign relationships with the extended family to include parenting and grandparenting roles.
- Expand family life into the community through various activities.
- Validate the family philosophy of life. The philosophy is tested when the child brings home new ideas and talks about different lifestyles he or she encountered, forcing the family to re-examine patterns of living.

CRITICAL THINKING

The Smiths are a blended family. In what ways might their tasks be similar to, or different from, the ones listed above?

These tasks are manifested differently by families from various cultural backgrounds; those who are homeless, live in poverty, or are migrants; or those who live in war-torn or Third World countries. As you care for families and assist them to meet these tasks, consider the uniqueness of the family situation.

Adoptive families have the same developmental tasks as other families. An issue for adoptive parents, however, is how to help their adopted child or children feel part of the family, especially if adoption occurs at an age when the child remembers the process.

Table 10-3 describes the adopted child's perception of adoption during the school years and how adoptive parents may respond. Prepare parents for when the adopted child may initiate search for the birth parent. Jenkins describes the reasons for the search and how the adoptive parents can help.[41]

The adopted child especially struggles with identity issues because of uncertainties about the past, especially when the child is of different racial or ethnic origin than parents. Parents must remain open to the children's questions, sustain an accepting and open atmosphere, expect turbulence, and help him or

her find other supportive adults. Adoption is not a constant issue; but parents cannot ever completely retreat from it.[42–45] Adoptive families need professionals who understand child development, behaviour management, and the psychological issues for children who have undergone separation and loss. Ongoing supports such as workshops and networks can also be of tremendous assistance to adoptive families.[46] Several authors describe feelings of the adopted child and various issues to be resolved.[47,48]

Relationships Outside the Family

As the child's social environment widens, other individuals begin to function as role models and to influence the child. The child strives for independence and establishes meaningful relationships with peers, teachers, and other significant adults. These relationships provide the child with new ideas, attitudes, perspectives, and modes of behaviour. Although the parents remain role models, the influence of the family and the time spent with family diminish. Through contacts with the peer group, the child acquires a basis for assessing the parents as individuals and learns that parents can make mistakes.

Schneider, a Canadian researcher, investigated the friendships of children considered socially withdrawn by their school peers. The videotaped data showed the withdrawn children to be somewhat restricted in their verbal communication with their friends. They were less competitive with their friends, than were friends in a comparison group. In dyads consisting of one withdrawn and one nonwithdrawn child, the withdrawn child perceived the relationship as characterized by greater closeness and helpfulness than did the nonwithdrawn friend. Despite some signs of inhibited behaviour within the friendship context, withdrawn children seem to have access to close friendship of high quality.[49] It is important to indicate

TABLE 10-3
Adopted Child's Perceptions and Suggested Parental Responses

Age	Child's Perception	Suggested Parental Response
5–7	Begins to grasp full notion of adoption, that parents are not blood relatives, and that most children live with biological parent(s) Feels sense of loss	Emphasize that child is important to them and was chosen. Answer questions comfortably and naturally. Explain it is normal for child to have mixed emotions about adoption.
8–11	Fantasizes and wonders about birth parents Realizes he or she is different from nonadopted children Wants to question parents about adoption but fears appearing disloyal or ungrateful Feels grief and goes through mourning process Frequently asks questions about why birth parents relinquished him or her, parents' appearance, and whether there are siblings	Discuss the adoption openly, when appropriate, to help the child vent curiosity and feelings. Help child accept fact that he or she is different and emphasize other differences as well. Answer questions truthfully. Do not criticize or overpraise birth parents. Adjust depth of answer to age of child. Realize children who are not adopted also fantasize that they are.

that peer rejection was not a variable in this study. Children are adaptable to their environment and usually gravitate to an acceptable niche for themselves.

The schoolchild has a growing sense of community that changes with increased mobility and independence and added responsibility. His or her understanding broadens to include a sense of boundaries, distance, location, and spatial relationships of resources and organizations, demographic characteristics, and group identity.

You are in a key position to listen to and explore with families their concerns about being parents, achieving the expected developmental tasks, and adjusting to the growing and changing child as he or she interacts with parents, siblings, other relatives, peers, and other adults outside the home. At times you may validate their approach to a given situation. At other times you may help them clarify their values so they can, in turn, better guide the child. Such practical suggestions as how to plan more economically a nutritious meal or handle sibling rivalry can help a distraught parent feel and become more effective.

Your ability to assess beyond the obvious and to help the family use community resources effectively to meet basic needs is often the first step in promotion of both physical and emotional health.

CRITICAL THINKING

What are some criteria that children might use to choose their friends?

PHYSIOLOGIC CONCEPTS

The following information is pertinent to assessment and health promotion strategies. Share this information with families.

Physical Characteristics

The *principles of growth* or *growth patterns* are comparable across cultures, generally. For example, progression of maturation of body organ systems is similar in all cultural groups. The child between six and 12 years old exhibits considerable change in physical appearance. Growth during this stage of development is hypertrophic (cells increase in size) instead of hyperplasic (cells increase in number). The growth rate is usually slow and steady, characterized by periods of accelerations in the spring and fall and by rapid growth during preadolescence.[50–56]

Weight, Height, and Girth

These measurements vary considerably among children and depend on genetic, environmental, and cultural influences.

Most Asian children born and raised in Canada or the U.S. are larger and taller than those children born and raised in Asian countries because of differences in diet, climate, and social milieu.[57]

The *average schoolchild grows* 5 to 6 cm (2 to 2.5 inches) per year to gain 30 to 60 cm (1 to 2 feet) in height by age 12. A *weight gain* of 2 to 3.5 kg (4 to 7 pounds) occurs per year. The average weight for a six-year-old boy is 21.5 kg (48 pounds), and

the average height is 117 cm (46 inches). By age 12, the average child weighs approximately 40 kg (88 to 90 pounds) and is more than 150 cm (59 inches) tall. By age 12, the child has usually attained 90% of adult height.

During the *juvenile* or *middle childhood period*, girls and boys may differ little in size; their bodies are usually lean, with narrow hips and shoulders. Although the amount of muscle mass and adipose tissue is influenced by muscle use, diet, and activity, males usually have more muscle cells, and females have more adipose tissue. The muscles are changing in composition and are growing at a rapid rate becoming more firmly attached to the bones. Muscles may be immature in regard to function, resulting in children's vulnerability to injury stemming from overuse, awkwardness, and inefficient movement. Muscle aches may accompany skeletal growth spurts as developing muscles attempt to keep pace with the enlarging skeletal structure. Ossification, the formation of bone, continues at a steady pace. The schoolchild loses the pot-bellied, swayback appearance of early childhood. Abdominal muscles become stronger; the pelvis tips backward and posture becomes straighter.[58–63]

Neuromuscular Development

The *brain* of the child is very active; studies reveal that from age four to puberty, glucose metabolism by brain cells is twice that of the adult brain. Thus the child is capable of processing new information readily.[64]

By age seven the brain has reached 90% of adult size. The growth rate of the brain is greatly slowed after age seven, but by age 12 the brain has virtually reached adult size. Memory has improved. The child can listen better and make associations with incoming stimuli.

Myelinization is complete. *Neuromuscular changes* are occurring along with skeletal development. Neuromuscular coordination is sufficient to permit the schoolchild to learn most skills he or she wishes.

Refer to Table 10-4 for a summary of neuromuscular development from six to 12 years of age.[65–70]

Cardiovascular System

The *heart* grows slowly during this age period; the left ventricle of the heart enlarges. After seven years of age, the apex of the heart lies at the interspace of the fifth rib at the midclavicle line. Before this age, the apex is palpated at the fourth interspace just to the left of the midclavicle line. By age nine, the heart weighs six times its birth weight. By puberty, it weighs ten times its birth weight. Even though cardiac growth does occur, the heart remains small in relation to the rest of the body. Because the heart is smaller proportionately to body size, the child may tire easily. Sustained physical activity is not desirable. The schoolchild should not be pushed to run, jog, or engage in excessively competitive sports such as football, hockey, and racquetball.[71–76]

Hemoglobin levels are higher for Caucasian than black 10- to 15-year-olds. In all likelihood, racial differences in hemoglobin levels during childhood exist independent of nutritional values. Racial differences are consistent with those for infants, preschool children, teenagers, pregnant women, and athletes, unrelated to nutritional variables.[77]

TABLE 10-4
Neuromuscular Development in the Schoolchild

Age (Yr)	Characteristic
6	High activity level but clumsy
	Moves constantly: skips, hops, runs, roller skates
	Can do manipulative skills: hammer, cut, paste, tie shoes, and fasten clothes
	Grasps pencil or crayon, makes large letters or figures
	Can throw with proper weight shift and step
	Walks chalk mark with balance
	Tandem gait
	Girls are superior in movement accuracy
	Boys are superior in forceful, less complex activity
7	Lower activity level; enjoys quiet and active
	Pedals a bicycle
	Prints sentences, reverses letters less frequently
	Spreads with a knife
	Can balance on one foot without looking
	Can walk 5-cm-wide balance beam
	Can hop and jump accurately into small squares
	Can do accurate jumping jack exercise
8	Moves energetically but with grace and balance
	Enjoys vigorous activity
	Improved coordination
	Can engage in alternate rhythmic hopping in 2-2, 2-3, or 3-3 pattern
	Faster reaction time
	More skillful at throwing because of longer arm, girls can throw small ball 1.2 m
	Better grasp of objects
	Begins cursive writing rather than printing, better small muscle coordination
	Has 5.5 kg (12 pound) of pressure in grip strength
9	Less restless
	Bathes self
	Refined eye–hand coordination, skilled in manual activities
	Draws a 3-dimensional geometric figure
	Enjoys models
	Uses both hands independently
	Spaces words and slants letters when writing
	Strives to improve coordination and perfect physical skills, strength, and endurance
	Boys can run 5 m (16.5 feet) per second
	Boys can throw a small ball 25 m (70 feet)
10	More energetic, active, restless movements
	Finger drumming or foot tapping
	Balances on one foot for 15 seconds
	Can judge and intercept pathway of small ball thrown from a distance
	Girls can run 5.25 m (17 feet) per second
11–12	Standing broad jump of 1.5 m (5 feet) is possible for boys, 15 cm (6 inches) less for girls
	Standing high jump of 1 m (3 feet) possible by age 12
	Can catch a fly ball
	Skillful manipulative movements nearly equal to those of adult
	Physical changes preceding puberty begin to appear

CRITICAL THINKING

What are several factors that promote cardiovascular fitness?

Vital Signs

Vital signs of the schoolchild are affected by size, sex, and activity. Temperature, pulse, and respiration gradually approach adult norms with an average *temperature* of 36.7° to 37°C (98° to 98.6°F), *pulse rate* of 70 to 80 per minute, resting pulse rate of 60 to 76 per minute, and *respiratory rate* of 18 to 21 per minute. The average *systolic blood pressure* is 94 to 112, and average *diastolic blood pressure* is 56 to 60 mm Hg. As respiratory tissues achieve adult maturity, *lung capacity* becomes proportional to body size. Between the ages of five and ten, the respiratory rate slows as the amount of air exchanged with each breath doubles. Breathing becomes deeper and slower. By the end of middle childhood, the lung weight will have increased almost ten times. The ribs shift from a horizontal position to a more oblique one; the chest broadens and flattens to allow for this increased lung size and capacity.[78–82]

Head

The growth of the *head* is nearly complete; head circumference measures proximately 53 cm (21 inches), and attains 95% of its adult size by the age of eight or nine. The sinuses strengthen the structured formation of the face, reduce the weight of the head, and add resonance to the voice. The child loses the childish look as the face takes on features that will characterize him or her as an adult. Jaw bones grow longer and more prominent as the mandible extends forward, providing an extended chin and a place into which *permanent teeth* can erupt. Girls lose teeth earlier than boys; deciduous or baby teeth are lost and replaced at a rate of four teeth per year until approximately age 11 or 12. The "toothless" appearance may produce embarrassment for the child. The first permanent teeth are six-year molars that erupt by age seven and are the key teeth for forming the permanent dental arch. Evaluation for braces should not be completed until all four 6-year molars have appeared. The second permanent molars erupt by age 14, and the third molars (wisdom teeth) come in as late as age 30. Some persons' wisdom teeth never erupt (Figure 10–1). When the first permanent central incisors emerge, they appear too large for the mouth and face. Generally the teeth of boys are larger than those of girls.[83–88]

Many governments and health organizations, including Health Canada, the Canadian Public Health Association, the Canadian Dental Association, the Canadian Medical Association, and the World Health Organization, endorse the fluoridation of drinking water to prevent tooth decay.[89,90] Health Canada works in collaboration with the provinces and the territories to maintain and to improve drinking water quality. Together, both levels of government have developed *Guidelines for Canadian Drinking Water Quality* (see Chapter 2). These guidelines are reviewed and revised periodically to take into account new scientific knowledge.[91]

Drinking water that meets quality guidelines does not usually need extra treatment. The following are several steps parents can take to keep fluoride intake within safe limits:

- Do not give fluoridated mouthwash or mouth rinses to children under six years of age, because they might swallow it.

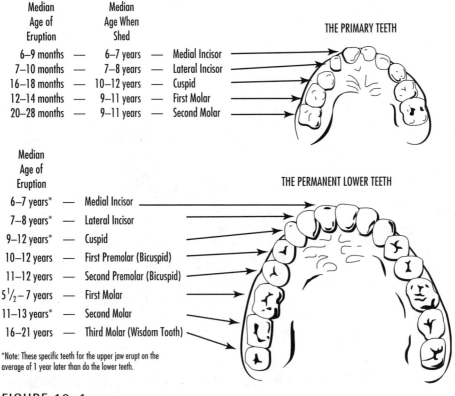

Median Age of Eruption	Median Age When Shed	
6–9 months	6–7 years	Medial Incisor
7–10 months	7–8 years	Lateral Incisor
16–18 months	10–12 years	Cuspid
12–14 months	9–11 years	First Molar
20–28 months	9–11 years	Second Molar

THE PRIMARY TEETH

Median Age of Eruption	
6–7 years*	Medial Incisor
7–8 years*	Lateral Incisor
9–12 years*	Cuspid
10–12 years	First Premolar (Bicuspid)
11–12 years	Second Premolar (Bicuspid)
5½–7 years	First Molar
11–13 years*	Second Molar
16–21 years	Third Molar (Wisdom Tooth)

THE PERMANENT LOWER TEETH

*Note: These specific teeth for the upper jaw erupt on the average of 1 year later than do the lower teeth.

FIGURE 10–1

Normal tooth formation in the child.

- Talk to the dentist before using a fluoride supplement or a fluoridated mouthwash.
- Do not take fluoride supplements if the drinking water is already fluoridated.
- Be informed. The Canadian Dental Association and the Canadian Paediatric Society have made recommendations on the use of fluoride supplements in communities where the water is not fluoridated.
- Make certain that children use no more than a pea-size amount of toothpaste on their toothbrush, and teach them not to swallow the toothpaste.
- Children under six years of age should be supervised while brushing, and children under the age of three should have their teeth brushed by an adult without using toothpaste.

Children who live in areas with high fluoride content in the drinking water may demonstrate **fluoride mottling** (*brownish permanent discolouration*) of the teeth in late childhood and adolescence.[92]

CRITICAL THINKING

What evidence can you think of to support the notion of a gender difference about brushing teeth?

Vision

The shape of the *eye* changes during growth, and the normal farsightedness of the preschool child is gradually converted to 20/20 vision by age eight. By age ten the eyes have acquired adult size and shape. Binocular vision is well developed in most children at six years of age; peripheral vision is fully developed. Girls tend to have poorer visual acuity than boys, but their colour discrimination is superior. Large print is recommended for reading matter and regular vision testing should be part of the school health program.[93]

Gastrointestinal System

Secretion, digestion, absorption, and excretion become more efficient. Maturity of the gastrointestinal system is reflected in fewer stomach upsets, better maintenance of blood sugar levels, and an increased stomach capacity.[94,95]

Urinary System

The urinary system becomes functionally mature during the school years. Between the ages of five and ten, the *kidneys* double in size to accommodate increased metabolic functions. Fluid and electrolyte balance becomes stabilized, and *bladder capacity* is increased, especially in girls. *Urinary constituents* and specific gravity become similar to those of an adult; however, 5% to 20% of school-age children have small amounts of albuminuria.[96,97]

Immune System

Lymphoid tissues reach the height of development by age seven, exceeding the amount found in adults. The body's ability to localize infection improves. Enlargement of adenoidal and tonsillar lymphoid tissue is normal, as are sore throats, upper respiratory infections, and ear infections, which are caused by the excessive tissue growth and increased vulnerability of the mucous membranes to congestion and inflammation. The *frontal sinuses* are developed near age six. Thereafter, all sinuses are potential sites for infection. Immunoglobulins G and A reach adult levels by age nine, and the child's immunologic system becomes functionally mature by preadolescence.[98–100]

Prepubertal Sexual Development

During the *preadolescent* or *prepuberty period*, both males and females develop preliminary characteristics of sexual maturity. This period is characterized by the growth of body hair, a spurt of physical growth, changes in body proportion, and the beginning of primary and secondary sex characteristics. They demonstrate physical changes such as increased weight and height, vasomotor instability, increased perspiration, and active sebaceous glands. There is an increase in fat deposition approximately one year before the height spurt. These fat deposits last approximately two years or until skeletal growth and muscle mass increase. Females have more subcutaneous fat deposits, and the fat is lost at a slower rate, accounting for the fuller appearance of the female figure.[101–106]

The girl's growth spurt begins as early as eight years; the average is ten, and maximum height velocity is reached around 12 years. The boy's growth spurt begins near 12 years; maximum height velocity is reached by approximately 14 years. The male grows approximately 10 cm (4 inches) per year for two-and-a-half years and then begins a slower rate of growth. The female grows an average of 7.5 cm (3 inches) per year until menarche begins. For both males and females, the growth spurt begins in the hands and feet and progresses to the calves, forearms, hips, chest, and shoulders; the trunk is the last to grow appreciably.[107–111]

As sebaceous glands of the face, back, and chest become active, acne (pimples) may develop. These skin blemishes are caused by the trapping of collected sebaceous material under the skin in small pores. The preadolescent and later the adolescent are concerned with their appearance; these blemishes cause considerable embarrassment. The young person and the family may resort to numerous remedies, such as visits to skin specialists or use of sun lamps, diets, makeup, lotions, and creams. Basically, the skin should be kept clean. If the problem persists, a dermatologist should be seen. To prevent the youth's withdrawal from social contact, the parents and youth should be encouraged to seek medical attention as early as possible after acne occurs.[112] Acne is further discussed in Chapter 11.

For a summary of physical changes, refer to the boxes entitled "Physical Changes in Girls during Prepuberty" and "Physical Changes in Boys during Prepuberty."

Teach parents about the physical and growth characteristics of the school-age child and the importance of nutrition, rest, immunizations, healthful activity, and regular medical and dental care. The rest of the chapter refers to variables that influence physical health.

CRITICAL THINKING

What steps can you take to promote the emotional well-being of a child with acne?

Physical Changes in Girls during Prepuberty

- Increase in transverse diameter of the pelvis
- Broadening of hips
- Tenderness in developing breast tissue and enlargement of areola diameter
- Axillary and body sweating
- Change in vaginal secretions from alkaline to acid pH
- Change in vaginal layer to thick, grey, mucoid lining
- Change in vaginal secretion flora from mixed to Döderlein's lactic acid–producing bacilli
- Appearance of pubic hair from 8 to 14 years (hair first appears on labia and then spreads to mons, adult triangular distribution does not occur for approximately two years after initial appearance of pubic hair)

These physical changes for females are listed in the approximate sequence of their occurrence

Sources: Bee, H., Lifespan Development (2nd ed.). New York: Longman, 1998; Gormly, A., Lifespan Human Development (6th ed.). Fort Worth: Harcourt Brace College Publishers, 1997; Papalia, D., S. Olds, and R. Feldman, Human Development (7th ed.). Boston: McGraw-Hill, 1998; Seifert, K., R. Hoffnung, and M. Hoffnung, Lifespan Development. Boston: Houghton Mifflin, 1997; Sigelman, C., Life-Span Human Development (3rd ed.). Pacific Grove, CA: Brooks/Cole, 1999; Wong, D., Whaley and Wong's Nursing Care of Infants and Children (6th ed.). St. Louis: C.V. Mosby, 1999.

Physical Changes in Boys during Prepuberty

- Axillary and body sweating
- Increased testicular sensitivity to pressure
- Increase in size of testes
- Changes in colour of scrotum
- Temporary enlargement of breasts
- Increase in height and shoulder breadth
- Appearance of lightly pigmented hair at base of penis
- Increase in length and width of penis

The physical changes for males are listed in the approximate sequence of their occurrence

Sources: Bee, H., Lifespan Development (2nd ed.). New York: Longman, 1998; Gormly, A., Lifespan Human Development (6th ed.). Fort Worth: Harcourt Brace College Publishers, 1997; Papalia, D., S. Olds, and R. Feldman, Human Development (7th ed.). Boston: McGraw-Hill, 1998; Seifert, K., R. Hoffnung, and M. Hoffnung, Lifespan Development. Boston: Houghton Mifflin, 1997; Sigelman, C., Life-Span Human Development (3rd ed.). Pacific Grove, CA: Brooks/Cole, 1999; Wong, D., Whaley and Wong's Nursing Care of Infants and Children (6th ed.). St. Louis: C.V. Mosby, 1999.

Physical Assessment of the School-Age Child

Information will be gained from the child, the parents or caretakers, or both when assessing the child.

A child may be better at drawing than at explaining what is wrong. For example, when asked to draw a big circle where it hurts, the child can normally identify the part if given a simple outline drawing of a child.

The child over age ten may wish to talk to the health care provider without the parent present. Being alert to the child's chronologic and developmental stage and his or her relationship with parents or caretakers will guide you in interviewing. Where the child lives (house or apartment, rural or urban area), how much personal space he or she has (own room, own bed), parents' marital situation, presence or absence of siblings, what is usually eaten, the amounts of exercise and rest in 24 hours, who cares for the child after school if parents are working, and how he or she spends free time are all important in assessing the health status.

When doing a review of systems, remember to use words the child understands. For example, instead of asking if the child has ever experienced any otitis problems, simply ask as follows: Do your ears ever ache? Can you always hear when people talk to you?

In assessing skin, remember that the school-age child is subject to allergic contact dermatitis, warts, herpes type 1, ringworm, and lice. When seeing any rash, a thorough history is necessary to determine the diagnosis and treatment.[113,114]

Understanding that visual function is more than reading the 20/20 line on a Snellen chart will help you suggest a more comprehensive visual examination when a child is experiencing difficulty with school work. Children and their parents do not always react predictably when there is a need for corrective lenses. Some children may feel self-conscious with their peers when wearing glasses. Parents may react as if the child's visual problem were a flaw and will deny it, stating that they are sure the child will outgrow the problem, ignore the information, or even go from doctor to doctor in search of reassurance.

If you are able to provide accurate information, using the principles of therapeutic communication, it will be exceedingly valuable to a child and family who are having difficulty adjusting to the need for therapy for a visual impairment. (This also holds true when therapy or a corrective device is needed on another body area.)

When assessing a child's hearing and ears, remember that hearing should be fully developed by age five. By age seven, most children should speak clearly enough to be understood by adults. If either of these factors seems deficient, a thorough investigation into congenital or inherited disorders and how this deficiency affects daily activities and communication is in order.

In the young child, because the ear canal slants up, pull the auricle down, but not back as you would in an adult, when using the otoscope. Also, the ear canal is short in the young child, so take care not to insert the ear tip too far. The otoscope should be controlled so that if the young child moves suddenly, you can protect the eardrum from being contacted by the otoscope. The cone of light is more indistinct in a child than in an adult.[115]

Keep in mind the following as you continue assessment of the child's body systems: (1) if you think you hear fluid in the lungs, check the child's nose because sounds caused by nose fluid can be transmitted to the lungs; (2) an S_3 sound and sinus arrhythmia are fairly common in children's heart sounds; (3) a child's liver and spleen usually will enlarge more quickly than an adult's in response to disease; (4) the bladder is normally found much higher in a child than in an adult, and the kidneys can more often be palpated; (5) the genitalia should be inspected for congenital abnormalities that may have been overlooked and for irritation, inflammation, or swelling; and (6) developmental guidelines must be used to assess the nervous system, specifically language development, motor and sensory functions, and cerebral function.[116–118]

In the last decade musculoskeletal and posture problems, especially scoliosis detection, have gained wide attention. **Scoliosis,** *lateral curvature of the spine,* is more common in girls than in boys and is of two types, functional and structural. Ask the child to bend over and touch the toes without bending the knees and keeping the palms of the hands together. If the child has functional scoliosis, the external curve will disappear with this exercise; if it is structural; the curve will remain and sometimes become more pronounced. Early diagnosis is extremely important to arrest this problem.[119,120] Refer the child and family to an orthopedic specialist. If scoliosis is not corrected early in life, it can result in mobility problems, obstructive pulmonary disease, and problems with body image later in life.

CRITICAL THINKING

What questions can you realistically ask the schoolchild about health conditions within the family?

Nutritional Needs

The school years are important regarding eating habits. Meeting the nutritional requirements of the school-age child requires larger amounts of the same food needed by the preschool child. Growth during prepuberty is slow and steady, with gradual increases in height and weight.[121] With the introduction of school into one's routine, the child's meal pattern will likely change. Even though children may prepare their own breakfast, parents should try to eat breakfast with their children as with other meals. Stockmyer found that beneficial effects on nutritional intake occur when children eat dinner with their family.[122]

During the school years, children become more responsible in making their own choices about what they eat. Children have built-in cues—like hunger, feeling full, thirst, and taste—to help them decide what and when to eat. Do you recall making your own snacks? Parents and significant caregivers struggle to make certain they help children to make good choices while respecting the child's ability to make his or her own decisions.[123]

Canada's Food Guide to Healthy Eating encourages eating and enjoying different foods from each food group every day. This selection helps children to meet their nutrient needs every day. Children eat mainly from the following four food groups:

- Grain products, such as whole-grain and enriched products, should be chosen most often.
- Vegetables and fruit, especially dark green and orange vegetables as well as orange fruit, should be chosen more often.
- Milk products, such as lower-fat products, are more important.
- Meat and alternatives, such as leaner meats, poultry, and fish, as well as dried peas, beans, and lentils should be chosen more often.

For *Canada's Food Guide to Healthy Eating,* visit http://www.hcsc.gc.ca/ hpfb-dgpsa/onpp-bppn/food_guide_rainbow_e.html.

Other foods—foods that are not part of the four main food groups—can also add energy and some nourishment. To promote variety in foods, children can try food from other cultures. Doing so can help them to learn about their friends and the world around them.[124] Children must be encouraged to drink water to quench their thirst. In fact, children need more water during hot weather and when they are playing hard. Most beverages (e.g., milk, juices, soft drinks) and many foods (such as fruit) are good sources of water.[125]

If children are healthy, growing well, and are eating a variety of foods, they are not likely to need a vitamin-mineral supplement. However, an increase in calcium needs occurs prior to puberty. This need is one of the reasons why the *Food Guide* recommends that children increase the number of servings of milk products to three or four per day.[126]

Nutritional assessment is determined by obtaining a history of the child's food intake; looking at the general appearance and skin colour and turgor; correlating height and weight; measuring subcutaneous tissue; checking for dental caries, allergies, and chronic illness; testing hemoglobin and hematocrit levels; and determining physical, cognitive, emotional, and social well-being.

NARRATIVE VIGNETTE
Nutritional Hurdles

You have two school-age children and an infant. Last week your family orthodontist placed braces on the teeth of the older two children. The orthodontist instructed you and the children that they could not eat raw fruits or vegetables, but starches are acceptable provided the teeth are brushed immediately after eating. Brushing after lunch at school is easily arranged. However, you wish to prepare snacks for the children to take to school to have after school before hockey practice twice weekly; but brushing at that time is a problem for them.

1. List foods from each group of the *Canada Food Guide* that your children could take for their after-school snack.

2. How will you alter the snacks to maintain a variety?

Eating Patterns

It is important to *discuss the child's eating needs and patterns with parents so that they can provide a diet with adequate caloric intake and nutrients.* Culture determines the type of foods eaten, when certain foods are to be eaten, and the manner in which they are consumed. The many dietary variations must be assessed for nutritional adequacy.[127] By age eight, children have increased appetites; by age ten, their appetites are similar to those of adults. Despite increasing appetites, children seldom voluntarily interrupt activities for meals. Television, sports, and other activities compete with mealtimes. Parents should be encouraged to establish a consistent schedule for meals and to allow their school-age child to participate in the meal planning. The schoolchild of six or seven is capable of learning about healthful eating and of helping plan and prepare meals. Such activities develop a healthy sense of industry and independence in the child if they are not overdone.

Mealtime continues to cause dissension within most families. When mealtime becomes a time of stress, digestive problems, poor eating habits, or a temporary aversion to food may occur. Making a fuss over eating certain foods may cause the child to reject them more strongly. Experience and time will improve eating patterns, as shown in Table 10-5.[128]

Food preferences and dislikes become strongly established during the school years; however, by age eight the child will try new or previously disliked foods. Food likes and dislikes are often carried over from the eating experiences of the toddler and preschooler. In addition, it is easy for the schoolchild, influenced by peers, television commercials and other forms of advertisement, and the availability of junk food, to avoid nutritious foods and to fill up on empty calories.

CRITICAL THINKING

How effective do you believe parental practices to be regarding adequate nutrition?

Diet is influenced by a child's activities. If the child has been active all day, he or she will be hungry and ready to eat. On the other hand, if the child has had limited activity or emotional frustrations during the day, he or she may have no appetite. The schoolchild has more freedom to move without parental supervision and often has small amounts of money to spend on candy, soft drinks, and other treats. Peer influence will frequently determine the child's lunch. Schools have attempted to satisfy current eating preferences of this age group by offering a la carte selections such as French fries, hot dogs, pizza, and salads as well as balanced meals. Total and saturated fat and sodium content should be reduced in both school lunches and home meals.

TABLE 10-5
Summary of Eating Patterns of Schoolchildren

6 Years	7 Years	8 Years	9 Years	10 Years	11 Years	12 Years
Has large appetite	Has extremes of appetite	Has large appetite	Has controlled appetite	Goes on eating sprees	Has controlled appetite	Has large appetite
Likes between-meal and bedtime snacks	Improves table manners	Enjoys trying new foods	Eats approximately an adult meal	Likes sweet foods	Improves table manners when eating in a restaurant	Enjoys most foods
Is awkward at table	Is quieter at table	Handles eating utensils skilfully	Acts more adult-like	Criticizes parents' table manners	Enjoys cooking	Has adult-like table manners
Likes to eat with fingers	Is interested in table conversation	Has better table manners away from home	Becomes absorbed in listening or talking	Has a lapse in control of table manners at times		Participates in table discussions in adult manner
Swings legs under table, often kicking people and things	Leaves table with distraction			Enjoys cooking		
Dawdles						
Criticizes family members						
Eats with better manners away from family						

Share the following suggestions with parents to improve nutrition and mealtime:[129]

1. Create an environment of respect, love, acceptance, and calm.
2. Make food attractive and manageable.
3. Establish basic rules regarding table etiquette and table language, topics of conversation, and behaviour. Provide a rest period before meals.
4. Have a firm understanding with the child that play and television do not take precedence over eating properly; keep television and the telephone at a minimum.
5. Between-meal snacks are necessary and enjoyed and do not interfere with food intake at meals if eaten an hour or longer before mealtime. Milk, cheese, fresh fruits and vegetables, peanut butter, and fruit juices are desirable snacks for both general nutritional needs and dental health.
6. Breakfast is crucial for providing the child with sufficient calories to start the day. The child who attends school without breakfast frequently exhibits fatigue and poor attention.
7. With a comfortable environment and adults eating the food on the table, the intake is likely to be adequate for the child, because the parents are role models.

Undernutrition in children can be manifested in delayed growth, underweight, fatigue, lassitude, restlessness, irritability, and poor school performance and work output. Anorexia and digestive disturbances, such as diarrhea and constipation, signal improper use of nutrients. Poor muscular development may be evidenced by a child's posture—rounded shoulders, flat chest, and protuberant abdomen. Prolonged undernutrition may cause irregularities in dentition and may delay epiphyseal development and puberty. See the box entitled "Subjective Global Assessment for Nutritional Status."

It is often surprising and somewhat disappointing to realize the effects of hunger on children in Canada. McIntyre and her colleagues examined the prevalence of hunger among

Subjective Global Assessment for Nutritional Status

Normal	Malnourished
HAIR: Shiny, firm in the scalp	**HAIR:** Dull, brittle, dry, loose; falls out
EYES: Bright, clear pink membranes; adjust easily to darkness	**EYES:** Pale membranes; spots; redness; adjust slowly to darkness
TEETH and GUMS: No pain or cavities, gums firm, teeth bright	**TEETH and GUMS:** Missing, discoloured, decayed teeth; gums bleed easily and are swollen and spongy
FACE: Good complexion	**FACE:** Off-colour, scaly, flaky, cracked skin
GLANDS: No lumps	**GLANDS:** Swollen at front of neck, cheeks
TONGUE: Red, bumpy, rough	**TONGUE:** Sore, smooth, purplish, swollen
SKIN: Smooth, firm, good colour	**SKIN:** Dry, rough, spotty; îsandpaperî feel or sores; lack of fat under skin
NAILS: Firm, pink	**NAILS:** Spoon-shaped, brittle, ridged
BEHAVIOUR: Alert, attentive, cheerful	**BEHAVIOUR:** Irritable, apathetic, inattentive, hyperactive
INTERNAL SYSTEMS: Heart rate, heart rhythm, and blood pressure normal; normal digestive function; reflexes, psychological development normal	**INTERNAL SYSTEMS:** Heart rate, heart rhythm, or blood pressure abnormal; liver, spleen enlarged; abnormal digestion; mental irritability, confusion; burning, tingling of hands, feet; loss of balance, coordination
MUSCLES and BONES: Good muscle tone, posture; long bones straight	**MUSCLES and BONES:** "Wasted" appearance of muscles; swollen bumps on skull or ends of bones; small bumps on ribs; bowed legs or knock-knees

Canadian children. In doing so, they studied the characteristics of, and coping strategies used by families with children who were experiencing hunger.[130] The data originated from the first wave of data collection for the National Longitudinal Survey of Children and Youth conducted in 1994. The data included 13 439 randomly selected Canadian families with children aged 11 years or under. The researchers found that hunger was experienced by 1.2% (206) of the families in the survey. The survey sample represented a population of 57 000 Canadian families. In addition, they found that single-parent families, families relying on social assistance, and off-reserve Aboriginal families were overrepresented among those experiencing hunger. Hunger coexisted with the mother's poor health and activity limitation and the poor health of children. Parents tend to offset the needs of their children by not taking food themselves.[131]

Overnutrition and overweight are rarely caused by metabolic disturbances. Obesity is sometimes defined as the condition of an *individual who is 20% or more above ideal weight*. The concept of body mass index (BMI), rather than weight alone, is currently used to determine whether or not an individual is obese.[132] Obesity is the most frequent nutritional disorder of children in developed countries. In Canada, the prevalence of obesity has tripled from 1981 to 1996.[133] In addition, childhood obesity can have serious social and emotional effects that may carry into adulthood.[134] Prevention of childhood obesity, through early nutrition education and established exercise habits, is important. The Weight Realities Division of the Society for Nutrition Education developed guidelines for obesity prevention programs that encourage a health-centred, rather than a weight-centred approach. This approach focuses on the whole child, physically, mentally, and socially.[135] The focus is on living actively, eating in normal and healthful ways, and developing a nurturing environment that helps children recognize their own worth and respects cultural footways and family traditions.[136]

Undernutrition and overnutrition may have the same causative factors: the child may be reflecting food habits of other family members; the parents and child may displace unrelated anxieties on food and mealtime; or eating may serve as a reward or punishment by both parents and child. In some cultures, being overweight is considered a sign of health and family affluence. In other cultures, obesity is considered unsightly and unhealthy.[137]

You can help parents learn about adequate nutrition for their child as well as what behaviour to expect at each age. You can also aid teachers as they plan lessons on nutrition. For example, learning activities for the schoolchild could include visiting grocery stores, dairies, or farms as well as taking part in tasting parties and playing store. They could plan menus, examine food labels, cook various foods, and taste them. Such activities are unlimited.

Rest and Exercise

Review the child's rest and exercise needs with parents. At the same time, you may have an opportunity to discuss with parents how they are meeting their own needs for rest and exercise and how the parents and child can engage in activities that are mutually interesting and healthful.

Hours of sleep needed depend on such variables as age, health status, and the day's activities. Schoolchildren usually do not need a nap. They are not using up as much energy in growth as they were earlier. A six-year-old usually requires approximately 11 hours of sleep nightly, but an 11-year-old may need only nine hours.[138] The schoolchild does not consciously fight sleep but may need firm discipline to go to bed at the prescribed hour. Sleep may be disturbed with dreams and nightmares, especially if he or she has considerable emotional stimulation before bedtime.

Exercise is essential for muscular development, refinement of coordination and balance, gaining strength, and enhancing other body functions such as circulation, aeration, and waste elimination. Regular physical activity at this age, and thereafter, helps to prevent coronary artery disease, hypertension, obesity, and type 2 diabetes in future years.[139]

Over half of Canadians aged five to 17 are not active enough for optimal growth and development. The term "active enough" is equivalent to an energy expenditure of at least 8 kilocalories per kilogram of body weight per day.[140] The most reported physical activity of children five to 12 is bicycling, followed by swimming, playing on swings, using playground equipment, and then walking. In this age group, the next most popular activities are winter activities such as tobogganing and skating. Girls are more likely to participate in social dancing, skating, gymnastics, or ballet. Meanwhile, boys are more likely to participate in team sports such as soccer, hockey, or baseball.[141]

Health Canada recognized that the rapid increase in overweight and obesity, combined with low levels of physical activity, represent a serious threat to the health of Canadian children and youth.[142] Health Canada and the Canadian Society for Exercise Physiology initiated the development of *Physical Activity Guides for Children and Youth* that were launched in 2002.[143] For people to order the guides free of charge, Health Canada has set up a toll-free telephone service at 1-888-334-9769. The guides are available at http://www.healthcanada. ca/paguide. The guides recommend that inactive children and youth increase the amount of time they currently spend being physically active by at least 30 minutes per day and decrease the time they spend watching TV, playing computer games, and surfing the Internet—by at least 30 minutes per day.[144] This increase in physical activity should include a combination of moderate activity (skating, or riding a bike) with vigorous activity (running and playing soccer). The guidelines recommend that inactive children and youth accumulate this increase in daily physical activity in periods of at least five to ten minutes each.[145]

CRITICAL THINKING

What are the main consequences of obesity for the school child? How can these consequences be overcome?

CRITICAL THINKING

What criteria would you include in developing an exercise program for school children in the community?

Health Promotion and Health Protection

Immunizations

Immunization is one of the most significant measures for protecting children from serious illness and death resulting from vaccine-preventable diseases.[146] See Table 7-6 on page 328 for routine immunization schedules for infants and children.

Bigham and Hoefer, researchers from British Columbia, conducted a population-based analysis using communicable disease and vaccine associated adverse events (VAAEs) that are routinely collected in British Columbia and other provinces and territories.[147] They considered four universal childhood immunization programs in British Columbia: measles, rubella, paralytic poliomyelitis, and invasive Hemophilias influenza type b (Hib). They found that after implementing universal programs, the average incidence of reported cases decreased 90% to 100% over a five-year period.[148] These benefits were sustained or strengthened over time. The rates of reported serious VAAEs were low. The researchers conclude that, overall, this study affirms the remarkable effectiveness of four universal childhood immunization programs and a high degree of safety associated with immunization.[149]

Some parents may have concerns about immunizations. A health professional has a responsibility to listen and try to understand the parent's concerns, fears, and beliefs about vaccination. Halperin indicates that an eight-step approach to addressing the issue is effective. See the box entitled "Eight-Step Approach to Respond to Parents Unsure about Immunization."[150] Many sources of information exist for parents. One such reference is *Your Child's Best Shot*, written by Dr. Ronald Gold and published by the Canadian Paediatric Society in 1997 (available in both English and French).

Eight-Step Approach to Respond to Parents Unsure about Immunization

1. Listen, evaluate, and categorize
2. Recognize legitimate concerns
3. Provide context
4. Refute misinformation
5. Provide valid information
6. Recognize that it is the parents' decision
7. Educate about potential consequences
8. Make a clear recommendation

The Canadian Nurses Association has written an article called "Nurses and Immunization—What You Need to Know" for all nurses. The Canadian Immunization Awareness Program (CIAP), a coalition of health care organizations, which includes the Canadian Nurses Association (CNA), the Canadian Nursing Coalition for Immunization, and the Canadian Public Health Association (CPHA), has identified common misconceptions about immunizations. One such misconception is that of complacency. The fact is that immunization programs have been so successful at preventing serious disease that many people have become complacent. People

believe that vaccine-preventable diseases have been eliminated from Canada. However, with an increasing number of people travelling the globe, diseases can easily be brought back to Canada.[151]

Nurses play a vital role in promoting and delivering immunization programs across Canada. Consider your immunization. Are you up to date? What is the status of your family's immunization? These are important questions for you to consider and to act upon.

CRITICAL THINKING

How would you respond to an older person who questions you about the benefits of a flu shot?

Safety Promotion and Injury Control

Injuries are the leading cause of death for Canadian children and youth between the ages of one and 19 years. For children over the age of four, injuries cause more deaths than all other causes of death combined.[152]

About 50 Canadian children and adolescents die each year from bicycle-related injuries; and 75% of all bicycle-related deaths are due to head injuries.[153] Leblanc and his colleagues conducted a study in which trained observers, who had a direct view of oncoming bicycle traffic, recorded helmet use, sex, and age group of cyclists in Halifax. They found that the rate of helmet use rose dramatically after legislation was enacted. Furthermore, the proportion of cyclists with head injuries in 1998–99 was half that in 1995–96.[154] Howard states that more Canadian children die of road traffic accidents than of any other cause. The nonuse and misuse of child restraints is common and leads to preventable severe injuries or death.[155] Visit the Transport Canada site at http://www.tc.gc.ca/roadsafety/childsafety/menu.htm for *child restraints* and *booster cushion* notices. Lapner and his colleagues found that proper seatbelt restraints reduce the morbidity involved in motor vehicles. Discussing safe travel with parents may be the health professional's most important child health promotion activity. In addition to counselling, health professionals could choose to be involved in advocacy, public education campaigns, legislation, research, and the treatment of injuries.[156]

Drkulec and Letts studied injury patterns of snowboarding trauma in children. They found that 79% of the injuries were to the upper extremity, whereas 7% were to the lower extremity. They concluded that the predominance of snowboarding injuries of the upper extremity seen in children differs significantly from those in adults in whom lower injuries are more common.[157] It is important that health professionals be aware of the types of injuries that occur and know the importance of instruction on the use of proper equipment, risk avoidance, and falling techniques for novice snowboarders.[158] For example, Wesner evaluated the impact that the Think First Saskatchewan school visit program had on students' knowledge of brain and spinal cord injury prevention. She found that the program statistically improved self-reported knowledge of the students receiving the Think First message.[159]

During the first 17 years of life, a major health concern for First Nations and Inuit people is injury. According to the

First Nations and Inuit Regional Health Survey (FNIRHS), 13% of First Nations and Inuit individuals will have broken a bone by the time they are 17; 4% will have incurred a serious head injury; 3% will have been seriously burned; 2% will have experienced frostbite; and 3% will have almost drowned.[160] Bristow and her team of researchers analyzed the drowning data of the Manitoba Paediatric Death Review Committee to identify drowning risk factors and potential prevention strategies. Their results indicated that the highest mortality rates regarding drowning were found in First Nations children, followed by all boys, and then toddlers who are one to four years old.[161] In summary, the death rate for Aboriginal children, as a result of injuries, is much higher than that of the total population of Canadian children.[162]

Some children apparently are *accident-prone*. They suffer more accidental injuries than the overall childhood population. Although the causative factors have not been completely determined, children who are overreactive, restless, impulsive, hostile, and immature are frequently found in this group.[163]

Parents should be encouraged to provide supervision and attention, and to repeat frequently, even to children who are not accident-prone, that caution is necessary. The child forgets when involved in play; conceptual thinking and judgment are not well developed. Consequently, the child does not foresee all dangers.

Accident prevention should be taught and enforced in school and at home. You must promote safety by helping parents and children identify and avoid hazards. The school-age child has increasing cognitive maturity, including improved ability to remember past experiences and anticipate probable outcomes of his or her actions. This makes the child a good candidate for safety instructions.

Safety education should include information about the hazards of risk taking and improper use of equipment. Water safety and survival skills should be taught with basic swimming skills at an early age. Families who go boating must teach related safety measures to their children.[164]

CRITICAL THINKING

If you were asked to develop a community program on water safety to prevent drowning, what would be your first few steps?

Farm children are at risk for accidental injury or death when they accompany or assist parents with farm work. *Teach farm parents the following rules to reduce hazards*:[165]

- Do not allow children as extra riders on equipment.
- Do not allow children to play with idle machinery.
- Leave any equipment that might fall, such as front-end loaders, in the down position.
- When self-propelled machinery is parked, brakes should be locked and keys removed from the ignition.
- Always leave a tractor power-takeoff unit in neutral.
- When starting machinery—and especially when reversing it—know where the children are.
- Maintain machinery in good repair, particularly protective shields and seat belts.
- Do not permit children to operate machinery until they have completed safety training.

- Fence farm ponds and manure pits.
- Place fixed ladders out of reach, or fit with a special barrier; store portable ladders away from danger areas.
- Shield dangerous machinery components and electric boxes and wiring and place out of easy reach or fit with locking devices.
- Place warning decals on all grain bins, wagons, and trucks.
- Maintain lights and reflectors for all equipment used on roads.
- Do not expect children to work with farm animals or with machinery that is beyond their maturity physically or mentally.

Meal preparation can be fun for the school-age child, but the hazards of sharp knives, hot stoves, microwave ovens (the health effect of microwave radiation leakage is still unknown) and hot liquids must be kept in mind. Supervise the use of matches or flammable chemicals, and teach the child the proper behaviour if clothing becomes ignited. A family-designed fire escape plan should be initiated and practised monthly.

Most boys and girls love to climb; adults should teach them how to climb in the safest possible way. Explain the dangers involved in climbing trees, electric poles, water towers, silos, and other structures. Instruct the child in the proper use of playground equipment and in the need to pick up toys from the floor to prevent falls.

Instruct parents to keep potentially dangerous products in properly labelled receptacles. Educate the child about the dangers of taking nonprescription drugs, chemicals. Gun accidents are common during the school-age period. Parents who have a gun should keep it under lock and place the key in a childproof location. Children of this age should be taught safety rules concerning guns.

Reinforce any teaching that takes place in the home. Books, films, and creation of a mock situation can all supplement your verbal instruction. You and the parents will repeat the same cautions endlessly. Yet, caution and concern can be overdone. When a child is overly anxious about his or her welfare, tension can lead not only to accident proneness but to being hurt worse when he or she does encounter danger. In the face of danger, panic prevents clear thinking and skillful action. In addition, overcaution stifles independence, initiative, and maturing. It is important to realize the necessity of shifting responsibility to the child with increasing age.

Correction of health problems is essential, as they may be a cause for injuries, illness, or difficulties with schoolwork or peers. As a nurse you have a responsibility to strengthen the school health program in your community through direct services; teaching the board of education, teachers, parents, and students about the value and use of such a program despite costs; and working for legislation to finance and implement programs that do more than first-aid care. A school health program should supervise not only the child's physical health, but also emotional, mental, and social health.

If there are chronically ill or disabled students in school, special preparation should be given to the teachers, the students, and the parents. You can promote understanding of the child and his or her condition, of the child's need to reach individual potential, and of a total rehabilitation program. Several references will be helpful.[166,167]

In summary, the recognition of injuries as a leading cause of death in children has resulted in extensive research and the generation of a considerable amount of comprehensive information on this issue.[168] Health professionals must be aware, not only of the statistics related to injuries in children but of health promotion strategies to prevent such injuries and to impart vital information to parents and significant caretakers.

Common Health Problems: Prevention and Treatment

Although the child should now remain basically healthy, health problems do exist. Teach parents about expected illnesses. School-age children get sick about one-half as often as preschoolers and about twice as much as their parents.[169] Inform parents of the need to treat both acute and chronic conditions.

Respiratory conditions (colds, sore throats, and earaches) account for more than 50% of the reported acute illnesses among children in this age group. *Asthma,* a persistent congestion in the lungs, is increasing in incidence, possibly related to environmental conditions, and it is a major health problem in both Canada and the U.S.[170] *Infective and parasitic diseases* (scabies, impetigo, ringworm, and head lice) are of concern because of their health threat to the child and to others. *Diseases of the digestive tract* (stomachaches, peptic ulcers, colitis, diarrhea, and vomiting) may have a psychosocial and a physiologic cause. Visual and hearing impairment, sickle cell anemia, asthma, hyperactivity, epilepsy, migraine headaches, hypertension, juvenile diabetes mellitus, and obesity are *chronic health problems* that may affect the school-age child. The child may have been born with a congenital anomaly that can be only partially corrected or a disease such as hemophilia that needs continuing treatment. A considerable number of schoolchildren have *risk factors that in adults are predictive of coronary heart disease:* hypertension, increased serum cholesterol and triglycerides, and obesity. The elementary school population may also be the main reservoir of *infectious hepatitis A,* for schoolchildren often have a mild undiagnosed disease that is spread person to person.[171–175]

Because of the short urethra, girls are prone to *urinary infection;* this may be diagnosed by reddened genitals, a feeling of burning on urination, and abnormal appearance and chemical analysis of the urine. Normal urinary output from age six to 12 ranges from 500 mL to the adult output of 1500 mL daily. Pinworms accompany urinary tract infections in approximately 50% of the cases.[176]

The seven-year-old has fewer illnesses but may complain of *fatigue* or *muscular pain.* It is common to call these "growing pains"; however, this is not accurate, because growing is not painful. Tension, overactivity or exertion, bruising, or injury may cause the leg pains. Pains in the knees with no physical signs of exertion signs are also common in school-age children. Such pains usually occur late in the day or night and disappear in the morning. Children with persistent leg pains should be referred to a physician.

Visual impairments that occur in the younger child may be undetected and untreated until the child attends school. Visual acuity may not develop normally. For more information, see the box entitled "Signs and Symptoms Indicating Defective Vision in Schoolchildren."[177,178] It is essential that visual problems be corrected.

Table 10-6 summarizes other common health problems, their definitions, symptoms and signs, and prevention or treatment measures.[179,180]

Signs and Symptoms Indicating Defective Vision in Schoolchildren

Behaviour

- Attempts to brush away blur; rubs eyes frequently; frowns, squints
- Stumbles frequently or trips over small objects
- Blinks more than usual; cries often or is irritable when doing close work
- Holds books or small playthings close to eyes
- Shuts or covers one eye, tilting or thrusting head forward when looking at objects
- Has difficulty in reading or in other schoolwork requiring close use of the eyes; omits words or confuses similar words
- Exhibits poor performance in activities requiring visual concentration within arm's length (e.g., reading, colouring, drawing); unusually short attention span; persistent word reversals after second grade
- Disinterested in distant objects or fails to participate in games such as playing ball
- Engages in outdoor activity mostly (e.g., running, bicycling), avoiding activities requiring visual concentration within arm's length
- Sensitive to light
- Unable to distinguish colours
- Steps carefully over sidewalk cracks or around light or dark sections of block linoleum floors
- Trips at curbs or stairs
- Poor eye–hand coordination for age, excessively hard-to-read handwriting, difficulty with tying shoelaces or buttoning and unbuttoning

Appearance

- Crossed eyes (iris of one eye turned in or out and not symmetric with other eye)
- Red-rimmed, encrusted, or swollen eyelids
- Repeated sties
- Watery or red eyes

Complaints

- Cannot see blackboard from back of room
- Blurred or double vision after close eye work
- Dizziness, headaches, or nausea after close eye work
- Itching or burning eyes

Sources: Hoole, A., C. Pickard, R. Ouimette, J. Lohr, and W. Powell, Patient Care Guidelines for Nurse Practitioners (5th ed.). Philadelphia: J.B. Lippincott, 1999; Wong, D., Whaley and Wong's Nursing Care of Infants and Children (6th ed.). St. Louis: C.V. Mosby, 1999.

TABLE 10-6
Common Health Problems of Schoolchildren

Problem	Definition	Symptoms/Signs	Prevention/Treatment
Accommodative esophoria	Eyes converge excessively in response to accommodation	Close work becomes exhausting and overwhelming	Eyeglasses and taking "eye breaks" recommended.
Otitis externa	Inflammation of the external auditory canal and auricle	Pain in ear aggravated by moving the auricle; exudate in ear canal	Prevention: Keep instruments out of ears. Keep dirty water out of ear. Use acetic acid (2%) solution in ear after swimming. After the fact, use antibiotic or steroid drops.
Serous otitis media	Accumulation of nonpurulent fluid in middle ear	Fullness and crackling in ear; decreased hearing	Administer decongestants (questionable help).
Allergic rhinitis	Allergic reaction affecting nasal mucosa (and sometimes conjunctiva)	Clear, thin nasal discharge; breathes through mouth; often does "allergic salute" (rubs nose upward)	Find offending irritant or antigen and try to eliminate. Administer antihistamines. Obtain workup by allergist if problem persists.
Asthma	Disease of lungs characterized by partially reversible airway obstruction, airway inflammation, and airway hyperresponsiveness; caused by hyperreactivity of the tracheobronchial tree to chemical mediators	Wheezing, cough, dyspnea, anxiety, restlessness	Try to stay away from allergens, if known. Avoid being around those with upper respiratory infections; avoid overexertion, rapid temperature or humidity changes, air pollutants, emotional upsets. Follow NAEP (National Asthma Education Program) step-care approach described by Boynton et al.[181] for appropriate timing of essential medications.
Herpes type I	Vesicular eruption of skin and mucous membranes above the umbilicus (usually mouth)	Soreness of mouth from eruption of mucosa; inflammation and swelling; sometimes fever and enlarged lymph glands (sub-mandibular)	Apply Zovirax ointment to slow down severity. Drink adequate fluids. Use saline solution mouthwash. Administer antipyretic. Isolate from susceptible persons.
Contact dermatitis	Vesicular formation on skin, usually from poison ivy or poison oak	Itching and formation of vesicles, sometimes on most body parts	Apply cold compresses and drying lotion. Sometimes administer cortisone-based oral medicine or injections. Teach how to avoid plants.

(continued)

TABLE 10-6 *(continued)*
Common Health Problems of Schoolchildren

Problem	Definition	Symptoms/Signs	Prevention/Treatment
Tinea corporis (ringworm of non-hairy skin)	Superficial fungal infection involving face, trunk, or limbs	Red patch areas that scale and are oval in shape; usually asymptomatic or mildly itchy; no systemic signs	Apply a topical antifungal daily for 2 or 3 weeks.
Tinea capitis (ringworm of the head)	Fungal infection involving scalp	Same as Tinea corporis	Apply fungal cream persistently. Sometimes it is necessary to shave hair.
Warts	Intradermal papillomas	Usually appear as common (on hands or fingers) or plantar (on feet)	Dichloroacetic acid will often dissolve them. Other removal methods are available from dermatologist.
Pediculus humanus capitis (head lice)	Infestation of head, hair, scalp	Itching scalp; see nits or ova as little dots attached to base of hairs	Shampoo with approved medication. Apply antihistamine for itching. Comb out any remaining ova-nits. Boil all head care items.
Mumps	Viral disease characterized by acute swelling of salivary gland, especially the parotid	Anterior ear pain; headache; lethargy; anorexia; vomiting; complication orchitis (*inflammation of one or both testes*)	Prevention: obtain vaccine. Use only supportive treatment such as antipyretics (not Aspirin products) and encourage fluid intake.
Diabetes mellitus type I (formally called juvenile diabetes)	Inherited disease with metabolic component that causes elevated blood sugar and vascular component that causes effects on eyes and kidneys	Increased urination; increased thirst and hunger; weight loss and fatigue	Obtain workup by appropriate health care practitioner. Follow diabetic diet and exercise recommendations. Administer insulin.
Fifth disease (erythema infectiosum)	Mild viral illness caused by human parvovirus B19; no ongoing harm to child but maternal infection can cause spontaneous abortions and stillbirths	Three-stage exanthemas: (1) slapped cheek appearance; (2) maculopapulary rash on trunk and extremities; looks lacy; (3) rash has evanescence and recrudescence	If it is a school-related breakout, expect a 25% infection rate. Stay away from pregnant women. There is no specific treatment, only symptomatic, i.e., acetaminophen for aches. Stay away from sun, which can exacerbate rash.
Hand-foot-and-mouth disease	Contagious viral disease caused by Coxsackie virus A	Abrupt fever; vesicular lesions of the mouth, palms of the hands, and soles of feet; anorexia	As it is highly contagious, keep isolated until temperature is normal for 24 hours. Treat symptomatically; saline mouth rinse; acetaminophen *(continued)*

TABLE 10-6 *(continued)*
Common Health Problems of Schoolchildren

Problem	Definition	Symptoms/Signs	Prevention/Treatment
			for temperature elevation; fluids; tepid baths.
Pityriasis rosea	An acute, self-limited, presumably viral disease, which produces a characteristic rash	Classic lesion on trunk, looks like a Christmas tree; starts with "mother spot" that is scaly, salmon-coloured, and spreads peripherally	There is no need to isolate. Expect rash to last as long as 4 months. Use symptomatic treatment such as cool compress, calamine lotion, Benadryl (if pruritis). Exposure to sunlight will relieve itching and shorten duration of rash.

Rabies, an *acute infectious disease characterized by involvement of the central nervous system, resulting in paralysis and finally death,* is fortunately not a common disease but comes from a common problem: the biting of a human by a mammal. Prevention is in keeping the child away from unfamiliar animals, particularly ones that act agitated, in seeing that all pets are properly vaccinated, and in taking steps to get pre-exposure immunization for high-risk children—those living or visiting in countries where rabies is a constant threat.

Increasingly, the ill effects of *smoking and drug and alcohol abuse* are emerging as a regular health problem. These habits are influenced by the habits of parents, siblings, and peers. In addition to the ill effects caused by smoking, children in families with cigarette smokers have an increased rate of respiratory conditions and cancer from secondary smoke. These small children have an increased number of days per year when their activities are restricted because of illness.[182]

Emphasize to adults that *more effective than organized educational attempts is the influence of significant adults, those who take a personal interest in the child and who set an example:* such as parents who neither smoke, drink, use drugs nor give cigarettes, alcohol, drugs to their children. *Equally important,* or more so, *is the peer group; leaders of the peer group who have positive health habits should be used as models.* Peer communication is also effective for initiating hygienic habits. You may have a role in working with the peer group.

CRITICAL THINKING

If you were asked to teach a group of school children in a community centre about the hazards of substance abuse, what topics would you address?

Determinants of positive health behaviour in a study of 260 nine- and ten-year-old boys and girls indicated that age and sex of the child, parental education, and family size influenced self-esteem and personal perception of health. Boys and girls in the fourth grade differed in their reported health habits; girls scored higher than boys in health behaviours, willingness to report symptoms, and self-concept. These results may reflect socialization patterns and expected role behaviours of men and women in our culture. Intrinsic motivation for health increases with age and during the school years. Children from larger families demonstrated higher self-esteem but were more extrinsically motivated. Children from families with higher maternal education had higher motivation for healthful practices. This study indicates that *interventions to teach health promotion to children must consider family assessment and the child's self-esteem and motivational levels, and must foster a positive personal responsibility in the child for healthful practices,* such as healthy snacks.[183] Further, it is *essential to consider cultural differences in definitions of disease prevention and health promotion practices.*[184]

You *can promote healthy behaviour and design and implement health promotion interventions.* Traditional sites (schools, clinics) and nontraditional sites (shelters, social service programs, correctional institutions, shopping malls, religious institutions, and work and recreational settings) in rural and urban areas are places to implement health promotion programs and teaching.

PSYCHOSOCIAL CONCEPTS

Share the following information about the schoolchild's cognitive, emotional, and moral-spiritual development with parents and teachers to guide assessment and promote health.

Cognitive Development

The schoolchild has a strong curiosity to learn, especially when motivation is strengthened by interested parents and opportunities for varied experiences in the home and school.

Learning, behaviour, and personality are complex issues and are not easily explained by one theory. This section uses information from a number of theorists. Refer to Chapter 5 for a review of how the major schools of theorists explain the development of learning, behaviour, and personality.

Pattern of Intellectual Development

Children manifest a **cognitive style,** *the characteristic way in which information is organized and problems are solved.* The style varies from child to child, but there are four major cognitive styles:[185]

1. *Analytic.* Examine minute details of objects or events.
2. *Superordinate.* Observe for shared attributes of objects or similarities of events.
3. *Functional-relational.* Objects or events are linked because they have interactional value.
4. *Functional-locational.* Objects or events have a shared location.

Older children are more likely to use analytic and superordinate cognitive styles.

In addition to cognitive style, children differ in their **conceptual tempo,** *the manner in which they evaluate and act on a problem.* Tempo may be either **impulsive,** *where the first idea is accepted and hurriedly reported without consideration for accuracy or thoughtfulness,* or **reflective,** *where a longer period is used to consider various aspects of a situation.* Reflective children are more likely to be analytic than are impulsive children.[186]

Certain kinds of questions or statements help the child learn to think more analytically and reflectively:[187]

- Why? Give an explanation.
- If that is so, what follows? What is the cause of _____?
- Aren't you assuming that _____?
- How do you know that?
- Is the point you were making that _____?
- Can I summarize your point as _____?
- Is this what you mean to say?
- What is your reason for saying that?
- What does that word mean?
- Is there another way of looking at _____?
- Is it possible that _____?
- How else can we view this? How else can we approach this situation?

The pattern of intellectual development can be traced through the school years.[188–191]

In North American culture the six-year-old is supposed to be ready for formal education. The child in grade one is frequently still in the preoperational stage. See Table 10-7 for a summary of cognitive abilities of the child from ages six to 12.[192–198]

At approximately age 7 the child enters the stage of **concrete operations,** *which involves systematic reasoning about tangible or familiar situations and the ability to use logical thought to analyze relationships and structure the environment into meaningful categories.* The child must have interactions with concrete materials to build understanding that is basic for the next stage.[199,200] Their mental operations work poorly with abstract ideas—ones not apparent in the real world.[201]

The following operations are characteristic of this stage:[202–206]

- **Classification.** *Sorting objects in groups according to specific and multiple attributes* such as length, size, shape, colour, class of animals, and trademark. Schoolchildren can identify which kind of Ford is approaching on the highway. Usually one characteristic is focused on first; then more characteristics are considered.

- **Seriation.** *Ordering objects according to decreasing or increasing measure* such as height, weight, and strength. The child knows A is longer than B, B longer than C, and A longer than C.

- **Nesting.** *Understanding how a subconcept fits into a larger concept.* For example, a German shepherd is one kind of dog; a reclining chair and a dining room chair are both chairs.

- **Multiplication.** *Simultaneously classifying and seriating,* using two numbers together to come out with a greater amount.

- **Reversibility.** *Returning to the starting point or performing opposite operations or actions with the same problem or situation.* The child can add and subtract and multiply and divide the same problems. A longer row of clips can be squeezed together to form a shorter row and vice versa; the child realizes the number of clips has not changed.

- **Transformation.** *Ability to see the shift from a dynamic to static or constant state, to understand the process of change, and to focus on the continuity and sequence, on the original and final states.* For example, the child realizes or anticipates how a shorter row of pennies was shifted to become a longer row or the gradual shift in level of fluid in a container as it is poured into another container and the increasing level of fluid in the second container.

- **Conservation.** *Understanding transformation conceptually and that a situation has not changed, to see the sameness of a situation or object despite a change in some aspect, and that mass or quantity is the same even if it changes shape or position.* There is an order to conservation; first number, followed by length, liquid, and mass, followed by weight. Piaget used the term *horizontal decalage* (meaning development with a stage) to describe the gradual mastery of logical concepts.[207] Three concepts contribute to this operation:[208]

1. *Identity.* A lump of clay rolled into different shapes is the same clay; six paper clips moved from a 6-cm line to an 8-cm line remain six paper clips.
2. *Reversibility.* Water in boiled form is vapour, which can return to water and freeze. It is still the same amount of water; nothing is lost in the process. Operations can be reversed; their effects can be nullified.
3. *Reciprocity.* A change of a mass of clay in one direction is compensated for by a change in another direction, but the total mass remains the same. A small, thick ball of clay can be flattened to be large and thick; but no clay material was added or taken away.

- **Decentring.** *Coordination of two or more dimensions, or the ability to focus on several characteristics simultaneously.* For example, space and length dimensions can be considered;

TABLE 10-7
Cognitive Characteristics of the School-Age Child

Age	Cognitive Ability
6	Thinking is concrete and animistic
	Beginning to understand semi-abstract concepts and symbols
	Defines objects in relation to their use and effect on self
	May not be able to consider parts and wholes in words at the same time
	Likes to hear about his past
	Knows numbers
	Can read
	Learning occurs frequently through imitation and incidental suggestion and also depends on opportunities
	May not be able to sound out words; may confuse words when reading, such as *was* and *saw*
	High correlation between ability to converse and beginning reading achievement; may have vocabulary of 8000 to 14 000 words when reading, if assisted with language
7	Learns best from interaction with actual materials or visible props
	Learning broad concepts and subconcepts, e.g., car identified as Ford or Chevrolet, based on memory, instruction, or experience
	A number of mental strategies or operations are learned
	Becoming less egocentric, less animistic
	Better able to do cause–effect and logical thinking
	More reflective; has deeper understanding of meanings and feelings
	Interested in conclusions and logical endings
	Attention span lengthened; may work several hours on activity of interest
	More aware of environment and people in it; also interested in magic and fantasy
	Understands length, area, or mass
	Sense of time practical, detailed; present focus; plans the day
	Knows months, seasons, years
	Serious in inventing, enjoys chemistry sets
8	Less animistic
	More aware of people and impersonal forces of nature
	Improvises simple activities
	Likes to learn about history, own and other cultures, geography, science, and social science
	Intellectually expansive; inquiries about past and future
	Tolerant and accepting of others
	Understands logical reasoning and implications
	Learns from own experience
	Extremely punctual
	Improvises simple rules
	Can read a compass
9	Realistic in self-appraisal and tasks
	Reasonable, self-motivated, curious
	Needs minimal direction
	Competes with self
	Likes to be involved with activities and complex tasks
	May concentrate on project for 2 or 3 hours
	Plans in advance; wants successive steps explained and wants to perfect skills
	Focuses on details and believes in rules and laws (they can be flexible), as much as luck or chance
	Enjoys history

(continued)

Age	Cognitive Ability

TABLE 10-7 *(continued)*
Cognitive Characteristics of the School-Age Child

Tells time without difficulty
Likes to know length of time for task
Likes to classify, identify, list, make collections
Understands weight

10
Is matter-of-fact
Likes to participate in discussions about social problems and cause and effect
Likes a challenge
Likes to memorize and identify facts
Locates sites on a map
Makes lists
Easily distracted; many interests and concentrates on each for a short time
Greater interest in present than past

11
Curious but not reflective
Concrete, specific thinking
Likes action or experimentation in learning
Likes to move around in the classroom
Concentrates well when competing with one group against another
Prefers routine
Better at rote memorization than generalization
Defines time as distance from one event to another
Understands relationships of weight and size

12
Likes to consider all sides of a situation
Enters self-chosen task with initiative
Likes group work but more inner motivated than competitive
Able to classify, arrange, and generalize
Likes to discuss and debate
Beginning formal operations stage, or abstract thinking
Verbal formal reasoning possible
Understands moral of a story
Defines time as duration, a measurement
Plans ahead, so feels life is under own control
Interested in present and future
Understands abstractness of space
Understands conservation of volume

the younger child would consider only one or the other. When 12 paper clips are spread from 6 to 12 cm, the child realizes the clips are spread and there are not more clips.

- **Combination.** *Ability to combine several tasks or operations at once, to see the regularities of the physical world and the principles that govern relationships among objects.* Perceptions alone become less convincing than a logical understanding of how the world operates. For example, a sunset on the ocean looks like the sun is sinking into the water; science teaches that what we see is a result of the earth's rotation on its axis.[209]

CRITICAL THINKING

What specific school and home experiences are likely to influence children's performance on Piaget's concrete-operational tasks?

These operations increase in complexity as the child matures from an empirical to logical orientation. The child can look at a situation, analyze it, and come up with an answer without purposefully going through each step. For example, if two rows of coins have been spread out, the child does not have to count the coins. He or she realizes that nothing was added to or subtracted from the rows, so each row still has the same number.

The child learns and can recall associations between sequences and groupings of events. At first he or she makes associations within a certain context or environment; later memory is used to transfer these associations to different contexts or environments. The child also rehearses; in the time between a learning experience and a memory test or application of learning, he or she goes over mentally what has been learned.[210]

You can discuss the child's changing cognitive abilities with parents and ways they can contribute to the cognitive achievement. If parents do not understand that certain cognitive behaviour is age-appropriate, their interactions with and guidance of the child may be less effective.

Cognitive development and an increasing understanding of implications and consequences and of cause-effect relations may be a factor in the changing *fearfulness* of the child. As a nurse, remember that the school-age child has great fear of body injury, disease, separation from loved ones, death, excess punishment (some diagnostic and treatment procedures seem like punishment), and doing wrong actions. In your practice you can help offset the child's fears. Inform parents to take their child's fears seriously and not to force their children to "be brave." A child who is scared is really scared. In fact, telling children that it is okay to be scared is comforting to them.[211]

CRITICAL THINKING

John is a school-age child being admitted to hospital for the surgical removal of a brain tumour. The parents tell you that John fears the surgery. How can you help to alleviate a few of his fears?

Concept of Time
The concept of time evolves during the early school period. See Table 10-8 for a summary of how the schoolchild develops a concept of time.[212–215]

You can help parents understand that their school-age children do not have adult concepts of time. The mother who is distraught because her six- or seven-year-old constantly dawdles in getting ready for school can be helped by understanding the child's concept of time. The mother must still be firm in direction but not expect the impossible. She can look forward to improvement in the eight-year-old.

Understanding maturing time concepts will also aid you as you explain the sequence of a procedure to the schoolchild in the doctor's office, school, clinic, or hospital.

Spatial Concepts
Spatial concepts also change with more experience. The six-year-old is interested in specific places and in relationships between home, neighbourhood, and an expanding community. He or she knows some streets and major points of interest. By age seven the sense of space is becoming more realistic. The child wants some space of his or her own such as a room or portion of it. The heavens and various objects in space and in the earth are of keen interest.[216,217]

For the eight-year-old, personal space is expanding as the child goes more places alone. He or she knows the neighbourhood well and likes maps, geography, and trips. He or she

TABLE 10-8
School-Age Child's Concepts of Time

Age	Conceptualization of Time
6	Time counted by hours; minutes disregarded Enjoys past as much as present; likes to hear about his or her babyhood Future important in relation to holidays Duration of episode has little meaning
7	Interested in present; enjoys a watch Sense of time practical, sequential, detailed Knows sequence of months, seasons, years Plans days; understands passage of time
8	Extremely aware of punctuality, especially in relation to others More responsible about time
9	Tells time without difficulty Plans days with excess activities; driven by time Wants to know how long a task will take to complete Interested in ancient times
10	Less driven by time than the 9-year-old Interested primarily in present Able to get to places in time on own initiative
11	Feels time is relentlessly passing by or dragging More adept at handling time Defines time as distance from one event to another
12	Defines time as duration, a measurement Plans ahead to feel in control Interested in future as well as present

understands the compass points and can distinguish right and left on others as well as self.[218]

Space for the nine-year-old includes the whole earth. He or she enjoys pen pals from different lands, geography, and history. For the ten-year-old, space is rather specific, the place where things such as buildings are. The 11-year-old perceives space as nothingness that goes on forever, a distance between things. He or she is in good control of getting around in the personal space.[219,220]

The 12-year-old understands that space is abstract and has difficulty defining it. Space is nothing, air. He or she can travel alone to more distant areas and understands how specific points relate to each other.[221,222]

Encourage the parents to discuss spatial concepts with the child to facilitate abstract reasoning. Pontious[223] and Webb[224] give practical suggestions for using Piaget's concepts in care and teaching of children.

The box entitled "Categories of Concepts Developed During the School Years" summarizes other concepts formulated at this time.

Categories of Concepts Developed During the School Years

- **Life:** Is aware that movement is not sole criterion of life.
- **Death:** Accepts death as final and not like life. Thinks of death as an angel or bogeyman. Thinks personal death can be avoided if one hides, runs fast, or is good. Traumatic situations arouse fear of death. By age 10 or 11, realizes death is final, inevitable, and results from internal processes. Belief in life after death depends on religious teachings.
- **Body functions:** Has many inaccurate ideas about body functions until taught in health class. Needs repetitive sex education. Becomes more modest for self but interested in seeing bodies of adults. Performs complete self-care by nine years.
- **Money:** Begins to understand value of coins and bills.
- **Self:** Clarifies ideas of self when sees self through eyes of teachers and peers and compares self with peers. By 11 or 12 years, considers self to be in brain, head, face, heart, and then total body.
- **Sex roles:** Has clear concept of culturally defined sex role and that male role is considered more prestigious.
- **Social roles:** Is aware of peers' social, religious, and socioeconomic status. Accepts cultural stereotypes and adult attitudes toward status. Group conscious.
- **Beauty.** Judges beauty according to group standards rather than own aesthetic sensibilities.
- **Comedy:** Has concept of comedy or what is funny influenced by perception of what others think is funny.

Multiple intelligences, rather than one intelligence exist. The **Triarchic Theory of Intelligence** proposed by Robert Sternberg *incorporates three realms of cognition.* This comprehensive theory views intelligence as a product of inner and outer forces.[225] The *first realm concerns how thinking occurs as well as the main components of thinking. Based on the information-processing model,* thinking includes skills at coding, representing, combining information, planning, and self-evaluation in problem solving. *The second realm concerns how individuals cope with experiences, how they respond to novelty in solving new problems, or how quickly they adjust to a new form of the task. The third realm of intelligence concerns the context of thinking*—the extent to which children adapt to, alter, or select environments supportive of their abilities.[226–228]

The **Theory of Multiple Intelligences** proposed by Howard Gardner *presents factors that reflect the influence of culture and society on intellectual ability.* It provides yet another view of how information-processing skills underlie intelligent behaviour.[229] Multiple intelligences take the following forms:[230–232]

1. *Language skill.* The child speaks fluently, learns new words easily, memorizes easily.
2. *Musical skill.* The child plays one or more musical instruments, sings, discerns subtle musical effects, and has a sense of timing or rhythm.
3. *Local skill.* The child organizes objects and concepts, and performs well at mathematics.
4. *Spatial skill.* The child can find the way around easily without getting lost, more so than other children of the same age.

Schoolchild Development

Sarah, age ten, and Joshua, her six-year-old brother, are visiting their grandmother, aunt, uncle, and cousins for the day. Sarah is thin, with narrow shoulders and hips and little adipose tissue, although she has considerable muscle mass.

A luncheon is being held for her grandmother's birthday, and Sarah is eager to help her aunt and cousins prepare the food, set the table, and make party favours. Sarah and Megan, her nine-year-old cousin, divide the nuts and candies into party cups to set at each person's plate. They do this systematically and logically, using the concepts of seriation and classification, so that each person receives an identical number of candies and nuts. This is typical of the concrete operations stage of cognitive development.

Sarah and Megan go to play school in Megan's room where there are a toy chest, dolls, bookshelves, and chalkboard. Sarah plays the teacher, writing multiplication tables on the board and talking to Megan and to pretend students. She demonstrates concrete transformations as she solves multiplication problems. Sarah pretends the class is being bad and reprimands them as a teacher would. In this behaviour she demonstrates understanding of relationships between various steps in a situation. It is apparent that Sarah's teacher is a role model for her; this is common among school-age children.

Sarah asks Megan for advice on solving the problems and on reprimanding the pretend class. This exchange of information is typical of the syntaxic mode of communication and consensual validation that is observed in the schoolchild. By incorporating Megan's ideas and answers, she shows that she cares about Megan's thoughts.

1. What activities might Sarah have carried out to exemplify principles of conservation?
2. In what ways has Sarah demonstrated emotional intelligence?

5. *Kinesthetic or body balance skill.* The child is sensitive to the internal sensations created by body movements, and easily learns dancing and gymnastics.
6. *Intrapersonal and interpersonal skills.* The child has an understanding of self and others that is accurate and promotes empathy. The child relates easily to others and can handle social encounters.

Gardner's list of abilities has yet to be firmly grounded in research. However, his ideas have been significantly challenging to reawaken the debate over a unitary, versus multifaceted, human intelligence.[233]

CRITICAL THINKING

Compare and contrast "core knowledge" as explained in Sternberg's Triarchic Theory of Intelligence and in Gardner's Theory of Multiple Intelligence.

Entering School

School entry is a crisis for the child and family, for behaviour must be adapted to meet new situations. The school experience has considerable influence on the child because he or she is in formative years and spends much time in school. School is society's institution to help the child:

1. Develop the fullest intellectual potential and a sense of industry.
2. Learn to think critically and make judgments based on reason.
3. Accept criticism.
4. Develop social skills.
5. Cooperate with others.
6. Accept other adult authority.
7. Be a leader and follower.

The child who attends a school with children from various ethnic or racial backgrounds, or with children who have immigrated will learn not only about cultures, but possibly several languages, firsthand (Figure 10–2). The course of instruction should be such that every child has a sense of successful accomplishment in some area. Not only school promotes these cognitive and social skills, however. The home and other groups (e.g., peer or organized clubs) are important in their own way for intellectual and social development and for promoting a sense of achievement and industry.

Various actions, such as teaching the child his or her address and full name, independence in self-care, and basic safety rules, help prepare the child for school. The parent or classroom teacher (and the nurse in the health care setting) can *stimulate the child's learning* in the following ways:

- Let each child's success be measured in terms of improved performance.
- Structure for individuation, not for convergence. Avoid having all learning activities structured so that there is only one right answer.
- Provide activities that are challenging, not overwhelming.
- Arrange for the child to accomplish individual activities in the company of peers, when appropriate, as peer interaction provides encouragement and assistance.
- Demonstrate problem-solving and thinking behaviour to serve as a model for the child.[234]
- Use a multisensory teaching approach.
- Include content and experiences that promote understanding of various cultures.[235–237]

There is increasing societal pressure to accelerate the child in the educational process. Piaget contends that optimum comprehension results from numerous experiences over time. Studies of schoolchildren show that a child can quickly learn a specific and advanced task but often with limited retention and transfer. Further, apparent shifts from concrete

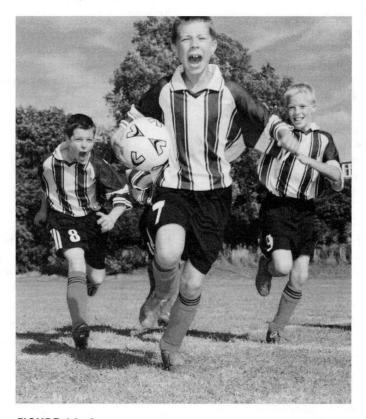

FIGURE 10–2

Exposure to a variety of peers and learning to work and play cooperatively are important for the school-age child.

to formal operations may result from experiences unrelated to education. Direct verbal instruction and use of **cognitive conflict** (*getting the child to question perceptions*) can result in acquisition of conservation abilities, but transfer apparently is limited. Success at learning tasks of increasing complexity depends on levels and interactions of sub skills already possessed by the learner. A variety of experiences and teaching methods increase comprehension, learning, and transfer, which promote acceleration to the next cognitive level. Piecemeal acceleration often results in distorted or incomplete conceptual development that may hamper future thinking.[238–240]

Research shows that certain skills are more easily learned at a certain age. Foreign language and geometry can be more easily learned by younger children; a second language can be learned from age one. Introducing music in preschool and continuing during the school years helps to train the brain for higher forms of thinking and reasoning, including spatial intelligence. Children are capable of far more at a younger age than schools generally realize.

The *teacher–pupil relationship* is important, for it is somewhat similar to the parent–child relationship. The child needs from the teacher a wholesome friendliness, consideration, fairness, sense of humour, and a philosophy that encourages his or her maturity. The teacher should have a thorough understanding of child development.

Most schools today have a *culturally diverse student body;* however, Caucasian perspectives usually prevail. Students benefit when educators understand their unique culture; however, *there are many intracultural, socioeconomic, geographic, generational, religious, and individual differences among families and children.*[241]

Teachers may *foster personal understanding of cultural differences* through the following measures:

- Listening to the behaviour as well as the words of the child
- Emphasizing that each person is unique and worthy of respectful behaviour, regardless of perceived differences
- Reading stories, books, and articles about the history, life patterns, and achievements of people from various cultures and religions
- Having bulletin board displays that commemorate the special days or historical leaders for each cultural group represented in the classroom
- Encouraging parents from various culture groups to come to the classroom, bring artefacts that are important or representative, and discuss commonly held beliefs or practices for the specific cultural group
- Encouraging children to find similarities as well as differences among the cultural and religious groups represented in the classroom

Problems of the family and child are brought into sharp focus when the child enters school. The teacher sees many difficulties: the loneliness of an only child; the pain of the child with divorce or death in the family; the negative self-image of the child who is not as physically coordinated or intellectually sharp as his or her peers; the child with dyslexia or learning difficulties; the child with separation anxiety or **school phobia,** *fear of or refusal to attend school.* School phobia or separation anxiety can be an indicator of a larger medical problem or it can be nothing more than a normal child with a temporary conflict.[242,243]

In addition, help parents to realize that the *child's ability to learn and achieve in school is affected by factors other than intellectual ability.* For example, at home parents should maintain an atmosphere with ample praise and encouragement. Times for parent and children to play together should be frequent, and the provision of opportunities for stimulation and learning through hobbies, games, and outings to parks and libraries should be equally important and a part of family life. Parents should stress the importance of learning. They should monitor school assignments and stay in touch with the child's teachers.[244] Typically, Canadian parents have been deeply involved in the education of their children. When parents come to parent–teacher conferences and get involved in attending school events, children are more strongly motivated, their self-esteem is better, and they adapt and adjust more satisfactorily to the learning activities in school.[245]

In Canada, according to the National Longitudinal Survey of Children and Youth (NLSCY), although the majority of children are succeeding at school, girls are more likely than boys to do "very well." Further, research is needed to identify the specific reasons behind such gender differences among school-age children.[246] Researchers and others are concerned about the education of Aboriginal children. Hamilton found that supporting culturally based curricula and sharing with non-Aboriginal students is important if negative stereotypes are to be erased and replaced with respectful knowledge and understanding.[247]

CRITICAL THINKING

As a health professional, what can you do about the education needs of students with Aboriginal heritage?

Too much pushing by parents for the child to be a success, perfect in physical skills, the most intellectual, or a hard worker can backfire. The pressure that is generated may be so intense that the child eventually does not succeed at anything. Perfectionist, highly successful, career-focused, or professionally focused parents are apt to push the child too much. Certain signs and symptoms are clues. The *perfectionist child* manifests:[248,249]

- Extreme concern about appearance.
- Avoidance of tasks, play, or school because of fear of failure.
- Dawdling or procrastinating on easy tasks to avoid harder ones or working so slowly on projects that creativity is lost.
- Jealousy and envy of the apparent success and perfection of others.
- Wanting to do something for which the child has no ability or talent.
- Low tolerance for mistakes (e.g., the boy who wins the race may feel he was not successful because he did not set any records).

If these behaviours are present, teach the parents to work on relaxing themselves and the child and developing a sense of tolerance and humour. You may be their counsellor, or you may refer them to counselling.

Education in Canada is the responsibility of the provinces and territories. In Canadian schools, the intellectual assessment of children, together with achievement test results, are no longer routinely used to assess students.[250] The critics of achievement tests state that although these tests are viewed as indicators of what children learn in school, they are very similar to IQ tests.[251]

Goleman's theory of emotional intelligence has added a considerable measure to researchers' understanding of intelligence and achievement.[252] Snow states that emotional intelligence is the ability to manage oneself and one's relationships effectively.[253] Emotional intelligence has three components: (1) awareness of one's own emotions, (2) the ability to share one's emotions in an appropriate manner, and (3) the capacity to channel emotions in the pursuit of one's worthwhile goals.[254] In essence, Snow indicates that with the effective application of one's emotional intelligence it is considerably more possible to achieve one's potential.[255]

CRITICAL THINKING

How can parents assist in the development of emotional intelligence in their school-age children?

10-1 BONUS SECTION IN CD-ROM

School Difficulty

This section gives the reader an overview of IQ testing in the U.S., coupled with results from a study by Fordham and the American Association of University Women.

A *classroom with diversity* in the children's intellectual ability, skills, and personality is helpful to the child; he or she learns about the real world. A small percentage of disabled or maladjusted children in a classroom will not adversely affect the educational process of the normal child. Putting the exceptional child in a normal classroom, however, may not make him or her feel normal; he or she still is perceived and perceives self as different. The exceptional child may need special classes to get the help needed; teachers cannot be expected to specialize in all areas of education, and large classrooms prevent teachers from spending the necessary time with the child who has learning disabilities.

The **gifted child** is *characterized by superior education and consumption of information and by outstanding ability to produce information, concepts, and new forms, and to perform consistently at a higher level than most children of the same age.* The gifted child demonstrates to a greater extent than other children the many types of intelligence: logical-mathematical, linguistic, musical, spatial, body-kinesthetic, interpersonal, and intrapersonal. The child is adept at problem solving and problem finding. The gifted child is considered educationally exceptional, and the child's full intellectual, creative, and leadership potential may be neglected if:

1. Parents are not attuned to the child's abilities and needs.
2. Parents or teachers are threatened by the gifted child who grasps concepts more quickly than they.

3. Parents do not value cognitive, creative, or leadership abilities.
4. The child is not given freedom to explore and be different.
5. The school system does not have a program suited for his or her abilities.

Often the gifted child is misunderstood. Research indicates, however, that gifted students have higher self-esteem than others and are more popular with their peers than other children.[256]

Yet, the gifted child may not excel or be ahead of the norm in all dimensions. The child may be intellectually ahead of chronological age but may be behind in physical growth and coordination, emotional development, or social skills. The inconsistency inherent in lack of developmental synchrony may be difficult for parents, teachers, and peers to accept; their response may cause lower self-esteem or withdrawal from others. You can be instrumental in fostering empathy for the child and an individualized program to enhance development and competency.[257]

Encourage parents to respect the individual interests and talents of their child. If parents are not intimidated by the child's unusual interests and behaviour, they will not fear deviations from neighbourhood patterns and thereby not crush budding interests or creativity. That is perhaps the essence of raising a gifted child—to facilitate, provide opportunity, let alone, not hold back or insist that something be done a certain way. **Home schooling** is conducted by some parents who believe the present public school system is inadequate to teach their children the needed skills. They are usually well-educated professionals and wish to teach their own children at home.

There are established curricular plans for the grade level and academic year with subject content, suggestions for teaching, and evaluation methods. The parent(s) have a choice, depending on cost factors and perceived needs and interests of the child. Often all the parents and children in a locale who are enrolled in home schooling gather periodically for social events to foster social skills in and friendships among the children. Parents, or groups of parents, may also plan field trips to enhance the child's education—for example to museums, parks, and historical sites.

When you work with these parents, help them realize the importance of curricular integrity, that if the child graduates from a home school program, he or she is expected to have achieved a certain standard. Further, emphasize the child's need for friendships and interaction with people from diverse backgrounds. Explore whether the child will have access to regular physical educational activity, playing a musical instrument or choral singing, and to art classes. Explore whether the parent(s) will be able to consistently engage the child in learning activities and monitor the necessary testing or evaluation. Several authors explore various facets of this movement.[258–260]

CRITICAL THINKING

What are the advantages and disadvantages of home schooling?

The *chronically ill child* poses unique problems for the school and parents. Ray explains that acquiring the knowledge, skills, and organization necessary to raise a child with a chronic health condition presents many challenges. Beyond that, a heavy demand is placed upon family resources as well. She presents a model—Parenting and Childhood Chronicity (PACC)—that was developed in an interpretive study with 43 parents of 34 children (aged 15 months to 16 years) with various chronic conditions.[261] Ray indicates that the care required for the child with a chronic condition, as described under three sections of the PACC model, includes medical care, parenting plus, and working the systems. The PACC provides a comprehensive framework for assessing areas of responsibility and concern for families; and it can provide a visual aid for conveying the full scope of responsibilities faced by parents of children with chronic conditions.[262]

Chronic illnesses extract a heavy toll on children and their parents or significant caregivers. For example, a diagnosis of childhood cancer poses challenges to the stability and adaptive functioning of the entire family setting.[263] In fact, Woodgate states that childhood cancer is described by families as an extremely overwhelming phenomenon to experience and that both physical and mental suffering become part of their daily lives.[264] Hypertension is an underrecognized clinical entity in children that poses huge management concerns.[265]

In a study, Harris and his team of researchers described disease patterns among children in an isolated community and compared them with patterns found among other Aboriginal and non-Aboriginal Canadian children.[266] They

---

EVIDENCE-BASED PRACTICE

Fathers' Experience of Parenting a Child with Juvenile Rheumatoid Arthritis

Family life in Western society has undergone many changes over the past century, but the implications of these changes for men are not fully understood. Whereas men's roles and achievements in the public sphere have been well documented, their private lives, particularly their identities as husbands and fathers, have been far less studied. Although fathers are assumed to be an integral part of family life, they have emerged as a focus of interest from an academic perspective relatively recently.

One domain in which fathers' experience is not well understood is in families of children who have a chronic health condition. Although a family-centred approach (i.e., family as primary unit of care) is advocated in pediatric health care literature, it has not translated into an understanding of the actual experience of fathers and the way they interpret their role.

The researcher examined the experience of fathers who have a child with juvenile rheumatoid arthritis (JRA). He used grounded theory methodology, in which 22 fathers participated in semi-structured interviews, and developed a substantive theory of fathers' experience that addresses the impact of their child's JRA, their adaptational responses, and the meanings they associated with their experiences. Fathers were profoundly affected, perceived their child's condition as a catalyst for meaningful involvement, experienced many emotions, and sought to adopt a positive approach to making sense of their child's condition. Fathers' efforts to be strong for others resulted in an overreliance on self-support strategies, particularly during periods of stress. Given the nature of fathers' experience and the extent of their involvement, greater attention by health care practitioners to fathers' adaptation is indicated.

Practice Implications

The findings from this study might be transferable in a manner consistent with qualitative research and used to sensitize clinicians about possible patterns of experience among fathers. Used in this way, the findings point to a number of potential considerations for clinicians:

1. Fathers are profoundly affected in multiple ways by their child's condition. Some fathers will welcome the opportunity to talk about their experience. This might be challenging for clinicians because fathers can be reluctant to disclose their more intense feelings in the presence of their partner, because doing so might be seen by them as undermining their ability to be a support for their partner. Fathers, therefore, might initially need some privacy to discuss their feelings.

2. The related finding that fathers attempted to be positive and pragmatic by addressing the things that could be changed to improve conditions for their child might mask their own underlying needs and be misinterpreted by clinicians as their not wanting or needing support for their feelings and reactions.

3. Fathers' reported willingness to be unpopular with the team if they feel a need to advocate for their child might bring them into greater conflict with the team. There was evidence that fathers perceived this responsibility as part of their protective role. Understanding this behaviour in the context of the couple relationship and the way partners co-construct their respective roles, rather than solely as an individual characteristic (e.g., unreasonable, difficult, hostile, angry), might provide a helpful vantage point.

4. Based on the many ways in which fathers are involved, consideration of their role should be part of any overall assessment plan. Increased efforts might be needed to ensure that service delivery strategies reach fathers and are truly accessible to them.

5. Providing quiet places for reflection and prayer might be particularly appreciated given the value that fathers in this study and elsewhere appear to place on prayer during stressful times.

6. Given that fathers' responses appear to be different from but often related to mothers' responses, it suggests the value of a family systems approach to understanding families as the unit of care.

Source: McNeill, T., Fathers' Experience of Parenting a Child with Juvenile Rheumatoid Arthritis, Qualitative Health Research, 14, no. 4 (2004), 526–545. Used with permission.

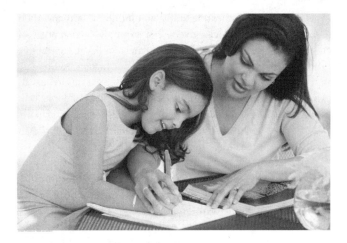

FIGURE 10–3

Parents nurture their children by providing support and encouraging their efforts and activities.

found that the illnesses most frequently seen in Aboriginal children are respiratory tract infections and skin conditions.

Because childhood obesity in Canada has become increasingly prevalent over the past two decades, the risk factors for cardiovascular disease and type 2 diabetes have been associated with increased levels of body fatness in youth.[267]

In spite of chronic illnesses, the child's learning remains greatly important. Professionally, you should help parents to understand that they are responsible for their child's behaviour and learning. The box entitled "Suggestions for Parents about Children's Homework" summarizes how parents can assist the child. The children must do their own growing and developing and only through their own motivation (Figure 10–3).

Intellectual Needs of the Hospitalized Child

You can *help meet the hospitalized child's needs and educate the child and parents.* A hospital tour, if it can be prearranged, helps the child feel acclimated during illness when his or her energy reserve is low. Because the child is beginning logical thought, he or she needs simple information about the illness to decrease the fear of the unknown and promote cooperation in the treatment plan. He or she needs to handle and become familiar with the equipment used. Heiney[268] describes practical ways to help the child deal with painful procedures. Wong[269] is also a thorough reference.

The child who must spend long periods in the hospital needs to learn about the outside world. Some hospitals take chronically ill children to the circus, athletic events, and restaurants. Teachers are also employed so that the child can continue with formal education.

Communication Patterns

Many factors influence the child's communication pattern, vocabulary, and diction. Some of these factors have been

---

Suggestions for Parents about Children's Homework

Do:

- Let your children know you believe they can do well. Encourage self-evaluation.
- Minimize time spent watching television.
- Help your children organize. Encourage them to do the most difficult task first.
- Talk and read to your children.
- Go to your children's school and volunteer.
- Encourage outside activities and having friends at home.
- Work with your children's teachers and let the teacher know you understand and are supportive.
- Insist on good eating habits.
- Plan activities with your children.
- Be a good example.

Do not:

- Dwell on the negative by criticizing.
- Allow the television to be your babysitter.
- Do homework for the children.
- Leave them to their own devices.
- Forget to encourage verbal exchange.
- Push them to have every minute scheduled or send them off to play.
- Criticize and interfere with everything you do not understand.
- Allow constant eating.
- Send them off without you to family functions (e.g., school plays, pot-luck dinners).
- Say, "Do as I say and not as I do."

---

referred to in previous chapters. Influences include:

1. Speech and verbal and nonverbal communication pattern of parent(s), siblings, other adults such as teachers and peers.
2. Attitudes of others toward the child's effort to speak and communicate.
3. General environmental stimulation.
4. Opportunity to communicate with a variety of people in a variety of situations.
5. Intellectual development.
6. Ability to hear and articulate.
7. Vocabulary skills.
8. Contact with television or other technology such as computers, the Internet, and video games.[270,271]

The six-year-old has command of nearly every form of sentence structure and can understand from 8000 to 14 000 words. The child experiments less with language, using it more as a tool and less for the mere pleasure of talking than during the preschool period. Now language is used to share in others' experiences. He or she also swears and uses slang to test others' reactions. The child enjoys printing words in large letters.[272–274]

At seven, the child can print several sentences, and at eight he or she is writing instead of printing. By nine, the child participates in family discussions, showing interest in family activities and indicating individuality. Verbal fluency has improved, and common objects are described in detail. Writing skill has improved; he or she usually writes with small, even letters. By ten, he or she can write for a relatively long time with speed. The preadolescent may seem less talkative, withdrawing when frustrated instead of voicing anger. Sharing feelings with a best friend is a healthy outlet.[275-277]

As the child shares ideas and feelings, he or she learns how someone else thinks and feels about similar matters. The child expresses self in a way that has meaning to others, at first to a chum and then to others. Thus he or she is validating and expanding vocabulary, ideas, and feelings. The child learns that a friend's family has similar life patterns, demands of the child, and frustrations. He or she learns about self in the process of learning more about another. The child recalls what has happened in the past, realizes how this has affected the present, and considers what effect present acts will have on future events. The child uses **syntaxic, or consensual, communication** *when he or she sees these cause-and-effect relationships in an objective, logical way and can validate them with others.*[278] By sixth grade, the child who has had opportunity to learn may have a vocabulary 10 to 20 times that of the six-year-old.[279]

Canada is a bilingual country where both English and French have equal status, rights, and privileges at the federal level.[280] Statistics Canada reports that in the 2002–03 school year, nearly 2 million students took courses in French as a second language.[281] A large body of carefully conducted research shows that bilingualism has positive consequences for development. That is, children who are fluent in two languages are advanced in cognitive development. Bialystok states that bilingualism helps with reading achievement, as the child is more conscious of some aspects of language sounds.[282] Many students taught in French immersion programs become functionally competent in both French and English, and they gain a special appreciation of the French-Canadian culture.[283]

CRITICAL THINKING

What did you learn in your French immersion program?

Convey love and caring, not rejection, when you talk with children. Love is communicated through nonverbal behaviour such as getting down to the child's eye level and through words that value feelings and indicate respect. Children understand language directed at their feelings better than at their intellect and the overt action.

Effects of Television and the Internet on the Child

According to the Vanier Institute of the Family, Canadian children between the ages of two and 11 watch approximately 18 hours of television per week, or 2.57 hours daily.[284] Video and computer games are becoming more popular for children and youth. In 2000, 4.7 million Canadian households were connected to the Internet, and 71% of households reported at least one person in the home regularly used the Internet at least seven times daily.[285] To find out how the Internet is influencing the lives of Canadian children and the degree of awareness parents have regarding its influences, the Media Awareness Network (MNet) conducted two benchmark surveys, one in 2000 with parents and the other in 2001 with children and youth. The results indicated that Canadian children and youth

are big users of the Internet and that 53% of the parents believe they are on top of the situation. However, according to Swift and Taylor, parents need to go online with their children and learn what they do.[286]

Television and movies, video and computer games, and the Internet exert a powerful influence on a child's communication and behaviour patterns.

Parents must help children select educational programming because it can:[287,288]

1. Present information about specific topics that add to understanding of the world in general.
2. Present positive images of people from various ethnic groups or people who are disabled.
3. Depict positive social behaviour and cultural values such as work, sacrifice, and goal-setting.
4. Convey positive ethical messages about the value of family life, friendship, and commitment to relationships.
5. Feature women and men in positions of authority or performing heroic acts.
6. Present and reinforce techniques associated with various sports or exercise routines.
7. Present information.

Teach parents that, increasingly, research indicates that seeing violent, sexually seductive programs or pornographic material on television or in films has long-term negative effects on children. Review Table 10-9 with them.[289-299] Heavy television viewing is associated with lower school achievement. Teachers report that more children are entering school with decreased imaginative play and creativity and increased aimless movement, low frustration level, poor persistence and concentration span, and confusion about reality and fantasy. Rapid speech and constantly changing visuals on television prevent reflection. The child does not learn correct sentence structure, use of tenses, or the ability to express thought or feeling effectively. The result may be a child who is unable to enunciate or use correct grammar and who is vague in the sense of time and history and cause-and-effect relationships.[300,301]

The violence in television programming is graphic, explicit, realistic, and intensely involving. It affects both children and adults but children more so because they have less ego control. Children act out more directly what they see and hear.

Aggressive actions lead to a heightened level of arousal of the viewer's aggressive tendencies, bringing thoughts, feelings, memories, and action to consciousness, causing outwardly aggressive behaviour. Even fast-paced programming arouses aggressive impulses.[302]

Many programs directly or indirectly teach violent behaviour, showing specifically how to carry out violent acts. It is not unusual when arson, rape, hostage taking, suicide, or homicide is described on the evening news on television to have, either locally or nationally, a number of such incidents repeated within a few days. The live and explicit portrayals of violence suggest that aggression and violence are normal, justified, and rewarded. Realistic or punitive consequences of violent behaviour are not shown. The viewer gets the idea and forms an attitude over time that aggressive or violent behaviour should be used to solve problems, that it is normal or courageous to be

TABLE 10-9
Negative Effects of Television

1. Promotes passive rather than active learning
2. Increases passivity from continual overstimulation
3. Encourages low-level, nonconceptual thinking
4. Takes time away or distracts from more creative and stimulating activity; reduces creativity and creative fantasy of the child
5. Encourages short attention span and hyperactivity through its use of snappy attention-getting techniques
6. Causes lack of understanding or comprehension of what is seen or inability to grasp consequences of behaviour because of fast pace of programming
7. Causes loss of interest in less exciting but necessary classroom or home activities
8. Creates a desire for the superficial rather than depth of information; teaches superficial judgments
9. Creates uncertainty about what is real and unreal in life and family
10. Creates a confusion of values
11. Promotes a desire for unhealthy products such as high-sugar and high-salt snacks, other products not normally used by the family, or toys or other products that may be unhealthy or dangerous
12. Interferes with correct pronunciation of words, vocabulary use, reading comprehension, and spelling achievement
13. Promotes sedentary lifestyle and snacking rather than participation in play, sports, physical exercise, community events discussion, or activities with parents
14. Increases aggressive behaviour because of program content, loud music, fast pace, and camera tricks
15. Increases passive acceptance of aggressive behaviour toward people as a way to solve problems
16. Becomes a way to keep the child occupied—a passive babysitter
17. Increases suspicion of others, fears, and anxiety
18. Competes with parents, school, and peers as a socializing agent
19. Promotes passivity and withdrawal from direct involvement in real life
20. De-emphasizes complexity of life with simplistic plots, fast action, no lasting consequences, no visual or cognitive depth
21. Conveys unrealistic and stereotyped view of men and women and sex roles; women usually portrayed as sex objects, ornamental, young, with limited speaking and/or problem-solving behaviours
22. Emphasizes overt sexual behaviour; portrays nudity, perversions, homosexuality, and sometimes pornographic content
23. Fosters increased incidence of aggressive and violent behaviour
24. Promotes excessive fears about war, about walking in one's own neighbourhood, about the "violent" world, and about the police who use only force
25. Increases emotional problems, including conduct disorders and post-traumatic stress disorder (nightmares, flashbacks, paranoia, poor concentration, impaired attachment to people)

violent, that violence is rewarded or socially acceptable, and that the violent person is the hero with whom to identify. Aggressive behaviour is expected in interactions and is used as a response in peer interactions and when frustrated. The world is viewed as dangerous; aggressive behaviour is a way to protect self.[303] Further, continual viewing of violence desensitizes the person to violence in general; it is no longer a noteworthy act in the home or society. Even worse, television violence shows inequality and domination; the most frequent victims are women, elders, and children.[304–307]

Violence on television makes children more aggressive, and aggressive children prefer violent television. Like Canada, the U.S. and South Africa are also reporting increased homicide rates 10 to 15 years after television viewing became widespread.[308]

Discuss with parents the need *to limit the amount of television viewing (two hours a day);* do alternative activities with their children; screen what their children are viewing; and work to reduce the trend to more violent and pornographic programming. Parents can be more vigilant about programs their children watch. Television programming can be improved. Networks and advertisers, of course, hope that parents will disregard research findings that make-believe violence makes for real violence in many settings. As long as violence on television is profitable, programming will contain violence. Parents can rebel: writing letters to stations, writing letters to advertisers, and refusing to buy the products advertised. This is a significant area of life that affects the child's and the family's physical, emotional, cognitive, social, and spiritual health.

In essence, interaction with parents and others and real experiences, not passive observations, help the child learn to work through conflicts of development and to solve problems.

CRITICAL THINKING

What effects can television advertisements have on children's social behaviour?

Play Patterns

The following information can be used to educate parents and children and to plan health promotion programs.

Peer Groups

Peer groups, including the gang and the close chum, provide companionship, shared time, conversation, and activity with a widening circle of persons outside the home. They are extremely important to the school-age child. Between the ages of seven and nine, children usually form close friendships with peers of the same sex and age. Later in this age group, peers are not necessarily of the same age. Functions of the peer group are listed in Table 10-10.

Children must earn their membership in the peer group, and being accepted by one's peers and belonging to a peer group are major concerns for this age group. Many factors determine a child's acceptance, including attractiveness and friendliness. Most children find acceptance with at least one or two peers; rejection and loneliness are always a risk. Children may be rejected because they are either too aggressive or too passive. Being an outsider carries all the risks that are implied if the peer group functions cannot be attained. Effects of not being a peer group member can be corrected through having a chum, as explained in a later section, or may set the foundation for either a shy, withdrawn personality or an overtly assertive or aggressive personality that tries to manoeuvre into groups. These effects may still be evident in adulthood.[309]

Play Activities

Play activities change with the child's development. From age six to eight, he or she is interested chiefly in the present and in the immediate surroundings. Because he or she knows more about family life than any other kind of living, the child plays house or takes the role of various occupational groups with which there is contact: mail carrier, firefighter, carpenter, nurse, occupational therapist, and teacher. Although the child is more interested in playing with peers than parents, the six- or seven-year old will occasionally enjoy having the parent as a "child" or "student." This allows the child to have imaginary control over the parent and also allows the parent to understand how the child is interpreting the parent or how the child perceives the teacher.

Both sexes enjoy some activities in common, such as painting, cutting, pasting, reading, collecting items such as baseball cards or stamps, simple table games, television, digging, riding a bicycle, construction sets or models, puzzles, kites, running games, team sports, rough and tumble play, skating, and swimming. Again, the parent can sometimes enjoy these activities with the child, especially if the parent has a special talent the child wishes to learn. The child imitates the roles of his or her own sex and becomes increasingly realistic in play.

By age eight, collections, more advanced models, the radio, art materials, "how to" books, farm sets, and train sets are favourite pastimes, and loosely formed, short-lived clubs with fluctuating rules are formed.

The schoolchild, usually near eight or nine years of age, enjoys computerized and electronic games, which give a sense of control and power; of being a peer with, or even superior to, the adult; of challenge and inventiveness; and an enjoyment of complexity and expandability. The computer can be a tool for robot thinking or for development of thought; for passivity or releasing aggressive impulses or creativity; for play or for learning. Computer and video toys can help the schoolchild understand the nature of systems and control of information—skills needed in the adult world. Let the child take the lead in when to move into computer games. Further, some schoolchildren will prefer reading, painting, playing an instrument, doing crafts, camping, or playing sports to working with computers. These skills and what these activities teach are as essential to the workplace as the ability to operate a computer.

At approximately age ten, sex differences in play become pronounced. Each sex is developing through play the skills it will later need in society; this is manifested through the dramatizing of real-life situations. The child's interest in faraway places is enhanced through a foreign pen pal and through travel.

From age nine to 12, the child becomes more interested in active sports but continues to enjoy quieter activity. He or she wants to improve motor skills. The child may enjoy carpentry or mechanic's tools, advanced models or puzzles, arts and crafts, science projects, music, dance, cameras and film, and camping. Adult-organized games of hockey, softball, football, or soccer lose their fun when parents place excessive emphasis on winning. The hug from a teammate after scoring a goal means more than just winning.

Throughout childhood, girls compare favourably with boys in strength, endurance, and motor skills, and in late childhood, girls are physically more mature than boys. At about age 12, girls

TABLE 10-10
Functions of the School-Age Peer Group

- Reinforces gender role behaviour
- Accepts those who conform to social roles
- Provides an audience for developing self-concept, self-esteem, and unique personality characteristics
- Provides information about the world of school and neighbourhood, games, dress, and manners; decreases egocentrism
- Provides opportunity to compete and compare self to others of same age
- Develops a personal set of values and goals; conformity is expected
- Teaches rules and logical consequences; punishes members who disobey rules
- Provides opportunity to test mastery in a world parallel to adult society, with rules, organization, and purposes
- Provides emotional support during stressful or crisis points in a member's life
- Protects against other peers who may threaten, bully, or intimidate, or actually harm if the member were alone

begin to perform less well than boys on tests of physical skills; they run more slowly, jump less far, and lift less weight if they are given no physical training. The traditional poorer performance is probably the result of gender expectations about behaviour. Athletic activity is attractive to both boys and girls and is becoming more accessible to girls than in the past.[310,311]

Gang Stage

Help parents understand the importance of the gang stage. You can work with the gang to promote health. You may also work with gangs to promote positive behaviour.

In preadolescence, the gang becomes important. A **gang** is a *group whose membership is earned on the basis of skilled performance of some activity, frequently physical in nature. Its stability is expressed through format symbols, such as passwords or uniforms.* Gang codes take precedence over almost everything. They may range from agreement to protect a member who smoked in the boys' washroom at school to boycotting a school dance. Generally, gang codes are characterized by collective action against the mores of the adult world. In the gang, children discharge hostility and aggression against peers rather than adults and begin to work out their own social patterns without adult interference. Unfortunately, some gangs do turn their hostility against other youths or adults. When this occurs, the pattern is laid for delinquent behaviours;[312] however, these groups are not necessarily offenders against the law. Gang formation is loosely structured at first, with a transient membership that cuts across all social classes. Early gangs may consist of both boys and girls in the same groups. Later, gangs separate by sex.

Data from the National Longitudinal Survey of Children and Youth (NLSCY) indicate that a significant proportion of school-aged children in Canada are either bullies (14%) or victims (5%). There are a higher percentage of boys compared to girls involved in bullying. Children who bully display other antisocial behaviours such as physical aggression, indirect aggression, and hyperactivity. Along with the immediate effects of bullying and victimization, this behaviour has long-term consequences for all those involved—bullies and victims.[313] It is important to stop bullying at a young age and strive to create a peaceful and safe environment for everyone. The Government of Canada's National Strategy on Community Safety and Crime Prevention was launched in 1998 and strives to intervene early in the lives of young people to address issues of antisocial behaviour before they become more serious problems.[314]

CRITICAL THINKING

How might you help teachers reduce bullying during the school years?

Chum Stage

The chum stage occurs around nine or ten years of age and sometimes later when affection moves from the peer group and gang to a **chum**, a *special friend of the same sex and age.* This is an important relationship because it is the child's first love attachment outside the family, when someone becomes as important to him or her as self. Initially, a person of the same sex and age is easier than someone of the opposite sex to feel concern for and to understand. The friend becomes an extension of the child's own self. As he or she shares ideas and feelings, the child learns a great deal about both self and the chum. Self-acceptance of uniqueness increases acceptance of others so that the child of this age is very sociable, generous, and sympathetic, enjoys differences in people, and is liberal in ideas about the welfare of others. It is also through the chum relationship that the child learns the syntactic mode of communication described earlier, for he or she learns to validate word meanings in talking with the chum. Thus ideas about the world become more realistic. Loyalty to the chum at this age may be greater than loyalty to the family.[315] **Altruism**, a *concern for others in various situations,* is an ability to respond to others' happiness and distress, to develop intimate associations, including with individuals of the opposite sex, and a sensitivity and concern for all humanity.[316,317]

The chum stage has homosexual elements, but it is not an indication of homosexuality. It provides the foundation for later intimacy with an individual of the opposite sex and close friends of both sexes. If the child does not have a chum relationship, he or she has little capacity for adolescent heterosexuality or adult intimacy. According to Sullivan, fixation at this level results in homosexuality.[318]

Help parents understand the importance of the chum stage. The chum stage fosters emotional health.

Tools of Socialization

Teach parents that competition, compromise, cooperation, and beginning collaboration are progressive tools that the schoolchild uses in accomplishing satisfying relationships with peers.[319] If a child is not relating well with peers, you may conduct a *group assertiveness training program* to effectively increase social and assertive behaviour through reinforcement procedures, relaxation techniques, guided imagery, and behaviour contracts.

Competition *comprises all activities that are involved in getting to a goal first, of seeking affection or status above others.* When the child is competing, he or she has rigid standards about many situations, including praise and punishment. For example, regardless of the circumstance, the child believes that the same punishment should be given for the same wrongdoing. He or she cannot understand why a three-year-old sibling should not be punished in the same way for spilling milk on the kitchen floor. Similarly, the child thinks he or she should be praised for dressing self as much as the three-year-old is. *The child accepts adult rules as compulsory and rigid; he or she experiences a* **morality of constraint.**

Compromise, a *give-and-take agreement,* is gradually learned from peers, teachers, and family. The child becomes less rigid in standards of behaviour. **Cooperation**, an *exchange between equals by adjusting to the wishes of others,* results from the chum relationship with its syntactic mode of communication.[320] Through the **morality of cooperation** the *child begins to understand the social implications of acts.* He or she learns judgment through helping make and carry out rules. **Collaboration**, *deriving satisfaction from group accomplishment rather than personal success,* is a step forward from cooperation and enables experimentation with tasks and exploration of situations.[321]

If a child does not learn how to get along with others, future socialization will be inhibited. For example, if a person is fixated at the competition level and does not learn how to compromise or cooperate, he or she is hard on self and is a hard person with whom to live. Eventually the person derives satisfaction only from competing but fails to enjoy the accomplishment, the end product.

Guidance and Discipline

In guidance, parents should invite confidence of the child as a parent, not as a buddy or pal. The child will find pals among peers. In the adult, he or she needs a parent. The atmosphere should be open and inviting for the child to talk with the parents, but the child's privacy should not be invaded. The parents should see the child as he or she is, not as an idealized extension of them.

The schoolchild has a rather strict superego and also uses many rituals to maintain self-control. He or she prefers to initiate self-control rather than be given commands or overt discipline, and stability and routine in his or her life provide this opportunity. You can talk with parents about methods of guidance and the importance of not interfering with behaviour too forcefully or too often. The child needs some alternatives from which to choose so that he or she can learn different ways of behaving and coping and be better able to express self later. Research indicates that preadolescent girls perceive their mothers as more supportive but also more punitive than their fathers. Boys who are less warmly treated by their parents are more responsive to social or peer influences than girls, which has implications for later antisocial behaviour.[322–324]

For some parents, guiding a child can be a problem. They will ask, "When, what kind, and how much should you punish a child?" "How do you handle guilt or hostile feelings that often accompany discipline?" You are in a position to help parents learn the value of positive guidance techniques.[325,326]

Guidance at this age takes many other and less dramatic forms. A mother can turn the often harried "getting back-to-school clothes" experience into a pleasant lesson in guidance. She can accompany the child on a special shopping trip in which he or she examines different textures of material, learns about colour coordination, understands what constitutes a good fit, and appreciates how much money must be spent for certain items. This principle can be carried into any parent–schoolchild guidance relationship such as learning responsibility for some household task or earning, handling, and saving money.

Emotional Development

The schoolchild consolidates earlier psychosocial development and simultaneously reaches out to a number of identification figures, expands interests, and associates with more people. Behavioural characteristics change from year to year. Table 10-11 summarizes and compares basic behaviour patterns,

TABLE 10–11
Assessment of Changing Behavioural Characteristics in the Schoolchild

6 Years	7 Years	8 Years
Self-centred	Self-care managed	Expansive personality but fluctuating behaviour
Body movement, temper outbursts release tension	Quiet, less impulsive, but assertive	Curious, robust, energetic
Behavioural extremes; impulsive or dawdles, loving or antagonistic	Fewer mood swings	Rapid movements and response; impatient
Difficulty making decisions; needs reminders	Self-absorbed without excluding others; may appear shy, sad, brooding	Affectionate to parents
Verbally aggressive but easily insulted	Attentive, sensitive listener	Hero worship of adult
Intense concentration for short time, then abruptly stops activity	Companionable; likes to do tasks for others	Suggestions followed better than commands
Security of routines and rituals essential; periodic separation anxiety	Good and bad behaviour in self and others noted	Adult responsibilities and characteristics imitated; wants to be considered important by adults
Series of three commands followed, but response depends on mood	High standards for self but minor infractions of rules: tattles, alibis, takes small objects from others	Approval and reconciliation sought, feelings easily hurt
Self-control and initiative in activity encouraged when adult uses counting to give child time ("I'll give you until the count of 10 to pick up those papers")	Concern about own behaviour, tries to win over others' approval	Sense of property; enjoys collections
Praise and recognition needed	Angry over others' failure to follow rules	Beginning sense of justice but makes alibis for own transgressions
		Demanding and critical of others
		Gradually accepts inhibitions and limits

(continued)

TABLE 10–11 *(continued)*
Assessment of Changing Behavioural Characteristics in the Schoolchild

9 Years	10 Years
More independent and self-controlled	More adult-like and poised, especially girls
Dependable, responsible	More self-directive, independent
Adult trust and more freedom without adult supervision sought	Organized and rapid in work; budgets time and energy
Loyal to home and parents; seeks their help at times	Suggestions followed better than requests, but obedient
More self rather than environmentally motivated; not dependent on but benefits from praise	Family activities and care of younger siblings, especially below school age, enjoyed
More involved with peers	Aware of individual differences among people, but does not like to be singled out in a group
Own interests subordinated to group demands and adult authority	Hero worship of adult
Critical of own and others' behaviour	Some idea of own assets and limits
Loyal to group; chum important	Preoccupied with right and wrong
Concerned about fairness and willing to take own share of blame	Better able to live by rules
More aware of society	Critical sense of justice; accepts immediate punishment for wrongdoing
	Liberal ideas of social justice and welfare
	Strong desire to help animals and people
	Future career choices match parents' careers because of identification with parents
	Sense of leadership

11 Years	12 Years
Spontaneous, self-assertive, restless, curious, sociable	Considerable personality integration; self-contained, self-competent, tactful, kind, reasonable, less self-centred
Short outbursts of anger and arguing	Outgoing, eager to please, enthusiastic
Mood swings	Sense of humour; improved communication skills
Challenges enjoyed	More companionable than at 11; mutual understanding between parents and child
On best behaviour away from home	Increasingly sensitive to feelings of others; wish good things for family and friends; caught between the two
Quarrelsome with siblings; rebellious to parents	Others' approval sought
Critical of parents, although affectionate with them	Childish lapses, but wishes to be treated like adult
Chum and same-sex peers important; warm reconciliation follows quarrels	Aware of assets and shortcomings
Secrets freely shared with chum; secret language with peers	Tolerant of self and others
Unaware of effect of self on others	Peer group and chum important in shaping attitudes and interests
Strict superego; zeal for fairness	Ethical sense more realistic than idealistic
Future career choices fantasized on basis of possible fame	Decisions about ethical questions based on consequences
Modest with parents	Less tempted to do wrong; basically truthful
	Self-disciplined, accepts just discipline
	Enthusiastic about community projects

although individual children will show a considerable range of behaviour. Cultural, health, and social conditions may also influence behaviour.[327–332]

CRITICAL THINKING

What health problems might affect emotional development in a child?

Developmental Crisis

The psychosexual crisis for this period is industry versus inferiority. **Industry** is *an interest in doing the work of the world, the child's feeling that he or she can learn and solve problems, the formation of responsible work habits and attitudes, and the mastery of age-appropriate tasks.*[333] The child has greater body competence and applies self to skills and tasks that go beyond playful expression. The child gets tired of play, wants to participate in the real world, and seeks attention and recognition for effort and concentration on a task. He or she feels pride in doing something well, whether a physical or cognitive task. A sense of industry involves self-confidence, perseverance, diligence, self-control, cooperation, and compromise rather than only competition. There is a sense of loyalty, relating self to something positive beyond the moment and outside the self. Parents, teachers, and nurses may see this industry at times as restlessness, irritability, rebellion toward authority, and lack of obedience.

The danger of this period is that the child may develop a sense of **inferiority,** *feeling inadequate, defeated, unable to learn or do tasks, lazy, unable to compete, compromise, or cooperate,* regardless of his or her actual competence.[334] See the box entitled "Consequences of Inferiority Feelings" for a summary of behaviours and traits of the child, and later the adult, if this stage is not resolved. If the child feels excessively ashamed, self-doubting, guilty, and inferior from not having achieved the developmental tasks all along, physical, emotional, and behavioural problems may occur. Sometimes opposite behaviour may occur as the person tries to cope with feelings of being no good, inferior, or inadequate. The person might immerse self in tasks. If work is all the child can do at home and school, he or she will miss out on a lot of friendships and opportunities in life, now and later, and eventually become the adult who cannot stop working.

Stress is experienced by the school-age child. Often stress response occurs from the demands placed on the child in relation to school achievement or for extracurricular performance, or the fear of violence during transportation or at school may predominate. One study indicated three major areas of stress:[335]

- Actual or anticipated loss of loved ones, pets, or space, such as home, school, and neighbourhood
- Threats to self; situations of anger, fear, aggression, or violence against self or personal belongings; threats to personal safety
- Feelings of being hassled; extra responsibility or restrictions; sibling relations; peer relations; other stresses: violence in the home; abuse; divorce

Table 10-12 lists signs of stress that can be observed in the classroom and school.

Relaxation methods and stress management can be taught to children through individual and group counselling, play therapy, and use of art and music. Several authors are helpful resources.[336–340]

There are sharp differences in how children bear up under such stress as abuse or divorce. Some children are **vulnerable** to stressors; *they are sensitive to or drawn in by the events around them. They become nervous, withdrawn and feel inferior. Some are illness-prone* and slow to develop. Other children are **resilient:** *They shrug off the stressors, thrive, and go on to be industrious, have high self-esteem, and as adults, lead highly productive lives.* True, some children are born with an innately easygoing temperament and handle stressors better than do children with a nervous, overreactive disposition. Children who have robust, sunny personalities are lovable and readily win affection, which further builds self-esteem and an identity. Resilient children are likely to have a number of protective factors, but the key is a basic, consistent, lasting, trusting relationship with an adult who is supportive and who is a beacon presence from infancy on.[341–345]

Vulnerable children, if placed in the right environment, become productive and competent adults. They need help to find a solid relationship—neighbour, teacher, relative—until they find at least one such adult. Then they distance self from the conflictual or abusive home, at least emotionally.[346–350] *Basic health* and *social and educational programs must be provided* to assist the child to adapt to the extent possible, now and in future adult life.[351–353] When the child's environment is overwhelmingly stressful, extra support and love are especially important. If the child is facing multiple stressors, it is more difficult for outside intervention to help the child. The more the risk factors, the worse is the outcome for the child, regardless of the intervention.

Teach parents that they can contribute to a sense of industry and avoid inferiority feelings by not having unrealistic expectations of the child and by using the suggested guidance and discipline approaches. They can encourage peer activities and home responsibilities, help the child meet developmental crises, and give recognition to his or her accomplishments and unique talents.

Consequences of Inferiority Feelings

- Does not want to try new activities, skills
- Is passive, excessively meek, too eager to please others
- Seeks attention; may be "teacher's pet"
- Is anxious, moody, depressed
- Does not persevere in tasks
- Is very fearful of bodily injury or illness
- Does not volunteer to do tasks alone, always works with another on tasks
- Isolates self from others, withdraws from peers
- Tries to prove personal worth, a "good worker" with directives or assistance
- Lacks self-esteem unless praised considerably
- Is overcompetitive, bossy
- Insists on own way, experiences difficulty with cooperation or compromise
- May immerse self in tasks to prove self, gain attention
- Acts out to prove self; lying, stealing, fire setting
- Displays extreme antisocial behaviour, destructive or aggressive acts
- Manifests illnesses associated with emotional state: enuresis, complaints of fatigue
- In adulthood, is unable to pursue steady work or become involved in life tasks as expected
- May become "workaholic"; in adulthood, is unable to engage in leisure

CRITICAL THINKING

What are some activities a parent can pursue with a child at home that could contribute to a sense of industry?

TABLE 10-12
Signs of Stress Observed at School

Physical Signs

1. Morning stomachaches, leg cramps
2. Frowning, squinting, clenched jaw, facial expressions reflecting misery
3. Mixes cursive and manuscript, lower- and upper-case letters when writing
4. May invert, omit, or substitute letters and words
5. Laborious writing, tiring easily when writing
6. Frequent erasures, hates writing activities
7. Negotiates to minimize writing assignments
8. Alert and attentive to noises and distractions not associated with learning task
9. Misses teacher instruction, directions
10. Needs directions repeated, instruction repeated
11. Reading is difficult
12. Falls asleep during the school day
13. Nail biting, throat-clearing, coughing, eye-blinking, incontinent of urine at school, bed-wetting at home
14. Exhaustion from performing school tasks
15. Low resistance to illness
16. Absenteeism
17. Relieves tension through constant physical activity

Emotional Signs

1. Seeks adult approval and reassurance
2. Needs a lot of praise
3. Needs immediate feedback and response from teacher
4. Fear of making a mistake, does not volunteer
5. Lacks confidence
6. Fears getting hurt
7. Withdraws from touch
8. Does not seek to try new things, does not take risks
9. Cannot readily change activities

10. Loses place in lessons
11. Daydreams
12. Often gives the right answer to the wrong question
13. Fears getting hurt
14. Cries easily
15. Picked on by classmates
16. Behaviour at school is acceptable, but parents report bad behaviour at home

Intellectual Signs

1. Inconsistent performance
2. Trouble keeping up the pace
3. Trouble completing assignments within the time limit
4. Has potential, but does not apply self
5. Loses the "low-grade" papers
6. Parents blame teacher for not challenging the child

Social Signs

1. Favourite at-home activity is watching television
2. Passive, apathetic, no initiative at school
3. Does not fit in with peer group
4. Avoids other children, tries to remain anonymous
5. Tries to annoy other children
6. Has few friends, feels uncomfortable in social situations
7. Does not take responsibility for not having assignments, makes excuses
8. Feels hurt and left out, may become angry or jealous of classmates
9. Can be a class bully
10. May show off in one area
11. Seeks out younger children to play with
12. Afraid to take risks
13. Avoids competition
14. Prefers to play alone

Self-Concept, Body Image, and Sexual Development

Self-concept and body image are affected by cultural, ethnic, or racial background; gender; grade level of the child; parents' education; history of illness; and type of illness. Until the child goes to school, self-perception is derived primarily from the parents' attitudes and reactions toward him or her. The child who is loved for what he or she is learns to love and accept self.

The child with a positive self-concept likes self and others; believes that what he or she thinks, says, and does makes a difference; believes he or she can be successful and can solve problems; and expresses feelings of happiness.

Younger children use mostly surface or visible characteristics to describe themselves. At about age eight the child describes the self with less focus on external characteristics and more on enduring internal qualities and is more realistic. Because of concern with appearance or body image, children may try to lose weight, influenced by the ultra-thin models in the media. Mothers exert a strong influence over their daughters' weight-control efforts.[354]

A negative self-image causes the child to feel defensive toward others and self and hinders adjustment to school and academic progress. Children with a low self-concept show more social withdrawal, academic difficulties, and inappropriate attention seeking than children with a high self-concept.[355–357]

At school the child compares self and is compared with peers in appearance and motor, cognitive, language, and social skills. If he or she cannot perform as well as other children, peers will perceive the child negatively, and eventually he or she will perceive self as incompetent or inferior because self-image is more dependent on peers than earlier in childhood.

Schoolchildren are frequently cruel in their honesty when they make derogatory remarks about peers with limitations or disabilities.

Parents, teachers, and health care professionals can contribute to a positive self-esteem and competence in performance by emphasizing the child's positive, healthy characteristics and reinforcing the child's potential. You can be instrumental in fostering a healthy relationship.

The teacher (or nurse) can intervene when derogatory remarks are made among classmates. The teacher may move a child into another work or play group appropriate for his or her ability or explain to peers in simple language the importance of accepting another who is at a different developmental level. Meanwhile, the teacher should encourage the child who has the difficulty. Thus the school experience may either reinforce or weaken the child's feeling about self as a unique, important person, with specific talents or abilities. If he or she is one of 30 children in a classroom and receives little attention from the teacher, self-concept may be threatened.

The *child's body image* is very fluid. Schoolchildren are more aware of the internal body and external differences. They can label major organs with increasing accuracy; heart, brain, and bones are most frequently mentioned, along with cardiovascular, gastrointestinal, and musculoskeletal systems. The younger child thinks that organs change position, and organ function, size, and position are poorly understood. Organs such as the stomach are frequently drawn at the wrong place (this may reflect the influence of television ads). Children generally believe that they must have all body parts to remain alive and that the skin holds in body contents. Consider the effect of injury or surgery on the child. This is an excellent age to teach about any of these inaccuracies.

Table 10-13 shows how aspects of the child's view of self change through the school years.[358,359]

TABLE 10-13
Assessment of Changing Body Image Development in the Schoolchild

6 Years	7 Years	8 Years
Is self-centred	Is more modest and aware of self	Redefines sense of status with others
Likes to be in control of self, situations, and possessions	Wants own place at table, in car, and own room or part of room	Subtle changes in physical proportion; movements smoother
Gains physical and motor skills	Has lower-level physical activity than earlier	Assumes many roles consecutively
Knows right from left hand	Does not like to be touched	Is ready for physical contact in play and to be taught self-defence mechanisms
Regresses occasionally to baby talk or earlier behaviour	Protects self by withdrawing from unpleasant situation	Is more aware of differences between the sexes
Plays at being someone else to clarify sense of self and others	Dislikes physical combat	Is curious about another's body
Is interested in marriage and reproduction	Engages less in sex play	Asks questions about marriage and reproduction; strong interest in babies, especially for girls
Distinguishes organs of each sex but wonders about them	Understands pregnancy generally; excited about new body in family	Plays more with own sex
May indulge in sex play	Concerned he or she does not really belong to parents	
Draws a man with hands, neck, clothing, and six identifiable parts	Tells parts missing from picture of incomplete man	
Distinguishes between attractive and ugly pictures of faces		

9 Years	10 Years
Has well-developed eye–hand coordination	Is self-conscious about exposing body, including to younger siblings and opposite-sex parent
Enjoys displaying motor skills and strength	Is relatively content with and confident of self
Cares completely for body needs	Has perfected most basic small motor movements
Has more interest in own body and its functions than in other sexual matters	Wants privacy for self but peeks at other sex
Asks fewer questions about sexual matters if earlier questions answered satisfactorily	Asks some questions about sexual matters again
	Investigates own sexual organs
	Shows beginning prepubertal changes physically, especially girls

(continued)

TABLE 10-13 *(continued)*
Assessment of Changing Body Image Development in the Schoolchild

11 Years	12 Years
States self is in heart, head, face, or body part most actively expressing him or her	Growth spurt; changes in appearance
Feels more self-conscious with physical changes occurring	Muscular control almost equal to that of adult
Mimics adults; deepening self-understanding	Identifies self as being in total body or brain
Masturbates sometimes; erection occurs in boys	May feel like no part of body is his or hers alone but like someone else's because of close identity with group
Discusses sexual matters with parents with reticence	Begins to accept and find self as unique person
Likes movies on reproduction	
Feels joy of life with more mature understanding	

Self-concept, body image, and sexuality development are interrelated and are influenced by parental and societal expectations of and reactions to each gender. You can assist parents in promoting a positive self-concept and body image. During latency, boys and girls are similar in many ways, but differences are taught. Girls reportedly are less physically active, but they have greater verbal, perceptual, and cognitive skills than boys. Girls supposedly respond to stimuli—interpersonal and physical, including pain—more quickly and accurately than boys. They seem better at analyzing and anticipating environmental demands; thus their behaviour conforms more to adult expectations, and they are better at staying out of trouble. Innate physiologic differences become magnified as they are reinforced by cultural norms and specific parental behaviours. Stereotypes are changing, however. Girls can cope with aggression and competition just as boys can.[360,361]

Early physical education activities teach general coordination, eye–hand coordination, and balance, basic movements that carry over into all movement and sports. Rigorous conditioning activities such as gymnastics are suggested for achieving high levels of physical fitness for prepubertal girls and will improve agility, appearance, endurance, strength, feelings of well-being, and self-concept.

CRITICAL THINKING

What initial steps could you take in the development of a community-based physical activity program for school-age children?

Sexuality Education

Sexual health is a major aspect of personal health that affects people at all ages and stages in their life. Canada focuses on enhancing sexual health and on reducing sexual problems among various groups in our society.[362] Health Canada's *Canadian Guidelines for Sexual Health Education* emphasizes the importance of assisting youth with the information, motivation, and skills needed to make informed and responsible sexual decisions.[363]

Wackett and Evans describe the first reported evaluation of family life/sexual health education program for elementary school students in Canada.[364] The program, called Choices and Changes, was designed following the concepts in the *Canadian Guidelines for Sexual Health Education*, and it was presented to students in the fourth through seventh grades in a school in Whitehorse, Yukon. They found that the program increased the motivation and personal insights of students regarding sexuality.[365]

CRITICAL THINKING

You have been asked to address a grade six class on sexuality education. What issues would you be sure to include in developing your presentation?

10–2 BONUS SECTION IN CD-ROM

Sexuality Education

The definition of sexuality education is provided with guidelines for parents.

Adaptive Mechanisms

The schoolchild is losing the protective mantle of home and early childhood and needs order and consistency in life to help cope with doubts, fears, unacceptable impulses, and unfamiliar experiences. *Commonly used adaptive mechanisms* include ritualistic behaviour, reaction formation, undoing, isolation, fantasy, identification, regression, malingering, rationalization, projection, and sublimation. Assess for these behaviours. Help parents understand the adaptive mechanisms used by the child and how to help the child use healthy coping mechanisms.

Ritualistic behaviour, *consistently repeating an act in a situation,* wards off imagined harm and anxiety and provides a feeling of control. Examples include avoiding stepping on cracks in the sidewalk while chanting certain words (so as not to break mother's back), always putting the left leg through trousers before the right, having a certain place for an object, or doing homework at a specific time.

Reaction formation, undoing, and isolation are related to obsessive, ritualistic behaviour. **Reaction formation** is used frequently in dealing with feelings of hostility. The child may unconsciously hate a younger brother because he infringes on the schoolchild's freedom, but such impulses are unacceptable to the strict superego. To counter such unwanted feelings, the child may become the classic example of a caring, loving sibling.

Undoing is *unconsciously removing an idea, feeling, or act by performing certain ritualistic behaviour.* For example, the gang has certain chants and movements to follow before a member who broke a secret code can return. **Isolation** is a *mechanism of unconsciously separating emotion from an idea because the emotion would be unacceptable to the self.* The idea remains in the conscious, but its component feeling remains in the unconscious. A child uses isolation when he or she seems to talk very objectively about the puppy that has just been run over by a truck.

Fantasy *compensates for feelings of inadequacy, inferiority, and lack of success* encountered in school, the peer group, or home. Fantasy is necessary for eventual creativity and should not be discouraged if it is not used excessively to prevent realistic participation in the world. Fantasy saves the ego temporarily, but it also provides another way for the child to view self, thus helping him or her aspire to new heights of behaviour.

Identification is seen in the hero worship of teacher, scoutmaster, neighbour, or family friend, someone whom the child respects and who has the qualities the child fantasizes as his or her own.

Regression, *returning to a less sophisticated pattern of behaviour,* is a defence against anxiety and helps the child avoid potentially painful situations. For example, he or she may revert to using the language or behaviour of a younger sibling if the child feels that the sibling is getting undue attention.

Malingering, *feigning illness to avoid unpleasant tasks,* is seen when the child stays home from school for a day or says he or she is unable to do a home task because he or she does not feel well.

Rationalization, *giving excuses when the child is unable to achieve wishes,* is frequently seen in relation to schoolwork. For example, after a low test grade, the response is, "Oh well, grades don't make any difference anyway."

Projection is seen as the child says about a teacher, "She doesn't like me," when really the teacher is disliked for having reprimanded him or her.

Sublimation is a major mechanism used during the school years. The child increasingly *channels sexual and aggressive impulses into socially acceptable tasks* at school and home. In the process, if all goes well, he or she develops the sense of industry.

Use of any and all of these mechanisms in various situations is normal, but overuse of any one can result in a constricted, immature personality. If constricted, the child will be unable to develop relationships outside the home, to succeed at home or school, or to balance work and play. Achieving a sense of identity and adult developmental tasks will be impaired.

Child in Transition

The school-age child is especially affected by a geographic move if he or she is just entering or is well settled into the chum stage. The child cannot understand why he or she cannot fit into the new group right away. Because routines are so important to the schoolchild, he or she is sometimes confused by the new and different ways of doing things. The parents will need to consult with the new school leaders about their child's adjustment.

Share the following ideas with parents.

1. If a family can include the schoolchild in the decision about where to move, the transition will be easier.

2. Ideally, the whole family should make at least one advance trip to the new community. If possible, the new home and town should be explored, and the child should visit the new school so that he or she can establish mentally where he or she is going.

3. Writing to one of the new classmates before the actual move can enhance a feeling of friendship and belonging.

4. If the child has a special interest such as gymnastics or dancing, contact with the new program can form another transitional step.

5. When parents are packing, they are tempted to dispose of as many of the child's belongings as possible, especially if they seem babyish or worn. They should *not do this.* These items are part of the child, and they will help him or her feel comfortable and at home during adjustment to a new home and community.

6. Sometimes parents in the new community are reticent about letting their children go to the new child's house. The new parents should make every attempt to introduce themselves to the new playmates' parents, assuring them that the environment will be safe for play; or parents can have a get-acquainted party for the few children who are especially desired as playmates or chums.

7. Just as the family initiated some ties before they moved, similarly, they keep some ties from the previous neighbourhood. If possible, let the child play with old friends at times. If the move has been too far for frequent visits, allow the child to call old friends occasionally.

8. If possible, plan a trip back so that some old traditions can be revived and friends can be visited. The trip to the old neighbourhood will cement in the child's mind that "home" is no longer there but in the new location.

9. The parents must accept as natural some grieving for what is gone. Letting the child express his or her feelings, accepting these feelings, and continuing to work with the above suggestions will foster the adjustment.

Foster adjustment through noticing the new child, watching his or her behaviour, working with the teacher and peers, and contacting parents if necessary.

Moral-Spiritual Development

You can assist parents in understanding the importance of their role and that of peers, school, and even literature and the media in moral and spiritual development. If you care for a child over a period, you will also contribute to this development.[366–368]

The child is learning many particulars about his or her religion, such as Allah, God, Jesus, prayer, rites, ancestor worship, life after death, reincarnation, heaven, and hell, all of which are developed into a religious philosophy and used in interpretation of the world. These ideas are taught by family, friends, teachers, church, books, radio, and television.

The child of six can understand God as creator, expects prayers to be answered, and feels the forces of good and evil with the connotation of reward and punishment. The six-year-old believes in a creative being, a father figure who is responsible for many things such as thunder and lightning. The adult usually interjects the natural or scientific explanation. Somehow the child seems to hold this dual thinking without contradiction. The adult's ability to weave the supernatural with the natural will affect the child's later ability to do so. Robert Coles discusses his studies of spiritual development in children. Most children, even those from an atheistic background, develop a concept of God and are likely to believe in God; however, children may not discuss their views if they fear ridicule or rejection from a secular society.[369]

The developing schoolchild has a great capacity for reverence and awe, continues to ask more appropriate questions about religious teaching and God, and can be taught through stories that emphasize moral traits. The child operates from a simple framework of ideas and will earnestly pray for recovery and protection from danger for self and others. In prepuberty the child begins to comprehend disappointments more fully and realize that his or her answers to problems or desires to change the world quickly are not always possible.[370] He or she realizes that self-centred prayers are not always answered and that no magic is involved.

The schoolchild can be in the conventional stage of moral development, according to Kohlberg.[371,372] Beliefs about right and wrong have less to do with the child's actual behaviour than with the likelihood of getting caught for transgression and the gains to derive from the transgression. Other factors that influence moral development include the child's intelligence, ability to delay gratification, and sense of self-esteem. The child with high self-esteem and a favourable self-concept is less likely to engage in immoral behaviour, possibly because he or she will feel more guilty with wrongdoing. Thus, moral behaviour may be more a matter of strength of will or ego than of strength of conscience or superego. Morality is not a fixed behavioural trait but rather a decision-making capacity. The child progresses from an initial premoral stage, in which he or she responds primarily to reward and punishment and believes rules can be broken to meet personal needs, through a rule-based highly conventional morality, and finally to the stage of self-accepted principles.[373,374]

Part of moral development is the ability to follow rules. Unlike the preschooler who initiates rules without understanding them, the seven- or eight-year-old begins to play in a genuinely social manner. Rules are mutually accepted by all players and are rigidly followed. Rules come from some external force such as God and are believed timeless. Not until the age of 11 or 12, when the formal operations level of cognition is reached, does the child understand the true nature of rules—that they exist to make the game possible and can be altered by mutual agreement.

Moral development is related to self-discipline and empathy, and how this is taught varies with the culture.

Developmental Tasks

Although the schoolchild continues working on past developmental tasks, he or she is confronted with a series of new ones:[375]

- Decreasing dependence on family and gaining some satisfaction from peers and other adults
- Increasing neuromuscular skills so that he or she can participate in games and work with others
- Learning ways to communicate with others realistically
- Becoming a more active and cooperative family participant
- Giving and receiving affection among family and friends without immediately seeking something in return
- Learning socially acceptable ways of getting money and saving it for later satisfactions
- Learning how to handle strong feelings and impulses appropriately
- Adjusting the changing body image and self-concept to come to terms with the masculine or feminine social role
- Discovering healthy ways of becoming acceptable as a person
- Developing a positive attitude toward his or her own and other social, racial, economic, and religious groups

The accomplishment of these tasks gives the schoolchild a foundation for entering adolescence, an era filled with dramatic growth and changing attitudes. Your support, teaching, and guidance can assist the child in this progression.

HEALTH CARE AND NURSING APPLICATIONS

Your role in caring for the school-age child and family has been described in each section of the chapter. Assessment, using knowledge about this era that is presented in this chapter, is the basis for *nursing diagnosis*. Nursing diagnoses that may be applicable to the schoolchild are listed in the box entitled "Selected Nursing Diagnoses Related to the School-Age Child." It is important to emphasize that wellness diagnoses are also important to develop as a plan of care for the school-age child and his or her family.[376] Interventions may involve measures that promote health (e.g., immunization or control of hazards); teaching, support, counselling, or spiritual care with the child or family; or direct care measures to the ill child. Your understanding of the child developmentally will enable you to give holistic care—care that includes physiologic, emotional, cognitive, social, and spiritual aspects of the person.

CRITICAL THINKING

What wellness diagnoses could you develop for a school-age child?

Selected Nursing Diagnoses Related to the School-Age Child

Pattern 1: Exchanging

Altered Nutrition: More than Body Requirements
Altered Nutrition: Less than Body Requirements
Altered Nutrition: Risk for More than Body
 Requirements
Risk of Injury
Risk for Trauma
Impaired Skin Integrity
Altered Dentition

Pattern 2: Communicating

Impaired Verbal Communication

Pattern 3: Relating

Impaired Social Interaction
Social Isolation
Risk for Loneliness
Altered Family Processes

Pattern 4: Valuing

Spiritual Distress

Pattern 5: Choosing

Ineffective Individual Coping
Impaired Adjustment
Health-Seeking Behaviours
Sleep Pattern Disturbance
Diversional Activity Deficit
Bathing/Hygiene Self-Care Deficit
Dressing/Grooming Self-Care Deficit
Altered Growth and Development

Pattern 6: Moving

Impaired Physical Mobility
Fatigue

Pattern 7: Perceiving

Body Image Disturbance
Self-Esteem Disturbance
Sensory/Perceptual Alterations
Hopelessness
Powerlessness

Pattern 8: Knowing

Knowledge Deficit

Pattern 9: Feeling

Pain
Dysfunctional Grieving
Anticipatory Grieving
Anxiety
Fear

Other NANDA diagnoses are applicable to the ill school-age child.

Source: North American Nursing Diagnosis Association, NANDA Nursing Diagnoses Definitions & Classification 1999–2000. *Philadelphia: North American Nursing Diagnosis Association, 1999.*

INTERESTING WEBSITES

CHILD AND FAMILY CANADA

http://www.cfc-efc.ca
This public education site, established by 50 nonprofit organizations, provides quality, credible resources on children and families.

DIVISION OF IMMUNIZATION & RESPIRATORY DISEASES

http://www.hc-sc.gc.ca/pphb-dgspsp/dird-dimr/
Brought to you by Health Canada, this site presents comprehensive information on immunizations and respiratory diseases in an easy-to-navigate format.

SAFE KIDS CANADA: INJURY PREVENTION PROFESSIONALS

http://www.safekidscanada.ca/ENGLISH/IP_PROFES-SIONALS/IP_Professionals.html
Information on this site is for individuals who work in injury prevention, such as public health nurses, firefighters, police officers, daycare providers, and others. The site is updated on a regular basis.

HEALTHY ACTIVE LIVING FOR CHILDREN AND YOUTH

http://www.caringforkids.cps.ca/healthy/healthyactive.htm
The Canadian Paediatric Society launched a national strategy on healthy active living for children and youth. Here you'll

Considerations for the Schoolchild and Family in Health Care

- Family and cultural background and values, the school, the support systems available, community resources
- Parents' ability to guide the child, to help the child develop coping skills and gain necessary competencies
- Relationships between family members
- Behaviours that indicate a parent (or parents), or another significant adult, such as a relative or teacher, is perpetuating abuse, neglect, or maltreatment
- Relationships between the family, school, and other community organizations (church, clubs) and resources
- Physical growth patterns, characteristics and competencies, nutritional status, and rest/sleep and exercise patterns that indicate health and are within age norms for the school-age child
- Growth spurt and secondary sex changes in prepubescence that indicate normal development in the boy or girl; self-concept and body image development related to physical growth
- Nutritional requirements greater than those for the adult
- Immunizations, safety education, and other health promotion measures
- Cognitive characteristics and behavioural patterns in the preschool child that demonstrate curiosity and concrete operations (concept formation, realistic thinking, and beginning social and moral value formation)
- Educational/school programs, demonstration of development of cooperation, compromise, and collaboration as well as competition
- Communication patterns; effect of television, computer, or the other media on communication, learning, and behaviour
- Overall appearance and behavioural patterns at home, school, and in the community that indicate development of industry, rather than inferiority
- Use of adaptive mechanisms that promote a sense of security, assist the child with relationships, promote realistic control of anxiety and age-appropriate emotional responses in the face of stressors
- Behavioural patterns that indicate ongoing superego development and continuing moral–spiritual development
- Behavioural patterns and characteristics that indicate the child has achieved developmental tasks
- Parental behaviours that indicate they are achieving their developmental tasks.
- Learning basic adult concepts and knowledge to be able to reason and engage in tasks of everyday living

find information, resources, and links that you can use in your practice with your patients and their families, and in your community.

SUMMARY

1. The schoolchild grows at a steady pace and continues physical growth and cognitive, emotional, social, and moral–spiritual development.

2. The growth spurt at prepuberty or preadolescence accelerates and influences development in all dimensions. Sexual identity is strengthened.

3. Relationships with parents, siblings, peers, and other adults change and influence development in all dimensions.

4. The child is learning to get along with a variety of people in diverse settings.

5. Family is especially important as a base, while peer relations develop in their significance.

6. The chum of the same sex is a major support; and he or she is vital in psychological, self-concept, and social development.

7. The child meets many challenges, faces and overcomes insecurities, and develops competence that indicates industry and development of concrete operations.

8. School, home, and community provide the avenues for development in all dimensions.

9. The box entitled "Considerations for the Schoolchild and Family in Health Care" summarizes what you should consider in assessment and health promotion with the schoolchild. The family is included.

ENDNOTES

1. Canadian Institute of Child Health, *The Health of Canada's Children* (3rd ed.). Ottawa: CICH, 2000.
2. *Ibid.*
3. Martin-Matthews, A., *Aging and Families: Ties over Time and Across Generations,* in N. Mandell and A. Duffy, eds., *Canadian Families: Diversity, Conflict and Change* (pp. 311–337). Toronto: Thomson Nelson, 2005.
4. Canadian Institute of Child Health, *op. cit.*
5. Séguin, L., Q. Xu, L. Potvin, M-V Zunzunegui, and K.L. Frohlich, Effects of Low Income on Infant Health, *Canadian Medical Association Journal,* 168, no. 12 (2003), 1523–1538.
6. Martin-Matthews, *op. cit.*
7. Levine, M., Childhood Neurodevelopmental Dysfunction and Learning Disorders, *The Harvard Mental Health Letter,* 12, no. 1 (1995), 5–6.
8. Newman, B., and P. Newman, *Development Through Life: A Psychosocial Approach* (7th ed.). Belmont, CA: Brooks/Cole, 1999.
9. Papalia, D., S. Olds, and R. Feldman, *Human Development* (7th ed.). Boston: McGraw-Hill, 1998.
10. Bee, H., *Lifespan Development* (2nd ed.). New York: Longman, 1998.
11. Gormly, A., *Lifespan Human Development* (6th ed.). Fort Worth: Harcourt Brace College Publishers, 1997.
12. Papalia et al., *op. cit.*
13. Sigelman, C., *Life-Span Human Development* (3rd ed.). Pacific Grove, CA: Brooks/Cole, 1999.
14. Cloutier, R., and G. Alain, Family Transitions Related to Parental Separation, *Canadian Journal of Community Mental Health,* Special Supplement, no. 4 (2002), 5–11.
15. *Ibid.*
16. Statistics Canada, *Census: Families and Households Profile,* Website: http://www12.statcan.ca/english/census01/products/analytic/companion/fam/contents.cfm, August 2004.
17. Canadian Council on Social Development, *Aboriginal Children in Poverty in Urban Communities,* Website: http://www.ccsd.ca/pr/2003/aboriginal.htm, July 2004.
18. Child & Family Canada, *Canada's Kids: Thriving? Or Just Surviving?* Website: http://www.cfc-efc.ca/docs/vanif/00000899. htm, August 2004.
19. *Ibid.*
20. Campaign 2000, *Honouring Our Promise, Meeting the Challenge to End Child and Family Poverty,* Website: http://www.campaign2000.ca/rc/rg03/NOV03reportCard.pdf, August 2004.

21. Macionis, J.J., and L.M. Gerber. *Sociology* (4th Canadian ed.). Toronto: Pearson Education Canada, 2002.

22. Campaign 2000, *Honouring Our Promise, Meeting the Challenge to End Child and Family Poverty.*

23. Health Canada, *Because Life Goes On … Helping Children and Youth Live with Separation and Divorce: A Guide for Parents,* Website: http://www.mentalhealthpromotion.com, August 2004.

24. *Ibid.*

25. *Ibid.*

26. Wallerstein, J., and S. Blakeslee, *Second Chances: Men, Women, and Children a Decade After Divorce.* New York: Ticknor & Fields, 1989.

27. Garbarino, J., E. Guttmann, and J. Seeley, *The Psychologically Battered Child: Strategies for Identification, Assessment and Intervention.* San Francisco: Jossey-Bass, 1987.

28. Burgess, A., C. Hartman, and S. Kelley, Assessing Child Abuse: The TRIADS Checklist, *Journal of Psychosocial Nursing and Mental Health Services,* 28, no. 4 (1990), 6–14.

29. Childhood Sexual Abuse and Eating Disorders, *The Harvard Mental Health Letter,* 11, no. 10 (1995), 7–8.

30. Garbarino, J., *Children in Danger.* New York: Jossey-Bass, 1992.

31. Osofsky, J., The Effect of Exposure to Violence on Young Children, *American Psychologist,* 50 (1995), 782–788.

32. Polk-Walker, G., What Really Happened? Incidence and Factor Assessment of Abused Children and Adolescents, *Journal of Psychosocial Nursing,* 28, no. 11 (1990), 17–22.

33. Zimmerman, M., W. Wolbert, A. Burgess, and C. Hartman, Art and Group Work: Interventions for Multiple Victims of Child Molestation (Part I), *Archives of Psychiatric Nursing,* 1 (1987), 33–39.

34. Zimmerman, M., W. Wolbert, A. Burgess, and C. Hartman, Art and Group Work: Interventions for Multiple Victims of Child Molestation (Part II), *Archives of Psychiatric Nursing,* 1 (1987), 40–46.

35. Hunt, C. *Active Safe Routes to School.* Ottawa: Canadian Institute of Child Health, 1999.

36. *Ibid.*

37. Canada Safety Council, *Children Home Alone,* Website: http://www.safety-council.org/info/child/alone.html, June 2004.

38. *Ibid.*

39. *Ibid.*

40. Duvall, E., and B. Miller, *Marriage and Family Development* (6th ed.). New York: Harper & Row, 1984.

41. Jenkins, A., When Your Child Searches for a Birth Parent, *Home Life,* May (1991), 37–40.

42. Gormly, *op. cit.*

43. Newman and Newman, *op. cit.*

44. Rosenberg, M., *Growing Up Adopted.* New York: Bradbury Press, 1989.

45. Smith, E., Unique Issues of the Adopted Child, *Journal of Psychosocial Nursing and Mental Health Services,* 34, no. 7 (1996), 29–39.

46. Child & Family Canada, *Adoption: So Many Issues, So Little Understanding,* Website: http://www.cfc-efc.ca/docs/vanif/00000063.htm, August 2004.

47. Rosenberg, *op. cit.*

48. Smith, *op. cit.*

49. Schneider, B.H., A Multi-method Exploration of the Friendships of Children Considered Socially Withdrawn by School Peers, *Journal of Abnormal Child Psychology,* 27, no. 2 (1999), 115–119.

50. Bee, *op. cit.*

51. Gormly, *op. cit.*

52. Papalia et al., *op. cit.*

53. Seifert, K., R. Hoffnung, and M. Hoffnung, *Lifespan Development.* Boston: Houghton Mifflin, 1997.

54. Sherwen, L, M. Scolevena, and C. Weingarten, *Maternity Nursing Care of the Childbearing Family* (3rd ed.). Norwalk, CT: Appleton-Lange, 1999.

55. Sigelman, *op. cit.*

56. Wong, D., *Whaley and Wong's Nursing Care of Infants and Children* (6th ed.). St. Louis: C.V. Mosby, 1999.

57. Andrews, M., and J. Boyle, *Transcultural Concepts in Nursing Care* (3rd ed.). Philadelphia: Lippincott, 1999.

58. Bee, *op. cit.*

59. Gormly, *op. cit.*

60. Papalia et al., *op. cit.*

61. Seifert et al., *op. cit.*

62. Sigelman, *op. cit.*

63. Wong, *op. cit.*

64. Bee, *op. cit.*

65. *Ibid.*

66. Gormly, *op. cit.*

67. Papalia et al., *op. cit.*

68. Seifert et al., *op. cit.*

69. Sigelman, *op. cit.*

70. Wong, *op. cit.*

71. Bee, *op. cit.*

72. Gormly, *op. cit.*

73. Papalia et al., *op. cit.*

74. Seifert et al., *op. cit.*

75. Sheline, J., B. Skipper, and W. Broadhead, Risk Factors for Violent Behavior in Elementary School Boys: Have You Hugged Your Child Today? *American Journal of Public Health,* 84 (1994), 661–663.

76. Wong, *op. cit.*

77. Nicklas, T., et al., Racial Contrasts in Hemoglobin Levels and Dietary Pattern Related to Hematopoiesis in Children: The Bogalusa Heart Study, *American Journal of Public Health,* 77, no. 10 (1987), 1320–1323.

78. Bee, *op. cit.*

79. Papalia et al., *op. cit.*

80. Seifert et al., *op. cit.*

81. Sigelman, *op. cit.*

82. Wong, *op. cit.*

83. Bee, *op. cit.*

84. Gormly, *op. cit.*

85. Papalia et al., *op. cit.*

86. Seifert et al., *op. cit.*

87. Sigelman, *op. cit.*

88. Wong, *op. cit.*

89. Health Canada, *It's Your Health,* Website: http://www.hc-sc.gc.ca/english/iyh/environment.fluroides.html, August 2004.

90. Royal College of Dental Surgeons of Ontario, *Policy Statement, Water Fluoridation,* Website: http://www.rcdso.org/pdf/policy_statements/policy_fluoridation.pdf, August 2004.

91. Health Canada, *It's Your Health.*

92. Butler, W., V. Segreto, and E. Collins, Prevalence of Dental Mottling in School-aged Lifetime Residents of 16 Texas Communities, *American Journal of Public Health,* 75 (1985), 1408–1412.

93. Papalia et al., *op. cit.*

94. *Ibid.*

95. Wong, *op. cit.*

96. Papalia et al., *op. cit.*

97. Wong, *op. cit.*

98. Gormly, *op. cit.*

99. Papalia et al., *op. cit.*

100. Wong, *op. cit.*

101. Bee, *op. cit.*

102. Gormly, *op. cit.*

103. Papalia et al., *op. cit.*

104. Seifert et al., *op. cit.*

105. Sigelman, *op. cit.*

106. Wong, *op. cit.*

107. Gormly, *op. cit.*

108. Papalia et al., *op. cit.*

109. Seifert et al., *op. cit.*

110. Sigelman, *op. cit.*

111. Wong, *op. cit.*

112. *Ibid.*

113. Boynton, R., E. Dunn, and G. Stephens, *Manual of Ambulatory Pediatrics* (3rd ed.). Philadelphia: J.B. Lippincott, 1994.

114. Hoole, A., C. Pickard, R. Ouimette, J. Lohr, and W. Powell, *Patient Care Guidelines for Nurse Practitioners* (5th ed.). Philadelphia: J.B. Lippincott, 1999.

115. Hoole et al., *op. cit.*

116. Boynton et al., *op. cit.*

117. Hoole et al., *op. cit.*

118. Wong, *op. cit.*

119. Hoole et al., *op. cit.*

120. Wong, *op. cit.*

121. Peckenpaugh, N.J. *Nutrition Essentials and Diet Therapy* (9th ed.). St. Louis: Saunders, 2003.

122. Stockmyer, C., Remember When Mom Wanted You Home for Dinner? *Nutrition Reviews,* 59, no. 2 (2001), 57–61.

123. Health Canada, Office of Nutrition Policy and Promotion, *Canada's Food Guide—Focus on Children 6–12 Years: Background for Educators and Communicators,* Website: http://www.hc-sc.gc.ca/hpfb-dgpsa/onpp-bppn/focus_child_e.html, July 2004.

124. Health Canada, Office of Nutrition Policy and Promotion, *Canada's Food Guide—Focus on Children 6–12 Years: Background for Educators and Communicators.*

125. *Ibid.*

126. *Ibid.*

127. Andrews and Boyle, *op. cit.*

128. Wilson, M., and M. Lagerborg, The Best Part of Dinner, *Focus on the Family,* August (1994), 12–14.

129. Wilson and Lagerborg, *op. cit.*

130. McIntyre, L., S.K. Connor, and J. Warren, Child Hunger in Canada: Results of the 1994 National Longitudinal Survey of Children and Youth, *Canadian Medical Association Journal,* 163 (2000), 1429–1433.

131. McIntyre et al., *op. cit.*

132. Lefrançois, G.R., *Of Children: An Introduction to Child and Adolescent Development* (9th ed.). Toronto: Nelson Thomson Learning, 2001.

133. Tremblay, M.S., and J.D. Willms, Secular Trends in the Body Mass Index of Canadian Children, *Canadian Medical Association Journal,* 163 (2000), 1429–1433.

134. Wong, *op. cit.*

135. Society for Nutrition Education, Guidelines for Childhood Obesity Prevention Programs: Promoting Healthy Weight in Children, *Journal of Nutrition Education and Behavior,* 35, no. 1 (2003), 1–4.

136. Society for Nutrition Education, *op. cit.*

137. Andrews and Boyle, *op. cit.*

138. Wong, *op. cit.*

139. American Academy of Family Physicians, *Summary of Policy Recommendations for Periodic Health Examination.* Washington, DC: Author, 1999.

140. Health Canada, *Canada's Physical Activity Guide for Children and Youth,* Website: http://www.hc-sc.gc.ca/hppb/paguide/child_youth/youth/activityStats.html, August 2004.

141. Health Canada, *Canada's Physical Activity Guide for Children and Youth.*

142. *Ibid.*

143. *Ibid.*

144. *Ibid.*

145. *Ibid.*

146. Heurter, H., K. Breen-Reid, L. Aronson, D. Manning, and E.L. Ford-Jones, Childhood Immunization: How Knowledgeable Are We? *Canadian Nurse,* 99, no. 4 (2003), 27–31.

147. Bigham, M., and M. Hoefer, Comparing Benefits and Risks of Immunization, *Canadian Journal of Public Health,* 92, no. 3 (2001), 173–177.

148. Heurter et al., *op. cit.*

149. Bigham and Hoefer, *op. cit.*

150. Halperin, S.A., How to Manage Parents Unsure About Immunization, *The Canadian Journal of Continuing Medical Education,* 1 (2000), 62–75.

151. Canadian Nurses Association, Nurses and Immunization—What You Need to Know, *Nursing Now,* no. 12 (November 2001), 1–4.

152. Bolaria, B.S., and R. Bolaria, Inequality, Family, and Child Health, in B.S. Bolaria and H.D. Dickinson, eds., *Health, Illness, and Health Care in Canada* (3rd ed, pp. 247–253.). Toronto: Nelson Thomson Learning, 2002.

153. LeBlanc, J.C., T.L. Beattie, and C. Culligan, Effect of Legislation on the Use of Bicycle Helmets, *Canadian Medical Association Journal,* 166, no. 5 (2002), 592–595.

154. *Ibid.*

155. Howard, A., Automobile Restraints for Children: A Review for Clinicians, *Canadian Medical Association Journal,* 167, no. 7 (2002), 769–773.

156. Lapner, P.C., M. McKay, A. Howard, B. Gardner, A. German, and M. Letts, Children in Crashes: Mechanisms of Injury and Restraint Systems, *Canadian Journal of Surgery,* 44, no. 6 (2001), 445–449.

157. Drkulec, J.A., and M. Letts, Snowboarding Injuries in Children, *Canadian Journal of Surgery,* 44, no. 6 (2001), 435–439.

158. *Ibid.*

159. Wesner, M., An Evaluation of Think First Saskatchewan: A Head and Spinal Cord Injury Prevention Program, *Canadian Journal of Public Health,* 94, no. 2 (2003), 115–120.

160. Canadian Institute of Child Health, *The Health of Canada's Children: A CICH Profile* (3rd ed.). Ottawa: CICH, 2000.

161. Bristow, K.M., J.B. Carson, L. Warda, and R. Wartman, Childhood Drowning in Manitoba: A 10-Year Review of Provincial Paediatric Death Review Committee Data, *Paediatric Child Health,* 7, no. 9 (2002), 637–641.

162. MacMillan, H., C. Walsh, and E. Jamieson, *Children's Health,* Ottawa: First Nations and Inuit Regional Health Survey National Steering Committee, 1999.

163. Wong, *op. cit.*

164. *Ibid.*

165. We Kill Too Many Farm Kids, *Successful Farming,* February (1989), 18A–18P

166. Spradley, B.W., *Community Health Nursing: Concepts and Practice* (3rd ed.). Glenview, IL: Scott, Foresman/Little Brown, 1990.

167. Wong, *op. cit.*

168. Bolaria and Bolaria, *op. cit.*

169. Seifert et al., *op. cit.*

170. Hoole et al., *op. cit.*

171. American Academy of Family Physicians, *op. cit.*

172. Boynton et al., *op. cit.*

173. Cox, R., Speaking Out for Those "Loud Black Girls," *American Association of University Women Outlook,* 91, no. 4 (1998), 8–11.

174. Hoole et al., *op. cit.*

175. Wong, *op. cit.*

176. Hoole et al., *op. cit.*

177. *Ibid.*

178. Wong, *op. cit.*

179. Boynton et al., *op. cit.*

180. Hoole et al., *op. cit.*

181. Boynton et al., *op. cit.*

182. Wong, *op. cit.*

183. Farrand, L., and C. Cox, Determinants of Positive Health Behavior in Middle Childhood, *Nursing Research,* 42 (1993), 208–213.

184. De Santis, L., and J. Thomas, The Immigrant Haitian Mothers' Transcultural Nursing Perspective on Preventive Health Care for Children, *Journal of Transcultural Nursing,* 2, no. 1 (1991), 2–15.
185. Gormly, *op. cit.*
186. *Ibid.*
187. *Ibid.*
188. *Ibid.*
189. Papalia et al., *op. cit.*
190. Piaget, J., *The Equilibration of Cognitive Structures: The Central Problem of Intellectual Development* (Transl. by T. Brown and K.J. Thampy). Chicago: University of Chicago Press, 1985.
191. Wadsworth, B., *Piaget's Theory of Cognitive and Affective Development: Foundations of Constructivism* (5th ed.). New York: Longman, 1996.
192. Gormly, *op. cit.*
193. Papalia et al., *op. cit.*
194. Piaget, J., and B. Inhelder, *The Psychology of the Child.* New York: Basic Books, 1969.
195. Piaget, J., and B. Inhelder, *Memory and Intelligence.* New York: Basic Books, 1973.
196. Piaget, *The Equilibration of Cognitive Structures: The Central Problem of Intellectual Development.*
197. Wadsworth, *op. cit.*
198. Webb, P., Piaget: Implications for Teaching, *Theory Into Practice,* 19, no. 2 (1980), 93–97.
199. Wadsworth, *op. cit.*
200. Webb, *op. cit.*
201. Berk, L.E., and E.A. Levin, *Child Development* (Canadian ed.). Toronto: Pearson Education Canada, 2003.
202. Piaget and Inhelder, *The Psychology of the Child.*
203. Piaget and Inhelder, *Memory and Intelligence.*
204. Piaget, *The Equilibration of Cognitive Structures: The Central Problem of Intellectual Development.*
205. Pontious, S., Practical Piaget: Helping Children Understand, *American Journal of Nursing,* 82, no. 1 (1982), 115–117.
206. Webb, *op. cit.*
207. Gormly, *op. cit.*
208. *Ibid.*
209. Newman and Newman, *op. cit.*
210. Wadsworth, *op. cit.*
211. Health Canada, *Helping Your Child Cope—Responding to the Stress of Terrorism and Armed Conflicts,* Website: http://www.hc-sc.gc.ca/pphb/dgspsp/publicat/oes-bsu-02/child_e.html, September 2004.
212. Gormly, *op. cit.*
213. Piaget and Inhelder, *The Psychology of the Child.*
214. Piaget and Inhelder, *Memory and Intelligence.*
215. Piaget, *The Equilibration of Cognitive Structures: The Central Problem of Intellectual Development.*
216. Seifert et al., *op. cit.*
217. Wadsworth, *op. cit.*
218. *Ibid.*
219. Gormly, *op. cit.*
220. Wadsworth, *op. cit.*
221. Gormly, *op. cit.*
222. Wadsworth, *op. cit.*
223. Pontious, *op. cit.*
224. Webb, *op. cit.*
225. Berk and Levin, *op. cit.*
226. Seifert et al., *op. cit.*
227. Sternberg, R., *Thinking and Problem Solving.* San Diego: Academic Press, 1994.
228. Sternberg, R., and R. Wagner (eds.), *Mind in Context: Interactionist Perspectives in Human Intelligence.* New York: Cambridge University Press, 1994.
229. Berk and Levin, *op. cit.*
230. Gardner, H., *Frames of Mind: The Theory of Multiple Intelligences* (2nd ed.). New York: Basic Books, 1993.
231. Gardner, H., *Multiple Intelligence: Theory in Practice,* New York: Basic Books, 1993.
232. Seifert et al., *op. cit.*
233. Berk and Levin, *op. cit.*
234. Webb, *op. cit.*
235. Andrews and Boyle, *op. cit.*
236. Duncan, G., Racism as a Developmental Mediator, *The Educational Forum,* 57 (Summer 1993), 360–370.
237. Sandhu, D., and J. Rigney, Culturally Responsive Teaching in U.S. Public Schools, *Kappa Delta Pi Record,* 31, no. 4 (1995), 157–162.
238. Gormly, *op. cit.*
239. Newman and Newman, *op. cit.*
240. Webb, *op. cit.*
241. Manning, M., and L. Barath, Appreciating Cultural Diversity in the Classroom, *Kappa Delta Pi Record,* 27, no. 4 (1991), 104–110.
242. Papalia et al., *op. cit.*
243. Wong, *op. cit.*
244. Child & Family Canada, *Middle Childhood (6–12 years old),* Website: http://www.cfc-efc.ca/docs/vocfc/00000798.htm, June 2004.
245. Bee, H., D. Boyd, and P. Johnson, *Lifespan Development* (Canadian ed., Study Edition). Toronto: Pearson Education Canada, 2005.
246. Canadian Institute of Child Health, *op. cit.*
247. Hamilton, D., Preparing for the People to Come: Secwepemc Activism in British Columbia, *Journal of Living,* 26 (2002), 28–37.
248. Seifert et al., *op. cit.*
249. Sigelman, *op. cit.*
250. Bee et al., *op. cit.*
251. *Ibid.*
252. Goleman, D. *Working with Emotional Intelligence.* New York: Bantam Books, 1998.
253. Snow, J.L., Looking beyond Nursing for Clues to Effective Leadership, *Journal of Nursing Administration,* 31, no. 9 (2001), 440–443.
254. Bee et al., *op. cit.*
255. Snow, *op. cit.*
256. Seifert et al., *op. cit.*
257. *Ibid.*
258. Papalia et al., *op. cit.*
259. Rakestraw, J., and D. Rakestraw, Home Schooling: A Question of Quality, an Issue of Rights, *The Educational Forum,* 55, no. 1 (1990), 67–77.
260. Richoux, D., A Look at Home Schooling, *Kappa Delta Pi Record,* 23, no. 4 (Summer 1987), 118–121
261. Ray, L.D., Parenting and Childhood Chronicity: Making Visible the Invisible Work, *Journal of Pediatric Nursing,* 17, no. 6 (2002), 424–438.
262. Ray, *op. cit.*
263. Wilkins, K., Sibling Adaptation to the Family Crisis of Childhood Cancer, *Canadian Oncology Nursing Journal,* 13, no. 1 (2003), 46–48.
264. Woodgate, R.L., Children's Cancer Symptom Experiences: Keeping the Spirit Alive in Children and Their Families, *Canadian Oncology Nursing Journal,* 13, no. 3 (2003), 142–150.
265. Fernandes, E., and B.W. McCrindle, Diagnosis and Treatment of Hypertension in Children and Adolescents, *Canadian Journal of Cardiology,* 44 (September 2000), 1869–1877.
266. Harris, S.B., R. Glazier, K. Eng, and L. McMurray, Disease Patterns among Canadian Aboriginal Children, *Canadian Family Physician,* 44 (September 1998), 1869–1877.
267. Ball, G.D.C., and L.J. McCargar, Childhood Obesity in Canada: A Review of Prevalence Estimates and Risk Factors for

Cardiovascular Diseases and Type 2 Diabetes, *Canadian Journal of Applied Physiology*, 28, no. 1 (2003), 117–140.

268. Heiney, S., Helping Children through Painful Procedures, *American Journal of Nursing*, 91, no. 11 (1991), 20–24.

269. Wong, *op. cit.*

270. Gormly, *op. cit.*

271. Papalia et al., *op. cit.*

272. Gormly, *op. cit.*

273. Papalia et al., *op. cit.*

274. Sigelman, *op. cit.*

275. Gormly, *op. cit.*

276. Papalia et al., *op. cit.*

277. Sigelman, *op. cit.*

278. Sullivan, L., The Biological Message for Models of Learning, *Kappa Delta Pi Record*, Fall (1993), 29–32

279. Gormly, *op. cit.*

280. Berk and Levin, *op. cit.*

281. Office of the Commissioner of Official Languages, *A Look at Bilingualism*, Website: http://www.ocol-clo.gc.ca/symposium/documents/brochure/brochure_e.html, September 2004.

282. Bialystok, E., and J. Herman, Does Bilingualism Matter for Early Literacy? *Language and Cognition*, 2 (1999), 35–44.

283. Berk and Levin, *op. cit.*

284. Vanier Institute of the Family, *Did You Know*, Website: http://www.vifamily.ca/library/dyk/dyk.html, September 2004.

285. Canadian Paediatric Society, Healthy Active Living for Children and Youth, *Paediatrics and Child Health*, 7, no. 5 (2002), 339–345.

286. Swift, C., and A. Taylor, The Digital Divide—A New Generation Gap: Parental Knowledge of the Children's Internet Use, *Paediatric Child Health*, 8, no. 5 (2003), 275–278.

287. DeMoss, B., Do You Know What Your Children Are Watching? *Focus on the Family*, August (1994), 2–4.

288. Piaget, *The Equilibration of Cognitive Structures: The Central Problem of Intellectual Development*.

289. Bee, *op. cit.*

290. DeMoss, *op. cit.*

291. Fordiani, T., Have You Read a Fairy Tale Lately? *Kappa Delta Pi Record*, Spring (1995), 116–119.

292. Gormly, *op. cit.*

293. Grube, J., and L. Wallach, Television Beer Advertising and Drinking Knowledge, Beliefs, and Intentions Among School Children, *American Journal of Public Health*, 84 (1994), 254–259.

294. Lego, S., Children Killing Children, *Perspectives in Psychiatric Care*, 34, no. 3 (1998), 3–4.

295. Newman and Newman, *op. cit.*

296. Papalia et al., *op. cit.*

297. Seifert et al., *op. cit.*

298. Sigelman, *op. cit.*

299. Violent Crimes Linked to Early Childhood Factors, *The Menninger Letter*, 3, no. 7 (1995), 7.

300. DeMoss, *op. cit.*

301. Newman and Newman, *op. cit.*

302. *Ibid.*

303. *Ibid.*

304. Gormly, *op. cit.*

305. Newman and Newman, *op. cit.*

306. Seifert et al., *op. cit.*

307. Sigelman, *op. cit.*

308. Bee, *op. cit.*

309. Newman and Newman, *op. cit.*

310. Papalia et al., *op. cit.*

311. Seifert et al., *op. cit.*

312. Wong, *op. cit.*

313. Government of Canada, *Bullying and Victimization among Canadian School Children*, Website: http://www11.sdc.gc.ca/en/ cs/sp/arb/publications/research/1998-000130/pag02.shtml, September 2004.

314. Public Safety and Emergency Preparedness, *Bullying in Canada*, Website: http://www.prevention.gc.ca/en/library/publications/ fact_sheets/bullying/, June 2004.

315. Sullivan, H.S., *The Interpersonal Theory of Psychiatry*. New York: W.W. Norton, 1953.

316. Gormly, *op. cit.*

317. Sullivan, *op. cit.*

318. *Ibid.*

319. *Ibid.*

320. *Ibid.*

321. *Ibid.*

322. Gormly, *op. cit.*

323. Newman and Newman, *op. cit.*

324. Papalia et al., *op. cit.*

325. Mackey, W., *Fathering Behaviors: The Dynamics of the Man-Child Bond*. New York: Plenum Press, 1985.

326. Phillips, A., *The Trouble with Boys*. New York: Basic Books, 1995.

327. Andrews and Boyle, *op. cit.*

328. Gormly, *op. cit.*

329. Newman and Newman, *op. cit.*

330. Papalia et al., *op. cit.*

331. Seifert et al., *op. cit.*

332. Sigelman, *op. cit.*

333. Erikson, E., *Childhood and Society* (2nd ed.). New York: W.W. Norton, 1963.

334. Erikson, *op. cit.*

335. Jacobson, G., The Meaning of Stressful Life Experiences in Nine-to-Eleven-Year-Old Children: A Phenomenological Study, *Nursing Research*, 43 (1994), 95–99.

336. Murphy, E., *God Cares When I Don't Feel Good*. Elgin, IL: David C. Cook, 1987.

337. Murphy, E., *God, You Fill Us Up With Joy: Psalm 100 For Children*, Elgin, IL: David C. Cook, 1987.

338. Murphy, E., *The Early Development of Sibling Relationships in Child-bearing Families*. San Francisco: University of California, 1989.

339. Zimmerman et al., Art and Group Work: Interventions for Multiple Victims of Child Molestation (Part I).

340. Zimmerman et al., Art and Group Work: Interventions for Multiple Victims of Child Molestation (Part II).

341. Bee, *op. cit.*

342. Gormly, *op. cit.*

343. Papalia et al., *op. cit.*

344. Werner, E., *Vulnerable but Invincible*. New York: Adams-Bannister-Cox, 1989.

345. Werner, E., *Against the Odds*. New York: Adams-Bannister-Cox, 1990.

346. Bee, *op. cit.*

347. Gormly, *op. cit.*

348. Papalia et al., *op. cit.*

349. Werner, *Vulnerable but Invincible*.

350. Werner, *Against the Odds*.

351. Bee, *op. cit.*

352. Werner, *Vulnerable but Invincible*.

353. Werner, *Against the Odds*.

354. Papalia et al., *op. cit.*

355. Bee, *op. cit.*

356. Papalia et al., *op. cit.*

357. Sigelman, *op. cit.*

358. Gormly, *op. cit.*

359. Newman and Newman, *op. cit.*

360. *Ibid.*

361. Wong, *op. cit.*

362. Health Canada, *Canadian Guidelines for Sexual Health Education*, Website: http://www.hc-sc.gc.ca/pphb-dgspsp/publicat/cgshe-1dnemss/cgshe_toc.htm, April 2004.

363. *Ibid.*

364. Wackett, J., and L. Evans, An Evaluation of the *Choices and Changes* Student Program: A Grade Four to Seven Sexual Health Education Program Based on the *Canadian Guidelines for Sexual Health Education, The Canadian Journal of Human Sexuality,* 9, no. 4 (2000), 265–273.

365. *Ibid.*

366. Murphy, *God Cares When I Don't Feel Good.*

367. Murphy, *God, You Fill Us Up With Joy: Psalm 100 For Children.*

368. Murphy, *The Early Development of Sibling Relationships in Child-bearing Families.*

369. Coles, R., *The Spiritual Life of Children.* Boston: Houghton Mifflin, 1990.

370. Schulman, M., *Moral Development Training:. Strategies for Parents, Teachers, and Clinicians.* Menlo Park, CA: Addison-Wesley, 1985.

371. Kohlberg, L., Development of Moral Character and Moral Ideology, in Hoffman, M.L., ed., *Review of Child Development Research,* Vol. 1. New York: Russell Sage, 1964, pp. 383–432.

372. Kohlberg, L., Stages of Moral Development as a Basis for Moral Education, in Beck, C.M., Crittenden. B.S. and Sullivan, E.V., eds., *Moral Education: Interdisciplinary Approaches.* New York: Paulist Press, 1972, p. 23ff.

373. Kohlberg, Development of Moral Character and Moral Ideology.

374. Kohlberg, Stages of Moral Development as a Basis for Moral Education.

375. Duvall and Miller, *op. cit.*

376. Stolte, K.M., *Wellness: Nursing Diagnosis for Health Promotion.* Philadelphia: Lippincott, 1996.

Chapter 11

ASSESSMENT AND HEALTH PROMOTION FOR THE ADOLESCENT AND YOUTH

For some, adolescence is short; for others,
adolescence extends many years.

Ruth Beckmann Murray

OBJECTIVES

STUDY OF THIS CHAPTER WILL ENABLE YOU TO:

1. Examine the impact of adolescence on family life and the influence of the family on the adolescent.

2. Explore with the family its developmental tasks and ways to achieve these tasks while giving positive guidance to the adolescent.

3. Compare and contrast, to those that occurred in preadolescence, the physiological changes and needs, including nutrition, exercise, and rest, of early, middle, and late adolescence.

4. Dialogue with parents about the cognitive, self-concept, sexual, emotional, and moral-spiritual aspects of the development of the adolescent, including various ways in which the family can support their healthy progress.

5. Identify examples of adolescent peer-group dialect and their use of leisure time. Discuss how knowledge of these issues can be used in your health-promotion activities and teaching.

6. Explore the developmental crisis of identity formation with the adolescent and the parents, the significance of achieving this crisis for ongoing maturity, and ways to counteract influences that interfere with identity formation.

7. Describe the developmental tasks of adolescence and how the adaptive mechanisms commonly used assist the adolescent in achieving them.

8. Assess and work effectively with an adolescent in all types of settings.

9. Discuss the challenges of the transitional period to young adulthood and your role in facilitating the transition from late adolescence into young adulthood.

10. Identify common health problems of the adolescent, factors that contribute to them, and your role in contributing to the adolescent's health.

How can I best describe my son? He is 13 years old but could pass for 16 physically and mentally. He has the physique of a football player and appears to grow taller each day. His general knowledge is superior because he watches television for at least two hours a day, scans the morning and evening papers, and listens to the radio periodically during the day. He is full of contradictions; for example, he talks about love, but a hug or sign of affection from his mother will send him running to his room.

PERSPECTIVES ON ADOLESCENCE

Adolescence is a long developmental stage, and because it differs cross-culturally, it is the most difficult to define. It is like old age in North America, for each population is considered something of a burden and unable to contribute much to society. In Canada and the United States children are physiologically maturing at an earlier age than previously. The increase in adult height and the change in age at which physical maturation occurs are called a secular growth trend. This trend is attributed to improved nutrition and health practices. Along with early maturation, the developmental era is being extended because of social, economic, employment, industrial, technological, and family changes. For some people adolescence ends in the teens, but for most the period ends in the mid-20s.[1–4] Certainly in some cultures when puberty occurs, rites of passage signal adulthood. Some cultures practise female circumcision, which mutilates the external genitalia and carries a number of health risks. Others encourage the male to perform acts of bravery. Some cultures expect certain types of behaviour at a specific age.

DEFINITIONS

In the past many people equated puberty and adolescence; they are now considered separate components. Puberty is preceded by prepuberty (discussed in Chapter 10).

Puberty is the *state of physical development between ten and 14 years for females and 12 and 16 years for males when sexual reproduction first becomes possible with the onset of* **spermatogenesis** *(production of spermatozoa) and* **menstruation** *(onset of menses.)* Common law usually fixes puberty at 12 years for females and 14 years for males. **Pubarche** refers to the *beginning development of certain secondary sex characteristics that precedes the actual onset of physiologic puberty.* Some define puberty as a process involving a number of physical changes over a period that culminates in menstruation and spermatogenesis. The female may be unable to conceive for one to two years after **menarche**, the *first menstrual period,* and the male is usually sterile for a year or more after ejaculation first occurs.

Some studies, however, have shown that some males become fertile at the onset of pubertal development.[5–8]

Adolescence is the *period in life that begins with puberty, and extends for eight to ten years or longer, until the person is physically and psychologically mature, ready to assume adult responsibilities and be self-sufficient because of changes in intellect, attitudes, and interests.*[9,10] Exceptions occur; some people never become psychologically mature. This definition does not reflect the individuality of the adolescent.

Preadolescence is the *stage of prepuberty.* These children are a part of the school-age population.

Early adolescence *begins with puberty and lasts for several years* (11 or 12 to 13 or 14 for females and 12 or 14 to 16 for males). The growth spurt focuses attention on self and the task of becoming comfortable with body changes and appearance. The teen tries to separate from parents; the dependency–independency struggle is shown by less involvement in family activities (and chores, if possible), criticism of the parents, and rebellion against parental and other adult discipline and authority. Conformity to and acceptance of peer-group standards and peer friendships are gaining in importance. The peer group usually consists of same-sex friends; however, the adolescent has an increased interest in the opposite sex. Group activities with peers are popular.[11–14]

Middle adolescence *begins when physical growth is completed and usually extends from age 13 or 14 to 16 for females and 14 or 16 to 18 or 20 for males.* The major tasks during this period are achievement of ego identity, attainment of greater independence, interest in the future and career planning, and establishment of a heterosexual relationship. Peer-group allegiance, at a peak in 15- to 16-year-olds, is manifested by clothing, food, and other fads, preferred music, and common jargon. Experimentation with adult-like behaviour and risk taking is common in an attempt to prove self to peers. Sexual experimentation often begins now (or earlier) as a result of social exploration and physical maturation. Changes in cognitive functioning may first be evident in that the person moves to more abstract thinking, returning to more concrete operations during times of stress.[15–18]

Late adolescence *may occur from approximately 18 to 25 years of age.* The person has usually finished adolescent rebellion, formed his or her views, and established a stable sense of self. The youth is not fully committed to one occupation and questions relationships to existing social, vocational, and emotional roles and lifestyles. He or she may be a student or an apprentice.[19] Lack of economic freedom may be a concern and prolong dependence on parents. The value system is being clarified; issues of philosophy, religion, life and death, and ethical decisions are being analyzed. The peer group has lost its primary importance, and the youth may take the final step in establishing independence from parents by moving away from home. More adult-like friendships begin between late adolescents and their parents as the earlier family turbulence subsides. At the same time there is more individual dating and fewer group activities with friends; often the first emotionally intimate relationship develops with a member of the opposite sex. At that point the person is developmentally a young adult, having made the transition from adolescence.

He or she is more realistically aware of strengths and limits in self and others.

FAMILY DEVELOPMENT AND RELATIONSHIPS

Discuss the developmental tasks and how to achieve them with the family. Generally speaking, the developmental tasks for a family at this time involve maintaining a grasp on the facets of life that continue to have meaning while striving for a deeper awareness and understanding of the present situation.

Developmental Tasks

The overall family goal at this time is to allow the adolescent increasing freedom and responsibility to prepare him or her for young adulthood.

Although each family member has personal developmental tasks, the family unit as a whole also has developmental tasks. They include the following:

- Provide facilities for individual differences and needs of family members
- Work out a system of financial responsibility with the family
- Establish a sharing of responsibilities
- Re-establish a mutually satisfying marriage relationship
- Strengthen communication within the family
- Rework relationships with relatives, friends, and associates
- Broaden horizons of the adolescent and parents
- Formulate a workable philosophy of life as a family

CRITICAL THINKING

What are some of the family-related developmental tasks you can expect to arise in the blended family?

Traditional Family Relationships

Discuss the following information and the points in the box entitled "Communicating with Your Teen" with parents. Help them understand the interaction between parents and offspring. The home should provide an accepting and emotionally stable environment for the adolescent. The home situation affects later marital adjustments and the type of parent he or she will become.

During early adolescence the teen typically remains involved in family activities and functions. Gradually family relationships change, and the adolescent develops social ties and close relationships outside the family. The family's beliefs, lifestyles, values, and patterns of interaction may influence the development of these relationships, as can the socioeconomic level of the parents. It is during middle and late adolescence that the most severe changes occur in the parent–child relationship (see box entitled "The Adolescent's View of Parents").[20] The relationship must evolve from a dependency status to mutual affection, equality, and autonomy. This process of achieving independence usually creates family turmoil, conflict, and ambivalence as both parents and adolescent learn new roles. The emancipation process must be gradual. Parents should gradually increase the teenager's responsibilities and allow privileges formerly denied. The adolescent wants to make independent decisions and to have increased freedom of movement. At the same time, he or she wants financial support, food, and safe sanctuary. Parents must resist granting instant adult status when the child reaches teen years and instead remember that the adolescent needs to be independent yet dependent. Although he or she protests, the teen values parental restraints if the restraints are reasonable. The adolescent feels more self-confident in exploring the environment if reasonable limits are imposed. Parents should listen to their adolescent's viewpoints concerning restrictions. Views may offer hints about the readiness for more independence and freedom.[21,22]

CRITICAL THINKING

What is your view regarding the notion that adolescence is typically a time of strife between the parents and adolescent?

The Adolescent's View of Parents

Ages 13–14

- No longer sees parents as all-powerful
- Feels parents love him or her but do not necessarily understand him or her
- Becomes attached to adults other than parents
- Continues dependence on parents and seeks their emotional support

Ages 15–18

- Continues need for parental support in self-evaluation of power and worth
- Continues selective process of self-identity by choosing various aspects of parental behaviour, feelings, and values
- Tends to gain autonomy through respect and continued affection for parents rather than through rebellious behaviour

Most ambivalent and negative behaviour in the adolescent stems from self-perceived external restrictions. Teenagers may fight for grownup privileges that they never use—the actual battle is more important than the privilege. Disagreements and conflicts about sexual behaviour, dress, drugs, school performance, homework, friendships, family car, telephone privileges, manners, chores and duties, money, and disrespectful behaviour frequently disrupt family harmony.[23,24]

In addition to other conflicts, the teen must also work through feelings for the parent of the opposite sex and unravel the ambivalence toward the parent of the same sex. He or she reworks some of the sex identity and family triangle problems that remain from the preschool era. In an attempt to resolve this ambivalence, the adolescent may strive to be as different as possible from the parent of the same sex. Frequently affection is turned to an adult outside the family—teacher, relative, family friend, neighbour, mentor, clergy person, or someone in public life. "Crushes" or "idol worship" of this nature are very common; they are usually brief and may occur once, twice, or on numerous occasions. Idolizing another adult person causes the adolescent to want to please that person; therefore, the adolescent's actions and language may change when the idolized person is present. Frequently the adolescent identifies so completely with this person that he or she absorbs some of the person's adult characteristics into the personality. These relationships are not harmful to the adolescent unless the person who is chronologically an adult still feels confused and rebellious toward society and fosters immaturity. On the contrary, an adult outside the family usually will be more objective than the parent and can help the adolescent grow toward psychological maturity. Parents are experiencing sexuality changes at the same time: They are facing middle age and menopause and are concerned with self-perceived decreased sexual attractiveness and potency.

During this period parents may believe they are not as important to the adolescent as before. The adolescent complains that parents are old-fashioned and "out of it." He or she may appear hostile and resent parental authority and guidance. The teen seeks to find flaws in parental behaviour and may try to build barriers between self and the parents to prove independence. The adolescent is critical, argumentative, and generally remote with both parents; a previously close and confiding relationship with the parents is lost. In their presence the adolescent may ridicule parents. This rejection is not consistent; response to parents varies with mood changes. At times the relationship can be close and positive; the adolescent may actually support the parents in the presence of peers.[25,26]

In addition to dealing with a loss of authority, parents are faced with other stresses. They are forced to redefine past child–parent relations and rethink their own values. Parents may also be forced to evaluate their own career choices as their adolescent begins vocational pursuits. Competition between parents and the teen may exist; parents may actually admit to not liking the adolescent. They may be anxious to relinquish financial, physical, and emotional childrearing responsibilities to increase their own freedom.

Changing Directions in Family Relationships

For some teens, there is little family life, not even discord. Sixty-three percent of teens are in households where both parents work outside of the home. Many teens help care for younger siblings and juggle part-time work with school and home responsibilities. At least half have lived through their parents' divorce. Loneliness, isolation, and craving attention from parents are major issues, and they create a vacuum for an intense peer culture. If parents and adults abdicate power, teenagers come up with their own rules.

Although many teens use the computer to send instant messages or e-mail, visit chat rooms, download songs, or do homework, increasingly, some teens are in their own secret world. The computer and Internet, video games, and no-holds-barred music are creating new worlds unknown to adults. New technologies and the entertainment industry, combined with changes in family structure, have isolated parents and other adults from teens. Many teens have a reality that excludes parents and adults. Teens are often unsupervised with the technology, looking at what they please. They often do not get an adult perspective on stimulation to which they are exposed. Teens have less access to parents and more access to potentially damaging information and more opportunity for damaging behaviour. Stresses that frequently produce family discord in North America grow out of conflicting value systems between the parent's and the child's generations. Today's adolescents are a generation born with technology (and place less emphasis on people skills) that has brought remote corners of the world into their homes and minds and has fostered questioning instead of reliance on authority. Grant states that a growing concern exists about whether or not the exposure of teenagers to sexual content in the media has an effect on their sexual attitudes and behaviours.[27]

Parents need help to see that the adolescent is a product of his or her time and the teen is reflecting what is happening socially. Further, teens may be confused by their parents' behaviour. Some grow up with little parental supervision. Some are in single-parent or stepparent families. In some families, a parent may announce that he or she is bisexual or homosexual, or the teen may turn to alternate sexual orientation.[28–31]

Parental and adolescent response to the ambivalence and conflicts of this period varies. Parents may adhere to rules and the status quo to bolster their own security or cultural traditions rather than change for the offspring's benefit. Parents may overprotect. Others may be reluctant to admit that their child is establishing an independent lifestyle. If the adolescent has come from a family that has provided past opportunities to learn responsibility, self-reliance, skills, and self-respect, he

or she will make a smoother transition from childhood dependency to adulthood independence. If parents have been too liberal, overly permissive, or uninterested, the adolescent will have more difficulty adjusting because the past lacked structure and a system of standards or values. He or she has no point of reference other than peers to determine if the behaviour is suitable and decisions are appropriate.[32–34]

Fortunately some parents trust their offspring to live the basic values they taught, although at times behaviour may appear differently. They work at being communicative and flexible, yet supportive, following suggestions such as those in the box entitled "Communicating with Your Teen." They accept that the adolescent may be as large as an adult but still behave childishly at times. The parents' behaviour is adult-like: they are a model for their offspring. If the parent–child relationship has been close in the past, it can remain close now in spite of superficial problems and responses.

A factor that may affect parent–adolescent communication and relationships is the *stepfamily, adoptive family,* or *foster family structure.* Often, these adolescents struggle with whether they really belong to the family (see Chapter 4). The adopted and foster child may search for the birth parent(s). Adoptive parents should cooperate rather than feel threatened. Because of the proliferation of divorce, single-parenting, and stepfamilies, these adolescents may display varying behaviours. In one study, Mahon and her colleagues examined differences in anger, anxiety, and depression between early adolescents from divorced families and early adolescents from intact families. They concluded that early adolescents from divorced families reported higher levels of anger as compared with their counterparts from intact families.[35]

Abuse, Neglect, and Maltreatment

Careful screening and *astute communication skills are essential.* You must establish a relationship and interview the adolescent

Communicating with Your Teen

- Make time for listening and talking.
- Create a beginning and an ending to the day.
- Respect the teen's privacy; do not insist on her or his disclosure.
- Do not judge or shame; state facts and recognition of differences.
- Say "thank you" and "please" as appropriate.
- Be generous with honest praise.
- Apologize when it is appropriate.
- Let the teen make choices and the inevitable mistakes.
- Talk about ways to cope with the consequences of unwise decisions.
- Avoid lectures, preaching, talking down, or sarcasm.
- Use open-ended questions, such as "How was your day?"
- Speak to feelings, "you look frustrated," or reflect back feelings that are disclosed.
- Nurture mealtime conversation; turn off the television, radio, computer, and stereo.

- Plan family times that emphasize casual talk.
- Take advantage of driving time, especially when you are alone with the teen, to talk. The need for the parent who is driving to keep "eyes on the road," avoiding eye contact, often helps exploration of sensitive issues.
- Welcome their friends; engage them in conversation, often through activity.
- Use "I" statements. If you have a plan, be open about it (e.g., a shopping trip).
- Keep the teen and self in perspective.
- Criticize the behaviour, not the person.
- Talk about one issue at a time; do not bring in past events or behaviour unrelated to the current topic.
- Make requests in a neutral, kind tone of voice, assertively but not commandingly.

Parental Behaviour Characteristics of Psychological Maltreatment of the Adolescent

Rejecting

- Refuses to acknowledge changing social roles and to move to autonomy and independence
- Treats adolescent like a young child
- Subjects adolescent to verbal humiliation and excess criticism
- Expels youth from family

Isolating

- Tries to prevent youth from participating in organized and informal activities outside the home
- Prohibits adolescent from joining clubs or after-school activities
- Withdraws youth from school to work or perform household tasks
- Punishes youth for engaging in normal social activity such as dating

Terrorizing

- Threatens to expose youth to public humiliation such as undressing youth, forcing encounter with police or stay in jail

- Threatens to reveal intensely embarrassing characteristics (real or fantasized) to peers or adults
- Ridicules youth in public regularly

Ignoring

- Abdicates parental role
- Shows no interest in youth as person or in activities; refuses to discuss adolescent's activities, plans, interests
- Concentrates on activities or relationships that displace adolescent from affections

Corrupting

- Involves youth in more intense or socially unacceptable forms of sexual, aggressive, or substance abuse behaviour; forces youth into prostitution
- Rewards aggressive or scapegoating behaviour toward siblings, peers, or adults
- Encourages trafficking in illicit drug use or alcohol use or in sex rings

Source: Garbarino, J., E. Guttmann, and J. Seeley, The Psychologically Battered Child: Strategies for Identification, Assessment, and Intervention. San Francisco: Jossey-Bass, 1987. Copyright 1986. Adapted by permission of Jossey-Bass, Inc., a subsidiary of John Wiley & Sons, Inc.

alone. Then you are more likely to learn of physical, sexual, and psychological abuse (maltreatment) or neglect.

Abuse, neglect, and maltreatment occur to numerous adolescents, although health care professionals may not be alert to physical and psychological cues. The adolescent who is physically abused may be present in the emergency room with some of the same kinds of injuries that are seen in the younger child (see Chapters 4, 6, 7, and 9). Sometimes bruises and lacerations are concealed from peers, teachers, and health care providers by cosmetics and clothes.

Maltreatment of the adolescent is demonstrated by the behaviours described in the box entitled "Parental Behaviour Characteristics of Psychological Maltreatment of the Adolescent." Other authors describe physical, psychological, and sexual abuse.[36-42]

Research in Canada with 16 refugee children and 16 children of battered women (aged 10 to 17 years) revealed parallels and common themes in their stories: pain, suffering, feelings of betrayal, uncertainty about the enemy, lack of sense of peace, and finding unexpected resources. Both groups of children used creative strategies to survive physical, emotional, social, and cultural violence.[43]

CRITICAL THINKING

As a health professional, how can you help reduce maltreatment of the adolescent?

PHYSIOLOGIC CONCEPTS

Influences on Physical Growth

The precise physiologic cause for the physical changes characteristic of this period is unknown. It appears that the hypothalamus, probably in some way related to brain maturation, initiates the pubertal process through secretion of neurohumoral releasing factors. These neurohumors stimulate the anterior pituitary gland to release gonadotrophic hormones, somatotropic hormone (STH) or growth hormone (GH), thyroid-stimulating hormone (TSH), and adrenocorticotropic hormone (ACTH). The amygdala in the limbic system also apparently changes function and promotes hormonal production.[44,45]

Gonadotrophic hormones (follicle-stimulating hormone [FSH] and luteinizing hormone [LH]) stimulate the gonads to mature and produce sex hormones. FSH stimulates the ovaries in females to produce estrogen and the development of seminiferous tubules in males; LH stimulates the Leydig cells in the testes to produce testosterone. Growth and development of the adrenal cortex and stimulation of the secretion of androgens are promoted by ACTH. These androgens are responsible for producing secondary sex characteristics. Deoxyribonucleic acid (DNA) synthesis and hyperplastic cell growth, particularly of the bones and cartilage, are stimulated by STH. Under the influence of TSH, thyroxin secretion is slightly increased during the pubertal period. Thyroxin levels increase to meet body metabolic needs.[46–49]

Both male and female hormones are produced in varying amounts in both sexes throughout life. During the prepubescent years, the adrenal cortex secretes a small amount of sex hormones; however, it is the sex hormone production that accompanies maturation of the ovaries and testes that is responsible for the physiologic changes observed in puberty. Physiologic changes in the male are produced by androgens, whereas large amounts of estrogens produce the changes in the female. Both forms of gonadal hormones stimulate epiphyseal fusion by repression of the pituitary growth hormone, thus slowing physical growth at the end of puberty.

Physical Characteristics

You can be very helpful in teaching the adolescent and in helping parents understand what they should teach their children. They both need realistic information about these subjects and an opportunity for discussion. Additional information can be obtained from the local library or health association, doctor, religious leader, counsellor, or personal product companies.

Growth

Adolescence is the second major period of accelerated growth (infancy was the first). The adolescent growth spurt occurs approximately two years earlier in the female than in the male.

Changes in appearance occur, and growth is likely to be asymmetrical (Asynchronous Principle of Development). The nose, lips, and ears often grow larger before the head increases in size. Weight is likely to be gained before height increases occur. The girl is likely to gain in cumulative volume of fat; the boy tends to drop fat tissue. There is a steady increase in strength. Late-maturing individuals tend to be taller than their peers in late adolescence.

During the years of the growth spurt, females grow 6 to 12.5 cm (2.5 to 5 inches) and gain 3.5 to 4.5 kg (8 to 10 pounds); males average 7.5 to 15 cm (3 to 6 inches) and gain 5.5 to 6.5 kg (12 to 14 pounds). In the initial phase of the growth spurt, the increase in height is due to lengthening of the legs; later, most of the increase is in the trunk length. The total process of change takes approximately three years in females and four years in males.[50–53] Between age 15 and 18, girls and most boys are approaching full adult size and appearance. The teen is more physically stable, and body equilibrium is being re-established. The person is less awkward and handles his or her body more efficiently.[54] Every system of the body is growing rapidly, but physiologic changes occur unevenly within the person.

Sexual Development

Four physical characteristics define puberty for most adolescents as they observe themselves and each other.[55–59]

Females

- Height spurt: ages 8 to 17; peak age, 12
- Menarche: ages 10 to 16; average age, 12.5
- Breast development: ages 8 to 18
- Pubic and underarm hair: ages 11 to 14

Males

- Height spurt: ages 10 to 20; peak age, 14
- Penile development: ages 10 to 16
- Testicular development: ages 9 to 17
- Pubic, facial, underarm, and chest hair: ages 12 to 16

Menarche is the indicator of puberty and sexual maturity in the female. Ovulation usually occurs 12 to 24 months after menarche. The onset of menarche varies among population groups and is influenced by heredity, nutrition, health care, and other environmental factors. In Canada and the U.S., the average age of onset is 12.3 to 12.6 years. Research on the onset of menarche has revealed conflicting results. Some researchers have shown a relationship between the height and weight of a girl and menarche.[60] Onset of menarche also varies from country to country: in Sweden, 12.9 years; in Italy, 12.5 years; in Africa, 13.4 to 14.1 years.

Secondary sex characteristics in the female begin to develop in prepuberty (see Chapter 10) and may take two to eight years for completion. Breast enlargement and elevation occur; areola and papillae project to form a secondary mound. Axillary and pubic hair grows thicker, becomes darker, and spreads over the pubic area.[61–65]

Spermatogenesis (**sperm production**) and seminal emissions mark puberty and sexual maturity in the male. The first ejaculate of seminal fluid occurs approximately one year after the penis has begun its adolescent growth, and **nocturnal emissions,** *loss of seminal fluid during sleep,* occur at approximately age 14.[66,67]

Secondary sex characteristics in the male also begin in prepuberty (see Chapter 10) and may take two to five years for completion. Changes in body shape, growth of body hair, muscle development, changes in voice and complexion, and stronger body odours may continue to develop until 19 or 20 or even until the late twenties. The penis, scrotum, and testes enlarge; the scrotum reddens; and scrotal skin changes texture. Hair grows at the axilla and base of the penis and spreads over the pubis. Body hair generally increases, especially facial hair. The voice deepens.[68–72]

Sex hormones are *biochemical agents that primarily influence the structure and function of the sex organs and appearance of specific sexual characteristics.* **Androgens** are *hormones that produce male-type physical characteristics and behaviours.* **Estrogens** are *hormones that produce feminine characteristics.* **Progesterones** are *female hormones that prepare the uterus to accept a fetus and maintain the pregnancy,* and may have other functions in the body as well. All three sex hormones are in both sexes. Androgens are in greater amounts in males; the other two hormones are in greater amounts in females.[73,74] More information about the function of sex hormones can be obtained in any physiology text.[75]

The 28-day menstrual or reproductive cycle is controlled by an intricate feedback system involving (1) the hypothalamus, which audits the level of the hormones in the bloodstream; (2) the anterior lobe of the pituitary and its hormones, FSH and LH; (3) the ovaries and their hormones, estrogen and progesterone; and (4) the interplay between the ovarian hormones and FSH and LH.[76–78]

At the onset of the cycle, when the estrogen level is lowest, the shedding of the endometrial (lining of the uterus) occurs. The hypothalamus, because of the low estrogen level, stimulates the pituitary gland to release FSH, which causes maturation of one of the ovum-containing ovarian or graafian follicles and increased production of estrogen. This is the time of the highest level of estrogen in the bloodstream. In response to estrogen, the endometrium begins to thicken to prepare to receive a zygote if fertilization occurs.[79–82]

In response to the high level of estrogen, the anterior pituitary releases LH. The sudden increase in LH triggers **ovulation,** *release of the mature ovum,* from the follicle, which happens approximately 14 days after the onset of the cycle. The LH moves to the ruptured follicle, which causes development of the glandular corpus luteum. This produces both estrogen and progesterone, which, when acting together, cause the glands of the endometrium to prepare further for the nourishment of a possible zygote.[83–86]

If fertilization of the ovum by a sperm cell does not occur, the ovum deteriorates. The pituitary stops production of both FSH and LH, and the corpus luteum becomes dormant and atrophies. The resulting drop in estrogen and progesterone levels stimulates the shedding of the endometrial lining, which consists of blood, mucus, and tissues, or the menstrual discharge. Menstruation lasts three to five days. The cycle then begins anew.[87,88] **Primary dysmenorrhea,** *painful menstruation occurring without any evidence of abnormality in the pelvic organs,* may occur. The cause is unknown, but endocrine factors, natural pain processes, and psychological factors have all been considered. Various analgesics have been used for this condition through the years. More recently the nonsteroidal anti-inflammatory agents have been used with some success. Some women find that adherence to a certain diet, such as one with decreased caffeine and sugar and increased protein intake, and exercise habits may decrease symptoms. Heat to the painful area may be palliative.[89]

In the male the hormonal system for reproductive behaviour is much simpler because there is no cyclical pattern. The male gonads, the testes, produce sperm continuously and secrete androgens. The major androgen is testosterone.[90]

Just as FSH promotes the development of the ovum in the female, FSH promotes the development of sperm in the male. A continuous level of sperm production takes place in the seminiferous tubules inside the testes. The secretion of LH (also called interstitial cell-stimulating hormone [ISCH]) stimulates the Leydig cells lying between these tubules to secrete the androgen.[91]

Musculoskeletal System

Structural changes—growth in skeletal size, muscle mass, adipose tissue, and skin—are significant in adolescence. The skeletal system grows faster than the supporting muscles; hands and feet grow out of proportion to the body; and large muscles develop faster than small muscles. Poor posture and decreased coordination result. Males and females differ in skeletal growth patterns; males have greater length in arms and legs relative to trunk size, in part because of a prolonged prepubertal growth period in boys. (Males are also clumsier than females.)

Males also have a greater shoulder width, a difference that begins in prepuberty. Ossification of the skeletal system occurs later for boys than girls. In girls, estrogen influences ossification and early unity of the epiphyses with shafts of the long bones, resulting in shorter stature. Muscle growth continues in males during late adolescence because of androgen production. Muscle growth in females is proportionate to growth of other tissue. Adipose tissue distribution over thighs, buttocks, and breasts occurs predominantly in females and is related to estrogen production.[92–95]

Skin

The skin texture changes. Sebaceous glands become extremely active and increase in size. Eccrine sweat glands are fully developed, are especially responsive to emotional stimuli, and are more active in males. Apocrine sweat glands also begin to secrete in response to emotional stimuli.[96] Because facial glands are more active, **acne** (*pimples*) emerges.

Cardiovascular System

The *heart* grows slowly at first compared with the rest of the body, resulting in inadequate oxygenation and fatigue. The heart continues to enlarge and blood volume to increase until age 17 or 18. Systolic *blood pressure* and pulse pressure increase; blood pressure averages 100 to 120/50 to 70. *Pulse* rate averages 60 to 68 beats per minute. Females have a slightly higher pulse rate and basal body temperature and lower systolic pressure than males.

Hypertension is increasing in adolescents, in males, in obese persons, and in those with a family history of hypertension. Higher systolic pressure occurs in urban dwellers; higher diastolic pressure has been seen in those who smoked and lacked regular exercise.

Routine hypertension screening should be done. The upper limit for normal blood pressure in individuals from 11 to 17 years old is 130/90.[97–99]

Respiratory System

The respiratory system also grows slowly relative to the rest of the body, contributing to inadequate oxygenation. Respiratory rate averages 16 to 20 per minute. Males have a greater shoulder width and chest size, resulting in greater respiratory volume, greater vital capacity, and increased respiration. The male's lung capacity matures later than that of the female, which is mature at 17 or 18 years.[100]

Blood Components

Red blood cell mass and hemoglobin concentration increase in both sexes because of increased hormone production. Hematocrit levels are higher in males; platelet count and sedimentation rate are increased in females, and white blood cell count is decreased in both sexes. Blood volume increases more rapidly in males.

Gastrointestinal System

The gastrointestinal system matures rapidly from 10 to 20 years. By age 21 all 32 *teeth* have usually appeared. The third molars may not erupt until later; extraction may be necessary.

If the person resides in an area with inadequate fluoride supply (less than 0.6 ppm), fluoride supplementation may be necessary to prevent dental cavities. Toothpaste with added fluoride should be used. *Stomach capacity* increases to approximately more than 900 mL (1 quart), up to 1500 mL, which correlates with increased appetite as the stomach becomes longer and less tubular; increased gastric acidity occurs to facilitate digestion of the increased food intake. *Intestines* grow in length and circumference. Muscles in the stomach and intestinal wall become thicker and stronger. Elimination patterns are well established and are related to food and fluid intake. The *liver* attains adult size, location, and function.[101]

Fluid and electrolyte balance changes reflect changes in body composition in terms of bones, muscle, and adipose tissue. Percentage of body water decreases, reaching adult levels. Approximately 60% of the male's total body weight is fluid, compared with 50% in the female; the difference is caused by the greater percentage of muscle mass in the male. Exchangeable sodium and chloride decline; intracellular fluid and body potassium levels rise with the onset of puberty. Again, because of their greater muscle mass, males have a 15% higher potassium concentration.[102]

Urinary System
Urinary bladder capacity increases; the adolescent voids up to 1500 mL (1.5 quarts) daily. Renal function is like that of the adult.[103]

Special Sense Organs
The eyeball lengthens, increasing the incidence of myopia in early adolescence. Auditory acuity peaks at 13 and from that age on, hearing acuity gradually decreases. Sensitivity to odours develops at puberty; the female's increased sensitivity to musk-like fragrances may be related to estrogen levels.[104]

Unique Differences
Racial differences in physical development exist, although adult statures are approximately the same. For example, black boys and girls attain a greater proportion of their adult stature earlier. Skeletal mass is greater in the black person; using Caucasian norms means that bone loss could go undetected. Because of the changing body, the adolescent needs information about the normality of anatomic and physiologic changes in addition to sex education. Adults should be cautioned not to pass on superstitions and taboos (e.g., that girls must rest and not participate in social or sport activities or that they should not take showers during menstruation). The adolescent male must be told that the release of spermatic fluid through nocturnal emissions is *not* the result of disease or punishment for masturbation or sexual daydreaming.

If the parents are knowledgeable about pubertal growth changes, they can predict coming physical changes based on how the teen presently looks, which can be reassuring to the child whose onset of puberty is delayed. This may be more difficult in one-parent families, as the man or woman is less equipped to understand and help the opposite-sex child.

CRITICAL THINKING

What are some beliefs of the adolescent regarding their pubertal growth changes in the Western culture as compared to non-Western cultures?

Physical Assessment of the Adolescent

Regular physical examinations should be encouraged. Useful references to help guide your assessment and formulate a health history are Boynton et al.,[105] Hoole et al.,[106] and Roye.[107] Uphold and Graham[108] and Dillon[109] are also thorough references.

The *examination is conducted much as for the adult;* however, it is *crucial that the examiner knows and understands the special emotional needs, developmental changes, age and maturation level of the person, and physiologic differences* specific to adolescence. Roye discusses methods for and barriers to communication with and education of the adolescent.[110] Health assessment of the early adolescent is presented by Manning.[111] Several authors give information on how to promote physical and emotional comfort while gathering the necessary evidence during a pelvic examination, including after rape.[112–116]

Honest and genuine interest in the adolescent and not "speaking down" as though the young person is a child are essential. Confidentiality and trust are key issues. Be sure to express honestly to the teen what part of the interview and examination can be kept in strict confidence and what may need to be shared. Specific age of the person and the nature of the findings determine these factors. Above all, do not say, "This is completely confidential," only to say later, "I believe we better share that."

Physical complaints and emotional symptoms may relate to underlying problems of drug abuse, alcoholism, sexual uncertainties and stress, date rape, pregnancy or fear of pregnancy, fear of or actual sexually transmitted disease, depression, family or peer adjustment problems, school problems, or concerns about future plans.

Because the adolescent may be extremely shy about his or her body, every effort must be made to protect privacy within the confines of the situation. With the advent of the female nurse practitioner conducting examinations on male patients, the traditional "embarrassment roles" are switched. Much has been written on the conduct of the male examiner with the female patient but not on the reverse. The younger the adolescent male is, in terms of sexuality development, the more concern he has about a female examiner seeing and touching his body parts that are considered private. The female examiner ought to provide proper draping and emphasize the touching as little as possible. She may make the preliminary statement, "It is important that I palpate your scrotum to detect…. I know this is a tender area and I will proceed as quickly as possible while being thorough in my exam."

The blood pressure should be at adult levels. The athlete in training may have a slower pulse rate than his or her peers.

Pallor, especially in girls, should be a clue to check hemoglobin levels.

The teen needs frequent dental visits because most have caries. Many young adolescents whose parents have insurance for the service or have sufficient funds have orthodontic work in progress.

Because myopia seems to increase during these years, increased reading and study encourage eyestrain. Many teens are now being fitted with contact lenses.

Although breast neoplasms are not common to this age group, females should be taught breast self-examination. Also, the girl should not be surprised if there is some asymmetric development. Some increase in breast tissue can also be expected in adolescent males. Excessive growth should be referred for evaluation. Both male and female breasts should be examined.

The heart should be found at the fifth left intercostal space as in the adult, and most functional murmurs should be outgrown. Serum cholesterol and triglyceride levels should be obtained if there is a family history of cardiovascular disease and preventive dietary and exercise regimens should be discussed.

Striae may be found on the abdomen of females because of the rapid weight gain and loss experienced by fad diets followed by return to overeating.

The examiner should be acutely aware not only of the pattern of sexual development of both males and females, but of the concerns and questions that may be voiced. The presence of the testes in the scrotum is of primary importance because undescended testicles at this age can mean sterility. Papanicolaou (Pap) smears and pelvic examinations are done when the adolescent becomes sexually active. These procedures, done for the first time followed by explanations and as much gentleness as possible, can set a positive tone for future examinations.

Some have suggested that urine cultures be taken periodically on females between the ages of 15 and 18 because of the number of asymptomatic urinary infections.

Scoliosis is common in teenagers, so a close look for asymmetry of the musculoskeletal system is essential, and any severe, persistent pain in the long bone area should also be referred.

CRITICAL THINKING

What do you need to consider as you address the personal hygiene habits of an adolescent?

Improving the health habits and quality of life of adolescents is important for community health nurses.[117] In fact, developing health promotion programs that are attractive to teenagers can be a major challenge. For example, in a rural Nova Scotia school district the teens were brought into the design and implementation of the Teens for Healthy Living Project. One of the most important implications for nurses that arose from the program is that nurses who are involved in planning and delivering health promotion programs for youth need to do so in collaboration with the teens.[118] Based on the longitudinal National Population Health Survey which included 1493 adolescents aged 12 to 19 years, Vingilis and her colleagues examined the factors that predict adolescents' concepts of their health. The study suggests that adolescents' appraisals of their heath are shaped by their overall sense of functioning, which includes physical health and nonphysical health dimensions—such as lifestyle, behaviours, and personal and socioeconomic factors.[119]

Nutritional Needs

Physical, emotional, and social change characterize the time of adolescence. Adolescent girls may be at risk for inadequate energy and nutrient intake, especially of calcium and iron.[120] Because of a desire to be thin, many adolescent girls may excessively restrict their energy intake. That is, to achieve weight loss, adolescent girls may deliberately skip meals, eat on the run, and adopt other irregular eating behaviours, including disordered eating. McVey and her colleagues examined the prevalence of dieting and negative eating habits among 2279 females (aged 10 to 14 years) in southern Ontario. They found that those with elevated ChEAT (Children's version of the Eating Attitudes Test) scores of 20 or higher were significantly more likely than those with lower scores to be engaged in dieting and other extreme weight-control measures. They state that the results suggest that unhealthy dieting behaviours are reported in girls as young as ten years of age.[121] On the other hand, boys usually have large appetites and consume a lot of food.[122] A few practical considerations to use with adolescents include:

- Assess whether their eating patterns follow *Canada's Food Guide to Healthy Eating* (see http://www.hc-sc.gc.ca/nutrition).
- Identify adolescent girls who may be restricting their food consumption in order to be thin. Advise them on healthy eating patterns that promote healthy growth and development.
- Teach an integrated approach to healthy eating, active living, and the building of a positive self-concept.
- Encourage a healthy eating pattern according to *Canada's Food Guide to Healthy Eating*, which emphasizes foods rich in iron and calcium.
- Provide factual and realistic information about body size to counteract social pressures to attain an unrealistic body weight.
- If you suspect an adolescent has an eating disorder or a problem with substance abuse, refer him or her to appropriate agencies in your community.[123]

In the development of nutrition intervention programs for teens, it is important to consider their culture and ethnic backgrounds, recognizing that food habits may differ.[124]

In summary, adolescents need good nutrition, both to grow to their full potential and to decrease the risk of obesity and chronic diseases that come both in adolescence and later life. The Food Habits of Canadians Study provided data on the important food sources of energy and nutrients in a sample of Canadian teenagers. Results from the survey of 178 teenagers found that a high intake of nutrient-poor foods, particularly high-sugar beverages, was a major problem.[125] The food the teenagers frequently consumed were cakes, cookies, carbonated beverages, salty snacks, and other poor-nutrient foods. Some nutrient-dense foods such as eggs, fish, and organ meats were notable in their absence or low consumption.[126] This high intake of nutrient-poor foods and high-sugar beverages is a concern. We certainly need health promotion programs for girls during the preadolescent phase that will avert disordered eating behaviours.[127]

Underweight and overweight are probably the two most common, but most overlooked, symptoms of malnutrition. *Assess the adolescent; teach both the adolescent and the parents to foster good health.*

CRITICAL THINKING

Develop a nutritional program for presentation to a grade ten class that focuses on food groups and menu selection.

11-1 BONUS SECTION IN CD-ROM
Nutritional Needs

This section outlines nutritional guidelines for adolescents in the United States.

Underweight

Underweight can be caused by an inadequate intake of calories or poor use of the energy. It is often accompanied by fatigue, irritability, anorexia, and digestive disturbances such as constipation or diarrhea. Poor muscular development evidenced by posture and hypochromic anemia may also be observed. In children and adolescents growth and development may be delayed. Even with the recommended dietary intakes, malabsorption of protein, fat, or carbohydrate can result in undernutrition. Underweight may be a symptom of an undiagnosed disease.[128,129] The most severe form of underweight is seen in individuals with anorexia nervosa and bulimia. You may be the first person to assess these conditions in the adolescent. A study by Jones and her colleagues examined disturbed eating attitudes and related behaviours of females, 12 to 18 years of age, from a large school-based population in Ontario. It was found that disordered eating attitudes and behaviours were present in over 27% of girls in that age group, and such behaviours tended to increase gradually throughout adolescence.[130]

Anorexia nervosa is a *syndrome,* occurring usually in females between the ages of 12 and 18, although onset may occur in the 20s and 30s, *in which the person voluntarily refuses to eat, presumably because of lack of hunger but related to distorted body image and conflictual relationships.* Refer to the box entitled "Signs and Symptoms of Anorexia Nervosa."[131,132]

Men may also suffer from this disease but may be even more reticent than women to reveal symptoms or seek treatment.[133]

Bulimia may be associated with anorexia nervosa and is a *syndrome characterized by voluntary restriction of food intake followed by extreme overeating and self-induced purging, such as vomiting, laxative abuse, and excess exercise.* Refer to the box entitled "Signs and Symptoms of Bulimia."[134,135]

Anorexia nervosa is more common than bulimia among adolescents, although the latter is increasing in incidence. Often both syndromes exist together. Impaired physiological and psychological functioning, disturbed body image, confused or inaccurate perceptions about body functions, and a sense of incompetence, depression, anger, and helplessness are present in all anorectic and bulimic clients.[136,137] There are several theories about causation and dynamics of anorexia nervosa.[138–141]

Signs and Symptoms of Anorexia Nervosa

- Refusal to eat or eating only small amounts yet feeling guilt about eating; excuses about not eating; inability to tolerate sight or smell of food
- Denial of hunger (hunger becomes a battle of wills) but preoccupation with food (plays with food when eating; collects recipes)
- Intense fear of becoming obese, even when underweight; refusal to maintain body weight; compulsive exercise and weighing
- Large (at least 20% to 25%) weight loss with no physical illness evident
- Abuse of laxatives or diuretics; frequent trips to bathroom, especially after meals
- Distorted body image; perception of self as fat even when below normal weight
- Vital sign changes: bradycardia, hypotension, hypothermia
- Interruption of normal reproductive system processes in females: at least three consecutive menses missed when otherwise expected to occur
- Malnutrition adversely affecting (1) the skeleton, causing decalcification, decreased bone mass, and osteoporosis; (2) muscular development; and (3) cardiac and liver function, arrhythmia, and (4) body metabolic functions, which may decrease as a result of liver involvement
- Skin dry, pale, yellow-tinged; presence of lanugo; hair loss
- Enlargement of brain ventricles, with shrinkage of brain tissue surrounding them; depression, irritability
- Apathy, depression, low motivation, poor concentration
- Regular use of loose-fitting clothing

Signs and Symptoms of Bulimia

- Binge eating—consumption of excessively large amount of food—followed by self-induced vomiting or laxative and/or diuretic abuse (at least twice weekly); secretive eating; frequent trips to bathroom, especially after eating
- Fear of inability to stop eating voluntarily
- Feeling of lack of control over the eating behaviour during eating binges
- Preoccupation with food and guilt about eating
- Weight fluctuations and fluid and electrolyte imbalances due to binges, fasts, and vomiting/laxatives
- Use of crash diets to control weight
- Weakness, headaches, fatigue, depression, dizziness
- Orthostatic hypotension due to fluid depletion
- Scars on dorsum of hand from induced vomiting
- Loss of tooth enamel and esophageal and gastric bleeding in vomiters
- Chest pain from esophageal reflux or spasm
- Parotid gland enlargement in vomiters; swollen or infected salivary glands
- Increased peristalsis, rectal bleeding, constipation if laxative abuser
- Menstrual irregularities
- Bursting blood vessels in eyes
- Red knuckles from forced vomiting
- More time alone or cooking

The person usually is treated on an outpatient basis; however, hospitalization, with nutritional support and intense psychotherapy, is recommended when loss of 25% or more of body weight leaves the person physically, emotionally, and socially compromised to the point of being in a life-threatening situation. The anorectic person should be hospitalized if there is a low serum electrolyte or fluid level; depression with suicidal thoughts or attempts; substantial disorganization of the family; or failure of outpatient treatment. These criteria also apply to the bulimic person; the additional criterion is spontaneous induced purging after binges. Hospitalization may also be helpful in defusing parent–adolescent tensions and the resultant power struggle and in preventing suicide.[142–144]

The *goals of treatment for the anorectic and bulimic client* are to:

1. Maintain normal weight.
2. Treat the hypokalemia and metabolic alkalosis.
3. Prevent physiological complications.
4. Change attitudes toward food.
5. Develop more effective coping skills to overcome the underlying conflicts.

The approach is holistic. *Treatment involves* any of the following methods: *behaviour modification and insight-oriented, supportive, individual, group, family therapy.*[145,146] A resource to be considered seriously is the National Eating Disorder Information Centre (NEDIC). This is a Toronto-based non-profit organization whose philosophy is to promote healthy lifestyles. It encourages clients to make informed choices based on accurate information. The national toll-free number for NEDIC is 1-866-NEDIC-20 (1-866-633-4220). (Also see the Interesting Websites section at the end of this chapter.)

Both the family and the adolescent need therapy. *Goals of family therapy* include:

1. Reducing pathogenic conflict and anxiety within the family relationships
2. Becoming more aware of and better at meeting each other's emotional needs
3. Promoting more appropriate role behaviour for each sex and generation
4. Strengthening the capacity of the adolescent and family as a whole to cope with various problems[147,148]

CRITICAL THINKING

How can you help a friend who you realize is bulimic?

Overweight

The World Health Organization (WHO) states that obesity is presently a blatantly visible—yet much neglected—public health problem.[149] Paradoxically, together with undernutrition, an escalating global epidemic of overweight and obesity—"globesity"—is becoming prevalent over many parts of the world. The WHO Global Strategy on Diet, Physical Activity, and Health identifies diet and physical inactivity as leading causes of illness and death. It recommends that governments adopt policies to fight against obesity, heart disease, and other

diet-related health problems.[150] The prevalence of overweight and obesity is commonly assessed by using the body mass index (BMI). The BMI is defined as the weight in kilograms divided by the square of the height in metres (kg/m^2). A BMI greater than 25 kg/m^2 is defined as overweight and a BMI over 30 kg/m^2 as obese.

CRITICAL THINKING

If an adolescent is 14 years old, weighs 55 kg, and is 160 cm tall, what is his BMI? Would he be classified as obese?

Obesity is a widespread problem in Canada. Research indicates that obesity is not just a problem for Canadian adults, but is also having a serious impact on children's health. For example, obese children and adolescents have a greater occurrence of hypertension, and they show high cholesterol levels.[151] Fernandes and McCrindle of Toronto's Hospital for Sick Children reviewed the recent recommendations of the Task Force on Blood Pressure Control in Children. They restricted the search criteria to studies with a primary focus of blood pressure for subjects 18 years old or younger. They concluded that hypertension is underrecognized in children. Further, clinical management is directed toward secondary causes, and, in general, cardiovascular risk reduction is aimed at dietary modification, increased exercise, and attainment and maintenance of ideal body weight.[152]

Katzmarzyk states that Canada has recently experienced a major epidemic of obesity; in fact, the population prevalence of obesity more than doubled between 1985 and 1998. In 1998, the problem was nationwide, meaning that it did not appear to be limited to one province or region.[153] Hanley and his colleagues conducted a study to evaluate the prevalence of pediatric overweight and associated behavioural factors in a Native Canadian community with high rates of adult obesity and type 2 diabetes. They concluded that pediatric overweight is a harbinger of future diabetes risk and indicates a need for programs targeting primary prevention of obesity in children and adolescents.[154]

Dr. Kim Raine, a professor and the director at the Centre for Health Promotion Studies at the University of Alberta, wrote a report on overweight and obesity in Canada, which was commissioned by the Canadian Population Health Initiative of the Canadian Institute for Health Information. The report concluded that we need precise knowledge of the determinants and the root causes of obesity.[155] The application of a population health perspective to the problem of obesity may provide timely insight into the potential means of addressing this critical issue. The aspects that are most clearly established are the behavioural determinants of obesity—excess energy intake via overconsumption of food coupled with decreased energy expenditure. However, what is less understood are the environmental and social determinants of those behaviours, and the best ways to change them.[156] It is important to note that the lack of available Canadian data on the environmental determinants of food consumption and physical activity patterns poses limitations to providing evidence-based policy options.[157] However, a comprehensive school health program would help to manage weight among overweight children and adolescents. The prevention of obesity can begin at the individual and interpersonal levels. Health Canada's Vitality program is a strategy that promotes healthy eating, active living, and positive concept of both self and body image.[158]

CRITICAL THINKING

What schools in your area have a nutritional program to initiate healthy eating patterns? What can you do as a health professional to support such a program?

In caring for an obese adolescent the nurse needs to obtain a thorough health history and have knowledge of the adolescent's health practices regarding nutrition.

Based on such an assessment, *the following suggestions, if followed, can help most obese adolescents lose weight*:[159]

- Consciously ask self before eating, "Am I really hungry?"
- Eat only at mealtimes and at the table; avoid snacks. To lose half a kilogram weekly, dietary intake must be reduced by 500 calories daily.
- Count the mouthfuls, cut food into small pieces, and eat slowly to eat less. Set down eating utensils between each bite of food.
- Keep a food diary, with the goal of reinforcing the adherence to the traditional food groups and avoiding empty calories.
- Engage in planned, regular exercise such as bicycle riding, walking the dog, gardening, yard work, callisthenics, or swimming.
- Maintain proper posture and an overall attractive appearance.

Families should be given the following suggestions to help the adolescent achieve weight loss:[160]

- Limit purchases and cooking and baking of carbohydrate foods or snacks.
- Remove tempting snacks such as candy and cookies from the home.
- Ban eating in front of the television or reading while eating.
- Make dining at the table a pleasant time.
- Avoid using food as reward or punishment.
- Serve food in individual portions on the plate rather than in bowls on the table to avoid second helpings, and serve food on smaller plates.
- Praise even a small weight loss; avoid nagging.
- Participate in physical activity with the adolescent when possible.

Further, reinforce the permanence of new food habits and achievement of weight loss through your continued guidance and realistic praise. The key to successful treatment may be in improving the adolescent's self-image. If emotional problems exist, you will need to counsel the adolescent or refer him or her to an appropriate source. Regardless of the methods of treatment used, parental understanding and cooperation are needed, and you are one member of the health team with whom both parents and the adolescent can discuss their concerns. Your ability to listen, to discuss, to teach, and to refer, when necessary, can help the adolescent prevent or overcome

the health hazard of obesity. You can also work with the school system to establish daily physical exercise programs that stimulate the teen to remain physically active, give dietary instructions, check weight, and provide low-calorie refreshments or low-carbohydrate snacks.

More information on types, effects, and treatment of obesity can be found in various references.[161–165]

Exercise, Play, and Rest

Over half of Canadians aged five to 17 are not active enough for their optimal growth and development. The term "active enough" is equivalent to energy expenditure of at least eight kilocalories per kilogram of body weight per day. Only 40 percent of adolescent boys and 30 percent of adolescent girls are considered active enough.[166] However, according to the 1998 Adolescent Health Survey, the majority of youth in British Columbia participated in at least one extracurricular activity.[167] Participation in extracurricular activities may enhance the lives of young people by expanding their social networks, by exposing them to new experiences, or by helping them to acquire new skills.[168]

The most popular activities among children aged five to 12, such as bicycling, remain popular among adolescents. However, the proportion of teenagers participating in each activity is usually lower.[169] Some of the more popular activities among teenagers include skiing, volleyball, golf, tennis, basketball and snowboarding. It is important to note that 51% of Canadian children aged five to 17 rely on inactive modes of transportation to get to and from school.[170]

Health Canada has developed guidelines to increase physical activity in youth. For more information, visit http://www.healthcanada.ca/paguide.

CRITICAL THINKING

In what ways, if any, do cultural influences bear on exercise habits in the adolescent?

Exercise and rest must be balanced for the adolescent to have a healthy body, and they appear to be related to other health habits. One study examined the association between physical activity and other health behaviours in a sample of 11 631 high-school students in the United States. Teens who scored low in physical activity were likely to engage in cigarette smoking, marijuana use, less fruit and vegetable consumption, more television watching, failure to wear a seatbelt, and lower academic performance.[171]

Exercise and Play Activities

Three types of play predominate in this age group: cooperative play, exemplified in games; team play, exemplified in sports; and construction play, exemplified in hobbies. All of these types of play can promote growth in the adolescent.[172,173]

Help parents and teens realize that competitive activities prepare young people to develop a process of self-appraisal that will last them throughout their lives. Learning to win and to lose can also be important in developing self-respect and concern for others. Physical activities provide a way for adolescents to enjoy the stimulation of conflict in a socially acceptable manner. Participation in sports training programs in junior and senior high schools can also help decrease the gap between biological and psychosocial maturation while providing exercise. Some form of physical activity should be encouraged to promote physical development, prevent overweight, formulate a realistic body image, and promote peer acceptance. Being an observer on the sidelines will not fulfill these needs.

CRITICAL THINKING

How can you initiate a physically active program for an adolescent who is hospitalized for depression?

Rest and Sleep

During adolescence bedtime becomes variable; the adolescent is busy with an active social life. The teen is expending large amounts of energy and functioning with an inadequate oxygen supply because the heart and lungs do not enlarge rapidly enough at the time of growth spurt. Both contribute to fatigue and need for additional rest. In addition, protein synthesis occurs more readily during sleep. Because of the growth spurt during adolescence, protein synthesis needs are increased.[174,175] Increased rest may also be needed to prevent illness.

Limit setting may be necessary to ensure adequate opportunities for rest. Rest is not necessarily sleep. A period spent with some quiet activity is also beneficial. Every afternoon should not be filled with extracurricular activities or home responsibilities, and when there is school the next morning, the adolescent should be in bed at a reasonable hour.

PSYCHOSOCIAL CONCEPTS

The following information will guide assessment and teaching of the adolescent and the parents.

Cognitive Development

Parents sometimes underestimate the cognitive abilities of the adolescent. Help them work with the adolescent from an intellectual and creative perspective. Parents can learn from adolescents, just as adolescents learn from parents. Help the adolescent learn how to use cognitive skills in a way that will not antagonize parents.

Formal Operations Stage

Tests of mental ability indicate that adolescence is the time when the mind has great ability to acquire and use knowledge. One of the adolescent's developmental tasks is to develop a workable philosophy of life, a task requiring time-consuming abstract and analytic thinking and inductive and deductive reasoning. Yet, according to media reports, many teens read at fourth-grade level or are functionally illiterate.

The adolescent uses available information to combine ideas into concepts and concepts into constructs, develop theories, and look for supporting facts; consider alternate solutions to problems; project his or her thinking into the future; and try to categorize thoughts into usable forms. He or she is capable of highly imaginative thinking, which, if not stifled, can evolve into significant contributions in many fields—science, art, music. The adolescent's theories at this point may be oversimplified and lack originality, but he or she is setting up the structure for adult thinking patterns, typical of Piaget's period of formal operations. The adolescent can solve hypothetical, mental, and verbal problems; use scientific reasoning; deal with the past, present, and future; appreciate a wide range of meanings and complex issues, and understand causality and contrasting features. The formal operations period differs from concrete operations in that a much larger range of symbolic processes and imagination, along with memory, and logic are used.[176] A few of Piaget's ideas on formal operational thought are being challenged. There is much more individual variation in formal operational thought than Piaget envisioned.

In North America the emphasis in education and the work world is on logical, analytical, critical, and convergent thinking. The goals of these linear thinking processes are precision, exactness, consistency, sequence, and correctness of response. The source of such thinking is the left hemisphere of the brain. Yet original concepts do not necessarily arise from logical thinking. Thinking that is creative or novel is marked by exploration, intentional ambiguity, problem solving, and originality. Creativity is a multivariate mental process, divergent, intuitive, and holistic in nature; its source is the right hemisphere of the brain. It is an intellectual skill in which the person creates new ideas rather than imitating existing knowledge.

Creativity, problem-solving ability, and cognitive competence can be encouraged when the educational process requires the following:[177,178]

- Written assignments that necessitate original work, independent learning, self-initiation, and experimentation
- Reading assignments that emphasize questions of inquiry, synthesis, and evaluation rather than factual recall
- Opportunity for females as well as males to gain skills in all facets of computer sciences and technology
- Group work to encourage brainstorming or exposure to creative ideas of others
- Oral questions that are divergent or ask for viewpoints during lectures
- Tests that include both divergent and convergent questions that engage the student in reflective, critical, and exploratory thought (questions should become increasingly complex in nature; ideally the questions are worded so that there is not just one right answer but answers that can be innovative and express thoughtfulness)
- A creative atmosphere, whereby the learner is autonomous, self-reliant, internally controlled, and self-evaluated (the curriculum emphasizes process, and the teacher provides a supportive atmosphere and recognizes creativity; in such an environment one would observe puzzlement and frustration but also eagerness, humour, laughter, and enjoyment related to the task at hand)

In addition, students cannot learn unless they are assured of an environment that feels safe, supportive and is as free as possible from the threats of bullies or the fear of system violence. Several strategies can be implemented:[179]

- Collaboration between administrators, teachers, and parents
- Development of a school safety plan to ensure a gun-free school
- Work with churches and other support groups or organizations in the community
- Establishment of a crisis management team to handle crises and their media coverage

The adolescent does not always develop intellectual potential by staying in school. Students drop out of school for a variety of reasons.[180–182] Dropping out has many negative consequences, including unemployment, welfare dependency, and problems with the law. For example, providing special classrooms for the teen during pregnancy and after delivery so that she can bring the baby for daycare while she attends class is one way to prevent school dropouts in that population.

Sexual Harassment and Adolescent Bullying in School and with Peers

Sexual harassment is prevalent in schools and in the workplace in Canada. A 1994 study by the Ontario Secondary School Teachers' Federation reported that over 80 percent of young women and 45 percent of young men that were surveyed had been sexually harassed by another student, while 20 percent had been sexually harassed by school staff.[183] Some behaviours reported were having sexual rumours spread about oneself; being the recipient of gestures, jokes, or looks; or being called gay or lesbian. Tutty and Bradshaw state that some sexual harassment prevention programs are available as early as grade five; but most such programs are offered to high-school students. The goal of these programs is to increase knowledge about sexual harassment—how it affects individuals and the school community, what attitudes and dynamics support this problem, and what strategies can be used to cope with harassment.[184]

Approximately 23 percent of Canadian young people in grades six through ten reported that they had bullied others.[185] Those who bully are at risk for developing antisocial behaviour such as criminality in adulthood. Bullying, characterized as a negative physical or verbal action that has hostile intent, causes distress to victims, is repeated over a period of time, and involves a power differential between bullies and their victims.[186] The use of power and aggression early in life can form a basis for sexual harassment, dating aggression, domestic violence, and child or elder abuse. Adolescents vary in their involvement in bullying, and different levels of support and intervention are required. Students who bully would benefit from a prevention program that is directed at all students. Students who are involved, at least occasionally, in bullying may experience negative effects from their actions and they may require school intervention and mediation.[187]

CRITICAL THINKING

What information would you deem necessary for developing a prevention program for adolescents who bully?

Peer-Group Influences

The **peer group**, or *friends of the same age*, influences the adolescent to a greater extent than parents, teachers, popular heroes, religious leaders, or other adults. Because peer groups are so important, the adolescent has intense loyalty to them. Social relationships take precedence over family and counteract feelings of emptiness, isolation, and loneliness. Significance is attached to activities deemed important by peers. Peers serve as models or instructors for skills not yet acquired. Usually some peers are near the same cognitive level as the learner; their explanations may be more understandable. When student peers of varying cognitive levels discuss problems, less advanced students may gain insights and correct inaccuracies in thinking. The more advanced students also profit; they must think through their own reasoning to explain a concept.[188]

The *purposes* of the peer group include promoting:[189–192]

- A sense of acceptance, prestige, belonging, approval
- Opportunities for learning how to behave
- A sense of immediacy, concentrating on the here-and-now, what happened last night, who is doing what today, what homework is due tomorrow
- A reason for *being* today, a sense of *importance right now*, and not just dreams or fears about what he or she might become in some vague future time
- Opportunities to learn behaviour related to later adult roles
- Role models and relationships to help define personal identity as he or she adapts to a changing body image; more mature relationships with others, and heightened sexual feelings

---

11–2 BONUS SECTION IN CD-ROM

Psychosocial, School, and Parent Factors Associated with Smoking among Early Adolescent Boys and Girls

This is the first study to report an association between peer influence and smoking for boys. Positive parenting practices protect young people from smoking.

Peer-Group Dialect

This dialect is a communication pattern seen in the adolescent period. Slang is one of the trademarks of adolescence and may be considered a **peer-group dialect.** *It is a language that consists of coined terminology and of new or extended interpretations attached to traditional terms.*

Slang is used for various reasons. It provides a sense of belonging to the peer group and a small, compact vocabulary for a teenager who does not want to waste energy on words. Slang also excludes authority figures and other outsiders and permits expression of hostility, anger, and rebellion. Unknowing adults do not understand the digs given with well-timed pieces of slang. Other adults sense the flippancy of underlying feelings but to their chagrin can do little other than try to understand. By the time they learn the meanings of the current terms, new meanings have evolved.

You can help parents understand the purposes of teenage dialect and the importance of not trying to imitate or retaliate verbally. In addition, encourage parents to enter into discussion with their teenager to understand him or her and the teen-age dialect more fully.

Use of Leisure Time

Leisure time with the peer group is important for normal social development and adjustment. The adolescent spends an increasing amount of time away from home, either in school, in other activities, or with peers, as he or she successfully achieves greater independence. School is a social centre, even though abstract learning is a burden to some students. In school, students seek recognition from others and determine their status within the group, depending on success in scholastic, athletic, or other organizations and activities.

Dating Pattern

Dating is one use of leisure time and is influenced greatly by the peer group but also varies according to the culture and social class and religious and family beliefs. Dating prepares the adolescent for intimate bonds with others, marriage, and family life. The adolescent learns social skills in dealing with the opposite sex, in what situations and with whom he or she feels least and most comfortable, and what is expected sexually.

When dating begins, the emphasis is first on commonly shared activities. Later the emphasis includes a sharing, close relationship. Similarly, dating may start with groups of couples, move to double dates, and finally involve single couples. With each step, the adolescent learns more about and feels more comfortable with the opposite sex. He or she also learns personal acceptability to others. Going steady has become popular because it provides a readily available partner for social activities, but it can be detrimental if it stops the adolescent from searching for the qualities he or she wants in a future mate or involves date rape or sexual experimentation that he or she is unprepared to handle. Further the male is more likely to be the one to force regular sexual intercourse.[193]

Banister and her colleagues conducted an ethnographic study to explore the health-related concerns within dating relationships. Their sample consisted of 40 female adolescents aged 15 and 16.[194] The results, from a health care point of view, suggested that unequal power dynamics in their dating relationships place girls at a disadvantage with serious consequences for their health. Difficulty in expressing their needs and desires within the intimate relationship made the participants sensitive to social isolation, substance misuse, and individual and social tolerance of violence.[195] These researchers conclude that nursing professionals should seriously consider the value of providing health information and care to female adolescents in a group format. That is, nurses seem particularly suited to be able to establish the type of group environments in which adolescents feel safe to expose the high level of vulnerability they experience in their everyday life.

As you work with adolescents, assess the stage of peer-group development and dating patterns. A few years will make a

considerable difference in attitudes toward the opposite sex. *Build your teaching on current interests and attitudes.* The same age groups in different localities may also be in different stages. Adolescents from another culture may sharply contrast in pattern with North American adolescents. For example, in Egypt the male is not supposed to have any intimate physical contact with the female until marriage. In North America, certain physical contact is expected.

Leisure Activities

Sports, dancing, hobbies, reading, listening to the radio, CDs, tapes, or stereo, talking on the telephone, daydreaming, experimenting with hairstyles, cosmetics, or new clothes, and just loafing have been teenagers' favourite activities for decades. Riding the all-terrain vehicle or motorcycle, driving and working on cars, using the computer, watching television, playing video games, and attending movies and concerts are also popular. Political activism draws some youth; various causes rise and then fade in interest as the youth matures. "Everybody's doing it" is seemingly a strong influence on the adolescent's interests and activities. Others participate in activities, such as camera club, French club, or yearbook projects, because of personal talents or interests.

Many parents consider a party in the home for a group of teenagers a safe use of leisure time. This is undoubtedly true if parents and other adults are on the premises and can give guidance as needed and if the parents are not themselves supplying the teens with alcohol and drugs. The latter sometimes happens; however, parents rationalize by saying that they prefer their youngster to be at home (or at a friend's home) if they are using or abusing alcohol and drugs. They may even drive home teens who are unsafe to drive. Usually, however, drug and alcohol parties are hosted by teens when parents are out of town; teenagers chip in for beer for an "open" party (any number of people may attend). When behaviour becomes boisterous, police are often called by the neighbours, but they find the situation difficult to handle because there is no responsible authority figure on the premises. The police in one community give the following *guidelines to help parents and teens host and attend parties.* You may wish to share these suggestions with parents:

- Parents should set the ground rules before the party to express feelings and concerns about the party, ask who will attend and whether adults will be present, and learn what is expected of their adolescent. The address and phone number of the host should be known by the parents of the teens who are attending.
- Notify neighbours that you will be hosting a party, and encourage your teen to call or send a note to close neighbours notifying them of the party and asking them to let the family know if there is too much noise.
- Notify the police when planning a large party. They can protect you, your guests, and your neighbours. Discuss with the police an agreeable plan for guest parking.
- Plan to have plenty of food and nonalcoholic beverages on hand.
- Plan activities with your teenager before the party so that the party can end before guests become bored (three to four hours is suggested as sufficient party time).

- Limit party attendance and times. Either send out invitations or have the teenager personally invite guests beforehand. Discourage crashers; ask them to leave. Open-house parties are difficult for parents and teenagers to control. Set time limits for the party that enable guests to be home at a reasonable time, definitely before a legal curfew.

- A parent should be at home during the entire time of the party. The parent's presence helps keep the party running smoothly; it also gives the parent an opportunity to meet the teenager's friends. Invite other adults to help supervise.

- Decide what part of the house will be used for the party. Pick out where your guests will be most comfortable and you can maintain adequate supervision. Avoid having the bedroom area as part of the party area.

- Do not offer alcohol to guests under the age of 18 or allow guests to use drugs in your home. Be alert to the signs of alcohol or drug use.

- Do not allow any guest who leaves the party to return to discourage teenagers from leaving the party to drink or to use drugs elsewhere and then return to the party.

- Guests who try to bring alcohol or drugs or who otherwise refuse to cooperate with your expectations should be asked to leave. Notify the parents of any teenager who arrives at the party drunk or under the influence of any drug to ensure his or her safe transportation home. Do not let anyone drive under the influence of alcohol or drugs.

- Teenagers frequently have parties at homes when parents are away. Typically, the greatest problems occur when parents are not at home. Tell your neighbours when you are going to be out of town.

- Many parties occur spontaneously. Parents and teens should understand before the party that these guidelines are in effect at all parties. If, despite your precautions, things get out of hand, do not hesitate to call the local police department for help.

- Emphasize to parents the importance of their being role models through minimum drinking of alcoholic beverages or use of drugs.

The teenager may also feel more secure when the parent is actively interested in knowing where he or she will be and what he or she will be doing even though rebellion may ensue. Parents should be awake or have the teen awaken them when arriving home from a party. This is a good sharing time. Peers are important, but if peer activity and values are in opposition to what has been learned as acceptable, the adolescent feels conflict. Explore with parents the adolescent's need for constructive use of leisure time and the importance of participation in peer activities. You may be involved in implementing constructive leisure activities.

For some teenagers there is little leisure time. They may have considerable home responsibility, such as occurs in rural communities, or work to earn money to help support the family. Other youths are active in volunteer work. Ideally, the adolescent has some time free for personal pursuits, to stand around with friends, and to sit and daydream.

CRITICAL THINKING

What health promoting activities would you suggest are suitable for the adolescent during leisure time?

Emotional Development

Emotional Characteristics

Emotional characteristics of the personality cannot be separated from family, physical, intellectual, and social development. Emotionally, the adolescent is characterized by mood swings and extremes of behaviour (Table 11-1). Refer to the box entitled "Major Concerns of Teenagers"; these concerns contribute to emotional lability and identity confusion.[196–199] Emotional development requires an interweaving and organization of opposing tendencies into a sense of unity and continuity. This process occurs during adolescence in a complex and truly impressive way to move the person toward psychological maturity.

TABLE 11-1
Contrasting Emotional Responses of Adolescents

Independent Behaviours	Dependent Behaviours
Happy, easygoing, angry, loving, gregarious, self-confident, sense of humour	Sad, irritable, unloving, withdrawn, fearful, worried
Energetic, self-assertive, independent	Apathetic, passive, dependent
Questioning, critical or cynical of others	Strong allegiance to or idolization of others
Exhibitionistic or at ease with self	Excessively modest or self-conscious
Interested in logical or intellectual pursuits	Daydreaming, fantasizing
Cooperative, seeking responsibility, impatient to be involved or finish project	Rebellious, evading work, dawdling, ritualistic behaviour, dropout from society
Suggestible to outside influences, including ideologies	Unaccepting of new ideas
Desirous for adult privileges	Apprehensive about adult responsibilities

Major Concerns of Teenagers

- Their appearance
- Divorce of parents
- Having good marriage and family life
- School performance
- Choosing a career; finding steady employment
- Being successful in life
- Having strong friendships; how others will treat them
- Paying for university or college
- Making lots of money
- Finding purpose and meaning in life
- Contracting AIDS
- Drug and alcohol use by self, friends
- Hunger and poverty
- Societal violence

Sources: Bee, H., Lifespan Development (2nd ed.). New York: Longman, 1998; Gormly, A., Lifespan Human Development (6th ed.). Fort Worth: Harcourt Brace College Publishers, 1997; Newman, B., and P. Newman, Development Through Life: A Psychosocial Approach (7th ed.). Belmont, CA: Brooks/Cole, 1999; Papalia, D., S. Olds, and R. Feldman, Human Development (7th ed.). Boston: McGraw Hill, 1998.

Share this information with parents and the adolescent. Through using principles of communication and crisis intervention and through your use of self as a role model you will be able to help the adolescent work through identity diffusion and achieve a sense of ego identity and an appropriate sense of independence.

We regularly hear of the rebellious, emotionally labile, egocentric adolescent but do not stereotype all adolescents into that mould. Many, perhaps more than we know of, can delay gratification, behave as adults, and have positive relationships with family and authority figures.

Developmental Crisis

The psychosexual crisis of adolescence is identity formation versus identity diffusion: "Who am I?" "How do I feel?" "Where am I going?" "What meaning is there in life?" **Identity** means that an *individual believes he or she is a specific unique person;* he or she has emerged as an adult. **Identity formation** *results through synthesis of biopsychosocial characteristics from a number of sources, for example, earlier sex identity, parents, friends, social class, ethnic, religious, and occupational groups.*

A number of influences can interfere with identity formation:

- Telescoping of generations, with many adult privileges granted early so that the differences between adult and child are obscured and there is no ideal to which to aspire
- Contradictory value systems of individualism versus conformity in which both are highly valued and youth believe that adults advocate individualism but then conform
- Emphasis on sexual matters and encouragement to experiment without frank talking about sexuality with parents or significant caregivers

- Increasing emphasis on education for socioeconomic gain, which prolongs dependency on parents when the youth is physically mature
- Rapid changes in the adolescent subculture and all of society, with emphasis on conforming to peers.

CRITICAL THINKING

What may be other relevant influences that interfere with identity formation?

According to a recent worldwide survey of parents, children throughout the world have similar behaviour problems. The random sample consisted of 13 000 children, ages six to 17 years, in 12 countries: Australia, Belgium, China, Germany, Greece, Israel, Jamaica, the Netherlands, Puerto Rico, Sweden, Thailand, and the United States. Overall, geographical and cultural differences accounted for only 8% to 11% of individual differences in the scores. Puerto Rican and Jamaican children were more likely to internalize problems with anxiety, depression, and social withdrawal. American, German, and Swedish children were more likely to externalize problems by showing aggression, delinquency, and hyperactivity. In all cultures, boys showed more externalizing and had higher problem behaviours than girls.[200]

Identity formation implies an *internal stability, sameness, or continuity, which resists extreme change and preserves itself from oblivion in the face of stress or contradictions.* It implies emerging from this era with a sense of wholeness, knowing the self as a unique person, feeling responsibility, loyalty, and commitment to a value system. There are three types of identity, which are closely interwoven: (1) **personal,** or **real, identity**— *what the person believes self to be;* (2) **ideal identity**—*what he or she would like to be;* and (3) **claimed identity**—*what he or she wants others to think* he or she is.

Identity formation is enhanced by having support not only from parents but also from another significant adult who has a stable identity and who upholds sociocultural and moral standards of behaviour. If the adolescent has successfully coped with the previous developmental crisis and feels comfortable with personal identity, he or she will be able to appreciate the parents on a fairly realistic basis, seeing and accepting both their strengths and shortcomings. The values, beliefs, and guidelines they have given him or her are internalized. The adolescent needs parents less for direction and support; he or she must now decide what acceptable and unacceptable behaviour really is.

Students from different ethnic and racial backgrounds have unique needs and ways of adapting to stressors and unique aspects of the developmental crisis of identity formation. Some may feel isolated and alienated in relation to mainstream culture values. Parents, teachers, and health care professionals can help these teens work through values and cognitive and emotional conflicts.

Identity diffusion *results if the adolescent fails to achieve a sense of identity.* He or she feels self-conscious and has doubts and confusion about self as a human being and his or her roles in life. With identity diffusion, he or she feels impotent, insecure, disillusioned, and alienated. Identity diffusion is manifested in other ways as well, as listed in the box entitled

"Negative Consequences of Identity Diffusion." The real danger of identity diffusion looms when a youth finds a negative solution to the quest for identity. He or she gives up, feels defeated, and pursues antisocial behaviour because "it's better to be bad than nobody at all." Identity diffusion is more likely to occur if the teenager has close contact with an adult who is still confused about personal identity and who is in rebellion against society.

Negative Consequences of Identity Diffusion

- Feels she or he is losing grip on reality
- Feels fragmented; lacks unity, consistency, or predictability with self
- Feels impatient but is unable to initiate action
- Gives up easily on a task; feels defeated
- Vacillates in decision making; is unable to act on decisions
- Is unable to delay gratification
- Appears brazen or arrogant, sarcastic
- Is disorganized and inconsistent in behaviour; avoids tasks
- Fears losing uniqueness in entering adulthood; displays regressive behaviour; acts out behavioural extremes to attract attention
- Has low self-esteem, negative self-concept, low aspirations
- Is unable to pursue academic or career plans; may drop out of school
- Isolates self from peers; is unable to relate to former friends or significant adults
- Feels cynical, disillusioned, excessively angry or suspicious
- Engages in antisocial or illegal behaviour; acts out sexually
- Seeks association with gang, cult, or negative community or media leader

The identity-seeking processes are even more diffused or abnormal if the child has encountered repeated stresses, such as abuse, neglect, or terror. Such experiences cause physical changes in the brain. The steady flood of stress chemicals keeps the person in a fight–flight pattern of behaviour (see Chapter 5), which results in the impulsive aggression that is seen in some teens. Any stimulus can increase the level of stress hormones and reaction, because the nervous system is highly reactive to anything perceived as a stressor. If parents and other adults are not available, supportive, or empathic, the youth may decide to "take things" into his or her own hands.[201,202]

In the process of achieving identity and committing to goals in life, the person may have experienced **identity moratorium,** a *time of making no decisions but a rethinking of values and goals,* which is part of identity crisis and a step beyond *identity diffusion,* when *the person has not begun to examine his or her own life's meaning and goals.* In some cultures, identity formation is not a task for the individual. Rather, **identity foreclosure** exists: *the goals, values, and life tasks have been established by the parents and the group, and the individual is not allowed to question or examine them. He or she is expected to follow the pattern set by the elders;* usually the roles are related to sex and socioeconomic or caste status.

Help parents to work with the adolescent who feels identity diffusion. Emphasize that parents must never give up trying to form a loving bond with offspring, showing attention and empathy and stimulating participation and emotional feelings in the teen, whether they are a nuclear, stepparent, or single-parent family. *Refer parents to counselling services* when needed to overcome the teen's neurological and behavioural vulnerability, just as you would refer patients to an allergist for asthma.

CRITICAL THINKING

Acne may cause an adolescent considerable amount of stress. What are ways you can help an adolescent to maintain the quest for his or her identity until acne therapy is successful?

Self-Concept and Body Image Development

Development of self-concept and body image is closely akin to cognitive organization of experiences and identity formation. The adolescent cannot be viewed only in the context of the present; earlier experiences have an impact that continues to affect him or her. The earlier experiences that were helpful enabled the adolescent to feel good about the body and self. If the youngster enters adolescence feeling negative about self or the body, this will be a difficult period.

Jungwee Park examined factors associated with adolescent self-concept and the impact of adolescent self-concept on psychological and physical health and health behaviours in young adulthood.[203] The data came from the household cross-sectional (1994–95) and longitudinal (1994–95 to 2000–01) components of Statistics Canada's National Population Health Survey. A portion of the results indicated that self-concept tends to be low among girls compared with boys; and a strong self-concept has a positive long-term effect on girls' perceived health.[204] Is it surprising to you that, cross-sectionally in the same study, the adolescent self-concept was associated with household income and emotional support?

Various factors influence the adolescent's self-concept, including:[205–207]

1. Age of maturation
2. Degree of attractiveness
3. Name or nickname
4. Size and physique appropriate to sex
5. Degree of identification with the same-sex parent
6. Level of aspiration and ability to reach ideals
7. Peer relationships
8. Culture

The rapid growth of the adolescent period is an important factor in body image revision. Girls and boys are sometimes described as "all legs." They are often clumsy and awkward. Because the growth changes cannot be denied, the adolescent is forced to alter the mental picture of self to function. Physical changes in height, weight, and body build cause a change in self-perception to the adolescent. To some male adolescents, the last chance to get taller is very significant.

The body is part of one's inner and outer world. Many of the experiences of the inner world are based on stimuli from the external world, especially from the body surface. Therefore the adolescent focuses attention on body surface. He or she spends a great deal of time in front of mirrors and in body hygiene rituals, grooming, and clothing. These are normal ways for the early adolescent to integrate a changing body image. If the teen does not seem to care about appearance, he or she may have already decided, "I'm so ugly, so what's the use?"

If the adolescent does have a disability or defect, peers and adults may react with fear, pity, revulsion, or curiosity. The adolescent may retain and later reflect these impressions, as a person tends to perceive self as others perceive him or her. If the adolescent develops a negative self-image, motivation, behaviour, and eventual lifestyle may also be inharmonious and out of step with social expectations.

By late adolescence, self-image is complete, self-esteem should be high, and self-concept should have stabilized. The person feels autonomous but no longer believes he or she is so unique that no one has ever experienced what he or she is currently experiencing. The older adolescent no longer believes everyone is watching or being critical of his or her physical or personality characteristics. Egocentricity has declined. Interactions with the opposite sex are more comfortable, although awareness of sex is keen.

Your understanding of the importance of the value the adolescent places on self can help you work with the adolescent, parents, teachers, and community leaders. Your goal is to avoid building a false self-image in the adolescent; rather, help him or her evaluate strengths and weaknesses, accept the weaknesses, and build on the strengths. You will have to listen carefully to the adolescent's statements about self and his or her sense of future. You will have to sense when you might effectively speak and work with him or her and when silence is best. Share an understanding of influencing factors on body image and self-concept development with parents, teachers, and other adults so that they can positively influence adolescents.

You may wish to use a therapeutic group such as reality therapy or rational thinking group, using cognitive restructuring exercises to help adolescents think more positively about themselves and reduce anxiety. Small group sessions outside the regular classroom have been found effective in enhancing self-concepts of junior high students. Group sessions can focus on personal and social awareness and how to cope with age-related problems.

CRITICAL THINKING

Observe adolescents at a movie theatre or shopping mall. What actions do you see that denote the adolescents are struggling to gain self-identity?

Sexual Development

Sexuality *encompasses not only the individual's physical characteristics and the act of sexual intercourse but also the following:* (1) *search for identity as a whole person,* including a sexual person; (2) *role behaviour of men and women;* (3) *attitudes,* *behaviours, and feelings toward self, each sex, and sexual behaviour;* (4) *relationships, affection, and caring between people;* (5) *the need to touch and be touched;* and (6) *recognition and acceptance of self and others as sexual beings.*[208,209] One of the greatest concerns to the adolescent is sexual feelings and activities. Because of hormonal and physiologic changes and environmental stimuli, the adolescent is almost constantly preoccupied with feelings of developing sexuality.

Sexual desire is under the domination of the cerebral cortex. Differences in sexual desire exist in young males and females, and desire is influenced by cultural and family expectations for sexual performance. The female experiences a more generalized pleasurable response to erotic stimulation; but she does not necessarily desire coitus. The male experiences a stronger desire for coitus because of a localized genital sensation in response to erotic stimulation, which is accompanied by production of spermatozoa and secretions from accessory glands that build up pressure and excite the ejaculatory response. The male is stimulated to seek relief by ejaculation.[210,211]

Menarche is experienced by the girl as an affectively charged event related to her emerging identity as an adult woman with reproductive ability. Menarche may be perceived as frightening and shameful by some girls; previous factual sex education does not necessarily offset such feelings. Often information in classes is not assimilated because of high anxiety in the girl during the class. Often the girl will seek advice from her mother regarding menarche (see the Interesting Websites section at the end of this chapter).

Family and cultural traditions are needed to mark the menarche as a transition from childhood to adulthood. Menarche is anticipated as an important event, but in North America no formal customs mark it, and no obvious change in the girl's social status occurs. The girl may get little help from her mother, other female adults, or peers in working through feelings related to menarche. Often menses is perceived as an excretory function, and advertisements treat it as a disease.

Nocturnal emissions are often a great concern for the boys but are also a sign of manhood.

Both sexes are concerned about development and appearance of secondary sex characteristics, their overall appearance, their awkwardness, and their sex appeal, or lack of it.

The most common form of sexual outlet for both sexes, but especially males, is **masturbation,** *which is the manipulation of the genitals for sexual stimulation.* Public education about the normality of masturbation is reducing guilt about the practice and fears of mental or physical illness.

Intercourse is increasing among adolescents. Premarital sexual activity is often used as a means to get close, sometimes with strangers, and may result in feelings of guilt, remorse, anxiety, and self-recrimination. The feelings associated with the superficial act may be damaging to the adolescent's self-concept and possibly to later success in a marital relationship. Adolescent males and females often report that the initial coitus was not pleasurable. The number of pregnant teenage females who are not marrying is significantly increasing, which has implications for the future care and well-being of the baby and implications for future intimate relations of the teenage girl. A wide variety of sexual experience before marriage may cause the person to feel bored with a single partner later.[212]

Evans and her colleagues assessed 539 teens in one Ontario city to identify knowledge about and use of birth control, comfort in discussing sexual health, and preferred sites, providers, and methods of service delivery. They concluded that becoming sexually active and using birth control appears to be maturational. Since teens were not comfortable talking with teachers, mall-based clinics may provide an alternative service for teens that require information about sexual activity and birth control.[213]

Canada focuses on enhancing sexual health and reducing sexual problems among various groups, including adolescents. The *Canadian Guidelines for Sexual Health Education*, published by the authority of the Minister of Health, are intended to unite and guide individuals and professionals working in the area of sexual health education and health promotion.[214] These guidelines are grounded in evidence-based research within a Canadian context.

CRITICAL THINKING

A shy 14-year-old girl you are caring for in a hospital setting informs you that she is concerned because she has not menstruated yet. How would you counsel her?

Other countries are also having their problems with teenage sexuality. Recently, however, Western permissiveness has crept in, especially among the teenagers in the larger cities. Pregnancy among girls from 14 to 18, with a rash of self-induced abortions, has caused leaders to insist on some sex education for their youth. Small pilot programs, sponsored jointly by government and church groups in connection with African educators, are making some impact at the secondary-education level.

Adaptive Mechanisms

The **ego** is the *sum total of those mental processes that maintain psychic cohesion and reality contact; it is the mediator between the inner impulses and outer world.* It is that part of the personality that becomes integrated and strengthened in adolescence and has the following functions:

- Associating concepts or situations that belong together but are historically remote or spatially separated
- Developing a realization that one's way of mastering experience is a variant of the group's way and is acceptable
- Subsuming contradictory values and attitudes
- Maintaining a sense of unity and centrality of self
- Testing perceptions and selecting memories
- Reasoning, judging, and planning
- Mediating among impulses, wishes, and actions and integrating feelings
- Choosing meaningful stimuli and useful conditions
- Maintaining reality

When a strong ego exists, the person can do all these tasks. He or she has entered adulthood psychologically. Adolescence provides the experiences necessary for such maturity.

Ego changes occur in the adolescent because of broadening social involvement, deepening intellectual pursuits, close peer activity, rapid physical growth, and social role changes, all of which cause frustrations at times. **Frustration** is the *feeling of helplessness and anxiety that results when one is prevented from getting what one wants.* Adaptive mechanisms leading to resolution of frustration and reconciling personal impulses with social expectations are beneficial because they permit the self to settle dissonant drives and to cope with strong feelings.[213] All adaptive mechanisms permit one to develop a self, an identity, and to defend the self-image against attack. These mechanisms are harmful only when one pattern is used to the exclusion of others for handling many diverse situations or when several mechanisms are used persistently to cope with a single situation. Such behaviour is defensive rather than adaptive, distorts reality, and indicates emotional disturbance.

The adaptive mechanisms used in adolescence are the same ones used (and defined) in previous developmental eras, although they now may be used in a different way. *Compensation,* a form of compromise, *sublimation,* and *identification* are particularly useful because they often improve interaction with others. They are woven into the personality to make permanent character changes, and they help the person reach appropriate goals.

Teach parents that adaptive abilities of the adolescent are strongly influenced by inner resources built up through the years of parental love, esteem, and guidance. The parents' use of adaptive mechanisms and general mental health will influence the offspring. Are the parents living a double standard? Has the teenager seen the parents enjoy a job well done or is financial reward the key issue? Do the parents covertly wish the teenager to act out what they could never do?

Even with mature and nurturing parents, the adolescent will at times find personal adaptive abilities taxed. But the chances for channelling action-oriented energy and idealism through acceptable adaptive behaviour are much greater if parents set a positive example.

Moral–Spiritual Development

According to Kohlberg,[215] the adolescent probably is in the conventional level most of the time; however, the adolescent may at times show behaviour appropriate to the second stage of the preconventional level or the first stage of the postconventional level.

The early adolescent typically is in the conformist stage; structure and order of society take on meaning for the person, and rules are followed because they exist (analogous to Kohlberg's conventional level). The late adolescent is in the conscientious stage, in which the person develops a set of principles for self that is used to guide personal ideals, actions, and achievements. Rational thought becomes important to personal growth (analogous to Kohlberg's postconventional level, stage 1). The young adolescent must examine parental moral and religious verbal standards against practice and decide if they are worth incorporating into his or her own life. He or she may appear to discard standards of behaviour previously accepted, although basic parental standards likely will be maintained. In addition, he or she must compare the religious versus the scientific views. Although moral-spiritual views of sensitivity, caring, and commitment may be prevalent in family teaching, the North American adolescent is also a part of the scientific, technologic, industrial society that emphasizes achievement, fragmentation, and regimentation. Often adolescents will identify with one of the two philosophies. These two views can be satisfactorily combined, but only with sufficient time and experience, which the adolescent has not had.

Gilligan has found a difference between adolescent males and females in moral reasoning. Males organize social relationships in a hierarchical order and subscribe to a morality of rights. Females value interpersonal connectedness, care, sensitivity, and responsibility to others. Thus, adolescent males and females view the dating relationship differently and approach aggressive or violent situations from a different perspective.[216] Other authors describe how our society interferes with development of moral standards or behaviour so that neither Kohlberg's nor Gilligan's theory seems applicable.[217–225]

If the adolescent matures in religious belief, he or she must comprehend abstractions. Often when he or she is capable of the first religious insights, the negativism tied with rebellion to authority prevents this experience.

Help parents and adolescents realize that the adolescent who does find strength in the supernatural, who can rely on a power greater than self, can find much consolation in this turbulent period of awkward physical and emotional growth. If he or she can pray for help, ask forgiveness, and believe he or she receives both, a more positive self-image develops. In this period of clique and group dominance, the church is a place to meet friends, to share recreation and fellowship, and to sense a belonging difficult to find in some large high schools. Several authors discuss the importance of parents and teachers: their faith, prayers, and efforts to focus on spiritual and moral formation, not just physical and intellectual development.[226,227]

Recent experiments show that a Socratic approach, which promotes moral development and clarifies values, produces fruitful results that have not been achieved by simply handing down rules of conduct. You can be instrumental in working with parents and teachers to use the Socratic approach and other value clarification exercises.

CRITICAL THINKING

How can you engage an adolescent to talk openly about his or her belief system?

Late Adolescence: Transition Period to Young Adulthood

In some cultures parents select schooling, occupations, and the marriage partner for their offspring. North American adolescents, however, are usually free to make some or all of these decisions.

By the time the teen is in grade 11 or 12, he or she should be thinking about the future. There are many options: whether to pursue a mechanical or academic job; to attend some form of higher education; to live at home or elsewhere; to travel; to marry soon, later, or not at all; to have children soon, later, or

not at all. Answers to these questions will influence the adolescent's transition into young adulthood.

Establishing a Separate Residence

This step is one marker of reaching young adulthood. The late adolescent often spends less time at home and prepares for separation from parents. If there is intense intrafamily conflict, if the adolescent feels unwanted, or if the adolescent is still struggling with dependence on parents or identity diffusion, a different mode of separation may occur.

In an effort to find self and think about the future or to escape abuse, incest, or other home problems, the adolescent may become either a walkaway or a runaway. The **teen walkaway** *leaves home before finishing high school or before reaching legal age; however, parents generally know where the child is and are resigned to the child's new living arrangements.* The **teen runaway** *leaves home without overt notice and his or her whereabouts are unknown to parents, friends, or police.* Some who walk away may continue high school or get some type of job while living with relatives, friends, or a boyfriend or girlfriend. The problem with the walkaway is that the adolescent can achieve developmental tasks better in a stable family situation in which parents continue to give support and assist him or her as necessary while treating the offspring in an adult manner. If the newly found living situation is unstable or emotionally unsupportive or if the adolescent has no means of financial support, he or she may be forced into prostitution or juvenile offences.

You may have an opportunity to discuss residence situations with the adolescent. If you can get to the person before he or she walks or runs away, help him or her consider the intolerability of parental demands and the family situation. Discuss alternative ways of handling the problem. You may contact a high-school counsellor or potential employer. Although either the walkaway or runaway situation should be avoided if possible, the teen should be encouraged to report incest or abuse so that the teen's parents and other siblings can receive proper therapy and an appropriate, healthy living situation can be found for the teen.

Health care is a problem for adolescent runaways. Health concerns include pregnancy, sexually transmitted infections, prostitution, alcohol abuse, and child maltreatment and incest. The following intervention strategies should be instituted when they are in treatment:

1. Clarification of the health care provider's attitudes and values
2. Establishment of trust
3. Use of effective interviewing skills
4. Ability to provide maximum medical treatment and information when the client presents self for care
5. Establishment of foundations for future interactions and care

Career Selection

This selection has often been haphazard. High-school counsellors often do more record keeping than realistic guiding toward career choices. Often youth are influenced by parental wishes or friends' choices. Because of changes in societal role expectations for men and women, jobs or postsecondary study programs that were once considered exclusively "male" or "female" are now open to both. Although these changes are positive, understand that the selection is more varied and thus more confusing to adolescents. You can guide them to testing resources in which their skills and interests are measured and jobs are recommended. You may direct them to members of various professions who can tell them about their jobs

Occupation represents much more than a set of skills and functions; it is a way of life. Occupation provides and determines much of the physical and social environment in which a person lives, his or her status within the community, and a pattern for living. Occupational choice is usually a function or a reflection of the entire personality, but the occupation, in turn, plays a part in shaping the personality by providing associates, roles, goals, ideals, mores, lifestyle, and perhaps even a spouse.

For many youth the university years are a time to consider various careers, to decide what type of people to associate with and imitate, and to measure self against others with similar aspirations.

Although university or college attendance and the pursuit of a profession are still the ideal of many, growing emphasis and opportunity exist for vocational and technical training. Many will enter jobs right out of high school.

You can be a key person in helping adolescents clarify values and attitudes related to occupational selection and in talking with parents about their concerns.

Defining a Self-Identity

Emotional and moral–spiritual development may take on a special significance if the adolescent period is extended into the 20s because of a vocational or university education. Instead of settling into the tasks coexistent with a partnership, job, and family, the adolescent has a period in which a great deal of thinking can be accomplished. He or she has passed the physically awkward stage so that time and energy formerly spent in making the transition into physical adulthood can be turned toward philosophy of life and self-awareness.

Developmental Tasks

The following developmental tasks should be met by the end of adolescence:

- Accepting the changing body size, shape, and function and understanding the meaning of physical maturity
- Learning to handle the body in a variety of physical skills and to maintain good health
- Achieving a satisfying and socially accepted feminine or masculine role, recognizing how these roles have similarities and distinctions
- Finding the self as a member of one or more peer groups and developing skills in relating to a variety of people, including those of the opposite sex
- Achieving independence from parents and other adults while maintaining an affectionate relationship with them

- Selecting an occupation in line with interests and abilities (although the choice of occupation may later change) and preparing for economic independence
- Preparing to settle down, frequently for marriage and family life or for a close relationship with another, by developing a responsible attitude, acquiring needed knowledge, making appropriate decisions, and forming a relationship based on love rather than infatuation
- Developing the intellectual and work skills and social sensitivities of a competent citizen
- Desiring and achieving socially responsible behaviour in the cultural setting
- Developing a workable philosophy, a mature set of values, and worthy ideals and assuming standards of morality

How you interact with the adolescent or teach other adults to interact with him or her, will contribute to the adolescent's maturity.

CRITICAL THINKING

What may be some good developmental tasks for an adolescent who is mentally challenged?

HEALTH CARE AND NURSING APPLICATIONS

Scope of the Health Care and Nursing Role

Your role in caring for the adolescent may be many-faceted. An assessment is needed; knowledge from this chapter and relationship and communication principles described in Chapter 5 may be useful in gaining information from a client or family who may be hesitant to disclose about self. *Nursing diagnoses* that may be applicable to the adolescent are listed in the box entitled "Selected Nursing Diagnoses Related to the Adolescent." Wellness diagnoses should also be developed to reinforce motivational levels of the adolescent positively. Interventions that may involve direct care to the ill adolescent or that involve various health promotion measures are described in the previous or following sections.

A mature and maturing body and an immature emotional state make the adolescent a source of misunderstanding, fear, and laughter. Mood swings, rebellious behaviour, and adherence to colourful fads baffle many adults, who then cannot look beyond the superficial behaviour to identify health needs. Yet health care needs of today's adolescents are great.

Many adolescent girls become pregnant each year, and many adolescents will run away from home. A significant number of youths will die from motor vehicle and other accidents, unintended gunshot wounds, and homicide and suicide.[228] Other health problems abound, including sexually transmitted infections, substance abuse, chronic illness, and obesity and nutritional deficiency (the latter two previously discussed). Although the scope of this book does not allow discussion of needs assessment and intervention for adolescents

Selected Nursing Diagnoses Related to the Adolescent

Pattern 1: Exchanging

Altered Nutrition: More than Body Requirements
Altered Nutrition: Less than Body Requirements
Altered Nutrition: Risk for More than Body Requirements
Risk for Infection
Risk for Injury
Risk for Trauma
Impaired Skin Integrity
Altered Dentition

Pattern 2: Communicating

Impaired Verbal Communication

Pattern 3: Relating

Impaired Social Interaction
Social Isolation
Risk for Loneliness
Altered Family Processes
Altered Sexuality Patterns

Pattern 4: Valuing

Spiritual Distress
Potential for Enhanced Spiritual Well-Being

Pattern 5: Choosing

Ineffective Individual Coping
Impaired Adjustment
Defensive Coping
Ineffective Denial
Decisional Conflict
Health-Seeking Behaviours

Pattern 6: Moving

Activity Intolerance
Fatigue
Sleep Pattern Disturbance
Diversional Activity Deficit
Altered Growth and Development

Pattern 7: Perceiving

Body Image Disturbance
Self-Esteem Disturbance
Chronic Low Self-Esteem
Situational Low Self-Esteem
Personal Identity Disturbance
Sensory/Perceptual Alterations
Hopelessness
Powerlessness

Pattern 8: Knowing

Knowledge Deficit

Pattern 9: Feeling

Pain
Dysfunctional Grieving
Anticipatory Grieving
Risk for Violence: Directed at Others
Risk for Violence: Self-Directed
Post-Trauma Response
Anxiety
Fear

Other NANDA diagnoses are applicable to the ill adolescent.

Source: North American Nursing Diagnosis Association, NANDA Nursing Diagnoses Definitions & Classification 1999–2000. Philadelphia: North American Nursing Diagnosis Association, 1999.

with physical disabilities, you may wish to consult several authors for information.[229–232]

Health Promotion and Health Protection

Immunizations

Your actions and teaching in relation to immunizations are important for the teenager's health now and in the adult years.

Immunizations are a part of health protection for the adolescent, although they may be overlooked during that time of life. You should take a careful health history

The first priority is to ensure that children receive the recommended series of doses, including the school leaving dose at 14 to 16 years of age.[233] See Table 7-6 on page 328 for immunization schedules at different ages. Physicians play an extremely important role in the identification of individuals in need of immunization.

According to the Canadian Nurses Association, immunizations are a way of exercising our immune systems, triggering what is already there to fight against disease. Within the primary health care approach to nursing, nurses know that disease prevention, coupled with health promotion practices, is the best way to achieve a healthy population.[234]

CRITICAL THINKING

Bob is an adolescent who tells you that vaccines cause many harmful side effects, illnesses, and even death; how will you respond to Bob?

NARRATIVE VIGNETTE
Wellness Diagnosis

In your class today, on health promotion through the life span, you are discussing the importance of wellness diagnoses being incorporated into nursing care plans. During the lively discussion the main focus comes to centre on assessing a combination of the client's strengths, concerns, and lifestyle patterns because such an approach provides the nurse with a foundation upon which to develop a variety of interventions to enhance health and wellness. For your assignment, you are given a case study of Roland. You are asked to respond to the questions immediately.

Case Study

You are the school nurse and are expected to see each student. Roland is a 16-year-old who is taking drama in high school.

He wants to be an actor. One member of the small group of friends he socializes with a lot is a girl in whom he has a growing interest. Roland really wants to ask this girl for a date. He is becoming tidier in his personal hygiene and appearance. Roland knows a lot about computers and he is even thinking of becoming a computer programmer—until the right acting job comes up. He spends much time reading about different computers and software.

Questions

1. What two assessment questions will you ask Roland?
2. Develop two wellness nursing diagnoses for Roland.

Nurses do have opportunities to work with adolescents who are well.[235] It is necessary that wellness diagnoses be developed in order to guide care that focuses on strengths of the adolescent client rather than on problems only.

Safety Promotion and Accident Prevention

In Canada, injuries are the biggest contributors to premature death among the on-reserve First Nations population, at a rate of four times that of the general Canadian population.[236] Injuries are one of the most prominent health problems that young people face during their school-aged years, and they are the leading cause of death among youth.[237] It is interesting to note that diverse activities are associated with injuries among youth. However, the results of a recent survey demonstrate clearly that sports are the cause of injuries in all grades and for both genders.[238] Team contact sports (such as hockey and football), noncontact sports (such as basketball), and individual sports (such as cycling) can often lead to serious injuries. Improving the safety of school and sports-related environments and enhancing first aid are necessary.[239]

CRITICAL THINKING

As a health professional, how can you advocate for the safety of sports-related environments?

Accidents, homicide, and suicide are responsible for approximately 75% of all deaths between the ages of 15 and 24; the incidence is higher for males. *Motor vehicle accidents* account for nearly half of the deaths of adolescents between the ages of 16 and 19 (over 30% of all deaths in persons 15 to 24 years). Motor vehicle accidents are more common among young drivers who use alcohol, marijuana, and other drugs while driving.[240–246] One of the biggest adolescent–parent hurdles comes with learning to drive. The adolescent needs to learn this skill; yet the arguments between parents and their children concerning how to drive, what vehicle to drive, and

where to go or not to go often keep parents in a state of anxiety and children in a state of rebellion.

Head and spinal cord injuries, skeletal injuries, abrasions, and burns may all result from an accident involving a car, motorcycle, motor scooter, moped, all-terrain vehicle, snowmobile, mini-bike/motor scooter, or from the work site.[247] Sports-related accidents such as drowning; football, hockey, gymnastic, and soccer injuries; and firearm mishaps are also common. Contusions, dislocations, sprains, strains, overuse syndromes, and stress fractures occur frequently.[248,249] In the adolescent, the epiphyses of the skeletal system have not yet closed, and the extremities are poorly protected by stabilizing musculature. These two physical factors, combined with poor coordination and imperfect sport skills, probably account for the numerous injuries.[250]

In the United States, homicide is the second leading cause of death in the 15- to 24-year-old group and is the leading cause of death among non-Caucasian youths in this age group. Handguns are the most frequently used weapons.[251,252] Use of weapons in schools is a national concern, but intentional injury and death to others as a leisure activity, with no remorse involved, is a way of life for some adolescent criminals.[253–258]

Suicide, the third leading cause of death, is discussed later in this chapter. (Non-motor-vehicle injuries are the fourth leading cause of death.)[259,260]

As a group, adolescents represent one of the nation's largest underserved populations. Characteristic feelings and behaviours contribute to many of the health problems and must be considered in assessment and care.

A review of the leading causes of mortality and morbidity among teens shows that nearly all contributory behaviours can be categorized into the following seven areas:[261]

1. Heightened sense of sensation-seeking and risk-taking
2. Behaviours that result in unintentional and intentional injuries
3. Drug and alcohol use

4. Tobacco use
5. Sexual behaviours that cause sexually transmitted diseases, including HIV infection, and unintended pregnancies
6. Inadequate physical activity
7. Dietary patterns that cause disease

Safety Education

As an informed citizen in the community or in relation to your job, you can initiate and teach in safety programs with the school, church, clinic, industry, Red Cross, or other civic organizations. If you do not teach, you can insist on qualified and objective instruction. Safety courses, including driver education, knowledge of safety programs in the community, instruction in water safety, routine safety practices, and emergency care measures should be required for every adolescent. Many accidents and deaths could be avoided if the adolescent were better equipped to handle the new freedom.

Parents and youths should be informed about the risks, the exercise, and prestige value involved with certain sports and privileges. The importance of a physical examination before participation and how to prevent sports injuries should be emphasized.[262]

Because of the sports activities in which adolescents are involved, they may sometimes experience musculoskeletal chest pain, minor strains or sprains to a joint, and minor ankle strain. You should know how to advise for these conditions.

Musculoskeletal chest pain *arises from the bony structures of the rib cage and upper-limb girdle, along with the related skeletal muscles.* Age does not automatically rule out heart-related problems. Although musculoskeletal pain is usually aggravated by activity that involves movement or pressure on the chest cage rather than by general exertion (such as stair climbing), a thorough lung and cardiac examination is merited. Applying heat to the area (unless it is a fresh injury), resting the area, and taking an antipyretic can be recommended.[263]

Minor strains and sprains to a joint involve a *mild trauma that results in minimal stretching of involved ligaments and contusion of the surrounding tissues.* The treatment is known as RICE: rest, ice, compression, elevation of the affected joint. Use an ice pack for 24 to 36 hours; local heat can then be used if needed. Because of the risk of Reyes Syndrome, Tylenol (acetaminophen), if tolerated, can be used for its analgesic and anti-inflammatory effects.[264]

A **minor ankle sprain** involving *stretching of the ligament without tearing* can be treated in the same way as minor strains and sprains with the addition of an elastic bandage and possibly keeping weight off the ankle longer than 24 to 36 hours through the use of crutches.[265]

Common Health Problems: Prevention and Treatment

Health care for the adolescent includes attention to a schedule of health screening measures, immunizations, counselling, and high-risk categories. Several references describe how to conduct physical assessments with the adolescent.[266–273]

In addition to the hazards of accidents, teenage pregnancy, and obesity, other health problems are also apparent among adolescents. Table 11-2 summarizes definitions, symptoms and signs, and prevention and treatment for common conditions.[274–276] Discuss prevention of these problems with adolescents and parents.

Neoplasms, both benign and malignant, are a major cause of death.[277] Females exposed to diethylstilbestrol (DES) in utero should be watched closely for adenocarcinoma of the vagina. Males exposed to DES in utero have an increase in urinary tract abnormalities and a higher incidence of infertility.[278] Dysplasia of the cervix, a precursor of cervical carcinoma, is a sexually transmitted disease that is occurring with increased frequency in adolescent females. Sexually active females should receive annual Pap smears and be taught breast self-examination. Testicular cancer, Hodgkin's disease, and certain bone cancers are not uncommon in this age group.[279,280] Males should be taught testicular self-examination.

Allergic dermatitis, cysts, and keloid formation of the earlobes are also seen with more frequency, as ear piercing has become popular. Inner ear damage from exposure to rock music is increasing and can be assessed by pure tone audiometry. The adolescent is also subject to postural defects, fatigue, anemia, and respiratory problems.

Chronic Illness in Adolescents

Chronically ill children constitute increasing numbers of those who are hospitalized, and advances in technology and medical practice also enable some children and adults to live longer with chronic conditions. With some chronic illnesses, such as diabetes, the issues may revolve around mealtime routines, adherence to medication or treatment schedules, daily bodily care, use of the family car, family rules, and being on one's own at parties. Death is not imminent; a change in lifestyle for the entire family is. The family unit, with its unique parenting style, marital satisfaction, and parental self-esteem, will have an impact on the offspring. Illness brings the stress of pain, body mutilation, and body image changes and possible death. Chronic illness adds stressors: lifestyle changes, dependency on others, developmental delay, failure to master expected social roles and developmental tasks, a drain on emotional resources, disruption of the family system, and financial difficulties.[281,282]

Adolescents have a particularly difficult time dealing emotionally with chronic illness because they feel different from and set apart from peers, may have fewer peer relationships and activities in which they can participate; and thereby have a disruption of the social support system. Psychosocial problems can lead to social disabilities that far outweigh the effects of the physical illness.[283–285]

Positive coping in the ill adolescent is associated with independent behaviours, peer contact, school achievement, and participation in normalization activities. Negative coping centres around fear, withdrawal, regression, use of symptoms for secondary gain in various ways, and low self-esteem.[286–288]

Mothers tend to bear the brunt of caring for the chronically ill child. Usually mothers, rather than fathers, suffer loss of

TABLE 11-2
Common Health Problems of Adolescents

Problem	Definition	Symptoms/Signs	Prevention/Treatment
Hordeolum (stye)	Localized infection of sebaceous gland on eyelid margin	Painful, reddened swelling on eyelid; sometimes drainage	Apply hot compresses. Administer antibiotic drops.
Epistaxis (nose bleed)	Spontaneous bleeding from nose caused by ruptured blood vessel	Bleeding from nose	Prevent dry and cracking nasal mucosa by keeping humidity level sufficient. If nose bleeds, sit with head slightly forward and pinch nostrils for at least 15 minutes. Use cold compresses.
Acne vulgaris	Comedones, pimples, and cysts formed from increased activity of sebaceous glands	"Blackheads," "whiteheads," and additional lesions, especially on face, chest, back	Use good hygiene techniques and cleansing agents. Apply topical preparations. Administer oral medications.
Dental caries and gingivitis	Decay of teeth and disease of gums	Broken, dark teeth; bleeding inflamed gums	Use good dental hygiene. Check periodically with a dental hygienist for education and treatment.
Aphthous stomatitis	Recurrent small painful ulcers in the oral mucosa, "canker sores"; unknown etiology, *not* herpes simplex	Burning and tingling before eruption; recurrent painful lesions from 1 to 10 mm; oval, shallow, light yellow or grey with erythematous border	Prevention: None is known. Use Kenalog in Orabase or other topical anaesthetic. Use tetracycline/Benadryl mouthwash.
Tinea cruris	Ringworm of the groin, "jock itch," superficial fungal infection of the groin	Rash and soreness on groin and inner aspects of thighs; may include scrotum, gluteal folds, buttocks	Eliminate sources of heat and friction. Bathe daily; dry thoroughly. Wear cotton underwear. Use antifungal cream and Domeboro solution compresses.
Tinea pedis (athlete's foot)	Fungal infection affecting feet, especially toe webs	Intense itching; cracking; peeling	Soak feet and dry well. Apply antifungal agent. Wear clean cotton socks.
Infectious mononucleosis	Condition caused by Epstein-Barr virus	Fever, sore throat, enlarged lymph nodes; general malaise; enlarged spleen; sometimes jaundice	Treat symptoms; use rest (mono), increased fluid intake, antipyretic, good nutrition.
Hepatitis A virus	Inflammation of hepatocytes of liver caused by viruses, bacteria, drugs, chemicals; transmitted	Fatigue, anorexia, swollen glands; aversion to smoking (if smokes); short incubation period: 15–45 days	Prevention: Stay in good physical condition, hand washing. If condition develops, prevent transfer. Treat symptoms.

(continued)

TABLE 11-2 *(continued)*
Common Health Problems of Adolescents

Problem	Definition	Symptoms/Signs	Prevention/Treatment
	via fecal contamination of food or water with subsequent close person-to-person contact (25% of hepatitis cases)		
Hepatitis B virus (HBV) infection	Transmitted via blood, primarily parentally, although person-to-person contact possible (50% of hepatitis cases)	Prodromal stage: 2–20 days; jaundice phase: 2–8 weeks; recovery phase: 2–24 weeks	Vaccine is available; take recommended precautions. Treat symptoms. Avoid complications.
Hepatitis C virus (HCV) (non-A, non-B) infection, and other types (D = HDV, E = HEV)	Diagnosed by deduction (25% of hepatitis cases)	Hepatitis symptoms; history of transfusion (HDV); history of fecal-oral route (HEV); some serologic markers	Treat symptoms.
Rocky Mountain spotted fever	Acute febrile disease caused by *Rickettsia rickettsii*; passed to human by bite of infected tick	Symptoms start in 2 days to 2 weeks: headache, fever, rash on hands and feet, pain in back and leg muscles	Prevention: Be aware of problem and appropriate removal of ticks. Treatment: Administer tetracycline.
Lyme disease	Tick-borne disease introduced by the spirochete *Borrelia burgdorferi* from animal host to human (ticks are only 1–2 mm)	Early (3 or 4 days after bite): ring-like rash at bite site (approximately 10 cm in diameter) then secondary lesion, flu-like symptoms, sometimes cardiac problems (10%); in 4 weeks, neurological problems (in 15%); in 6 weeks to 1 year, arthralgias and synovitis (in 50%)	Administer antibiotic (doxycycline). Provide rest and healthy diet. Treat symptoms. Prevent through education.

social life. Some fathers exclude themselves from care of the disabled child and from the family, which contributes to poor marital adjustment and relationship difficulties with the children.

Nurses are the health providers in the most critical position to assess coping strategies of the chronically ill individual and the family and to assist the family with physical care, to cope with the impact of the chronic illness, and to practise stress management.[289,290]

Suicide

Suicide ranks as the third most frequent cause of death in adolescents.[291–298] Suicide in adolescents is frequently reported as an accidental death. Motor vehicle accidents, drug and alcohol overdose, firearm accidents, and even homicides can be disguised suicides.[299] Psychological, social, and physiologic stressors are the apparent causes for the rising number of suicides. Television dramatizations on the nightly news or in movies of teenage suicides appear to contribute to an increased wave of teenage suicide attempts and successes.[300]

Adolescents who attempt suicide often come from families who have nonproductive communication patterns, inconsistent positive reinforcement behaviours, and a high level of conflict or child abuse. Suicides occur in rich and poor, urban and rural families. In Canada, the First Nations on-reserve population have double the rate of suicidal deaths compared to the general Canadian population. For Nunavut, where 85 percent of the population is Inuit, the rate of deaths by suicide is over six times the Canadian rate.[301] Boothroyd and her colleagues carried out a case-control study of 71 people who died by suicide, between 1982 and 1996, among the Inuit in northern Quebec, and 71 population-based living control subjects matched for sex, community of residence, and age within one year. The results indicated that most of the case subjects were single males aged 15 to 24 years. The two principal means of suicide were hanging and gunshot. It is interesting to note that about 33% had been in contact with medical personnel in the month before their death.[302] Furthermore, the case subjects were significantly more likely than the control subjects to have received a lifetime psychiatric diagnosis and to have had a history of psychiatric symptoms.[303]

Females are now using forms of suicide usually associated with males. The males, however, are more successful, more violent, and less likely to give warning before the suicidal act.[304,305] Pinhas and her colleagues examined whether or not gender-role conflicts influenced the suicidal behaviour of adolescent girls. Gender-role conflict is defined as psychological or social difficulty arising when individuals have internalized characteristics other than those ascribed to their sex. They concluded that gender-role conflict plays an important role in the suicidal behaviour of girls.[306]

Frequently, physical fatigue contributes to the emotional stress that precipitates a suicide attempt. Most adolescents have short bouts with suicidal preoccupations in the presence of these stresses. Sometimes even a small disappointment or frustration can lead to an impulsive suicidal attempt. Often the impulsive acts are committed to force parents to pay attention to the adolescent's pleas for help and get needs met. Because the adolescent often feels great ambivalence toward parents, he or she rejects parents and yet solicits love, sometimes by attempting suicide. In reality, the parents may be giving all the love they can. In other situations, the adolescent may be experiencing (1) an intense sense of loss, external or internal, real or imagined, that is believed to be permanent, or (2) anger at parents, teachers, or another significant person. Hurting self is a way to get even and make the other sorry for not treating the person right. Death is not seen as irreversible. If there is a history of family suicide, the adolescent may attempt reunion with the deceased, often on the anniversary of the suicide. Other reasons for suicide are discussed in several resources.[307–313]

Signs of suicide are often subtle to detect, but a composite of behaviours should be a clue that the teen is experiencing severe stress. See the box entitled "Warning Signs for Suicide and Interventions in Adolescents" for a list of behaviours associated with or indicators of suicide attempts.[314,315] Do not be afraid to ask if the youth has thought of suicide. The stressed person welcomes this query and the fact that you are taking the statements and behaviour seriously.

The suicidal adolescent may be a loner at school and feel unable to meet scholastic expectations of parents. School performance often drops; there may be frequent absences. If peers state that a friend is suicidal, investigate their concerns. No threat should be ignored. Depression is found in two-thirds of suicidal adolescents; depression may be masked by a variety of symptoms, signs, or behaviour.[316]

Rarely does the adolescent plan a suicide because he or she really wants to die. At times, however, when death is desired, the adolescent is engaging in self-destructive behaviour as a punishment for guilt over actions or thoughts that he or she has committed or experienced. Ten percent of adolescents who attempt suicide make further attempts within a year.[317,318]

Screen for emotionally distressed adolescents and be available to listen to and *ask about their problems. Take a careful history to identify the underlying stresses.* Refer to several references for guidelines in assessing family and school indicators, personality traits, and danger signs.[319–322] If you believe you are unable to handle the situation, discuss it with the teen and refer him or her to a guidance counsellor, nurse therapist, clergy, school psychologist, or private or school physician or psychiatrist. Frequently the adolescent will turn to an adult with whom he or she has had a personal relationship or sees as an advocate for teens. This relationship may help the adolescent through the present crisis. You can accept, support, inform, and serve as an advocate for teens, working with parents and adolescents.[323,324]

Follow-up care with the family and adolescent after suicidal gestures is important. Some adolescents who attempt suicide ultimately do commit suicide.

If the adolescent makes a suicide attempt, crisis intervention is essential after the necessary medical and physical care is given (see Chapter 5). The goals, once life is assured, are to help the person work through feelings that led to and resulted from the suicide attempt, feel hope, identify the problem, see alternative ways of handling it, and mobilize supportive others to continue caring contact with the client. The family needs your support and help in working through their feelings of anxiety, shame, guilt, and anger. Murray and Huelskoetter describe effective intervention for the suicidal person and **postvention,** *care of the surviving family, friends, and peers of a successful suicide victim.*[325]

CRITICAL THINKING

If you identify an adolescent contemplating suicide in your neighbourhood, what are the resources you can use for referral?

Alcoholism and Alcohol Abuse

In Canada, Hotton and Haans conducted an analysis of the prevalence of substance use among young adolescents. They used data from the 1998–99 National Longitudinal Survey

Warning Signs for Suicide and Interventions in Adolescents

Loss of Someone or Something Important

(The greater the number of losses in a short period, the higher the risk)
- Death
- Divorce
- Move to new school or geographic location
- Job
- Self-esteem related to poor relationship or loss of status
- Prolonged family disruption
- Pet
- Health

Feelings and Behaviours of Depression

- Change in daily habits
- Changed eating or sleeping patterns
- Lack of energy; fatigue; weakness; extreme lethargy
- Problems of concentration; slow speech or movements
- Drop in grades or work performance
- Neglecting appearance more than usual
- Lack of friends or interests
- Truancy at school or poor work attendance
- Increase in drug or alcohol use; excessive smoking
- Appearing sad, angry, sullen, irritable most of time; mood swings
- Accident proneness
- Increase in promiscuity
- Continuous acting out that masks other behaviour
- Negative self-concept; feeling unloved, rejected, guilty, hopeless

Statements about Suicide

- Direct or indirect statements about a plan
- Thought + Action = Suicide Attempt or Success

Behavioural Actions or Changes

- Subtle or abrupt, different than norm
- History of suicide attempts
- Giving away prized possessions
- Withdrawal from activities and friends
- Writing, art work, or talking about suicide and death
- Accident proneness
- Crying for no apparent reason
- Depressed mood quickly lifts
- Vague physical complaints
- Listening only to music about death

High Risk Symptoms

- A clear plan with time and details, using a lethal method
- Intoxication with drugs or alcohol
- Anniversary of the death of a loved one by suicide
- Auditory hallucinations telling the teen to die
- Extreme isolation and no support systems
- Feelings of hopelessness, helplessness, and worthlessness
- A previous suicide attempt using a lethal method and continued suicide ideation

Interventions

- Determine lethality
- Encourage communication with family, teachers, or other supportive adults
- Encourage appropriate expression of feeling, especially guilt and anger
- Use self-esteem building activities
- Encourage positive statements about self
- Assist the child to cope with the situation that is causing despair or sense of helplessness

---

of Children and Youth. Analysis is based on a cross-sectional file from 4296 respondents aged 12 to 15 years.[326] The main results indicated that drinking to intoxication and drug use were more common among 14- and 15-year-olds than among 12- and 13-year-olds. The odds of drinking to intoxication and drug use were highest among adolescents whose friends used alcohol or drugs or were often in trouble, who reported low commitment to school, or whose parents had a hostile and ineffective parenting style.[327] Boyle and his colleagues used data from the Ontario Health Survey to examine within-family influences on the use of tobacco, alcohol, and marijuana in households with offspring aged 12 to 24 years. They concluded that the treatment and prevention of substance use (and abuse) among adolescents and young adults might be enhanced by including a family focus, especially where there are two or more siblings at home.[328] Williams and Chang from the Addiction Centre Adolescent Research Group in Calgary reinforce that for treatment, outpatient

family therapy appears superior to other forms of outpatient treatment.[329]

Alcohol intake among adolescents has greatly increased in recent years, and it is the most common psychoactive drug used by adolescents. Statistics vary with the geographic area and researcher.

In the U.S. in 1998, about 81% of high-school seniors experimented with alcohol, compared with 65% who tried marijuana. The average age of beginning alcohol intake has dropped from 14 to 12 years. Alcohol intake peaks around ages 18 to 22. In late adolescence, on university and college campuses and in the community, heavy episodic or binge drinking is a problem for students who are of legal drinking age and those who are not. Over 40% are classified as **binge drinkers,** *males who had five or more drinks in a row and females who had four or more drinks in a row at least once in the previous two weeks.* These individuals drink to get drunk. However, 22% of college students are abstainers.[330,331]

Alcohol is a factor in the leading cause of death, which is motor vehicle accidents, for 15- to 20-year-olds. Intoxicated drivers are risk takers as they experience their "high" or "rush." They are less likely to use seatbelts; 71% of the young drivers involved in fatal passenger vehicle accidents in 1997 were not using seatbelts. Some of these accidents are suicidal or homicidal in intent.[332,333]

A number of *factors contribute to underage drinking and college binge drinking:*[334-336]

1. A need to feel mature or defend against depression or anxiety
2. Lack of enforcement of underage drinking laws, even though most jurisdictions restrict sale of alcohol to minors
3. Advertising and marketing in which drinking is glamorized
4. Promotion practices that attract young consumers, in which alcohol is seen as a way to gain gratification and avoid problems
5. Peer pressure and social and cultural beliefs that encourage underage drinking, especially in street gangs, fraternities, sororities, and other social groups
6. School policies, practices, and norms that encourage underage drinking and college binge drinking
7. Parental drinking patterns

Medical hazards of alcohol abuse are numerous. All body systems may eventually become involved because of the toxic effects of alcohol, including the following conditions:[337-341]

- Gastritis (nausea, vomiting, headache, gastric pain; may vomit blood or ropy, thick mucus)
- Pancreatitis (severe abdominal pain, nausea, vomiting)
- Hepatitis (fever, jaundice, abdominal edema, ankle and foot edema, tenderness in area of liver)
- Gastric and duodenal ulcers (vomiting of blood, severe pain, indurate abdomen; obstruction and perforation of stomach or intestine may occur)
- Impotency (inability to achieve or sustain erection)
- Neuritis (tingling, burning, itching, numbness, weakness, and finally paralysis of limbs if untreated)
- Fatty liver (enlarged liver on palpation; symptoms of hepatitis may persist)
- Cirrhosis (weight loss, chronic nausea, vomiting, weakness; impotency; abdominal pain; bloated, indurate abdomen; hemorrhage; seventh leading cause of death)
- Esophageal varices (varicose veins of the esophagus; internal hemorrhage may cause death)
- Degeneration of cerebellum (permanent loss of motor coordination, unsteady walk, tremors)
- Esophageal cancer (difficulty swallowing, sense of blockage behind sternum)
- Delirium tremens (withdrawal from alcohol causes tremors, sweating, nausea, insomnia, confusion, delusions, hallucinations, and convulsions; may be fatal in 10% of patients)
- Birth defects (fetal alcohol spectrum disorder; infant is underweight, has small brain and head size, may have cleft palate and congenital heart defect; slow growth in childhood; slower mental development)

In addition to vehicle accidents, suicides, homicides, and medical illness, *various other health problems, injuries, or death may result* from alcohol abuse, including (1) fire deaths; (2) choking on foods; (3) freezing to death; (4) drowning; (5) accidental asphyxiations, and (6) falls.[342-344]

Social problems, which may in turn cause physical and emotional health problems (and death), that arise from alcohol abuse include child and spouse abuse and homicide (a large percentage of violent crimes involve alcohol). Alcohol use is one of the best predictors for early sexual activity and failure to use contraception. More than any other single factor or substance of abuse, alcohol use is implicated in unplanned pregnancy, sexually transmitted infections, and HIV infection.[345]

Avoid lecturing to adolescents about the hazards of drinking and driving and the medical effects of drinking. *Help the person to clarify values about healthful activities* and see the detrimental effects of drinking—physically, emotionally, mentally, and socially. Point out people who have suffered the ill effects of excessive alcohol intake. Teach adolescents how to identify hazards and to act responsibly to avoid injury to themselves and others.

Care of the alcoholic person and family is complex; specific measures vary with the stage of alcoholism and manifestations of the disease.[346-348]

A number of *strategies are being tried to reduce underage and binge drinking. You can be an advocate for such strategies, as follows:*[349]

1. Work with local bars to eliminate promotions that encourage excessive teen drinking.
2. Encourage local police to ensure stricter controls on alcohol sales so that retailers do not sell to individuals under the legal age for drinking.
3. Work with universities to eliminate alcohol sales at the stadium and alcohol advertising at its athletic programs and events.
4. Encourage stricter controls on alcohol sales, advertising, and promotions and banning home delivery.
5. More media attention to teens who do not drink or who engage in light-to-moderate drinking to reduce peer pressure to drink.
6. Work for effective online screening and blocking technologies for preventing youth access to alcohol and tobacco-related websites.

CRITICAL THINKING

As a health professional, what would be your recommendations for effective programming to prevent and to reduce substance abuse among youth?

Conditions Associated with Sexual Activity

Sexual decision making and premarital coitus were controlled in the past by family, social, and religious rules and restrictions. Today sexual activity is almost completely regarded as an individual responsibility. Because of the emotional and social characteristics of adolescents, the individual may have neither the readiness or desire to engage in sexual activity nor the decision-making skills and ego strength to behave counter to the peer group in order to abstain. There is not much educational help for the adolescent to develop the necessary decision-making or value-clarification skills or the emotional strengths to be autonomous or to avoid what is perceived as expected behaviour. The areas related to the adolescent sexual activity that influence health are those involving sexually transmitted diseases, the use of contraceptives, pregnancy, abortion, and incest. A careful history is essential.

SEXUALLY TRANSMITTED DISEASES

Sexually transmitted diseases (STDs) are *infections grouped together because they spread by transfer of infectious organisms from person to person during sexual contact, through sexual intercourse, oral sex, or anal sex.*

Sexually transmitted diseases are a public health epidemic and a major problem because of high communicability. Reports of new cases represent only a percentage of those affected.[350-353] Enormous human suffering, the cost of hundreds of millions of dollars, and the tremendous demands on health care facilities all result. The problem is rooted in ignorance, apathy, and neglect. Women and children bear an inordinate share of the problem—sterility, ectopic pregnancy, fetal and infant deaths, birth defects, and mental retardation. Cancer of the cervix may be linked to the sexually transmitted herpes II virus. Some of the specific reasons for the increase in recent years include changing sexual patterns, changing attitudes, and cultural mores regarding sexual behaviour, lack of understanding about STDs, the feeling of "it can't happen to me," breakdown of the family unit, increased mobility within the population, and the widespread use of contraceptives. *Adolescents have many reasons for wanting to be sexually active, including to:*

1. Enhance self-esteem
2. Have someone care about them
3. Experiment

CONTROVERSY DEBATE

You Tell Him, Please

Rebecca, a 15-year-old adolescent, comes to the Women's Health Clinic for her first visit. Her boyfriend, John, is with her. Rebecca informs the nurse that she has been having unprotected sex with John for a while now. She goes on to say that she loves John, but does not know if she could ever tell him that he must wear a condom. She thinks that John does not believe in using condoms; and she does not wish to offend him by mentioning the subject to him. She pleads with you to speak to him privately about contraceptive measures.

1. What will be your initial response to Rebecca?
2. How will you initiate a dialogue about sexual health education with the couple?
3. What objectives will you set for yourself to educate this couple in sexual matters?

4. Be accepted by peers
5. Feel grown up
6. Be close and touched by another
7. Feel pleasure or have fun
8. Seek revenge
9. Determine normality
10. Love and be loved
11. Gain control over another.[354-359]

It is probable that all cases of STDs are not reported. AIDS is discussed primarily in Chapter 12. Table 11-3 compares the causes, common symptoms, prognosis, and treatment of gonorrhoea, syphilis and herpes genitalis, to assist you as you assess and care for clients.[360-365] Other sexually transmitted diseases include vaginitis, genital warts, and pubic lice. Vaginitis can be grouped into four categories—candidal, trichomonal, nonspecific, and chlamydia—that may or may not be related to sexual activity.

TABLE 11-3			
Comparison of Gonorrhea, Syphilis, and Herpes Genitalis			
	Gonorrhoea	Syphilis	Herpes Genitalis
Cause	*Neisseria gonorrhoea*	*Treponema pallidum*	Herpes simplex virus, type 2 (HSV-2)
Incubation	3–9 days	10–90 days; average, 3 weeks	Several days to 3 weeks
Symptoms	Male: asymptomatic at times, including when organism lodged rectally; urethritis–thin, watery, white urethral discharge, becoming purulent, dysuria Female: asymptomatic in 60% to 90% of cases, including when organism lodged rectally;	Male and female: Stage 1 (primary): chancre—solitary, indurate, painless, ulceration on genitalia 10–28 days after sexual contact; lesion occasionally on mouth, nipples, anus; lesion healing within 4 to 6 weeks;	Male and female: Beginning infectious stage: after intercourse with infected partner, itchy, tingling, numb, when virus beneath skin Active infectious symptomatic stage: blister-like sores that ulcerate on skin, mucous

(continued)

TABLE 11-3 *(continued)*
Comparison of Gonorrhea, Syphilis, and Herpes Genitalis

	Gonorrhoea	Syphilis	Herpes Genitalis
	dysuria and vaginal discharge common symptoms; vaginal trichomoniasis present in 50% of cases Both sexes: gonococcemia, systemic gonorrhea, with skin lesions, malaise, fever, tachycardia	treponemes multiplying rapidly Stage 2 (secondary): rash covering skin, mouth, and genitalia (red-copper on white skin, grey-blue on black skin; red rash on palms and soles); hair loss; eyes and ears inflamed; lymphadenitis, low-grade fever; sore throat; pain from bone involvement; albuminuria; liver and spleen enlarged, jaundice, nausea; blood test positive after 5 weeks Stage 3 (latent): symptoms gone in 2–6 weeks; symptoms possibly absent from a few months to a lifetime; blood test positive; person is noninfectious, but possible for syphilitic pregnant woman to give birth to congenitally syphilitic child Stage 4 (tertiary): complications after 3 to 30 years in 30% of untreated cases; symptoms affecting heart, blood vessels, brain, spinal cord, eyes, skin, and bones; blood test positive *Note:* Symptoms from all stages may be present at once Other names: syph, the pox, bad blood	membranes, vagina, cervix, penis, anal area; fever, headache, muscle aches, general malaise, vaginal discharge, enlarged lymph glands; dyspareunia (painful intercourse); lesions heal in 5–7 days but are sites for secondary infection; symptoms last several weeks Infectious dormant stage: lesions heal; no symptoms, blisters within vagina or urethra may go undetected; may be transmitted sexually at this time Recurring symptomatic stage: usually recurrence of repeated painful attacks because virus remains dormant near base of spine between attacks; duration of time between attacks varies; may be precipitated by emotional stress, ovulation, onset of menses, poor diet, excess sun or wind, lack of sleep, friction from clothes
Prognosis	Male: usually treated successfully Female: sterile Both sexes: arthritis, endocarditis No immunity to future infections Reinfection common	Can be treated successfully; no immunity; transmitted to fetus via placenta unless mother treated before 16 weeks' gestation If untreated: aortic aneurysm, heart failure; complete or partial paralysis or crippling; personality changes; blindness, gumma, lesions of granulation tissue, causing tissue breakdown and impaired circulation; pain from bone involvement; convulsions	Incurable. Complications: herpes keratitis, eye infection (results from rubbing eye after touching herpes sore); repeated attacks and blindness possible Females: five times more likely to develop cervical cancer Pregnant women: pregnancy often ends in spontaneous abortion, stillbirth, prematurity, neonatal infection, or death; fetal infection may occur in utero Infant: virus transmitted through

(continued)

TABLE 11-3 *(continued)*
Comparison of Gonorrhea, Syphilis, and Herpes Genitalis

	Gonorrhoea	Syphilis	Herpes Genitalis
		Death: congenital syphilis or death for fetus	placenta or by direct contact at birth; 50% chance of being born with disease unless delivered by caesarean section; 75% of infected neonates are blind or have brain damage; death may occur
Treatment	Aqueous penicillin Some drug-resistant strains of organisms are developing	Penicillin G benzathine or procaine penicillin	Aseptic technique in care of patient; cleansing lesions with soap and water; use of drying medications Experimental drugs reported to reduce symptoms Antibiotics for secondary infection Incurable, but Zovirax suppresses signs and symptoms Psychological counselling Prevention of further spread by avoiding any contact with genitals and sexual intercourse while lesions are present unless male wears condom

Other sexually transmitted diseases are described in Table 11-4 to assist you in assessment and treatment, as well as prevention.[366–371]

CRITICAL THINKING

Prepare a nursing care plan for an adolescent who has chlamydia.

Contraceptive Practices

In Canada, new advances in contraceptive methods are making it possible for Canadians to have access to a broad range of options. However, the new and comprehensive *Sex Sense* written by the Obstetricians and Gynaecologists of Canada states that youth and adults are unaware of the dangers of unprotected sex.[372] This book provides answers to questions about today's contraceptive methods and the best protection from sexually transmitted infections and HIV/AIDS (visit http://www.sogc.org/sexsense/tips.htm).

Contraception, or **birth control**, is the *use of various devices, chemicals, or abortion to prevent or terminate pregnancy.* The adolescent may choose contraception to avoid pregnancy while continuing sexual activity. Contraceptive practices used in North America are summarized in Table 11-5 and additional information may be obtained from various references at the end of this chapter.[373–381] Although contraceptives may prevent pregnancy (and sexually transmitted diseases, when the

contraceptive device is a condom), they have unwanted side effects or disadvantages. *The only way to avoid both pregnancy and the unwanted side effects is sexual abstinence.* Your approach and the structure of the health care environment are critical to the teenager's adherence to instructions about contraceptive practices or abstinence.

Some youth, however, do not use contraceptives for the following reasons:

1. Misconceptions or ignorance about them
2. Inability to secure appropriate contraceptives
3. Inability to plan ahead for their actions
4. Belief that using contraceptives marks them as promiscuous
5. Rebelliousness

Males are less likely to recognize risk of pregnancy as a result of sexual activity, have less information about contraceptives, and are less supportive of contraceptive use than females. The attitude of the male may indeed influence the female toward sexual activity without contraceptive use, even though she realizes the hazards and wishes to avoid them.[382,383]

CRITICAL THINKING

What are some ways health care professionals can promote a better understanding of, and compliance with, practices related to family planning?

TABLE 11-4
Other Sexually Transmitted Diseases

Problem	Definition	Symptoms/Signs	Prevention/Treatment
Candidal vaginitis	Inflammatory process caused by a common skin fungus, *Candida albicans*	Copious cheesy vaginal discharge, intense vulval inflammation and itching or burning	May be related to diabetes, use of antibiotics, birth control pills, bath oil, lack of moisture-absorbing underpants, or sexual intercourse; use cool compresses, vaginal antifungal cream
Trichomonal vaginitis (trichomoniasis)	Inflammatory process caused by the common flagellate parasite, *Trichomonas vaginalis*	Frothy, bubbly, greenish-yellow, foul-smelling vaginal discharge; minimal inflammation, some itching	Oral medication if nonpregnant; vaginal cream if pregnant
Nonspecific or bacterial vaginitis	Inflammation caused by more than one bacteria, but especially *Gardnerella vaginalis*	Small amount of yellowish-white vaginal discharge with "fishy" smell; moderate itching	Douche; vaginal cream or oral medication, with sexual partner also being treated
Chlamydia	Infection caused by an intracellular parasite, *Chlamydia trachomatis*	Vaginal discharge or pelvic inflammatory disease in women; can cause sterility, urethritis, epididymitis, painful and frequent urination or infertility in men; conjunctivitis or pneumonia in infants	Antibiotic treatment
Genital warts	Growth caused by human papillomas virus, appearing 1–3 months, or longer, after contact	Seen on foreskin and penis in males and on perineum and vaginal mucosa in females	Repeated topical application followed by sitz bath
Pubic lice or "crabs"	Infests genital region after contact with a person, clothes, towels, or bedding that is infested with *Phthirus pubis*	Intense itching; nits may be seen on hair shafts; small black dots (probably excreta) may be visible in pubic hair; occurs 4–5 weeks after contact	Application of gamma benzene hexachloride 1% cream or lotion; repeat application in 7–10 days; treat sexual contacts; oral antihistamines for itching

Adolescent Pregnancy

Adolescent pregnancy has been on the decline in Canada and most U.S. states since the mid-1990s.[384] In Canada, the teenage pregnancy rate was 42.7 pregnancies for every 1000 women aged 15 to 19 in 1997, the lowest rate in 10 years.[385] Older teenagers are more likely than their younger counterparts to be sexually active, which is reflected in higher pregnancy rates. At ages 18 and 19, the 1997 rate was 68.8 pregnancies for every 1000 women, compared with 25.5 for those aged 15 to 17.[386] Wackett states that in the Yukon Territory, teen pregnancy in the late 1990s was almost 40% lower than in the

1980s.[387] The United States has one of the highest teenage pregnancy rates in the Western world.

Unintended pregnancy causes much human misery—for the pregnant teen and her family and often for the offspring. Effects on the teen father are less well known.[388–390]

Various factors influence whether the adolescent becomes pregnant. Although some pregnancies may be accidental, four *other themes may underlie the mask of "accident"*:

1. Self-destruction or self-hate
2. Rebellion, anger, hate, reverse aggressiveness toward parents and authority

TABLE 11-5
Contraceptive Measures: Effectiveness and Disadvantages

Name	Description	Effectiveness	Disadvantages
Oral contraceptives	Pills used to chemically suppress ovulation; new low-dose pill available, with one-tenth amount of hormones, thus fewer side effects	Highly effective, 2 pregnancies in 100	Fewer serious effects than previously seen; screen for nausea, edema, weight gain, depression, anemia, yeast infections, blood clots, myocardial infarction, liver cancer; smokers have increased triglycerides, total cholesterol, and lipoproteins and greater cardiovascular disease risk
Intrauterine device (IUD)	Metal coil inserted in uterus, preventing implantation of fertilized ovum	Very effective, 5 pregnancies in 100	Cramping and bleeding between periods, heavy periods, anemia, perforation of uterus, pelvic infection
Spermicidal chemicals	Chemical substances inserted in vagina before intercourse	Less effective, 5 to 24 pregnancies in 100; effective if used with diaphragm	Irritation of penis or vagina
Billings's ovulation method	Changes in cervical discharge show presence of ovulation	Very effective when followed and abstinence maintained during fertile time	Accurate observation by the woman is necessary
Diaphragm	Small occlusive device inserted over cervix before intercourse	Very effective when properly placed and checked often	Irritation of cervix; aesthetic objections
Condom	Occlusive device placed over penis before ejaculation	Effective when properly used, 9 to 10 pregnancies in 100	Aesthetic objections; possibly impaired sensation in male
Rhythm	Abstinence of intercourse before and during ovulation; increased body temperature during fertile days	Less effective, 5 to 24 pregnancies in 100	Pregnancy unless menstrual periods regular, ovulation closely observed, and abstinence adhered to
Prostaglandins	Chemicals that regulate intracellular metabolism administered parenterally or orally for contraception or to induce abortions	Effectiveness uncertain	Nausea, vomiting, diarrhea, and pelvic pain
Luteinizing hormone-releasing hormone (LHRH)	Daily injection of hormone decreases sperm; substance inhibits pituitary gland's release of hormone that controls ovulation and spermatogenesis	In women, 98% effective; useful in men and women	Experimental; data on men still limited

(continued)

TABLE 11-5 *(continued)*
Contraceptive Measures: Effectiveness and Disadvantages

Name	Description	Effectiveness	Disadvantages
Injections	150 mg injection of a progestogen, medroxyprogesterone acetate (Depo-Provera); 200-mg injection of a progestogen, Norigest	Injections 98% effective for 3 months	Intermittent vaginal bleeding
Implants	Levo-Norgestrel (progestin) inserted via silicone rubber, matchstick-size tubes into woman's arm	Implants last 5 years; continual release of synthetic hormone inhibits ovulation, thickens cervical mucus, and impedes sperm passage; removed if woman desires pregnancy	Contraindicated in women with liver disease, breast cancer, blood clots, unexplained vaginal bleeding. Side effects: headaches, dizziness, nervousness, nausea
Hysterectomy	Surgical removal of uterus; usually done for pathologic condition of uterus rather than for sterilization only	Completely effective; ovum and hormonal production unchanged; menstruation ceases	Mortality rate higher than after tubal ligation; possible postoperative complications; irreversible procedure
Tubal ligation	Surgical interference with tubal continuity and transport of an ovum	Effectiveness depending on type of procedure done, 0.5 to 3 pregnancies in 100; ovum maturation, menstruation, and hormonal production unchanged	Occasional recanalization (fallopian tube ends regrowing together) causing fertility; adhesions, infection, or swelling of tubes postoperatively
Vasectomy	Surgical severing of the vas deferens (sperm duct) from each testicle	Effectiveness depending on type of procedure done; failure rate low; less expensive and time consuming and easier to obtain than female sterilization; no risk to life; no effect on hormone production of testes or sexual functioning	Bleeding, infection, and pain postoperatively in 2%–4%; occasional recanalization of severed ends of vas deferens causing fertility; uncertain reversibility

Note: A combination of contraceptive practices may be used by the couple.

Factors Influencing Incidence of Adolescent Pregnancy

Developmental Factors

- Low self-esteem
- Need to be close to someone; to relieve loneliness
- Recent experience of significant loss or change
- Early physical sexual maturation
- Egocentrism
- School-dropout or truancy, school underachiever
- Personal fable (feeling that "it won't happen to me")
- Responsiveness to peers' sexual behaviour
- Independence from family
- Need to prove own womanhood
- Denial of personal sexuality or sexual behaviour
- Self-punishment for earlier sexual activity or pregnancy for which teen feels shame, guilt

Societal Factors

- Variety of adult sexual behaviour values
- Implied acceptance of intercourse outside of marriage

- Importance of involvement in heterosexual relationships stressed by the media
- Inadequate access to contraception
- Access to public financial support for teen parents and offspring

Family and Friends

- Difficult mother–daughter relationship
- Desire to break symbolic tie between self and mother
- Lack of religious affiliation
- Mother, sister, or close relative pregnant as teen
- Sexually permissive behaviour norms of the larger peer group
- Sexually permissive behaviour of close friends; immediate peer group sexually active
- Inadequate communication in heterosexual relationships
- Fulfillment of mother's prophecy if she expects such behaviour
- History of sexual abuse or incest
- Few, if any, girlfriends
- Older boyfriend
- Substance abuse or use in family or peer group

---

3. Lack of responsibility for self and personal behaviour, related to identity diffusion or confusion

4. Plea for attention and help, either from parents, the boy involved, or others.

Other factors and combinations of factors may also contribute to the teenage girl's becoming pregnant; the box entitled "Factors Influencing Incidence of Adolescent Pregnancy" summarizes them.[391–393]

The early adolescent is not physically, socially, emotionally, educationally, or economically ready for pregnancy or parenthood. The late adolescent is physically mature but may not be ready for pregnancy emotionally, socially, or economically. These latter factors override the biological advantages of early pregnancy and may account, in part, for health care not being sought during pregnancy. In turn, health providers often do not understand the needs underlying adolescents' behaviour and thereby fail to provide the necessary services.

Neonatal risks associated with teenage maternity are not uniform but are common. The risks vary by age of the adolescent mother, amount of prenatal care, and ethnic identification.

Risks are highest for 11- to 14-year-old teens. Early fertility implies early menarche, which is associated with short stature, a risk factor for poor neonatal outcome. The excessive rates of short gestation, low birth weight, and neonatal mortality may result from a variety of physiologic consequences of environmental or sociocultural disadvantage, not primarily from biological developmental limits.[394,395]

The late adolescent male is more likely to be involved in the pregnancy and be supportive to the girl than his younger counterpart. The more mature the adolescent girl and boy when they become parents, the more likely they will manifest positive parenting characteristics described in Chapter 7. The younger the adolescent, the more likely it is that negative

parenting behaviours will occur. Often the adolescent parent expects behaviour beyond the developmental ability of the baby, which creates intense frustration and anger that result in child abuse or neglect. *You may be able to assess these behaviours and intervene with support, teaching, and counselling.* The ultrasound procedure and education using visual aids can foster attachment feelings.[396] Agencies that have adolescent pregnancy programs should provide both teen fathers and mothers with parenting classes and child development information.

A major problem in adolescent parenting is that many teenage girls who become mothers have themselves come from single-parent homes or homes in which active participation by the father is lacking. Further, the teenage father often gives no real support—emotional or financial. The maternal grandmother is the one who is expected to raise the child. If she cannot, the adolescent single parent is likely to lack the emotional maturity or knowledge to demonstrate positive parenting characteristics. If the teenage couple marries, divorce often occurs within the first or second year so that the baby is in a single-parent home.

There are ways to help the teenage mother be a more effective and loving mother and also feel more secure and comfortable with parenting. Having a warm, caring woman visit the teen in her home during the infancy stage to assist with infant care, model nurturing child care, explain normal development, and encourage expression of the mother's feelings of frustration and anxiety improves the teen's parenting behaviour. In addition, a drop-in centre where the teen can take her baby for a few hours to be free of child care for a while and to gain emotional support and information is also a useful community support. The teen parent needs multiple supports from family, school, peers, church, the media, the community, and the legal system. Check the Interesting Websites section

EVIDENCE-BASED PRACTICE

The Home Environment of Métis, First Nations, and Caucasian Adolescent Mothers: An Examination of Quality and Influences

The purpose of this study was to compare maternal psychosocial, situational, and home-environment characteristics of Métis/First Nations and Caucasian adolescent mothers and to explore the role of psychosocial situational variables in shaping the home environment. This longitudinal exploratory study compared maternal psychosocial, situational, and home-environment characteristics at four weeks and at 12 to 18 months after birth for a convenience sample of 71 Métis, First Nations, and Caucasian adolescent mothers. The combined group of Métis/First Nations mothers had significantly higher infant-care emotionality scores than the Caucasian mothers at four weeks. The Caucasian mothers scored considerably higher on quality of the home environment; a refined multiple regression model containing infant-care emotionality, education level of the infant's maternal grandmother, ethnicity, and enacted social support explained 49% of the variance, with significant influences being infant-care emotionality and grandmother's education level.

The high number of infants born to Canadian adolescent mothers and the negative consequences of this parenting situation for the child underscore the need to better understand influences on adolescent mothering. Infants parented by adolescent mothers are at greater risk for negative parenting, health, and developmental outcomes than infants with mothers over 19 years of age. In 1994 alone, 24 700 infants were born to mothers between 15 and 19 years of age in Canada. The adverse social effects associated with adolescent parenting have been shown to endure even into adulthood.

An examination of the home environmental influences for Aboriginal adolescent mothers is especially critical, as this group is particularly likely to live in poverty. In fact,

Canada's Aboriginal population scores well below the general population on the Human Developmental Index, at levels similar to those of developing countries. The development rating for Aboriginal people living off reserves is similar to that for residents of Trinidad and Tobago (ranked 35th globally), while those living on reserves are only marginally better off than Brazilians (ranked 63rd).

Practice Implications

The findings from this study have implications for nurses caring for adolescent mothers and their infants in community, primary care, and acute care settings.

1. Economic factors have a greater effect than maternal age or ethnicity on the quality of cognitive stimulation in the home.
2. Nurses can assist adolescent mothers, especially those in low-income groups, to develop mothering practices that promote infant care.
3. Nurses who are aware that poverty is associated with numerous physical, social, cognitive, and emotional problems can refer adolescent mothers to early-intervention programs that focus on health promotion strategies and training in infant care.
4. Métis/First Nations adolescent mothers may be considered at special risk due to socioeconomic conditions and negative home environments.
5. The nurse may act as an advocate for health care and child care policies.
6. An appropriate goal for contemporary maternal-infant/child nurses is to develop a model of nursing care that helps mothers of various cultures to promote their infant's health.

Source: Secco, M.L., and M.E.K. Moffatt, The Home Environment of Métis, First Nations, and Caucasian Adolescent Mothers: An Examination of Quality and Influences, Canadian Journal of Nursing Research, 35, no. 2 (2004), 106–126. Used with permission from CJNR.

in Chapter 7 for some resources for new parents. In Canada, many government-sponsored child and family programs exist, such as parental-leave benefits and Canada Child Tax Benefit—a tax-free monthly payment based on family income.

Abortion

Abortion is a method of terminating a pregnancy through expulsion or extraction of the fetus, usually for economic, emotional, or social reasons. Poor women who economically cannot take care of another child may resort to this form of birth control when they believe they cannot possibly meet the demands of parenting. Abortion carries risks to the physical and psychological health of the female, although the legal abortion is statistically safer than the illegal abortion. More widespread use of abstinence or contraception, however, would reduce the need for abortion. You may be involved in helping

the female who is pregnant, the parents, and even the father of the baby to determine their values and feelings about remaining pregnant versus having an abortion. Give full information, including the effects of abortion and alternatives, be nonjudgmental, and listen. More people are choosing to keep the baby rather than have an abortion. Abortion rates dropped during the 1990s.[397]

In Canada, the number of teenagers having abortions has stabilized. Among women 18 and 19, who accounted for the majority of teenage pregnancies (nearly two-thirds in 1997), the live births outnumbered abortions.[398]

CRITICAL THINKING

What resources in your community are available for a pregnant adolescent who is contemplating an abortion?

Incest

A universal taboo in all cultures is incest, *sexual intercourse between persons in the family too closely related to marry legally.* Incest has been present at epidemic levels for some time but is now being admitted more freely by victims as they speak of the resultant emotional and physical pain.[399]

In your assessment be aware that adolescent, either male or female, is at risk for incest or for youth prostitution. The child and adolescent will tell you if you pick up the initial verbal cues or ask if he or she has been the victim of such activity. The risk to boys is not as well documented as that to girls but may be equally common, with either the mother or the father as the abuser. Incestuous relations usually begin when the child is young and continue through adolescence. Incest may involve stepparents or stepsiblings, grandparents, or uncles or cousins.

In incestuous families, the man is often the sole economic support. The female partner or mother often is isolated. The family does not have visitors. The daughter singled out for the sexual relationship is usually spared the beatings or other abuse given other family members, but she clearly understands what happens if she incurs the man's displeasure. Incestuous men are described as family tyrants but, when confronted with the behaviour, will appear pathetic, meek, bewildered, and ingratiating. Instead, with the health care professional, the man will attempt to gain the professional person's sympathy and deny, minimize, or rationalize his behaviour.[400–403]

Inexperienced professionals may incorrectly blame the mother for the incest; however, typically the mother is working outside of the home, is ill or disabled and cannot effectively care for herself or her children. Incestuous men do not assume maternal caretaking roles when the female partner is disabled. Rather they expect the eldest daughter to assume the "little mother" role for housework and child care responsibilities. The daughter's sexual relationship with the male often evolves as an extension of her other duties. When the oldest daughter becomes resistant, the male often turns his attention to the next daughter or nieces, stepchildren, or granddaughters. The male continues to demand sexual activity with the partner during this time; it is his choice if he limits sexual activity only to the daughters.[404,405]

The main obstacle to obtaining a history of incest is the clinician's reluctance to ask about it. False accusations of sexual abuse or incest are rare; however, the girl commonly retracts a true allegation because of family pressure.[406]

Discovery of incest is a family crisis. *Immediate reporting to authorities and crisis intervention is essential.* Typically the behaviour has been going on many years, and the family's defences are organized around preservation of the incest secret. Disclosure interrupts patterns of functioning. Suicide and runaway behaviour are likely at this time as the offspring is being segregated and driven out of the family.[407]

An active, directive, even coercive approach is necessary. Treatment requires ongoing cooperation between the therapist, law enforcement, and child protective services. It may be necessary to remove the offspring from the home to ensure safety. This intervention, however, reinforces the couple's bonding against the offspring. It is preferable to have the man leave during this period. (He may be imprisoned for a time.)

All family members need intensive support. *Crisis support for the offspring* involves the following:

- Reassure the adolescent (or child) that there are protective adults outside of the family that believe his or her story and will not allow further exploitation to occur.
- Praise the adolescent (or child) for the courage to reveal the incest secret.
- Assure the offspring that he or she is not to blame for the incest and that he or she is helping, not hurting, the family by seeking outside help.
- Tell the offspring explicitly that many children retract their initial complaint because of pressure or fear; encourage him or her not to do so, with the assurance he or she will not be abandoned by authorities if he or she does.

Crisis support for the mother involves encouragement and assistance to do the following:

- Continue to believe the offspring, even if this is painful.
- Resist the tendency to bond with the husband against the offspring.
- Talk about her feelings of shame, guilt, anger, fear, and inadequacy.
- Explore ways she can handle the issues of survival and seek needed help.
- Obtain treatment for health problems.

Group treatment for the mother, father, and offspring is more effective than family or individual therapy alone. Individual therapy can be combined with group therapy. Family therapy may be used in the late stages of treatment. The best motivator for the offender to remain in therapy is the court mandate. Self-help activities can supplement other therapy. Restoration of the incestuous family centres on the mother–daughter relationship. Safety for the daughter comes first. Help the mother feel strong enough to protect herself and her children. Ensure that the daughter feels safe. Help her turn to her mother and other adults for protection.

Destructive effects of incest continue into adult life, long after contact has ceased. Adult women are now more likely to talk about prior incest. They may have persistent and often severe impairments in self-esteem, intimate relationships, and sexual functioning. Incest victims also have a higher-than-normal risk for repeated victimization (battering and rape). Marriage to an abusive spouse, with potential repetition of abuse in the next generation, is a frequent outcome. Incest occurs between siblings and may have consequences similar to those described. Less is known about the psychological effects of incest between siblings.

Rape and *other sexual abuse* may be part of the adolescent's experience as a victim. Burgess and colleagues[408] describe three types of sex rings: child sex initiation rings, youth prostitution rings, and syndicated pornography and prostitution rings. Be aware that sex rings may exist in your area. Work with law enforcement for their removal.

As you work with sexual assault victims, be aware of various types of assault and entanglements that exist so that you can better detect verbal and nonverbal cues, give immediate assistance, and refer the person (and parents) to receive the necessary medical and legal assistance.[409–415]

CRITICAL THINKING

What strategy would you use with an adolescent who states that she has been sexually assaulted?

Drug Abuse Problems

The problem of drug abuse (illicit and prescription) continues to intensify. It is an epidemic with serious consequences for future generations. A major problem is the increasing number of infants born with addiction to one or several drugs (see also Chapter 6). Every age group takes a certain amount of medication at one time or another.[416–420] Usually these drugs are taken for therapeutic reasons; however, reports show that schoolchildren, adolescents, and young adults are increasingly using drugs that cause dependence and toxicity.[421,422] In Canada, the increasing use of Ritalin to control children and youth who are diagnosed as attention deficit disorder results in much of the drug ending up on the street.[423]

Drug abuse is the *use of any drug in excess or for the feeling it arouses.* A **drug** is a *substance that has an effect on the body or mind.* Excessive use of certain drugs causes **drug dependence,** a *physical need or psychological desire for continuous or repeated use of the drug.* **Addiction** is *present when physical withdrawal symptoms result if the person does not repeatedly receive a drug and can involve* **tolerance,** *having to take increasingly larger doses to get the same effect.*

Reasons for drug abuse are many:

1. Curiosity
2. Peer pressure
3. Need to overcome feelings of insecurity and aloneness and to be a part of the group
4. Need for acceptance
5. Easy availability
6. Imitation of family
7. Rebellion, escape, or exhilaration
8. Need for a crutch
9. Unhappy home life
10. Sense of alienation or identity problem
11. Attempt at maturity or sophistication

Gradually the drug subculture replaces interest in family, school, church, hobbies, or other organizational activity. The beliefs and attitudes of the drug subculture are learned from experienced drug users and are fortified by certain rock-and-roll songs and stars.[424]

Drug abuse and addiction affect all socioeconomic, ethnic, and racial groups. Entire communities are affected. In large cities much of the drug trade also involves street gangs, which have become ghetto-based drug trafficking organizations. Even rural communities are affected. When drug abuse is the presenting problem, the accessibility and ability to buy drugs, subcultural acceptance of their use, and at least a relative immunity from legal consequences do not motivate behavioural change. Total community effort is needed to stop or prevent the problem.

Ingestion of alcohol and illicit drugs depresses the cerebral cortex, a still immature reasoning and intellectual centre in the teens, and releases inhibitions in the limbic system, the centre of love, pleasure, anger, pain, and other emotions. The limbic system seeks instant and constant gratification or stimulation and contributes to the adolescent's sense of boredom. Thus some adolescents go to extremes in seeking alcohol, hard drugs, hard rock, and aggressive outlets. See the box entitled "Signs and Symptoms of Drug Abuse among Adolescents."[425,426]

Therapy is usually entered into as a result of family pressure—or a crisis event such as attempted suicide or arrest. The behaviour and illness of the young drug abuser control the entire family, causing family illness. Parents must regain control of their home, forcing the youth to face the illness by seeking treatment. Love and care in a family are essential, but that alone will not cure the drug abuse problem or the craziness that results in a family in which a member is a drug abuser. Nor will parental strictness solve the problems. Professional treatment should be obtained in a centre that treats the whole person and family, using an interdisciplinary team approach and that provides after-discharge care to the person and family. Intensive treatment over time to the entire family system creates the attitude change that is essential for remaining healthy and functional and for ongoing maturity. A combination of drug detoxification, methadone maintenance, and emotional, cognitive, didactic, and experiential therapies is helpful to reduce symptoms and work through underlying character and interactional pathology.

If after discharge the adolescent returns to his or her drug-using friends, there will be a return to drug abuse and all the consequences. The change in attitudes, self-concept, and body image must be total enough so the person feels like a new person and is strong enough in that identity that the new self is maintained in the face of the inevitable peer, school, family, and other stressors. The ability to give up aspects of the old self and maintain the new identity begins with treatment, but can be accomplished only with love, support, and encouragement from family and other loved ones. *The person must feel that he or she is gaining more than what is being lost to maintain the changes begun in treatment and to move forward in maturity.* To remain drug-free involves more than just "saying no" or a one-time seminar. Support groups in the school, church, and community for teens who do not want to use alcohol or drugs are essential to prevent the loneliness and ostracism some teens feel when they go against peers. Illicit drug trade can be stopped best by community action, which reduces supply to individuals.

Accurate information on the nature and extent of substance use and associated problems is a critically important basis for prevention program development.[427] The Canadian Community Epidemiology Network on Drug Use supports a number of communities in developing a profile of drug use. Each community in the network brings together local experts, such as treatment specialists, to contribute quantitative and qualitative information relevant to local needs.[428]

Table 11–6 and Table 11–7 (see page 518) will assist you in assessing the specific signs (objective evidence) and symptoms (subjective evidence) resulting from commonly abused drugs, as well as give information pertinent to intervention. Often the youth is taking a mixture of these drugs, as use of any of them is likely to increase use of other drugs. Assessment becomes more complex. At times neither the person nor

Signs and Symptoms of Drug Abuse among Adolescents

- Decrease in quality of schoolwork without a valid reason. (Reasons given may be boredom, not caring about school, or not liking the teachers.)
- Personality changes; lack of empathy; becoming more irritable, less attentive, less affectionate, secretive, unpredictable, uncooperative, apathetic, depressed, withdrawn, hostile, sullen, easily provoked, insensitive to punishment
- Less responsible behaviour; not doing chores or school homework; school tardiness or absenteeism; forgetful of family occasions such as birthdays
- Change in activity; lack of participation in family activities, school or church functions, sports, prior hobbies, or organizational activities
- Change in friends; new friends who are unkempt in appearance or sarcastic in their attitude; secretive or protective about these friends, not giving any information
- Change in appearance or dress, in vocabulary, in music tastes to match those of new friends, imitating acid, thrasher, heavy metal, or industrial rock-and-roll stars
- More difficult to communicate with; refuses to discuss friends, activities, drug issues; insists it is all right to experiment with drugs; defends rights of youth, insists adults hassle youth; prefers to talk about bad habits of adults
- Rebellious, resistant to authority, antisocial behaviour, persistent lying; seeks immediate gratification; feels no remorse

- Irrational behaviour, frequent explosive episodes; driving recklessly; unexpectedly stupid behaviour
- Loss of money, credit cards, cheques, jewellery, household silver, coins from the home, when losses cannot be accounted for
- Addition of drugs, clothes, money, CDs, or stereo equipment suddenly found in the home
- Presence of whisky bottles, marijuana seeds or plants, hemostats, rolling papers, drug buttons, and marijuana lead buttons; also may be unusual belt buckles, pins, bumper stickers, or T-shirts and magazines in the car, truck, or home
- Preoccupation with the occult, various pseudo-religious cults, Satanism, or witchcraft; evidence of tattoo writing of 666, drawing of pentagrams on self or elsewhere, or misrepresentation of religious objects
- Signs of physical change or deterioration, including pale face, dilated pupils, red eyes; chewing heavily scented gum; using heavy perfumes; using eyewash or drops to remove the red; heightened sensitivity to touch, smell, or taste; weight loss, even with increased appetite (marijuana smoking causes the "munchies"—extra snacking)
- Signs of mental change or deterioration, including disordered thinking or illogical patterns, decreased ability to remember or to think in rapid thought processes and responses; severe lack of motivation

Sources: Boyd, M., and M. Nihart, Psychiatric Nursing. *Philadelphia: Lippincott, 1998; Seifert, K., R. Hoffnung, and M. Hoffnung,* Lifespan Development. *Boston: Houghton Mifflin, 1997; Uphold, C., and M. Graham,* Clinical Guidelines in Family Practice *(2nd ed.). Gainsville, FL: Barmarrae Books, 1994.*

friends know for sure what drugs have been used. Various authors provide information on drug abuse.[429–435]

Not included in the table are "designer drugs," one of the newer and more dangerous types of drugs, which are chemical variants of popular drugs that can be produced in a simple "lab." Because the chemical content varies with every "batch," intoxication or overdose is very hard to treat and the drugs' effects are unpredictable.

Because the use of cocaine (or crack) is a serious health and social problem, a discussion in addition to the information in Table 11-6 is presented.

Cocaine is an *alkaloid extracted from the leaves of the coca bush, which grows mainly in the eastern slope of the Andes Mountains in Peru and Bolivia.* It is sold on the streets as a hydrochloride salt; it is a fine, white crystalline powder. Freebase cocaine resembles rock candy chunks. Street cocaine is diluted with cornstarch, talcum powder, sugar, amphetamines, and quinine. Its cocaine content is usually 5% to 50%; it may be 80%. Cocaine is taken by (1) snorting (inhaled through a straw or a rolled-up dollar bill or coke spoon), (2) freebasing (smoked in a small water pipe filled with rum instead of water), or (3) mainlining (intravenous injection).[436–438]

Cocaine creates tolerance and is addicting because of the sense of stimulation (rush) that comes from activation of nerve cells in the brain that release dopamine. The sense of pleasure or good feeling is so great that the person develops a stronger

compulsion for cocaine each time he or she uses it; addiction results. Chronic cocaine use blocks the ability of the brain cells to release dopamine without increasing amounts of cocaine. The person feels terrible without the drug. Finally, there is the **kindling effect:** *a small amount of cocaine can trigger unexpectedly severe dopamine reactions,* resulting in seizures or bursts of psychotic behaviour.[439,440]

Physical changes that occur from cocaine use are:[441]

- *Cardiovascular:* tachycardia, arrhythmias, hypertension
- *Respiratory:* nasal stuffiness, tachypnea, shortness of breath, runny nose
- *Musculoskeletal:* twitching, tremors, weight loss
- *Gastrointestinal:* nausea, constipation, anorexia
- *Genitourinary:* difficult urination, impotency
- *Dermatologic:* pallor, cold sweats
- *Ophthalmologic:* dilated pupils, blurred vision
- *Central nervous system:* fever, insomnia, fatigue, headache, seizures
- *Reproductive:* abnormal spermatozoa

Medical hazards that result from cocaine use include the following:[442]

- Nasal septum and mucous membrane destruction from inhalation
- Bronchitis, with infection, hemorrhage, and blocking of the respiratory tract from inhalation of foreign particles

- Respiratory failure from vasoconstriction of blood vessels in the lung, cyanosis, shortness of breath, dyspnea, pulmonary edema, respiratory collapse, and death

- Cardiac arrhythmias, tachycardia, myocardial infarction, cardiac arrest, sudden death

- Seizures from freebasing and mainlining, which cause strong, explosive stimulation; convulsions, which may result in death

- Phlebitis from repeated injections in the veins; resulting thrombus can cause an embolus, causing myocardial infarction, pulmonary embolism, renal embolism, or cerebrovascular accident

- Endocarditis from mainlining with bacteria-contaminated needles, causing infection of heart valves (fatality rate is 50%)

- Hepatitis from mainlining with blood-contaminated needles, causing tender, enlarged liver, jaundice (repeated attacks can be fatal)

- Brain abscess from mainlining with bacteria-contaminated needles, causing fever, convulsions, paralysis, and possible death

- AIDS from mainlining with needles contaminated with HIV-infected blood (75% of all intravenous addicts have been exposed to the virus, 5% to 10% or more will develop the fatal disease)

Crack or **rock** is an *extremely potent, highly addictive, inhalant form of cocaine.* It is beige or slightly brown, white or yellowish white, and it is sold in pellet-sized chips called "rocks" or in small plastic vials, in an envelope, or in foil wrap. It can be smoked using a glass pipe or a tin can; the user inhales the vapour from the heated crack. It may be mixed with marijuana or tobacco, or it may be mixed with PCP (angel dust), which is called "space blasting," or with other drugs. Some users smoke in a "base house," "crack house," or "rock house" in which the person pays a fee to use the house, pipes, and torches. The well-to-do individual may use crack in his or her suburban or urban home.[443]

The frightening aspect about *crack* is that *the person may become addicted the first time of use or in a matter of weeks.* The addiction is as powerful as heroin addiction. The intense high feeling is produced in four to six seconds and lasts five to seven minutes. The high is followed by an intensely uncomfortable low feeling so that the person will do anything to get more crack. The person may become violent toward friends or family; may become paranoid or psychotic, or may commit suicide. Death may occur because of heart or respiratory failure. The first dose may cost only a few dollars, but a binge that lasts one to three days and is repeated weekly may cost thousands of dollars. Crack becomes the most, the only, important thing in life, so that all other aspects of life suffer: family relations, friendship, jobs, emotional status, social status, ability to think or behave rationally, personal hygiene or self-care, activities of daily living. If the user is a pregnant woman, there is risk of miscarriage, stillbirth, an addicted baby, impaired physical and mental development in the child, or respiratory failure or strokes in the baby.[444–447]

CRITICAL THINKING

What may be some health promoting strategies for a group of adolescents who are contemplating using crack?

Nursing Role in Health Promotion

The adolescent is between childhood and adulthood. Allow him or her to handle as much personal health care and business as possible, yet be aware of the psychosocial and physical problems with which he or she cannot cope without help. Watch for hidden fears that may be expressed in unconventional language. Today's adolescent, because of improved communications, knows more about life than did former generations. He or she is bombarded with information but does not have the maturity to handle it. Do not assume that because of apparent sophistication he or she understands the basis of health promotion. The adolescent may be able to discuss foreign policy but think that syphilis is caught from toilet seats.

Some teenagers, especially those with understanding and helpful families, go through adolescence with relative ease; it is a busy, happy period. But the increases in teenage suicide and in escape activities, such as drugs and alcohol, speak for those who do not have this experience. Adolescents are looking for adults who can be admired, trusted, and levelled with and who genuinely care. Parents are still important as figures to identify with, but the teenagers now look more outside the home—to teachers, community, and national leaders. They idealize such people, and if the leaders are found to be liars or thieves, their idealism turns to bitterness. As a nurse, you will be one of the community leaders with the opportunity, through living and teaching health promotion, to influence these impressionable minds.

Counselling the Adolescent for Health Promotion

Help the teen and family clarify values, beliefs, and attitudes that are important and be more analytic in thinking: these are first steps in bringing behaviour into congruence and to reduce a sense of conflict. Value clarification exercises may be helpful.

Teach the adolescent effective decision-making skills so that the person learns how to develop a plan of action toward some goal. The decision-making model involves (1) defining the problem; (2) gathering and processing information; (3) identifying possible solutions and alternatives of action; (4) making a decision about action; (5) trying out the decision; (6) evaluating whether the decision, actions, and consequences were effective or desirable; (7) rethinking other alternate solutions with new information; and (8) acting on these new decisions. Some teens and parents may resist health promotion suggestions.[448,449]

Promote warm, accepting, supportive nonjudgmental feelings and honest feedback as the adolescent struggles with decisions. Help him or her make effective choices by fostering a sense of self-importance (he or she is a valuable and valued individual). Helping the person look ahead to the future in terms of values, goals, and consequences of behaviour can strengthen a sense of what is significant in life and a resolve to live so the values find goals and are fulfilled and positive consequences are achieved.

TABLE 11-6
Summary of Legal and Illegal Drugs Related to Nursing Assessment and Intervention

Drug Type/Name	Street Names	Action & Duration	Administration	Desired Effect	Physical & Emotional Effects/Complications
Narcotics Opiates; opium, morphine, heroin, codeine Synthetic non-opiates; Methadone, Demerol, Darvon, Percodan, Percoset	Snow, stuff, H, junk, smack, scag, dreamer	Central nervous system depressant 3–24 hours Addicting	Oral; smoked; sniffed; injected under skin (skin popping); intramuscular (IM); intravenous (IV); cough medicine containing codeine	Euphoria Prevention of withdrawal discomfort	Drowsiness, sedation, nodding stupor. Eye and nose secretions. Euphoria. Relief of pain. Impaired intellectual functioning and coordination. Constricted pupils that do not respond to light. Excessive itching. Poor appetite. Constipation. Urinary retention. Loss of sexual desire, temporary impotence or sterility. Slow pulse and respiration(s); hypotension. Death from overdosage caused by respiratory and cardiovascular depression and collapse. Severe infection at injection sites (needle marks and tracks)
Barbiturates Nembutol, Seconal, Amytal, Fiornal, Tuinol, Phenobarbital	Sleepers, downers, goofballs, redbirds, yellow jackets, heavens, red devils, barbs	Central nervous system depressant 1–16 hours Can be lethal with alcohol	Oral or injected IM or IV	Relaxation and euphoria	Relief of anxiety and muscular tension, relaxation, sleep. Respirations slow, shallow. Slowed reactions. Euphoria. Impaired emotional control, judgment, and coordination. Irritability. Apathy. Confused. Poor hygiene. Slurred, slow speech. Poor memory. Weight loss. Liver, brain, kidney damage from long-term use. Death from overdose. Psychosis, possible convulsions, or death from abrupt withdrawal of barbiturates

Tolerance Potential	Physical Dependence	Psychological Dependence	Withdrawal Characteristics	Nursing Care
Yes	High Controlled substance	High	Abdominal pain. Muscle cramps, tremors, spasms. Nausea, vomiting, diarrhea. Lacrimation, watery eyes. Goose bumps, sweating, chills. Hypertension, tachycardia, increased respirations. Anxiety, irritability, depression. Craving for drugs	(1) Observe for symptoms of withdrawal and report to physician. (2) Give medications prescribed to suppress withdrawal symptoms. (3) Monitor for vital signs at least qid for first 72 hours following admission. (4) Carry out nursing measures to promote safety, general health, and sense of security. (5) Observe and take precaution for seizure activity. (6) Promote general health and sense of security.
Yes	Moderate Controlled substance	Moderate	Nausea, vomiting, diarrhea. Bleeding. Tremors. Diaphoresis. Hypertension or hypotension. Temperature above 99.6°F. Irritability, hostility, restlessness, agitation. Sleep disturbance. Impaired cognitive function. Acute brain syndrome. Seizures.	(1) Observe for withdrawal symptoms and report to physician. (2) Give prescribed medication to suppress symptoms. (3) Provide calm, quiet, safe environment, as free of external stimuli as possible, for acute or severe withdrawal symptoms. (4) Observe for insomnia and nightmares and provide nursing measures to promote sleep.

(continued)

TABLE 11-6 *(continued)*
Summary of Legal and Illegal Drugs Related to Nursing Assessment and Intervention

Drug Type/Name	Street Names	Action & Duration	Administration	Desired Effect	Physical & Emotional Effects/Complications
Sedatives Doriden, Chloral hydrate, Methaquolone, Placidyl		Central nervous system depressant 3–4 hours Can be lethal with alcohol	Oral	Sleep Relaxation	May be same effect as barbiturates but not as severe
Minor tranquilizers Valium, Librium, Miltown, Equanil		Central nervous system depressant 3–4 hours	Oral or injected IM or IV	Sense of calm	Relieve anxiety. Varied onset and duration of effect according to preparation and administration.
Inhalants (Glue sniffing, aerosols, airplane glue, amyl nitrate, nitrous oxide, any spray, including paint)		Central nervous system depressant 1–3 hours	Inhaled through tubes, glue smears on paper or cloth	Intoxication, relaxation, euphoria	Excess nasal secretion. Watering of eyes. Tinnitus. Diplopia. Poor muscular control, lack of coordination. Appears dreamy, blank, or drunk. Impaired perception and judgment. Possibility of violent behaviour. Sleepy after 35 to 45 minutes or unconscious. Damage to lungs, nervous system, brain, liver. Death through suffocation, choking, or overdose.

Tolerance Potential	Physical Dependence	Psychological Dependence	Withdrawal Characteristics	Nursing Care
Yes	Controlled substance	Yes	Anxiety. Insomnia. Tremors. Delirium. Convulsions.	(1) Observe and treat if taken in suicide attempt. (2) Provide environment for safety and sleep. (3) Teach measures to promote sleep and rest.
Yes	Controlled substance	Yes	Anxiety. Irritability. Poor concentration.	(1) Observe for withdrawal symptoms or if a suicide attempt and treat. (2) Provide calm safe environment. (3) Teach stress management. (4) Promote general health.
Yes	No	Yes	Withdrawal symptoms have not been recorded	(1) Emergency care for respiratory damage or neurological complication. (2) Provide for safety. (3) Implement other nursing measures related to presenting symptoms, especially if this drug has been used in combination with others.

(continued)

TABLE 11-6 *(continued)*
Summary of Legal and Illegal Drugs Related to Nursing Assessment and Intervention

Drug Type/Name	Street Names	Action & Duration	Administration	Desired Effect	Physical & Emotional Effects/Complications
Stimulants Amphetamines; Dexedrine, Methedrine, Methamphetamine ("crystal meth")	Pep pills, uppers, A, speed, dexies, bennies, lid poppers	Central nervous system stimulant. Varies in duration of action	Oral or injected under skin or IV	Sense of well-being Alertness, feelings of activity and increased initiative. Excitation. Over-confidence	Giggling, silliness, talkativeness. Rapid speech. Dilated pupils. Hypertension, dizzy, tachycardia. Loss of appetite, loss of weight. Diarrhea, Extreme fatigue. Dry
Cocaine	Leaf, snow, coke, speedballs, flake, gold dust, crack, smack, blow Rock Fire Crack Ice	2–4 hours Crack immediate Depression and exhaustion can last several days	Cocaine sniffed, snorted, IV, or smoking (freebasing)		mouth, bad breath. Chill, sweating, increased muscle tension; shakiness, tremors, restlessness. Irritability. Confused, grandiose thinking. Deep depression. Mood swings. Aggressive behaviour. Paranoid ideas which may persist. Feelings of persecution. Delusions. Hallucinations. Panic. Toxic psychosis. Possible seizures. Tachycardia may cause heart damage or heart attack. Death from cardiac damage, hypertensive crisis, paralysis of respiratory centre, fatigue or overdose.
Caffeine (Found in tea, coffee, and tablet form, including many over-the-counter drugs.)	Kiddie dope (caffeine, ephedrine, phenylopropa-nolamine), black beauty, speckled eggs, speckled birds, pink heart, 20–20's, blue and clears, green and clears	Central nervous system stimulant. Cardiac stimulant 2–4 hours High similar to amphetamines	Oral	A "pick-up"; to increase alertness and decrease fatigue. More rapid, clearer flow of thoughts	Restlessness. Disturbed sleep or insomnia. Nausea, abdominal distension. Myocardial stimulation, palpitation, and tachycardia. Large amounts have led to irrational or hysterical behaviour and, very large doses, cardiac standstill. Stimulates gastric secretions. Raise BMR by 10%. Diuretic.

Tolerance Potential	Physical Dependence	Psychological Dependence	Withdrawal Characteristics	Nursing Care
Yes	Yes	High	Tremors. Neurological hyperactivity. Paranoia. Assaultive behaviour. Irritability. Depression. Possible suicidal behaviour or psychotic reaction. Tachycardia, hypertension. Oversensitivity to stimuli. Insomnia. Intense craving	(1) Observe for symptoms of withdrawal and report to physician. (2) Give medication as prescribed to suppress agitated state and prevent exhaustion. (3) Take precautions for staff and client safety according to client's paranoia and depression. (4) Monitor vital signs at least qid for first 72 hours following admission. (5) Provide calm, nonthreatening, quiet environment and sense of security. (6) Provide for sleep and nutrition. (7) Cocaine—observe for chronic nosebleed and perforated nasal septum. (8) Detoxification. (9) Teach stress management, alternate leisure activities.
Yes Develops quickly	Strongly possible	Yes	In moderate heavy users, there may be headache, irritability, nervousness, tremors, lethargy	(1) Introduce substitute decaffeinated beverage (2) Provide for general health needs and teaching (3) Observe for caffeinism: irritability, tremors, tics, insomnia, sensory disturbance, tachypnea, arrhythmias, diuresis, and GI distress.

(continued)

TABLE 11-6 *(continued)*
Summary of Legal and Illegal Drugs Related to Nursing Assessment and Intervention

Drug Type/Name	Street Names	Action & Duration	Administration	Desired Effect	Physical & Emotional Effects/Complications
Hallucinogens Synthetic D-lysergic acid (LSD) 4-methyl-2 (STP, DOM) Phencyclidine (PCP) Dimethyltryptamine (DMT) Natural cactus (mescaline, peyote) Mushroom (psilocybin)	Acid, Big D, sugar, trips, cubes Serenity, tranquility, peace Businessman's special	Hallucinogenic, varies: LSD 10–12 hours; STP 6–8 hours Mescaline 12–24 hours	Primarily oral; some are inhaled or injected	Insight. Distortion of senses Exhilaration Increased energy	Severe hallucinations, feelings of persecution and detachment. Amnesia. Incoherent speech. Laughing, crying. Exhilaration, depression, or panic alternates with sense of invulnerability. Suicidal or homicidal tendencies. Suspicious. Impaired judgment. Cold, sweaty hands and feet; shivering, chills. Vomiting. Weight loss. Irregular breathing. Exhaustion. Dilated pupils. Hypertension. Brain damage from chronic use. Accidental death. Flashbacks. May intensify psychosis; long-lasting mental illness has resulted. Symptoms may persist for an indefinite period after discontinuation of drug.
Nicotine (Found in cigarettes, cigars, pipe and chewing tobacco, and snuff)		Variable action. Central nervous system toxin. Can act as stimulant or depressant: 15 minutes–2 hours	Smoked, sniffed, chewed	Calmness, sociability	Can have stimulating and/or calming effect. Factor in lung cancer, coronary artery disease, circulatory impairment, peptic ulcer, and emphysema.

IM, intramuscular; IV, intravenous; qid, four times daily

Source: Adapted from Boyd, M., and M. Nihart, Psychiatric Nursing. *Philadelphia: Lippincott, 1998; Evans, K., and J. Sullivan,* Treating Addicted Survivors of Trauma. *New York: Guilford Press, 1995; Murray, R., and M.M. Huelskoetter,* Psychiatric/Mental Health Nursing: Giving Emotional Care *(3rd ed.). Norwalk, CT: Appleton & Lange, 1991.*

Tolerance Potential	Physical Dependence	Psychological Dependence	Withdrawal Characteristics	Nursing Care
				(4) Teach cognitive methods and stress management techniques to reduce fatigue, promote alertness.
Yes	Yes	Probable	Severe apprehension, fear, or panic. Perceptual distortions and hallucinations. Hyperactivity. Diaphoresis. Tachycardia	(1) Have someone who is close to client stay with client at all times to provide support and comfort. (2) Provide nonthreatening environment with subdued, pleasant stimuli. (3) Provide orientation and diversion to pleasant experiences. (4) Avoid use of sedative/ tranquilizers, if possible. (5) Monitor vital signs. (6) Provide for general health needs. (7) Teach stress management and cognitive methods to increase energy, insight, feelings of health, and life satisfaction. (8) Teach alternate leisure activities.
Yes	Yes	Yes	Headache. Anorexia, irritability, nervousness. Decreased ability to concentrate. Craving for cigarette. Energy loss. Fatigue. Dizziness. Sweating. Tremor and palpitations	(1) Provide support. (2) Explore behavioural changes necessary to quit smoking as well as provide information as to available self-help groups (3) Provide for general health needs. (4) Teach smoking cessation program.

TABLE 11-7
Summary of Marijuana Drugs Related to Nursing Assessment and Intervention

Drug Type/Name	Street Names	Action & Duration	Administration	Desired Effect	Physical & Emotional Effects/ Complications
Marijuana (cannabis), *Indian hemp*, which produces varying grades of hallucinogenic material; *hashish*, pure cannabis resin, the most powerful grade from leaves and flowering tops of female plants; *ganja*, less potent preparation of flowering tops and stems of female plant and resin attached to them; *bhang*, least potent preparation of fried mature leaves and flowering tops of male and female plants; *THC* in fat part of cell prevents nutrients from crossing cell membranes; RNA production and new cell growth reduced; *all* cell function interfered with	Joints, reefer, pot, grass, weed Acapulco Gold The Sticks Hash	Mixed: central nervous system depressant and stimulant. Great variance in duration 2–12 hours THC is fat-soluble, absorbed especially by brain cells and reproductive organs. Builds in the brain; 2 cigarettes per week for 3 months causes personality change. Impairment during nonintoxicated state remains when smoking persists over months	Smoked or swallowed	Euphoria Relaxation Increased perception Escape	**Nervous system** Stored in fat portion of cells; remains in brain 6 weeks after cessation of smoking Speech comprehension, ability to express ideas, and ability to understand relationships impaired because of damage to the cerebral cortex Memory, decision making, handling complex tasks, ability to concentrate or focus impaired because of effects on cells in the hypocampus and cerebrum Emotional swings, depression, pessimism, irritability, low frustration tolerance, and temper outbursts because of cell damage in limbic system Does not learn adaptive skills or how to cope with stressors Lack of motivation, fatigue, moodiness, depression, inability to cope, loss of interest in vigorous activity or all previously enjoyed activities occur because of THC effects on various parts of the brain; failure to continue in emotional development

Tolerance Potential	Physical Dependence	Psychological Dependence	Withdrawal Characteristics	Nursing Care
Yes	Yes	Yes	Heavy smokers report irritability, restlessness, loss of appetite, sleep disturbance, sweating, tremor, nausea, vomiting, and diarrhea, hyperacidity. Ability for memory, thinking, learning, concentration is impaired.	(1) Not usually admitted to acute care settings unless this drug has been used in combination with others, so that a mixed effect occurs. (2) Implement nursing measures listed above under *Hallucinogens*. (3) Likely to see increasing number of children and adolescents with physical effects from chronic use or injuries from accidents; appropriate medical and surgical nursing care should be given. (4) Teach stress management and cognitive methods to relax, cope with stressors, and increase life satisfaction. (5) Explore alternate leisure activities.

(continued)

TABLE 11-7 *(continued)*
Summary of Marijuana Drugs Related to Nursing Assessment and Intervention

Drug Type/Name	Street Names	Action & Duration	Administration	Desired Effect	Physical & Emotional Effects/ Complications
					Insomnia because of damage to cells in the hypothalamus
					Vision blurred and irregular visual perception because of damage to cells in the occipital areas
					Body coordination, maintenance of posture and balance, ability to perform sports or drive a car impaired because of damage to cells in the cerebellum
					Respiratory system
					Upper respiratory infections common because of destruction to mucosal cells from the smoke (more destructive than tobacco smoke)
					Sinusitis, inflammation of the lining of one or more of the sinuses from nasal infection
					Bronchitis, with low-grade fever, chest pain, chronic cough, and yellow-green sputum, common because of inflammation to the bronchial tree caused by smoke inhalation
					Lung cancer more likely because of the numerous chemicals in marijuana (smoking three to five joints a week is equivalent to smoking 16 cigarettes daily for 7 days a week)

Drug Type/Name	Street Names	Action & Duration	Administration	Desired Effect	Physical & Emotional Effects/Complications
					Emphysema and chronic obstructive pulmonary diseases from long-time smoking and deep inhalation; lung function permanently damaged
					Cardiovascular system
					Cardiac arrhythmias and tachycardia related to the dose of THC absorbed (one joint immediately raises heart rate by as much as 50%)
					Hypertension, which may contribute to aneurysm formation or cardiovascular accident, common
					Myocardial infarction possible
					Congested conjunctiva associated with hypertension
					Reproductive system
					Infertility in males from moderate to heavy use because production of testosterone is reduced and low sperm production or production of abnormal sperm occurs
					Impotence, inability to ejaculate sperm
					Gynecomastia, enlarged breast formation, in puberty when secondary sex characteristics are being developed (lower testosterone level causes fat deposits around the breast tissue)
					Hirsutism in females, with increased androgen production resulting in male secondary sex characteristics (increased hair growth on face and arms, deeper voice), irregular menstrual cycles, serious acne, and lack of development of female secondary sexual characteristics
					Infertility in the female because of damage to the ova; menstrual cycle irregularity
					Pregnancy, if present when marijuana is smoked, endangers the embryo and fetus, increasing chance of congenital defects and fetal mortality because THC crosses the placental barrier
					Lactation, if breastfeeding while smoking marijuana, endangers baby's health because THC transfers through breast milk
					Immune system suppressed; prone to infections
					Endocrine system impaired for 11-to 16-year-olds
					Marijuana combined with PCP causes psychosis; if taken with other substances, effect of each drug multiplied

Source: Adapted from Boyd, M., and M. Nihart, Psychiatric Nursing. *Philadelphia: Lippincott, 1998; Evans, K., and J. Sullivan,* Treating Addicted Survivors of Trauma. *New York: Guilford Press, 1995; Newman, B., and P. Newman,* Development Through Life: A Psychosocial Approach *(7th ed.). Belmont, CA: Brooks/Cole, 1999; Murray, R., and M.M. Huelskoetter,* Psychiatric/Mental Health Nursing: Giving Emotional Care *(3rd ed.). Norwalk, CT: Appleton & Lange, 1991; Seifert, K., R. Hoffnung, and M. Hoffnung,* Lifespan Development. *Boston: Houghton Mifflin, 1997.*

CASE SITUATION
Adolescent Drug Abuse

Jess, 17, was taken for treatment to an adolescent chemical abuse unit. "My parents, when they put me in (the hospital), they thought I was just drinking and using pot. When they got my tox screen back, my mom almost fainted."

The drug-screening analysis showed that marijuana, Valium, Demerol, Dilaudid, and codeine all had been ingested within a week. "All I did was live to get high—and, I guess you could say, get high to live," he said.

"I used to work at the home of a doctor who had a medicine cabinet full of everything anybody could dream of. He had a bunch of narcotics and stuff, and I thought I was in heaven. But I could go out right now and get drugs in about 15 minutes if I wanted. People, they're waiting for you to buy it. Around [age] 10, I started drinking a little bit—just tasting it, and getting that warm feeling. The first time I got high, I was 12, and I loved it. There wasn't no stopping me then. I got high all I could. I used to wake up and think, 'How can I get high today?'"

His friends put pressure on him to try other drugs. "I told myself I'd never do any pills, never drop any acid, but those promises went by the wayside." He first took Quaaludes in the ninth grade and dropped acid that year at a concert. Soon he was drinking a lot and taking speed and Valium and other depressants.

"If I drank any beer, I'd want another one. If I got drunk, I'd want to get high; if I got high, I'd want to get pills. When I started out, I thought it was just cool, and that feeling was great. Instead of dealing with normal, everyday problems, I'd run off and get high. It got so I was picking fights just so I could stomp out of the house and get high."

He became a connoisseur. "I didn't buy dope at school. There's no good dope at school."

He also became more difficult to handle at home and at school, "I started fighting a lot with my parents. My grades dropped. I got into fistfights at school. I was real rebellious. I usually was high during class.

"I think it was real obvious to my teachers, because of the way I dressed and the way I acted in class. All the guys I hung around with had real long hair, moccasin boots, heavy metal T-shirts, and leather pants.

"I was pretty much an A student, and they [grades] dropped to low Cs and Ds. I was really withdrawing into myself.

"I wasn't myself when I was stoned. For years, I didn't even know how to feel (emotions). I've left home a few times.

"One time I was on LSD and I took a razor blade and cut my leg up. I still have the scars from that. I blanked out a lot. I'd come home beaten-up looking, and didn't know why."

Jess spent eight weeks in treatment and now says he's been straight for over a year.

"It's a dependency," he said. "There's no way to eliminate it. You just try to control it. If I smoked a joint today or took a drink, I'd be right back."

Jess agrees with other former addicts: part of the problem is the naïveté of the parents.

"My parents, when I started getting in trouble, weren't going to admit it." Advice for parents who uncover a drug problem is simple: "Get some help. Not just for your kids, but for the parents and siblings also, because the whole family gets crazy. It's a family disease.

"I'll have to be on the lookout for the rest of my life to avoid falling back into drug use. I've learned just to be myself, and people will like me—and I never would have believed that before."

QUESTIONS

1. What could have been a motivating factor for Jess to go to the treatment centre?
2. What principles would you use as a guide for effective programming to prevent and reduce the harmful effects of substance abuse among youth?

Both individual and group counselling are useful. In the group setting, the adolescent may be asked to bring a close friend or parent to share the experience. Some concerns and conflicts, however, are best worked through with the individual. Group sessions are effective for the following reasons:[450]

- The person realizes concerns, feelings, and sense of confusion are not unique to him or her.

- Experiences and successful solutions to problems can be shared with others who are at different points of development.

- Ideas and roles can be tried out in the group before being tried in real life.

- Values can be clarified and decisions made with support and feedback from others.

Care Related to Sexuality

Personal Attitudes. First examine personal attitudes toward yourself as a sexual being, the sexuality of others, family, love, and changing mores regarding sexual intercourse before you do any sex education through formal or informal teaching, counselling, or discussion. The adolescent may be trying to understand another kind of sexual experience in his or her own family. For example, a number of adolescents have to deal with the formerly hidden primary sexual orientation of their parents. Either parent may, during this time, announce a same-sex preference, so in addition to the adolescent's working out his or her own sexual identity, the identity of the parent must be reworked. Your astute assessment, case finding, and ability to refer the adolescent elsewhere are still major contributions toward helping him or her stay healthy. The rapport necessary to work with the adolescent in any area is something to which the teen is highly sensitive, and if he or she has no rapport with the family, your attitudes are crucial.

Promoting Education. You can promote education about sexuality, family, pregnancy, contraceptives, and sexually transmitted diseases through your own intervention and by working with parents and school officials so that objective, accurate information can be given in the schools. Most adults favour sex education in school and on television as a way to reduce the problem of teenage pregnancy.

Perhaps most important, you can *encourage the teenager and family to talk together and can teach the parents* how and what to teach, where to get information, and the significance of formal sex education beginning in the home.[451–453]

Care and Counselling. You may work directly with a pregnant teenager or one with a sexually transmitted infection. That person needs your acceptance support, and confidentiality as you do careful interviewing to learn his or her history of sexual activity, symptoms, and contacts. Use effective interviewing, communication, and crisis intervention as discussed in Chapter 5 and by other authors.[454,455]

Information is needed about the type of disease, symptoms, contagious nature, consequences of untreated disease, and where to get treatment. In all of these diseases, both male and female partners (along with any other person who has had sexual contact with these partners) should be treated by medication and use of hygiene measures and by counselling and teaching. You are in a key position to determine signs and symptoms and to help make a differential diagnosis.

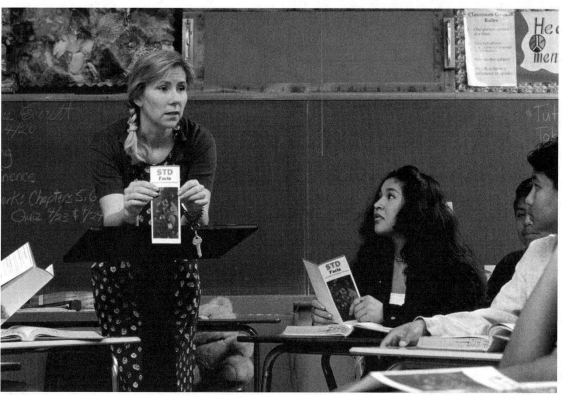

FIGURE 11–1

Nurses should encourage adolescents to discuss health concerns and provide teaching for the issues that are important to this age group.

The girl wants to find out whether she is pregnant and talk about personal feelings, family reactions, and what to do next. Explain what services are available and answer her questions about the consequences of remaining pregnant, keeping or placing the baby for adoption, or terminating pregnancy.

An adolescent girl may want to know about methods of abortion and services available. Reputable abortion clinics do counselling before the abortion so that the girl does not regret her decision, but you can begin counselling. The questions you raise and guidance you give can help her make necessary decisions and avoid complications.[456]

Reforming the Present Health Care System. Reforming the present health care system seems essential, because

present public health services are frequently incapable of kindly or completely handling the problems resulting from adolescents' sexual activity, because of policy, philosophy, understaffing, or underfinancing. You can participate in change by working through your professional organization and as an informed citizen. You can promote a deeper awareness of the adolescent as an individual with unique needs and work to extend education and counselling services, including peer-group counselling and teenage advisory boards. Further, you can help establish community services to work with the adolescent or youth in a health care crisis. The disabled adolescent also requires special care and teaching.

CRITICAL THINKING

What resources in your community are available for a disabled adolescent?

Working with the Drug Abuser and Alcoholic

Personal Attitudes. You must work through your attitudes about drug use and abuse to assess the person accurately or intervene objectively. Why does a drug problem exist? Do you believe drugs are the answer to problems? How frequently do you use drugs? Do you use amphetamines or barbiturates? Have you ever tried marijuana, LSD, or heroin? What are the multiple influences causing persons to seek answers through use of illegal drugs? What are the moral, spiritual, emotional, and physical implications of excessive drug use, whether the drugs are illegal or prescribed? What treatment do drug abusers deserve? How does the alcoholic differ from the drug abuser?

An accepting attitude toward the drug abuser and alcoholic as a person is essential while at the same time you help him or her become motivated and able to cope with stresses without relying on drugs or alcohol. You will need to use effective communication and assessment, but because these problems are complex, you need to work with others. Various references at the end of this chapter, which were cited previously, provide more detailed information to aid you in your care.

Members of society impose heavy responsibilities on the young adult. With your intervention, some adolescents who could not otherwise meet these forthcoming demands will exert a positive force in society.

Knowledge. Knowledge about drugs—current ones available on the street, their symptoms and long-term effects, legislation related to each—is necessary for assessment, realistic teachings, and counselling. Also learn about the effects of alcohol. Know local community agencies that do emergency or follow-up care and rehabilitation with drug abusers and alcoholics.

Help teenagers understand that problems of drug abuse and alcoholism can be avoided in several ways. They must get accurate information and make decisions based on knowledge rather than on emotion, have the courage to say "no," and know and respect the laws. They must also participate in worthwhile, satisfying activities, have a constructive relationship with parents, and recognize that the normal, healthy person does not need regular medication except when prescribed by an authorized practitioner. Help teens realize the unanticipated consequences of drug and alcohol abuse: loss of friends; alienation from family; loss of scholastic, social, or career opportunities; economic difficulties; criminal activities; legal penalties; poor health; and loss of identity rather than finding the self.

INTERESTING WEBSITES

"TALK TO ME"
SEXUALITY EDUCATION FOR PARENTS

http://www.phac-aspc.gc.ca/publicat/ttm-pm/ index.html
"Talk To Me" is a sexual education program designed to help parents to talk to their children about sexuality. It has been developed with emphasis on teenage perspectives. The intent of the program is to make parents more aware of adolescent needs and difficulties related to sexuality, to develop their communication skills, and to help them become more knowledgable and more "askable" parents.

SEXUAL HEALTH AND
SEXUALLY TRANSMITTED INFECTIONS

http://www.phac-aspc.gc.ca/std-mts/faq_e.html
This is a "Sexual Health Info Centre" that provides information on bacterial vaginosis, chlamydia, genital herpes, hepatitis B, human papillomavirus, gonorrhea, HIV/AIDS, pelvic inflammatory disease, syphilis, trichomoniasis, yeast infections, and more.

THE NATIONAL EATING DISORDER
INFORMATION CENTRE

http://www.nedic.ca
This Toronto-based, nonprofit organization provides information and resources on eating disorders and weight preoccupation. NEDIC has a philosophy that promotes healthy lifestyles and encourages clients to make informed choices based on accurate information. They do not promote dieting or other behaviours that limit the full expression of our humanity.

CANADIAN ADOLESCENTS
AT RISK RESEARCH NETWORK

http://educ.queensu.ca/~caarrn
This is a Queen's University–led research program funded by the Canadian Population Health Initiative to study adolescent health. Find studies and national and international data on adolescent health in seven key areas: bullying, sexual health, injuries, school culture, disability and chronic conditions, social capital, and obesity and physical activity.

HEART AND STROKE FOUNDATION OF CANADA

http://ww1.heartandstroke.ca/Page.asp?PageID=24
Unhealthy lifestyles threaten children's hearts. Overweight children could be three to five times more likely to suffer a heart attack or stroke before they reach the age of 65, warn the Heart and Stroke Foundation (HSF) and the Canadian Cardiovascular Society (CCS). This is just one example of the type of information available at this site.

SUMMARY

1. Adolescence is the final period of rapid physical growth, as well as considerable cognitive and emotional change.
2. Relationships with the family remain basically important, but the peer group is dominant and exerts considerable influence on the adolescent's behaviour.
3. This is the time during which the individual works to develop his or her identity or sense of uniqueness, to become independent of and separate from parents while retaining basic ties and values.
4. Because of the many available options, determining one's identity, value systems, and career or life path can

be difficult, take time, and sometimes be detoured by various societal forces of acquired habits, such as substance abuse.

5. A number of health problems may arise in the physical, psychological, or social dimensions.

6. The box entitled "Considerations for the Adolescent and Family in Health Care" summarizes what you should consider in assessment and health promotion.

7. The home situation affects emotional and physical health, adaptive ability, school performance, social skills, later job and marital adjustment, and the type of citizen and parent the adolescent will become.

Considerations for the Adolescent and Family in Health Care

- Family, cultural background and values, support systems, and community resources for the adolescent and family
- Parents as identification figures, able to guide and to allow the adolescent to develop his or her own identity
- Relationship among family members or significant adults and its impact on the adolescent
- Behaviours that indicate abuse, neglect, or maltreatment by parents or other significant adults
- Physical growth patterns, characteristics and competencies, nutritional status, and rest, sleep, and exercise patterns that indicate health and are within age norms for the adolescent
- Completion of physical growth spurt and development of secondary sex characteristics that indicate normal development in the male or female; self-concept and body image development and integration related to physical growth
- Nutritional requirements greater than for the adult
- Immunizations, safety education, and other health promotion measures
- Cognitive development into the stage of formal operations, related value formation, ongoing moral–spiritual development, and beginning development of philosophy of life
- Peer relationships, use of leisure time
- Overall appearance and behavioural patterns at home, school, and in the community that indicate positive identity formation, rather than role confusion or diffusion, or negative identity
- Use of effective adaptive mechanisms and coping skills in response to stressors
- Behavioural patterns in late adolescence that indicate integration of physical changes; cognitive, emotional, social, and moral–spiritual development, effective adaptive mechanisms
- Behavioural patterns and characteristics that indicate the adolescent has achieved developmental tasks
- Parental behaviour that indicates they are achieving their developmental tasks

ENDNOTES

1. Bee, H., *Lifespan Development* (2nd ed.). New York: Longman, 1998.
2. Gormly, A., *Lifespan Human Development* (6th ed.). Fort Worth: Harcourt Brace College Publishers, 1997.
3. Newman, B., and P. Newman, *Development Through Life: A Psychosocial Approach* (7th ed.). Belmont, CA: Brooks/Cole, 1999.
4. Sigelman, C., *Lifespan Human Development* (3rd ed.). Pacific Groves, CA: Brooks/Cole, 1999.
5. Bee, *op. cit.*
6. Dorn, L.D., et al., Perceptions of Puberty: Adolescent, Parent, and Health Care Personnel, *Developmental Psychology,* 26, no. 2 (1990), 322–329.
7. Gormly, *op. cit.*
8. Papalia, D., S. Olds, and R. Feldman, *Human Development* (7th ed. Boston: McGraw Hill, 1998.
9. Newman and Newman, *op. cit.*
10. Wong, D., *Whaley and Wong's Nursing Care of Infants and Children* (6th ed.). St. Louis: C.V. Mosby, 1999.
11. Gormly, *op. cit.*
12. Papalia et al., *op. cit.*
13. Sherwen, L., M. Scolovena, and C. Weingarten, *Maternity Nursing Care of the Childbearing Family* (3rd ed.). Norwalk, CT: Appleton & Lange, 1999.
14. Wong, *op. cit.*
15. Gormly, *op. cit.*
16. Newman and Newman, *op. cit.*
17. Sherwen et al., *op. cit.*
18. Wong, *op. cit.*
19. Newman and Newman, *op. cit.*
20. Sigelman, *op. cit.*
21. Gormly, *op. cit.*
22. Wong, *op. cit.*
23. Gormly, *op. cit.*
24. Newman and Newman, *op. cit.*
25. McLanahan, S., and G. Sandefur, *Growing With a Single Parent.* Cambridge: Harvard University Press, 1994.
26. Newman and Newman, *op. cit.*
27. Grant, C., Teens, Sex, and the Media: Is There a Connection? *Paediatric Child Health,* 8, no. 5 (2003), 285–286.
28. McGown, A., How to Help Your Lesbian Teenager, *Journal of Psychosocial Nursing,* 31, no. 8 (1993), 48.
29. McLanahan and Sandefur, *op. cit.*
30. Newman and Newman, *op. cit.*
31. Ryan, C., D. Futterman, and K. Stine, Helping Our Hidden Youth, *American Journal of Nursing,* 98, no. 12 (1998), 37–41.
32. Burke, V., Pump up Your Parental Influence, *Believer's Voice of Victory,* June (1997), 22–23.
33. French, S., C. Perry, G. Leon, and J. Fulkerson, Weight Concerns, Dieting Behavior, and Smoking Initiation Among Adolescents: A Prospective Study, *American Journal of Public Health,* 84 (1994), 1818–1820.
34. Newman and Newman, *op. cit.*
35. Mahon, N.E., A. Yarcheski, and T.J. Yarcheski, Anger, Anxiety, and Depression in Early Adolescence from Intact and Divorced Families, *Journal of Pediatric Nursing,* 18, no. 4 (2003), 267–273.
36. Davies, J., and M. Frawley, *Treating the Adult Survivor of Childhood Sexual Abuse: A Psychoanalytic Perspective.* New York: Basic Books, 1994.
37. Evans, K., and J. Sullivan, *Treating Addicted Survivors of Trauma.* New York: Guilford Press, 1995.
38. Garbarino, J., *Children in Danger.* New York: Jossey-Bass, 1992.
39. Gillis, A., Teens for Healthy Living, *Canadian Nurse,* June 1996, 26–30.
40. Polk-Walker, G., What Really Happened? Incidence and Factor Assessment of Abused Children and Adolescents, *Journal of Psychosocial Nursing,* 28, no. 11 (1990), 17–22.
41. Warren, J., F. Gary, and J. Moorhead, Self-reported Experiences of Physical and Sexual Abuse Among Runaway Youths, *Perspectives in Psychiatric Care,* 30, no. 1 (1994), 23–28.
42. Wong, *op. cit.*
43. Berman, H., Stories of Growing Up Amid Violence by Refugee Children of War and Children of Battered Women Living in Canada, *IMAGE: Journal of Nursing Scholarship,* 31, no. 1 (1999), 52–63.

44. Guyton, A., *A Textbook of Medical Physiology* (9th ed.). Philadelphia: W.B. Saunders, 1996.
45. Wong, *op. cit.*
46. Fenstermacher, K., and B. Hudson, *Practice Guidelines for Family Nurse Practitioners.* Philadelphia: Saunders, 1997.
47. Guyton, *op. cit.*
48. Sherwen et al., *op. cit.*
49. Wong, *op. cit.*
50. Gormly, *op. cit.*
51. Papalia et al., *op. cit.*
52. Sherwen et al., *op. cit.*
53. Wong, *op. cit.*
54. Papalia et al., *op. cit.*
55. Bee, *op. cit.*
56. Gormly, *op. cit.*
57. Papalia et al., *op. cit.*
58. Seifert, K., R. Hoffnung, and M. Hoffnung, *Lifespan Development.* Boston: Houghton Mifflin, 1997.
59. Sigelman, *op. cit.*
60. Wong, *op. cit.*
61. Guyton, *op. cit.*
62. Seifert et al., *op. cit.*
63. Sherwen et al., *op. cit.*
64. Dorn et al., *op. cit.*
65. Wong, *op. cit.*
66. Sherwen et al., *op. cit.*
67. Wong, *op. cit.*
68. Gormly, *op. cit.*
69. Papalia et al., *op. cit.*
70. Seifert et al., *op. cit.*
71. Sherwen et al., *op. cit.*
72. Wong, *op. cit.*
73. Sherwen et al., *op. cit.*
74. Wong, *op. cit.*
75. Guyton, *op. cit.*
76. *Ibid.*
77. Sherwen et al., *op. cit.*
78. Wong, *op. cit.*
79. Guyton, *op. cit.*
80. Papalia et al., *op. cit.*
81. Sherwen et al., *op. cit.*
82. Wong, *op. cit.*
83. Guyton, *op. cit.*
84. Papalia et al., *op. cit.*
85. Sherwen et al., *op. cit.*
86. Wong, *op. cit.*
87. Sherwen et al., *op. cit.*
88. Wong, *op. cit.*
89. *Ibid.*
90. Guyton, *op. cit.*
91. *Ibid.*
92. Gormly, *op. cit.*
93. Papalia et al., *op. cit.*
94. Seifert et al., *op. cit.*
95. Sigelman, *op. cit.*
96. Papalia et al., *op. cit.*
97. French et al., *op. cit.*
98. Papalia et al., *op. cit.*
99. Wong, *op. cit.*
100. *Ibid.*
101. *Ibid.*
102. *Ibid.*
103. *Ibid.*
104. *Ibid.*
105. Boynton, R., E. Dunn, and G. Stephens, *Manual of Ambulatory Pediatrics* (3rd ed.). Philadelphia: J.B. Lippincott, 1994.
106. Health Risks, *Women's Health Advocate Newsletter,* 2, no. 11 (1996), 2–3.
107. Roye, C., Breaking Through to the Adolescent Patient, *American Journal of Nursing,* 95, no. 12 (1995), 19–23.
108. Uphold, C., and M. Graham, *Clinical Guidelines in Family Practice* (2nd ed.). Gainsville, FL: Barmarrae Books, 1994.
109. Dillon, P.M. *Nursing Health Assessment: Clinical Pocket Guide.* Philadelphia: F. A. Davis, 2004.
110. Roye, *op. cit.*
111. Manning, M., Health Assessment of the Early Adolescent: Challenges and Clinical Issues, *Nursing Clinics of North America,* 25, no. 4 (1990), 823–831.
112. Heiney, S., Helping Children through Painful Procedures, *American Journal of Nursing,* 91, no. 11 (1991), 20–24.
113. Muscari, M., The First Gynecologic Exam, *American Journal of Nursing,* 99, no. 1 (1999), 68–69.
114. Muscari, M., Rebels with a Cause: When Adolescents Won't Follow Medical Advice, *American Journal of Nursing,* 98, no. 12 (1998), 28–35.
115. Roye, *op. cit.*
116. Sharts-Hopko, N., STDs in Women: What You Need to Know, *American Journal of Nursing and Special Women's Health Issue,* 97, no. 4 (1997), 5–7.
117. Gillis, A., Teens for Healthy Living, *The Canadian Nurse,* 92, no. 6 (1996), 26–30.
118. *Ibid.*
119. Vingilis, E.R., T.J. Wade, and J.S. Seeley, Predictors of Adolescent Self-Rated Health, *Canadian Journal of Public Health,* 93, no. 3 (2002), 193–197.
120. Health Canada, *Nutrition for a Healthy Pregnancy—National Guidelines for the Childbearing Years,* Website: http://www.hc-sc.gc.ca//hpfb-dgpsa/onpp-bppn/national_guidelines_05c_e.html, September 2004.
121. McVey, G., S. Tweed, and E. Blackmore, Dieting among Preadolescent and Young Adolescent Females, *Canadian Medical Association Journal,* 170, no. 10 (2004), 1559–1561.
122. Rodwell Williams, S., and E.D. Schlenker, *Essentials of Nutrition & Diet Therapy* (8th ed.). St. Louis: Mosby, 2003.
123. Health Canada, *Nutrition for a Healthy Pregnancy—National Guidelines for the Childbearing Years.*
124. Rodwell Williams and Schlenker, *op. cit.*
125. Philips, S., L. Jacobs Starkey, and K. Gray-Donald, Food Habits of Canadians: Food Sources of Nutrients for the Adolescent Sample, *Canadian Journal of Dietetic Practice and Research,* 65, no. 2 (2004), 81–84.
126. *Ibid.*
127. McVey et al., *op. cit.*
128. French et al., *op. cit.*
129. Wong, *op. cit.*
130. Jones, J.M., S. Bennett, M.P. Olmstead, M.L. Lawson, and G. Rodin, Disordered Eating Attitudes and Behaviours in Teenaged Girls: A School-Based Study, *Canadian Medical Association Journal,* 165, no. 5 (2001), 547–558.
131. Tierney, L., S. McPhee, and M. Papadakis, *Current Medical Diagnosis & Treatment, 1999* (38th ed.). Stamford, CT: Appleton & Lange, 1999.
132. Wong, *op. cit.*
133. Tierney et al., *op. cit.*
134. Gormly, *op. cit.*
135. Tierney et al., *op. cit.*
136. French et al., *op. cit.*
137. Tierney et al., *op. cit.*
138. French et al., *op. cit.*
139. Fritz, T., and M. Barbie, What Are the Warning Signs for Suicidal Adolescents? *Journal of Psychosocial Nursing,* 31, no. 2 (1993), 37–40.
140. Newman and Newman, *op. cit.*

141. Tierney et al., *op. cit.*
142. French et al., *op. cit.*
143. French, S., C.M. Story, B. Downs, M. Bronick, and R. Blum, Frequent Dieting Among Adolescents: Psychosocial and Health Correlates, *American Journal of Public Health,* 85 (1995), 695–701.
144. Wong, *op. cit.*
145. Tierney et al., *op. cit.*
146. Wong, *op. cit.*
147. Boyd, M., and M. Nihart, *Psychiatric Nursing.* Philadelphia: Lippincott, 1998.
148. French et al., *op. cit.*
149. World Health Organization, *Nutrition and Health Development,* Website: http://www.who.int/nut, September 2004.
150. World Health Organization, *Global Strategy on Diet, Physical Activity and Health, Obesity and Overweight,* Website: http://www.who.int/hpr/NPH/docs/gs_obesity.pdf, September 2004.
151. Canadian Institute for Health Information, *Improving the Health of Canadians.* Ottawa: Canadian Institute for Health Information, 2004.
152. Fernandes, E., and B.W. McCrindle, Diagnosis and Treatment of Hypertension in Children and Adolescents, *Canadian Journal of Cardiology,* 16, no. 6 (2000), 801–811.
153. Katzmarzyk, P.T., The Canadian Obesity Epidemic, 1985–1998, *Canadian Medical Association Journal,* 166, no. 8 (2002), 1039–1040.
154. Hanley, A.J.G., S.B. Harris, J. Gittelsohn, T.M.S. Wolever, B. Saksvig, and B. Zinman, Overweight among Children and Adolescents in a Native Canadian Community: Prevalence and Associated Factors, *The American Journal of Clinical Nutrition,* 71, no. 3 (2000), 693–700.
155. Raine, K.D., *Overweight and Obesity in Canada: A Population Health Perspective.* Ottawa: Canadian Institute for Health Information, 2004.
156. *Ibid.*
157. *Ibid.*
158. Health Canada, *The Vitality Approach: A Guide for Leaders,* Ottawa: Health Canada, 2000.
159. French et al., *op. cit.*
160. *Ibid.*
161. Boyd and Nihart, *op. cit.*
162. French et al., *op. cit.*
163. *Ibid.*
164. Uphold and Graham, *op. cit.*
165. Wong, *op. cit.*
166. Health Canada, *Canadian Physical Activity Levels for Children and Youth,* Website: http://www.hc-sc.gc.ca/english/media/releases/2002/2002_25bk3.htm, September 2004.
167. Canadian Institute of Child Health, *The Health of Canada's Children* (3rd ed.). Ottawa: CICH, 2000.
168. *Ibid.*
169. Health Canada, *Canadian Physical Activity Levels for Children and Youth.*
170. *Ibid.*
171. Pate, R., G. Heath, M. Dowde, and S. Trost, Associations Between Physical Activity and Other Health Behaviors in a Representative Sample of U.S. Adolescents, *American Journal of Public Health,* 86, no. 11 (1996), 1577–1581.
172. Gormly, *op. cit.*
173. Wong, *op. cit.*
174. Guyton, *op. cit.*
175. Wong, *op. cit.*
176. Wadsworth, B., *Piaget's Theory of Cognitive and Affective Development: Foundations of Constructivism* (5th ed.). New York: Longman, 1996.
177. Gender Gaps: How Are Our Schools Doing? *Missouri in Motion–Newsletter of the American Association of University Women of Missouri,* Winter (1999), 1, 7.
178. Papalia et al., *op. cit.*
179. Dill-Schreiber, V., *A Peaceable School: Cultivating a Culture of Non-violence.* Bloomington, IN: Phi Delta Kappa, 1997.
180. Manning, *op. cit.*
181. McLanahan and Sandefur, *op. cit.*
182. Papalia et al., *op. cit.*
183. Tutty, L.M., and C. Bradshaw, Violence against Children and Youth: Do School-based Prevention Programs Work?, in C.A. Ateah and J. Mirwaldt, eds., *Within our Reach: Preventing Abuse across the Lifespan* (pp. 47–53). Winnipeg: Fernwood, 2004.
184. *Ibid.*
185. Canadian Adolescents at Risk Research Network, *Fact Sheet: Adolescent Bullying,* Website: http://www.educ.queensu.ca/~caarrn, September 2004.
186. *Ibid.*
187. *Ibid.*
188. Webb, P., Piaget: Implications for Teaching, *Theory into Practice,* 19, no. 2 (1980), 93–97.
189. Gormly, *op. cit.*
190. Papalia et al., *op. cit.*
191. Seifert et al., *op. cit.*
192. Sigelman, *op. cit.*
193. Attachment Needs May Lead to Date Rape, *The Menninger Letter,* 3, no. 9 (1995), 2.
194. Banister, E.M., S.L. Jakubec, and J.A. Stein, "Like, What Am I Supposed to Do?": Adolescent Girls' Health Concerns in Their Dating Relationships, *Canadian Journal of Nursing Research,* 35, no. 2 (2003), 17–33.
195. *Ibid.*
196. Bee, *op. cit.*
197. Gormly, *op. cit.*
198. Papalia et al., *op. cit.*
199. Seifert et al., *op. cit.*
200. Alfons, A., M. Crijnen, J. Ackenbach, and F. Verhulst, Comparisons of Problems Reported by Parents of Children in 12 Cultures: Total Problems, Externalizing, and Internalizing, *Journal of the American Academy of Psychiatry,* 36, no. 9 (1997), 1269–1277.
201. Constantino, J., Breaking the Cycle of Violence, *Outlook: Washington University Alumni Magazine,* Winter (1997), 24–25.
202. Eron, L., What Becomes of Aggressive School Children, *Harvard Mental Health Letter,* 14, no. 10 (1998), 8.
203. Park, Jungwee, Adolescent Self-Concept and Health into Adulthood, *Health Reports,* 14 (2003), suppl.
204. *Ibid.*
205. Newman and Newman, *op. cit.*
206. Murray, R., and M.M. Huelskoetter, *Psychiatric/Mental Health Nursing: Giving Emotional Care* (3rd ed.). Norwalk, CT: Appleton & Lange, 1991.
207. Muscari, M., When to Worry About Adolescent Angst, *American Journal of Nursing,* 98, no. 3 (1998), 22.
208. Murray and Huelskoetter, *op. cit.*
209. Sherwen et al., *op. cit.*
210. Newman and Newman, *op. cit.*
211. Wong, *op. cit.*
212. *Ibid.*
213. Evans, S.J., B.L. Wright, L. Goodbrand, J.P. Kilbreath, and J. Young, Teen Sexuality: Reaching Out in the Malls, *Canadian Journal of Public Health,* 93, no. 1 (2002), 47–51.
214. Health Canada, *Canadian Guidelines for Sexual Health Education,* Ottawa: Minister of Public Works and Government Services Canada, 2003.
215. Kohlberg, L., Moral Stages and Moralization: The Cognitive Development Approach, in Lickera, T., ed., *Moral Development and Behavior.* New York: Holt Rinehart & Winston, 1976.
216. Muuss, R., Carol Gilligan's Theory of Sex Differences in the Development of Moral Reasoning During Adolescence, *Adolescence,* 23, no. 89 (1988), 229–243.

217. Buckley, T., Academic Excellence Is Not Enough: The Moral Formation of Our Students, *Conversations,* Number 11 (Spring, 1997), 26–27.
218. Burke, *op. cit.*
219. Constantino, *op. cit.*
220. Dill-Schreiber, *op. cit.*
221. Eron, *op. cit.*
222. Guyton, *op. cit.*
223. McCoy, B., and G. Boutre, Excluding the Black Male in School and Society, *Kappa Delta Pi Record,* 31, no. 4 (1995), 172–176.
224. Shepherd, B., When Moms Pray, *Focus on the Family,* August (1999), 3–5.
225. Webster, D., P. Gainer, and H. Champion, Weapon Carrying among Inner-city Junior High Students: Defensive Behavior vs. Aggressive Delinquency, *American Journal of Public Health,* 85 (1995), 1604–1608.
226. Buckley, *op. cit.*
227. Shepherd, *op. cit.*
228. Wong, *op. cit.*
229. Clemen-Stone, S., D.G. Eigsti, and S.L. McGuire, *Comprehensive Family and Community Health Nursing* (4th ed.). St. Louis: Mosby-Year Book, 1995.
230. Hoole, A., C. Pickard, R. Ouimette, J. Lohr, and W. Powell, *Patient Care Guidelines for Nurse Practitioners* (5th ed.). Philadelphia: J.B. Lippincott, 1999.
231. Uphold and Graham, *op. cit.*
232. Wong, *op. cit.*
233. Health Canada, *Canadian Immunization Guide, Sixth Edition.* Ottawa: Minister of Public Works and Government Services, 2002.
234. Canadian Population Health Initiative, *Improving the Health of Canadians.* Ottawa: Canadian Institute for Health Information, 2004.
235. Stolte, K.M. *Wellness: Nursing Diagnosis for Health Promotion,* Philadelphia: Lippincott, 1996.
236. Canadian Population Health Initiative, *op. cit.*
237. *Ibid.*
238. Canadian Adolescents at Risk Research Network, *Fact Sheet: Adolescent Injuries,* Website: http://www.educ.queensu.ca/~caar-rn, September 2004.
239. *Ibid.*
240. Bee, *op. cit.*
241. Clemen-Stone et al., *op. cit.*
242. Escobedo, L., J. Chorba, and R. Waxweiler, Patterns of Alcohol Use and the Risk of Drinking and Driving Among U.S. High School Students, *American Journal of Public Health,* 85 (1995), 976–978.
243. Gormly, *op. cit.*
244. Papalia et al., *op. cit.*
245. Sigelman, *op. cit.*
246. Wong, *op. cit.*
247. Parker, D., W. Carl, L. French, and F. Martin, Characteristics of Adolescent Work Injuries Reported to the Minnesota Department of Labor and Industry, *American Journal of Public Health,* 84 (1994), 606–611.
248. Fenstermacher and Hudson, *op. cit.*
249. Hoole et al., *op. cit.*
250. Wong, *op. cit.*
251. Webster et al., *op. cit.*
252. Wong, *op. cit.*
253. Bee, *op. cit.*
254. Haberman, M., and V. Dill, Commitment to Violence Among Teenagers in Poverty, *Kappa Delta Pi Record,* 31, no. 4 (1995), 148–156.
255. McCoy and Boutre, *op. cit.*
256. Papalia et al., *op. cit.*
257. Dorn et al., *op. cit.*
258. Webster et al., *op. cit.*
259. Bee, *op. cit.*
260. Dorn et al., *op. cit.*
261. Papalia et al., *op. cit.*
262. Muscari, M., Preventing Sports Injuries, *American Journal of Nursing,* 98, no. 7 (1998), 58–59.
263. Hoole et al., *op. cit.*
264. *Ibid.*
265. *Ibid.*
266. Boynton et al., *op. cit.*
267. Hoole et al., *op. cit.*
268. Manning, *op. cit.*
269. Heiney, *op. cit.*
270. Muscari, Rebels with a Cause.
271. Roye, *op. cit.*
272. Ryan et al., *op. cit.*
273. Wong, *op. cit.*
274. Boynton et al., *op. cit.*
275. Hoole et al., *op. cit.*
276. Tierney et al., *op. cit.*
277. *Ibid.*
278. *Ibid.*
279. *Ibid.*
280. Wong, *op. cit.*
281. Hauser, S., J. DiPlacido, A. Jacobson, J. Willett, and C. Cole, Family Coping With an Adolescent Chronic Illness: An Approach and Three Studies, *Journal of Adolescence,* 16, no. 3 (1993), 305–329.
282. Keller, C., and R. Nicolls, Coping Strategies of Chronically Ill Adolescents and Their Parents, *International Disability Studies,* 13, no. 4 (1991), 138–140.
283. Fenstermacher and Hudson, *op. cit.*
284. Hauser et al., *op. cit.*
285. Keller and Nicolls, *op. cit.*
286. Hauser et al., *op. cit.*
287. Keller and Nicolls, *op. cit.*
288. Muscari, When to Worry About Adolescent Angst.
289. Keller and Nicolls, *op. cit.*
290. Wong, *op. cit.*
291. Gormly, *op. cit.*
292. Grossman, D., C. Milligan, and R. Deyo, Risk Factors for Suicide Attempts Among Navajo Adolescents, *American Journal of Public Health,* 81, 2 (1991), 870–874.
293. Hawton, K., *Suicide and Attempted Suicide among Children and Adolescents.* Beverly Hills, CA: Sage, 1990.
294. Papalia et al., *op. cit.*
295. Seifert et al., *op. cit.*
296. Sigelman, *op. cit.*
297. Uphold and Graham, *op. cit.*
298. Sigelman, *op. cit.*
299. Papalia et al., *op. cit.*
300. Newman and Newman, *op. cit.*
301. Canadian Population Health Initiative, *op. cit.*
302. Boothroyd, L.J., L.J. Kirmayer, S. Spreng, M. Malus, and S. Hodgins, Completed Suicides among the Inuit of Northern Quebec, 1982–1996: A Case-Control Study, *Canadian Medical Association Journal,* 165, no. 6 (2001), 749–755.
303. *Ibid.*
304. Gormly, *op. cit.*
305. Grossman et al., *op. cit.*
306. Pinhas, L., H. Weaver, P. Bryden, N. Ghabbour, and B. Toner, Gender-Role Conflict and Suicidal Behaviour in Adolescent Girls, *Canadian Journal of Psychiatry,* 47, no. 5 (2002), 473–476.
307. Gormly, *op. cit.*
308. Grossman et al., *op. cit.*
309. Hawton, *op. cit.*

310. Muscari, The First Gynecologic Exam.
311. Wong, *op. cit.*
312. Seifert et al., *op. cit.*
313. Dorn et al., *op. cit.*
314. Boyd and Nihart, *op. cit.*
315. Wong, *op. cit.*
316. *Ibid.*
317. Boyd and Nihart, *op. cit.*
318. Grossman et al., *op. cit.*
319. Clemen-Stone et al., *op. cit.*
320. Hawton, *op. cit.*
321. Muscari, When to Worry About Adolescent Angst.
322. Wong, *op. cit.*
323. Ryan et al., *op. cit.*
324. Wong, *op. cit.*
325. Murray and Huelskoetter, *op. cit.*
326. Hotton, T., and D. Haans, Alcohol and Drug Use in Early Adolescence, *Health Reports,* 15, no. 3 (2004), 9–19.
327. *Ibid.*
328. Boyle, M.H., M. Sanford, P. Szatmarie, K. Merikangas, and D.R. Offord, Familial Influences on Substance Use by Adolescents and Young Adults, *Canadian Journal of Public Health,* 92, no. 3 (2001), 206–209.
329. Williams, R.J., and S.Y. Chang, A Comprehensive and Comparative Review of Adolescent Substance Abuse Treatment Outcome, *Clinical Psychology: Science and Practice,* 7, no. 2 (2000), 138–166.
330. Binge Drinking Still a Major Problem on Campus, *Advances,* Issue 1 (1999), 4.
331. RWJF Programs Tackle Underage and Binge Drinking. *Advances,* Issue 1 (1999), 1–2.
332. Binge Drinking Still a Major Problem on Campus.
333. RWJF Programs Tackle Underage and Binge Drinking.
334. Binge Drinking Still a Major Problem on Campus.
335. Escobedo et al., *op. cit.*
336. RWJF Programs Tackle Underage and Binge Drinking.
337. Boyd and Nihart, *op. cit.*
338. Guyton, *op. cit.*
339. Murray and Huelskoetter, *op. cit.*
340. Tierney et al., *op. cit.*
341. Uphold and Graham, *op. cit.*
342. Clemen-Stone et al., *op. cit.*
343. Escobedo et al., *op. cit.*
344. Tierney et al., *op. cit.*
345. RWJF Programs Tackle Underage and Binge Drinking.
346. Boyd and Nihart, *op. cit.*
347. Evans and Sullivan, *op. cit.*
348. RWJF Programs Tackle Underage and Binge Drinking.
349. *Ibid.*
350. Bee, *op. cit.*
351. Papalia et al., *op. cit.*
352. Seifert et al., *op. cit.*
353. Sigelman, *op. cit.*
354. Bee, *op. cit.*
355. Clemen-Stone et al., *op. cit.*
356. Newman and Newman, *op. cit.*
357. Papalia et al., *op. cit.*
358. Seifert et al., *op. cit.*
359. Sigelman, *op. cit.*
360. Bee, *op. cit.*
361. Hoole et al., *op. cit.*
362. Seifert et al., *op. cit.*
363. Sharts-Hopko, *op. cit.*
364. Sigelman, *op. cit.*
365. Uphold and Graham, *op. cit.*
366. Bee, *op. cit.*
367. Hoole et al., *op. cit.*
368. Seifert et al., *op. cit.*
369. Sharts-Hopko, *op. cit.*
370. Sigelman, *op. cit.*
371. Uphold and Graham, *op. cit.*
372. Society of Obstetricians and Gynaecologists of Canada, *Canadian Guide about Sexuality and Contraception,* Website: http://www.sogc.org/sexsense/index.htm, September 2004.
373. Boyd and Nihart, *op. cit.*
374. Clemen-Stone et al., *op. cit.*
375. Hoole et al., *op. cit.*
376. Sigelman, *op. cit.*
377. Seifert et al., *op. cit.*
378. Sherwen et al., *op. cit.*
379. Tierney et al., *op. cit.*
380. Uphold and Graham, *op. cit.*
381. Wong, *op. cit.*
382. Clemen-Stone et al., *op. cit.*
383. Sharts-Hopko, *op. cit.*
384. Statistics Canada, *The Daily,* Teenage Pregnancy, Website: http://www.statcan.ca/Daily/English/001020/d001020b.htm, September 2004.
385. *Ibid.*
386. Health Canada, *Canadian STD Guidelines,* Website: http://www.hc-sc.gc.ca/hpb/lcdc/bah, September 2004.
387. Wackett, J., Factors Affecting Yukon Teen Pregnancy Decline in the Mid and Late 1990s, *Journal of Obstetrics and Gynaecology in Canada,* 24, no. 11 (2002), 889–893.
388. Clemen-Stone et al., *op. cit.*
389. Sherwen et al., *op. cit.*
390. Wong, *op. cit.*
391. Buckley, *op. cit.*
392. Clemen-Stone et al., *op. cit.*
393. Wong, *op. cit.*
394. Sherwen et al., *op. cit.*
395. Wong, *op. cit.*
396. Colucciello, M., Pregnant Adolescents' Perceptions of Their Babies Before and After Realtime Ultrasound, *Journal of Psychosocial Nursing,* 36, no. 11 (1998), 12–19.
397. Ventura, S., S. Curten, and T. Mathews, *Teenage Births in the United States, National and State Trends, 1990–1996, National Vital Statistics System.* Hyattsville, MD: National Center for Health Statistics, 1998.
398. Statistics Canada, *The Daily,* Teenage Pregnancy.
399. Bee, *op. cit.*
400. Polk-Walker, *op. cit.*
401. Boynton et al., *op. cit.*
402. Sherwen et al., *op. cit.*
403. Wong, *op. cit.*
404. Gormly, *op. cit.*
405. Seifert et al., *op. cit.*
406. *Ibid.*
407. Gormly, *op. cit.*
408. Burgess, A., and H.J. Birnbaum, Youth Prostitution, *American Journal of Nursing,* 82, no. 5 (1982), 832–834.
409. Webb, *op. cit.*
410. Burgess and Birnbaum, *op. cit.*
411. Burke, *op. cit.*
412. Davies and Frawley, *op. cit.*
413. Murray and Huelskoetter, *op. cit.*
414. Polk-Walker, *op. cit.*
415. Wong, *op. cit.*
416. Boyd and Nihart, *op. cit.*
417. Clemen-Stone et al., *op. cit.*
418. Fenstermacher and Hudson, *op. cit.*
419. Sherwen et al., *op. cit.*
420. Wong, *op. cit.*

421. Clemen-Stone et al., *op. cit.*

422. Gormly, *op. cit.*

423. Schissel, B. The Pathology of Powerlessness: Adolescent Health in Canada, in B.S. Bolaria and H.D. Dickinson, eds., *Health, Illness, and Health Care in Canada* (3rd ed., pp. 265–273). Toronto: Nelson Thomson Learning, 2002.

424. Seifert et al., *op. cit.*

425. Boyd and Nihart, *op. cit.*

426. Seifert et al., *op. cit.*

427. Health Canada, *Preventing Substance Abuse Problems among Young People: A Compendium of Best Practices.* Ottawa: Minister of Public Works and Government Services Canada, 2001.

428. *Ibid.*

429. Boyd and Nihart, *op. cit.*

430. Clemen-Stone et al., *op. cit.*

431. Evans and Sullivan, *op. cit.*

432. Gormly, *op. cit.*

433. Murray and Huelskoetter, *op. cit.*

434. Seifert et al., *op. cit.*

435. Wong, *op. cit.*

436. Boyd and Nihart, *op. cit.*

437. Clemen-Stone et al., *op. cit.*

438. Gormly, *op. cit.*

439. Boyd and Nihart, *op. cit.*

440. Guyton, *op. cit.*

441. Boyd and Nihart, *op. cit.*

442. *Ibid.*

443. Seifert et al., *op. cit.*

444. Boyd and Nihart, *op. cit.*

445. Seifert et al., *op. cit.*

446. Sherwen et al., *op. cit.*

447. Wong, *op. cit.*

448. Muscari, Rebels with a Cause.

449. Ryan et al., *op. cit.*

450. Murray and Huelskoetter, *op. cit.*

451. Pate et al., *op. cit.*

452. Clemen-Stone et al., *op. cit.*

453. Murray and Huelskoetter, *op. cit.*

454. Boyd and Nihart, *op. cit.*

455. Murray and Huelskoetter, *op. cit.*

456. *Ibid.*

Part 4

THE DEVELOPING PERSON AND FAMILY: YOUNG ADULTHOOD THROUGH DEATH

CHAPTER 12

ASSESSMENT AND HEALTH PROMOTION FOR THE YOUNG ADULT

CHAPTER 13

ASSESSMENT AND HEALTH PROMOTION
FOR THE MIDDLE-AGED PERSON

CHAPTER 14

ASSESSMENT AND HEALTH PROMOTION
FOR THE PERSON IN LATER ADULTHOOD

CHAPTER 15

DEATH, THE LAST DEVELOPMENTAL STAGE

Chapter 12

ASSESSMENT AND HEALTH PROMOTION FOR THE YOUNG ADULT

*When I was a child I spoke as a child, I understood
as a child, I thought as a child, but when I became
a man, [an adult], I put away childish things.*

I Corinthians 13:11

*To keep the lamp burning, you have to keep
putting oil in it.*

Mother Teresa

OBJECTIVES

STUDY OF THIS CHAPTER WILL ENABLE YOU TO:

1. Discuss young adulthood as a developmental crisis and explain how the present young adult generation differs from earlier generations.

2. Explore with middle-aged and older adults ways to be helpful to young adults.

3. List the developmental tasks of the young adult's family, and describe your role in helping families to meet these tasks.

4. Assess the physical characteristics of a young adult.

5. Disclose findings from sex behaviour research when asked for information about sexuality.

6. Teach nutritional requirements to the young adult male and female, including the pregnant and lactating female.

7. Identify various body rhythms, and give examples of body rhythms that maintain adaptation.

8. Examine factors that influence biological rhythms and illness, and the nonsynchrony that may result.

9. Discuss nursing measures to assist the person's maintenance of normal biological rhythms during illness.

10. Compare and contrast the stages of the sleep cycle, effects of deprivation of the different stages of sleep, and sleep disturbances that occur.

11. Discuss with the young adult his or her need for rest, sleep, exercise, and leisure.

12. Assess emotional characteristics, self-concept and body image, and adaptive mechanisms of a young adult, and determine nursing implications for each.

13. Examine the meaning of intimacy versus isolation.

14. Compare and contrast lifestyle options and their influence on the health status of the young adult and your plans for his or her care.

15. Describe how cognitive characteristics, social concerns, and moral, spiritual, and philosophical development influence the total behaviour and well-being of the young adult.

16. List the developmental tasks of the young adult, and describe your role in helping him or her achieve them.

17. Assess a young adult who has one of the health problems described in this chapter, write a care plan, and work effectively with him or her to enhance health status.

Childhood and adolescence are the periods for growing up; adulthood is the time for settling down. The changes in young adulthood relate more to sociocultural forces and expectations and to value and cognitive changes than to physical development. The young adult generally has more contact with people of different ages than previously in history. This experience tends to influence the young adult toward a more settled viewpoint.

The young adult is expected to enter new roles of responsibility at work, at home, and in society and to develop values, attitudes, and interests in keeping with these roles. The young adult may have difficulty simultaneously handling work, school, marriage, home, and childrearing. He or she may work primarily at one of these tasks at a time, neglecting the others, which then adds to the difficulties.

The definition, expectations, and stresses of young adulthood are influenced by socioeconomic status, urban or rural residence, ethnic and educational background, various life events, and the historical era. This generation of young adults is unique. They have experienced economic growth and related abundance of material goods and technology, rapid social changes, and sophisticated medical care. They have never known a world without the threat of nuclear war, pollution, overpopulation, and threatened loss of natural resources. Instant media coverage of events has made the world a small and familiar place. Changes in the role of women, the decreasing birth rate, and increasing longevity are modifying the timing of developmental milestones in many people.

Generation X is a recently identified group of young adults in North America. They are well educated and have the means to achieve the upper-middle-class lifestyle; however, they differ from the dominant culture in some ways. They are concerned about the quality of family life and divorce rates, and want the job to accommodate to family values. They speak of promoting social equality, preserving parks, and improving the environment, but also want to get by with the status quo when possible. They say they want to "get back to basics." They desire to avoid risks and may feel paralyzed by the social problems around them. Overall, this young adult generation makes demands that may create discomfort or conflict for older generations.[1–3]

Further, the person who is 25 or 30 (the young-young adult) works at developmental tasks differently from the person who is 35, 40, or 45 (the old young adult).

CRITICAL THINKING

What are some characteristics that define Generation X?

FAMILY DEVELOPMENT AND RELATIONSHIPS

The major family goal is the reorganization of the family into a continuing unity while releasing maturing young people into lives of their own. Most families actively prepare their children to leave home.

Use the following information for assessment and health promotion with young adults and their family members. You can help parents understand that, although they are releasing their own children, new members are being drawn into the family circle through their offspring's marriage or close relationships. That the young adult is ready to leave home indicates the parents have done their job. Use the following knowledge to teach and counsel families as they work through concerns about family relationships.

Family Relationships

In Canada and the United States, the young adult is expected to be independent from the parents' home and care, although if the person has an extended education, he or she may choose to remain living with the parents to save expenses. Sometimes the young adult does not leave the parents' home as quickly as parents would like. With the increasing number of separations and divorces, the tight job market, and increasing apartment rental rates, the young adult child may move back home, sometimes with children.

Often family expenses are at a peak during this period as parents pay for education and weddings or finance their offspring while they establish their own home or profession. Young adults will earn what they can, but they may not be able to be financially independent even if they are no longer living at home. Both parents may work to meet financial obligations. As young adult offspring establish families, parents should take the complementary roles of letting go and standing by with encouragement, reassurance, and appreciation.

Often the main source of conflict between the parents and young adult offspring is the difference in philosophy and lifestyle between the two generations. The parents who sacrificed for their children to have a nice home, material things, education, leisure activities, and travel may now be criticized for how they look, act, and believe. In fact, the young adult may insist that he or she will *never* live like the parents.

Help the parents resolve within themselves that their grown children will not be carbon copies of them. The parents, however, can secretly take solace in knowing that usually the basic values they instilled within their children will remain their basic guidelines, although outward behaviour may seem different. (Often behaviour will not be that much different.) This becomes evident as the young adult becomes middle-aged. Help the parents to realize the importance of their acceptance and understanding of their offspring and of not deliberately provoking arguments over ideologies.

The parents need help in providing a secure home base, both as a model for the young adult and to reduce feelings of threat in the younger children. Although the parents are withstanding the criticism of their grown children, they must remain cognizant that younger children in the home will be feeling conflict, too. The parents are still identification models to them, but young children and adolescents value highly the attitudes and judgments of young adult siblings, who, in turn, can have a definite influence on younger children. The parents can help the younger children realize that there are many ways to live and that they will encourage each to find his or her own way when the time comes.

Gradually the parents themselves must shift from a household with children to a couple again as the last young adult establishes a home. Family structure, roles, and responsibilities change, and use of space and other resources change.

Family Developmental Tasks

In summary, the following tasks must be accomplished by the family of the young adult. Your listening, teaching, and counselling may help the family to meet these tasks:

- Rearrange the home physically and reallocate resources (space, material objects) to meet the needs of remaining members.
- Meet the expenses of releasing the offspring and redistribute the budget.
- Redistribute the responsibilities among grown and growing children and finally between the husband and wife or between the adult members living in the household on the basis of interests, ability, and availability.
- Maintain communication within the family to contribute to harmony and happiness while remaining available to young adult and other offspring.
- Enjoy companionship and sexual intimacy as a couple while incorporating changes.
- Widen the family circle to include the close friends or spouses of the offspring and the entire family of in-laws.
- Reconcile conflicting loyalties and philosophies of life.

CRITICAL THINKING

What are some developmental tasks of the family when a recently divorced young adult son or daughter comes back home with three children?

PHYSIOLOGIC CONCEPTS

Use the following information to teach the young adult and in your assessment and health promotion intervention.

Physical Characteristics

Although body and mind changes continue through life, most physical and mental structures have completed growth when the person reaches young adulthood. Changes that occur during adult life are different from those in childhood; they occur more slowly and in smaller increments.

Young adulthood is the life era when most people are in their peak for strength, energy, and endurance.[4]

Weight and Height

Females have usually reached full height by 17 or 18 years; males are usually full height by 21 years; some grow another inch before age 25.[5] Norms denote a set standard of development or the average achievement of a group; however, an average adult person has never really been described. Each person is an individual, and normal values cover a wide range of healthy individuals. Height and weight depend on many factors: heredity, sex, socioeconomic level, geographic area, food habits and preferences, level of activity, and emotional and physical environments. Weight loss or gain is unpredictable in this age group; and norms for height and weight are difficult to determine.

In Canada, the concept of weight classification has a broader meaning than solely that of body weight.[6] The *Canadian Guidelines for Body Weight Classification in Adults* provides a scheme for classifying weight as measured by the body mass index (BMI), according to the level of health risk. The BMI is an index of weight to height (kg/m^2).[7] It is considered to be the most useful indicator of health risks associated with being underweight, overweight, or obese. The waist circumference (WC) is positively correlated with abdominal fat and is an independent indicator of health risk associated with abdominal obesity.[8] The BMI does not, however, provide an indication of the distribution of fat in the body, and research has shown that excess fat in the abdominal area is associated with an increased risk to health. The information derived from the application of the weight classification system can help to guide policy decisions as well as provide a tool for the evaluation of public health intervention programs.[9]

The 2003 Canadian body weight classification categorizes BMIs between 25.0 and 29.9 as "overweight" and is associated with increased health risk. A BMI of 30 and over reflects obesity and is associated with a high to extremely high risk of developing health problems. These categories are in accordance with the World Health Organization (WHO) weight classification system.[10] The "obese" category was further subdivided by WHO into Obesity Class I (BMI of 30.0–34.9), Obesity Class II (35.0–39.9), and Obesity Class III (40.0 and over). This differentiation has been adopted in the 2003 Canadian body weight classification system.[11]

Obesity is not only a public health concern but it is also a medical, legislative, environmental, and societal concern.[12] According to the Canadian Health Survey, obesity rates have almost tripled in the past few decades, increasing to 15% of total health expenditures in 2000–2001.[13] Overweight and obesity are known risk factors for type 2 diabetes, stroke, heart disease, hypertension, gallbladder disease, and certain types of cancer, osteoarthritis, and sleep apnea.[14] Psychological disorder is also a risk factor of obesity and must be taken into consideration.[15]

CRITICAL THINKING QUESTION

How do you account for "obesity epidemic"?

You can calculate the BMI as follows:

1. ***Convert body weight to kilograms.***
   (1 kilogram = 2.2 pounds)

   Body weight (pounds) ÷ 2.2 = weight (kilograms)
   Example: 132 pounds ÷ 2.2 = 60 kilograms

2. ***Convert height to meters.***
   (1 meter = 39.37 inches)

   Height (inches) ÷ 39.37 = height (meters)
   Example: 65 inches ÷ 39.37 = 1.65 meters

3. ***Calculate BMI.***

   Weight (kg) ÷ height $(m)^2$ = BMI
   Example: 60 kg ÷ (1.65 m × 1.65 m) = 22.03 BMI

4. ***Check BMI against risk for health problems related to body weight.***

CRITICAL THINKING

What are health promotion activities to pursue for someone who has abdominal obesity?

Musculoskeletal System

Skeletal growth for the young adult is completed by age 25, or sooner, when the epiphyseal line calcifies and fuses with the main shaft of the long bones. The vertebral column continues to grow until the individual reaches age 25; 3 to 5 mm may be added to an individual's height. Smaller leg bones, the sternum, pelvic bones, and vertebrae attain adult distribution of the red marrow by approximately 25 years of age. By the early 40s, the bones will have lost some mass and density. The process begins earlier in women. With increasing age, the cartilage in all joints has a more limited ability to regenerate itself. Normally, posture is erect.[16,17]

Body systems are functioning at their peak efficiency, and the individual has reached optimum physiologic and motor function and stamina. Muscle growth is complete at age 30. Peak muscle strength is attained, and maximum physical potential occurs between the ages of 19 and 30. It is during young adulthood that most athletes accomplish their greatest achievements. After this peak period, a 10% loss of strength occurs between the ages of 30 and 60; this loss usually occurs in the back and leg muscles. A person can maintain peak performance through the 30s and much of the 40s, however, with regular exercise and dietary moderation.[18–20]

Skin

The skin of the young adult is smooth, and skin turgor is taut. Acne usually disappears because sex hormones have less influence on secretion of oils from sebaceous glands of the skin. In late young adulthood the skin begins to lose moisture, becoming more dry and wrinkled. Smile lines and lines at the corners of the eyes are usually noticeable.[21]

Cardiovascular System

Maximum physical potential is reached in young adulthood so far as muscles and internal organs are concerned. *Heart* and *circulatory* changes occur gradually with age, depending on exercise and diet patterns. During young adulthood, the total blood volume is 70 to 85 mL/kg of body weight. Maximum cardiac output is achieved and peaks between 20 and 30 years of age. Heart rate averages 72 beats per minute; the blood pressure gradually increases, reaching 100 to 120 mm Hg systolic and 60 to 80 mm Hg diastolic. Heart and blood vessels are fully mature, and cholesterol levels increase. Arteries become less elastic. Hemorrhoids and other varicose veins may become health problems, especially in the childbearing woman. Maintaining normal *blood pressure* (120/80 is considered optimal, normal range is below 140/90) reduces risk for later heart disease and strokes.[22,23]

Respiratory System

Since birth, the lungs have increased in weight 20 times.[24,25] Breathing becomes slower and deeper, 12 to 20 breaths per minute. The maximum breathing capacity decreases between ages 30 and 60. Breathing rate and capacity will differ according to the size of the individual. Larger people have a slower rate.

Gastrointestinal System

The *digestive organs* function smoothly during this period of life. Stomach capacity is 2000 to 3000 mL. The amount of ptyalin decreases after 20 years of age, and digestive juices decrease after 30 years of age. *Dental maturity* is achieved in the early 20s with emergence of the last four molars (wisdom teeth).[26,27] Some people must have their wisdom teeth removed because they become impacted and cause pain.

Neurologic System

The *brain* continues to grow into adolescence and young adulthood and reaches its maximum weight and size during adulthood. Mature patterns of brain wave activity do not appear until age 20; maturation continues to age 30. Nerve conduction velocity is at maximum functional capacity.[28,29]

Visual and auditory sensory perceptions should be at their peak. Gradually during young adulthood the lenses of the eyes lose elasticity and begin to have difficulty changing shape and focusing on close objects; however, by age 30 the changes are seldom sufficient to affect function of the eye. Women in this age group can detect high auditory tones better than men.[30,31] Some young adults wear corrective glasses, contact lenses, or hearing aids. Assess for them when you are giving emergency care, especially if the person is unconscious, so that they are not lost or the person does not suffer eye or ear injury.

Information on how to remove contact lenses from another person's eyes can be obtained from your local optometry association, optometrist, or ophthalmologist.

Endocrine System

Adrenal secretion of cortisol decreases approximately 30% over the entire adult life span. Because plasma cortisol levels remain constant in young adulthood the person maintains good response to stress. **Basal metabolic rate** (*body's consumption of oxygen*) is at maximum functional capacity at age 30 and then decreases gradually, which is related to decrease in the mass of muscle tissue (primarily large oxygen consuming tissue). A gradual decrease in *thyroid hormone* is an adjustment to the progressively slower rate at which it is broken down and removed from the blood. The blood level of thyroxine (T_4) falls approximately 15% over the adult life span. The blood level of tri-iodothyronine (T_3), the active thyroid hormone, declines only when the person is ill and not eating. In women *estrogen* and *progesterone* levels fluctuate. Changes are indicated by the monthly menstrual cycle.[32,33]

Sexuality and Sexual Development

Sexual Maturity

Sexual maturity for men is usually reached in the teens, but their sexual drive remains high through young adulthood. In healthy women menstruation is well established and regular by this time. Female organs are fully matured; the uterus reaches maximum weight by age 30. The woman is well equipped for childbearing. The optimum period for reproduction is between 20 and 30 years of age. The Leydig cells, source of male hormones, decline in number after age 25.[34,35]

Sexuality may be defined as a *deep, pervasive aspect of the total person, the sum total of one's feelings and behaviours, the expression of which goes beyond genital response.* Sexuality includes **sex identity,** *the sense of self as male, female, bisexual (feeling comfortable with both sexes), homosexual, or ambivalent (transsexual).* Sex identity also includes **sex role,** *what the person does overtly to indicate to self and others maleness, femaleness, bisexuality, or ambivalence.* Throughout the life cycle, physiologic, emotional, social, and cultural forces condition sexuality. Today's society offers many choices in sexual behaviour patterns.

You will encounter four basic values taken by young adults toward sexuality: absolutist, hedonistic, relativistic, and relational. The **absolutist or procreation position** *states that sexuality exists for the purpose of reproduction.* The **hedonistic** or **recreational sex view** *has pleasure and pursuit as its central value* and is interested in ultimate fulfillment of human sensual potentials. The **relativistic** or **situational position** is *based on research and has become the basis for the new morality, which says that acts should be judged on the basis of their effects.* The **relational,** or **person-centred, position** *views sexual activity as a natural extension of intimate relationships.*[36] You will have your private set of values, but you must recognize that others' values may be, to them, as valid as yours.

During adulthood a number of sexual patterns may exist, ranging from heterosexuality, bisexuality, and homosexuality to masturbation and abstinence. Few people are totally homosexual or heterosexual; most people feel attracted or sexually responsive at some time to both sexes. Within each of these patterns the person may achieve a full and satisfactory life or be plagued with lack of interest, impotence, or guilt. Young adulthood is the time to reap the rewards or disasters of past sex education. Changes in sexual interest and behaviour occur through the life cycle and can be a cause of conflict unless the partners involved can talk about their feelings, needs, and desires. Many misunderstandings arise because of basic differences between the male and female in sexual response. The more each can learn about the other partner, the greater will be the chance of working out a compatible relationship for successful courtship, marriage, and intimacy. The person cannot assume that the partner knows his or her wishes or vice versa. Each must declare his or her needs.

CRITICAL THINKING

How does homophobia develop in society? What health promotion strategies might be used to prevent homophobia in a community?

Sexuality Education

Often the popular literature promotes misinformation, and you should be prepared to give accurate information. Because people feel freer now to discuss sexual matters, you may be questioned frequently by the person recuperating from an illness, by the partner, after delivery, or by the healthy young adult who feels dissatisfied with personal knowledge or sexual pattern. Various references provide in-depth information on this subject.[37,38]

The following are facts that you can teach young adults based on current research:[39–42]

- Sexual mores and norms vary among ethnic and cultural groups, socioeconomic classes, and even from couple to couple. Sexual activity that is mutually satisfying to the couple and not harmful to themselves and others is acceptable.
- Sexual activity varies considerably among people in relation to sex drive, frequency of orgasm, or need for rest after intercourse.
- Various factors and feelings are as influential on men as on women in determining sexual expression. Sexual function, especially in men, is not an uninhibited, mechanical, automatic act requiring only appropriate stimulus and intact physical equipment.
- Heterosexual intercourse is a reproductive act, but people do not engage in sexual intercourse only for reproduction. *Many sexual acts are nongenital in nature but involve people sharing touch, affection, and pleasure.*
- The more sexually active person maintains the sex drive longer into later years.
- The human sexual drive has no greater impact on the total person than any other biological function. Sex is *not* the prevailing instinct in humans, and physical or mental disease does not result from unmet sexual needs.

- Erotic dreams that culminate in orgasms occur in 85% of all men at any age and commonly in women, increasing in older women.
- The woman is not inherently passive and the man aggressive. Maximum gratification requires that each partner is both passive and aggressive in participating mutually and cooperatively in sexual intercourse.
- Women have as strong a sex desire as men, sometimes stronger.
- Women have greater capacity than men with regard to duration and frequency of orgasm. The female can have several orgasms within a brief period.
- Female orgasm is normally initiated by clitoral stimulation, but it is a total body response rather than clitoral or vaginal in nature.
- The woman may need stimulation to the clitoris other than that received during intercourse to achieve orgasm. Some studies show that a large percentage of women regularly do not have orgasm in sexual intercourse. Overall sexual response is enhanced for the women when there is warm, loving behaviour from the partner before, during, and after intercourse, when foreplay between partners increases arousal, and when she has worked through strict parental admonitions against touching self, enjoying her body, masturbation, or sexual intercourse.
- Simultaneous orgasm of both partners may be desired but is an unrealistic goal and occurs only in the most ideal circumstances. It does not determine sexual achievement or satisfaction.
- No physiologic reason exists for abstinence during menses as menstrual flow is from the uterus, no tissue damage occurs to the vagina, and the woman's sex drive is not necessarily diminished.
- No relationship exists between penile size and ability of the man to satisfy the woman, and little correlation exists between penile and body size and sexual potency. The women's reaction to penile size or her feelings with penile penetration, however, do affect the man's ability for orgasm and satisfaction.
- No single most accepted position for sexual activity exists. Any position is correct, normal, healthy, and proper if it satisfies both partners.
- Achievement of satisfactory sexual response is the result of interaction of many physical, emotional, developmental, and cultural influences and of the total relationship between man and woman.
- Chronically ill or disabled persons learn to live with physical changes and to adapt to express their sexual interests. Underlying fantasies, anxiety, guilt, attitudes toward self, and history of relationships with people affect sexual functioning.
- Decreased sexual desire may be related to physical or emotional illness, prescribed medications, use of alcohol or other drugs, changed behaviour in the partner, or fatigue from the stress and demands of employment or professional life—for either men or women.
- Making love and having sex are not necessarily the same, although ideally they occur together.

Additionally, you may wish to share the following information. In the normal male, spermatozoa are produced in optimum numbers and motility when ejaculation occurs two or three times weekly. A decreased or increased frequency of ejaculation is associated with deceased number of sperm.[43]

Menstruation is a part of sexuality in women. Periods of emotional stress, either happy or upsetting, can cause irregular menses.

CRITICAL THINKING

What do you think attitudes about sexuality will be in the next 25 years?

12–1 BONUS SECTION IN CD-ROM

Human Sexual Response

This section touches on the research findings of the sexual behaviour studies of Masters and Johnson during the late 1970s and early 1980s.

Premenstrual Phenomena

Premenstrual syndrome (PMS) *is a group of signs and symptoms occurring approximately a week before, and associated with, hormonal changes and fluid retention:* mild cerebral edema and edema of fingers, feet, thighs, legs, hips, breasts, abdomen, and around the eyes. However, Erlick Robinson states that the PMS symptoms that most often bring women to their doctors for help are irritability, depression, and agitation.[44] The box entitled "Common Signs and Symptoms of Premenstrual Syndrome" lists physiologic symptoms and signs and emotional reactions that are reported by some women. Symptoms are more likely to appear or increase as women enter their 30s or reach age 40. No simple cause has been identified; several mechanisms for pathogenesis have been described.[45,46] PMS is not the same as **dysmenorrhea,** *painful or severely uncomfortable menstruation.*[47]

Not all these signs and symptoms appear together; they are variable in degree, and they decrease after menses begins.[48–51] *Be empathic to the woman* who describes these symptoms or feelings. *Help the spouse and other family members* recognize their significance, the importance of medical treatment and that their caring and reduction of stress may contribute to a decrease in symptoms.

Treatment for PMS may be symptomatic. It is advisable to combine treatment with a healthy lifestyle. For example, dietary measures and aerobic exercise are suggested.[52–54] In addition, relaxation techniques and cognitive therapy help clients to reframe their attitude towards PMS.[55] Self-help literature can also help women feel that they have control over their bodies.

Teach women that the following measures can offset symptoms:[56–58]

- Consume less caffeine in beverages, colas, and over-the-counter drugs and less sugar, alcohol, and salt, especially during the premenstrual period.

Common Signs and Symptoms of Premenstrual Syndrome

Physiologic Symptoms and Signs

- Fatigue, increased need for sleep
- Appetite change, craving for salty or sweet foods
- Abdominal distension, swollen hands or feet, puffy eyes
- Headache or backache
- Breast tenderness, swelling, increased nodularity just before menstrual period
- Weight gain
- Nausea
- Constipation or diarrhea
- Acne or hives
- Dizziness
- Menstrual cramps
- Clumsiness
- Sex drive changes
- Thirst
- Proneness to infection
- Lower alcohol tolerance

Psychological Reactions

- Apprehension or anxiety
- Confusion
- Forgetfulness
- Frequent crying
- Indecisiveness
- Irritability
- Restlessness
- Mood swings
- Sadness or depression
- Suspiciousness
- Tension
- Withdrawal
- Difficulty with concentration

- Eat four to six small meals a day rather than two or three meals to minimize the risk of hypoglycemia that accompanies PMS.

- Snack on complex carbohydrates, such as fresh fruits, vegetable sticks, and whole wheat crackers, which provide energy without excessive sugar.

- Drink six to eight glasses of water to help prevent fluid retention by flushing excess salt from the body.

- Limit fat intake (especially in red meats), which increases levels of hormones that cause breast tenderness and fluid retention. Choose dairy products low in fat.

- Eat more whole grains, nuts, and raw greens, which are high in vitamin B, magnesium, and potassium, and add vitamin B_6 and calcium to reduce symptoms.

- Develop a variety of interests, including maintaining exercise routines, so that focus is not on self and body symptoms during this period.

■   Walk and perform other physical exercise at least four times weekly to reduce symptoms of mood swings, increased appetite, crying, breast tenderness, craving for sweets, fluid retention, and depression (exercise raises beta-endorphin levels, which in turn increase feelings of well-being and improve the glucose tolerance curve).

■   Get extra rest and use relaxation techniques, meditation, and massage. Treat yourself to a relaxing and creative activity.

■   Discuss your feelings with family and friends so that they can be more understanding of your behaviour.

■   Join a self-help group to hear other ideas on how to more effectively cope with symptoms.

Premenstrual syndrome is not the same as **premenstrual dysphoric disorder (PMDD).** PMDD is rare (3% to 5% of menstruating women) and *involves a pattern of severe, recurrent symptoms of depression and other negative mood states in the last week of the menstrual cycle and markedly interferes with daily living.* PMS occurs in 8% to 10% of women and is less disabling.[59]

CRITICAL THINKING

What is your knowledge of complementary therapies and/or homeopathic remedies in assisting women who are experiencing PMS?

Ovulation

Share the following information about ovulation, especially with couples who desire **natural family planning.** Ovulation normally occurs in every menstrual cycle but not necessarily mid-cycle. The ovum is capable of being fertilized for 24 hours after ovulation. Sperm survive in the female reproductive tract for three to four days.

The mucus cycle by which to predict ovulation is as follows. It begins with menstruation. The period is usually followed by a few "dry days," variable in number, when no mucus is seen or felt. As the ovum begins to ripen, some mucus is felt at the vaginal opening and can be seen if the woman wipes the vaginal area with toilet tissue. This mucus is generally yellow or white, but definitely opaque and sticky. When the blood estrogen level (derived from the ripening ovum) reaches a critical point, the glands of the cervix respond with different mucus. This fertile mucus starts out cloudy and is not sticky and becomes very clear, like raw egg white. After ovulation, progesterone causes the abrupt cessation of the clear, slippery, fertile mucus and produces its own mucus, which is sticky, much less preponderant, and sometimes not present at the vagina. Progesterone prepares the uterine lining for the reception of the egg if the egg has been fertilized. *Usually the egg is ovulated within 24 hours of the peak of wetness,* but this interval may be as long as 48 hours or even longer in some women. Although the sticky mucus does not allow a sperm to live very long, the sperm could possibly survive long enough to reach a freshly ovulated egg through a lingering fertile mucus channel. If this method will be used to avoid pregnancy, there should be abstinence from intercourse from the beginning of the slippery fertile mucus until the height of wetness ("peak day" when there may be so much wetness that mucus is not seen but moisture is noted on the underclothing) *plus a full 72 to 96 hours* to ensure that the ovum will not be impregnated.[60] (See Figure 12–1.)

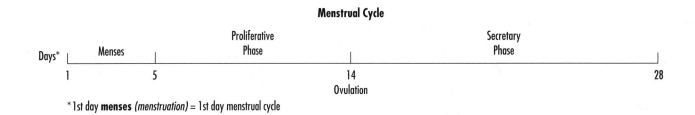

Menstrual Cycle

Days* | Menses | | Proliferative Phase | | Secretary Phase |
1   5   14   28
                                   Ovulation

*1st day **menses** *(menstruation)* = 1st day menstrual cycle

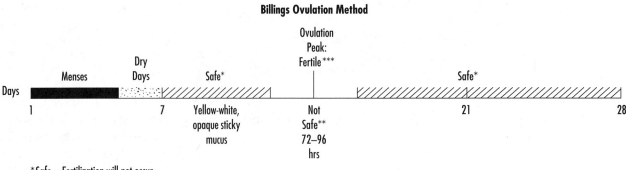

Billings Ovulation Method

Days

Menses | Dry Days | Safe* | Ovulation Peak: Fertile*** | Safe* |
1   7   Yellow-white,   Not   21   28
                   opaque sticky   Safe**
                   mucus   72–96
                                        hrs

*Safe = Fertilization will not occur.
**Not Safe = Fertilization can occur.
***Fertile Mucus: Clear, slippery, like raw egg white,
          Peak of secretions, moisture felt.

FIGURE 12-1

Relationship of menstrual cycle to use of Billings Ovulation Method (natural family planning).

Because the lifetime of the sperm depends on the presence of the fertile mucus, all genital contact between the partners must be avoided. The first drop of semen (the one that escapes before ejaculation) has the highest concentration of sperm. The average ejaculation of about 1 teaspoon of semen contains 200 to 500 million sperm. A woman can conceive even if only one drop of semen touches her external genital organ; sperm are powerful, and the mucus is equally potent.

Teach that spotting or bleeding may occur between menses and may be associated with ovulation, a cervical polyp, post-intercourse in the presence of cervicitis, or carcinoma. Any abnormal pattern of bleeding should be investigated by a gynecologist.

Sexual Dysfunctions

Sexual dysfunctions affect both male and female for various reasons. Several authors provide additional information on sexual dysfunctions.[61–63] Your education and referral can assist couples in obtaining effective diagnosis and treatment.

12–2 BONUS SECTION IN CD-ROM

Research Abstract: Differences in Cortisol, a Stress Hormone, in Women with Turmoil-Type Premenstrual Symptoms

This research abstract provides insight into the type of research being conducted on premenstrual syndrome (PMS).

Variations in Sexual Behaviour

The identity crisis that occurs during adolescence may not be completely resolved by the time the person enters young adulthood chronologically. Identity confusion may lead to confusion over sexual identity and may precipitate homosexual and heterosexual experimentation and arouse homosexual fears and curiosity.

Homosexuality. **Homosexuals** are people who are regularly aroused by and who engage in sexual activity with members of their own sex. Being a **homosexual man** (gay) or a **homosexual woman** (lesbian) was accepted by many ancient cultures and is becoming more socially accepted in North America today. A trend exists in the general population toward more accepting attitudes of gays and lesbians.[64] Particularly among the religious, the less educated, and the older generations, a core of our society still remains opposed to same-sex marriage and same-sex family formation.[65] However, even among those who are favourable to the change, questions still remain. One such question, for example, regarding same-sex marriages is directed toward quality of homosexual unions.

In Canada, political and legal changes are occurring so that there can be no criticism of homosexuality. In a number of Western countries, the legal age of consent for homosexual intercourse is being lowered from 18 to 16 or 14.

Many theories attempt to explain the causes of homosexual behaviour: genetic, biochemical, developmental, and emotional. A number of factors may be involved.[66,67] However, *homosexual experiences are a part of normal growth and development in childhood and early adolescence.* Most people can report having had a close emotional attachment, with or without sexual contact, with a peer or adult that involved sexual feelings. Although the chum stage involves a very close emotional experience, it may include some fondling or exploration between the two chums. If the person is rejected by, or is uncomfortable with, persons of the opposite sex, he or she may receive the greatest acceptance (friendship) from others of the same sex. That reinforces the homosexual preference.

Studies show that these individuals love and care for each other, and are friends with and care for those who are straight. They are responsible citizens to the same extent as are straight or heterosexual people. Developmental tasks for the couple during the childbearing and childrearing experience are also similar to those of heterosexual couples, although there may be more planning for the child and their relationship. Gays and lesbians can be nurturing parents to their children if at some point they decide to leave a heterosexual marital relationship (or mixed-orientation relationship) for a stable gay or lesbian relationship.

The process of **coming out** *(openly disclosing one's homosexual orientation)* occurs in four stages, as follows:

1. Recognition of being homosexual happens as early as age four or as late as adolescence, or later. This time of trying to find self can be lonely, confusing, and painful.
2. Getting to know other homosexuals and establishing romantic and sexual relationships with them. This diminishes feelings of isolation and improves self-image.
3. Telling family and friends may not be done at all, or at least not for a long time. This revelation can bring disapproval, rejection, and conflict.
4. Complete openness involves telling colleagues, employers, and anyone else. In this stage, there is healthy acceptance of their sexuality and the self.[68]

Parents, and the spouse, if the gay man was married, are likely to blame themselves when the man discloses his sexual preference. The feelings of the parents are described by Blum in the article "What Made Troy Gay?"[69] Another interesting article, which explores the experience of disclosing HIV infection to family members, is by Anne Katz ("Mom, I Have Something to Tell You").[70]

Sexual orientation in men is largely innate and influenced by heredity. The genes that drive homosexuality are inherited from mothers. In one study among identical twins, if one brother was gay, the other brother was gay 52% of the time. Among fraternal twins, the rate was 22%. The numbers were nearly the same for lesbians. No one knows how the genes that determine homosexuality work.[71]

Some scientists theorize that in males a testosterone release starts around age four that organizes brain cells toward the opposite sex orientation. Genes in homosexual boys prompt the same urge in a different direction. Further, environmental or cultural triggers cannot be ruled out.[72,73]

There is no evidence that a mother's specific personality or the quality of family life influence sexual preferences. Gay men are more likely to have more distant relationships with their fathers; perhaps the fathers sensed and rejected their gay sons.[74,75]

People who identify themselves as homosexual evidence a complexity and diversity of lifestyles, interests, problems, and relationships comparable to those of heterosexuals. There is also a wide spectrum of emotional experience on the homosexual–heterosexual continuum. Contrary to the stereotype, sexual intercourse is not the predominant concern; meaningful relationships with love and companionship are the key.[76,77]

Both male and female homosexuals vary widely in their emotional and social adjustment, just as heterosexuals do. Some people demonstrate a homosexual orientation only under extreme conditions, such as imprisonment. Some have their total life adjustment dominated by homosexuality and live in a homosexual subculture. For some, sexual behaviour is only an aspect of their total life experience; they may remain discreet and secretive about their homosexuality. Others seek out the organization Exodus International, which ministers to gays and lesbians who seek heterosexual activity, to marry, and to have families.[78]

The lesbian has not been studied as much as the gay man. It is still more socially acceptable for two women to live together in one household than for two men. There may also be less societal fear of gay women than of gay men. As a result, less is known about their feelings, reactions, lifestyles, or health problems. The Society of Gynaecologists and Obstetricians in Canada (SOGC) has developed a policy statement on Lesbian Health Guidelines.[79] This statement was reviewed and approved by the Social and Sexual Issues Committee and was also approved by the Council of the SOGC. The policy statement says that for the lesbian client to receive appropriate and quality care, her sexual orientation and lifestyle must be known and understood by her health care providers. Education is the first step toward improving care for lesbian clients; the final step is the enlightenment of attitudes toward sexuality among health care providers.[80]

The occurrence among homosexuals of sexually transmitted infections, such as pediculosis, gonorrhea, syphilis, urethritis, anorectal warts and infection, herpes genitalis, AIDS, intestinal infections, shigellosis, and hepatitis, has been publicized. The rapidly increasing incidence of AIDS has caused some homosexuals to change their sexual practices, to limit the number of sexual partners, or to increase use of condoms. Heterosexual partners also get these diseases through sexual intercourse, and not all homosexuals get them.

It is essential that you convey a **nonjudgmental attitude** toward the person who is gay or lesbian. Often this person feels discriminated against by health care providers. This person may be a business executive, minister, inventor, health care professional, delivery person, artist, homemaker, or parent with children.

Parents of homosexual offspring are often not considered, but they may also need help in coping with the homosexuality. Parents of gay or lesbian offspring may feel too embarrassed to talk about their feelings; some believe that they have lost a child; some grieve at the prospect of not having a grandchild;

some fear meeting a same-sex lover. Acceptance of the fact that their child is a homosexual may be a long time in coming, but most parents eventually reach that point. Listen to their feelings and concerns; help them focus on a wholesome relationship; caution against punitive behaviour toward the offspring; and refer them to a counsellor to work through spiritual and emotional conflicts related to the situation.

CRITICAL THINKING

How do gays and lesbians develop their self-identity in today's society?

Sexual Experimentation Outside Marriage. Sexual activity outside marriage may include homosexuality, group sexual experiences, premarital intercourse, cohabitation, or infidelity. The idea of finding a compatible partner through *extramarital* sexual intimacy is unfounded. Yet, in this time of high divorce rates, such activity is not unusual.

Various factors contribute to infidelity: the need to prove masculinity or femininity; difficulty in maintaining a steady and continuing relationship; feelings of insecurity, rejection, or jealousy; and a sense of loss when heightened passions of the initial stages of love do not remain constant. The strains that infidelity places on the marital relationship are damaging for most people. Staying married to one person and living with the frustrations, conflicts, and boredom that any close and lengthy relationship imposes requires constant work by both parties.

Cohabitation, *a consensual informal union between two persons of the opposite sex who live together without being married,* is not unusual. Sometimes the person may have had no siblings or no siblings of the opposite sex, and the person wants the experience of living with someone of the opposite sex who would be like a sibling. In such a situation both work to keep the relationship asexual. Most decide to marry or separate within two years.[81]

Young adults sometimes live together in an effort to avoid some of the problems they saw in their parents' marriage or to test the degree of the partner's commitment before actually becoming married. Those goals may be achieved for some, but the danger is that one partner may take the commitment very seriously and the other may use the situation only as a convenient living arrangement. Rather than replacing marriage, cohabitation is considered by many to be a stage before marriage.[82] The 2001 Canadian Census showed that an increasing proportion of couples choose to live common-law, and the trend toward common-law relationships was strongest in Quebec.[83] Cohabitants have rights and legal obligations similar to those of married couples, including property rights, eligibility and entitlements to health insurance, pension plans, and inheritance.[84]

Cohabitation varies from culture to culture, depending on traditional customs and socioeconomic pressures. In some cultures, cohabitation remains an alternative to marriage.[85]

CRITICAL THINKING

In what ways do you think that cohabitation, compared to a nuclear family, affects the health status of its members?

Personal Attitudes

Pangman and Seguire state that sexuality provides the opportunity to express affection, admiration, and affirmation of one's body and its functioning.[86] In fact, sexuality not only encompasses the whole individual, but it serves as a reference frame in relation to others. To incorporate human sexuality into health care and nursing practice, *you must accept your own sexuality and understand sexuality as a significant aspect of development.* Then you can acknowledge the concerns of the clients, recognize your strengths and limits in working with people who have sexual concerns, help clients cope with threats to sexuality, and counsel, inform, or refer them as indicated.

Supporting, caring, and nurturing are nursing behaviours. Feeling positively toward someone can help you give effective care. If you have negative feelings about someone, you can deal with these feelings if you can recognize the possible reasons for your feelings. Actually, when you begin to understand another person, most likely you will find that person interesting; even if that person might not be an individual you would choose for a friend. The patient may express sexual behaviour by brushing against you, trying to feel breasts or hips, or referring to sexual topics in conversation. Recognize the behaviour as an energy outlet or as a way to validate himself or herself as a person. If the patient is observed masturbating, do not make a joke of this discovery. Realize that this is an acceptable sexual release and provide privacy. However, if a patient or client becomes obnoxious in either words or actions, tell him or her that such behaviour is not appropriate.

CONTROVERSY/DEBATE

How Do I Handle This Situation?

You are a clinical practitioner on a rehabilitation ward in a large hospital. One of your clients is a 16-year-old male who lost his legs below the knees due to a train accident. Lately, he has been making lewd sexual comments and gestures at you when you provide basic care. Yesterday you became so frustrated by him that you did not complete his basic care. You have been trying to cope by avoiding eye contact and ignoring his remarks. You are reluctant to confront the client directly because the doctor in charge is the client's uncle. To make matters worse, the client has informed you that he will report you to his uncle (the doctor) for not completing his basic care if you make a formal report of his behaviour to management. It is anticipated that this client will remain on your unit for at least several weeks while he becomes adapted to his prostheses.

1. If you had the opportunity to start over with this client, what would you do differently at the beginning of your interactions to avoid this situation?

2. Now that you are in the situation, however, how will you handle it from here on?

Sexuality Assessment

Follow these guidelines when you are taking a sexual history:

- Ensure privacy and establish confidentiality of statements.
- Progress from topics that are easy to discuss to those that are more difficult to discuss. For example, ask questions such as: What does sexuality mean to you? Has your illness changed the way you see yourself?[87]

Sexuality assessment includes a history as well as the gynecologic examination, breast screening, Papanicolaou (Pap) smear in the female and a genital-rectal examination in the male

Klingman discusses the following general assessment plan:[88]

1. Breast self-examination by the woman monthly after age 19 or 20. Clinical breast exam:
   a. Every three years for women ages 19 or 20 to 40.
   b. Annually for women over age 40.

2. Mammogram:
   a. Every other year for women between age 40 and 50.
   b. Annually after age 50.

Klingman discusses in-depth examination of the female external genitalia and the internal genitalia, the Pap smear procedure and result categories, and the recto-vaginal examination.[89] She also discusses in-depth assessment of the male.[90] Her description covers the physical procedure, comfort and emotional considerations, and normal findings:

- Ask the person how he or she acquired sexual information before asking about sexual experience.
- Precede questions by informational statements about the generality of the experience, when appropriate, to reassure the person and reduce anxiety, shame, and evasiveness.
- Observe nonverbal behaviour while you listen to the person's statements.
- Do not ask questions just to satisfy your curiosity.

The following are *topics to include in the sexual history:*

- How sex education was obtained
- Accuracy of sex education
- Menstrual history if female or nocturnal emission history if male
- Past and present ideas on self as a sexual being, including ideas on body image, masturbation, coitus, childbirth, parenting
- Sexual experiences—with men, women, or both
- Number of partners in past year
- Use of condoms: when started, consistency of use
- Ability to communicate sexual needs and desires
- Partner's (if one exists) sexual values and behaviour
- Sexual partners who have AIDS
- History of sexually transmitted disease of self or partner(s)

If necessary, use several interviews to obtain information and be sure to include any specific questions or concerns that the person voices. Respect the person's desire not to talk about sexual matters and moral, spiritual, or aesthetic convictions. Know the terminology and have a nonjudgmental attitude when the person talks about sexuality concerns. Your matter-of-fact attitude helps the adult feel less embarrassed. Be aware of how illness and drugs can affect sexual function. Do not assume that chronic or disabling disease or mutilating surgery ends the person's sexual life.

Give accurate information and counselling when the person or family asks questions or indicates concerns. You may wish to prepare instructional units for a specific teaching plan to share with patients with various conditions, especially chronic diseases, and with their families to help them better understand how to meet sexual needs. Give information related to pursuit of sexual activity rather than personal advice or judgment. Know community resources for consultation or referral when necessary.

12–3 BONUS SECTION IN CD-ROM

Energy Expenditure for Activity

This section gives the reader information regarding caloric intake and it provides a way to determine daily energy needs for the body.

Physical Fitness and Exercise

According to the 2000–01 Canadian Community Health Survey, 56% of Canadians (20 years of age and older) are inactive, accumulating on average less than 1.5 metabolic equivalent (METs) of physical activity daily.[91] This amount of physical activity could be achieved through walking a total of half an hour a day. Of the remainder, 24% are classified as moderately active, and 20% are active.[92] One MET is the caloric need per kilogram of body weight per hour of activity divided by the caloric need per kilogram per hour at rest.[93]

Health Canada, in partnership with the Canadian Society for Exercise Physiology, has developed *Canada's Physical Activity Guide to Healthy Active Living*.[94] Canadians wanted a valid and practical guide, similar to *Canada's Food Guide to Healthy Eating*, that would help them judge how much physical activity they needed to achieve better health.[95] The guide addresses three types of activities: (1) endurance activities that help one's heart, lungs, and circulatory system to stay healthy; (2) flexibility activities that help one move easily, keeping muscles relaxed and joints mobile; and (3) strength activities that help one's muscles and bones stay strong, improve posture, and help to prevent diseases such as osteoporosis.[96] (See http://www. healthcanada.ca/paguide.) The guide also provides a wide variety of physical activities to help people have more energy, move more easily, and get stronger.

CRITICAL THINKING

How would you begin to develop a program of physical activity for a group of young adults who are physically disabled?

As a matter of interest, jogging makes joints in good condition stronger. Jogging as a regular form of exercise can aggravate old injuries of the back, hips, knees, and ankles because it puts as much as five times normal body weight on lower joints and extremities. Jogging can cause abnormal wear on joints and muscles. The person who jogs must also engage in exercise for the upper extremities and other muscles. Weight-lifting can strengthen. Aerobic exercise, brisk walking, jumping rope, and bicycling may actually be better exercise than jogging. These activities promote bone building, thickness, and strength, and increase circulation throughout the body.[97]

Swimming is probably the best overall activity because it increases strength and endurance and stimulates heart and blood vessels, lungs, and many muscle groups without putting excess stress on the person because of less gravity pull in the water. Further, swimming keeps joints supple, aids weight loss or weight control, and reduces hypertension. Perhaps more important, it is an enjoyable activity, either alone or with others.[98]

Regular physical activity has been viewed as a natural tranquilizer, for it reduces anxiety and muscular tension. Some studies show that regular physical exercise improves a number of personality characteristics, correlating with composure, extroversion, self-confidence, assertiveness, persistence, adventurousness, and superego strength.[99,100]

Exercise periods are frequently not planned by young adults. Some will get abundant exercise in their jobs, but many will not. Those who do not can check with the local YMCA or YWCA organizations, community recreation departments, continuing education departments of community colleges, or

Suggestions for an Exercise Program

- Get pre-exercise physical examination that includes the feet.
- Make exercise a part of your lifestyle: errands, stairs instead of elevator, parking distance.
- Start in small increments, keep it fun, and avoid injury.
- Avoid exercising for two hours after a large meal and eating for one hour after exercising.
- Avoid exercise in extremes of weather.
- Include at least 10 minutes of warm-up and cool-down exercises in an exercise program.
- Use proper equipment, footwear, and clothing when exercising.
- Post goals, pictures of the ideal self, and notes of encouragement in a readily seen place for self-encouragement.
- Use visualization daily to picture successful attainment of exercise benefit (e.g., looking toned or graceful, ideal weight).
- Keep records of weekly measures of weight, blood pressure, and pulse.
- Focus on the rewards of exercise; keep a record of feelings and compare differences in relaxation energy, concentration, and sleep patterns.
- Work with a peer or join a structured exercise class, running club, or fitness centre. Spend more time with people dedicated to wellness.
- Stop exercising or at least slow down and consult with a practitioner if any unusual, unexplainable symptoms occur.
- Reward self for working toward exercise goals and for attaining them. For example, after a month in an exercise program, buy a new pair of running shoes or treat yourself to a special wish.

Principles of Body Mechanics

- The wider the base of support and the lower the centre of gravity, the greater is the stability of the object.
- The equilibrium of an object is maintained as long as the line of gravity passes through its base of support.
- When the line of gravity shifts outside the base of support, the amount of energy required to maintain equilibrium is increased.
- Equilibrium is maintained with least effort when the base of support is broadened in the direction in which movement occurs.
- Stooping with hips and knees flexed and the trunk in good alignment distributes the work load among the largest and strongest muscle groups and helps to prevent back strain.
- The stronger the muscle group, the greater is the work it can perform safely.
- Using a larger number of muscle groups for an activity distributes the work load.
- Keeping centre of gravity as close as possible to the centre of gravity of the work load to be moved prevents unnecessary reaching and strain on back muscles.
- Pulling an object directly toward (or pushing directly away from) the centre of gravity prevents strain on back and abdominal muscles.
- Facing the direction of movement prevents undesirable twisting of spine.
- Pushing, pulling, or sliding an object on a surface requires less force than lifting an object, as lifting involves moving the weight of the object against the pull of gravity.
- Moving an object by rolling, turning, or pivoting requires less effort than lifting the object, as momentum and leverage are used to advantage.
- Using a lever when lifting an object reduces the amount of weight lifted.
- The less the friction between the object moved and surface on which it is moved, the smaller is the force required to move it.
- Moving an object on a level surface requires less effort than moving the same object on an inclined surface because the pull of gravity is less on a level surface.
- Working with materials that rest on a surface at a good working level requires less effort than lifting them above the working surface.
- Contraction of stabilizing muscle preparatory to activity helps to protect ligaments and joints from strain and injury.
- Dividing balanced activity between arms and legs protects the back from strain.
- Variety of position and activity helps maintain good muscle tone and prevent fatigue.
- Alternating periods of rest and activity helps prevent fatigue.

commercial gymnasiums and health salons for exercise programs appropriate to their lifestyles and physical conditions. Refer to the boxes entitled "Suggestions for an Exercise Program" and "Principles of Body Mechanics."

Sex Differences

Women and men sometimes share the same physical exercise activities; sometimes interests and energy levels are different, and partners may engage in exercise activities separately. Women may have as much endurance as men, especially with training, but there are some physiologic differences that account for differences in performance in physical exercise activities or athletic events.

Men have greater upper-body strength, primarily because of their longer arms, broader shoulders, and higher muscle-fibre counts. Muscle can be conditioned by exercise, but muscle-fibre count cannot be increased. Whether men exercise or not, their muscle fibres gain bulk from the hormone testosterone. In men, the heart and lungs, which average 10% larger than those of women, provide more powerful and efficient circulation. The delivery of oxygen to men's muscles, a factor crucial to speed, is further enhanced by the higher concentration of hemoglobin in the blood. Finally, the longer limbs provide them with greater leverage and extension.

The aspects of female physiology that result in women's athletic advantages are not as self-evident as in males. A woman's body contains an average of 9% more adipose tissue than a man's body. This tissue is deposited not only on the thighs, buttocks, and breasts, but in a subcutaneous layer that covers the entire body. It is this adipose tissue that makes the women more buoyant and better insulated against cold, both of which are advantages in long-distance swimming. (The record for swimming the English Channel—7 hours, 40 minutes—is held by a woman, Penny Dean.) Body adipose tissue may also be one of the reasons few female runners report the pain and weakness that most male runners encounter. The body is conditioned to call on stored fats once its supply of glycogen, which fuels the muscles, has been exhausted. As women have greater reserves of body fat, they are able to compete in an athletic event longer. Women perspire in smaller amounts and less quickly than men. Perspiring is the body's way of avoiding overheating. Yet women may tolerate heat better than men. Not only can body temperature rise in a woman several degrees higher before she begins to sweat, but women sweat more efficiently because of the even distribution of their sweat glands. In women, **vascularization,** *capacity for bringing blood to the surface for cooling,* is also more efficient. The woman has certain structural advantages for all types of running and swimming events. In swimming, narrower shoulders offer less resistance through water. Even at identical heights (and ideal weights), female bodies are lighter than male bodies, leaving them with less weight to carry while running.[101]

CRITICAL THINKING

How does physical activity aid women in the prevention of chronic disease?

12-4 BONUS SECTION IN CD-ROM

Physical Fitness

This section will provide the reader with information on physical fitness.

12–5 BONUS SECTION IN CD-ROM

Levels of Exercise

This section provides the reader with different activities for various intensity levels.

Foot Care

Emphasize the importance of foot care in an exercise program. The feet, during walking, will meet the surface at one to two times the body weight and at up to three times its weight when running. Proper shoe fit, which includes heel height, stability, and cushion, wedge support, and forefoot cushion, must be considered. Also, proper-fitting and absorbent socks are important, along with proper washing and careful drying of feet after exercise.[102]

Nutrition

Canada's Food Guide to Healthy Eating helps one to make wise food choices.[103] (See http://www.hc-sc.gc.ca/nutrition.) The guide is based on the following guidelines from Health Canada:

- Enjoy a variety of foods.
- Emphasize cereals, breads, other grain products, and vegetables and fruit.
- Choose lower-fat dairy products, leaner meats and food prepared with a small amount or no fat.
- Achieve and maintain a healthy body weight by enjoying regular physical exercise and healthy eating.
- Limit salt, alcohol, and caffeine.

It is important that the right balance of food and activity helps one stay healthy at a healthy body weight.

CRITICAL THINKING

What is your understanding of "sports drinks"?

12–6 BONUS SECTION IN CD-ROM

Normal Nutrition

This section informs the reader about the food groups and provides information on the nutritional needs of pregnant women.

Nutrition Assessment

Incorporate nutritional status into nursing assessment and the health history. Ask questions related to the following list to guide your assessment with the person or family:

- Knowledge of nutrients, food groups, balanced diet, and their relationship to health
- Knowledge of nutrient requirements at present level of growth and development and whether nutrient needs are being met
- Associations with food and how they influence food and eating patterns
- What increases or decreases appetite
- Cultural background, including religious beliefs, ethnic patterns, and geographic area, and how these beliefs influence food intake and likes and dislikes
- Relationship of lifestyle and activity to food intake
- Income level and food buying power; influence of income on dietary habits
- Knowledge of alternatives to high-cost foods
- Usual daily pattern of intake: times of day, types, amounts
- Which is main meal of the day
- Eating environment
- Special diet requirements
- Food allergies
- Relationship of eating patterns of family or significant others to individual's habits and patterns
- Medications and methods used to aid digestion and nutrition intake; influence of other medications on nutritional intake
- Condition of teeth and chewing ability
- Use, condition, and fit of dentures
- Types of food individual has difficulty chewing or swallowing
- Condition of oral cavity and structures
- Disabilities that interfere with nutritional intake
- Assistance or special devices needed for feeding

Information may be given on ways to maintain energy and nutrition (see the box entitled "First-Rate Snack Pack").

Nutrition and Disease Relationships

Although overt clinical symptoms of *vitamin or mineral deficiencies* are seldom observed in most North Americans, you will see individuals and families in whom you suspect inadequate nutrition. Pallor; listlessness; brittle, dull nails and hair; dental caries; complaints of constipation and poor resistance to common infections; and being over- or underweight suggest a need for a complete diet history.[104]

Your assistance will be sought when dietary problems occur during early pregnancy, usually the transitory nausea and vomiting, commonly called *morning sickness*. Physiologic and psychological factors contribute to this condition. Small frequent meals of fairly dry, easily digested energy food, such as carbohydrates, are usually tolerated. Separating intake of liquids and solids and drinking flavoured or carbonated beverages instead of plain water may also help. Constipation resulting from pressure of the expanding uterus on the lower portion of the intestine occurs in later pregnancy. Increased fluid intake and use of dried fruits, fresh fruits and juices, and whole-grain cereals should induce regularity of elimination. Laxatives should be avoided unless prescribed by a physician.

First-Rate Snack Pack

Air-popped popcorn seasoned with herbs
Bagels
Breadsticks
Broth-based soups
Cereals, low-sugar, low-fat
Cocoa, low-sugar, low-fat
English muffins
Fresh fruit
Frozen fruit juice bars
Gingersnaps
Graham crackers
Low-fat or nonfat frozen yogurt
Matzo
Milk shake of low-fat milk and frozen fruit
Pita chips with salsa
Plain nonfat yogurt with fruit and cinnamon or other seasonings
Pretzels
Raw vegetables
Rice cakes
Rye crisps or rice cakes thinly spread with peanut butter or
    low-fat cheese
Sorbet
Tabbouleh
Unsalted nuts
Vanilla wafers
Vegetables marinated in vinegar or dipped in low-fat yogurt
    and seasoned with herbs
Whole-wheat crackers and cereals
Zwiebach crackers

*Source: Adapted from Health Information Card, Supplement to
Health, Health Magazine, Boulder, Co: 1999.*

CRITICAL THINKING

A young woman informs you that to avoid morning sickness she has a diet cola for breakfast and a pizza for dinner. How would you respond to her?

12–7 BONUS SECTION IN CD-ROM

Recommended Nutritional Intake for Young Adults

This table provides recommended nutritional intake for young adults in the U.S.

Obesity

In Canada, obesity is a problem. We are a society that is preoccupied with losing weight and we spend billions of dollars a year on weight loss products and services. Strychar states that governmental and nongovernmental organizations, as well as industry, need to join forces to ensure a safe and healthy environment for the Canadian population.[105]

Vegetarianism

Vegetarianism has grown popular with young adults, but it is not new. Certain religious groups (e.g., the Seventh-Day Adventists) have been effectively practising a form of vegetarianism for years. In addition to religious reasons, people are vegetarians for moral reasons (opposed to killing animals for food), for economic reasons (cannot afford animal protein), and for health reasons (may believe that a significant amount of animal food is detrimental or that a large amount of plant food is beneficial). Young adults probably fall mainly into the last category.

People who consider themselves vegetarians range from those who eat limited amounts of meat, milk products, or fish and animal products to vegans who eat only vegetables, fruits, legumes, nuts, and grains. Ovovegetarians consume eggs, and lactovegetarians consume milk products in addition to plant foods. It is generally considered that all vegetarians avoid all foods of animal origins.[106]

Gross nutrient deficiencies are rare among lacto-ovovegetarians, as they adapt to reduced intakes of certain nutrients, such as iron and calcium.[107] Energy intake is generally lower among vegetarians than among omnivores, but it is usually adequate. Vegetarians frequently have a body mass index lower than that of omnivores.[108]

Depending on the extent of the vegetarian's dietary restrictions, certain precautions must be taken to maintain an adequate intake of required nutrients (Figure 12–2).[109] If animal proteins, eggs, or milk are inadequate in the diet, the person may need supplementary calcium, iron, zinc, and vitamins B_2 and B_{12}. Vegetarians are at a high risk of inadequate intake of vitamin B_{12}. In Canada, although vitamin B_{12} fortification is permitted in meat analogues such as tofu burgers, often these foods are not fortified. It is very important to read food labels.[110] Soy milk fortified with vitamin D can supply that vitamin. Iron supplements may be needed, even if enriched grain products are used.[111–113] It appears that the increased availability of fortified foods makes dietary planning somewhat easier for those who are vegetarians.

CRITICAL THINKING

In what ways does Health Canada support vegetarian diets?

Cultural Influences on Nutrition

Black people are frequently lactose-intolerant; the level of consumption of dairy products is low and calcium intake must be monitored (see Chapter 6). *Foods, cooking patterns, and ingredients based in Africa, the Caribbean, and the southern U.S.* are popular with some blacks. These foods are economical and are well seasoned with salt and fat. For example, chitlins are made by scrubbing pig intestines, boiling them with vinegar several hours until tender, and serving them with spicy hot sauce. Collard, turnip, and mustard greens contain fibre, calcium, and vitamin A. However, if overcooked, foods may lose fibre and nutrition, especially if the **pot liquor,** *the cooking liquid,* is discarded. The dietary fat and salt intake may create health problems, especially for the pregnant woman.[114]

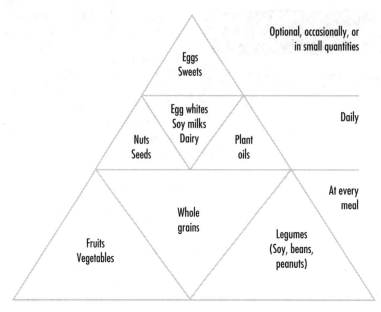

This diet pyramid, developed by researchers at Harvard and Cornell universities, can be used as a guide for planning a well-balanced vegetarian diet.

FIGURE 12-2

Vegetarian diet pyramid.

Source: Vegetarianism: Should You or Shouldn't You? Harvard Health Letter, *24, no. 10 (1999), 7.*

To the *American Indian,* food has religious, cultural, tribal, social, and family meanings. Tribal/nation specific rules may be followed to maintain health or balance. Three staples are considered basic or sacred by most of the 550 recognized tribes or nations in the U.S: corn, squash, and beans. Many American Indians are lactose-intolerant. Depending on the geographic area and tribe, game, fish, berries, roots, wild greens, and fruits are important food sources. Lack of accessibility or refrigeration may limit consumption of meat and fresh fruits and vegetables. If nonperishable foods are the bulk of the diet, they may be deficient in key nutrients and too high in refined sugar, cholesterol, fat, and calories. Diets on some reservations supply less than two-thirds of the recommended calories, calcium, iron, iodine, riboflavin, and vitamins A and C. Diets tend to be high in carbohydrates, saturated fat, sodium, and sugar.[115]

These cultural food traditions affect women during pregnancy, for example, causing anemia or affecting fetal development (see Chapter 6). Some women believe cravings must be satisfied by eating nonfood substances, as in pica (see Chapter 6), or in following other folklore. One example is to avoid eating craved-for strawberries, because it is believed they will cause a red birthmark. *Teach about the importance of certain nutrients and foods to the baby's and mother's health. Explore foods that are acceptable to her, analyze their nutritional content,* and *emphasize the importance of their intake.* You also can share up-to-date information, for example, that high levels of calcium in green leafy vegetables, such as spinach, chard, and beet greens and other foods cannot be absorbed because calcium is bound to oxalic acid.[116]

Cultural food patterns also affect the woman's postpartal diet. *Latino* and *Asian women* may prefer to avoid cold foods (certain fruits, vegetables, and juices) for one to two months after delivery because they are believed to slow the flow of blood and prevent emptying of the uterus.[117]

NARRATIVE VIGNETTE
Cultural Patterns and Food

In your health promotion class on Food Habits and Cultural Patterns, you have been asked to select a person of a cultural background different from your own. You have selected a Filipino family to interview. Use the following questions as a beginning guideline for the interview. Record the family responses and bring them to class.

1. What foods and preparation practices are used specifically by you?
2. What dietary practices do you use to promote health?
3. What, if any, food rituals are followed in the culture?

For assistance, check Purnell and Paulanka.[118]

Nutrition Education

You may be able to advise young adults about nutrition in a variety of settings. Keep in mind the basic foods as you suggest a diet pattern, and adjust your information to the vegetarians or those who have allergies or specific ethnic or cultural preferences. These suggestions, if followed, will contribute to nutritional health:[119–122]

- Keep a specific record of intake for one week to determine eating patterns.
- Increase consumption of fruits, vegetables, and whole grains. Eat a variety of foods.
- Decrease consumption of foods or beverages high in refined sugars; instead drink more water and fruit juices.
- Do not add salt to foods during cooking or at the table and avoid snack foods with visible salt or foods prepared in brine; instead use herbs, spices, and lemon for seasoning.
- Decrease consumption of foods high in total fat and animal fat and partially replace saturated fats (beef, pork, butter, fatty meats), whether obtained from animal or vegetable sources, with polyunsaturated fats (fish, poultry, veal, lean meats, margarine, vegetable sources).
- Substitute low-fat and nonfat milk for whole milk and low-fat dairy products for high-fat products (except for young children). Limit cholesterol intake to less than 300 mg daily.
- Reduce use of luncheon or variety meats (e.g., sausage, salami).
- Use skim or low-fat milk and cheeses instead of whole milk and cream.
- Avoid deep fat frying; use baking, boiling, broiling, roasting, and stewing, which help remove fat.
- Avoid excessive intake of any nutrient or food as excess consumption of, and in turn deficiency of, any substance can contribute to disease.
- Avoid more than a minimum intake of alcohol.

Keep in mind the young adult who may need suggestions on economical but nutritious foods. Using powdered skim milk, less expensive cuts of meat, and home-cooked cereals does not sacrifice nutrition but does save money.

Teach about the need for fibre in the diet, which can prevent constipation and help reduce the incidence of cancer of the colon, diverticulosis, appendicitis, gallstones, and heart disease. Some fibres contribute to constipation if they are not diluted with substantial amounts of water.[123–125] Teach about the adverse effects of caffeine.[126] Effects of caffeine can be detrimental to health. Warn also that herbal teas may contain strong drugs that can cause severe problems.

Hospitalized young adults may be suffering from nutritional deficiencies resulting from a specific diet. Be aware that hospital-induced malnutrition exists. Patients whose meals are withheld because they are undergoing various diagnostic tests or treatments, especially over a long period, are candidates for this problem.

CRITICAL THINKING

Outline the nutritional principles you would discuss with a client who is an athlete.

Biological Rhythms

Rhythms occur throughout the life cycle of each individual. From the time of birth different body structures and functions develop rhythmicity at different rates. By the time the individual reaches young adulthood, biological rhythms are established by body chemistry and by the suprachiasmatic nucleus, a tiny cluster of cells buried deep in the brain. **Biological rhythms** are *self-sustaining, repetitive, rhythmic patterns found in plants, animals, and humans.* The rhythms are found throughout our external and internal environment and can be exogenous or endogenous.

Exogenous rhythms *depend on the rhythm of external environmental events,* such as seasonal variations, lunar revolution, and the night-and-day cycle that function as time givers. These events help to synchronize internal rhythms with external environmental stimuli and establish an internal time pattern or biological clock.

Endogenous rhythms such as sleep-wake and sleep-dream cycles arise *within the organism.* Endogenous and exogenous rhythms are usually synchronized. Many internal rhythms do not readily alter their repetitive patterns, however, even when the external stimuli are removed. For instance, when a person shifts to sleeping by day and waking at night, as frequently happens with nurses, a transient or temporary desynchronization occurs. Body temperature and adrenal hormone levels are usually low during the sleep cycle. With the shift in sleep and waking, the person is awake and making demands on the body during the usual sleep period. Three weeks may be needed before internal rhythms adapt to the shift. A similar period of desynchronization occurs when a person makes a flight crossing time zones.

Within any 24-hour period, physiologic and psychological functions reach maximum and minimum limits. When a physiologic function approaches a high or low limit, the body's feedback mechanisms attempt to counterregulate the action. *This form of endogenous rhythm that reoccurs in a cyclic pattern within a 20- to 28-hour period, even when external factors are held constant, is a* **circadian rhythm.** Body temperature, blood pressure, pulse, respirations, urine production, and hormone, blood sugar, hemoglobin, and amino acid levels demonstrate this rhythmic pattern. Similar variations or rhythms in the levels of alertness, fatigue, tenseness, and irritability can also be demonstrated. *When rhythms reach their maximal level or peak,* they are **in-phase.** *When various rhythms peak at different times,* they are **out-of-phase.**[127]

In humans mental efficiency and performance apparently are related to the rhythms of body temperature and catecholamine excretion in the adult. The body temperature rises and drops by approximately 2°F (or 1°C) over each 24-hour period. The body temperature begins to decline near 10 p.m., is lowest on awaking, gradually rises during the morning, levels off in the afternoon, and then drops again in the evening (Figure 12–3). The level of adrenocortical hormone secretion appears correlated with body temperature rhythms and the individual's state of alertness and wakefulness. The level of adrenocortical hormones rises early in the morning, peaks around the time we typically awaken, and then drops to a low

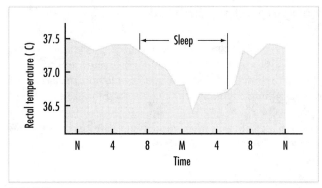

FIGURE 12–3

Diurnal cycle of temperature variations.

Source: Berger, K.J., and M.B. Williams, Fundamentals of Nursing: Collaborating for Optimal Health. *Stamford, CT: Appleton & Lange, 1992, p. 446.*

point by late evening.[128] Usually the best mental and physical performances coincide with peak temperature, and the least desirable performances coincide with intervals of lowest body temperature. In addition, studies have shown that the lowest excretory rates of epinephrine in day-active people correlate with the time of maximum fatigue and poorest performance. Physical strength crests at different times of the day.

Researchers have theorized that many disasters have resulted from failure to consider human biology. For example, at the nuclear accident at Three Mile Island, the three young men in the control area worked on a shift system called slow rotation— days for a week, evenings for a week, and late nights for a week. At the time of the disasters at Bopal and Chernobyl, people were working unusual shifts. Work schedules that have changing shift rotation cause a desynchronization of circadian rhythms, altering performance levels.

Circadian Rhythms in Illness

An interrelationship exists between circadian rhythms and mental or physical illness. The pattern of living taught by the culture also affects body rhythms. A few examples of how circadian rhythms influence the health of young adults are presented next.[129–134]

Diagnostic cues are influenced by biological rhythms. Observing the integration of the body's rhythms (or lack of such integration) can be used to determine the person's health status. Diagnosis and treatment of some illnesses can be determined from the study of circadian rhythms or biological time. In some instances the illness alters the pattern of circadian rhythm. Other illnesses show exaggerated or decreased symptoms at a particular biological time. Blood pressure and temperature values, laboratory findings, and biopsy specimens for cell study differ according to the biological time of day. For instance, growth hormone levels in the blood are highest during the night hours; therefore routine blood values taken at 8 a.m. will not give a total picture. The percentage of red blood cells drops approximately 4.5% late at night; a decrease in red blood cells of 5% prompts blood transfusions in some hospitals. Concentrations of white blood cells peak in the morning and early afternoon.[135] Ambiguous laboratory findings, the need for repeated medical tests, and the potential for unnecessary medical therapies can be avoided if the person's normal biological rhythms are considered first.

Rhythmic time cycles appear to influence many aspects of human life. Births and deaths occur more frequently at night and during the early morning. Persons with ulcers and allergies suffer more in the nighttime and in spring; allergic responses, including asthmatic attacks, occur more frequently at night and in the early morning hours. There are certain yearly peaks in the number of suicides, psychotic episodes, and accidents. Eventually knowledge about circadian rhythms and biological time may serve as a major tool in preventive health programs.

Depression has a number of causes but may be directly related to biological rhythms of depressed people. Altered biochemical rhythms, diurnal (daytime) mood swings, and altered sleep cycles have been noted. Researchers have hypothesized that abnormalities of sleep patterns in some types of depression are due to abnormal internal phase relationships of circadian rhythms. The circadian rhythm of rapid eye movement (REM) sleep may occur abnormally early. Depressed persons usually experience insomnia or periods of predawn wakefulness. Their sleep cycles are shortened and fragmented, and they are easily disturbed by environmental changes. Successful treatment frequently comes in the form of antidepressant drugs that slow biological clocks (e.g., lithium carbonate) or speed biological clocks (e.g., imipramine).[136]

Various mental functions and the emotional, behavioural, and autonomic responses associated with them depend on certain chemicals secreted at the synapses of the neurons in specific pathways of the brain. Several brain neurotransmitters (norepinephrine, dopamine, serotonin, and acetylcholine) undergo cyclic changes in amount of chemical present. These fluctuations are thought to be related factors concerned with periodicity and emotion.[137]

Cells in almost every tissue of the body divide or reproduce in circadian rhythm. Normal cells show intervals of accelerated reproductive activity. In human beings, for example, skin and liver cells are more active at night. Cancer cells do not reproduce at the same rate as normal cells; abnormal mitosis (cell reproduction) rhythms and, in many instances, a complete lack of circadian rhythms have been reported. Further, timing has been found crucial for surgical treatment or chemotherapy of cancer patients; recovery is linked to time of day of the treatment.

Research suggests that people who are desynchronized or constantly consuming foods and drugs that change the phase of their circadian rhythms may be a high-risk group for cancer.[138] *Health teaching* should include the need to decrease the intake of coffee, tea, and certain barbiturates that may be carcinogens.

Adrenal hormone production is cyclic in humans. For persons on schedules of diurnal activity and nocturnal sleep, the blood and urine concentrations of adrenocorticosteroid hormones drop at night and rise to their highest level in early morning. The course of the adrenal cycle may also be followed by measuring the eosinophil (white blood cell) level; eosinophils decrease as the blood level of adrenal hormones increases.

Light is probably the synchronizer of the adrenocorticosteroids rhythm. This factor has implications for people who are night workers or who have varying degrees of blindness. Because adrenal hormones control other circadian rhythms within the body, knowledge of their cycle is important in the study and treatment of numerous conditions.

Low blood levels of adrenal hormones affect the nervous system and cause increased sensitivity to sounds, tastes, and smell. Sensory acuity reaches its maximum at the time of lowest steroid levels. A sudden drop in acuity occurs in the early morning as steroid levels begin to rise. A person is therefore better able to detect taste, smell, or sound at the end of the day. Daily fatigue from lack of sleep and neuro-logically related symptoms associated with adrenal insufficiency (Addison's disease) may be related to low levels of adrenal hormones.

Adrenal rhythm is also important in handling certain allergies. Sensitivity to histamine follows a circadian rhythm: it peaks near evening or night when adrenocorticosteroids are reaching their lowest levels. Nasal congestion from hay fever, skin reactions from drug sensitivity and breathing crises in asthma patients occur more frequently during the evening or night. Suggest to individuals with hay fever and asthma that they do their gardening and weeding in the morning when their adrenocorticosteroids levels are at their highest.

CRITICAL THINKING

Keep a daily log of your routines. What do you conclude from this log?

Nursing Assessment and Intervention

Nursing care should be planned with biological rhythms in mind. Because our cyclic functioning is synchronized with environmental stimuli, physiologic disequilibrium occurs whenever we are confronted with environmental or schedule changes. Transient desynchronization may occur whenever a person is exposed to the hospital or nursing home stimuli. New noise levels; lighting patterns; schedules for eating, sleeping, and personal hygiene; and unfamiliar persons intruding on the person's privacy may all contribute to this desynchronization. Disturbed mental and physical well-being and increased sub-jective fatigue reflect the conflict between the internal time pattern and external events. Several days usually are required before the person adapts to the environment and thereby regains synchronization—normal biological rhythms.

You can control some external factors, such as meals, baths, and various tests; make them more nearly similar to the patient's normal (outside) routine; and lessen the stress to which the patient is subjected. Obtaining and using a nursing history con-stitutes one method of lessening this stress.

Your *nursing history* should be directed at getting infor-mation about the patient's pre-illness or pre-hospitalization patterns for sleep, rest, food and fluid intake, elimination, and personal hygiene. The questionnaire developed by Alward and Monk is a useful guide. Do you consider yourself a "day" per-son or a "night" person? Do you feel cheerful when you first wake up? What time of day do you feel most alert? What hours do you prefer to work? Why do you prefer these hours? How do you feel when something causes you to change your routine? Answers to these questions will provide you informa-tion about the patient's daily patterns. Once this information has been obtained, nursing actions can be initiated that sup-port these established patterns and possibly prevent total dis-ruption of body rhythms during hospitalization.

After the patient has been hospitalized for a few days, cer-tain objective data are available that will assist you in deter-mining a rough estimate of the person's circadian patterns. The routine graphic record supplies information about the patient's vital signs. Using this source, you might be able to identify peaks and lows in blood pressure, pulse, or temperature curves. Also, an intake and output record that shows both the time and the amount voided will aid in determining the patient's daily urinary-excretory pattern. In addition to the post-admission nursing history, a daily log of sleep and waking hours, meal-times, hunger periods, voiding and defecation patterns, diur-nal moods, and other circadian rhythms recorded for 28 days before hospitalization can help determine the person's cyclic patterns. Diagnostic tests and certain forms of medical and nursing therapy can then be appropriately prescribed by using the person's own baseline rhythm measurements. Determination of each patient's rhythms before, during, and after hospitaliza-tion or illness eventually will be possible when more sim-plified, economic, and accurate measurement devices are available.

The *client's medication schedule* can also reflect your understanding of biological rhythms. Drug effectiveness can be altered by the time of day that the particular drug is admin-istered. Digitalis (a cardiac glycoside) is several times more effective when administered in the early morning than when administered at other times. The dosage of analgesics needed to relieve pain during the evening or the dark hours is higher than that needed during the daytime. Sensitivity to pain increases in the evening.[139]

One area of **chronopharmacology** (*study of cellular rhythms in relationship to drug therapy*) that has been researched extensively is the relationship of adrenocortical function and corticosteroid drug administration. The secre-tion of corticosteroids by the adrenal cortex has a 24-hour rhythm, with the highest corticosteroid values expected after the usual time of awakening. When corticosteroids are admin-istered daily or on alternate days, adrenal suppression and pos-sibly growth disturbance can be minimized by timing to the circadian crest in adrenocortical function. Morning doses of prednisolone (a glucocorticoid) are less likely to cause alterations in the rhythmic pattern of urinary excretion than twice-daily divided doses or a single dose in the late evening.

Circadian rhythms are also important factors in determining drug toxicity. A distinct 24-hour rhythm of vulnerability or resistance to drugs has been identified. Before setting a drug's toxic level, both the person's biological clock and the drug dosage must be considered. At present, problems exist in determining toxicity levels. Research guidelines do not consider the circadian rhythms of the animals being tested. Nocturnal animals are tested in the daytime; animals are tested before they have had time to adjust to a new laboratory environment; animals are tested in light and dark cycles that are not regulated; and animals whose feeding schedules are not fixed and recorded are tested. All these factors can cause altered rhythms in animals and altered vulnerability or resistance to the drug being tested.

In the future, as knowledge of the internal clock increases, you, the nurse, will find yourself altering drug administration times to suit the person's biological time. Perhaps you will be in charge of a master computer that, after analyzing information about each person's biological clock, will send the appropriate medication dose at the appropriate time.

Vital signs routine should be based on circadian rhythm patterns rather than on tradition or convenience of the agency staff. Both internal and skin temperatures show a systematic rise and fall over a 24-hour period, a cycle difficult to alter in normal adults. Body temperature usually peaks between 4 and 6 p.m. and reaches its lowest point around 4 a.m. in people who are active by day and sleep by night. When the internal temperature is normally peaking, other body functions such as pulse rate, blood pressure, and cardiac output (volume of blood pumped by the heart) are also changing. Pulse rate is high when the temperature is highest and drops during the night. The human heart rate will vary as much as 20 or 30 beats per minute in 24 hours. Blood pressure shows a marked fall during the first hour of sleep, followed by a gradual rise throughout the daily cycle, with a peak between 5 and 7 p.m. Cardiac output reaches minimum levels between 2 and 4 a.m., the period of lowest temperature findings.[140]

CRITICAL THINKING

What questions might researchers pose regarding the study of the internal clock in individuals?

Work Schedules

Work schedules should be developed with biological rhythms in mind. You can also establish your own circadian patterns to help you gain insight into physical feelings and behaviours and can use this information to plan your days to advantage. You might choose to cope with the most difficult patient assignment during the time of peak mental and physical performance, for example.

Nurses and many industrial and law-enforcement personnel are frequently required to change shifts every week or month. Night and rotating shift workers are at excessive risk for accidents and injuries on the job because of disrupted circadian rhythms. Sleep cycles are interrupted. There is difficulty in falling asleep, a shorter duration of sleep, poorer quality of sleep, and persistent fatigue. Alertness and other physiologic processes suffer. Eating habits are disrupted; diets are poorer; and digestion is interfered with. Constipation, gastric and peptic ulcers, and gastritis are more common. Social activities and interactions essential to physical and mental health are interrupted. Family life and relationships are interfered with; shift workers have difficulty fulfilling family and parental roles. Rotating shift assignments are thus relevant to the worker's health and quality of work performance. Altering the sleep–wake sequence requires time for the person to make adjustments and regain synchrony. Thurston, Tanguay, and Fraser state that a common eight-hour nursing rotation is based on one week per shift followed by a counterclockwise rotation to the previous shift (day shift to night shift, night shift to evening shift, and evening shift to day shift). They claim that this is the worst possible scene: just as the nurse is beginning to acclimate to the shift after one week, a second eight-hour phase shift is imposed. This change to a new shift is not unlike jet lag and requires the nurse to be alert on the new shift at a time when alertness is at its lowest. A preferred rotation would be in a clockwise direction (day to evening, evening to night, night to day), as it is easier to delay an internal clock than to advance it.[141]

If shift rotation cannot be eliminated, individuals should be required to rotate no more frequently than once a month. Consistently working at night allows a person to acquire a new sleep-wake rhythm. Therefore night work should be made more attractive to persons who can adapt to the shift and are willing to remain on it permanently. Those who cannot adapt should be exempt from rotation. The rigours of working shifts may be reflected in the fact that only a few individuals are able to maintain those hours over several years.[142]

Health teaching of any rotating-shift worker concerning the possible consequences of such a routine should not be overlooked. Night workers taking medications should be aware that the effects of medications may vary somewhat from those they usually experience when working days. The susceptibility to various degrees of drug metabolism occurs throughout the day but even more when a person is experiencing jet lag or the early phase of shift rotation. Individuals with a chronic illness such as diabetes, epilepsy, or hypertension and cardiac problems must consider these factors when they plan their medication regimen.

CRITICAL THINKING

What are a few safety concerns that may be inherent in a rotating-shift worker?

Rest and Sleep

Sleep is a *complex biological rhythm, intricately related to rest and other biological rhythms.* Help clients realize that such factors as emotional and physical status, occupation, and amount of physical activity determine the need for rest and sleep. For example, workers who alternate between day and night shifts frequently feel more exhausted and need more sleep than people who keep regular hours. Surgery, illness, pregnancy, and the postpartum state all require that the individual receive more sleep. Mothers of infants, toddlers, and preschoolers may need daytime naps.

Some young people find themselves caught in a whirlwind of activities. Jobs, social activities, family responsibilities, and educational pursuits occupy every minute. The young adult can adjust to this pace and maintain it for a length of time without damaging physical or mental health. The person may think he or she is immune to the laws of nature and can go long periods without sleep. If the person finds that he or she is not functioning well on a certain amount of sleep, the schedule should be adjusted to allow for more hours of rest. He or she also must be cognizant of the biological rhythms for rest and activity. Setting aside certain periods for quiet activities such as reading, sewing, watching television, and various hobbies is restful but not as beneficial as sleep.

Each person has his or her own sleep needs and cycle, and research is helping us better understand the different stages of sleep and the importance of sleep to well-being. The tradition that young adults should have seven to eight hours of sleep seems valid, although some get along fine with less. When left to the body's natural pace, the person is likely to sleep every 25 hours.

Normal Sleep Pattern

Sleep is a complex phenomenon.[143–149] The functional component of the brain stem that exerts influence on consciousness and the wake-sleep cycle is called the *reticular activating system (RAS).* The RAS activates the state of consciousness and functions as a deactivation mechanism to decrease alertness and to produce sleep. **Electroencephalograms (EEGs),** *recordings of brainwave activity,* vary with the awake and asleep states and at different intrasleep cycles (Figure 12–4). When a person is wide awake and alert, the EEG recordings show rapid, irregular waves. High-frequency beta and alpha waves predominate. As he or she begins to rest, the wave pattern changes to an **alpha rhythm,** *a regular pattern of low voltage; with frequencies of eight to 12 cycles per second.* During sleep, a **delta rhythm,** *a slow pattern of high voltage and one to two cycles per second,* occurs. At certain stages of sleep, **sleep spindles,** *sudden short bursts of sharply pointed alpha waves of 14 to 16 cycles per second,* and **K-complexes,** *jagged tightly peaked waves,* occur.

Sleep is divided into **NREM** (*non–rapid eye movement*) and **REM** stages. NREM sleep is divided into four stages—light to deep. REM sleep follows the deepest NREM sleep as the person ascends to stage II sleep and occurs before repeated descent through stages II, III, and IV.

In **NREM stage I sleep,** the *person makes a transition from wakefulness to sleep* in approximately five minutes. The alpha rhythm is present, but the waves are more uneven and smaller than in later stages. The person is drowsy and relaxed, has fleeting thoughts, is somewhat aware of the environment, can be easily awakened, and may think he or she has been awake. The pulse rate is decreased.

NREM stage II sleep is the *beginning of deeper sleep* and fills 40% to 50% of total sleep time. The person is more relaxed than in the prior stage but can be easily awakened. Sleep spindles and K-complexes appear in the brain waves at intervals.

NREM stage III sleep is a *period of progressively deeper sleep* and begins 30 to 45 minutes after sleep onset. EEG waves become more regular; delta (slow) waves appear; sleep spindles are present; muscles are more relaxed; vital signs and metabolic activity are lowered to basal rates; and the person is difficult to awaken.

NREM stage IV sleep is *very deep sleep, occurs approximately 40 minutes after stage I, and rests and restores the body physically.* This stage is as important as REM sleep; and it comprises 10% to 15% of sleep in healthy young adults. Delta waves are the dominant EEG pattern. The person is very relaxed and seldom moves, is difficult to arouse, and responds slowly if awakened. Physiologic measures are below normal. Sleepwalking and enuresis may occur during this

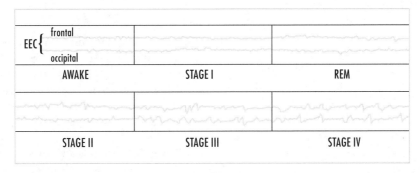

FIGURE 12–4

Changes in electroencephalogram tracing during sleep.

stage. After strenuous physical exercise, this stage is greatly needed. Deep sleep is less deep the last half of the night.

REM sleep is called *active, or paradoxic, sleep* and is the *stage of rapid eye movements and dreaming that occurs before descending to the deeper sleep of stages II, III, and IV.* This stage is of great importance. In REM sleep the EEG readings are active and similar to those of stage I sleep, but various physiologic differences from other sleep stages are present. These differences, in addition to rapid, side-to-side eye movements, are:

- Muscular relaxation and absent tendon reflexes, with occasional twitching, so that the body is in immobility-like paralysis
- Respiratory rate increased 7% to 20% alternating between rapid and slow with brief apneic periods
- Pulse rate irregular and increased 5%; cardiac output decreased
- Blood pressure fluctuations up to 30 mm Hg
- Body temperature lowers
- High oxygen consumption by the brain; change in cerebral blood flow
- Increased metabolism
- Blood may become thicker resulting from autonomic instability and temperature changes
- Increased production of 17-hydroxycorticosteroids, posterior pituitary hormones, and catecholamines
- Increased gastric secretions
- Penile erections in men of all ages

REM sleep occurs in 70- to 90-minute cycles that increase as the night progresses. Duration of REM sleep is longer and more intense just after minimum body temperature, around 5 a.m. It rests and restores mentally and is important for learning and psychological functioning. It allows for review of the day's events, categorizing and integrating of information into the brain's storage systems, and problem solving. During psychological stress this stage is vital. Dreams that occur during REM sleep allow for wish fulfillment and release of potentially harmful thoughts, feelings, and impulses so that they do not affect the waking personality.

In a seven- or eight-hour period the person will have 60- to 90-minute cycles of sleep descending from stage I to IV and back to REM sleep. After 10 to 15 minutes of REM sleep, the person again descends to stage IV. The person may ascend to REM sleep three to five times a night, but each time he or she spends a longer period in it. In the first third of the night, he or she spends more time in stage IV sleep; in the last third of the night more time is spent in REM sleep. Dreams in the early REM stages are shorter, are less interesting, and contain aspects of the preceding day's activities. As the night progresses, the dreams become longer, more vivid and exciting, and less concerned with daily life. Stages III and IV together constitute approximately 20% of sleep time until old age, when deep sleep almost disappears.

CRITICAL THINKING

What is your understanding of dreams?

Variations in Sleep Patterns

The percentage of time a person spends in sleep differs with age and with body temperature at the time of falling asleep. If the person's body temperature is at its high point in the biological rhythm, he or she will sleep two times longer than if the temperature is at a low point in the biological rhythm. REM sleep remains constant throughout adult life, constituting 20% to 25% of sleep, in contrast to 40% to 50% of sleep for babies. But the percentage of time spent in stage IV sleep decreases 15% to 30% with age so that the aged person sleeps less time and awakens more frequently. Elderly women's sleep patterns change approximately ten years later than men's patterns. The aged person's adjustment to sleep seems dependent on arteriosclerotic changes so that the alert aged person sleeps about the same as the young adult. The aged person with cerebral arteriosclerotic changes sleeps 20% less than the young adult.[150–152]

REM sleep is related to the onset of certain diseases. Convulsions are more likely to occur in the epileptic individual just before awakening, which is during REM sleep. Because the pulse is irregular during REM sleep, myocardial infarctions and arrhythmias are more likely to occur. Gastric secretion is increased during the REM state. The person with a peptic ulcer has more pain at these times.[153]

Sedatives, antidepressants, and amphetamines significantly decrease REM sleep. If the person continually takes a sedative, there is a gradual return to the usual amount of REM sleep. But when the drug is withdrawn, REM sleep is markedly withdrawn, causing insomnia and nightmares, irritability, fatigue, and sensitivity to pain, all of which persist up to five weeks. Thus sedatives should be given sparingly, including to the young adult, although different sedatives cause different effects, and effects differ from person to person. You should learn from the person if he or she is regularly on sedatives. If the person is, he or she must continue them to avoid withdrawal symptoms while receiving health care.[154–156]

If REM deprivation and the rebound of more REM sleep later occur because of administration of sedatives, the patient with any health problem, but especially cardiovascular disease, should have sedative administration stopped before discharge. At home the person will not have the close observation needed during the prolonged periods of REM sleep when myocardial infarction is more likely to occur. Further, in contrast to popular belief, alcoholic beverages should not be used to promote sleep. Alcohol speeds the onset of sleep but interferes with REM sleep, which may contribute to hangover feelings.

Sleep Deprivation

Sleep deprivation should be avoided by the young adult. The person may feel rested if he or she awakens after four or five hours of sleep, but there has been insufficient time for REM sleep. If the person is awakened frequently, the sleep cycle must be started all over again. See the box entitled "Physical and Psychological Changes with Sleep Deprivation" for more information.[157–163]

When the person decides to recover lost sleep by sleeping longer hours, he or she will spend more time in REM sleep. Twelve to 14 hours of sleep help to overcome brief periods of sleep deprivation. Studies indicate a minimum of five hours

Physical and Psychological Changes with Sleep Deprivation

Physical Changes

- Lack of alertness
- Feeling pressure on head
- Nystagmus; ptosis of eyelids
- Lack of coordination; tremors
- Slowed reflexes
- Fatigue
- Bradypnea
- Cardiac arrhythmias
- Poorer performance
- Increased errors; injury prone
- Physical discomfort; hypochondriasis

Psychological Changes

- Anxiety; insecurity; irritability
- Introspective; unable to respond to support from others; irritable
- Apathy; withdrawal; decreased motivation
- Depression
- Increased aggressiveness
- Suspiciousness
- Decreased mental agility; decreased concentration
- Decreased creativity
- Decreased spontaneity
- Illusions
- Decreased concentration
- Loss of creativity
- Poor judgment
- Memory failure
- Confusion; disorientation
- Hallucinations
- Bizarre behaviour; psychosis

sleep daily is needed and for most people seven to eight hours are needed to avoid sleep deprivation. After 48 hours of sleep loss, the body produces a stress chemical related structurally to LSD-25, which may account for behavioural changes. After four days of sleep deprivation, the body does not produce adenosine triphosphate (ATP), the catalyst for energy release, which may be a factor in fatigue. With total sleep deprivation, confusion, hallucinations, and psychosis occur.[164–167]

Thus the client, who needs all stages of sleep for physical and psychological restoration, *should not be awakened during the night if at all possible.* Observe the person before awakening by studying eye movements under the lids. If he or she is in REM sleep, wait a few minutes for it to end before awakening the person, as this is a short and important stage. Sleep has priority over taking vital signs, especially because the vital sign measurement is affected by the stage of sleep and therefore cannot be compared accurately to daytime measurements. As steroids are released during REM sleep, disturbance of REM sleep causes steroid release to be out of synchrony with other biological rhythms, affecting all areas of function in the person.

Being frequently awakened during the night such as happens to young parents with young children produces the same effects as sleeping fewer hours, even if the total length of time asleep is the usual amount. Blocks of uninterrupted sleep are a definite physical and psychological need.

Help parents work out a system that responds to baby's needs but also allows each parent to get as much uninterrupted sleep as possible. Use the above information on sleep stages and effects of sleep interruption and deprivation to teach the young adults.

CRITICAL THINKING

If a couple asked you to help them work out a system to respond to their baby's needs, where would you begin?

Sleep Disturbances

Many people do not get normal sleep daily. They either sleep too much or not enough, suffer night terrors, or stop breathing for a minute or two during sleep. The cost of sleep disorders is enormous; some people pay a great deal for pills and potions to maintain normal sleep.

Insomnia, *a disorder of initiating and maintaining sleep,* is sometimes a problem for young adults. **Primary insomnia** is *a sleep problem that exists in the absence of any major medical or psychiatric condition.* Other types of insomnia are **sleep onset** (*difficulty falling asleep*), **sleep maintenance** (*awakening in the middle of the night*), and **terminal insomnia** (*early-morning awakening*). Factors that may lead to insomnia include (1) disturbed circadian rhythms; (2) physical symptoms such as pain, dyspnea, and fever; (3) environmental disturbances; (4) emotional stress; and (5) stimulant drugs.[168–171] Depression is often associated with terminal insomnia.

Knowing the quantity and quality of sleep is useful in determining the existence of insomnia. Individual sleep requirements vary, and an individual's satisfaction with the length and quality of sleep is the basis for assessing the presence of insomnia.

You can help the insomniac by being an interested, calm listener and by suggesting that the following measures be tried:[172–176]

- Get enough exercise, at least 20 to 40 minutes, three to five days a week.
- Maintain a regular schedule of pre-bedtime relaxation, sleep, and wakefulness to keep biorhythms in synchrony.
- Reduce caffeine intake (coffee, tea, chocolate milk, soft drinks). Caffeine can remain in the blood for 20 hours.
- Avoid strenuous activity in the evening before retiring; instead rely on soothing but enjoyable stimuli such as a backrub for muscular and emotional relaxation, quiet music, warm bath, progressive relaxation to loosen tight muscles, or a nonstimulating book or hobby.
- Try a glass of warm milk, which contains l-tryptophan, a chemical that increases brain serotonin and induces sleep.
- Limit alcohol intake; it reduces quality of sleep by causing a light sleep and more wakening and reducing REM sleep.
- Limit cigarette smoking; nicotine causes the person to take longer to fall asleep, wake more often, and have less REM and deep NREM sleep.

- Avoid high-fat or hard-to-digest meals near bedtime; gastric secretions regurgitate into the esophagus, causing heartburn. This may be relieved by raising the head of the bed on blocks.
- Avoid medications that cause sleeplessness as a side effect.
- Improve the sleeping environment: make the bedroom dark, quiet, and as comfortable as possible so it is associated only with pleasurable feelings.
- Purposefully relax after going to bed. Stretch out, get comfortable, and let the body become heavy and warm. Avoid television or work tasks.
- If you lie awake worrying, about an hour ahead, write in a worry journal, making a list of worries and the next day's tasks. The journal is a place to put things while you sleep.
- Use pleasant imagery; let the mind "float."
- Sleep on your back on a firm mattress. When sleeping on your side, tuck a small pillow between your waist and the mattress to provide proper support. Sleeping on the abdomen is not recommended because the head is turned sharply to one side all night, affecting neck joints and the lower back. In addition, pressure on one side of the face can irritate the jaw. Sleeping with one arm under the pillow stresses the jaw and may interfere with circulation or pinch a nerve in the wrist.
- If not asleep in 20 minutes, get out of bed and go to another room. Stay calm. Do something boring or relaxing until you are sleepy.

Flemons states that sleep apnea is a common disorder that affects as many as 2% of adult females and 4% of adult males.[177] Sleep apnea refers to breathing cessation during sleep. It is the result of repetitive closure of the upper airway while the person sleeps. Although it is not a new problem, this sleep disorder has only recently been described.[178] Most individuals who suffer from this disorder are snorers. However, many will not suspect that they have the disorder because daytime signs and symptoms are not specific; and nocturnal symptoms often go unrecognized. Effective treatment for sleep apnea exists, but clients should be encouraged to have their condition diagnosed properly in a qualified sleep laboratory prior to deciding upon a therapeutic regimen.[179]

In summation, if the person complains of any sleep problems, the problems should be explored with the goal of eventual correction. Refer the person to a qualified sleep research centre so that, through electronic monitoring of the sleep cycle and close surveillance, the problem can be identified and treated.

PSYCHOSOCIAL CONCEPTS

The following information is relevant for assessments, teaching, and health promotion interventions.

Cognitive Development

Different learning abilities are required in different life stages. Youth is the time for acquisition; young adulthood is the time for achievement; middle age is the time for responsibility; and old age is the time for reintegration.

Theories about Cognitive Development

Cognitive theories are described here; refer also to Chapter 5. Erikson theorized that the basis for adult cognitive performance is laid during the school years when the child accomplishes the task of industry, learns how to learn and win recognition by producing and achieving, and learns to enjoy learning. The child learns an attitude that lasts into adulthood: how much effort a task takes and how long and hard he or she should work for what is desired or expected. The sense of industry is useful in adult life, both in coping with new experiences and in functioning as a worker, family member, citizen, and life-long learner.

Current researchers and theorists propose that learning continues throughout the adult years. The brain shows increasing myelinization through middle age, which permits more integrated modes of social response and stable or increasing intellectual functions.[180–182]

Becoming mature in young adulthood involves intellectual growth, becoming more adaptive and knowledgeable about self, forming values, and developing increasing depth in analytic and synthetic thinking, logical reasoning, and imagination. There are multiple and different intelligences besides academic aptitude, including leadership ability, creative and performing arts abilities, and ability to manage self, others, and a career. Further, developing social and interpersonal skills and personal friendships may have a powerfully maturing effect on intellectual skills.

Table 12–1 summarizes ego functions of the adult based on the analytic theory discussed in Chapter 5.[183] Table 12-2 will assist you in assessing reality thinking processes.

Influences on Learning

Influences differ somewhat from childhood to adulthood and include (1) level of knowledge in society generally, (2) personal values and perceptions and previously learned associations, (3) level of education, (4) available life opportunities, (5) interests, (6) participation by the person in the learning activity, (7) the learning environment, and (8) life experiences.[184–189] As a result of these influences, the person develops a preferred way of learning or cognitive style—a characteristic way of perceiving, organizing, and evaluating information.

Formal Operations Stage

The young adult remains in the formal operations stage, according to Piaget. The adult is creative in thought. He or she begins at the abstract level and compares the idea mentally or verbally with previous memories, knowledge, or experience. The person combines or integrates a number of steps of a task mentally instead of thinking about or doing each step as a separate unit. He or she considers the multiplicity and relativism of issues and alternatives to a situation, synthesizing and integrating ideas or information into the memory, beliefs, or solutions so that the end result is a unique product. Adult thought is different from adolescent thought in that the adult can differentiate among many perspectives and the adult is objective, realistic, and less egocentric. Thinking and learning are problem-centred, not just subject-centred. Reality is considered only a part of all that is possible. The person can imagine

TABLE 12-1
Major Ego (Cerebrum) Functions or Tasks of the Adult

1. **Reality testing**
   a. Distinguishes inner and outer stimuli
   b. Perceives accurately: time, place, and events that relate to self or are familiar
   c. Is psychologically minded and aware of inner states
   d. Has accurate sense of body boundaries

2. **Judgment**
   a. Anticipates probable dangers, legal limits, and social censure or disapproval of intended behaviours
   b. Is aware of appropriateness and consequences of behaviour
   c. Behaves in a way that reflects judgment

3. **Sense of reality of the world and self**
   a. Distinguishes external events that are real and those that are embedded in familiar context, such as déjà vu, trance-like states
   b. Experiences the body and its functions and one's behaviour as familiar, unobtrusive, and belonging to the self
   c. Develops a sense of individuality, uniqueness, self, self-esteem
   d. Develops a sense that the self is separate from the external environment

4. **Regulation and control of drives, affects, and impulses**
   a. Directs impulse expression to indirect forms of behavioural expression
   b. Balances delay and control behaviour
   c. Demonstrates frustration tolerance
   d. Maintains self-esteem independent of daily occurrences and other's opinions
   e. Does minimal acting out

5. **Interpersonal relationships**
   a. Relates to and invests in others, taking account of one's own needs
   b. Relates to others in an adaptive way and based on present mature goals rather than past immature goals
   c. Perceives others as separate rather than as an extension of self
   d. Sustains relationships over long period and tolerates absence of the person
   e. Lists own assumptions against objective data or other's opinion

6. **Thought processes**
   a. Sustains processes for attention, concentration, anticipation, concept formation, memory, and language
   b. Controls unrealistic, illogical, loose, or primitive thinking
   c. Thinks clearly
   d. Has no association or communication problems

7. **Adequate regression in the service of the ego**
   a. Relaxes perceptual and conceptual acuity and other ego controls with concomitant increase in awareness of previously preconscious and unconscious contents
   b. Increases adaptive potentials as a result of creative endeavours

8. **Defensive functioning**
   a. Uses adaptive mechanism for ideation and behaviour effectively
   b. Controls anxiety, depression, or other behavioural affects of weak defensive operations

9. **Stimulus barrier**
   a. Maintains a threshold for, sensitivity to, or awareness of stimuli that impinge on senses
   b. Uses active coping mechanisms in response to levels of sensory stimulation to prevent or minimize disorganization, avoidance, withdrawal

10. **Autonomous functions**
    a. Maintains function or prevents impairment of sight, hearing, intention, language, memory, learning, or motor function
    b. Maintains function or prevents impairment of habit patterns, learned skills, work routines, and hobbies

11. **Synthetic-integrative functioning**
    a. Reconciles or integrates potentially contradictory attitudes, values, affects, behaviour, and self-representations
    b. Relates together and integrates psychic and behavioural events, whether or not contradictory
    c. Identifies chronologic order of events
    d. Integrates good and bad aspects of self

12. **Mastery-competence**
    a. Is motivated with sufficient energy to meet daily demands
    b. Plans goal-directed behaviour
    c. Performs in relation to existing capacity to interact with and master the environment
    d. Expects success in performance of tasks
    e. Maintains autonomy
    f. Evaluates self and resources, as well as expectations of others
    g. Is open to and capable of change
    h. Has diversity of interests

Source: Adapted from Burgess, A., Psychiatric Nursing: Promoting Mental Health. *Stamford, CT: Appleton & Lange, 1997.*

TABLE 12-2
Assessment of Reality Testing Function of Ego (Cerebrum): Distinction between Inner and Outer Stimuli

1. **Maximal impairment**
   a. Hallucinations and delusions pervade
   b. Minimal ability to distinguish dreams from waking life
   c. Inability to distinguish idea, image, and hallucination
   d. Perception disturbed, e.g., moving objects appear immobile and vice versa

2. **Severe impairment**
   a. Hallucinations and delusions severe but limited to one or more content areas
   b. Difficulty distinguishing events as dream or reality

3. **Medium impairment**
   a. Illusions more common than hallucinations
   b. Aware of experiencing illusions others do not
   c. Projects inner states onto external reality more than having hallucinations or delusions

4. **Minimal impairment**
   a. Possible confusion about inner and outer states when awakening, going to sleep, or under severe stress

5. **No impairment**
   a. Distinguishes inner and outer stimuli accurately
   b. Denies external reality occasionally as part of adaptive behaviour
   c. Is aware whether events occurred in dreams or waking life
   d. Identifies source of thoughts and perceptions as being an idea or image and from internal or external source
   e. Distinguishes between inner and outer perceptions even under extreme stress
   f. Checks perceptions against reality automatically

and reason about events that are not occurring in reality but that are possible or in which he or she does not even believe. Hypotheses are generated; conjectures are deduced from hypotheses, and observations are conducted to disconfirm the expectations. The thought system works independent of its context and can be applied to diverse data. The person can evaluate the validity of a train of reasoning independent of its factual content. A concrete proposition can be replaced by an arbitrary sign of symbolic logic such as *p* or *q*. Probability, proportionality, and combining of thought systems occur.[190]

Arlin[191] proposed that some people continue to develop cognitively beyond the formal operations proposed by Piaget into a *fifth stage* of cognitive development that progresses through adulthood. The stage of formal operations describes strategies used in problem solving. The *problem finding stage*, or post-formal thought, goes beyond the problem-solving stage and is characterized by creative thought in the form of discovered problems, relativistic thinking, the formation of generic problems, the raising of general questions from ill-defined problems, use of intuition, insight, and hunches, and the development of significant scientific thought.

CRITICAL THINKING

Compare and contrast adult and adolescent thought. What is distinctive about adult thought?

There are *four criteria for post-formal thought*:

1. *Shifting gears.* Going from abstract reasoning to practical, real-world considerations.
2. *Multiple causality, multiple solutions.* Awareness that most problems have more than one cause and more than one solution and that some solutions are more likely to work than others.
3. *Pragmatism.* Ability to choose the best of several possible solutions and recognize criteria for the choice.
4. *Paradox recognition awareness.* A problem or solution has inherent conflict.

Sternberg, in his Triarchic Theory of Intelligence, stated that IQ tests do not measure creative insight and practical intelligence. He proposed *three elements of adult intelligence*:[192]

1. *Componential or analytic.* How efficiently people process information, solve problems, monitor solutions or evaluate results.
2. *Experiential, insightful.* How people approach novel and familiar tasks, compare new information to old, and think originally while automatically performing familiar operations.
3. *Contextual, practical.* How people deal with the environment, size up a situation, adapt to or change a situation, or find a new, more suitable setting.

The person may use different thinking for scientific operations, business transactions, artistic activities, and intimate interpersonal interactions. Thus mature thinkers can accept and live with contradictions and conflicts and engage in a number of activities. At times, however, the adult will of necessity do thinking typical of concrete operations. At times the adult may regress to the preoperational stage (some never get beyond this period), as shown by superstitious, egocentric, or illogical thinking. The adult may not have the ability to perform formal operations.

CRITICAL THINKING

In what kinds of situations in the health care delivery system would post-formal thought be most useful?

A further distinction in types of adult thinking separates the *managers,* those who have a better developed right brain and who synthesize data to see the overall picture, from the *planners,* those who have a better developed left brain and who analyze sequentially and look closely to the minute details. Women tend to have a better integrated brain and usually combine both manager and planner thinking.[193]

The young adult continues to learn both formally and informally to enhance cognitive and job skills and self-knowledge. Learning may be pursued in "on-the-job training," job-sponsored orientation courses, trade schools, college studies, or continuing education courses. Environmental stimulation is important in continued learning. Increasingly young adults are changing their minds about their life work and change directions after several years of study or work in the original field. Formal operations, or abstract thinking, appears to be linked to the content areas in which the person has extensive training. After concrete operations, a person may acquire abstract thinking in behavioural, symbolic, semantic, or figural content areas, depending on experience.[194,195] There are some age differences between younger and older adults according to research findings, but the influences on learning described earlier may be major factors in those differences.[196]

Gender Differences

Gender differences may be the result of bias in research. Cognitive ability in men and women has been considered unequal and has been described on the basis of different functions in each cerebral hemisphere, although brain structure is the same in men and women. The left hemisphere is dominant in 97% of people for language, logical reasoning, and mathematical calculation. The right hemisphere is nonverbal and mute: it knows but cannot tell what it knows without processing the knowledge through the left hemisphere. The right hemisphere processes spatial and visual abstractions, recognition of faces, body image, music, art forms, and intuitive, preconscious, and fantasy processes. At birth asymmetry in the left hemisphere is more marked in the male. Female infants have a somewhat larger area of visual cortex in the right hemisphere than male infants, which implies an anatomic advantage for nonverbal ideation. The female's brain matures earlier; thus the two hemispheres are more integrated in the female as indicated by less impairment of intellectual function in women who have suffered either right or left hemisphere damage. Males are more vulnerable to brain damage. Women use verbal strategies to solve spatial problems on tests because of the greater interplay between the two hemispheres of the brain. In adulthood, women are better able to coordinate activities of both hemispheres; thus they can think intuitively and globally. Men are better at activities in which the two hemispheres do not compete, such as problem solving and determining spatial relationships.

Nonconformity to sex-role stereotypes is positively related to IQ. The more assertive and active woman has greater intellectual ability and more interests. The less aggressive man focuses less on developing physique and develops intellectual ability and interests to a greater extent.

Cognitive abilities have often been related to personality traits and interpersonal orientation. Sex-role socialization has been related to cognitive style. Some researchers believe the level of information processing a person attains exerts a profound influence on personality and on ability to integrate and differentiate in problem solving.

Claims about sex differences in other cognitive abilities, such as creativity, analytic ability, and reasoning, also apparently are the result of differences in verbal, quantitative, or visual-spatial abilities or in opportunity to develop such abilities—in either sex.[197]

The confident young adult takes pride in being mentally astute, creative, progressive, and alert to events. He or she normally has the mental capacity to make social and occupational contributions, is self-directive and curious, and likes to match wits with others in productive dialogue.

Both men and women have similar basic needs, their own unique cognitive abilities and talents, and often unspoken ideas and feelings longing for self-expression. From young childhood on, both females and males should be considered cognitively capable to their maximum potential and should have the opportunity, including in the adult years, to meet that maximum potential.

CRITICAL THINKING

Give examples of the influence that culture has on the cognitive abilities of men and women.

Teaching the Adult

Information on cognitive development should be considered whenever you are teaching adults. Table 12-3 presents principles of learning. See also Table 1-16 for suggestions on teaching methods.[198–201] Avoid "canned" audiovisual presentations. Emphasize a sharing of ideas and experiences, role-play, and practical application of information. In some cases you will be helping the person to unlearn old habits, attitudes, or information to acquire new habits and attitudes.

If you teach illiterate young adults, you must compensate for their inability to read and write. Slow, precise speech and gestures and the use of pictures and audiovisual aids are more crucial than with literate adults. *Demonstration* and *return*

TABLE 12-3
Principles of the Learning Process

1. Learning is an active, self-directed process.
2. Learning is central to ongoing development and behavioural changes.
3. Learning is influenced by readiness to learn, abilities, potential to learn, and emotional state.
4. Learning is facilitated when the content or behaviours to be learned are perceived as relevant.
5. Learning proceeds from simple to complex and known to unknown.
6. Learning is facilitated when the learner has opportunities to take risks, test ideas, make mistakes, and be creative.
7. Learning is facilitated when the person has knowledge of progress and feedback that serves as a measure for further learning.
8. Learning transfer occurs when the person can recognize similarities and differences between past experiences and the present situation.
9. Learning is effective when it can be immediately applied.
10. Learning occurs best when the teaching methodology is relevant to the content to be learned.
11. Learning occurs best in an environment that is nonthreatening, comfortable, and free of distractions.
12. Learning occurs best and is continued when the learner feels satisfied and successful.

demonstration ensure learning. Do not underestimate the importance of your behaviour and personality as a motivating force, especially if some members of the person's family do not consider learning important.

Some adults have attention deficit hyperactivity disorder (ADHD). Modify your teaching strategies accordingly.[202]

CRITICAL THINKING

How would you modify your teaching strategy for a group of young adults who have attention deficit hyperactivity disorder?

Work and Leisure Activities

Although the following discussion focuses on work outside of the home, implying paid employment, we do not demean or overlook the young adult woman or man who chooses to stay at home and rear a family. *Homemaking and childrearing are essential and important work;* each is fatiguing and stressful in its own way. In fact, staying at home can be hazardous to health. The many noise and air pollutants or chemical toxins that come from appliances, building materials, cleaning products, and combinations of materials or supplies used in a home should be discussed (see Chapter 2).

Work Options and Attitudes

There are many work options and attitudes. For example, the young adult "workaholic" executive may put in 70 to 80 hours weekly at the job, think about the job most of the remaining hours, feel guilty when not working, and channel much anger and aggression through work. In contrast, a factory worker while feeding a certain part into the assembly line, may be planning what he or she will do after work—to this person work is only a means of livelihood. There are people who work long hours and who are highly involved in their work but who are not workaholics. They feel exhilarated about the flow of work, the challenge, their goals, and the use of skills involved, and they feel creative, active, and motivated. These feelings are more likely to come from work than leisure. These people contribute a great deal to the advancement of their vocation or profession generally and to the individuals they serve.

In addition to agricultural, skilled and semiskilled workers, blue-collar and white-collar workers, managerial or executive personnel, and professionals, a new classification exists—the knowledge worker. Because of expanding technology, rapid change, the burgeoning size of industries and megaindustries, and the knowledge explosion, the **knowledge worker** is *hired to do job planning and to create, innovate, and make decisions within the organization.* The ultimate goal of the knowledge worker is cost containment for the company, improved efficiency of the worker, a more marketable product, and a more willing buyer. You must cope with unanticipated changes, predict changes, and collaborate with others.

You may find the worker—all the way from the executive level to the delivery person—a victim of **substance abuse,** *ingesting excessive alcohol or drugs or engaged in pushing illicit drugs* on the job. Substance abuse is a response to stress, often job-related. The implications of substance abuse are grave,

including job errors, accidents to self or others, poor job performance, a product that does not meet standard results, and increased insurance and worker's compensation benefits to employees, all of which increases the cost of the product to the consumer. In addition, the lives of family, friends, and coworkers are affected. Work with the personnel director, safety director, employee assistance programs, administrative personnel, and the affected individual (and family if possible) to help the person get the necessary treatment needed.

Nurses may also suffer from substance abuse, but they are no more likely to have such problems than are other employees. Several authors write about understanding and assisting the colleague who is chemically dependent.[203–205] Refer also to the discussion of alcoholism and drug abuse later in this chapter.

CRITICAL THINKING

In your province or territory, what programs are made available by professional bodies for health practitioners who are chemically dependent?

The majority of young adult women are in the work force. Sometimes the job is a necessity (e.g., if she is single, divorced, and has children, or if her husband has only seasonal work or a low-paying job). Many women are working to maintain occupational skills, self-esteem, and independence.

Balancing work and family life responsibilities is often stressful for the woman who is a single parent, a divorced parent, or member of a two-career family. There is never enough time and often too much to do.[206–211] Some employers, to attract and keep competent workers, are offering flexible work schedules, job sharing, on-the-site daycare, and both paternity leave and extended maternity leave. These *suggestions can be shared with the parent who has the greatest responsibility for balancing home and work*:[212,213]

- Identify priorities. Discuss with the spouse, or the children if they are old enough, what tasks must be done, what can be delegated (either on the job or to a service company in the home), and who can take on which responsibilities to even the load.

- Allocate tasks. Design a system for assigning tasks, based on skill, age, availability, and fairness. Rotate tasks, if possible, or assign tasks that are especially requested.

- Speak up for yourself at home and on the job. Explore grievance channels if necessary.

- Use a support network. Family, friends, neighbours, and child care providers can be asked for assistance on a regular basis or for help in emergencies.

- Rechannel emotional investments. Having multiple roles gives an opportunity to excel in one realm if you have problems in another.

- Assess progress. Plan frequent review sessions to discuss effectiveness of the plan as well as problem areas in order to avoid resentments or rebellions.

Fellow employees must be aware that women often look differently at the same work situation and respond to different rewards in the workplace than men and that they bring a perspective and judgment level that is not based solely on competition and aggressiveness. Further, equipment or protective clothing that fits men may well be hazardous to women because of size, weight, muscle stretching involved, or poor fit. The employer can benefit from the qualities and expertise women bring to the work force. Technologic change will increasingly compete with a rising demand for human services, especially in health, law, and recreation. Technology can help free people for service work; however, in a technologic age, skills related to caring for or serving others are often neglected. *Regardless of the various attitudes about work, it remains a central part of the adult self-concept in most North Americans,* and a close relationship exists between occupational and family satisfaction. If the person is dissatisfied in either work or family life, he or she will try to compensate in the other.[214,215]

Because the nurse views the person holistically, you may be asked for assistance by the manager, executive-level employees, or the employers. They may find it difficult to understand the young adult worker who acts differently than the middle-aged or older worker; the behaviour of the young adult worker who has newly achieved an executive position may be poorly understood by employees who are middle-aged and near retirement. Help them understand that each generation of worker has a different value system and responds to different values and different motivational stimuli.

CRITICAL THINKING

How do Baby Boomers and members of Generation X view the world of work?

As a nurse, others will seek you out as someone who can assist with safety and health problems, listen to and counsel about job problems, help another make decisions pertinent to occupation, and assist in resolving conflicts related to the work setting or homemaker, career woman, and mother roles. Through your counselling and education role, you can assist both the individual employee and administrative or management personnel to realize the importance of feelings of self-respect in relation to employment. Management consultants have learned that low self-esteem and feelings of stress in the worker lowers productivity, morale, and profits. You can be instrumental in helping the work system promote workers' feelings of self-esteem and about the importance of their work.

You may also become an advocate for the woman who is undergoing sexual harassment on the job. Increasingly, women workers are gaining the courage to talk publicly about and to seek legal aid for sexual harassment in factories, mines, offices, migrant farm fields, and health care facilities.[216]

Each workplace must have policies and procedures established to handle complaints of harassment on the job. Ideally the work atmosphere should be such that, first, harassment would not occur, and second, everyone would be concerned about the problem and know how to handle it.

The problems of sexism and sexual harassment in the workplace and in society in general are not limited to North America. You must resolve your own job-related conflicts before you can help others. By using the above information and insights you gain from being a professional who works with and learns from many other people, you are indeed in a key position to assist the worker regardless of the setting. Several references assist in job self-assessment and ways to overcome job stress.[217–222]

Leisure

Some young adults are in pursuit of leisure.[223–227] As job hours per week are being cut (especially in automated jobs), the time for leisure increases. Additionally, the work ethic is decreasing in importance. Socialization of current young adults has fostered a leisure ethic.

Leisure is *freedom from obligations and formal duties of paid work and opportunity to pursue, at one's own pace, mental nourishment, enlivenment, pleasure, and relief from fatigue of work.* Leisure may be as active as backpacking up a mountain or as quiet as fishing alone in a huge lake. Some people never know leisure, and others manage an attitude of leisure even as they work. Various factors influence the use of leisure time: sex; amount of family, home, work, or community responsibilities; mental status; income and socioeconomic class; and past interests.

Maintaining friendships is a healthy use of leisure time. It takes time, self-disclosure, and sharing of interests to form friendships. Gradually, a sense of reliability and confidentiality grows as a core to the friendship. Some conflict may surface and is natural as intimacy deepens. In a world in which women juggle career, love, and family, time may limit the size of the friendship circle. Several close friendships should be made. Successful friendship combines the freedom to depend on one another with the freedom to be independent.

Doing volunteer work with a favourite charity or community group is a way to use non–work time that can promote a sense of leisure and enjoyment while simultaneously using skills and talents to improve life for others. The rewards are dual—to the self and to society. Help the client realize the importance of leisure as a part of balanced living. The young adult needs to develop a variety of interests as preparation for the years ahead to maintain physical and mental health.

CRITICAL THINKING

What are some of your leisure activities?

Emotional Development

Emotional development in young adulthood is an ongoing, dynamic process, an extension of childhood and adolescent developmental influences and processes. Development is still influenced by the environment, but the environment is different. The fundamental developmental issues continue as central aspects of adult life but in an altered form. Thus trust, autonomy, initiative, industry, and identity all are reworked and elaborated, based on current experiences. Young adulthood is a time when there is increased clarity and consistency of personality; a stabilization of self and identity; established preferences of interests and activities; increased coping ability; less defensiveness; decrease in youthful illusions, fantasy, and impulsiveness; more responsiveness to and responsibility for self and others; more giving than taking;

and more appreciation of surroundings. It is a time to develop expanded resources for happiness. Certainly adult experiences, lifestyle, and geographic changes can contribute to personality development and change. A major modifying variable is gender. Degrees of childhood passivity and dependency remained continuous for women but not for men.

In 1990, two psychologists, Salovey and Mayer, coined the term *emotional intelligence,* which refers to the ability to recognize and deal with one's own feelings and the feelings of others.[228] Strickland states that, according to Daniel Goleman, who popularized the concept, there are five components of emotional intelligence: self-awareness, self-regulation, motivation, empathy, and social skills.[229] Health care delivery systems that wish to thrive need leaders in the health professions who have high emotional intelligence.

CRITICAL THINKING

In what kinds of situations would emotional intelligence be most appreciated?

Theories of Emotional Development

Various theorists discussed in Chapter 5 also have research findings on which to base their beliefs about adult personality development. The findings of Gould, Sheehy, Levinson, and Erikson are discussed in the following pages.

Gould[230,231] describes life stages and key issues or tasks in late adolescence and young adulthood (Table 12-4). Gould believes there is an increasing need throughout adulthood to win permission from the self to continue development. The direction of change through adulthood is becoming more tolerant of self and more appreciative of the surrounding world. Although Gould does not list specific assumptions about adult development, he sees adulthood as a time of thoughtful confrontation with the self—letting go of an idealized image, the desire to be perfect, and acknowledging the realistic image of self and personal feelings. Conflicts between past and present beliefs are resolved. Through constant examination and reformulation of beliefs embedded in feelings, the person can substitute a conception of adulthood for childhood legacy and fantasies. Whereas children mark the passing years by their changing bodies, adults change their minds, deepen their insights about self, and mature emotionally.

Sheehy[232] believes that development occurs throughout adulthood and is influenced by external events or crises, the historical period, membership in the culture, and social roles and by the internal realism of the person—values, goals, and aspirations. Sheehy ties developmental stage in late adolescence and young adulthood to Erikson's development stage.

Levinson[233–236] studied only men in formulating a concept of adult developmental stages; however, he believes the stages are age linked and universal and, thus, should be applicable to women (Table 12-5). In each period biological, psychodynamic, cultural, social, and other timetables operate in only partial synchronization, which makes for developmental

TABLE 12-4
Gould's Developmental Stages of Adulthood

Stage	Age Range (yr)	Developmental Task
1	16–18	Pre-adulthood; desire to escape from parental control. May perceive self as adult in some cultures.
2	18–22	Leave family. Establish peer friendships.
3	22–28	Develop greater independence. Commit self to career and family.
4	28–34	Transition; question life goals. Re-evaluate marriage and career commitments.
5	34–43	Sense of time running out. Realign life goals.
6	43–53	Settle down. Accept personal life situation.
7	53–60	Accept past. Greater tolerance for others; general mellowing.

difficulties. The organizing concept of **life structure** *refers to a pattern of the person's life at a specific time* and is used to focus on the boundary between the individual and society. In its external aspects life structure *refers to roles, memberships, interests, conditions or style of living, and long-term goals.* In its *internal aspects,* life structure includes the *personal meanings of external patterns, inner identities, care values, fantasies, and psychodynamic qualities that shape the person.*

Developmental Crisis

According to Erikson, the psychosexual crisis is in intimacy versus self-isolation. **Intimacy** is *reaching out and using the self to form a commitment to and an intense, lasting relationship with another person or even a cause, an institution, or creative effort.* In an intimate experience there is mutual trust, sharing of feelings, and responsibility to and cooperation with each other. The physical satisfaction and psychological security of another are more important than one's own. The person is involved with people, work, hobbies, and community issues. He or she has poise and ease in the lifestyle because identity is firm. There is a steady conviction of who he or she is, a self-acceptance, and a unity of personality that will improve through life.

TABLE 12–5
Levinson's Theory of Early Adulthood

Era	Age Range	Life Structure
Pre-adulthood	0–22	Preparing for adulthood.
	17–22	Transition to early adulthood.
		Begin novice phase; person is guided out of adolescence.
Early adulthood	17–45	Combine social and occupational roles that are adapted to personality and skills.
	22–28	Enter young adulthood. Novice phase tasks:
		a. Form dream for life
		b. Establish or enter relationship
		c. Select occupation
		d. Establish love relationship
	28–33	Age 30 transition: reappraise life plan and modify it.
	33–40	Culminating life plans and structure for early adulthood: seek to realize goals.
	40–45	Transition to or preparation for midlife.

Intimacy is a situation involving two people that permits acceptance of all aspects of the other, self-disclosure, and a collaboration in which the person adjusts behaviour to the other's behaviour and needs in pursuit of mutual satisfaction.

A person's mental health is dependent on the ability to enter into a relationship and experience self-disclosure; in so doing, the support and maintenance of the relationship alleviates feelings of loneliness.

Women, more so than men, are concerned with relationships and are interested in the process rather than the product of something. They also recognize their vulnerability and can acknowledge the need to change more readily than men. Women self-disclose more easily than men. If a healthy balance between dependence and independence exists, social relationships and intimacy are maintained more easily, and the risk of experiencing loneliness and isolation decreases.

With the intimate person, the young adult is able to regulate cycles of work, recreation, and procreation (if chosen) and to work toward satisfactory stages of development for all offspring and the ongoing development of self and the partner.

CRITICAL THINKING

What factors within a relationship promote and maintain intimacy?

Love

Love is the feeling accompanying intimacy, and love and intimacy change over time[237] (Figure 12–5). The young adult often has difficulty determining what love is. A classic description of love as stated by the apostle Paul in I Corinthians 13:4–7 has been the basis for many statements on love by poets, novelists, humanists, philosophers, psychiatrists, theologians, and common people:

Love is patient and kind; love is not jealous or boastful; it is not arrogant or rude. Love does not insist on its own way; it is not irritable or resentful; it does not rejoice at wrong, but rejoices in the right. Love bears all things, believes all things, hopes all things, and endures all things.

One of the most important things the person can learn within the family as a child and adolescent is to love. By the time the person reaches the mid-20s, the person should be

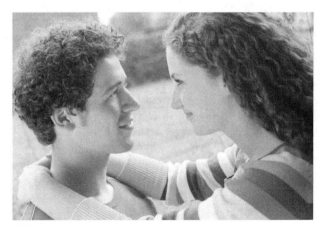

FIGURE 12–5

The principal developmental task of young adults is the formation of close relationships with significant others.

experienced in the emotion of love. If there was deprivation or distortion of love in the home when he or she was young, the adult will find it difficult to achieve mature love in an intimate relationship. By this time, the person should realize that one *does not fall* in love; one *learns* to love; one *grows* into love.

Intimacy and love are usually considered from an emotional perspective, with an expression in physical closeness. Michael Liebowitz, a psychiatrist at New York State Hospital Psychiatric Institute, studied the effect of love on brain chemistry. He divided love between men and women into two stages: (1) the attraction stage, characterized by giddiness, euphoria, optimism, and energy; and (2) the attachment stage, characterized by peaceful, secure, comfortable feelings. These two phases are caused by increased brain activity, he believes. In the attraction stage, phenylethylamine causes euphoria and increased sexual attraction. Eventually the brain's tolerance for this natural aphrodisiac dulls; less infatuation is felt. Then the attachment stage, with increased production of endorphins and feelings of well-being, occurs. This is an example of how the interpersonal situation influences brain chemistry and, in turn, influences behaviour.[238,239]

You will have many opportunities for discussions, individual and group counselling, and education on marriage, establishing a home, the relationship between spouses and the relationship between parents and children. When you help people sort through feelings about life and love, you are indirectly making a contribution to the health and stability of them and their offspring.

Marriage

Attachment is a concept that applies across the life span and is manifested in several layers of relationship in adulthood.[240] The socially accepted way for two people in love to be intimate is in marriage, a social contract or institution implying binding rules and responsibilities that cannot be ignored without some penalty. Marriage is endorsed in some form by all cultures in all periods of history because it formalizes and symbolizes the importance of family. Social stability depends on family stability. Marriage is more than getting a piece of paper.

There are norms in every society to prevent people from entering lightly into the wedded state (e.g., age limits, financial and property settlements, ceremony, witnesses, and public registration and announcement). One of the major functions of marriage is to control and limit sexuality and provide the framework for a long-term relationship between a man and a woman. Marriage gives rights in four areas: sexuality, birth and rearing of children, domestic and economic services, and property.[241]

The pattern and sequence of a person's life history influence whom, when, and why he or she marries. Apparently many people do not really know the person they are marrying and do not realize how greatly the partner's personality will influence their own. The problems of marital adjustment and family living have their roots and basis in the choice of the partner.[242]

Mates often choose each other on the basis of unconscious needs, which they strive to meet through a mate whose personality complements rather than replicates their own, or

out of fear and loneliness or on the basis of physical attraction. The person chooses someone for an intimate relationship whose lifestyle and personality pattern strengthen and encourage his or her own personal development.

Although the person tends to marry an individual who lives and works nearby and has similar social, religious, and racial backgrounds, an increasing number of mixed marriages are occurring, an outgrowth of more liberal social attitudes. A number of *factors influence the success of the marriage that crosses religious, ethnic, socioeconomic, or racial boundaries*:[243,244]

- Motive for marriage
- Faithfulness to the spouse; if one person engages in an extramarital affair, it is possible to repair the brokenness, but a feeling of mistrust may remain and is difficult to overcome
- Desire, commitment, and effort to bridge the gulf between the couple and their families
- Ability and maturity of the two people to live with and resolve their differences and problems
- Reaction of the parental families, who may secretly or openly support **homogamy** (*marriage between a couple with similar or identical backgrounds*)

There are *four patterns of marriage*:[245]

1. Traditional. The male is provider; the female is homemaker and mother.
2. Romantic. Sexual passion is the main focus.
3. Rescue. Marriage makes up for previous painful experiences.
4. Companionate. Relationship based on friendship and equal division of work and family roles.

CRITICAL THINKING

What are the benefits of marriage in today's society?

If young adults are to *establish a strong family unit* of their own and avoid in-law interference, their loyalties must be to their *own* family before either his or her family. The *following guidelines may be helpful*:[246]

- They should establish themselves as a collaborative pair in their own eyes and in the eyes of mutual friends and both families; spending time together.
- In-laws should not take priority over the spouse and home of the couple. If friends of either husband or wife are offensive to the partner, be prepared to minimize this friendship. Husband and wife together build new friendships.
- Working through intimate systems of communications that allow for exchange of confidences and feelings and an increased degree of empathy and ability to predict each other's responses.
- Planning ahead for a stable relationship and arriving at a consensus about how their life should be lived; being committed to each other.
- Be mindful of sensitive areas, those that are sources of irritation in each other's life. Each needs to *work* at coping with the other's idiosyncrasies or habits and try to meet the other's preferences to keep love in the relationship.

CASE SITUATION
Young Adult Development—Marriage and Commitment

James Chaney, 26 years old, received his bachelor's degree in nursing this year after combining full-time employment as an attendant at a local hospital and part-time school attendance for five years. He has recently accepted a position at the hospital as a nurse in the surgical intensive care unit. James and his wife, Mary, have been married for two years. Mary, 25 years old, is finishing her bachelor's degree in accounting while she continues employment with an insurance firm. James and Mary plan to wait a few years before starting a family as both realize the importance of graduate education in their fields. They would also like to move from their apartment to a home with more space and a yard.

To save money to achieve their future plans, both James and Mary work extra hours when asked. This has frequently interfered with their studies. They also find they have little time for leisure activities and less time together. Communication is sometimes in the form of memos posted on the refrigerator. Increasingly, the stresses of balancing school, work, and home demands have resulted in arguments, often over minor issues.

When a long-anticipated vacation must be cancelled because of unexpected expenses, James and Mary are disappointed and angry; however, they decide to plan a week of inexpensive activities in the local area that will allow them to spend time together uninterrupted. They decide to tell no one that they have remained at home. The resulting vacation is truly restful and meaningful as they share favourite activities and explore their dreams and goals for the future.

QUESTIONS

1. What do you think James and Mary could have done earlier to minimize, or avoid, the hardships they encountered?
2. To what extent do you agree, or disagree, that marital anger and conflict are necessary in an intimate relationship? What makes you think so?
3. What do you believe are the underlying strengths in each partner that enabled their conflict to be resolved? Was the resolution gender based?

- Giving each other positive reinforcement, expressing appreciation and affection, to release love rather than focus on problems.
- Manage money and material possessions or they will manage the couple. Money and things are important, but the focus in a relationship should be on the person.
- Maintain a spirit of courtship, spontaneity, and freshness to keep love in a marriage.
- Deal with crises in a positive way.

You may ask certain questions to ascertain readiness for marriage in the young adult or self. One such question is: Are you willing to take responsibility for your own behaviour? You can explore this question and other questions in premarital counselling or courses in family living.

CRITICAL THINKING

As a health professional, what would you ask a couple regarding their readiness for marriage?

Isolation, or **self-absorption,** is the *inability to be intimate, spontaneous, or close with another, thus becoming withdrawn, lonely, and conceited and behaving in a stereotyped manner.* The isolated person is unable to sustain close friendships. The person may not marry; there is avoidance of a need for a bond with another. If he or she does marry, the partner is likely to find personal emotional needs unmet while giving considerably of the self to the isolated, self-absorbed person.

You may counsel the self-absorbed person and help him or her achieve the tasks of intimacy. You may also be a role model of commitment to serving others. Use the principles of communication and relationship described in Chapter 4. Also, see the box entitled "Consequences of Isolation" for further description of behaviours and traits associated with isolation.

Consequences of Isolation

- Is pessimistic, distrustful, ruthless
- Is lonely; may rationalize why being alone is enjoyed
- Avoids close relationships, especially with person of the opposite sex
- Lives a façade
- Has experienced a number of unsuccessful relationships
- Insists on having own way in a relationship
- Lacks empathy for others; cannot see another's perspective
- Is naïvely childlike
- Is easily disillusioned, embittered, cynical
- Overextends self without any real interest or feeling
- Is unable to reciprocate feelings or behaviour in a relationship; makes demands but cannot give in a relationship
- Participates readily in encounter groups or forced fellowship to temporarily relieve loneliness, alienation
- Avoids real issues in life
- May be overtly friendly but drops a relationship when it becomes intimate; unable to sustain a relationship; may become engaged but never marry
- May spend considerable time on the computer or Internet but is actually alienated from people

Moral-Spiritual Development

The young adult may be in either the conventional or the postconventional level of moral development. In the postconventional level, he or she follows the principles defined as appropriate for life. There are two stages in this level. In both stages the person has passed beyond living a certain way just because the majority of people do. Yet in stage I of this level, the person adheres to the legal viewpoint of society. The person believes, however, that laws can be changed as people's needs change, and he or she is able to transcend the thinking of a specific social order and develop universal principles about justice, equality, and human rights. In stage II, the person still operates as in stage I but is able to incorporate injustice, pain, and death as an integral part of existence.

Kohlberg[247] espouses that the reason for the behaviour indicates the level of moral development and that for a person to be at any level, the reasons for behaviour should be consistent to the stage 50% of the time. Therefore it would appear difficult for the average young adult, concerned about family, achieving in a career, paying the bills, and so on, to be in the postconventional level. Although the person may follow principles some of the time, conflicting situations and demands arise. To be consistently in the postconventional level takes considerable ego strength, a firm emotional and spiritual identity, and a willingness to stand up to societal forces. It may take years of maturing before the adult can be that courageous and consistent in Western society.

Today's young adults have grown up with the influence of science and technology. As early as World War II, some prophesied that the children born then would be post-religious, disinterested in other worlds, and concerned only in the secular existence of the present. Although some young adults fit this description and others are rejecting the institutional church, many have retained a desire and ability to apply spiritual and moral principles in this world. Increasingly, parents with young children are joining a church or synagogue, seeking religion and a way to instil values in the children.

In young adulthood there is a humanizing of values and a trend toward relativism as conflicts are encountered. The person increasingly discovers the meaning of values and their relation to achievement of social purposes, and he or she brings both personal experiences and motives to affirm and promote a value system. The person's values, whatever they are, become increasingly his or her own and a part of a unified philosophy of life. At the same time, there is expanding empathy for others and their value systems.[248,249]

The spiritual awakening often experienced during adolescence, which might have receded with seeking of success, may now take on a more mature aspect as the young adult becomes firmly established in another life stage.

Several qualities contribute to a spiritually mature disposition. The disposition is:

- *Individualized and integrated.* The person translates the abstract knowledge into practical action. It helps him or her to reach goals and to attain harmony in various aspects of living.
- *Consistent.* It produces basic standards of morality and conduct.
- *Comprehensive, dynamic, and flexible.* It never stops searching for new attitudes and ideas. The person can hold ideas tentatively until confirmed or until evidence produces a more valid belief.

Because new and different ideas are always available, the mature disposition can continue for a lifetime. The person realizes that there is always more to learn. Root[250] discusses spiritual development in the current young adult generation and how they differ from parental generations.

One of the *dilemmas for the interfaith or intercultural couple* is what values and religion, if any, to follow in the home and to teach the children; how to celebrate holidays; what rituals and traditions to follow (e.g., Hanukkah or Christmas). Even when the couple makes a choice, there may be conflicts with relatives. The couple should learn as much as possible about each other's religion or culture and talk to their families and friends about their experiences. It is critical that each family group remain open and accepting of the other. In turn, the children can learn deeper dimensions of spirituality, moral values, and their cultural background.

Although spiritual development and moral development follow sequential steps and are often thought of simultaneously, there is no significant link between specific religious affiliation or education and moral development. Moral development is linked positively with empathy, the capacity to understand another's viewpoint, and the ability to act reciprocally with another while maintaining personal values and principles. Being with people who are at a higher moral level stimulates the person to ask questions, consider his or her actions, and move to a higher moral level.

CRITICAL THINKING

What are some of the differences in moral principles held by young adults from cultures different from your own?

Adaptive Mechanisms

The young adult seeks stability while he or she is adapting to new or changing events. When the young adult is physically and emotionally healthy, total functioning is smooth. Adaptation to the environment, satisfaction of needs, and social interaction proceed relatively effortlessly and with minimum discomfort. The young adult behaves as though he or she is in control of impulses and drives and in harmony with superego ideals and demands. He or she can tolerate frustration of needs and is capable of making choices that seem best for total equilibrium. The person is emotionally mature for this life stage.

Emotional maturity or intelligence is not exclusively related to physical health. Under stress, the healthiest people might momentarily have irrational impulses; in contrast, the extremely ill have periods of lucidity. Emotional health and maturity have an infinite gradation of behaviour on a continuum rather than a rigid division between healthy and ill. Concepts of maturity are generated by culture. What is normal in one society may be abnormal in another.

In coping with stress in the environment, the young adult uses any of the previously discussed adaptive mechanisms. Use of these mechanisms, such as *denial* and *regression,* becomes abnormal or maladaptive only when the person uses the same mechanism of behaviour too frequently, in too many situations, or for too long a duration.

Self-Concept and Body Image Development

Self-concept and body image, defined in Chapters 5 and 7 and discussed in each developmental era, are now redefined and expanded to fit the young adult perspective.

The *person's perception of self physically, emotionally, and socially, is based on:*

1. Reactions of others that have been internalized.
2. Self-expectations.
3. Perceived abilities.
4. Attitudes.
5. Habits.
6. Knowledge.
7. Other characteristics.

These factors affect self-concept and affect how that person will handle situations and relate to others. How the person behaves depends on whether he or she feels positively or negatively about self, whether the person believes others view him or her positively or negatively, and how he or she believes others expect the person to behave in this situation. The reactions of the family members, including spouse and partner, and the employment situation, are strong influences on the young adult's self-concept. Additionally, the person discloses different aspects of self to various people and in various situations, depending on needs, what is considered socially acceptable, reactions of others, and past experience with self-disclosure.[251–253]

Body image, a *part of self-concept, is a mental picture of the body's appearance integrated into the parietotemporal area of the cortex. Body image includes the surface, internal, and postural picture of the body and values, attitudes, emotions, and personality reactions of the person in relation to the body as an object in space, separate from others.* This image is flexible, subject to constant revision, and may not be reflective of actual body structure. Body image shifts back and forth at different times of the day and at different times in the life cycle.

Under normal conditions, the body is the focus of an individual's identity, and its limits more or less clearly define a boundary that separates the person from the environment. One's body has spatial and time sense and yields experiences that cannot be shared directly with others. A person's body is the primary channel of contact with the world, and it is a nucleus around which values are synthesized. Any disturbance to the body influences total self-concept.

Contributing Influences
Many factors contribute to the body image:[254]

- Parental and social reaction to the person's body
- The person's interpretation of others' reactions to him or her
- The anatomic appearance and physiologic function of the body, including sex, age, kinesthetic and other sensorimotor stimuli, and illness or deformity
- Attitudes and emotions toward and familiarity with the body
- Internal drives, dependency needs, motivational state, and ideals to which the person aspires

- Identification with the bodies of others who were considered ideal (a little bit of each person significant to the person is incorporated into the self-concept and personality)
- Perception of space and objects immediately surrounding the body such as a chair or car; the sense of body boundaries
- Objects attached to the body such as clothing, a wig, false eyelashes, a prosthesis, jewellery, makeup, or perfume
- Activities the body performs in various roles, occupations, or recreations

CRITICAL THINKING

What are a few other psychosocial factors in the health care system that contribute to one's perception of body image?

The kinesthetic receptors in the muscles, tendons, and joints and the labyrinth receptors in the inner ear inform the person about his or her position in space. By means of perceptual alterations in position, the postural image of the body constantly changes. Every new posture and movement is incorporated by the cortex into a **schema** (*image*) in relation to or in association with previously made schemata. Thus the image of the body changes with changing movements—walking, sitting, gestures, changes in appearance, and changes in the pace of walking.

Self-produced movement aids visual accuracy. When a person's body parts are moved passively instead of actively (e.g., sitting in a wheelchair instead of walking), perceptual accuracy about space and the self as an object in space is hindered. Athletes, ballet dancers, and other agile people are more accurate than most in estimating the dimensions of the body parts that are involved in movement. Activity appears to enhance sensory information in a way that passive movements do not. If a person undergoes body changes, he or she must actively explore and move the involved part to reintegrate it.

Self-Knowledge. How do you visualize your body as you walk, run, stand, sit, or gesture? How do you feel about yourself as you go through various motions? What emotions are expressed by your movements? How do you think others visualize you at that time? The message you convey about yourself to another may aid or hinder the establishment of a therapeutic relationship. You must be realistically aware of the posture and movement of your body and what they may be conveying to another.

Self-knowledge is not necessarily the same as knowledge gained about the self from others. Each person sees self differently from how others see him or her, although the most mature person is able to view self as others do. New attributes or ideas are integrated into the old ones, but all ideas received are not necessarily integrated. Before any perception about the self can affect or be integrated into one's self-concept, the perceptions must be considered good or necessary to the self. A person has definite ideas and feelings about his or her own body, what is satisfying and what is frustrating. What the person thinks of self has remarkable power in influencing behaviour and the interpretation of other's behaviour, the choice of associates, and goals pursued.

Body image in the adult is a social creation. Normality is judged by appearance and ways of using the body are prescribed by society. Approval and acceptance are given for normal appearance and proper behaviour. Self-concept continually influences and enlarges the person's world, mastery of and interaction with it, and ability to respond to the many experiences it offers. This integration, largely unconscious, is constantly evolving and can be identified in the person's values, attitudes, and feelings about self. The experiences with the body are interpreted in terms of feelings, earlier views of the self, and group or cultural norms.[255] *In the adult there is a close interdependence between body image and personality, self-concept, and identity.*

You need to remember and use information about self-concept and body image. Your feedback to others is important. If you are to help another elevate self-esteem or feel positively about his or her body, you must give repeated positive reinforcement and help the person overcome unrealistic guilt and shame. Saying something positive or recognizing abilities once or twice will not be enough. The self-concept, whether wholesome or not, is difficult to change, as the person perceives others' comments and behaviour in relation to an already established image to avoid conflict and anxiety within self. The person with a sense of trust, self-confidence, or positive self-concept is less threatened by others' ideas, remarks, or behaviour. He or she is more flexible, able to change, and admit new attributes to self.

Body Image Change in Illness

A wide variety of messages about the body are constantly fed into the self-image for rejection, acceptance with integration, or revision. You will see disturbances in the person's body image after loss of a body function, structure, or quality—teeth, hair, vision, hearing, breast, internal organs, or youth—that necessitate adjustment of the person's body image. Because the body image provides a base for identity, almost any change in body structure or function is experienced as a threat, especially in our society, where wholeness, beauty, and health are highly valued.

A threat to body image is related to the person's pattern of adaptation. The degree to which this loss of body control creates loss of customary control of self, physical environment, time, and contacts with others is very closely related to the degree of threat felt. To understand the nature of the threat, you must assess the pattern of adaptation, the value of this pattern for the person, and the usual coping mechanisms. The person with limited adaptive abilities, who easily feels helpless and powerless, will experience greater threat with a change in body structure or function.

CRITICAL THINKING

Discuss how gender and the effects of culture can affect the body image of a client who is physically disabled?

The Adult Undergoing Body Changes

Assessment. Assessment during illness, injury, or disability that necessitates eventual changes to self-image is often difficult because of the abstractness of self-image. But if you listen closely to the person, validate statements for less obvious meanings, and explore feelings with him or her you can gain considerable

information for worthwhile intervention. Assessment could include determining the person's response to the following:[256]

- Feelings about the self before and since the condition occurred
- Values about personal hygiene
- Values on beauty, self-control, wholeness, and activity
- Value of others' reactions
- Meaning of the body part affected
- Meaning of hospitalization, treatment, and care
- Awareness of extent of condition
- Effect of condition on person, roles, daily activities, family, and use of leisure time
- Perception of others' reaction to person with this condition
- Problems in adjusting to condition
- Mechanisms used in adapting to condition and its implication

Observation of the client must be combined with purposeful conversation. Observe movements, posture, gestures, and expressions as he or she answers your questions or talks about self to validate the consistency between what is said and what is meant.

Nursing Intervention. Measures to help someone with a threat to or change of body image involve assisting the person to reintegrate the self-view and self-esteem in relation to his or her condition. You can help the person in the following ways:[257]

- Encourage talking about feelings in relation to the changed body function or structure. Talking about feelings is the first step to reintegration of body image.
- Assist client, without pressure, to become reacquainted with self by looking at the dressing or wound, feeling the cast, bandage, or injured part, prostheses, or looking at self in mirror. The client who wants to "show the scar" should be allowed to do so. Reaction from you and the family can make a difference in how the person accepts the changed body.
- Provide opportunity for gaining information about the body, both the intact and changed parts, and its strengths and limits.
- Provide opportunity to learn mastery of the body, resume activities of daily care and living routines as indicated, move about, become involved with others, resume roles, and handle equipment.
- Give recognition for what the person can do. Avoid criticism, derogation, or a nonverbal reaction of disgust or shame.
- Help him or her see self as a whole person despite losses or changes.
- Encourage talking about unresolved experiences, distortions, or fears in relation to body image.

You will be encountering many young adults with body image distortions or changes as a result of accidental injuries, disease, weight gain or loss, pregnancy, or identity problems. You can make a significant contribution to the health of this person for the remainder of life by giving assistance through physical care, listening, counselling, teaching, and working with family and significant people important to his or her life. Your efforts are important for your own positive self-concept and for unbiased care of each person, thus promoting a positive self-concept.

CRITICAL THINKING

What are a few health promoting strategies for clients who are undergoing body changes?

Lifestyle Options

The increased pace of life has brought people an unparalleled degree of social alienation at all levels of society. Choosing a lifestyle very different from one's childrearing experiences is an attempt to ward off alienation and organize one's life around meaning. The young adult has many options. He or she may decide to base the style of living around age (the youth cult); work (the company man or woman executive); leisure (the surf bum); drugs; or marriage, partnership, and family.

Singlehood, *remaining unmarried and following a specific lifestyle,* is not new. Maiden aunts, bachelors, and single schoolteachers are traditional, as are those whose religion calls for singlehood. Others never marry but are in some form of committed relationship. But remaining unmarried is increasingly an option, either as an end in itself or as a newly prolonged phase of postadolescence.

The single person can accomplish the task of intimacy through emotional investment of self in others. Many are extroverts, have several very close friends with whom they share activities, have a meaningful career, and have a harmonious rather than conflictual relationship with parents.[258–261] On the other hand, the single person may be in emotional isolation, unable to establish a close relationship and alienated from self and others or may feel depressed about the life situation. However, most singles do *not* fit this description. For whatever reasons, the number of single people is on the rise, especially in the 20 to 34 age group.[262]

The single person may need help in resolving feelings about being a single person and validation about his or her choice. If the person is single because of isolation and self-absorption, mental health counselling may be needed, not for singlehood, but because of feelings about self and others. Several references give suggestions for managing alone.[263,264]

Family Planning:
The Expectancy Phase
and Parenthood

Parenthood is an option for the couple or a single person. Today, oral contraceptives for the female and more skilled vasectomy procedures for the male make it possible for couples to say: "We don't want children now," "We don't want children ever," or "We want to try to have two children spaced three years apart."

Information presented in Table 11-5 (pages 502–503) that summarizes contraceptives and various references at the end of this chapter will help you teach about all aspects of family planning. Chapter 4 provides information useful for understanding the family with whom you are working.

Reasons for Childbearing
The couple may have a child for a variety of reasons:

1. Extension of self
2. To offset loneliness
3. Sense of pride or joy
4. Psychological fulfillment of having a child
5. Having someone to love self
6. Attempt to hold a marriage together
7. Feeling of power, generated by ability to create life
8. Representation of wealth
9. To secure replacements for the work force
10. To have an heir for family name and wealth
11. Religious convictions

Whether the couple chooses to have only one child or more children is related to more than fertility and religious background. Lifestyle, finances, career, available support systems, and emotional maturity are factors.

Developmental Tasks for the Couple during the Expectant Stage
You are in a position to assist the couple in understanding the changes that childbearing will create and the following developmental tasks for this stage of family life:

- Rearrange the home to provide space, facilities, and supplies for the expected baby.
- Rework the budget and determine how to obtain and spend income to accommodate changing needs and maintain the family unit financially.
- Evaluate the changing roles, division of labour, how responsibilities of child care will be divided, who has the final authority, and whether the woman should continue working outside the home if she has a career or profession.
- Adapt patterns of sexual relationships to the pregnancy.
- Rework the communication system between the couple; explore feelings about the pregnancy and ideas about childrearing, and work to resolve the differences.
- Acquire knowledge about pregnancy, childbirth, and parenthood.
- Rework the communication system and relationships with family, friends, and community activities, based on the reality of the pregnancy and their reactions.
- Use family and community resources as needed.
- Examine and expand the philosophy of life to include responsibilities of childbearing and childrearing.

12–8 BONUS SECTION IN CD-ROM
Research Abstract

This study explores differences in paternal confidence between inexperienced and experienced fathers. Results indicate some differences and similarities between the two groups.

Developmental tasks that must be mastered during pregnancy and the intrapartum period to ensure readiness for the maternal role are:

1. *Pregnancy validation:* Accepting the reality of the pregnancy, working through feelings of ambivalence
2. *Fetal embodiment:* Incorporating the fetus and enlarging body into the body image
3. *Fetal distinction:* Seeing the fetus as a separate entity, fantasizing what the baby will be like
4. *Role transition:* After birth, an increasing readiness to take on the task of parenthood

A number of authors have researched transition to parenthood, feelings, symptoms, body image changes, and needs for social support during pregnancy. Events during pregnancy affect family functioning and child care after birth.[265]

CRITICAL THINKING

What are some advantages and disadvantages of choosing not to have children in today's society?

Father's Response. Some research indicates that attachment of the father to baby begins during pregnancy, rather than after birth, and that a strong marital relationship and vicariously experienced physical symptoms resembling pregnancy (and sometimes the couvade syndrome) strengthen attachment.[266]

Studies indicate a characteristic pattern of development of subjective emotional involvement in pregnancy among first-time expectant fathers. Three phases occur: announcement phase, moratorium, and focusing period.

The **announcement phase** is *when pregnancy is suspected and confirmed.* If the man desired the pregnancy, he shows desire and excitement. If he did not want the pregnancy, he shows pain and shock.

During the **moratorium period,** the *man suppresses thoughts about the pregnancy.* This period can last from a few days to months and usually ends when the pregnancy is obvious. This period is characterized by emotional distance, a feeling the pregnancy is not real, concentration on himself and other life concerns, and sometimes leaving home. The man's emotional distance allows him to work through ambivalence and jealousy of the woman's ability to bear a child, but his distance causes her to feel unloved, rejected, angry, and uncared for. Marital tension exists. Gradually the man faces the financial and lifestyle implications of the pregnancy. If he feels financially insecure, unstable with his partner, or wishes to extend the childless period, he resents pregnancy and spends a longer time in the moratorium stage. Most men eventually become enthusiastic about the pregnancy and baby when they feel the baby move or hear the heartbeat. If the man does not become enthusiastic and supportive, the couple may then be at risk for marital and parenting problems.

The **focusing period** occurs *when the man perceives the pregnancy as real and important in his life.* This begins at approximately 25 to 30 weeks' gestation and extends until labour onset. The man redefines himself as father; he begins to feel more in tune with and is more helpful to his wife. He begins to read or talk about parenting and child development,

notices other children, and is willing to participate in childbirth classes and purchasing baby supplies. He constructs a mental image of the baby, sometimes different from the woman's mental image of the baby. The circle of friends may change to those who have children. He may feel fear about the coming labour and birth and feel responsible for a successful birth. The man who participates in pregnancy and birth experiences greater closeness with the infant and spouse and heightened self-esteem and esteem for the spouse. The man's readiness for pregnancy may significantly influence emergence of father involvement. The man's unconscious feelings and his earliest memories of childhood play an important role in his emotional reaction and adjustment to pregnancy and childbirth.

Mother's Response. Certainly one would expect that an even stronger attachment would occur in the woman as she physically experiences the fetus and physical symptoms related to pregnancy and that her feelings for the child are stronger if she has a loving, supportive partner. Be aware also that some men have difficulty accepting the responsibility implied by a pregnant partner and do not want to be involved in child care.

Nursing Roles

An important decision for the expectant parents is whether to attend childbirth education classes. Encourage the pregnant woman and her partner to attend childbirth education classes during pregnancy. Insist that they be allowed to use the techniques and practical suggestions they learned during the labour and delivery process. The woman who is well supported during pregnancy experiences fewer complications during labour and delivery. The woman who has had childbirth education during pregnancy and can practise Lamaze techniques during labour uses less medication and is more likely to choose rooming-in with the baby.

Your support, acceptance, flexibility, helping the couple to use what they learned and practised in prenatal classes, letting them assume responsibility for decisions when possible, assistance to mother, and teaching during the postpartum period are crucial to family-centred care. Cultural considerations are important as well.[267]

Be aware that in contrast to the societal romanticized view of pregnancy and care of the pregnant woman, the *pregnant woman may be a victim of physical battering or abuse as well as emotional and mental abuse.* Sonkin, Martin, and Walker[268] described assessment of and intervention with the male batterer. Later in this chapter general information is given on spouse abuse and the male batterer.

The Health Surveillance and Epidemiology Division at Health Canada's Centre for Healthy Human Development have established the Canadian Perinatal Surveillance System (CPSS). The CPSS is guided by a steering committee composed of expert representatives of health professional organizations, consumer and advocacy groups, provincial and territorial governments, and Canadian and international specialists in perinatal health and epidemiology. The CPSS is part of Health Canada's efforts to strengthen Canada's national health surveillance capacity.[269] The CPSS has identified that the proportion of pregnant women reporting physical abuse is an important health indicator.[270] During pregnancy, physical abuse has been associated with adverse maternal and fetal health outcomes. More understanding of the epidemiology of physical abuse during pregnancy, including its frequency, risk factors, adverse maternal conditions and birth outcomes, could have important clinical and public health implications.[271] The early identification followed by intervention to prevent the abuse of pregnant women will go far to reduce the adverse outcomes.[272]

CRITICAL THINKING

What health promotion strategies would you advocate for women who may be victims of physical abuse during pregnancy?

Other Approaches to Parenthood

Some couples delay childbearing until they are in their 30s or early 40s. The woman may wish to pursue her education, a career, or a profession; the couple may choose to travel, start a business, become financially established, or have a variety of experiences before they settle down with one or two children. With genetic counselling, the surgical ability to undo vasectomy and tubal ligation, improved prenatal and neonatal care, and reduced risk of maternal or neonatal complications, pregnancy is safe for the mother in her 30s and even early 40s. Many of the risks of late parenthood are related to pre-existing disease, if any, rather than to late conception. Of equal concern are the emotional and social implications, especially after birth when the couple's life revolves around baby rather than work or earlier interests.

Maternal age does not affect maternal role behaviours, and the sense of challenge, role strain, and self-image in the mother role is similar during the first year for childbearing women of all ages. Mercer's study[273] of the process of maternal role attainment in three age groups (15–19, 20–29, and 30–42) over the first year of motherhood found that love for the baby, gratification in the maternal role, observed maternal behaviour, and self-reported ways of handling irritating child behaviours remained the same over the year.

The single person may desire to be a parent. The single woman may, through pregnancy or adoption, choose to have a child. More is being written about the single woman who decides to become a mother and remain single. Some are well-educated, professional women in their late 30s or 40s who believe they have no chance of becoming married, for various societal reasons, but who wish to have the experience of motherhood. Some single men who will not be biological fathers are also choosing to experience fatherhood through adoption. The woman may choose to remain single but maintain a relationship with the biological father or with a man who can act as father to the child. The man may have a close relationship with a woman who can assist in mothering, or he may decide to nurture alone.

You are in a key position to help the person as he or she thinks through why there is a wish to have a child and remain single. Who the support system will be who can act in the father or mother role to the child, the consequences of a single mother or father to the child during school years or adolescence, and the social, familial, and economic consequences of single parenthood should be discussed. Implications related to the cultural and religious background of the person must also be considered.

Family planning is sometimes made difficult by **infertility,** *inability to achieve pregnancy after one year of regular, unprotected intercourse or the inability to carry a pregnancy to a term, live birth.* Both partners should be given diagnostic tests together, as 50% of infertility factors are in women and 50% are in men. Infertility can create great psychological problems for the woman and man, between the couple, and between families of each partner. The problem becomes compounded by the increasing difficulty in adopting a local healthy baby in most communities, as more single mothers retain their babies. Artificial insemination and a surrogate mother are alternatives that may not always be acceptable to the couple.[274]

It is estimated that up to one in eight Canadian couples suffer from infertility. As a result, Canadians, now more than ever, are turning to assisted human reproduction (AHR) procedures to help them build their families.[275] Visit www.hc-sc.gc.ca/english/protection for relevant information regarding AHR. Health Canada's website specifies efforts in this area and provides links to other related sources of information. A note of interest is that the AHR legislation became law on March 30, 2004.

The couple who cannot biologically have a child may consider a **surrogate parent,** *a woman who, for a fee, will conceive through insemination, carry, and deliver a child for the woman who cannot conceive.* Many ethical concerns arise with this practice: the meaning of family, psychological effects on the surrogate and contracting parents, relationship between fetus and pregnant woman, the possibility that the child who is born may not meet the desires of the contracting parents, care of the deformed child, and effect on the child when he or she learns about the surrogate parent. Does the couple have a right to children by any means? What are the cultural, moral, and religious implications? Further, legal aspects are also tenuous. As of now, there are no answers, just many questions. You can help a couple considering the surrogate parent method work through the above issues and questions according to their spiritual, cultural, and family values and beliefs and their personal philosophies, values, and beliefs.

Developmental Tasks

The specific developmental tasks of the youth as he or she is making the transition from adolescence into young adulthood are discussed in Chapter 11 and can be summarized as choosing a vocation, getting appropriate education, establishing a residence, and formulating ideas about selection of a mate or someone with whom to have a close relationship.

For the young adult in general, the following tasks must be achieved, regardless of the station in life. You can assist young adults in meeting these developmental tasks through use of therapeutic communication principles, counselling, teaching, and crisis intervention:

- Accepting self and stabilizing self-concept and body image
- Acknowledging and resolving conflicts between the emerging self and conformity to the social order
- Establishing independence from parental home and financial aid

- Becoming established in a vocation or profession that provides personal satisfaction, economic independence, and a feeling of making a worthwhile contribution to society
- Learning to appraise and express love responsibly through more than sexual contacts
- Establishing an intimate bond with another, either through marriage or with a close friend
- Establishing and maintaining a home and managing a time schedule and life stresses
- Finding a congenial social and friendship group
- Deciding whether or not to have a family and carry out tasks of parenting
- Resolving changed relationship with the parental families

- Formulating a meaningful philosophy of life and reassessing priorities and values
- Becoming involved as a citizen in the community
- Achieving a more realistic outlook about other cultures, mores, and political systems

McCoy,[276] using the stages of development proposed by the life-stage theorists discussed earlier, formulated similar developmental tasks for each stage. These tasks are depicted in Table 12-6.

CRITICAL THINKING

What are some developmental tasks for the young adult who has chosen to remain single?

TABLE 12-6
Developmental Tasks and Outcomes for the Stages of Young Adulthood

Developmental Stage	Developmental Task	Outcome Sought
Becoming adults, ages 23–28	1. Select mate 2. Settle in work; begin career ladder 3. Parent 4. Become involved in community 5. Consume wisely 6. Own home 7. Socially interact 8. Achieve autonomy 9. Solve problems 10. Manage stress accompanying change	1. Successful marriage 2. Career satisfaction and advancement 3. Effective parents; healthy offspring 4. Informed, participating citizen 5. Sound consumer behaviour 6. Satisfying home environment 7. Social skills 8. Fulfilled single state, autonomy 9. Successful problem solving 10. Successful stress management; personal growth
"Catch-30," ages 29–34	1. Search for personal values 2. Reappraise relationships 3. Progress in career 4. Accept growing children 5. Put down roots; achieve "permanent" home 6. Solve problems 7. Manage stress accompanying change	1. Examined and owned values 2. Authentic personal relationships 3. Career satisfaction, economic reward, a sense of competence and achievement 4. Growth-producing parent–child relationship 5. Sound consumer behaviour 6. Successful problem solving 7. Successful stress management; personal growth
Midlife re-examination, ages 35–43	1. Search for meaning 2. Reassess marriage 3. Re-examine work 4. Relate to teenage children 5. Relate to aging parents 6. Reassess personal priorities and values 7. Fulfilled single state 8. Successful problem solving 9. Manage stress accompanying change	1. Coping with existential anxiety 2. Satisfying marriage 3. Appropriate career decisions 4. Improved parent–child relations 5. Improved child–parent relations 6. Autonomous behaviour 7. Adjust to single life 8. Solve problems 9. Successful stress management; personal growth

Source: Adapted from McCoy, V., Adult Life Cycle Tasks, Adult Continuing Education Program Response, Lifelong Learning in the Adult Years, October (1977), 16.

HEALTH CARE AND NURSING APPLICATIONS

Health Promotion and Health Protection

Your role in caring for the young adult may be many faceted. Assessment based on knowledge presented throughout this chapter is the basis for formulating nursing diagnoses. Nursing diagnoses that may be applicable to the young adult are listed in the box entitled "Selected Nursing Diagnoses Related to the Young Adult." Wellness diagnosis must also be considered for the young adult.[277] Young adulthood is a time when a shift occurs from developing one's own personal identity, even though that is still occurring to some degree, to making attachments to others resulting in intimate relationships. The need for human closeness and sexual fulfillment is paramount for many

---

Selected Nursing Diagnoses Related to the Young Adult

Pattern 1: Exchanging

- Altered Nutrition: More than Body Requirements
- Ineffective Family Coping: Compromised
- Family Coping: Potential for Growth
- Decisional Conflict
- Health Seeking Behaviours

Pattern 2: Communicating

- Impaired Verbal Communication

Pattern 3: Relating

- Impaired Social Interaction
- Social Isolation
- Risk for Loneliness
- Altered Role Performance
- Altered Parenting
- Risk for Altered Parenting
- Alcoholism
- Altered Family Process: Alcoholism
- Parental Role Conflict
- Altered Sexuality Patterns

Pattern 4: Valuing

- Spiritual Distress
- Potential for Enhanced Spiritual Distress

Pattern 5: Choosing

- Ineffective Individual Coping
- Impaired Adjustment
- Defensive Coping
- Ineffective Denial
- Ineffective Family Coping: Disabling

Pattern 6: Moving

- Fatigue
- Risk for Activity Intolerance

- Sleep Pattern Disturbance
- Diversional Activity Deficit
- Impaired Home Maintenance Management
- Altered Health Maintenance

Pattern 7: Perceiving

- Body Image Disturbance
- Self-Esteem Disturbance
- Chronic Low Self-Esteem
- Situational Low Self-Esteem
- Personal Identity Disturbance
- Sensory/Perceptual Alterations
- Hopelessness
- Powerlessness

Pattern 8: Knowing

- Knowledge Deficit

Pattern 9: Feeling

- Pain
- Chronic Pain
- Dysfunctional Grieving
- Anticipatory Grieving
- Risk for Violence: Directed at Others
- Risk for Violence: Self-Directed
- Post-Trauma Syndrome
- Rape Trauma Syndrome
- Anxiety
- Fear
- Altered Nutrition: Less than Body Requirements
- Altered Nutrition: Risk for More than Body Requirements
- Risk for Infection
- Risk for Injury
- Risk for Impaired Skin Integrity
- Altered Dentition
- Energy Field Disturbance

Other NANDA diagnoses are applicable to the ill young adult. See Stolte[279] for an explanation of the necessity of developing wellness diagnoses.

Source: North American Nursing Diagnosis Association, NANDA Diagnoses Definitions & Classification 1999–2000. *Philadelphia: North American Nursing Association, 1999.*

young adults.[278] Developing wellness diagnosis for the young adult fosters a holistic approach to care.

CRITICAL THINKING

Develop several wellness diagnoses for a young adult.

Health promotion interventions to assist the young adult and the family to meet physical, cognitive, emotional, social, and spiritual needs are described in the following, and in the previous, sections.

In your assessment and care of the person, it is impossible to calculate the exact probability of anyone developing disease. The following principles are a guide:[280]

1. *Genetic makeup or family history* is the strongest single determinant of risk. The Human Genome Project, an effort to identify and locate each of our 50 000 to 100 000 genes, may help better predict risk profile in the future.

2. *Magnitude* or *a slight elevation* (10% to 30%) in risk for a given disease has a minor effect on the person. A *marked increase* in risk (100%) would serve as an alarm.

3. *Repetition,* or *independently researched risk factors,* such as cigarette smoking, excess alcohol intake, obesity, sedentary lifestyle, and diet high in saturated fats, must be taken seriously as risks for everyone.

Immunizations

In Canada, all adults require maintenance of immunity to tetanus and diphtheria preferably with combined (Td) toxoids. The acceptable option for adult booster doses is to continue offering boosters of Td at ten-year intervals (at age 15, 25, 35 years) or, as a minimum, to review immunization status at least once during adult life (e.g., at 50 years of age). A single dose of Td should be offered to everyone who has not had one within the previous ten years.[281] Adults born before 1970 may be considered immune to measles. Adults born in 1970 and later, who do not have documentation of adequate measles immunization or who are known to be seronegative, should receive measles vaccine (given as MMR). For adults who have received one dose of measles vaccine, a second dose of vaccine would provide optimal protection. Priority for a second dose should be given to health care workers, college students, and travellers to areas where measles are epidemic.[282]

Most individuals born before 1970 may also be considered immune to mumps. Mumps vaccine (given as MMR) is recommended for young adults with no history of mumps. Rubella vaccine should be given to all female adolescents and women of childbearing age unless they have documented evidence of detectable antibody or documented evidence of vaccine. Combined measles, mumps, and rubella (MMR) vaccine is preferred. Universal immunization for hepatitis B is recommended in Canada.[283]

As an example, all undergraduate students enrolled in the Faculty of Nursing at the University of Manitoba must submit proof of immunization against the following diseases: measles and rubella, chicken pox (Varicella), hepatitis, and tuberculosis. It is the student's responsibility to review his or her immunization status annually and to update any outstanding immunization requirements.[284]

CRITICAL THINKING

What is the protocol to follow for the healthy management of a person following possible contact with rabies?

Common Health Problems: Prevention and Treatment

Physical Problems

Young adults in North America are typically healthy. Many have no disease. Some diseases could have been prevented by access to health care and adequate nutrition as well as immunization against six serious childhood diseases: polio, tetanus, measles, diphtheria, pertussis, and tuberculosis.[285] Health problems and risks, preventive behaviour, and response to illness are influenced by sex and lifestyle, as well as other factors. Table 12-7 summarizes common health problems encountered by the young adult.[286–290]

Acquired Immunodeficiency Syndrome. AIDS was defined by the Centers for Disease Control and Prevention (CDC) in 1987 as a *disabling or life-threatening illness caused by human immunodeficiency virus (HIV) and characterized by HIV encephalopathy, HIV wasting syndrome, or certain diseases resulting from immunodeficiency in a person with laboratory evidence for HIV infection or without certain other causes of immunodeficiency.*[291]

In Canada, AIDS was first identified in 1979 and became a reportable disease in 1982.[292] Since then, thousands of Canadians have been infected with HIV. Health Canada estimated that in 2003, 56 000 Canadians were living with HIV/AIDS, of whom 17 000 were not aware of their infection.[293] To date, no vaccine exists to prevent HIV infection; and no cure exists for the disease.

In 1990 Phase I of the National AIDS Strategy began. Significant progress was made in education, prevention, care, and treatment. In 1993, Phase II was launched.[294] This phase responded to the growing complexity of HIV/AIDS in Canada and the need for an extended commitment of time, funds, and energy. National surveillance systems were put into place; and guidelines for training health care professionals were developed. By the end of Phase II, Canadians could look back with pride at the progress that had been achieved. For example, there were 33% fewer new AIDS cases in 1996 than in 1995, and 36% fewer deaths related to HIV.[295] HIV infections were primarily concentrated in two population groups—gay men and people infected through blood supply. However, while progress had been made, the epidemic had spread to other populations including women. Aboriginal peoples and injection drug users remained a serious threat to some of the initially infected populations, particularly gay men.

In May 1998, the Canadian Strategy on HIV/AIDS was developed.[296] In September 2002, with the assistance of a stakeholder advisory committee, the federal minister of health initiated a review of the current federal role in the Canadian

TABLE 12-7
Common Health Problems for Young Adults

Problem	Definition	Symptom/Signs	Prevention/Treatment
Upper respiratory infection (URI) or common cold	Acute infection of the upper respiratory tract, lasting several days	General malaise; nasal stuffiness and discharge, mild sore throat, watery eyes; sometimes ear discomfort	If bacterial: antibiotic; otherwise, symptomatic treatment; antipyretic, antihistamine, decongestants
Influenza	Acute contagious viral illness often occurring in epidemics	Fever, malaise, myalgia, and respiratory symptoms; sometimes cough, rhinitis, and scattered rales	Prevention: immunization Treatment: antipyretic, increase fluid intake, rest; amantadine hydrochloride
Hypertension, essential (uncomplicated)	Persistent elevation of arterial blood pressure 150/100 but less than 200/110 present on three weekly determinations, without secondary cause found	Sometimes none; sometimes headache, dizziness, light-headedness	Appropriate lab workup along with other testing; diet; weight reduction; exercise; possibly medication
Mitral value prolapse	Insufficiency of valve to open and close appropriately	Usually in young adult female; chest pain, arrhythmias, palpitations, tachycardia, sense of fullness in neck and head, feeling faint, anxious	Medication, adequate rest; reduction of stress in life to extent possible
Iron deficiency anemia	Blood hemoglobin level ≤ 10 g/dL, compared with normal value of 12–16 g/dL (for women)	Usually caused by menses; sometimes no signs; fatigue, irritability, depression, weakness, dizziness, headache, pallor of skin and conjunctivae, brittle nails	Prevention: blood screen, iron-rich foods Treatment: iron preparation (ferrous sulphate)
Atopic dermatitis of adulthood	Dry, thickened skin, accentuating normal folds (different appearance than in infancy)	Hyperpigmentation, especially on flexor areas of extremities, eyelids, dorsi of hands and feet, and back of neck	Keeping skin dry in humid conditions; mild, non-drying soap; hydrocortisone cream
Folliculitis	Localized infection of hair follicle	Irritated area around hair follicle	Washing well; hot compresses
Furuncle (boil)	Infected area that has draining point	Raised red area with exudate	Hot compresses; antibiotics; sometimes incision and drainage
Carbuncle	Large group of furuncles with several draining points	Raised red area with multiple exudate areas	Hot compresses; antibiotics; incision and drainage
Urticaria (hives)	Allergic reaction, usually to drugs, food, inhalants, or insect bites	Itching, red raised welts, usually on trunk or extremities	Cool compresses; sometimes antihistamine or epinephrine; attempt to find offending agent
Scabies	Dermatitis caused by mite burrowing into skin and consequent allergic reaction		Lindane (Kwell) treatment (all sexual and household contacts too)

(continued)

TABLE 12-7 *(continued)*
Common Health Problems for Young Adults

Problem	Definition	Symptom/Signs	Prevention/Treatment
Simple diarrhea of adulthood	Gastrointestinal upset by viral infection, caused psychological disturbance, dietary changes, laxatives	Frequent loose, watery stools that are not greasy, bloody, or purulent	Clear liquid diet; anti-diarrhea preparation (e.g., loperamide hydrochloride [Imodium])
Cystitis	Inflammation of bladder (often seen in young adult women)	Dysuria, frequency, bladder spasms	Appropriate antibiotics after clean-catch urinalysis and culture; increased water intake (at least eight 8-oz [250 mL] glasses daily); sometimes antispasmodic medication
Acute pyelonephritis	Cystitis plus inflammation of kidneys and collection system	Dysuria, frequency, flank pain, chills, nausea, vomiting	Appropriate antibiotic treatment plus antipyretic and anti-nausea medicine if necessary
Chronic fatigue syndrome (CFS)	Debilitating fatigue that lasts at least 6 months	Eight of the following must persist or recur over 6 months: chills or low-grade fever; sore throat; tender lymph nodes; muscle pain and weakness; extreme fatigue; headaches; joint pain without swelling; neurological problems (confusion, memory loss); sleep disorders	Prevention: none known Treatment: adequate rest, nutritious diet, small amounts of exercise; rationing of energy; dealing emotionally with disease; possibly tricyclic antidepressants
Hepatitis B	Type of liver inflammation	Jaundice, malaise, may lead to liver cancer, cirrhosis, or death; some are carriers only	Immunization (series of 3 injections), rest, nutritious diet
Dental caries and periodontal disease	Tooth decay and bleeding, hypertrophied gums	Gradual receding of gums and bones and loss of teeth	Early dental checks and personal mouth care; proper diet
Lactose intolerance or milk malabsorption syndrome	Lactose (milk sugar) not hydrolyzed because of lack of appropriate amounts of the enzyme lactase	Severe abdominal discomfort and flatulence following direction of milk products	Products containing concentrated forms of the enzyme; also *Lacto-bacillus sp.* milk; avoid foods made with milk or milk products
Anxiety	Combination of fearfulness, nervousness, apprehension, and restlessness, often associated with family or personal crisis and sometimes with physical or mental illness	Loss of appetite, increased appetite, lack of sleeping ability; increased perspiration, "thumping of heart," headaches, weakness, fatigue, trembling	Supportive therapy, crisis intervention, some medicines for short term

(continued)

TABLE 12-7 *(continued)*
Common Health Problems for Young Adults

Problem	Definition	Symptom/Signs	Prevention/Treatment
Tension headache	Band-like pressure across forehead and around back of skull	Dull, aching pain with a feeling of tightness, tension in neck muscles	Reassurance, mild analgesics, occasionally a muscle relaxant, massage, manipulation, elimination of tension
Migraine headache	Vascular in origin: arterial spasm followed by dilation	Throbbing unilateral pain, sometimes preceded by **aura** (*inherent warning, usually visual*); sometimes nausea and vomiting	Try to rest when aura first appears, various medications, such as anti-inflammatory drugs and caffeine; rest in a dark room; nutrition; chiropractic care; biofeedback
Lyme disease	Infection caused by *Borrelia burgdorferi*, spirochete spread by bites of deer tick	Erythema migrans, red, raised circular rash that spreads and itches. Flu-like, vague symptoms If untreated: Arthritic symptoms (with swollen, painful joints). Neurological symptoms (paraesthesis, insomnia, lethargy). Heart symptoms (irregular pulse, faint, dizzy, short of breath). Psychological symptoms (mood changes, depression) Pregnancy may cause miscarriage.	In tick-infested areas: Walk along cleared surfaces, avoid tall grass and woods if possible. Avoid light-colour garments. Wear long-sleeved shirts, long pants tucked into socks, closed shoes. Use insect repellent. Shower as soon as possible after returning indoors from tick-infected area. If bitten by tick, remove immediately by grasping it close to skin, tug gently. Use flea and tick collars on pets, brush them after being outdoors. Mow weeds and grass around house. Antibiotic treatment.

Strategy on HIV/AIDS. The review, completed in June 2003, examined lessons learned over the five years since its initiation; and it identified current challenges. It defined the most appropriate federal role within the broader strategy and it proposed the allocation of federal funding for 2004 to 2008.[297] It is recommended that the increased funding be contingent on the establishment of five-year measurable goals and objectives for decreasing the number of new cases each year.[298]

The decline in the annual number of AIDS cases that started in 1995 is continuing. The rate of decline, however, has slowed and the curve is levelling off.[299] The number of deaths due to HIV/AIDS has also decreased.[300] It is interesting to note that the number of deaths has decreased more quickly than the incidence rate, indicating that people with HIV are progressing at a slower rate and that people with

AIDS diagnoses are living longer.[301] An alarming fact is that many Canadians do not know that they have HIV.

CRITICAL THINKING

What factors might contribute to the fact that people who have HIV or AIDS now tend to live longer?

AIDS will be a major global cause of death, if not the biggest killer in some countries,[302,303] because it is occurring in epidemic rates in some countries not previously affected. Africa, India, Thailand, and other countries in Southeast Asia, and countries in the former Soviet Union and Middle East now are experiencing HIV epidemics.[304]

AIDS is a devastating disease to the already disadvantaged who are often carrying other sexually transmitted diseases and who are often in the IV drug and crack-cocaine culture. These young adults have a resigned attitude about their diagnosis and mistrust of the conventional medical system. Thus, they often will not take the medicine suggested or will not cooperate in informing past or current sexual partners of their diagnosis.[305]

CRITICAL THINKING

How do you think the presence of AIDS will change sex and relationships?

The HIV virus attacks white blood cells (T-cells) and weakens the immune system. AIDS occurs when an HIV-infected person develops a life-threatening condition or the number of T-cells becomes dangerously low. T-cells regulate the body's immune system. If they are destroyed, the capacity to fight disease is gone. *HIV is transmitted through:*

1. Body fluids containing blood, semen, and vaginal secretions during unprotected vaginal, oral, or anal sex with an infected person.

2. Contaminated needle-sharing among injection drug users, or use of contaminated needles during tattooing or piercing body parts.

3. During pregnancy, birth, or breastfeeding, from the HIV-infected woman to baby.

4. Transfusions of infected blood or blood products before 1985 (since then, all blood has been tested), or use of blood-contaminated equipment.

5. Contact with open sores of an infected person.

Prevention of AIDS is dependent on not engaging in the above behaviours.[306–309]

Diagnosis can be determined in a person over four months of age by the HIV antibody test. The blood test reveals if the body has been exposed to virus and has produced antibodies to HIV. The test may be negative because the infected body has not produced enough antibodies for the test to detect. Retesting should be done in six months. A positive test is a sign of infection that can be spread to others. Research is being done on the use of saliva to do rapid HIV testing. Results to date are accurate.[310–312]

The tests cannot determine if the person will get AIDS or has AIDS, if newly infected. The antibodies are not protective, as is true with other diseases. It is suggested that large amounts of the virus are required to cause the infection. Co-factors may also be necessary for infection to occur, such as decreased immune system function, alcohol use, poor nutrition, inadequate rest or exercise, severe stress, or presence of other infection.[313–315]

The person with a positive test result should not donate blood, plasma, sperm, organs, or tissue. Pregnancy should be postponed (see Chapter 6). *Abstinence from sexual intercourse is the only sure way to avoid infecting another.* (Affection can be shown by massage or hugs.) If partners choose sex, a latex condom must be worn. The condom should not be used past the expiration date. Condoms are not foolproof and must be used as soon as the penis is erect. A water-based lubricant should be used for vaginal and anal sex. The condom must be carefully removed.[316–319]

HIV/AIDS may take up to ten years to be manifested in signs and symptoms. The following symptoms of AIDS are also caused by other conditions. *The warning symptoms include:*[320–322]

1. Painful, swollen lymph glands in the neck, armpits, or groin.

2. Persistent skin blotches or rashes, usually pink to purple, that grow in size, are harder than surrounding areas, and may appear in the mouth, nose, rectum, or other body sites.

3. Rapid weight loss of more than 5 kg within two months for no reason.

4. Recurrent fever or night sweats, lasting longer than one week.

5. Persistent dry cough, shortness of breath.

6. Persistent diarrhea.

7. Constant fatigue, malaise.

8. Recurring vaginal yeast infections; thrush or white coating on tongue.

9. Easy bruising.

10. Blurred vision, persistent headaches.

11. Mouth sores.

These symptoms may indicate early stages of the disease and may lead to complications and death.

HIV disease appears to have four relatively distinct stages in the young adult:

1. Early or acute period with flu-like and respiratory symptoms lasting a few weeks.

2. Middle or asymptomatic period of minor or no clinical problems lasting months or sometimes years.

3. Transitional, symptomatic period lasting an intermediate length of time.

4. Late or crisis period lasting months or occasionally years.

Mean time from infection to disease is eight years, and from disease to death, 18 months.[323,324]

Serious illnesses that occur with AIDS caused by a weakened immune system include:[325–328]

- *Pneumocystis carinii* pneumonia (PCP), a rare type and the major cause of death.

- Kaposi's sarcoma (KS), a rare form of malignant skin cancer and organ tumours.

- Infections of the nervous system.

- Opportunistic fungal, parasitic, and bacterial infections, including tuberculosis.

These infections can attack any body part and cause death.

Anti-retroviral treatment has reduced mortality, hospitalizations, and incidence of opportunistic infections for people with HIV infections. Thus, AIDS is considered a long-term chronic disease. Anti-retroviral treatment is expensive, associated with adherence to a complex medication schedule, and has a number of toxic and unpleasant side effects.[329]

Health care professionals are not immune. The Canadian Association of Nurses in AIDS Care (CANAC) is a national professional nursing organization committed to fostering excellence in HIV/AIDS nursing, promoting the health, rights, and dignity of persons affected by HIV/AIDS, and to preventing the spread of HIV infection.[330] The Canadian AIDS Treatment Information Exchange (CATIE) has teamed up with CANAC to provide an extensive resource centre for HIV/AIDS-related nursing information.[331]

The Canadian Nurses Association endorses implementation of policies and procedures requiring the use of standard precautions (previously called universal precautions).[332] The adherence to standard precautions is the appropriate and effective means to protect nurses, clients, and others from the spread of blood-borne pathogens. The adherence to standard precautions is ethically acceptable as it precludes the need to know the blood-borne pathogen status of nurses or clients, and further safeguards the rights of individuals for privacy and confidentiality of information.[333] In caring for all clients, whether or not their status regarding blood-borne pathogens is known, the nurse is guided by the values of the Code of Ethics for Registered Nurses. Nurses have the professional responsibility to regularly update their knowledge of blood-borne pathogen practices. That is, all practices related to the prevention, immediate exposure, testing, reporting, and the use and disposal of equipment are of particular importance. Nurses have a special responsibility, along with experts and other professionals, to develop clear policies and procedures based on current knowledge.[334]

CRITICAL THINKING

What would you do if your friend found out that he or she had HIV?

If hospital infection control practices are followed when health care providers care for patients with AIDS or work with their biological specimens, there is low risk of occupationally acquiring the opportunistic infections associated with AIDS, which are (1) HIV through serum conversion, (2) cytomegalovirus (CMV), or (3) hepatitis B virus (HBV) or herpes simplex virus type 2 (HSV-2). Seroconversion to HIV is most likely to follow a contaminated, hollow needle-stick injury. Health care professionals who use rubber gloves are effectively protected against transmission of HIV when the gloves are correctly fitted and worn and are intact. In addition, thorough hand washing is mandatory. A face mask should be worn when required. Sharp objects, if contaminated, should be carefully handled. Contaminated instruments should be sterilized or disposed of properly.[335–337]

You may care for the person with AIDS in the hospital, in his or her home, or in a special home designated for AIDS clients and families. You will be a resource to relatives, partners, and friends of AIDS clients. Care will be determined by body parts affected, mind set, and neurological and other physical and emotional symptoms and signs. Remember the extreme isolation and loneliness that most clients will experience as they deal with a disease with such stigma. Seek various educational tools.[338]

Considerable research is in progress on vaccines to immunize the body against the virus. Research continues on use of antiviral medications, gene therapies, and other anti-infective or anticancer drugs. It appears that the best way to treat HIV infection is with good nutritional support and a variety of potent medications that attack the virus in different biochemical ways in its life cycle. Tuberculin testing and administration

of influenza vaccine is essential to protect the person's health. Virtually all people with HIV infection will develop AIDS. However, with treatment, HIV infection can be slowed and the onset of AIDS delayed.[339] A vaccine is the only hope of stopping the pandemic.

Public education is the only way of dealing with this public health epidemic. New approaches to education must be tried, including teaching groups at schools, occupational sites, churches, gay bars, and gay or lesbian organizations. Television could be used to promote responsible sexual behaviour, including abstinence and use of condoms to prevent STDs. Further, some cities distribute free needles to drug users, using a monitoring system that is designed to prevent the spread of AIDS. This action appears to reduce sharing of needles between infected and noninfected drug users and provides a time for education.[340] However, educational programs that emphasize hope and not just fear and include social and community issues and disease facts are most effective.

It is essential to have access to accurate, up-to-date information on HIV/AIDS. Information that is reliable enables people at risk to change their behaviours to avoid HIV infection; and those living with HIV/AIDS can find help to learn about new treatments, to manage their health, and to improve their quality of life. The Canadian HIV/AIDS Information Centre is Canada's largest distributor of HIV/AIDS materials (see www.aidssida.cpha.ca).[341]

CRITICAL THINKING

What resources are available in your community regarding HIV/AIDS?

Tuberculosis. Malloy and Yiu state that this "old" disease has re-emerged.[342] It affects vulnerable populations such as the elderly, women, children, and those who are poverty stricken, homeless, or with immune deficiencies.[343] According to the Canadian Lung Association, there are three reasons why Canada has not managed to eliminate the disease: (1) the tuberculosis bacterium is a living organism in a constant fight to survive in its changing environment, and new strains of the bacteria adapt themselves to resist drugs; (2) people are immigrating from every area of the world, so the disease is brought to Canada from countries where drug treatments for tuberculosis are not readily available; and (3) a reservoir for tuberculosis exists among people considered "high risk" for infection (e.g., those with a weak immune system, or those living in communities without proper health services).[344] A Canadian study indicates that tuberculin screening programs would be less cost effective than anticipated because of high rates of client and provider noncompliance.[345,346]

After their first birthday, Aboriginal children are invited to clinics to be tested for tuberculosis. Meanwhile, school screening is conducted at schools on reserves when children are in the fourth grade.[347]

Accidents. In Canada, injury mortality increases over the adolescent years, and peaks for 20- to 24-year-olds. First Nations and Inuit people are at particularly high risk of injury.[348] The mortality rates associated with major vehicle traffic crashes are high across all age groups; but the highest rates are for youth between 15 and 24 years of age. Even though there has been a reduction in injury deaths associated with motor vehicle traffic crashes, automotive crashes still remain the leading cause of unintentional injury deaths among Canadians. It is interesting to note that when injury mortality rates are compared internationally, Canadian rates have been found to be higher than those for some other nations.[349]

CRITICAL THINKING

What job features are associated with higher rates of injury at work?

Malignancies. Cancer is the leading cause of premature death—or early death—in Canada. An estimated 145 500 new cases of cancer and 68 300 deaths were expected to occur in Canada in 2004.[350] Table 12-8 summarizes the types, incidence,

risks, signs and symptoms, and prevention and treatment measures for cancers found in young adults. Spencer-Cisek presents an overview of cancer prevention, risk assessment, screening criteria and specific measures, and detection of breast, cervical, ovarian, endometrial, prostate, colorectal, cutaneous, and oral cancers.[351]

Breast cancer is the most frequently diagnosed cancer in Canadian women.[352] Breast cancer is rare under the age of 25, but the risk increases steadily after the age of 30. *All young women should be taught and encouraged to do breast self-examinations,* as most breast cancers are first detected by the individual. In addition, a woman between 50 and 69 years of age should have a screening mammogram (a breast screening x-ray) at least once every two years based on personal risk factors and the advice of a health provider.[353] In recent years, screening programs and better treatment have

TABLE 12-8
Types of Cancer Found in Young Adults

Type	Risks, Symptoms, Signs	Prevention, Teaching
Oral cancer or cancer of mouth	Twice as high in men as in women; highest incidence in black males Colour changes in mouth; a sore in mouth that does not heal	Avoid smoking, alcohol, smokeless tobacco; have a through exam by a professional including lips, gingiva, buccal mucosa, palate, floor of mouth, tongue, and pharynx
Cervical cancer	Risk factors include early age at first intercourse, multiple sex partners, smoking, human papillomavirus infection, and diethylstilbestrol exposure Abnormal vaginal bleeding or abnormal discharge	Avoid risk factors listed; avoid smoking; have a Pap smear at recommended intervals
Breast cancer	Risk factors include age > 50 and first-degree relative history of breast cancer, first child born after age 30 or never had children Breast lump or thickening, bleeding from nipple	Breast self-exam, clinical breast exam, and mammography as indicated for age and time interval Research being done on drugs to reduce risk
Cancer of the testes	Increased incidence in males with history of cryptorchidism, gonadal digenesis, Klinefelter's syndrome, or in utero exposure to diethylstilbestrol Any mass in testicle	Teach person proper self-exam technique and recommend regular checks as part of periodic health exam
Skin cancer	Increased incidence in fair skin, sun exposure, severe sunburn in childhood, and familial conditions like dysplastic nevus syndrome A change in a mole or sore that does not heal	Advise against overexposure to sun by using appropriate sunscreens (at least SPF 15); wear protective clothing; examine skin for any changes; have periodic skin exam as part of regular health exam

helped decrease the number of women who die from breast cancer. Many women are hesitant to do breast self-examinations; fear, lack of knowledge, modesty, health orientation, education level, and age contribute to this reluctance. Women are likely to practise self-examination of the breasts if they have a positive self-concept, if they are aware of the benefits, if barriers are minimized, and if they perform other preventive health measures. Media coverage of someone who has successfully recovered from mastectomy increases the incidence of self-examination.[354-357] You should teach the information about breast self-examination described and depicted in Table 12-9.

CRITICAL THINKING

What are the risk factors of breast cancer?

TABLE 12-9
Breast Self-Examination (BSE)

There are many good reasons for doing breast self-examination (BSE) each month. One reason is that breast cancer is most easily treated and cured when it is found early. Another is that if you do BSE every month, it will increase your skill and confidence when doing the exam. When you get to know how your breasts normally feel, you will quickly be able to feel any change. Another reason, it is easy to do.

The best time to do BSE is right after your period, when breasts are not tender or swollen. If you do not have regular periods or sometimes skip a month, do BSE on the same day every month.

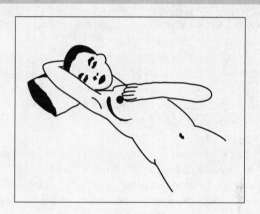

1. Lie down and put a pillow under your right shoulder. Place your right arm behind your head.
2. Use the finger pads of your three middle fingers on your left hand to feel for lumps or thickening. Your finger pads are the top third of each finger.
3. Press firmly enough to know how your breast feels. If you're not sure how hard to press, ask your health care provider. Or try to copy the way your health care provider uses the finger pads during a breast exam. Learn what your breast feels like most of the time. A firm ridge in the lower curve of each breast is normal.
4. Move around the breast in a set way. You can choose either the circle (A), the up and down line (B), or the wedge (C). Do it the same way every time. It will help you make sure that you've gone over the entire breast area, and remember how your breast feels each month.
5. Now examine your left breast using right-hand finger pads.
6. Repeat the examination of both breasts while standing, with one arm behind the head. You may want to do BSE while in the shower. If you find any changes, see your doctor right away.

Remember: BSE could save your breast—and save your life. Most breast lumps are found by women themselves, but, in fact, most lumps in the breast are not cancer. Be safe, be sure.

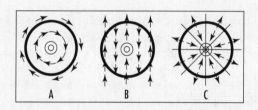

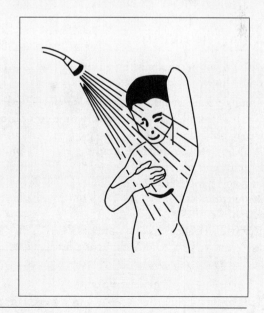

Source: How To Do Breast Self-Examination. No. 2088, Atlanta: American Cancer Society, 1998.

EVIDENCE-BASED PRACTICE

Women's Perceptions of Breast Cancer Screening and Education Opportunities in Canada

Breast cancer remains one of the leading causes of death among Canadian women. Early detection continues to provide women with increased treatment options and improved survival. A comprehensive breast assessment program to facilitate early detection includes breast self-examination (BSE), clinical breast examination (CBE), and mammography for selected population segments. While organized (government) screening opportunities exist in most provinces, especially for populations of high risk, participation rates have been lower than desired.

A large body of nursing literature has examined many aspects of breast screening and breast cancer. The vast majority of studies have been quantitative and have tended to focus on women who had already received a diagnosis of breast cancer, or represented particular ethnic populations.

The purpose of this study was to examine the perceptions of a random sample of Canadian women about breast health education and screening practices. The investigators wished to determine which opportunities for breast health education and screening women believed were available to them.

The participants were 63 women taken from a larger telephone survey involving 1224 women living in Canada. Questions in the follow-up interviews asked about knowledge of and satisfaction with specific breast education and screening opportunities in each woman's geographic area. Information was sought on factors that hindered or encouraged each woman's participation in breast screening

Nursing Implications

1. Examination of barriers to breast cancer screening identified in the study supports the notion that the meaning of the experience determines the motivation for participation in healthy behaviours. Cues to action, such as breast cancer in a family member or friend, acted as a barrier or a motivator, or both. Global cues, however, such as reminder cards, media attention, and marketing, were identified as motivating. Although barriers and motivators were mentioned by many women, it appeared that if the motivation was present, barriers were not a significant issue.

2. Teaching and attitudes of the nurses in the screening clinics were clearly a very positive aspect of the screening experience. While nurses may not always be readily identified as the first contact for health teaching, for these women, nurses were a credible and caring source of information.

3. Lack of information related to screening or to the opportunities to participate appeared to be a large issue.

4. Nurses may be so concerned about completing patient teaching that it is critical to the medical diagnosis that general health promotion topics such as breast health, may be far down on the priority list. Thus, nurses may inadvertently be guilty of contributing to the lack of cues to action related to breast cancer screening.

5. A cue to action need not be a major discussion or full-fledged teaching plan. Nurses have a unique opportunity to respond to people during informal "teachable moments." Such cues to action may pay large dividends in terms of increasing the motivators and raising the personal awareness of patients and clients.

Source: Leeseberg Stamler, L., B. Thomas, K. Lafreniere, and R. Charbonneau-Smith, Women's Perceptions of Breast Cancer Screening and Education Opportunities in Canada, Canadian Nurse, 97, no. 9, (2001), 23–27. Used with permission.

CRITICAL THINKING

How would you teach about breast cancer to women from culturally diverse backgrounds?

During young adulthood the man should be taught to examine his scrotum and penis regularly since **cancer of the testes** may occur and be detected by palpating unusual nodules.[358] Klingman describes in detail the examination of the penis, scrotum, rectum, and prostate, and detection of inguinal and femoral hernias.[359] Table 12-10 describes the self-examination and procedure. Teach the information about the examination.[360]

Teach clients about risks of cancer as described in the box entitled "Cancer Risks" and Table 12-11. Teach also *signs that should be considered suspicious* and reported to a physician:[361–364]

- Changes in a dark-colour mole or spot
- Pink or flesh-colour nodule that slowly grows larger
- Open or crusted sore that does not heal
- Red, rough patch, orange-peel skin, or bump that persists
- Mole that grows, changes, hurts, bleeds, or itches

TABLE 12-10
Procedure for Examination of the Scrotum and Penis

1. Perform the examination immediately after shower or a warm bath. Both the scrotum and examiner's hands should be warm.

2. Hold the scrotum in the palms of the hands and palpate with thumb and fingers of both hands. Examine in a mirror for swelling.

3. Examine each testicle individually, using both hands. Gently roll testicle between thumbs and fingers. (One testicle should be larger.)

4. Locate the epididymis (found on top of and extending down behind the testicle); it should be soft and slightly tender.

5. Examine the spermatic cord next; it ascends from the epididymis and has a firm, smooth, tubular texture.

6. Become familiar with the consistency of normal testicular structures so that changes can be detected.

- Mole that is larger in size than a pencil eraser and has irregular borders or variegated colours with shadings of red-white or blue-black
- Elevation or bulge in a mole that was flat
- Mole on the bottom of the feet or in an area of repeated trauma
- Changes in body contours

Dietary and other daily habits may contribute to risk for cancer. Table 12-11 lists risks for skin cancer. Risks for lung and hematopoietic cancers apparently are increased in adulthood after childhood exposure to parental smoking. Tell women that the incidence of breast cancer or fibrocystic disease is higher in those who consume increased amounts of caffeine. Consuming two or more cups of caffeinated coffee a day may be associated with increased risk of colon or bladder cancer.[365,366] Realize that some cultural groups are more prone to cancer. Environmental and cultural factors (e.g., diet [see Table 12-12], lifestyle stress, and exposure to pollutants) contribute significantly to increased incidence of cancer (see Chapter 2).[367–369] Hormones secreted by the brain and adrenal glands (e.g., cortisol) in response to emotional stress may inhibit the immune system and enhance growth of cancerous tumours. Stressful times often reduce the person's pursuit of healthy habits as well (e.g., exercise, nutrition), which may contribute to cancerous growth. Immune substances also affect activity of the hypothalamic-pituitary-adrenal axis, the endocrine system that regulates stress responses.[370–372] Physical, emotional, social, and spiritual circumstances are highly interdependent.

In summary, the consequences of a diagnosis of cancer for the young adult are great.[373] These individuals have most of the potentially great years of life ahead of them; and they may either spend decades living with the effects of the cancer diagnosis, or have tragically shortened lives with major repercussions on their families.[374]

Cancer Risks

Lifetime—Probability, over lifetime, of developing or dying from cancer

Relative—With exposure, strength of relationship between risk factors and a specific cancer influences development of cancer

All cancers involve malfunction of genes that control growth and division of cells

TABLE 12-11
Risk Factors for Melanoma and Other Skin Cancers

Severe sunburn in childhood (3 or more before age 14).

Fair skin that freckles easily.

Family history; parent or sibling, especially if family member had history of atypical moles. (Dermatologist examination recommended every 3 months).

Atypical moles that are benign between puberty and age 40 may be cancer precursors.

Chronic overexposure to intense sunlight.

Age: more common in young adults.

Appearance of lesion:

Asymmetrical;

Border irregular: ragged, notched, blurred;

Colour uneven: black, brown, or tan; areas of white, grey, red, or blue;

Diameter: changes in size.

Size of lesion: good prognosis if lesion invades skin no more than 0.75 mm deep (95% of patients survive 5 years; 90% survive 15 years); poorer prognosis if lesion is 1 mm deep or deeper (50% survive 5 years).

TABLE 12-12
Nutrition Guidelines to Reduce Cancer Risk

Daily Nutrition Factor	Protect Against These Cancers
Plant sources of food emphasized; 5 or more fruits and vegetable servings Several servings of cereals, rice, bread, other grains, pasta, beans.	Gastrointestinal, respiratory, and lung
Limit intake of high-fat foods, especially coconut oil, animal fats, and trans-fatty acids, found in artificially processed and packaged snacks.	Colorectal Prostate
Alpha linolenic fats or Omega-3 oils in tuna steak, mackerel, and sardines appear protective.	Endometrial
Monosaturated fats in peanuts, oils, and avocados appear safe.	Potentially all
Increase fibre content.	Colorectal
Limit caloric intake to maintain normal weight; avoid obesity.	Breast Endometrial Prostate Colorectal Kidney
Limit alcohol intake (especially in combination with tobacco smoking). (Resveratol in red wine and grape juice slows oxidative damage.)	Oral Esophageal Laryngeal Pancreatic Bladder Breast, potentially

CRITICAL THINKING

What are the implications for a family when the father, who is a young adult, has cancer?

Hepatitis C. In Canada, hepatitis C virus (HCV) is a significant public health problem.[375] Although the precise number of cases of HCV infection is unknown, it is estimated that approximately 240 000 Canadians carry the virus, and of these, only 30% are aware of their infection.[376] Hepatitis C is transmitted through blood or body fluids contaminated with the virus.[377] The most important risk factor associated with the transmission of HCV is the sharing of drug injection equipment. Unapparent parenteral exposure, such as tattooing, body piercing, and the sharing of personal hygiene items are presumed to be risk factors only if the instruments are contaminated with blood or body fluids.[378] However, according to a public health sentinel, 3% of new cases of hepatitis C (as presented in clinics in Calgary, Edmonton, Winnipeg, and Ottawa-Carleton) are associated with body piercing or tattooing.[379] The risk associated with blood transfusions and the use of blood products is markedly reduced as a result of the screening of blood donations.

An HCV-infected individual can help to protect the liver from further damage by reducing or eliminating use of alcohol; tobacco; and prescription, over-the-counter, and illicit drugs.[380] As a health professional, you should know that there is no vaccine against HCV. The key to prevention is a matter of eliminating, or minimizing, exposure to fluids or tissues potentially contaminated with HCV (including all blood- and tissue-borne pathogens).[381]

CRITICAL THINKING

What are other strategies to prevent hepatitis C?

Lifestyle and Physical Illness. Life is rooted in and organized around a person's changing culture and society, whether the changes are dramatic or subtle. Coping with extreme change taxes the person physically and psychologically and may be responsible for physical disease. *Research shows relationships between physical adaptation and illness and sociocultural experiences.* Death rates from cancer, diabetes, tuberculosis, heart disease, and multiple sclerosis for urban populations are inversely proportional to income, implying that stresses of poverty may be a cause of disease.[382,383]

The adult is most likely to fall ill when he or she is experiencing the "giving up–given up complex": feelings of lowered self-esteem, discouragement, despair, humiliation, depression, powerlessness to change or cope with a situation, imagined helplessness, loss of gratifying roles, sense of uncertain future, and memories of earlier periods of giving up. Apparently such feelings modify the capacity of the organism to cope with concurrent pathogenic factors. Biologically, the central nervous system fails in its task of processing the emergency defence system so that the person has a higher statistical tendency toward illness or death. Conversely, contentment, happiness, faith, confidence, and success are associated with health.[384–386]

Homeless individuals and families also have similar health care needs and problems (refer also to Chapter 1). Be attuned to cultural differences, including language difficulties,

definitions of health and illness, food preferences, lines of authority, health practices, job-related diseases, and general lifestyle of your clients.

Biofeedback. The young adult is likely to be interested in and benefit from biofeedback training, learning to control body functions once considered involuntary such as heartbeat, blood pressure, breathing, and muscle contractions (see Chapter 5 for further discussion). Learning biofeedback techniques is much like learning other skills of muscular coordination and physical activity. It involves controlled production of alpha waves, the brain waves typical of relaxation and reverie, the fringe of consciousness. Biofeedback has been used to treat a variety of conditions.[387–389]

Emotional Health Problems

Stress reactions, *physiologic and psychological changes resulting in unusually or disturbed adaptive behaviour patterns* and depression, including postpartum,[390] result when the young adult is unable to cope with the newly acquired tasks and responsibilities. Mate selection, marriage, childrearing, college, job demands, social expectations, and independent decision making are all stressors that carry threats of insecurity and possibly some degree of failure. Some of these stress reactions take the form of physical illnesses just described. Others take the form of self-destructive behaviour such as suicide, alcoholism, drug abuse and addiction, eating disorders, and smoking. Other stress reactions include abuse of spouse. **Self-destructive behaviour,** in the form of death by suicide, is increasing despite the many religious, cultural, and moral taboos. Thousands of people take their own lives or attempt suicide yearly.

Suicide. In Canadian Aboriginal communities, compared with the rest of the Canadian population, suicide and self-inflicted injuries are three times higher (six times higher for the 15-to-24 age group).[391] Aboriginal people are exposed to severe environmental hazards; industrial and resource development have polluted water and disrupted fish and game stock in many reserve communities. Although changes are occurring, disruptions in the quality of life are prevalent. Men are more likely than women to commit suicide. Women, however, are twice as likely as men to be depressed; and their depression lasts longer.[392]

Both physiologic and psychological factors influence the choice of method for suicide. Women tend to use less lethal methods such as Aspirin or barbiturate overdose; poisoning; or cutting the wrists. Men usually use the more lethal methods: gunshot wounds to the head or hanging. Women may see attempted suicide as a means of expressing aggression or manipulating relationships or events in the environment; therefore they select the less lethal methods. Degree of physical strength and the subconscious fear of disfigurement may also influence women's choice of methods.[393–395] Most of the time the person does not really desire death, but rather a way out of an apparently hopeless or intolerable situation.

Occupation is also an important factor in suicide rates. Professional groups such as dentists, psychiatrists, and physicians are considered high-risk groups, although the underlying causes for this are undetermined.[396,397] The required strenuous educational courses or the stressful demands and responsibilities of their positions may be factors.

Consider three factors when planning primary prevention of suicide among young adults. Educate the public about emotional needs of the person and early signs of suicide so that high-risk persons can be more easily identified by family and friends. To compensate for the effects of separating from home and encountering a variety of stressors, a close and significant relationship should be established between the high-risk person and a caring person. The person needs opportunity to talk through frustration, anger, and despair and to formulate life plans. Finally, encourage young adults to participate in group and extracurricular activities that prevent social isolation.

Nursing responsibility for the suicidal person extends to the industrial setting, clinic, general or psychiatric hospital, and general community. You are in contact with and in the position to identify persons who may be potential candidates for suicide: unwed mothers, divorcees, widows and widowers, alcoholics, the terminally ill, and depressed people. *Watch for signs of depression*:[398–400]

1. Expressions of overwhelming sadness, worthlessness, hopelessness, or emptiness

2. Complaints of sleep and gastrointestinal disturbances, lack of energy, or chronic illness

3. Decreased muscle tone with slumped shoulders, slowed gait, drooped faces

4. Decreased interest in work, personal appearance, religion, family and friends, or special events

5. Preference for being alone; self-occupied

6. Inability to carry out ordinary tasks or make simple decisions.

Once identified, these signs of depression must be communicated to others: friends, relatives, a physician, or other persons concerned with the potentially suicidal person.

The person is more prone to attempt suicide *when the depression is lifting* and energy is greater. Listen closely to the person who speaks of being alienated, in an impossible situation, or of the future looking bleak and unchangeable, even after saying the situation is improving. He or she is a high-risk suicidal candidate, as is the person who talks of suicide, who has made an attempt, who is in crisis, or who is an alcoholic or a drug abuser.[401–403]

Your responsibility in individual suicide prevention varies according to the setting, the source, and extent of distress. You will need to protect the person against self-destructive behaviour by reducing environmental hazards; but *emotional support is of greater importance while the person works through problems*. The principles of crisis intervention, therapeutic communication, and nurse–client relationship are discussed in psychiatric nursing texts.[404,405] Show the person verbally and nonverbally that someone—you—understands, respects, and cares about him or her.

CRITICAL THINKING

In working with a depressed client who has suicidal ideation and who may be overwhelmed by personal problems, what are ways to assist this client to cope?

Alcoholism. Alcoholism, a complex disease, is also a form of self-destructive behaviour. One suicide in every five is that of an alcoholic because alcoholism contributes to depression.[406,407] In addition, many alcoholics literally drink themselves to death or die as a result of physical debilitation or injuries sustained while under the influence of alcohol.

Alcoholism may occur during any life period. Male alcoholics outnumber female alcoholics; however, identification of female alcoholics is increasing yearly. The alcoholic's life span is shortened approximately 12 years, and most alcoholics show physical and cognitive complications because of their prolonged drinking. In addition, millions of dollars are lost yearly in business as a result of absenteeism, lowered work efficiency, and accidents.

Alcoholism is a disease with physiologic, psychological, and sociologic aspects. Excessive drinking causes physiologic addiction and psychological dependence. Not drinking causes mild to severe withdrawal symptoms. Alcohol is used to relieve worry and guilt, and it falsely leads to an increased sense of adequacy and sociability. In turn, the person becomes more anxious and guilty when learning of his or her behaviour while drinking. He or she drinks again to forget and deny. The vicious cycle becomes worse; behaviour, performance, and health deteriorate until he or she is forced to seek help or dies. References listed in the endnotes at the end of this chapter give more information on the causes, psychodynamics, symptoms, and treatment of alcoholism.[408–410] Alcoholism in nurse colleagues is a concern.

The same stress-producing situations that lead to suicide may also promote alcoholism in the young adult. Early case finding and early treatment are important in alcoholism, both for the ill individual and for the family members. A growing concern is the effect of the alcoholic parent on the development of children.[411–413] You can be active in both case finding and treatment.

Acceptance of the alcoholic as a sick person and providing support for those close to him or her are as important as the technical care you give during or after detoxification. You might write for the self-administered test for alcoholism that is available through the National Council for Alcoholism or Alcoholics Anonymous. A certain score indicates alcoholic tendencies.

Drug Abuse and Addiction. These are other forms of self-destructive behaviour. Drug abuse is increasing in the young adult, including all levels of workers, and abuse and addiction contribute to a number of other physical, emotional, and social health problems.

As with alcoholism, male addicts are more numerous than female ones. Symptoms of drug addiction differ with the type of drug, amount used, and personality of the user (see Table 11-6 on pages 510–516). Symptoms may also differ for the young adult at work; see the box entitled "Signs and Symptoms of Drug Abuse in the Young Adult" for a listing.

Treatment for drug abuse and addiction involves helping the person work through emotional problems, seeing that he or she has proper medical and nutritional regimens, helping him or her return to a community where the dangers of becoming addicted again are not too great, and helping him or her get involved in worthwhile work or activities. Several

Signs and Symptoms of Drug Abuse in the Young Adult

- Late to work frequently; late in producing assignments.
- Increased absenteeism (abusers miss twice as much work as nonabusing employees).
- Increased productivity in work for a short period (cocaine will cause some people to perform better than normal or more creatively for a short time; overachievement can be used to compensate for or cover up initial stages of abuse).
- Falling productivity, poorer quality work, disorganized thinking and work outcome, missed deadlines.
- Forgetfulness, failure to follow instructions properly and to carry out usual steps of a procedure.
- Personality change, increasing irritability, depression, suspicion.
- Chronic runny nose from cocaine inhalation or sniffing glue or other chemicals that cause irritation of the nasal mucous membrane; regular complaints of a cold.
- Napping or sleeping on the job.
- Accident proneness, clumsiness at work, poor gross or fine motor coordination on the job, reports of accidents in the auto or at home.
- Clandestine meetings and discussions with other employees (users become dealers for fellow employees and withdraw from supervisory staff).

references cover the many facts of multiple addictions and their assessment and intervention.[414–420]

Gambling. Gambling is a controversial topic in our society today. In recent years, provinces in Canada have expanded their gaming activities. Such activities raise much revenue for the province.[421] According to a gambling prevalence study by the Addictions Foundation Manitoba, 3.8% of the population of Manitoba is composed of problem gamblers, and 2.3% are probable pathological gamblers.[422] It appears that the rates of problem gambling in Manitoba are in the same range as other provinces that have video lottery terminals (VLTs) in locations outside casinos. Evidence indicates that problem gamblers may come from a family where addictions were present.[423] It is important for health professionals to offer resources for problem gamblers and their families in order to assist them with their problem.

CRITICAL THINKING

What resources are available in your community for the problem gambler?

Eating Disorders. Eating disorders (anorexia and bulimia) currently are identified more frequently in young adults. Refer to Chapter 11 for information also pertinent to the young adult who has this condition. Several authors provide helpful information.[424–427]

Smoking. Smoking is considered self-destructive behaviour because nicotine causes many harmful physiologic effects and is habit-forming.

Tobacco use is the most preventable cause of premature death and disability in North America. Smoking is most prevalent in young adults, ages 25 to 44. This may be because

90% of new smokers are teens and cigarette use on university and college campuses is increasing. Many people, even some with serious respiratory and vascular disorders, continue to smoke heavily despite the warnings from their physicians and about the harmful effects of smoking.

More women than men now smoke cigarettes. Smoking in younger women has significantly increased the number of cardiac deaths and the incidence of lung cancer in women. Other health problems are also attributed to smoking. Effects of smoking during pregnancy are discussed in Chapter 6. Additional problems are periodontal disease, carcinoma in situ of the cervix, chronic respiratory disease, and shortened life expectancy. Offspring of the person who smokes are subject to more respiratory infection and allergies.[428,429]

Various reasons are given for smoking: smoking is relaxing; it prevents nervousness and overeating; and it gives the person something to do with his or her hands in social gatherings. All these reasons may stem from internal tensions and may well be the young person's way of dealing with stress. If the pattern of smoking is not altered during the stage of young adulthood, it may be impossible for changes to be made later in life.

Chemicals found in cigarette smoke are also commonplace in many work environments. Thus the person who smokes may suffer double jeopardy. Further, the person who smokes has more occupational accidents and injuries and uses more sick time and health benefits.

Work with the young adult to reduce or stop cigarette smoking. To achieve this goal, you will have to do more than give information about health effects and morbidity and mortality rates. Explore his or her ideas of health and personal vulnerability to adverse effects from smoking. The social dynamics of smoking must also be considered. Realize that to give up

Health Effects of Smoking Cessation

1. Blood pressure and pulse start to normalize.
2. Temperature of hands and feet increase to normal within 2 hours.
3. Carbon dioxide level in blood returns to normal level in 4 hours.
4. Oxygen level in blood increases to normal in 8 hours.
5. Digestion improves in 8 hours.
6. Overall circulation improves in 24 hours.
7. Sense of smell and taste improve in 48 hours.
8. Lung function increases; coughing, congestion, and shortness of breath decrease in 72 hours.
9. Overall energy increases.
10. Lungs increase ability to clean themselves.
11. Risk of heart attack decreases and returns to baseline as non-smoker in 1 year.
12. Risk of other nicotine-related deaths decreases, e.g., heart attack, lung and other cancers, stroke, chronic obstructive lung disease.

Source: Lindell, K., and L. Reinke, Nursing Strategies for Smoking Cessation, ANA Continuing Education Independent Study Module, American Nurses Association, May 6, 1999, A1–A6.

Smoking Cessation Suggestions

- Keep a notebook of current and past success. Use the list as a reminder of your ability to succeed in new ventures.
- Identify a personal reason for quitting smoking other than because "It's bad for me,"
- Make a list of things that are personally pleasurable and choose one as a reward (instead of a cigarette) when feeling uncomfortable or bored.
- Make a list of reasons smoking began and compare it with a list of current reasons for smoking.
- Keep a log of each cigarette lit including the purpose; focus on smoking the cigarette and sensations occurring before and after smoking.
- Put cigarettes in an unfamiliar place.
- Every time you reach for a cigarette, ask "Do I really want this cigarette?" "Do I really need a cigarette?" "What can I do instead of smoking this cigarette?"
- Develop and practise responses to peer pressure to smoke.
- Smoke with the hand opposite that usually used.
- Buy cigarettes only by the pack, not by the carton.
- Buy different brands of cigarettes and avoid smoking two packs of the same brand in a row.
- Stay away from friends who smoke and from places where people smoke.
- End all meals with foods not associated with smoking (e.g., a glass of milk or half a grapefruit rather than a cup of coffee or a drink).
- Switch to noncaffeinated coffee or tea or bouillon.
- When using cigarettes as an energizer, substitute six small high-protein foods, sufficient sleep, a glass of milk, a piece of fresh fruit or vegetable juice, exercise or movement, or a relaxation exercise.

- Have carrot sticks, celery, or sunflower seeds ready to chew instead of smoking a cigarette.
- Eat more foods that leave the body alkaline such as vegetables, seeds, and fruits and reduce the urge to smoke.
- Write a list of stress enhancers; learn structured relaxation and stress reduction approaches to deal with each stressor.
- Use affirmations such as "I no longer smoke," "I can quit," "It's getting easier and easier to quit smoking," or "It's getting easier and easier to think about quitting smoking." Tell six people.
- Use deep breathing or breathe for centring when the urge for a cigarette appears.
- Work with a peer who can be called for positive feedback when the urge for a cigarette occurs. Be sure the peer is positive about ability to quit and does not nag or induce guilt.
- Ask friends and co-workers not to leave cigarettes around or offer them.
- When the urge for a cigarette occurs, picture the word "STOP" in big red letters.
- Ask for a hug instead of having a cigarette.
- Choose a time to stop smoking when peak mental or physical performance is not expected.
- Write a contract and sign it with a trusted person so continuing to smoke will prove embarrassing or will result in great loss.
- Read articles and books by people who have successfully quit smoking or helped others to do so.
- When feeling depressed, talk with people who have successfully quit smoking and ask for information about why they are glad they quit.
- Reward self at specified intervals for not smoking.

Sources: Edelman, C., and C. Mandle, Health Promotion Throughout the Lifespan (4th ed.). St. Louis: C.V. Mosby; Lindell, K., and L. Reinke, Nursing Strategies for Smoking Cessation, ANA Continuing Education Independent Study Module, American Nurses Association, May 6, 1999, A1–A6; New Aid for Smoking Cessation, Focus on Healthy Aging, 2, no. 1 (1999), 2; Pender, Health Promotion in Nursing Practice (3rd ed.). Norwalk, CT: Appleton & Lange, 1996.

smoking represents a loss. Help the person who is trying to stop smoking to acknowledge feelings of loss and grief related to giving up a part of self and social lifestyles. Instead of emphasizing that the person is "giving up" smoking, help the person verbalize feelings and identify what is being gained by a smoking cessation program. Give the person positive feedback for not smoking. Give the person time to change habits. If the person has smoked for many years, it is not easy to stop.[430] See the boxes entitled "Health Effects of Smoking Cessation"[431] and "Smoking Cessation Suggestions" for tips on the initiation, maintenance, and successful completion of a smoking cessation program.[432–435]

There are several smoking cessation aids on the market: the nicotine patch, nicotine gum, nicotine nasal spray, and an inhaler that looks like a hollow cigarette holder. The inhaler allows the user to mimic the hand-to-mouth ritual. Using an aid doubles the chance of quitting, but it is best used with some type of cessation behavioural program and a support program to address psychological dependence.[436] Because

nicotine is an addictive substance, it is possible to get addicted to the nicotine delivery systems designed for smoking cessation.

Spousal Violence
Battered or Abused Women. Statistics Canada's 1999 general Social Survey on Victimization, which collected demographic information, including marital status, family and household composition, and household income, indicated that spousal violence rates were highest among those whose partners were between 15 and 34 years of age; rates were highest among those whose partners were heavy drinkers, and whose partners were looking for work.[437] There has been significant research indicating that young couples are at an increased risk of spousal violence compared to older people.[438]

Family violence is a social and emotional health problem of all socioeconomic levels that has gained increasing public attention. Wife-beating has always been a problem: woman was the man's property and beating was accepted behaviour in some cultures. Traditionally the woman was too ashamed or too helpless to admit the problem or seek help. Further, no help existed. Efforts are being made in cities to make the police and legal system more aware of **abuse** or **battering**, *a symptom complex of violence in which a woman has received deliberate and severe injury more than three times from the husband or a man with whom she has a close relationship. It is a pattern of behaviour that seeks to establish power and control over another through fear and intimidation.* Further, attempts have been made to make the police and legal system more protective of the woman who has been treated violently, and more punitive to the violent man. Emergency shelters and safe homes for battered women and their children are increasingly being established in urban areas so that the woman who seeks help does not have to return home or be at home when the man who was released shortly after arrest returns home even more violent than before. Crisis telephone lines have been established and publicized by the media, and many women have memorized these numbers. In some communities rap sessions and referrals are available for battered women. Assistance to women seeking divorce is inadequate in most cities because of the cost and bureaucratic red tape.[439,440]

CRITICAL THINKING

What resources are available in your community for the women and children who are being abused?

You can work with other health and legal professionals to identify and overcome the problem of abused women. *Assessment of a family and woman suffering adult abuse often reveals the following typical characteristics:*[441–446]

- The family and the woman are isolated socially or physically from neighbours, relatives, and friends.
- The woman feels increasing helplessness, guilt, isolation, and low self-esteem. She feels trapped and has been forced to be dependent on the man.
- The woman may range in age from teens to old age and may suffer violent injury for months or years.
- The woman's educational and occupational status is often higher than that of the man.
- Most beatings begin early in marriage and increase in frequency and intensity over the decades.
- Most violence occurs in the evening, on weekends, and in the kitchen.
- Generally there are no witnesses.
- The woman is frequently unable to leave the home because of lack of money, transportation, a place to go, support people, or support agencies in the community. Further, she has learned helplessness behaviours and feels unable to try to escape.
- The injuries from abuse may not be visible, but if abuse is present, the woman usually talks about the problem freely when asked directly if abuse is occurring.
- With increasing incidence of abuse and the physical and emotional consequences of abuse, the woman becomes more passive, less flexible, less able to think logically, more apathetic, depressed, and possibly suicidal.

- Eventually the frustration, stress, and anger may be externalized into physical behaviour that is more than protective of the self or the children; she may in turn become violent to the point of killing the battering partner.

The Canadian Nurses Association Position Statement on Violence clearly states that violence is recognized as a social act involving a serious misdirection of power.[447] Nurses alone cannot manage nor eliminate violence. The approach must be multidisciplinary, multi-sectorial, and multifaceted. All professionals, including the private sector, unions, and governments, have strategic roles to play to ensure that legislation, education, research, administrative supports, and adequate resources are in play to deal with the impact of violence.[448]

Women remain in a threatening situation for many complex and interrelated reasons, as described in the box entitled "Reasons Why Women Are Unable to Leave a Violent Situation."[449] An astute assessment will uncover at least some of these characteristics and factors if present. The box entitled "Identification of Partner Abuse in the Health Care Setting" describes some "red flags" that can help you identify a battered adult in an emergency room or intensive care, occupational, or other medical setting.[450–455]

CRITICAL THINKING

What health promoting strategies could you offer a woman who informs you that her spouse is verbally abusive to her?

Several authors present helpful information on assessment and treatment of the rape victim.[456–459] Increasingly the literature is discussing *marital* (not just date) *rape* as a problem in young adulthood. Marital rape meets the criteria for criminal sexual conduct. The difference is that the rapist and his victim are married; thus the man may be immune from prosecution. Often the women have been child victims of sexual abuse or incest, and there are physical, psychosomatic, and emotional effects. Some of the content related to the abused or battered women applies in this situation. Often children in these marriages are also raped or molested.[460–463]

Incest, *sexual intercourse between biologically related persons,* is another form of battering that may affect either the man or the woman, but more commonly the woman. Incest is considered one form of sexual abuse, although adult family members may convey that incestual behaviour is normal.

Symptoms and problems in adulthood resulting from childhood sexual abuse and incest are:

- Chronic depression, hopelessness related to shame and guilt
- Drug and alcohol abuse
- Various physical complaints, including panic attacks, headaches, hysterical seizures
- Problems with trusting or intimate relationships with the opposite sex
- Character disorders, such as borderline or narcissistic states
- Multiple personality disorders
- Sexual dysfunction and gynecologic problems

Reasons Why Women Are Unable to Leave a Violent Situation

- Lacking economic independence and being without money
- Being forbidden to leave the house or visit or call others
- Fear of being alone, being unable to support self and children, or the man's finding and harming her after she left him (Personal safety is a continual issue.)
- Lacking emotional or social support (Often parents encouraged her to return to the abusive partner.)
- Believing that she is unworthy of anything better
- Having nowhere to go or being turned away from a public shelter
- Believing traditional norms related to women's role, marriage, religion, and violence; believing the woman is less than human
- Believing there are positive aspects of the relationship that are worth preserving; emotional dependency in the relationship
- Desiring a father for her children; wanting to protect the children from greater harm
- Feeling disbelief, sense of horror, and shock about the man's violent behaviour to her and denial or rationalizations that it would happen again
- Believing the man's promise that he will not hit again; thinking she can change him
- Finding the police unresponsive to calls for help (Many women have kept extensive records of the number of times legal action was taken with unsatisfactory results.)
- Taking responsibility for the violence, feeling guilty and that this behaviour is her fault (Often the man would say, "Look what you made me do.")
- Feeling helpless; being unable to counter the power, authority, and threats of the man (Often the women were forced out or locked out of the home in the middle of the night in winter without clothing or money.)
- Increasing force or violence, which was condoned by police or society, brought on by failing to comply with the husband's wishes or demands
- Relying on the sexual relation to punish him, to prevent battering, and to prove self-worth (Sexual enjoyment lessened as battering increased.)
- Wanting to protect the man's reputation in the community or in the job
- Having several small children and the related child care responsibility, often coupled with need to protect the children against the man's violence
- Fearing what would happen after leaving the home and man (welfare, homelessness, unemployment, single parenting); often there is a predictability about his behaviour versus the unpredictability of the future
- Introjecting the societal attitude that the victim is to blame
- Believing that all marriages are like this (violent), especially if the woman grew up in a violent home

Identification of Partner Abuse in the Health Care Setting

Multiple Injuries

- Multiple abrasions and contusions to different anatomic sites should alert health care providers. There are relatively few ways of sustaining such injuries.

Body Map

- Many incidents of abuse involve injury to the face, neck, chest, breasts, or abdomen, whereas most accidents involve the extremities.

Rape

- Most women are raped by a male intimate, and many times rape is yet another incident of ongoing physical abuse.

Severity of Injury

- Severity varies among abused victims. Presentation of medically insignificant trauma to the emergency service may alert medical personnel that ongoing assault and impending danger constitute the real emergency for which she is seeking aid.

Pregnancy

- Abused women are more likely to be beaten when pregnant. There is a higher rate of miscarriage among battered women.

Trauma History

- Frequent visits to the emergency department or physician.
- A history of trauma can be the key indicator! Both asking about previous injuries and looking at medical records are important. Records may indicate repeated visits and injuries to the same site.

Suicide Attempts

- Studies indicate that battering is a frequent precipitant of female suicide attempts; conversely, women who attempt suicide are likely to have a history of domestic violence.

Inconsistent Description of Injuries

- Injuries do not fit with the victim's description of the genesis of injury.

Vague and Nonspecific Complaints

- Complaints include, for example, anxiety, depression, and sleeplessness and many indicate intrafamilial crisis.

Heavy Use of Alcohol and Drugs

- Victims are more likely than nonvictims to use alcohol and drugs, and partners are much more likely to use alcohol and drugs excessively.

This problem is expected to affect more young adults in the future, based on the statistics currently of childhood sexual abuse and incest.[464–468]

Why do women leave the violent situation? Often the woman leaves when she feels suicidal but does not want to kill herself because of concern about the children's welfare; or the woman may fear for the life of the unborn child, if pregnant, or for the lives of her other children. Fear of being killed is a motivator; acknowledging that the situation will never improve is important. The shock of a particular beating or the horror of being beaten while pregnant may be the turning point. The woman realizes she has no power to make her partner change. At some point the woman may have received enough subtle or overt encouragement to leave or a new vision of what marriage and family life should be, coupled with a renewed sense of self-worth and the feeling she "doesn't have to take it anymore." The woman realizes the point at which the man no longer asks for forgiveness, shows no remorse (as he might have after the first beating), and usually denies he behaved violently. There comes a decision point, and then a plan may be made. Some women, however, leave abruptly to avoid being murdered.[469]

CRITICAL THINKING

What elements should be included in a safety plan for a woman who is being abused?

Women may or may not be in acute distress when they leave. Despite the desperate situations and the difficulty in finding aid, these women are not typically helpless. Generally, they continually scheme how to stop the battering, either by examining personal behaviour or planning ways to escape and how to get and keep some money. They take steps to please their partners and to satisfy their demands while protecting and caring for the children. Often they are the primary wage earner in the home. They may describe how they actively defended themselves; if they did not, it was not because they felt helpless but because other negative consequences or a worse beating would ensue.[470]

Typical adult and parental behaviour of the male batterer in order of incidence, according to the research by Sonkin, Martin, and Walker[471] is as follows:

1. Has battered a previous partner
2. Is employed, frequently under stress at work
3. Has children who have viewed the domestic violence and his battering behaviour
4. Was under the influence of alcohol or drugs at the last battering incident
5. Uses physical punishment on his children
6. Has been violent with others not in their family, outside the home
7. Has been violent both when under the influence and when not under the influence of drugs and alcohol
8. Has a family history of suicide (attempted and completed)
9. Has been violent only when under the influence of alcohol and drugs
10. Has been violent only when not under the influence of alcohol or drugs
11. Lacks close friends or someone with whom to talk

Psychological violence by the man against the woman can be categorized as follows:[472]

■ Explicit threats
■ Extreme controlling type of behaviour, taking her everywhere; saying when she must come home; knowing her whereabouts, companions, and life activities
■ Pathologic jealousy; continually questioning her about her behaviour; making accusations without cause; highly suspicious
■ Mental degradation; calling her names or telling her she is incompetent, stupid, and no good
■ Isolating behaviour; because of his jealousy, suspicion, and dependence, he controls the woman's behaviours so that she in turn becomes extremely isolated and dependent on him

The man who abuses the female partner has the following typical childhood history, in order of incidence, according to research by Sonkin, Martin, and Walker:[473]

1. Received physical punishment as a child
2. Saw his mother abused or treated violently by his father
3. Attacked one of the parents
4. Was physically abused as a child
5. Was sexually abused as a child

The male batterer comes from all walks of life and cultures. *Personality characteristics of the male abuse or perpetrator that are typical* include:

■ Denying of or minimizing the violent behaviour and its effects (The batterer may actually lose memory of the event because of his rage.)
■ Blaming the behaviour of the woman or others as the cause of the violent scenes
■ Periodic uncontrollable anger and rage, which is externalized into physical and verbal behaviour
■ Dependency on the partner as sole source of love, support, intimacy, and problem solving, resulting from the controlling and isolating behaviour that entwined him and the partner and children
■ Sense of alienation from others and society (He considers himself a loner and therefore his "own boss"—means he can do whatever he wants in his home.)
■ Jealousy of and suspiciousness of his partner, children, and finally everyone else
■ Low self-esteem; lack of confidence in his ability to keep his partner, lack of skill or ability to ask for what is wanted in a nonthreatening way

Some stresses predispose to family violence and male battering of the woman and children. These stresses are listed in the box entitled "Stresses that Predispose to Family Violence." You are in a position to:

1. Make a thorough and holistic assessment, using the prior content.
2. Provide necessary crisis and emergency care.
3. Encourage the abused woman to share her secret with you, another nurse, a social worker, confidante, or religious leader.
4. Educate the public and abused women about the myths of abuse, as described in the box entitled "Myths and Realities about Battered Women."[474–476]

Stresses that Predispose to Family Violence

- Financial pressures, low pay, high cost of living
- Family separation
- Geographic mobility, loss of friends, social supports, and familiarity
- Isolation and communication barriers
- Cultural differences; living in a strange environment or with unfamiliar customs, creating higher mutual dependence
- Lack of family support
- Living abroad such as in military families
- Inability to separate administrative or work roles from home life (Behaviour that is functional at work may not be at home.)
- Lack of privacy at work or at home
- Job pressures or competitiveness, lack of support from supervisor

5. Help her secure help from social service agencies, legal aid societies, counsellors, health centres, and the welfare office.
6. Encourage separation from her husband if her life is in danger.
7. Work with the individual woman to the extent possible for her to talk through her feelings of shame, guilt, embarrassment, anger, and fear.

8. Help her gain courage to make decisions, including decisions on how to protect herself and her children, how to leave her husband, and where to go.

CRITICAL THINKING

In assessing the family of a child who has been brought in with injuries, what behaviours by the parents might indicate possible child abuse?

CRITICAL THINKING

After reading the myths, take a moment to reflect on them. See if any other myth comes to mind. If it does, jot it down.

Group therapy and individual therapy are effective for the woman victim.[477–481] Group therapy may be more effective than individual therapy for the man as it helps him recognize angry and frustrated feelings in self, realize it is not acceptable to vent feelings through violent behaviour to the spouse, and learn alternate coping and behaviour patterns.[482–486] Intervention must take into account incest, marital rape, and battering. Work also with the children, if possible. Research shows that children (ages two to 12) of battered women have deep feelings of fear about safety and abandonment, anger, confusion, social isolation, and aggression. The children's play reveals conflicts about overpowering adults and identification with the same-sex parent; children

Myths and Realities about Battered Women

Myth 1: Battered Women Are a Small Percentage of the Overall Population.

- **Fact:** Domestic violence is one of the most underreported crimes. In the United States, the Federal Bureau of Investigation estimates that 60% of all married women experience physical violence by their husbands at some time during their marriage. There are an estimated 2 to 6 million female victims of family violence each year.

Myth 2: Battered Women Are Masochistic.

- **Fact:** Battered women are *not* masochistic. The prevailing belief has always been that only women who "liked it and deserved it" were battered; that women experienced some pleasure, often akin to sexual pleasure, from being beaten by the man they love. Because this is such a prevailing stereotype, many battered women begin to wonder if indeed they are masochistic.

Myth 3: Battered Women Are Crazy.

- **Fact:** Battered women are not crazy, although battering may contribute to mental illness. This myth places the blame for battering on the woman's negative personality characteristics and takes the focus off the batterer. Further, being abused and beaten may result in what apparently is abnormal behaviour—the woman's attempt to adapt.

Myth 4: Middle-Class Women Are Not Battered as Frequently or as Violently as Poorer Women.

- **Fact:** Women from lower socioeconomic classes are more likely to come in contact with community agencies, so their problems are more visible. Middle- and upper-class women often fear that disclosure will result in social embarrassment and harm to their own or their husband's career or that people will not believe them. This is often true when the husband is held in high esteem in the community.

Myth 5: Women from Ethnic or Racial Minority Groups Are Battered More Frequently than Caucasian Women.

- **Fact:** Studies show that battering crosses all ethnic lines, with no one group suffering more than another.

Myth 6: Battered Women Are Uneducated and Have Few Job Skills.

- **Fact:** Educational levels of battered women range from grade school through completion of professional and doctoral degrees. Many successful career women would be willing to give up their careers if to do so would eliminate battering. Changing jobs or staying home to ease the situation usually has no effect on their partner's behaviour, and sometimes battering worsens.

(continued)

Myths and Realities about Battered Women (continued)

Myth 7: Batterers Are Unsuccessful and Lack Resources to Cope with the World.

■ **Fact:** It has been suggested that men who feel less capable than women resort to violence. Contrary findings were reported in England, where the highest incidence of wife beating was among physicians, service professionals, and police. Affluent batterers include lawyers, professors, and salesmen. Many of these men donate a great deal of their time to community activities and could not maintain their involvement in these projects without the support of their wives.

Myth 8: Batterers Are People with Personality Disorders.

■ **Fact:** If batterers could simply be considered antisocial personalities, individual therapy could be used to differentiate batterers from other men. Unfortunately, it is not that simple. One trait they share is the ability to use charm as a manipulative technique. Manipulation, acting out of anger, exhilaration felt when they dominate and beat the woman, and denial of the behaviour are characteristic of people with personality disorders.

Myth 9: Police Can Protect Battered Women.

■ **Fact:** At most, only 10% of battered women call the police. Of those who did, many believe the police officers were ineffective. When the police left, the men continued the assault with vigour. In St. Louis, Missouri, a pro-arrest policy is improving police response to domestic violence. Several thousand women are murdered annually by male partners, often as a part of the battering act. At least one-half of the injuries presented by women at an emergency room are the result of battering. Battering may also be the basis for a suicide attempt.

Myth 10: Batterers Are Violent in All Their Relationships.

■ **Fact:** Most men who batter their wives are generally not violent in other aspects of their lives. Although being violent in public has definite, negative consequences, there are few consequences in domestic cases.

Myth 11: The Batterer Is Not a Loving Partner.

■ **Fact:** Batterers are often described by women during the honeymoon phase of the cycle of violence as fun-loving, playful, attentive, sensitive, exciting, and affectionate. The woman may describe some very positive characteristics in the man that cause her truly to love him.

Myth 12: Long-standing Battering Relationships Can Change for the Better.

■ **Fact:** Relationships that have rested on the man's having power over the woman are stubbornly resistant to an equal power-sharing arrangement. Even with the best of help, such relationships usually do not become battering-free.

Myth 13: Once a Batterer, Always a Batterer.

■ **Fact:** Batterers can be taught to change their aggressive responses; however, very few batterers are willing to get help. If the batterer does not get treatment and if he is divorced and then remarries, he is likely to batter the next woman he marries.

Myth 14: Battered Women Can Always Leave Home.

■ **Fact:** Many battered women have no place to go and no means of survival outside the framework of their marriage. They also may have small children to care for, whom they would not want to leave home alone with the father. Because battering weakens a woman's self-esteem, she may believe she is incapable of managing on her own.

Myth 15: Battered Women Are Weak and Come from a Bad Background.

■ **Fact:** Typically the battered woman in Hoff's study had a warm, loving relationship as a child with the mother and a negative, destructive relationship with the father. Not all battered women were abused as children. Women who experienced violence before they were battered by their mates showed resilience and strength. But long-standing abuse breeds self-degradation and despair so that a woman feels unworthy of the continued love of even her mother and unable to reach out for help. The battered woman should be considered a survivor type of person.

Myth 16: Battering May Occur Only Once or Infrequently and Could Be Predicted, and thus Prevented, by the Woman.

■ **Fact:** For most of the battered women in several studies, the violence was frequent, extended over time and often unexpected and included many similar incidents. Often violence occurred concomitantly with the man's rages, drunkenness, and/or financial insecurity and during the woman's pregnancy. Often each beating was worse than the previous one. Women consistently report doing everything possible to avoid violence; they try to second-guess the husband: "It's like walking on eggshells." Women have been socialized into the nurturing role, so they doggedly try to succeed in it as wife and mother, regardless of the circumstances. Further, society and medical and psychiatric services and professionals reinforce the belief that the woman's troubles are the result of her own inadequacies and failures (men are taught that the source of stress is other than self). Although the battered woman may think of hurting or killing the man as a punishment, the woman is often inhibited from such action by concern for the children, if present, and fear of consequences for self. Yet there have been times that the women retaliated; most women found that if they fought back, the man became even more violent.

are learning abnormal behaviour and roles that could be carried into their adult relationships and lifestyle.[487,488] You can also work with others to establish emergency centres or crisis phone lines for the woman and to exert pressure to reform the current legal and judicial system so it will be more equitable to women.

Social support and the meaning a person attaches to stressful events can influence whether the person becomes ill or remains healthy—physically and emotionally—in a situation. The battered woman who extricates herself from her violent situation has strengthened her ability to survive, to resolve crisis, and to move forward.

The problem of spouse abuse, like that of child abuse discussed in Chapters 6 and 9, violent television programming discussed in Chapter 10, and elder abuse discussed in Chapter 14, is part of overall societal violence. Each professional, as a citizen and health care provider, must work in whatever way possible to decrease violence, its cause, and its effects.[489–491] Check also with the resources in your area for information.

Hoff[492] describes the shelter experience for battered women and their children, the difficulties of poor and homeless women and children, the struggles of moving to a life without violence, the complexities of starting new relationships, and the effects on the children. Hoff calls the battered woman who removes herself from a violent situation not just a victim, but also a survivor. A five-year follow-up study of the women showed their continued resilience despite hardships. Most of the women still felt shock that someone who supposedly loved them beat them, but they also sensed victory, self-mastery, and recognition of their survival ability.

Social Health Problems

Divorce. **Divorce** is the *termination of marriage, preceded by a period of emotional distress in the marriage, separation, and legal procedures.* Divorce is a *crisis* for those involved and can affect society in general as well as the physical and emotional health of the persons involved.[493–496] Divorce is frequently a factor in poverty and homelessness.[497]

Some young people enter marriage to escape the problems of young adulthood. Marriage provides them with a ready-made role, and it supposedly solves the problem of isolation. If marriage takes place before the individual has developed a strong sense of identity and independence, however, intimacy cannot be achieved.

There is no question that divorce has greatly increased in Canada since 1968 when the divorce laws entered into effect. A seven-fold increase in divorce was experienced in 1987, when divorce rates peaked, and since then a five-fold increase occurred from 1968 to 1995.[498] Whether or not the rates will go up or down in the future depends largely upon demographic factors and on people's lifestyle and values.[499] For example, more and more young couples choose to cohabit; and as the children of divorce, who are at a higher risk of divorcing, enter into marriage, there are chances that divorce rates could rise again.[500] Statistics Canada states that couples who make it to their fifth year of marriage are less likely to break up.[501] After three consecutive years of increasing rates of divorce, the numbers dropped in 2001 and 2002.[502]

Marriage often breaks down because of the partners' inability to satisfy deep mutual needs in a close demanding relationship. One of the partners may be overly dependent and seek in the other a mother or father. Dependent behaviour may at first meet the needs of the more independent partner. But as the dependent person matures, the relationship is changed. If the stronger partner neither understands nor allows this change, divorce may follow.

Emotional deprivation in childhood is also a poor foundation for marriage. Children of divorce are more likely to get divorced and to see divorce as a way to resolve marital conflict. Separation from the father in early life has adverse effects for girls and boys, as well as teens.[503] The person from a home in which the parents' marital relationship was one of detachment or conflict or in which abuse or divorce occurred is poorly prepared for marriage. He or she has no healthy or loving marital model to follow. The person may try to model the marriage after another's happy marriage; however, the person learns most thoroughly that which is lived during childhood.

The divorce rate reflects the ease with which a divorce can be obtained. The lack of commitment to people and relationships when the going gets tough, seen also in other areas of life, and the dichotomy between the romanticized ideal of marriage and the reality of married life contribute to separation and divorce.

CRITICAL THINKING

What are some reasons for young adults to cohabitate?

When marriage fails and bonds are broken, aloneness, anger, mistrust, hostility, guilt, shame, a sense of betrayal, fear, disappointment, loss of identity, anxiety, and depression, alone or in combination, can appear both in the divorcee and the one initiating the divorce. Eventually there may be a feeling of relief. There must be an interval of adjustment to the physical and emotional loss. Second and subsequent remarriages can be successful, but they carry a higher risk of instability and are more likely to end in divorce because of:

1. The person's lack of ability to form a mutually satisfactory new relationship.
2. The past experiences, vulnerability, guilt, and insecurity that cannot be easily removed.
3. The hassles of her kids, his kids, and their kids.
4. Child and wife support.
5. Interference from the ex-spouse.

Psychological effects of divorce vary because of the following factors:

1. Family psychodynamics before divorce.
2. Nature of the marital break-up.
3. Relationship between the ex-spouses after the divorce.
4. Developmental age and coping skills of the children, if any, during the time of marital disharmony and divorce.
5. Coping skills of each ex-spouse.

If the offspring are adolescents, expression and control of aggressive and sexual impulses, dependency-independency issues, and deidealization of the parents, peer acceptance and social approval, and premature responsibilities of adulthood may intensify.[504–506]

Children, even 15 or more years later into adulthood, suffer from the consequences—emotional and social—of divorce. The problems of low self-esteem, depression, anxiety about intimacy and relationships, mistrust of others and close relationships, depression, guilt, and fantasies about the parents' reunion remain strong for many years. Thus some researchers believe it is critical for parents to work at resolving marital conflicts, to recommit to each other, and ultimately to improve the relationship and gain greater maturity. Health care professionals and society must provide support systems so that parents can work out their stresses in other than divorce courts.

CRITICAL THINKING

Discuss the impact of parental divorce on adult children.

If the divorce cannot be prevented, the parents and children should be given emotional support. (Mothers and children may also have to struggle to meet physical needs and may need help in getting financial support.) The losses must be resolved, a new identity must be formed, and the children involved should have the option of continued close relationships with both parents.[507–511]

Helping divorced women or men identify and pursue personal goals is important. Primary needs of divorced women are economic independence, education, managing parenting, maintaining friendships, establishing a partner relationship, and obtaining adequate housing, school, and environment for self and children. Goals for the man may be the same, although typically there is less economic difficulty.[512] Groups for children of divorcing and divorced parents can help the child work through the feelings of loss, anger, guilt, and ambivalence about relationships with parents and often, eventually, stepparents and stepsiblings. The key is for the parents to continue showing love to their children and to maintain open communication between them about the offspring.

Abortion. Surgical abortions in Canada have been a recognized medical procedure since it was removed from the Criminal Code in 1969.[513] From 1969 through to 1988, a Therapeutic Abortion Committee (TAC) was established at each hospital where abortions were performed, and women were obligated to apply to the TAC to have an abortion. In 1988 the Supreme Court of Canada declared the 1969 abortion law unconstitutional. About 40% of Canadians and Americans feel that women should have access to abortion for whatever reason they choose.[514] The vast majority (90% of Canadians) would allow abortion if there was a strong likelihood of a serious defect in the baby or if the pregnancy was the result of a rape. Only about 5% would prohibit abortion under any circumstances.[515]

As a nurse, you may experience considerable emotional turmoil unless you think through the abortion issue. Women or men seeking your counsel on this issue need to hear a professional presentation. If you feel incapable of this counsel, refer the person to someone who can counsel.

CRITICAL THINKING

What is your own opinion on the abortion issue?

Continuing Health Promotion

As a nurse, realize that the health state of the young adult and the type of health care sought are influenced by the person's background, knowledge, experience, philosophy, and lifestyle. Young adults with health problems might more readily seek care and information if they could find programs compatible with their expectations and lifestyles. You can initiate programs that are specifically aimed at young adults, as they seem to accept the treatment plan more readily when they understand the rationale and expected effects. Keep the previously discussed health problems and unmet physiologic needs in mind as you talk with young adults and plan and give care.

Young adulthood ends in the 40s when the person should have a stable position in society and the knowledge of what he or she can make out of life. Your efforts at teaching and counselling can enhance the young adult's awareness of health promotion and establish a program to make that position more stable.

Continuing Adjustments

One couple invited others to a celebration of their 25th wedding anniversary with the following words:[516]

We continue to adjust to each other, an adjustment that started 25 years ago, and will never stop because we each continue to grow and change. We will always be different.

Don't mistake it for a solid marriage. There is no such thing. Marriage is more like an airplane than a rock. You have to commit the thing to flight, and then it creaks and groans, and keeping it airborne depends entirely on attitude. Working at it, though, we can fly forever. Only the two of us know how hard it has been or how worthwhile.

Celebrate with us ...

INTERESTING WEBSITES

CANADIAN HIV/AIDS INFORMATION CENTRE

http://www.aidssida.cpha.ca/

The mandate of the Canadian HIV/AIDS Information Centre is to provide information on HIV prevention, care, and treatment to community-based organizations, health and education professionals, resource centres and others with HIV and AIDS information needs in Canada.

DIETITIANS OF CANADA

http://www.dietitians.ca/

This organization provides nutritional advice that is accurate, reliable, and trustworthy because it is based on science.

EGALE CANADA

http://www.egale.ca

This is a national organization dedicated to promoting the full acceptance of gay, lesbian, bisexual, and transgendered Canadians.

SEX INFORMATION AND EDUCATION COUNCIL OF CANADA

http://www.sieccan.org/

This national nonprofit organization was established in 1964 to foster public and professional education about human sexuality.

SUMMARY

1. Young adulthood is a time of stabilization. Physical growth is completed.

2. The person has established independence from parents but maintains a friendly relationship with them.

3. The person is settling into a committed intimate relationship and friendships and into career or profession.

4. The couple may choose to become parents or remain childless.

5. The person may choose to live a single lifestyle.

6. Development continues in the cognitive, emotional, social, and moral-spiritual dimensions. The philosophy of life is being formulated.

7. Behaviours, whether at home, on the job, at leisure or with family, friends, or strangers, are adaptive in response to stressors.

Considerations for the Young Adult in Health Care

- Cultural and family background, values, support systems, community resources
- Relationships with family of origin, extended family, family of friends or spouse
- Behaviours that indicate abuse by spouse or significant other
- Physical characteristics, nutritional status, and rest/sleep and exercise patterns that indicate health and are age-appropriate
- Integrated self-concept, body image, and sexuality
- Immunizations, safety education, and other health promotion measures used
- Demonstration of continued learning and use of formal operations and concrete operations competencies in cognitive ability
- Overall appearance and behavioural patterns that indicate intimacy rather than isolation
- Behavioural patterns that demonstrate a value system, continuing formation of philosophy of life, and moral-spiritual development
- Established employment, vocation, or profession, including homemaking and child care
- Behavioural patterns that reflect commitment to parenting, if there are children
- Relationships with work colleagues, coping skills for work stress
- Demonstration of integration of work and leisure and avoidance of physical or emotional illness
- Behavioural patterns and characteristics indicating the young adult has achieved developmental tasks

---

8. Stress effects may result in unhealthy habits or physical or emotional illness.

9. The box entitled "Considerations for the Young Adult in Health Care" summarizes what you should consider in assessment and health promotion of the young adult.

ENDNOTES

1. Burke, R., Generation X: Measures, Sex, and Age Differences, *Psychology Reports,* 74, no. 2 (1994), 555–562.
2. Giles, J., Generations, *Newsweek,* June 8 (1994), 62–68.
3. Root, W., *A Generation of Seekers.* San Francisco: Harper, 1993.
4. Papalia, D. and S. Olds, *Human Development* (3rd ed.). Boston: McGraw Hill, 1998.
5. Gormly, A., *Lifespan Human Development* (6th ed.). Fort Worth: Harcourt Brace College Publishers, 1997.
6. Health Canada, *Canadian References for Body Weight Classification in Adults,* Website: http://www.hc-sc.gc.ca/hpfb-dgspsa/onpp-bppn/weight_book_02_html, August 2004
7. *Ibid.*
8. *Ibid.*
9. *Ibid.*
10. *Ibid.*
11. *Ibid.*
12. Strychar, I., Fighting Obesity: A Call to Arms, *Canadian Journal of Public Health,* 95, no. 1 (2004), 12–14.
13. Statistics Canada, *The Daily,* Wednesday, May 8, 2002, Website: http://www.statcan.ca/Daily/English/020508/d020508a.htm.
14. Health Canada, *Canadian References for Body Weight Classification in Adults.*
15. *Ibid.*
16. Gormly, *op. cit.*
17. Papalia and Olds, *op cit.*
18. Gormly, *op. cit.*
19. Guyton, A., *Textbook of Medical Physiology* (9th ed.). Philadelphia: W.B. Saunders, 1996.
20. Papalia and Olds, *op. cit.*
21. *Ibid.*
22. Guyton, *op. cit.*
23. Papalia and Olds, *op. cit.*
24. Guyton, *op. cit.*
25. Papalia and Olds, *op. cit.*
26. Guyton, *op. cit.*
27. Papalia and Olds, *op. cit.*
28. Guyton, *op. cit.*
29. Papalia and Olds, *op. cit.*
30. Guyton, *op. cit.*
31. Papalia and Olds, *op. cit.*
32. Guyton, *op. cit.*
33. Papalia and Olds, *op. cit.*
34. Guyton, *op. cit.*
35. Papalia and Olds, *op. cit.*
36. Santrock, J. W., *Life Span Development* (6th ed.). Chicago: Brown & Benchmark, 1997.
37. Gormly, *op. cit.*
38. Papalia and Olds, *op. cit.*
39. Gormly, *op. cit.*
40. Masters, W., and V. Johnson, *The Human Sexual Response.* New York: Bantam, 1981.
41. Newman, B., and Newman, P., *Development Through Life: A Psychosocial Approach* (7th ed.). Belmont, CA: Brooks/Cole, 1999.
42. Papalia and Olds, *op cit*
43. Masters and Johnson, *op. cit.*
44. Erlick Robinson, G., The Problem with Premenstrual Syndrome, *Canadian Family Physician,* 48 (2002), 1753–1755.
45. Gormly, *op. cit.*

46. Uphold, C., and M. Graham, *Clinical Guidelines in Family Practice* (2nd ed.). Gainesville, FL: Barmarrae Books, 1994.
47. *Ibid.*
48. Lewis, L., One Year in the Life of a Woman with Premenstrual Syndrome: A Case Study, *Nursing Research,* 44 (1995), 111–115.
49. Mitchell, E., N. Woods, and M. Lentz, Differentiation of Women with Three Premenstrual Symptom Patterns, *Nursing Research,* 43 (1994), 25–30.
50. P.M.S.: It's Real, *Harvard Women's Health Watch,* 1, no. 11 (1994), 2–3.
51. Uphold and Graham, *op. cit.*
52. Duyff, R., *The American Dietetic Association's Complete Food & Nutrition Guide.* Minneapolis: Chronimed Publishing, 1998.
53. P.M.S.: It's Real.
54. Uphold and Graham, *op. cit.*
55. Erlick Robinson, *op. cit.*
56. Papalia and Olds, *op. cit.*
57. P.M.S.: It's Real.
58. Uphold and Graham, *op. cit.*
59. *Ibid.*
60. Guyton, *op. cit.*
61. American Psychiatric Association, *Diagnostic and Statistical Manual of Mental Disorders* (4th ed.). Washington, DC: American Psychiatric Association, 1994.
62. Sherwen, L., M. Scoloreno, and C. Weingarten, *Nursing Care of the Childbearing Family.* Norwalk, CT: Appleton-Lange, 1991.
63. Woodward, K., et al., A Time to Seek, *Newsweek,* December 17 (1990), 50–56.
64. Ambert, A-M, Vanier Institute of the Family, *Contemporary Family Trends, Same-Sex Couples and Same-Sex Parent Families: Relationships, Parenting and Issues of Marriage,* Website: http://www.vifamily.ca/library/cft/samesex.pdf, October 2004.
65. *Ibid.*
66. Isay, R., *Being Homosexual: Gay Men and Their Development.* New York: Farrar, Strauss, Giroux, 1990.
67. Young, M., Leaving the Lesbian Lifestyle, *Journal of Christian Nursing,* 8, no. 4 (1992), 11–13.
68. Papalia and Olds, *op. cit.*
69. Blum, D., "What Made Troy Gay?" *Health,* April 1998, pp. 82–86.
70. Katz, A., "Mom, I Have Something to Tell You"—Disclosing HIV Infection, *Journal of Advanced Nursing,* 25 (1997), 139–143.
71. Gormly, *op. cit.*
72. *Ibid.*
73. Papalia and Olds, *op. cit.*
74. Gormly, *op. cit.*
75. Papalia and Olds, *op. cit.*
76. Isay, *op. cit.*
77. Papalia and Olds, *op. cit.*
78. Young, *op. cit.*
79. Davis, V., and Social and Sexual Issues Committee Members, Lesbian Health Guidelines, *Journal of Society of Gynaecologists and Obstetricians in Canada,* 22, no. 3 (2000), 202–205.
80. *Ibid.*
81. Papalia and Olds, *op. cit.*
82. Mandell, N., and A. Duffy, Explaining Family Lives, in N. Mandell and A. Duffy, eds., *Canadian Families: Diversity, Conflict, and Change* (3rd ed., pp. 3–16). Toronto, Thomson, Nelson, 2005.
83. Statistics Canada, *Profile of Canadian Families and Households: Diversification Continues,* Website: http://www12.statcan.ca/english/Census01/Products/Analytic/companion/fam/pdf/96F0030XIE2001003.pdf, October 2004.
84. Mandell and Duffy, *op. cit.*
85. Papalia and Olds, *op. cit.*
86. Pangman, V.C., and M. Sequire, Sexuality and the Chronically Ill Older Adult: A Social Justice Issue, *Sexuality and Disability,* 18, no. 1 (2000), 49–59.
87. *Ibid.*
88. Klingman, L., Assessing the Female Reproductive System, *American Journal of Nursing,* 99, no. 8 (1999), 37–43.
89. *Ibid.*
90. Klingman, L., Assessing the Male Genitalia, *American Journal of Nursing,* 99, no. 7 (1999), 47–50.
91. Canadian Fitness and Lifestyle Research Institute, *Physical Activity Monitor,* Website: http://www.cflri.ca/cflri/pa/surveys/2-002surveys/2002survey.html, July 2004.
92. *Ibid.*
93. Taylor, B.V., G.Y. Oudit, and M.F. Evans, Walking or Vigorous Exercise? Which Best Helps Prevent Coronary Heart Disease in Women? *Canadian Family Physician,* 46 (2000), 316–318.
94. Health Canada, *Physical Activity Guide, Physical Activity Unit,* Website: http://www.hc-sc.gc.ca/hppb/paguide/intro.html, October 2004.
95. *Ibid.*
96. Canadian Society for Exercise Physiology, *Handbook for Canada's Physical Activity Guide to Healthy Active Living,* Ottawa: Health Canada, 1998.
97. Taylor et al., *op. cit.*
98. *Ibid.*
99. Papalia and Olds, *op. cit.*
100. Taylor et al., *op. cit.*
101. *Ibid.*
102 Fenstermacher and Hudson, *op. cit.*
103. Health Canada, *Using the Food Guide,* Ottawa: Minister of Public Works and Government Services Canada, 1997.
104. Williams, S., *Nutrition and Diet Therapy* (10th ed.). St. Louis: Times Mirror/Mosby, 1995.
105. Strychar, *op. cit.*
106. Health Canada, Office of Nutrition Policy and Promotion, *Nutrition for a Healthy Pregnancy—National Guidelines for the Childbearing Years,* Website: http://www.hc-sc.gc.ca/hpfb-dgpsa/onpp-bppn/national_guidelines_05b_e.html, July 2004.
107. *Ibid.*
108. *Ibid.*
109. Vegetarianism: Should You or Shouldn't You? *Harvard Health Letter,* 24, no. 10 (1999), 7.
110. Health Canada, Office of Nutrition Policy and Promotion, *Nutrition for a Healthy Pregnancy—National Guidelines for the Childbearing Years.*
111. Duyff, *op. cit.*
112. Taylor et al., *op. cit.*
113. Williams, S., *Nutrition and Diet Therapy* (10th ed.). St. Louis: Times Mirror/Mosby, 1995.
114. Andrews, M., and J. Boyle, *Transcultural Concepts in Nursing Care* (3rd ed.). Philadelphia: Lippincott, 1999.
115. Centers for Disease Control and Prevention General Recommendations on Immunization: Recommendations of the Advisory Committee on Immunization Practices (ACIP), *Morbidity and Mortality Weekly Report,* 43 (January 28, 1994), 23.
116. *Ibid.*
117. *Ibid.*
118. Purnell, L.D., and B.J. Paulanka, *Transcultural Health Care: A Culturally Competent Approach, Second Edition,* Philadelphia: F.A. Davis Company, 2003.
119. Duyff, *op. cit.*
120. Taylor et al., *op. cit.*
121. Uphold and Graham, *op. cit.*
122. Williams, S., *Nutrition and Diet Therapy* (10th ed.). St. Louis: Times Mirror/Mosby, 1995.
123. Duyff, *op. cit.*
124. More to Life than Just Lowering Your Cholesterol, *Tuft's University Diet and Nutrition Letter,* 13, no. 8 (1995), 2–3.

125. Williams, S., *Nutrition and Diet Therapy* (10th ed.). St. Louis: Times Mirror/Mosby, 1995.
126. Caffeine and Health: The Caffeine Connection, *Harvard Women's Health Watch,* 1, no. 8 (1994), 2–3.
127. Boyd, M. and M. Nihart, *Psychiatric Nursing: Contemporary Practice.* Philadelphia: Lippincott, 1998.
128. Sperling, M., and W. Berman, *Attachment in Adults: Clinical and Developmental Perspectives.* New York: Behavioral Science Book Science, 1994.
129. Boyd and Nihart, *op. cit.*
130. Fenstermacher, K., and B. Hudson, *Practice Guidelines for Family Nurse Practitioners.* Philadelphia: Saunders, 1997.
131. Guyton, *op. cit.*
132. Intrinsically Rewarding Work Relieves Workplace Stress, *The Menninger Letter,* 3, no. 7 (1995), 3, 5.
133. Santrock, *op. cit.*
134. Tierney, L., S. McPhee, and M. Papadakis, *Current Medical Diagnosis and Treatment, 1999* (38th ed.). Stamford, CT: Appleton-Lange, 1999.
135. Guyton, *op. cit.*
136. Boyd and Nihart, *op. cit.*
137. Guyton, *op. cit.*
138. *Ibid.*
139. Tierney et al., *op. cit.*
140. Santrock, *op. cit.*
141. Thurston, Norma E., Sharon M. Tanguay, and Kristin L. Fraser, Sleep and shift work I, *The Canadian Nurse,* 96, no. 9 (2000), 35–38.
142. Statistics Canada, *The Daily,* Thursday, July 25, 2002, Shift Work and Health, Website: http://www.statcan.ca/Daily/English?020725b.htm.
143. Bootzin, R., H. Lahmeyer, and J. Lilie, eds., *Integrated Approach to Sleep Management.* Washington, DC: American Nurses Association, 1994.
144. Gormly, *op. cit.*
145. Insomnia: Get a Good Night's Sleep, *Harvard Health Letter,* 24, no. 2 (1998), 1–3.
146. Integrating an Understanding of Sleep Knowledge Into Your Practice, *The American Nurse,* November/December (1994), 24–25.
147. Seifert, K., R. Hoffnung, and M. Hoffnung, *Lifespan Development.* Boston: Houghton Mifflin, 1997.
148. Sleep Disorders—Part I, *The Harvard Mental Health Letter,* 11, no. 2 (1994), 1–4.
149. Sleep Disorders—Part II, *The Harvard Mental Health Letter,* 11, no. 3 (1994), 1–
150. Bootzin et al., *op. cit.*
151. Sleep Disorders—Part I.
152. Sleep Disorders—Part II.
153. Integrating an Understanding of Sleep Knowledge Into Your Practice.
154. Bootzin et al., *op. cit.*
155. Integrating an Understanding of Sleep Knowledge Into Your Practice.
156. Uphold and Graham, *op. cit.*
157. Bootzin et al., *op. cit.*
158. Fenstermacher, and Hudson, *op. cit.*
159. Insomnia: Get a Good Night's Sleep.
160. Sleep Disorders—Part I.
161. Sleep Disorders—Part II
162. Tierney et al., *op. cit.*
163. Uphold and Graham, *op. cit.*
164. Bootzin et al., *op. cit.*
165. Guyton, *op. cit.*
166. Sleep Disorders—Part I.
167. Sleep Disorders—Part II
168. Bootzin et al., *op. cit.*
169. Sleep Disorders—Part I
170. Sleep Disorders—Part II
171. Uphold and Graham, *op. cit.*
172. Bootzin et al., *op. cit.*
173. Integrating an Understanding of Sleep Knowledge Into Your Practice.
174. Sleep Disorders—Part I
175. Sleep Disorders—Part II
176. Uphold and Graham, *op. cit.*
177. Flemons, W.W. Symptoms of Sleep Apnea, Sleep Apnea Society of Alberta, Website: http://www.sleep-apnea.ab.ca/symptoms.htm, July 2004.
178. *Ibid.*
179. *Ibid.*
180. Gormly, *op. cit.*
181. Newman and Newman, *op. cit.*
182. Papalia and Olds, *op. cit.*
183. Burgess, A., *Psychiatric Nursing: Promoting Mental Health.* Stamford, CT: Appleton & Lange, 1997.
184. Bee, H., *Lifespan Development* (2nd ed.). New York: Loengman, 1998.
185. Santrock, *op. cit.*
186. Newman and Newman, *op. cit.*
187. Papalia and Olds, *op. cit.*
188. Seifert et al., *op. cit.*
189. Sigelman, C., *Life-Span Human Development* (3rd ed.). Pacific Grove, CA: Brooks/Cole, 1996.
190. Wadsworth, B., *Piaget's Theory of Cognitive and Affective Development: Foundations of Constructivism* (5th ed.). New York: Longman, 1996.
191. Arlin, P., Cognitive Development in Adulthood: A Fifth Stage? *Developmental Psychology,* 11, no. 5 (1975), 602–606.
192. Sternberg, R., *Beyond IQ: A Triarchic Theory of Human Intelligence.* New York: Cambridge University Press, 1985.
193. Wadsworth, *op. cit.*
194. Papalia and Olds, *op. cit.*
195. Wadsworth, *op. cit.*
196. Papalia and Olds, *op. cit*
197. Gormly, *op. cit.*
198. Bailey, K., M. Hoepner, S. Jeska, S. Schneller, and C. Wolohan, The Nurse as an Educator, *Journal of Nursing Staff Development,* 11, no. 4 (1995), 206–209.
199. Bonheur, B.B., Creating a New Learning: The Story of Art and Prudent Art, *The Journal of Continuing Education in Nursing,* 25, no. 5 (1994), 209–212.
200. Burgess, *op. cit.*
201. Gormly, *op. cit.*
202. Bemporad, J., Psychotherapy for Adults with Attention Deficit Disorder, *The Harvard Mental Health Letter,* 14, no. 12 (1998), 4–5.
203. Broom, B., Impact of Marital Quality and Psychological Well-being on Parental Sensitivity, *Nursing Research,* 43 (1994), 138–143.
204. Burgess, *op. cit.*
205. Sullivan, E., Is Campus Drinking an Antecedent to Professional Impairment? *Journal of Professional Nursing,* 11, no. 1 (1995), 4.
206. Badgers, J., Tips for Managing Stress on the Job, *American Journal of Nursing,* 95, no. 9 (1995), 31–33.
207. Gormly, *op. cit.*
208. Hochschild, A., *The Time Bind,* New York: Metropolitan, 1997.
209. Kenney, E., Creating Fulfillment in Today's Workplace, *American Journal of Nursing,* 98, no. 5 (1998), 44–48.
210. Price, *op. cit.*
211. Stress and Work, *Harvard Women's Health Watch,* 2, no. 1 (1994), 1.
212. Badgers, *op. cit.*
213. Stress and Work.
214. Kenney, *op. cit.*
215. Papalia and Olds, *op. cit.*

216. Blumenthal, T., Harassment in the Workplace, *In Brief,* Issue No. 4 (April 1999), 1–2.

217. Alderman, L., How to Tell the Boss You're Getting Worked to Death—Without Killing Your Career, *Money,* May (1995), 41–42, 44.

218. Badgers, *op. cit.*

219. Cullen, A., Burnout: Why Do We Blame The Nurse? *American Journal of Nursing,* 95, no. 11 (1995), 23–27.

220. Intrinsically Rewarding Work Relieves Workplace Stress.

221. Newman and Newman, *op. cit.*

222. Stress and Work.

223. Alderman, *op. cit.*

224. Gormly, *op. cit.*

225. Newman and Newman, *op. cit.*

226. Papalia and Olds, *op. cit.*

227. Seifert et al., *op. cit.*

228. Papalia, Diane E., Sally Wendkos, and Ruth Duskin Feldman. *Human Development, Ninth Edition,* New York: McGraw Hill Higher Education, 2004.

229. Strickland, Donna, 2000. Emotional Intelligence: The Most Potent Factor in the Success Equation, *Journal of Nursing Administration,* 30, no. 3, 112–117.

230. Gould, R., Adults Life Stages Growth Toward Self-tolerance, *Psychololgy Today,* 8, no. 7 (February 1975), 74–78.

231. Gould, R., *Transformations: Growth and Change in Adult Life.* New York: Simon & Schuster, 1978.

232. Sheehy, G., *The Silent Passage: Menopause.* New York: Random House, 1992.

233. Levinson, D., *The Seasons of a Man's Life.* New York: Ballantine Books, 1978.

234. Levinson, D., et al., Periods in the Adult Development of Men: Ages 18 to 45, *Counseling Psychologist,* 6, no. 1 (1976), 21–25.

235. Levinson, D., A Conception of Adult Development, *American Psychologist,* 41 (1986), 3–13.

236. Levinson, D., A Conception of Adult Development, *American Psychologist,* 41 (1986), 3–13.

237. Papalia and Olds, *op. cit.*

238. Newman and Newman, *op. cit.*

239. Papalia and Olds, *op. cit.*

240. Sperling and Berman, *op. cit.*

241. Seifert et al., *op. cit.*

242. Papalia and Olds, *op. cit.*

243. Gormly, *op. cit.*

244. Papalia and Olds, *op. cit.*

245. *Ibid.*

246. Smalley, G., and J. Trent, *The Language of Love.* Colorado Springs, CO: Focus on the Family, 1998.

247. Kohlberg, L., *Recent Research in Moral Development.* New York: Holt, Rinehart & Winston, 1971.

248. Newman and Newman, *op. cit.*

249. Seifert et al., *op. cit.*

250. Root, *op. cit.*

251. Papalia and Olds, *op. cit.*

252. Seifert et al., *op. cit.*

253. Sigelman, *op. cit.*

254. Seifert et al., *op. cit.*

255. *Ibid.*

256. Price, B., Assessing Altered Body Image, *Journal of Psychiatric and Mental Health Nursing,* 2 (1995), 169–175.

257. Miller, K., Body Image Therapy, *Nursing Clinics of North America,* 26, no. 3 (1991), 727–736.

258. Gormly, *op. cit.*

259. Newman and Newman, *op. cit.*

260. Papalia and Olds, *op. cit.*

261. Seifert et al., *op. cit.*

262. Bee, *op. cit.*

263. Hoff, L., *People in Crisis: Understanding and Helping* (4th ed.). Redwood City, CA: Addison-Wesley, 1995.

264. Taylor et al., *op. cit.*

265. Smith-Battle, L., Change and Continuity in Family Caregiving Practices with Young Mothers and Their Children, *IMAGE: Journal of Nursing Scholarship,* 29, no. 2 (1997), 145–149.

266. Maloni, J., and M. Ponder, Fathers' Experience of Their Partner's Antepartum Bed Rest, *IMAGE: Journal of Nursing Scholarship,* 29, no. 2 (1997), 183–18.

267. Andrews and Boyle, *op. cit.*

268. Sonkin, D., D. Martin, and L. Walker, *The Male Batterer: A Treatment Approach.* New York: Springer, 1985.

269. Health Canada, *Canadian Perinatal Surveillance System: Physical Abuse during Pregnancy,* Ottawa: Her Majesty the Queen in Right of Canada, 2004.

270. Health Canada, *Perinatal Health Indicators for Canada: A Resource Manual,* Ottawa: Minister of Public Works and Government Services Canada, 2000.

271. Cokkinides, V.E., A.L. Coker, M. Sanderson, C. Addy, and L. Bethea, Physical Violence during Pregnancy: Maternal Complications and Birth Outcomes, *Obstetrics and Gynaecology,* 93, no. 5 (1999), 661–666.

272. *Ibid.*

273. Mercer, R., and S. Ferketich, Predictors of Family Functioning Eight Months Following Birth, *Nursing Research,* 39, no. 2 (1990), 76–81.

274. Uphold and Graham, *op. cit.*

275. Health Canada, *Health Protection, Assisted Human Reproduction,* Website: http://www.hc-sc.gc.ca/english/protection/reproduction/agency.html, August 2004.

276. McCoy, Y., Adult Life Cycle Tasks/Adult Continuing Education Program Response, *Lifelong Learning in the Adult Years,* October (1977), 16.

277. Stolte, Karen M. *Wellness: Nursing Diagnosis for Health Promotion.* Philadelphia: Lippincott, 1996.

278. *Ibid.*

279. *Ibid.*

280. Risk: What It Means to You, *Harvard Women's Health Watch,* 3, no. 3 (1995), 3–4.

281. Health Canada, *Canadian Immunization Guide* (6th ed.). Ottawa: Minister of Public Works and Government Services Canada, 2002.

282. *Ibid.*

283. *Ibid.*

284. University of Manitoba, Faculty of Nursing, Student Health, Website: http://www.umanitoba.ca/academic/faculties/nursing/staffarea/handbook/Section2/studenthealth.shtml, October 2004.

285. Many Deaths Preventable, Says WHO's First Global Health Survey, *The Nation's Health,* May/June (1995), 17.

286. Health Risks: Perception and Reality, *Harvard Women's Health Watch,* 1, no. 10 (1994), 1.

287. Health Risks, *Women's Health Advocate Newsletter,* 2, no. 11, (January 1996), 2–3.

288. Hoole, A., R. G. Pickard, R. Ouimette, J. Lohr, and W. Powell, *Patient Care Guidelines for Nurse Practitioners* (5th ed.). Philadelphia & Lippincott, 1999.

289. Obesity Insights, *Harvard Women's Health Watch,* 3, no. 2 (1995), 1.

290. Zlotniek, C., and M. Cassanego, Unemployment and Health, *Nursing and Health Care,* 13, no. 2 (1993), 78–90.

291. Tierney, L., S. McPhee, and M. Papadakis, *Current Medical Diagnosis and Treatment, 1999* (38th ed.). Stamford, CT: Appleton-Lange, 1999.

292. Shah, Chandrakant P. *Public Health and Preventive Medicine in Canada* (5th ed.). Toronto: Elsevier Saunders, 2003.

293. Health Canada, *HIV/AIDS, Ministerial Council on HIV/AIDS Annual Report 2003–2004,* Website http://www.hc-sc.gc.ca/hppb/hiv_aids/can_strat/ministerial/ap_03_04/2.htm/#strategy, October 2004.

294. *Ibid.*

295. *Ibid.*

296. House of Commons, *Strengthening the Canadian Strategy on HIV/AIDS*, Report of the Standing Committee on Health, Website: http://www.parl.gc.ca/infocomdoc/37/2/HEAL/Studies/Reports/healrp03/healrp03-e.pdf, October 2004.

297. Health Canada, *HIV/AIDS, Ministerial Council on HIV/AIDS Annual Report 2003–2004.*

298. House of Commons, *Strengthening the Canadian Strategy on HIV/AIDS*, Report of the Standing Committee on Health.

299. Health Canada, *Diseases & Conditions, AIDS*, Website: http://www.hc-sc.gc.ca/english/diseases/aids.htm, July 2004.

300. Shah, *op. cit.*

301. *Ibid.*

302. Strychar, *op. cit.*

303. Gray, J., The Difficulties of Women Living with HIV Infection, *Journal of Psychosocial Nursing*, 37, no. 5 (1999), 39, 43.

304. Papalia and Olds, *op. cit.*

305. Gray, J., The Difficulties of Women Living with HIV Infection, *Journal of Psychosocial Nursing*, 37, no. 5 (1999), 39, 43.

306. Scherer, P., How AIDS Attacks the Brain, *American Journal of Nursing*, 90, no. 1 (1990), 41–52.

307. Sherer, P., How HIV Attacks the Peripheral Nervous System, *American Journal of Nursing*, 9, no. 5 (1990), 66–70.

308. Tierney et al., *op. cit.*

309. Uphold and Graham, *op. cit.*

310. Scherer, How AIDS Attacks the Brain.

311. Scherer, How HIV Attacks the Peripheral Nervous System.

312. Tierney et al., *op. cit.*

313. Scherer, How AIDS Attacks the Brain.

314. Scherer, How HIV Attacks the Peripheral Nervous System.

315. Tierney et al., *op. cit.*

316. Scherer, How AIDS Attacks the Brain.

317. Scherer, How HIV Attacks the Peripheral Nervous System.

318. Sherman, D., Guest Editor, HIV/AIDS Update, *Nursing Clinics of North America*, 34, no. 1 (1999), 1–233.

319. Tierney et al., *op. cit.*

320. Scherer, How AIDS Attacks the Brain.

321. Scherer, How HIV Attacks the Peripheral Nervous System.

322. Tierney et al., *op. cit.*

323. Scherer, How AIDS Attacks the Brain.

324. Scherer, How HIV Attacks the Peripheral Nervous System.

325. Scherer, How AIDS Attacks the Brain.

326. Scherer, How HIV Attacks the Peripheral Nervous System.

327. Sherman, How AIDS Attacks the Brain.

322. Tierney et al., *op. cit.*

329. *Ibid.*

330. Canadian Association of Nurses in AIDS Care, Website: http://www.canac.org/english/WELCOME.htm, October 2004.

331. CATIE, Website: http://www.catie.ca/e/nurses/index.htm, October 2004.

332. Canadian Nurses Association, *Position Statement, Blood-Borne Pathogens*, Website: http://www.cna-aiic.ca/pages/policies/Blood-borne%20Pathogens_Nov%202000.pdf, October 2004.

333. *Ibid.*

334. *Ibid.*

335. Sherman, *op. cit.*

336. Tierney et al., *op. cit.*

337. Uphold and Graham, *op. cit.*

338. Boyd and Nihart, *op. cit.*

339. Tierney et al., *op. cit.*

340. Sherman, *op. cit.*

341. Health Canada, *Canadian Strategy on HIV/AIDS*, Website: http://www.hc-sc.gc.ca/hppb/hiv_aids/report03/wad6.html, October 2004.

342. Malloy, P., and L. Yiu, Communicable Diseases, in L. Leeseberg Stamler and L. Yiu, eds., *Community Health Nursing: A Canadian Perspective* (pp. 187–189). Toronto: Pearson Education Canada Inc., 2005.

343. *Ibid.*

344. CBC, News In Depth, *Tuberculosis*, Website: http://www.cbc.ca/news/background/tuberculosis/, July 2004.

345. Clemen-Stone, S., D. Eigsti, and S. McGuire, *Comprehensive Family and Community Health Nursing* (4th ed.). St. Louis: C.V. Mosby, 1995.

346. Many Deaths Preventable, Says WHO's First Global Health Survey.

347. Canada's Role in Fighting Tuberculosis, *Tuberculosis Prevention*, Website: http://www.lung.ca/tb/index.html, July 2004.

348. Health Canada, *National Statistics and Trends, Injury in Canada*, Website: http://www.injurypreventionstrategy.ca/downloads/HC_stat.pdf, October 2004.

349. *Ibid.*

350. Canadian Cancer Society, *General Cancer Stats*, Website: http://www.cancer.ca/ccs/internet/standard/0,2283,3172_14423_langId-en,00.html, October 2004.

351. Spencer-Cisek, P. Overview of Cancer Prevention, Screening, and Detection, *Nurse Practitioner Forum*, 9, no. 3 (1998), 134–146.

352. Canadian Cancer Society, *Breast Cancer Stats*, Website: http://www.cancer.ca/ccs/internet/standard/0,3182,3172_14435_langId-en,00.html, October 2004.

353. Health Canada, *It's Your Health, Reducing the Risk of Breast Cancer*, Website: http://www.hc-sc.gc.ca/english/iyh/diseases/breast_cancer.htm, October 2004.

354. American Cancer Society. *Cancer Facts and Figures—1997.* Atlanta: American Cancer Society, 1997

355. Bailey et al., *op. cit.*

356. Klingman, Assessing the Female Reproductive System.

357. Uphold and Graham, *op. cit.*

358. Klingman, Assessing the Female Reproductive System.

359. Klingman, L., Assessing the Female Reproductive System, *American Journal of Nursing*, 99, no. 8 (1999), 37–43.

360. Klingman, Assessing the Female Reproductive System.

361. Fenstermacher and Hudson, *op. cit.*

362. Melanoma: It's Affecting More and Younger Women: Here's What to Look For, *Women's Health Advocate Newsletter*, 4, no. 2 (1997), 1–2.

363. Tierney et al., *op. cit.*

364. Uphold and Graham, *op. cit.*

365. Caffeine and Health: The Caffeine Connection.

366. Hatherill, R., *Eat to Beat Cancer.* New York: St. Martin's Press, 1999.

367. Duyff, *op. cit.*

368. Hatherill, *op. cit.*

369. Health Canada, *Physical Activity Guide, Physical Activity Unit.*

370. Fenstermacher and Hudson, *op. cit.*

371. Guyton, *op. cit.*

372. Tierney et al., *op. cit.*

373. Marrett, L.D., J. Frood, D. Nishri, A-M Ugnat, and the Cancer in Young Adults in Canada (CYAC) Working Group, Cancer Incidence in Young Adults in Canada: Preliminary Results of a Cancer Surveillance Project, *Chronic Diseases in Canada*, 23, no. 2 (2002), 58–64.

374. *Ibid.*

375. Health Canada, *Special Report on Youth Piercing, Tattooing, and Hepatitis C: Trends and Findings*, Ottawa: Population and Public Health Branch, 2001.

376. *Ibid.*

377. Health Canada, *Population and Public Health Branch, Hepatitis C in Canada*, Website: http://www.hc-sc.gc.ca/pphb-dgspsp/publicat/ccdr-rmtc/01pdf/27s3e.pdf, July 2004.

378. *Ibid.*

379. Zou, S., M. Tepper, and A. Giulivi, Current Status of Hepatitis C in Canada, *Canadian Journal of Public Health,* 91S1 (2000), S10-S15.
380. Hepatitis C Society of Canada, *Hepatitis C in Depth,* Website: http://www.hepatitiscsociety.com/english/HepCInDepth.htm, July 2004.
381. *Ibid.*
382. Andrews and Boyle, *op. cit.*
383. Hoole et al., *op. cit.*
384. Boyd and Nihart, *op. cit.*
385. Burgess, *op. cit.*
386. Taylor et al., *op. cit.*
387. Boyd and Nihart, *op. cit.*
388. Burgess, *op. cit.*
389. Taylor et al., *op. cit.*
390. Postpartum Disorders, *The Harvard Mental Health Letter,* 14, no. 2 (1997), 1–4.
391. Bolaria, B.S., and R. Bolaria, Women's Lives, Women's Health, in B.S. Bolaria and H.D. Dickinson, eds., *Health, Illness, and Health Care in Canada* (3rd ed., pp. 169–173). Toronto: Nelson, Thomson Learning, 2002.
392. *Ibid.*
393. Boyd and Nihart, *op. cit.*
394. Burgess, *op. cit.*
395. Price, *op. cit.*
396. Boyd and Nihart, *op. cit.*
397. Burgess, *op. cit.*
398. Boyd and Nihart, *op. cit.*
399. Burgess, *op. cit.*
400. Hoff, *op. cit.*
401. Boyd and Nihart, *op. cit.*
402. Burgess, *op. cit.*
403. Hoff, *op. cit.*
404. Boyd and Nihart, *op. cit.*
405. Burgess, *op. cit.*
406. Boyd and Nihart, *op. cit.*
407. Burgess, *op. cit.*
408. Boyd and Nihart, *op. cit.*
409. Burgess, *op. cit.*
410. Kelleher, K., M. Chaffin, J. Hollenberg, and E. Fischer, Alcohol and Drug Disorders Among Physically Abusive and Neglectful Parents in a Community-based Sample, *American Journal of Public Health,* 84 (1994), 1586–1590.
411. Boyd and Nihart, *op. cit.*
412. Burgess, *op. cit.*
413. Evans, K., and J. Sullivan, *Treating Addicted Survivors of Trauma.* New York: Guilford Press, 1995
414. Boyd and Nihart, *op. cit.*
415. Burgess, *op. cit.*
416. Chen, K., and D. Kandel, The National History of Drug Use from Adolescence to the Mid-thirties in a General Population Sample, *American Journal of Public Health,* 85 (1995), 41–47.
417. Evans and Sullivan, *op. cit.*
418. Fenstermacher and Hudson, *op. cit.*
419. Gfroerer, J., and M. Brodsley, Frequent Cocaine Users and Their Use of Treatment, *American Journal of Public Health,* 83 (1993), 1149–1154.
420. Kelleher et al., *op. cit.*
421. Statistics Canada, *Family Violence in Canada: A Statistical Profile, 2004.* Ottawa: Minister of Industry, 2004.
422. *Ibid.*
423. *Ibid.*
424. Boyd and Nihart, *op. cit.*
425. Burgess, *op. cit.*
426. Miller, K., Compulsive Overeating, *Nursing Clinics of North America,* 26, no. 3 (1991), 699–705.

427. Tierney et al., *op. cit.*
428. Fenstermacher and Hudson, *op. cit.*
429. Tierney et al., *op. cit.*
430. Taylor et al., *op. cit.*
431. Loria, C., T. Bush, M. Carroll, A. Looker, et al., Macronutrient Intakes Among Adult Hispanics: A Comparison of Mexican Americans, Cuban Americans, and Mainland Puerto Ricans, *American Journal of Public Health,* 85 (1995), 684–689.
432. Canadian Fitness and Lifestyle Research Institute, Physical Activity Monitor.
433. Loria et al., *op. cit.*
434. New Aid for Smoking Cessation, *Focus on Healthy Aging,* 2, no. 1 (1999), 2.
435. Taylor et al., *op. cit.*
436. Lindell, K., and L., Reinke, Nursing Strategies for Smoking Cessation, *ANA Continuing Education Independent Study Module,* American Nurses Association, May 6, 1999, A1–A6.
437. Statistics Canada, *Family Violence in Canada: A Statistical Profile, 2004.*
438. Patterson, J. Spousal Violence, in *Family Violence in Canada: A Statistical Profile,* Canadian Centre for Justice Statistics. Ottawa: Statistics Canada, 2003.
439. Draucker, C., Impact of Violence in the Lives of Women: Restriction and Resolve, *Issues in Mental Health,* 18 (1997), 59–80.
440. Hoff, *op. cit.*
441. Burgess, A., W. Fehder, and C. Hartman, Delayed Reporting of the Rape Victim, *Journal of Psychosocial Nursing,* 33, no. 9 (1995), 21–29.
442. Draucker, *op. cit.*
443. Hoff, *op. cit.*
444. Ledray, L. and S. Arndt, Examining the Sexual Assault Victim: A New Model for Nursing Care, *Journal of Psychosocial Nursing,* 32, no. 2 (1994), 7–12.
445. O'Campo, P., A. Grelen, R. Faden, N. Xine, N. Kass, and N. Wang, Violence by Male Partners against Women During the Childbearing Years. A Contextual Analysis, *American Journal of Public,* 85 (1995), 1092–1097.
446. Sonkin et al., *op. cit.*
447. Canadian Nurses Association, *Position Statement, Violence,* Website: http://www.cna-aiic.ca/, October 2004.
448. *Ibid.*
449. Hoff, *op. cit.*
450. Boyd and Nihart, *op. cit.*
451. Burgess, *op. cit.*
452. Campbell, J., If I Can't Have You, No One Can: Murder Linked to Battery During Pregnancy, *Reflections,* Third Quarter (1999), 6–12.
453. Draucker, *op. cit.*
454. Hoff, *op. cit.*
455. Wright, J., A.G. Burgess, A.W. Burgess, G. McCrary, and J. Douglas, Investigating Stalking Crimes, *Journal of Psychosocial Nursing,* 33, no. 9 (1995), 38–46.
456. Boyd and Nihart, *op. cit.*
457. Burgess, *op. cit.*
458. Burgess, *op. cit.*
459. Ledray, *op. cit.*
460. Campbell, A., and P. Alford. The Dark Consequences of Marital Rape, *American Journal of Nursing,* 89, no. 7 (1989), 846–849.
461. Hoff, *op. cit.*
462. Holtzworth and Monroe, A., Marital Violence, *The Harvard Mental Health Letter,* 12, no. 2 (1995), 4–6.
463. O'Campo et al., *op. cit.*
464. Boyd and Nihart, *op. cit.*
465. Burgess, *op. cit.*
466. Draucker, *op. cit.*
467. Hoff, *op. cit.*

468. Sexual Abuse: The Longest Legacy, *Women's Health Advocate Newsletter,* 3, no. 4 (1996), 4–5.
469. O'Campo et al., *op. cit.*
470. Sexual Abuse: The Longest Legacy.
471. Sonkin, D., D. Martin, and L. Walker, *The Male Batterer: A Treatment Approach.* New York: Springer, 1985.
472. *Ibid.*
473. *Ibid.*
474. Draucker, *op. cit.*
475. Hoff, *op. cit.*
476. Miles, A., When Faith Is Used to Justify Abuse, *American Journal of Nursing,* 99, no. 5 (1999), 32–35.
477. Boyd and Nihart, *op. cit.*
478. Burgess, *op. cit.*
479. Campbell and Alford, *op. cit.*
480. Hoff, *op. cit.*
481. Sexual Abuse: The Longest Legacy.
482. Boyd and Nihart, *op. cit.*
483. Burgess, *op. cit.*
484. Draucker, *op. cit.*
485. Nikstaitis, G., Therapy for Men Who Batter, *Journal of Psychosocial Nursing,* 23, no. 7 (1985), 33–36.
486. Sonkin et al., *op. cit.*
487. Hall, L., B. Sachs, and M. Rayens, Mothers' Potential for Child Abuse: The Roles of Childhood Abuse and Social Resources, *Nursing Research,* 47, no. 2 (1998), 87–95.
488. Sachs, B., L. Holly, M. Lutenbacher, and M. Rayens, Potential for Abusive Parenting by Rural Mothers with Low-Birth-Weight Children, *IMAGE: Journal of Nursing Scholarship,* 31, no. 1 (1999), 21–25.
489. Campbell and Alford, *op. cit.*
490. Hoff, *op. cit.*
491. Wright, L., and M. Leahey, *Nursing Families: A Guide to Family Assessment and Intervention* (2nd ed.). Philadelphia: F.A. Davis, 1994.
492. Hoff, L., *Battered Women as Suvivors.* New York: Routledge, 1990.
493. Broom, *op. cit.*
494. Gormly, *op. cit.*
495. Papalia and Olds, *op. cit.*
496. Seifert et al., *op. cit.*
497. Newman and Newman, *op. cit.*
498. Child and Family Canada, *Divorce: Facts, Figures, and Consequences,* Website: http://www.cfc-efc.ca/docs/vanif/00005_en.htm, July 2004.
499. *Ibid.*
500. *Ibid.*
501. CNEWS, *Canada: Risk of Divorce Declines over Time: STATSCAN,* Website: http://cnews.canoe.ca/CNEWS/Canada/2004/05/04/pf-446835.html, July 2004.
502. *Ibid.*
503. Seifert et al., *op. cit.*
504. Gormly, *op. cit.*
505. Newman and Newman, *op. cit.*
506. Papalia and Olds, *op. cit.*
507. Gormly, *op. cit.*
508. Hoff, *op. cit.*
509. Newman and Newman, *op. cit.*
510. Papalia and Olds, *op. cit.*
511. Seifert et al., *op. cit.*
512. Newman and Newman, *op. cit.*
513. Fowler, D., and K.J. Trouton, Should Abortion Reporting Continue in Canada? *Canadian Journal of Public Health,* 91, no. 5 (2000), 396–397.
514. Macionis, J.J., and L.M. Gerber, *Sociology* (4th Canadian ed.). Toronto: Prentice Hall, 2002.
515. *Ibid.*
516. Heuermann, P., and J., Interview—Twenty-fifth Wedding Anniversary Invitation, August 1988, Des Moines, IA.

Chapter 13

ASSESSMENT AND HEALTH PROMOTION FOR THE MIDDLE-AGED PERSON

Forty is the old age of youth.
Fifty is the youth of old age.

Victor Hugo

OBJECTIVES

STUDY OF THIS CHAPTER WILL ENABLE YOU TO:

1. Explore with middle-aged persons ideas about their generation, lifestyle, and the conflict they see among generations.

2. Discuss the family relationships and sexual development of the middle-aged adult, conflicts that are to be resolved, and your role in helping the family work through issues and conflicts.

3. List the developmental tasks for the middle-aged family, and give examples of how these tasks can be accomplished.

4. Discuss the emotional, social, economic, and lifestyle changes usually encountered by the widow(er).

5. Describe the hormonal changes of middle age and the resultant changes in physical appearance and body image.

6. Discuss the nutritional, rest, leisure, work, and exercise needs of the middle-aged adult, factors that interface with achieving those needs, and your role in promoting their health.

7. Describe how the middle-aged adult's cognitive skills and emotional and moral development influence your nursing care practice.

8. Debate the developmental crisis of this era and its significance to social well-being.

9. Compare and contrast the behaviour of generativity, or maturity, and self-absorption, or stagnation, and related adaptive mechanisms.

10. Describe the developmental tasks for the middle-aged person and your role in helping him or her accomplish these tasks.

11. Explore with a middle-aged adult strategies to promote health.

12. Assess the body image, physical, mental, and emotional characteristics, and family relationships of a middle-aged person.

13. Plan and implement effective care to a middle-aged person.

Middle age does not exist in every country; it is attributed to improved nutrition, control of communicable disease, discovery and control of familial disease, and other medical advances. In North America, life has been stretched in the middle; what used to be old age is now middle age. Most non-Westernized and preindustrial cultures recognize only mature adulthood, followed by old age. In some countries, the average life span is shorter than the age span that constitutes middle age in North America.

Further, as the work structure and roles and technologic development become more complex, as family life and child-drearing patterns change toward smaller families and a longer post-parental period, the periods of childhood and youth are lengthened. Thus, middle age has become a distinct life period. New concepts of adulthood involve a change in definitions of gender and age roles. Midlife development implies growth of the personality to encompass some characteristics that had stereotypically been assigned to the opposite sex. Thus, biology diminishes its influence on much of what had been held to be immutably biological characteristics. Individuals may also work out more flexible adaptations. Middle adulthood is a time of widening social interest in which the family becomes increasingly oriented to its responsibility to the greater society.

Defining middle age is a nebulous task. Chronologically, **middle age** *covers the years of approximately 45 to 65 or even 70, but each person will also consider the physiologic age condition of the body and psychological age—how old he or she acts and feels.*[1,2] Many people today consider themselves young until nearly age 50 and middle-aged until around 70 years. Age assignment varies according to social class; the person living in poverty perceives the prime or midpoint of life to vary from the mid-20s to 40. People who were in their 50s at the millennium are called "the baby boomer generation." They have lived through an affluent era that has kept them young physically, and they perceive themselves as youthful and in control as they enter the second half of life.

Some couples in this age bracket may actually be middle-aged chronologically but be pursuing the developmental tasks of young adulthood. If the couple first has children or the person remarries and has stepchildren in the 40s, the couple will have teenagers in their late 50s or early 60s. They may have less time for middle-age tasks and may want to retire when their children need college money and are still living at home.

Because of changing demographics, an increasing number of North Americans are considered middle-aged. They earn most of the money, pay a major portion of the bills and most of the taxes, and make many of the decisions. Thus, the power in government, politics, education, religion, science, business, industry, and communication is wielded not by the young or the old, but by the middle-aged.

Middle age is a time of relatively good physical and mental health, new personal freedom, and maximum command of self and influence over the social environment. At work the person has increasing ability to make decisions, hold high-status jobs, and earn a maximum income. The person has expanding family networks and social roles.

In her book, *The Silent Passage: Menopause,* Gail Sheehy describes middle age and the post menopause as a time of health and zest, a "second adulthood" for women.[3] That also applies to middle-aged men.[4]

CRITICAL THINKING

Glance through a few fashion magazines. How are middle-aged men and women portrayed by the media?

FAMILY DEVELOPMENT AND RELATIONSHIPS

The following information will assist you in understanding the middle-aged family system in assessing and in promoting health.

Relationship with Children

The **generation gap,** the *conflict between parents and adolescents,* may have always existed to some degree. The experience of the parent generation, and therefore their values and expectations, differs from that of their offspring. Actually the generation lines are blurring. Some presently middle-aged adults, perhaps out of fear of their own mortality, are looking and acting more like their children. These adults would rather think of themselves as carefree, innocent, and young. The changing attitudes, values, behaviour, and dress of middle-aged persons reflect our cultural emphasis on youth and beauty, versus tradition and wisdom, and our more informal society. Yet, each generation is concerned about the other, although for different reasons. In fact, the younger and older generations can successfully combine efforts to work for legislation, policy changes, or social justice.

There is a difference in values and lifestyle between the early and late middle-agers (see Table 1-2). In contrast to the baby-boomers, the late middle-aged adult was born sometime between the late 1920s and early 1940s. Values and behaviour have been influenced by growing up with inadequate material resources after the Great Depression and during World War II and by rapid social and technologic changes that occurred after World War II and during the 1950s and 1960s. The generation gap may be as much between early and late middle-agers as between middle-agers and their offspring.

The nuclear family is no longer prominent in North America, and we mostly discount learning from elders. The offspring cannot be fully prepared for the future by the parent generation. Youth must develop new patterns of behaviour based

on the changing world, their own experience, and that of peers. The present affluence, emphasis on age differences and independence, blurring of sex differences, and insistence on a unique lifestyle that is characteristic of today's younger people add to the conflict for late middle-agers—both value conflicts and envy of the younger people. Youth's seeking of control over self and cultural institutions and living various lifestyle options may be better understood by younger middle-aged persons. Negative reactions of offspring to societal problems or to their parents' lifestyles reawaken in parents or late middle-agers some personal conflicts. They remember early personal commitments to ideals that became compromised over the years to fit narrower concerns. The addition of innate parental feelings of affection, admiration, and compassion for youth to the negative feelings produces ambivalence.[5]

Social mobility, *in which the child moves away from the social position, educational level, class, occupation, or ethnicity of parents,* causes offspring overtly to forsake parental teaching and seek new models of behaviour. The mass media and societal trends help to set standards and expectations about behaviour that may be counter to parental teaching or wishes. Rapid social changes and awareness that much about the future is unknown threaten established faiths and stimulate attraction to new ideologies and exceptional behaviour. This is particularly difficult for immigrant and refugee families.[6]

Discuss with middle-aged persons what they as adults have to offer their children. They are the only generation to ever know, experience, and incorporate such rapid technological and scientific changes into daily life and the job. They can give their offspring imaginative, innovative, and dedicated adult care, a safe and flexible environment in which children can be given support, feel secure, grow, and discover themselves and the world. Reaffirm that it is up to the parents to teach *not what* to learn but *how to learn, not what to be* committed to but the *value of commitment.* Explain to parents that research shows the continuity of values from generation to generation within a family. Typically the values of young adults are more similar to their parents' values than to those of other adults or peers. This is true in North American society as well as in other societies.[7] Help youth to ask questions adults do not think of but yet to trust their parents enough to work on the answers together. The middle-aged parent can be encouraged to listen and exchange information and ideas honestly and with a sense of humour. If the parent works to maintain open communication, the generation gap may be minimal. Your work with families can promote greater harmony.

Divorce of offspring is an increasing area of concern for middle-aged parents. The parents may feel shock (or relief if they did not like the child's spouse). They may believe that their effort and help in getting the child "out of the nest" through marriage or helping the couple set up a home were to no avail. This feeling may be especially strong if the divorced family member decides to live at the parents' home again. The parents may blame their child or the in-laws and may criticize the couple for not working on the marital problems as the middle-aged parents have done.[8–10]

If younger children are still at home, their needs and desires may be temporarily neglected because the emphasis is on the divorce crisis. Furthermore, the younger children may have to give back a room to the returning divorced brother or sister. The parents, in an attempt to make the divorced family member feel comfortable, may negate their own new patterns of freedom. If the divorced son or daughter is in a financial crisis, the parents' money may also go to help him or her instead of being used as originally planned. If the divorcing couple has children, additional strain will be added.

The divorce may not have a completely negative effect on the middle-aged parents. If the parents have a healthy self-esteem and an ability to proceed cautiously, they may help their offspring to gain the essential maturity that he or she was previously lacking. However, the crisis and stages of grief that accompany divorce and loss of a family member are still keenly felt.[11,12]

Young adults may return home to live with parents for reasons other than separation or divorce. Some new university graduates cannot find a job of their choice or are finding that their first jobs are not paying enough for them to cover high rents along with other costs of living, so they are living with parents until they can accumulate some money or can move to higher-income jobs. Some young adult children return home more than once until they finally become independent.

This may cause stress, as most middle-aged parents look forward to having children leave the home—the so-called "empty nest."[13–15] The middle-aged adult wants space, time, and financial resources to pursue personal, organizational, and civic goals rather than to continue child care responsibilities. Prolonged dependence of young adult offspring may also create conflict with grandparents and other children who are still at home.

The *grandparent role* has a different dimension in middle age than in later maturity, although people become grandparents during the middle-age era, or even in late young adulthood. The middle-aged person is not necessarily happy about being a grandparent, because that may indicate old age to them.

If the offspring has established his or her own home and has a family, grandparenthood is a happy status and role. The relationship to the grandchild is informal and playful; the child is a source of fun, leisure activity, and self-indulgence. Emphasis is on mutual satisfaction, authority lines are irrelevant, and the child is seen as someone for whom to buy gifts.[16–18] Because of the recent increases in the number of baby boomers becoming grandparents, grandparent–grandchild relationships have begun to receive more research attention.[19] For example, research findings suggest that regular interactions with grandparents usually leave children with fewer prejudices about old people.[20]

If the adult offspring is divorced and brings young grandchildren into the middle-aged adult's home or if the offspring is unmarried and has children, the sense of responsibility and loss of independence are heightened. The middle-aged woman, especially, may resent the demands and constraints placed on her by having young children, including grandchildren, in the home full-time. The carefree relationship is less likely if the grandchild lives in the home with the middle-aged person. Further, having extra children and grandchildren in the home interferes with the relationship with the spouse. Normal developmental tasks cannot be met. The return of

children to the home and the resultant demands may also serve to prevent the middle-aged woman from attempting to pursue new career goals.

In the case of divorce, the middle-aged grandparents wonder what their future relationship with their grandchildren will be. Relations may be strained between the in-laws as each family wonders how to interact with the other. Recent cordiality and affection may turn to anger and criticism. Currently, grandparents are raising their grandchildren because their children have died, are divorced, or are incapacitated through drugs or other devastating problems. The increase in the rate of divorce among Canadian families and in the number of children affected by divorce, has resulted in the emergence of "grandparents' rights groups" across the country.[21]

Increasingly you will be caring for middle-aged parents who are being threatened emotionally or are having social or financial problems because of their children's separation or divorce. Use the principles of crisis intervention described in Chapter 5, as well as principles of communication and crisis intervention described in other texts.[22–24] Parents should be cautioned to proceed carefully with financial assistance. The middle-aged grandparents may also need encouragement in securing visitation rights when divorce or death has severed the relationship. Help the middle-aged couple regain a sense of self-esteem, a sense of confidence in setting limits so that they can pursue their own life goals, and a method of working through decisions and problems with the young adult offspring.

CRITICAL THINKING

Talk to a few grandmothers and grandfathers. How do they see their role in grandparenting? From their statements, what do you conclude about grandparenting today?

Relationship with Spouse

Equally important as rearing the children and establishing wholesome affectional ties with them, and later with the grandchildren, is the middle-aged adult's relationship with the spouse.

A *happy marriage* has security and stability, although there are also struggles. The couple knows each other well; they no longer have to pretend with each other. Children can be a source of pleasure rather than concern, because conflicts that arose between partners about rearing or disciplining children vanish when the children leave home. Each knows that his or her way of life and well-being depend on the other. Each has become accustomed to the way of the other. There is increased shared activity, and the sexual relationship can be better than ever before. Because the middle-aged adult is likely to have roots firmly implanted in the community of choice, he or she is able to cultivate warm friendships with members of the generation and with parents, the family of the spouse, and families of married children.

Although there has been much discussion in the literature about the crisis of menopause and the "empty nest," menopause and middle age may bring both men and women an enriched sense of self and enhanced capacity to cope with life. The timing of the "empty nest" in the family life cycle depends on the person's (or the couple's) age when the last child was born.[25] The empty nest, in recent years, has become increasingly "cluttered." Adult children are remaining at home until later years, and some adult children are returning (sometimes several times) to the parental home. Therefore, rates of adult child–middle-aged parent(s) co-residency have increased in the last few decades.[26] These young adult children returning to the parental home are sometimes referred to as the boomerang kids.[27] Research indicates that the presence of boomerang kids does not negatively affect the marriages of middle-aged parents.[28] Mothers, in particular, are pleased to have their children back. However, boomerang kids can have a disruptive effect if they "bounce" back and forth several times. However, this pattern is not common.[29]

CRITICAL THINKING

Is the "cluttered empty nest" syndrome a fact or fiction in different cultural groups? State your rationale for your opinion.

Negative Marital Relationship

Negative, critical feelings can gradually erode what was apparently a happy relationship. At some point the husband and wife may feel they are each living with a stranger, although the potential still exists for a harmonious marriage. Their relationship is changing because they are changing. *Marital crisis may result from:*

1. Feelings of disappointment with self
2. Feeling depleted emotionally because of lack of communication with the spouse
3. Seeking rebirth or changing directions
4. Seeking escape from reality and superego pressures[30–33]

In contrast, *two factors are predictive of successful long-term marriages:* (1) congruence of perceptions between spouses of the marriage and each other and (2) sexual satisfaction.[34,35]

Often the woman and man overlook that they still do really love each other. They simply have to become reacquainted. It may be difficult for the middle-aged man and woman to "tune in" to each other because both are encountering problems peculiar to their own sex. The woman may equate ability to bear children with capacity to enjoy sexual relationships, although they have nothing to do with each other. Whereas the woman needs the man's support to reinforce her femininity, he too is undergoing a crisis; he believes that he is losing his vigour, virility, and self-esteem, which are products primarily of psychological reactions rather than physiologic inabilities.

The middle-aged person is an active sexual being. Physical changes in appearance and energy and the multiple stresses of daily living may result in an increased desire for physical intimacy and the need for reassurance of continuing sexual attractiveness and competency. Intercourse is not valued for procreation but for body contact, to express love and trust, and to reaffirm an integral part of the self-concept. The person may fear loss of potency and rejection by the partner, but talking with the spouse about feelings and preferences related to sexual activity can promote increased closeness.

Men and women differ in their sexual behaviour. Males reach their peak in their late teens and early 20s. Females peak in desire in the late 30s or 40s and maintain that level of desire and activity past the menopause into late middle age. The enjoyment of sexual relations in younger years, rather than the frequency, is a key factor for maintenance of desire and activity in women, whereas frequency of relations and enjoyment are important factors for men.[36–39]

Extramarital Relationship

Relationships with work colleagues may set the stage for an extramarital affair. Although divorce occurs during these years, the extramarital affair does not necessarily lead to the divorce courts. Divorce is major surgery, and the man may be reluctant to cut that much out of his life. Besides, he may find, having aroused the ardour of the younger woman, that he is no match for her physical demands. With increased consciousness of his age, he may return to his wife, particularly if she has in the meantime assessed her own situation, remained committed, and changed behaviour.[40–43]

In the community mental health setting you will increasingly work with troubled families who are contemplating divorce or who have experienced separation and divorce.

Reducing Marital and Partnership Stress

Helping the couple regain closeness and happiness is worth the effort, for the mature years can be regarded as the payoff on an investment of many years together, many problems shared, and countless expressions of love exchanged. Each knows that his or her way of life and well-being depend on the other, so there is a willingness to change outlook, habits, and lovemaking, if necessary, to enhance their marriage and partnership. You can promote such changes.

You may teach or counsel the middle-aged adult who is having difficulty in relating to his or her spouse or partner. Help the person determine, and then live out, the values of continuing to love and being patient and forgiving when the spouse or partner has been unfaithful. Facilitate a desire to change behaviour so that two people can grow together rather than apart. Work with the couple or refer them to counselling.

The following *guidelines for couples may help them reduce stress in the marriage or partnership:*

- Talk daily to each other about feelings so that small problems are solved continually, rather than allowing emotional tensions to accumulate, creating a breaking-point scene.
- Explore with each other feelings and ideas about possible, even if unlikely, life events that may occur—"what if" conversations. Such anticipatory problem-solving and critical thinking helps the couple expand the repertoire of ideas and behaviour so that if unexpected events occur, each will have more adaptive resources.
- Vary schedules and chores, family goals or expectations, and roles and rules, or make other periodic changes, just to stay comfortable with change and to be prepared to adapt if a crisis requiring flexibility occurs.
- Use each other as a resource. Talk to each other about individual problems, validate solutions, or ask each other

about options for dealing with problems. Each must be willing to disclose about self to the other and be willing to support and help the other.

■ Maintain contact with others, including the extended family and friends, who can help during a crisis. Sometimes the family does not exist or cannot be supportive; seek other resources such as a church or other support groups or networks.

■ In times of high stress or crisis, each should express the feelings of anger, grief, or helplessness to the other and to others who are caring. Expressing feelings about the circumstance, not about the spouse, allows conflict to surface and be handled.

■ Keep active with each other and with others. Doing so prevents feelings either of stagnation during routine times, or of helplessness during stressful times.

CRITICAL THINKING

What may be some other ways of reducing stress in same-sex marriages or partnerships?

Loss of Spouse

Widow(er)hood, the *status change that results from death of husband (or wife),* is a crisis in any life era, but it is more likely to occur first in middle age. The 2001 Canadian census data indicates that approximately 3% of men and 8% of women between the ages of 50 and 54 were widowed; by the age of 65 and over, these figures increase to 27% among men and 48% among women.[44]

The person who is about to become a widow(er) usually appreciates being able to participate in care of the spouse but must feel that the wife or husband will not suffer lack of care or support if a few hours are taken for rest. She or he needs someone to listen to feelings of anger, sadness, and guilt. You may be better able to listen, support, and encourage than family or friends. You can gently test reactions to determine if he or she is ready for the shock of death by offering to call a clergyperson or by asking if family members need to be prepared for deterioration of the spouse's condition. After death the person may linger on the nursing unit—a place of support—rather than leaving for home, a very empty place.

The person's reaction to death of a spouse depends on personality and emotional makeup, the relationship between the couple (how long they have been married, how long the mate has been ill), and religious, cultural, and ethnic background. It will also be determined by other factors that existed in the relationship; for example, there may be less sorrow, or even relief, if the dead spouse was abusive, or severely or chronically disabled, either physically or mentally.

The *loss of a spouse may mean many things:*

1. Loss of a sexual partner and lover, friend, companion, caretaker.

2. Loss of an audience for unguarded spontaneous conversation.

3. Loss of a "handy man," a helper, an accountant, plumber, or gardener, depending on the roles performed by the mate.

4. Financial problems, especially for the widow.

5. Secondary losses involving reduced income, which frequently means change in residence, environment, lifestyle, and social involvements.

6. Return to the workforce.

7. Giving up any number of things previously taken for granted.

The *widow* may be a threat to women with husbands; they perceive her as competition, and she is a reminder of what they might experience. With friends the widow is the odd person in number, so social engagements become stressful and are a constant reminder of the lost partner. The widow also becomes aware that she is regarded as a sexual object to men who may offer her their sexual services at a time when she has decreased sexual desires but a great need for companionship and closeness. Yet in contrast to assumptions, most widows are quite competent in managing their lives.[45]

Although the *widower* is more accepted socially, he too will have painful gaps in his life. If the wife concentrated on keeping an orderly house, cooking regular and nutritious meals, and keeping his wardrobe in order, he may suddenly realize that what he had taken for granted is gone. Even more significant is the loss if his wife was a "sounding board" or confidante in business matters and if she was actively involved in raising children still in the home.

Your contact with the widower(er) can help to resolve the crisis. Death of a husband in middle age is more common than that of a wife; you will encounter more widows. You can *assist the person in the following ways as you promote crisis resolution:*

1. Encourage the bereaved to talk about feelings, and help the widow(er) to find a supportive relationship.

2. Build up confidence and self-esteem in the widow(er) especially if he or she has lived a protected life.

3. Help her (or him) identify people other than the children who can assist with various tasks to avoid feelings of burden in any helper.

4. Encourage her (or him) to try new experiences, to expand interests, to join community groups, do volunteer work, seek new friends, and become a person in their own right.

5. Encourage getting a medical check-up and following practices of health promotion. Encourage self-care.

6. Inform her (or him) that books and articles can be useful to the widow(er).[46,47]

Caserta, Lund, and Rice have developed a Pathfinder Program that teaches widows and widowers many skills and promotes good self-care behaviours.[48] Some of the important topics in this intervention include stress management, immunizations, health screenings, medication management, physical and social activities, meal planning and preparation, and housekeeping skills.[49] In fact, learning new skills is one of the best ways to build self-esteem—at any age.

CRITICAL THINKING

If you were asked to develop a program for bereaved widow and widowers in the community, how would you begin?

The Gay Widower and His Partner's Family

You have been providing care to John, a gay middle-aged client who has just lost his partner of 20 years to cancer. John informs you that he is unable to attend his partner's funeral because the family has told John that he was not invited. John confides to you that he is quite depressed and is worried about his own future—both personally and professionally. He states that the family does not acknowledge that their son was gay or that he was living with another man for the past 20 years. John is aware that you know his partner's family well, as he has often seen you interact with them. From your discussions with the family, you know that they are ashamed of their son's gay lifestyle. John pleads with you to intervene on his behalf in an attempt to allow him to attend the funeral.

1. How do you respond initially to John?

2. How would you assist John to help him to build his self-esteem?

3. What strategies will you employ with this family?

Relationship with Aging Parents and Relatives

According to Chappell, Gee, McDonald, and Stones the "sandwich generation" refers to midlife families, especially women, who are caught between the care demands of children and the care demands of aging parents.[50] A study conducted by Rosenthal, Martin-Matthews, and Matthews used data from over 5000 persons who were 34 to 64 years of age in 1990. They distinguished between those who have a structural potential to be "sandwiched" (i.e., have a living parent, a dependent child, and a paying job) and those who in reality actually have an aging parent who needs their assistance and who also have competing intergenerational responsibilities.[51] Their results indicated 35 percent of women in their late 40s, and a much smaller proportion of women after the age of 50, have the structural potential for sandwiching. Among these women, the highest percentage in any group who provide assistance to a parent at least once a month is only 7 percent.[52] Thus, the actual element of sandwiching is not a common phenomenon.[53] In fact, caregiving to elderly parents tends to occur after the dependent children have left home. Martin-Matthews states that the notion of the sandwich generation is largely a myth.[54] However, the relatively few Canadians who become sandwiched between two generations do have a heavy burden.

CRITICAL THINKING

What are some life choices available for women who get caught or sandwiched between two generations?

Responsibility for Elderly Relatives

The following cultural trends affect the dilemma of caring for older dependent relatives:[55–58]

- Long-term societal emphasis on personal independence and social mobility of middle-aged and young adults, which creates physical separateness of generational households and new kinship patterns of intimacy at a distance
- Focusing on the dynamics of the marriage bond and socialization of young children, with the emphasis on affection, compatibility, and personal growth of each person in the nuclear family as the most important aspects of family life
- Longer life spans of older people and the problem of caring for the older generation when they become dependent

Filial responsibility is an *attitude of personal responsibility toward the parents that emphasizes duty, protection, care, and financial support,* which are indicators of the family's traditional protective function. Middle-class Caucasian culture in North America believes that good relationships between the aged and their adult children are dependent on the autonomy of the parents. They believe that a satisfactory role reversal between generations is not possible because the mores of society do not sanction it and both children and parents resent it. Yet, older persons do assist their children and younger family members in many ways and as long as possible. However, they are likely to expect children to assume responsibilities when they can no longer maintain their independence.

Families provide nurturance and companionship through:

1. Visits and telephone calls
2. Providing information
3. Assistance in decision making
4. Transportation
5. Assistance with shopping, laundry, and household chores
6. Immediate response to crisis
7. Being a buffer against bureaucracies
8. Help in searching out services
9. Facilitation for continuity of individual–bureaucracy relations

In many ethnic or racial cultures, structure and style for the younger generation(s) have evolved through an extended family system to provide support, assistance, protection, and mobility. Often inadequate family economic reserves and inadequate health insurance necessitate the middle-aged adult's having to be caregiver.

Middle-aged children of various racial and ethnic groups are more likely than Caucasians to provide a home for elderly parents or other relatives. There are some differences within groups. For example, elderly Japanese are more likely to live with spouse or alone than other Asian groups. Elderly Southeast Asians are more likely to live with family members.

Caregiver Role

Many issues related to caregiving and social support are important to Canadians.[59] Demographic changes (such as the aging population and the increasing life expectancy), family restructuring (such as delayed marriage and low fertility), and the prevalence of women in the labour force continue to affect the proportion of Canadians requiring and providing care. What is particularly new, however, is the dramatic rise in the proportion of the "oldest old" in our population.[60] Between 1991 and 2001, the number of seniors aged 80 years and over increased by more than 40%.[61] This suggests that a growing group of older adults is about to require care.

Ward-Griffin and Marshall state that a shift away from institutionalization has left the bulk of caregiving duties to family members and friends.[62] Various *factors that influence the caregiving role* include the following:[63–73]

■ Seriousness of the elder's health status
■ The caregiver–care recipient relationship and living arrangement
■ Duration of the caregiving experience
■ Other roles and responsibilities of the caregiver
■ Overall coping effectiveness of the caregiver
■ Caregiver sex and age
■ Number of generations needing care
■ Help and support from others—family or social agencies
■ Information needed to carry out tasks related to physical care of the parent

Meeting parents' dependency needs may have many diverse effects:[74–81]

■ Financial hardship
■ Physical symptoms such as sleeplessness and decline in physical health, especially in the primary caregiver
■ Emotional changes and symptoms in the caregiver and other family members, including frustration, inadequacy, anxiety, helplessness, depression, guilt, resentment, lowered morale, and emotional distance
■ Emotional exhaustion related to restrictions on time and freedom and increasing responsibility
■ A sense of isolation from social activities
■ Conflict because of competing demands, with diversion from care of other family members
■ Difficulty in setting priorities
■ Reduced family privacy
■ Inability to project future plans
■ Sense of losing control over life events
■ Interference with job responsibilities through late arrival, absenteeism, or early departure needed to take care of emergencies or even routine tasks
■ Interference with lifestyle and social and recreational activities

Thus the whole family and its relationships are affected.

The *caregiver role* is a major one, especially for the woman. In Canada, 14% of all women and 10% of all men provide informal care to family or friends.[82] It is interesting to note that men represent a substantial group of caregivers. However, relatively little is known about men's characteristics as caregivers. Taylor and Kopot conducted a study to examine men's experiences based on two major considerations: (1) the conceptualization of male spouses and sons providing care to individuals with Alzheimer's disease or related dementia and (2) participation in a male support group called the "Breakfast Club."[83] The researchers found that, as caregivers, men shared common perceptions of stress and burden. They learned from each other how to adapt to the ever-changing trajectory of Alzheimer's disease. Further, the support group was a successful intervention approach providing an opportunity for men to deal with their feelings in a safe, confidential, and supportive environment.[84]

CRITICAL THINKING

Compare and contrast the roles of formal and informal caregiving.

Interestingly, women who work provide as much caregiving as women who do not work outside the home. Nonemployed daughters provide more tangible help, but employed daughters contribute in other ways.[85–88] Some may reduce their working hours; others quit their jobs, especially if the aged parent lives with them. For some, adult day-care services may be available for the woman to use with elderly parents or relatives during the day while she is at work. Relations between husband and wife are affected because of financial or other help one person may give to the elderly parents, especially when done without consulting the other spouse. The needs of elderly parents may cause discord among their sons and daughters by recalling childhood rivalries and jealousies. A common phenomenon is when the middle-aged person resents those siblings who will not help care for the elderly parents or other relatives. Further, if the middle-aged adult believes he or she was not well cared for by the parents as a child, continued resentment, anger, or hate may inhibit a nurturing attitude or even minimum assistance.

Sometimes the adult child continues to care for the parent beyond physical and psychological means to do so, rather than to use formal support systems. Various dynamics are at work: (1) symbiotic ties, (2) gratification from being the burden bearer, (3) a fruitless search for parental approval that has never been received, and (4) expiation of guilt for having been a favourite child. The middle-aged adult may perceive caregiving as an acceptable permanent, full-time role that is altruistic and enhances self-esteem.

Over several decades the disciplines of social science and health care have explored the stress and burden of the major consequences of caregiving.[89] These scholarly articles and research studies enriched the understanding of caregiving, but did not yield a total picture of the process of becoming a caregiver.

Perry conducted a study on wives giving care to spouses with dementia. The grounded theory study describes the wives' experiences as a process of interpretive caring. Perry states that this process is neutral and allows for positive aspects of caring to be considered along with grief and frustration.[90] Another study, by Bar-David, was conducted to describe caregiver self-development through the caregiving journey.[91] Bar-David concludes that the caregiver's capacity for caring was found to be at the core; it unfolds in three phases: (1) development of caring capacity for the care recipient, (2) development of capacity for self-care, and (3) development of caring capacity for others. The four elements of caring capacity (perception, motivation, competency, and action) are expressed in relation to the care recipient, to the self, and to less familiar others.[92]

These studies reflect the positive aspects of caregiving. Health professionals need to focus on the strengths of the family in the caregiving situation. As well as assessing the burden of caregiving, it is necessary to explore the rewards the caregiver is experiencing.

One of the most difficult decisions when parents become aged and dependent concerns the housing arrangement. The older daughter usually is the one to take the dependent parent into her home. Or the unmarried adult child may move into the parent's home. When the parent(s) cannot manage living alone, the middle-aged person may not have the room to take the parent(s) into his or her home. Even if there is adequate space, if all members of the household are working, finding someone to stay during the day may be difficult, although such an arrangement or the use of adult daycare is less cost prohibitive than placing the parent who is in poor health in an institution. Most communities do not have adequate, or any, daycare facilities for elderly adults. Placing the parent(s) in an institution may be the only answer, but it is typically considered the last resort.

Health Care Role

You are in a key position to help the middle-aged adult work through the conflicts, feelings of frustration, guilt, and anger about the increased responsibility and past conflicts or old hurts from parents or siblings.

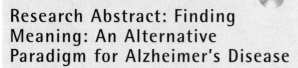

13–1 BONUS SECTION IN CD-ROM

Research Abstract: Finding Meaning: An Alternative Paradigm for Alzheimer's Disease

Learn about the experiences of caregivers who attend to Alzheimer's disease clients.

The middle-aged adult who verbally expresses great irritation typically also loves the older relative very much. Assist the middle-aged adult to gain a sense of satisfaction and rewards from the help he or she gives and a greater understanding of the person being helped. The generation gap and negative feelings that exist between the middle-aged adult and elderly person can be overcome with love, realistic expectations, a sense of forgiveness, and the realization that sometimes it is all right to say "No" to the demands of the elders. The rewards the caregiver experiences will assist the caregiver toward a desire to promote positive outcomes for the person cared for.

One study indicated that teaching the caregiver stress management and time management techniques may reduce the sense of burden more than participation in a support group.[93] Encouraging the caregiver to maintain other roles outside of caregiving and family roles may also increase the sense of caregiver well-being and health. Refer to a counsellor or spiritual leader if necessary. Counselling can promote a resolution of feelings that in turn fosters a more harmonious relationship between the middle-aged adult and parents.

CRITICAL THINKING

In what ways can you foster the creative abilities of family caregivers?

Further, outside resources can be used to support the adult child in the caregiving role. Often a little help will enable the person to make changes and use inner resources in a distressing situation. Having the caregiver keep a daily list of helping behaviours and of negative behaviours (not feelings) is a way of assisting the caregiver to see the role and behaviour in a positive light and to gain reinforcement from the caregiving because almost always the helping behaviours far outnumber the negative behaviours. Such a log can provide a base for talking with the adult child about the interaction with the parent and ways to resolve feelings and improve the interaction.

Policy analysts have attempted to address the cost borne by the caregiver. In particular, the issue of financial compensation for family members providing informal care to elderly relatives has been debated for some time in Canada and around the world.[94] One program that financially compensates family members for care of an elderly relative is the Nova Scotia Home Life Support.[95] The Canadian Caregiver Coalition's broad aim is to ensure the respect and support of family caregivers, and emphasize that they are not a substitute for public responsibility in health and social care (see the Interesting Websites section at the end of the chapter).

Death of Parents in Adulthood

A critical time for the adult is when both parents have died, regardless of whether the relationship between parent(s) and offspring was harmonious or conflictual. The first death of a parent signals finiteness and mortality of the self and of the other parent and other loved ones. Memories of childhood experiences are recalled. The person may wish deeply, even though simultaneously realizing it is impossible, to be able to relive some of those childhood days with the parent, to undo naughty behaviour, to be a good child just once more, to sit on the parent's lap and be cuddled one more time, to return to the relatively carefree days and to relive holidays. Further, more recent memories are recalled—the joys that were shared and the disharmonious times that are normal in any relationship but that are likely to engender guilt. There may be deep yearning to hold the parent one more time. Mourning may be done not only for the parent but for previously lost loved ones, and some mourning is in anticipation of future losses of the other parent, other beloved relatives and friends, and self. When the other parent dies, the adult is an orphan. Now he or she is no longer anyone's "little boy" or "little girl." The person may feel forlorn and alone, especially if there are few other relatives or friends. Sometimes there are no other living relatives and no sons so that the adult offspring represents the last of the family line. The person may question who and what will be remembered and by whom. This is a time of spiritual and philosophical searching whether or not the adult child is alone, has siblings, or has other relatives.

If there was conflict between the adult offspring and parents to the point of one-sided or mutual hate and lack of forgiveness, grief feelings may be denied or repressed or may be especially guilt-laden. Consequently, the mourning process is delayed and not resolved as effectively. There is a yearning that life experiences with the parent(s) could have been better or different, a wish that harsh feelings could have been smoothed, and sadness over what was never present more than sadness over what has been lost. The adult survivor may fear that he or she in turn may have similarly parented children, if any, and anxiety may arise about how the third generation will feel when their parents die. Will the scene and feelings be replayed? Can that be prevented? Certainly this can be a time for the adult to take stock, undo past wrongs with his or her children (and others), resolve old conflicts, and become motivated to move ahead into more harmonious relations with family members and others.

Throughout the period of parental loss, you may be a key person in helping the adult survivor or adult orphan relive, express, and sort out feelings; accept that any close relationship will not always go smoothly; and finally achieve a balance between happy, sad, and angry memories and feelings in regard to the parent(s). Finally, through such counselling, the person can mature to accept and like self and other significant persons better and to change behaviour patterns so that future relationships are less thorny.

Developmental Tasks

The following developmental tasks must be accomplished for the middle-aged family to survive and achieve happiness, harmony, and maturity:

- Maintain a pleasant and comfortable home.
- Assure security for later years, financially and emotionally.
- Share household and other responsibilities, based on changing roles, interests, and abilities.
- Maintain emotional and sexual intimacy as a couple or regain emotional stability if death or divorce occurs.
- Maintain contact with grown children and their families.
- Decrease attention on child care tasks and adapt to departure of the children.
- Meet the needs of elderly parents in such a way as to make life satisfactory for both the parents and middle-aged generations.
- Participate in community life beyond the family, recommitting energy once taken by child care.
- Use competencies built in earlier stages to expand or deepen interests and social or community involvement.

McCoy has formulated developmental tasks and their outcomes for the stages of middle age (Table 13-1).

You will have the opportunity and responsibility to help the middle-aged couple meet their developmental tasks.

TABLE 13-1
Developmental Tasks of Middle Age and Their Outcomes

Developmental Stage	Developmental Task	Outcome Sought
Restabilization, ages 44–55	Adjust to realities of work	Job adjustment
	Launch children	Letting go of parental authority
	Adjust to empty nest	Exploring new sources of satisfaction
	Become more deeply involved in social life	Effective social relations
	Participate actively in community concerns	Effective citizenship
	Handle increased demands of older parents	Better personal and social adjustment of elderly
	Manage leisure time	Creative use of leisure time
	Manage budget to support college-age children and ailing parents	Sound consumer behaviour
	Adjust to single state	Fulfilled single state
	Solve problems	Successful problem solving
	Manage stress accompanying change	Successful stress management, personal growth
Preparation for retirement, ages 56–64	Adjust to health problems	Healthier individuals
	Deepen personal relations	Effective social skills
	Prepare for retirement	Wise retirement planning
	Expand avocational interests	Satisfaction of aesthetic urge; broadening of knowledge; enjoyment of travel
	Finance new leisure	Sound consumer behaviour
	Adjust to eventual loss of mate	Adjustment to loss, fulfilled single state
	Use problem solving	Successful problem solving
	Manage stress accompanying change	Successful stress management, personal growth

Source: Modified from McCoy, V., Adult Life Cycle Tasks/Adult Continuing Education Program Response, Lifelong Learning in the Adult Years, October (1977), 16.

CRITICAL THINKING

What are some developmental tasks for the single middle-aged person?

PHYSIOLOGIC CONCEPTS

You are in a key position to help the middle-aged adult work through feelings about the meaning of midlife changes and ways to prevent or minimize their effects.

Physical Characteristics

The growth cycle continues with physical changes in the middle years, and different body parts age at different rates. One day the person may suddenly become aware of being "old" or middle-aged. Not all people decline alike. How quickly they decline depends on the stresses and strains they have undergone and on the health promotion measures that were maintained. If the person has always been active, he or she will continue with little slowdown. People from lower socioeconomic groups often show signs of aging earlier than people from more affluent socioeconomic groups because of their years of hard physical labour, poorer nutritional status, and lack of money for beauty aids to cover the signs of aging.[96]

Now the person looks in the mirror and sees changes that others may have noticed some time ago. Grey, thinning hair, wrinkles, coarsening features, decreased muscular tone, weight gain, varicosities, and capillary breakage may be the first signs of impending age.

Because a number of your clients will be middle-aged, you are in a key position to help them understand the physiologic changes that occur in middle age, work through feelings about these changes, reintegrate the body image, and find specific ways to remain as healthy as possible. Use the following information to assist you in listening, teaching, reaffirming a positive self-concept, and counselling.

Hormonal Changes

Female Climacteric. This is the era of life known as the *menopause* for the woman or the *climacteric* for either sex. The terms are often used interchangeably. The **menopause** is the *permanent cessation of menstruation preceded by a gradually decreasing menstrual flow*. The term **perimenopausal years** denotes a *time of gradual diminution of ovarian function and a gradual change in endocrine status from before the menopause through one year after the menopause*. The **climacteric** is the *period in life when important physiologic changes occur, with the cessation of the woman's reproductive ability and the period of lessening sexual activity in the male*. Basic to the changing physiology of the middle years is declining hormonal production.[97–101]

Contrary to myth (Table 13-2), depression or other symptomatology is neither inevitable nor clearly related to the perimenopausal or climacteric years.[102–104] Most women feel relieved or neutral about menopause; only a small percentage view it negatively. Attitudes toward menopause improve as women move from before to after menopause, and perception of health becomes more positive as menopause proceeds.[105–107] The most difficult part about the menopause or climacteric may be unclear as to what to expect. Myths abound and there are several conceptual views of menopause.

In North American culture, menopause is viewed primarily as a biomedical as well as a psychiatric view, but sociocultural and feminist views are found in the literature (Table 13-3).[108,109]

In the biomedical view, menopause is a cluster of symptoms or a syndrome. The ovarian failure, with a hormone deficiency, is the cause of various physical and psychological symptoms, such as hot flashes, vaginal atrophy, and depression. The syndrome can be treated by hormone replacement.[110]

In the psychiatric view, the changes of menopause cause anxiety and depression, which can be treated with psychotropic medication.[111] Women who think of menopause primarily in these terms may feel negative about themselves during the climacteric period, because the emphasis is on the body's deficiency or loss. Thus traditional homemakers in North America may experience greater difficulty with menopause because the reproductive role has passed.

In societies in which women rise in status after menopause or generally enjoy high status regardless of reproductive stage, a menopausal syndrome is nonexistent. A woman's perception of her menopause experience is largely her perception of the physical, social, and psychological changes she undergoes.[112,113]

The sociocultural view has emerged over several decades in reaction to the biomedical and psychiatric view, in response to the feminist movement, and especially in response to greater understanding of women from various cultures in North America or of women in other societies. In the sociocultural view, menopause has little or no effect on the woman. Instead, role changes or cultural attitudes toward aging are identified as the cause of any discomforts.[114]

Menopause is seen as a normal life event; even though some of the physical changes can be problematic. The sociocultural view explains the difference between North American women with severe menopausal symptoms and the absence of incapacitation during the menopause in women in other cultures. In other cultures, there is a role beyond the menopause.[115] In North America, most women and men, and a growing number of scientists, also see that there are life and roles beyond the menopause. A wellness approach is needed as a routine strategy for health promotion during this life event.

Table 13–3 lists assumptions about menopause from the biomedical and sociocultural perspectives.

Male Climacteric. This comes in the 50s or early 60s, although the symptoms may not be as pronounced as in the female climacteric. Sheehy describes the "**MANopause**" as *a five- to 12-year period during which males go through hormonal fluctuations and physical and psychological changes*.[116]

A man's "change of life" may be passed almost imperceptibly, but he usually notices it when he makes comparisons with past feelings and performance. A few men may even complain of hot flashes, sweating, chills, dizziness, headaches, and heart palpitations. Unlike women, however,

TABLE 13-2
Myths about the Menopause

Myth	Fact
1. Menopause is a deficiency disease and catastrophe.	1. Menopause is a normal developmental process.
2. Most women have serious disability during the menopause.	2. Most women pass through it with a minimum of distress. Some have no noticeable symptoms or reactions and simply stop menstruation.
3. Menopause is the end of life.	3. The average life expectancy for today's 50-year-old woman is 81 years; one-third of her life is postmenopausal. Postmenopause is a time of new zest.
4. Menopausal women are more likely to be depressed than other people (older men are handsome, distinguished, and desirable; older women are worn out and useless).	4. Menopausal depression in middle age is likely to be caused by social stressors: a. The double standard of aging b. Caregiver demands c. Loss of loved ones d. Loss of roles e. Other health problems (the decreased level of estrogen affects neurotransmitters that regulate mood, appetite, sleep, and pain perception)
5. Numerous symptoms accompany the menopause.	5. Predictable manifestations of menopause are: a. Change in menstrual pattern b. Transient warm sensations or vasomotor instability (hot flashes) to some degree (47%–85% of women) c. Vaginal dryness in some women
6. Hot flashes are "in the woman's head."	6. Vasomotor instability results from hemodynamic compensatory mechanisms. Until the body adjusts to less estrogen, hypothalamic instability causes dips in body's core temperature. The flash is the body's adaptive response to equalize peripheral and core temperatures through dermal heat loss.
7. The woman may have a heart attack during a hot flash.	7. The tachycardia that occurs during a flush is the body's adaptive response to skin temperature changes.
8. The woman loses sexual desire during and after the menopause.	8. Vaginal changes may cause some discomfort, which would reduce libido. Psychosocial concerns about the empty nest, partner's loss of sexual capacity, or expectation of loss of libido are more likely the cause than reduced estrogen.
9. The indicators of the menopause are the various symptoms women experience.	9. Women may have regular menstrual cycles with decreased estrogen levels; hot flashes may occur before the menopause begins.
10. Only women have to worry about osteoporosis.	10. By age 70, osteoporosis risk is equal in men and women.

men do not lose their reproductive ability, although the likelihood diminishes as age advances. The output of sex hormones of the gonads does not stop; it is merely reduced. Testosterone level usually is lower in the middle-aged man who has high stress, lowered self-esteem, and depression. Testosterone therapy should be used cautiously because administration may increase prostatic hypertrophy and cancer development.[117] Medications to increase a sense of virility are not the answer either. The physical and emotional changes may be indicative of other health problems. Thorough screening is advised.

Menopause. The average age for onset of menopause is 51; the usual range is between 45 and 55 years, although it may occur as early as age 35 in approximately 1% of women.[118] In the woman the process of aging causes changed secretion of follicle-stimulating hormone (FSH), which brings about progressive and irreversible changes in the ovaries, leading to the menopause and loss of childbearing ability. The primordial follicles, which contain the ovum and grow into vesicular follicles with each menstrual cycle, become depleted, and their ability to mature declines. Finally, ovulation ceases because all ova have either degenerated or been released. Thus, the cyclic

TABLE 13-3
Biomedical versus Sociocultural Assumptions about Menopause

Biomedical

1. Science, which is objective and precise, provides the true knowledge about a condition.
2. Women are products of their reproductive systems and hormones.
3. Women's behaviour is caused by their biology and hormones.
4. Menopause can be studied as biomedical variables, treatments, and outcomes.
5. Menopause is a disease that causes psychological distress, an outcome of the handicap of menstruation.
6. Women are considered medically old and socially useless when menopause occurs.
7. Norms of the male are the baseline for considering norms for the woman.
8. Menopause can be treated as a disease of decreased hormones.
9. Treatment will restore the woman to the premenopausal, and desirable, state.

Sociocultural

1. Science is an important model for research, but view of women is less negative than in the biomedical model.
2. The world, and therefore womankind, is dynamic and cannot be fully understood from experimental studies.
3. Social and cultural variables are basic to understanding people, their behaviour, and reactions to their bodies.
4. Attitudes, relationships, roles, and interactions are important variables in understanding people.
5. Positions of women and societal conditions contribute to women's reactions to the menopause.
6. The meaning of an event is critical to the person's reaction to the event.
7. There is no consistent relationship between the biochemical or physiologic processes and the person's perception of an event or behaviour.
8. *Menopause is a natural developmental phase, not a disease process,* based on changes in the endocrine system.
9. *Menopause is a part of natural life transitions,* and views include cultural ideas about life and nature.

production of progesterone and estrogen fails to occur and levels rapidly fall below the amount necessary to induce endometrial bleeding. (The adrenal glands continue to produce some estrogen.) The menstrual cycle becomes irregular; periods of heavy bleeding may alternate with amenorrhea for one or two years, eventually ceasing altogether.[119] Consistent

or regular excessive bleeding may be a sign of pathology, not of the approaching menopause.

The pituitary continues to produce FSH and luteinizing hormone (LH), but the aging ovary is incapable of responding to its stimulation. With the pituitary no longer under the normal cyclic or feedback influence of ovarian hormones, it becomes more active, producing excessive gonadotropins, especially FSH. A disturbed endocrine balance influences some of the symptoms of menopause. Although the ovaries are producing less estrogen and progesterone, the adrenals may continue to produce some hormones, thus helping to maintain younger feminine characteristics for some time.[120]

During the perimenopausal period (approximately five years) some discomforts may occur in a small percentage of women. Vasomotor changes cause hot flashes associated with chilly sensations, dizziness, headaches, perspiration, palpitations, water retention, nausea, muscle cramps, fatigability, insomnia, and paresthesia of fingers and toes. Many symptoms, including irritability, depression, emotional lability, and palpitations, are frequently attributed to menopause. Some women experience *no* symptoms, only a decrease, then cessation, of menses. The great majority of women experience no effect in their sexual relationships from the menopause. Most find menopause a time of integration, balance, liberation, confidence, and action.[121]

Difficulties experienced during menopause may be associated with concurrent life change or recent loss, or marital, psychological, or social stress. The cause of the symptoms apparently is more complex than simple estrogen deficit. Psychological factors such as anger, anxiety, and excitement are considered as important in precipitating hot flashes in susceptible women as conditions giving rise to excess heat production or retention such as a warm environment, muscular work, and hot food; however, the symptoms may arise without any clear psychological or heat-stimulating mechanism.[122]

The Heart and Stroke provides a Menopause Check List that women can complete online, print out, and take to the doctor (see the Interesting Websites section at end of the chapter).

CRITICAL THINKING

What health teaching episodes could you implement for women experiencing hot flashes?

Physical Changes. Table 13-4 summarizes physical changes that occur in middle age, physiological reasons for the changes and characteristics that are commonly seen, and implications for health promotion and client teaching.[123–132]

Hormone Replacement Therapy. In Canada for many years, women have been prescribed estrogen with or without progestin hormone replacement therapy to relieve some of the symptoms of menopause.[133] Recent scientific studies have identified significant risks associated with this therapy.

In 1991, the U.S. National Institutes of Health launched the Women's Health Initiative (WHI), a set of studies involving healthy postmenopausal women that were carried out in 40 U.S. centres. The WHI included a clinical trial to evaluate the risks and benefits of the two types of HRT (in pill form)

TABLE 13-4
Physical Changes and Characteristics of Middle Age and Health Promotion Implications

Body System or Physical Parameter	Change/Characteristic	Implications for Health Promotion
Endocrine and Reproductive Systems		

Women	Decline in production of neurotransmitters that stimulate hypothalamus to signal pituitary to release sex hormones
	Less estrogen synthesized
	No estrogen produced by ovaries; menses stops
	Aging oocytes (eggs) destroy necessary genetic material for reproduction
	Uterine changes make implantation of blastocyte unlikely
	Gradual atrophy of tissues:
	  Uterus and cervix become smaller
	  Vulvar epithelium thins
	  Labia majora and minora fatten
	  Vaginal mucosal lining thinner, drier, pale (20%–40% women; some never experience this)
	Natural lubrication during intercourse decreases
		Reproductive cycle is ended; this may represent sexual liberation or loss of femininity.
		Counsel about meaning of femininity.
		Support group may be helpful.
		Instruct in Kegel exercises.
		Hormone replacement therapy may be prescribed.
		Artificial (water-soluble) lubrication can be used during intercourse to reduce discomfort.
		Regular sexual intercourse maintains lubrication and elasticity of tissue.

	Neuroendocrine symptoms, such as hot flashes and night sweats followed by chilling, fatigue, nausea, dizziness, headache, palpitations, and paresthesias may occur.	Avoid precipitating factors such as hot drinks, caffeine, alcohol, stress, and warm environment. Counsel to stop smoking. Hormone replacement therapy may reduce symptoms.
Men	Testosterone production gradually decreases, which eventually causes: Degeneration of cells in tubules Production of fewer sperm More time needed to achieve erection Less forceful ejaculation Testes less firm and smaller	Sperm production continues to death, so man is capable of producing children. Premature ejaculation is less likely, which may contribute to more enjoyable intercourse. Practise Kegel exercises for firmer erections.
Basal Metabolism Rate (BMR)		
Minimum energy used in resting state	BMR declines 2% per decade Gradually reduces as ratio of lean body mass to adipose tissue decreases (metabolic needs of fat are less than for lean tissue)	If eating pattern is maintained, 3 to 4 pounds are gained per decade Fewer calories (2%) need to be consumed, even if the person exercises regularly, to avoid weight gain.
Weight	Gain should not occur; weight gain occurs if as many calories consumed as earlier: wider hips, thicker thighs, larger waist, and more abdominal mass	Overweight contributes to a number of health problems; crash diets should be avoided.

(continued)

TABLE 13-4 *(continued)*
Physical Changes and Characteristics of Middle Age and Health Promotion Implications

Body System or Physical Parameter	Change/Characteristic	Implications for Health Promotion
Integumentary System		
Sebaceous oil glands	Produce less sebum secretions, skin drier and cracks more easily More pronounced in women after menopause than in men of same age	Protect and lubricate skin with lotion or moisturizer. Avoid excess soap and drying substances on skin. Avoid excessive strong sun and wind exposure.
Sweat glands	Decrease in size, number, and function	Ability to maintain even body temperature is affected; dress in layers to maintain comfort.
Skin	Skin wrinkles, tissue sags, and pouches under eyes form because: Epidermis flattens and thins with age, collagen in dermis becomes more fibrous, less gel-like Elastin loses elasticity, causing loss of skin turgor Loss of muscle tone causes sagging jowls	Wrinkles are less apparent with use of moisturizer or lotion. Wrinkled appearance of skin is made worse by excess exposure to sun or sunburn; use sunscreen. Skin is more prone to injury; healing is slower. Use humidifier in home.
Women	Estrogen decrease gradually causes skin and mucous membranes to lose thickness and fluids; skin and mucous membranes thinner, drier, and begin atrophy Estrogen decrease gradually causes breasts to sag and flatten	Avoid burns and bruises. Use lotions. Maintain support with correctly fitted brassiere. Maintain erect posture.
Hair	Progressive loss of melanin from hair bulb causes grey hair in most adults by age 50; hair thins and growth slows; hair rest and growth cycles change	Slow hair loss by gentle brushing, avoiding excess heat from hair dryer, and avoiding chemical treatment.
Women	Estrogen decrease may gradually cause increased growth of facial hair Hair loss not as pronounced as in male	Accept change. Manage cosmetically.
Men	Testosterone decrease causes gradual loss of hair Hereditary male-pattern baldness occurs with receding hairline and monk's spot area on back of head	Accept change. Manage with styling, hairpiece, or hair transplant.
Muscular System		
	Slight decrease in number of muscle fibres; about 10% loss in muscle size from ages 30 to 60 Gradual loss of lean body mass	Physical exercise and fitness, proper nutrition, and healthy lifestyle can improve or sustain muscle strength during middle age.

(continued)

TABLE 13-4 *(continued)*
Physical Changes and Characteristics of Middle Age and Health Promotion Implications

Body System or Physical Parameter	Change/Characteristic	Implications for Health Promotion
	Muscle tissue gradually replaced by adipose unless exercise is maintained Most loss of muscle occurs in back and legs Grip strength decreases with age Gradual increase in subcutaneous fat	Variations in peak muscular activity depend on type of exercise.
Skeletal System		
	Gradual flattening of intervertebral disks and loss of height of individual vertebrae cause compression of spinal column	Maintain erect posture. Maintain adequate calcium intake (1000–1500 mg daily). Exercise maintains bone mass and joint flexibility, improves balance and agility, and reduces fatigue. Loss of height occurs in later life.
Men and women	At age 70, osteoporosis risk equal in men and women unless vitamin D has been taken to increase bone density	Vitamin D decrease risk of fractures.
Women	Estrogen reduction increases decalcification of bones, bone resorption, decreased bone density, and gradual osteoporosis Cultural differences: Caucasians and Asians more likely than Latinos and blacks to suffer bone porosity because their bones are less dense and they lose mass more quickly	Maintain exercise and calcium intake. Maintain erect posture. Maintain calcium and good nutrition intake. Teach safety factors; forearms, hips and spinal vertebrae are most vulnerable to fractures. Supplemental vitamin D and regular small amounts of exposure to sunlight improve calcium absorption. Avoid smoking, high alcohol intake, and high caffeine intake, all of which interfere with nutrition. Caffeine causes calcium loss. Women may eventually be 7.5 cm shorter if they have vertebral osteoporosis. Dowager's hump will form in cervical and upper thoracic area if osteoporosis occurs. Women who have taken oral contraceptives for 6 or more years have higher bone density in lumbar spine and femoral neck.
Neurologic System		
	Speed of nerve conduction, nerve impulse travelling from brain to muscle fibre, decreases 5% by age 50, and only 10% through life cycle Brain structural changes minimal; gradual loss of neurons does not affect cognition	Sensation to heat and cold and speed of reflexes may be impaired. Teach safety factors. Functional abilities are maintained, and learning from life experiences enhances functional abilities.

(continued)

TABLE 13-4 *(continued)*
Physical Changes and Characteristics of Middle Age and Health Promotion Implications

Body System or Physical Parameter	Change/Characteristic	Implications for Health Promotion
Vision	Average 60-year-old requires twice the illumination of 20-year-old to do close work Eyes begin to gradually change at about 40 or 50, causing **presbyopia** (*farsightedness*) Lens less elastic, loses accommodation Cornea increases in curvature and thickness, loses lustre Iris responds less well to light changes; pupils smaller Retina begins to lose rods and cones Optic nerve fibres begin to decrease	Wear brimmed hat and sunglasses that block UV rays to protect vision. Person eventually needs bifocals or trifocals to see small print or focus on near objects. Eyes do not adapt as quickly to darkness, bright lights or glare (implications for safety and night driving). More light is needed to see well.
Hearing	Auditory nerve and bones of inner ear gradually change Gradual decrease in ability to detect certain tones and certain consonants Loss of hearing from high-pitched sounds	Reduce exposure to loud work machinery or equipment; wear ear protectors. Reduce exposure to loud stereo, radio, or electronic music. Cross-cultural studies show our high-tech culture contributes to increasing and earlier impairment. Hearing aids, correctly chosen, or surgery may correct hearing impairment.

Voice
  Women
  Men
	Estrogen decrease gradually causes lower pitch of voice
	Testosterone decrease gradually causes higher pitch of voice	

Cardiovascular System	Efficiency of heart may drop to 80% between 30 and 50 Decreased elasticity in muscles in heart and blood vessels Decreased cardiac output Cardiovascular disease risk for women equal to that of men by age 70 because reduced estrogen causes lipid changes, increase in low-density lipoproteins (LDLs), decrease in high-density lipoproteins (HDLs), and gradual increase in total serum cholesterol.	Regular aerobic exercise maintains heart function and normal blood pressure. Inactivity affects system negatively. Quit smoking. Maintain healthy diet. Take regular low doses of aspirin. Maintain low-cholesterol diet.

(continued)

TABLE 13-4 *(continued)*
Physical Changes and Characteristics of Middle Age and Health Promotion Implications

Body System or Physical Parameter	Change/Characteristic	Implications for Health Promotion
Respiratory System		
	Gradual loss of lung elasticity	Regular exercise enhances respiratory efficiency.
	Thorax shortens	Inactivity affects system negatively.
	Chest cage stiffer	
	Breathing capacity reduced to 75%	
	Chest wall muscles gradually lose strength, reducing respiratory efficiency	
Urinary System		
Women	Glomerular filtration rate gradually decreases	Maintain adequate fluid intake; drink 8 glasses of water daily.
	Loss of bladder muscle tone and atrophy of supporting ligaments and tissue in late middle age causes urgent urination, possibly cystocele, rectocele, and urine prolapse.	Instruct in Kegel exercises as follows: Draw in perivaginal muscles (pubococcygeus muscle) and anal sphincter as if to control urination, without contracting abdominal, buttock, or inner thigh muscles. Maintain contraction for 10 seconds. Follow with 10 seconds of relaxation. Perform exercises 30–80 times daily.
Men	Hypertrophy of prostate begins in late middle age; enlarging prostate around urethra causes frequent urination, dribbling, and nocturia	Urinary stasis may predispose to infections. Drink adequate amount of water. Surgery may be necessary.

and to observe how they affected the incidence of heart disease, breast cancer, colorectal cancer, and fractures in postmenopausal women.[134] The trial was divided into arms:

- One arm involved more than 16 000 postmenopausal women aged 50 to 79 who had not had a hysterectomy. They took pills daily that were either a combination of estrogen and progestin or a placebo pill.

- The second arm involved more than 10 000 women who had received a hysterectomy and who took estrogen pills alone or a placebo.[135]

The safety monitoring board of the WHI recommended premature cessation of the combination Premarin/Provera arm and concluded that there were more risks than benefits among the group using the combined HRT.[136] That is, the risks of breast cancer and cardiovascular disease, although small, outweighed potential benefits (reduced incidence of osteoporotic fractures and the possibility of colorectal cancer) in these asymptomatic subjects.[137]

The WHI is a landmark study providing critical information on a variety of endpoints relating to the risks and benefits

of hormone replacement therapy (HRT).[138] The Society of Obstetricians and Gynaecologists of Canada (SOGC) recommend that women discuss their issues with their health professional so that they can make an informed choice about continuous combined HRT. The SOGC conclude that the best treatment for distressing menopausal symptoms is HRT. The alternative (nonhormonal) therapies are limited in their effectiveness, and safety has not been tested in a large-scale trial like the WHI study.[139] The SOGC indicates that continuous combined HRT should not be recommended routinely for all postmenopausal women because it does not appear to offer cardiovascular protection, and the slightly increased risk of coronary heart disease and breast cancer outweighs the benefits in asymptomatic women.[140] However, short-term use remains an option for osteoporosis prevention and may be considered in conjunction with benefits, risk, tolerability, and the costs of alternatives.

Lemay states that new mid-term and long-term randomized studies need to be conducted on women starting various formulations of HRT before the age of 60 to evaluate their impact on risk factors and events of cardiovascular disease.[141]

Humphries and Gill conclude that the use of HRT should be individualized, with the risks and benefits of HRT for each woman being taken into consideration.[142]

CRITICAL THINKING

What health-promoting strategies would you use to counsel a woman who is considering HRT?

Emotional Changes Related to Physical Changes. Depression, irritability, and a change in sexual desire may occur in response to physical changes and their meaning, but they do not automatically occur. Some women fear loss of sexual identity. Earlier personality patterns and attitudes are more responsible for the symptoms than the cessation of glandular activity. Women who had previous low self-esteem and life satisfaction are more likely to have difficulties with menopause. Reactions to menopause are consistent with reactions to other life changes, including other reproductive turning points such as puberty. Women with high motherliness scores and heavy investment in childbearing react more severely to the menopause.

Postmenopausal women generally take a more positive view than premenopausal women, agreeing that the menopause creates no major discontinuity in life and, except for the underlying biological changes; women have a relative degree of control over their symptoms and need not inevitably have difficulties. In general, menopausal status is not associated consistently with measurable anxiety in any group.

Women in various cultures experience menopause differently. A study of Japanese, American, and Canadian women revealed that Japanese women experience menopause differently than Western women. Fewer than 10% reported hot flashes and little or no physical or psychological discomfort. This was substantiated by physician survey. There is no Japanese term for "hot flash" although their language makes many subtle distinctions about body states. In Japan, menopause is regarded as a *normal* life event, *not* a medical condition requiring treatment, in contrast to beliefs in the United States and Canada. Hot flashes are rare among Mayan women, North African women in Israel, Navaho women, and Indonesian women.[143,144]

Cultural attitudes affect how women interpret physical sensations of menopause and their interpretation of menopause as a life event. Childbearing and nutritional practices may influence the experience of menopause. Mayan women, who are almost constantly pregnant or breast feeding, look forward to menopause as the end of a burden. Far Eastern diets (tofu, soybeans) have more phytoestrogens, an estrogen-like compound, which may lower premenopausal hormone levels. When natural estrogen levels fall, the phytoestrogens may act like estrogen in inhibiting menopausal symptoms. Further, Japanese women, the longest-lived women in the world, have a lower incidence of osteoporosis than Caucasian women in North America despite lower average bone mass. Japanese women are also about one-fourth as likely as North American women to die of coronary heart disease and breast cancer. Besides phytoestrogens in the diet, Japanese women eat well-balanced diets, exercise throughout life, and seldom smoke or drink.[145–147]

Nutritional Needs

In Canada, the *Food Guide to Healthy Eating* is recommended. The importance of getting enough calcium and vitamin D in the diet, along with exercise, is important.[148] Food is the best source of calcium. Milk, nonfat milk, almonds, and soybeans are a few foods that are high in calcium.[149] Vitamin D is also important because it helps the body absorb calcium from the diet. The Osteoporosis Society of Canada recommends that after the age of 50 women and men need about 800 IU (20 micrograms) per day.[150] Studies have shown that people who have no digestive problems and are eating according to *Canada's Food Guide to Healthy Eating* do not need magnesium supplements.

The body mass index (BMI) is the most useful indicator, to date, of health risks associated with being overweight or underweight. In the body weight classification system, categories of BMI are used to identify levels of health risk.[151] A BMI in the normal range has been shown in population-wide studies to be associated with the lowest relative risk of morbidity and mortality.[152]

Teach people to limit their intake of carbohydrates and foods with high fat, saturated fat, and cholesterol content, including the foods with "empty" calories, such as rich desserts, candies, fatty foods, gravies, sauces, and alcoholic and nondiet cola beverages. Substitute sparkling waters or reduced-calorie wines or beers; half the previous intake of alcoholic beverage is desirable. Intake of salty food should be limited; herbs, spices, and lemon juice can be used for flavouring. Overweight is not just a genetic factor[153–155] and should be avoided, because it is a factor in diabetes, cardiovascular and hypertensive disease, and problems with mobility, such as arthritis.

Plenty of fluids, especially water and juices, along with an adequate diet, will maintain weight control and vigour and help prevent "heartburn," constipation, and other minor discomforts caused by physiologic changes. Snacks of fibre and protein maintain energy. Equally important, the person should chew food well, eat smaller portions throughout the day to maintain a consistent metabolism, eat in a pleasant and unhurried atmosphere, and avoid eating when overtired.

Drinking too much coffee or tea can be a real problem in middle age. Intake should be limited to one or two cups daily, including decaffeinated forms, and be drunk between meals. The tannins in coffee and tea at mealtime can reduce the body's ability to absorb nutrients such as calcium. There may also be an association between coffee and high blood cholesterol levels. Coffee and tea, other than green tea, should be avoided if there is a family history of heart disease or if the person is overweight, eats a high-fat diet, and does not exercise.[156,157]

There is no evidence that use of commercial vitamin-mineral preparations is necessary unless they are prescribed by a physician because of clinical signs of deficiency and insufficient diet.

Joining self-help groups such as Weight Watchers or Take Off Pounds Sensibly (TOPS) is effective for many people. It is possible to change habits of overeating and to lose weight in middle age.

Teach the middle-aged person to avoid using extreme diets to decrease weight quickly and to avoid repeatedly losing weight that is then regained. Each gain–lose cycle reduces the total muscle mass with weight loss and increases body fat, as regained weight is in the form of adipose tissue. Adipose tissue burns fewer calories than muscle, so each round of dieting makes it more difficult to lose weight and maintain weight loss. Extreme low-calorie diets should also be avoided because with them, the basic metabolic rate becomes lower so that, even with restricted calories, little weight is lost. Thus, to lose weight it is essential to exercise—at least moderately (see Chapter 11)—and

eat a healthy high-fibre, low-fat diet. See the box entitled "Healthy Eating Plan for the Middle-Aged Adult" for some helpful suggestions.[158–160]

CRITICAL THINKING

Plan a daily menu for a week for a middle-aged person who lives alone.

Healthy Eating Plan for the Middle-Aged Adult

Go Nutrient Dense and High Fibre

- Buy cereals that give you a larger portion for the calories.
- Serve meals loaded with complex carbohydrates such as pasta, rice (brown for more fibre), barley, and potatoes.
- Be creative with your potato toppings—plain yogurt mixed with herbs, picante sauce, or melted low-fat cheese.
- Use meats such as lean beef and skinless turkey and chicken, not as the biggest part of the meal, but more as condiments. Serve them in 2- to 3-oz (50 to 80 g) portions.
- Use romaine lettuce in salads instead of the pale, anemic-looking variety. Romaine lettuce has approximately eight times more vitamin A and double the iron of iceberg lettuce.
- Serve an iron-rich plant food such as a legume or dried fruit with a vitamin C-rich food such as citrus fruit. Vitamin C helps your body use the iron more efficiently.
- Chop fruits and vegetables as little as possible, cook them just a short time, and minimize standing time. A number of vitamins are destroyed by air, light, and heat.
- Choose dark green and bright orange vegetables and fruits. They tend to have more nutrients than the paler plant foods. One half cup of cooked, chopped broccoli, for instance, has more than double the vitamin A and eight times more vitamin C than the same amount of lighter green beans.
- Choose plain, low-fat yogurt and add your own fruit.
- Steam foods rather than cook them in large amounts of water, which can leach away important nutrients.
- Select whole-grain products more often than refined ones.
- Try to avoid empty calories (those giving you few nutrients) such as those found in alcohol or in desserts such as cake and pie.
- Work more fibre into your meals with peas and beans: mix them with rice or pasta, use them in meatless chilli, or sprinkle them on salads.

Ease More Fish into Meals

- Try fish in your favourite meat and chicken recipes.
- Do not overcook fish. Cook fish for approximately 10 minutes per inch of thickness, be it on the grill, under the broiler, or in an oven preheated to 230°C (450°F).
- Be creative: serve fish and shellfish in soups, salads, stews, pasta, and stir-fry dishes.

Cut the Fat

- Reduce fat in the diet by eating ordinary foods and cutting back on just four things: fat used in prepared foods and in cooking, oils, red meats, and whole milk dairy products. These measures will reduce fat intake to approximately 20% of caloric intake.
- Avoid fried foods. Simulate the crunch of fried foods by oven frying. For instance, dip fish or chicken in egg whites and then in bread or cracker crumbs and bake on a nonstick cookie sheet at 150°–175°C (300°–350°F) until done; or slice potatoes into spears and bake in the oven at 175°C (350°F) for 30 minutes.
- Invest in a large nonstick frying pan that uses little or no oil when sautéing or pan-frying. Lightly coat regular pans and casseroles with nonstick vegetable spray.
- Experiment with low-fat, low-calorie flavour enhancers such as Dijon mustard, horseradish, chopped green or red peppers, onions, and seasonings such as tarragon, dry mustard, dill, and curry powder.
- Chill sauces, gravies, and stews ahead of time so the hardened fat can be skimmed from the surface.
- Make sauces without fat by slowly mixing cold liquid directly into the flour or cornstarch. Stir until smooth and bring to a boil, stirring frequently.
- Use evaporated skimmed milk instead of cream in coffee and recipes.
- In place of sour cream, use nonfat sour cream, low-fat or nonfat yogurt, or low-fat cottage cheese that has been mixed in a blender with a little milk and lemon juice.

Boost Milk Intake (without Drinking a Drop)

If your system is not lactose intolerant, but you prefer not to drink milk as a beverage:

- Sneak nonfat dry milk powder into anything you can: soups, sauces, casseroles, meat loaf, and stews. Add a few teaspoons of it to coffee; this blend will taste like café au lait.
- Treat yourself to low-calorie puddings made with skim or low-fat milk.
- Make milk-based soups with skim milk.
- Use a blender to make a low-fat milkshake with a few ice cubes, skim or low-fat milk, fresh fruit, and low-calorie sweetener.
- Experiment with fun flavourings in low-fat milk: vanilla, rum extract, or even cocoa with a little artificial sweetener.
- Have cold breakfast cereals with milk and fresh fruit.

Rest and Exercise

Teach that middle age is not a time when a person's body fails, but it is a period that requires better maintenance than was necessary in the earlier years.

Exercise

Exercise and erect posture may not increase longevity but they will enhance quality of life by keeping people healthy and independent (Figure 13–1). A combination of the following activities appears optimum: *consistent brisk walking*, stretching, weight bearing, bicycling, rowing, swimming, aerobics, and resistance activities.

The recommended amounts and duration of exercise varies with the author who is consulted. Moderate exercise of 30 to 45 minutes daily or 20- to 30-minute sessions daily of an intense level of exercise has the following *positive effects*:[161-165]

1. Maintains or improves strength (by as much as 170% with weight-lifting routines)

2. Maintains or improves muscle mass, which also stabilizes joints

3. Improves coordination and agility

4. Maintains body flexibility

5. Stimulates bone formation, increases bone density and size

6. Maintains collagen tissue elasticity, and prevents shortening of connective tissue. Stretching exercises, hatha yoga, and floor exercises put joints and muscles through range of motion.

7. Improves cardiovascular function and circulation, increases pulse rate between 85 and 120 beats per minute, which reduces heart disease risk by 30% to 50%

8. Promotes deeper respirations

9. Improves abdominal muscle tone and posture, aiding gastrointestinal function

10. Maintains weight or promotes weight loss by reducing percentage of body fat by "burning off" calories

11. Enhances immune function

12. Improves mental function and memory

13. Fosters positive self-concept, self-esteem, and life satisfaction

14. Reduces depressive mood, anger

Refer to Chapter 12 for additional information about exercises.

One of the most stable characteristics is *activity level*. Although there is a general and gradual decline in quickness and level of activity during the latter part of life, people who were most active among their age group during adolescence and young adulthood usually are the most active among their age group during middle and old age. It is almost as though each person has a physical and mental "clock" that runs at a fast or slow rate throughout life. The rate at which an individual's clock runs is reflected as well in various cognitive and personality characteristics.

The middle-aged adult invests considerable energy in occupational or professional, home, and organizational activity and in leisure time pursuits. He or she often has fine physical health. Although chronic disease is more prevalent than in the young, there is ordinarily good resistance to communicable diseases, superior emotional stamina, and a willingness to work despite minor illnesses. The person brings economy of effort, singleness of purpose, and perseverance to various roles.

Teach that, although physical changes do occur, adopting sedentary habits will not maintain health. Physical activity must be balanced with rest and sleep to keep the body posture and functioning at its optimum. Capacity for intense and sustained effort diminishes, especially if engaged in irregularly, but judicious exercise may modify and retard the aging process. In addition to the physical benefits, regular and vigorous exertion is an excellent outlet for emotional tensions. For people with sedentary jobs, doing back exercises (Figure 13–2) can prevent loss of muscle tone and discomfort.[166]

Teach about the value and precautions of exercise. The type of exercise does not matter as long as the person *likes* it and engages in it *regularly*, and it is *suitable* for personal strength and physical condition. The *middle-aged person should take certain precautions*: (1) gradually increase the exercise until it is moderate in strenuousness, (2) exercise consistently, and (3) avoid overexertion. Ten minutes after strenuous exercise, the heart should be beating normally again, respirations should be normal, and there should be no sense of fatigue. If the person is overweight, has a personal or family history of cardiovascular disease, or has led a sedentary life, new exercise routines should not be started until after a thorough physical check-up.[167] Using exercise as an overcompensation to prove youthfulness, health status, or prevent old age is pointless. The person may benefit from enrolling in an exercise program that is directed by a health professional.

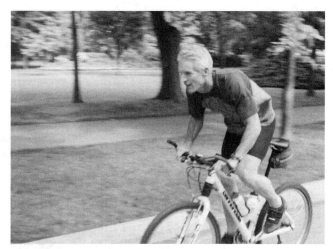

FIGURE 13-1

Middle-aged adults should be encouraged to participate in healthy behaviours such as exercising.

Given that back pain is unpredictable, a daily dose of preventive exercises will help keep your back strong. Here are several exercises you can do at home.

The first rule of exercising is to warm up. Shake out the arms and legs. Stretch the arms, reaching up with one, then the other. March in place for several minutes to circulate the blood and loosen leg muscles.

(1) The pelvic tilt can be done in any position. Lie on your back, knees bent, feet flat. Press your waist and lower back to the floor, tightening the abdominals, tucking the buttocks under the pelvis and relaxing the upper body. Release. Tuck again. Release. Repeat.

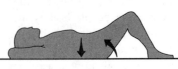

(2) Tightening the abdominal muscles will strengthen the back. Begin by lying on your back on a carpeted floor. Bend the knees and keep the feet flat on the floor. Arms are on the floor with palms down. Slowly bring one knee to your chest and face. Slowly return the leg, knee still bent, to the starting position. Repeat this exercise with each leg 5-10 times.

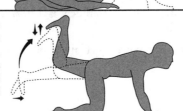

(3) Kneel on the floor on all fours. Extend the left leg out from the buttocks so that there is a straight horizontal line from the heel to the head. Now bend the knee so the bottom of the foot is facing the ceiling. Raise the leg carefully and evenly several times. Straighten the leg again and start over. Repeat with the opposite leg.

While the exercises illustrated here are considered comparatively safe, if you suffer from back or joint problems, extreme overweight, or chronic heart, circulation, or respiratory problems, check with your doctor or chiropractor before starting any exercise program. If any exercise selected becomes painful, stop immediately.

FIGURE 13–2

Back exercises for daily sitters.

Source: Back Protection for Daily Sitters, Staying Well Newsletter, May–June (1991), 2. Publication produced by The Foundation for Chiropractic Education and Research, Des Moines, Iowa.

CRITICAL THINKING

What activities would you plan for an exercise program for a middle-aged adult?

Foot balance, the *ability to alter one's position so that body weight is carried through the foot with minimum effort,* is essential to prevent strain, foot aches, and pain during exercise as well as when walking or standing. Foot imbalance may result from contracted toes, improper position, size or shape of one or more bones of the foot, weak or rotating ankles, muscle strain, weak ligaments, poor body posture, overweight, arthritis, injuries, and improperly fitted or shaped shoes. Treatment by a podiatrist consists of careful assessment of the posture and provision of balance inlays for insertion into the shoes.[168]

Foot problems may occur in middle age. Teach the person to observe for the following common signs of need for diagnostic evaluation and possible treatment:[169]

- Swelling of the feet and ankles
- Cramps in the feet and the calf while walking or at night
- Inability to keep the feet warm
- Loss of the fat tissue on the padded surfaces of the feet
- Chronic ulcers on the feet that fail to respond to treatment
- Absence of or bounding pulse in the arteries of the feet
- Showing of arteries in the foot on routine x-ray film
- Burning in the soles of the feet

Foot care should include the following:

- Clean the feet with soap and water at least once daily; dust with foot powder or cornstarch.
- Exercise the feet, extend the toes, and then flex rapidly for one or two minutes. Rotate the feet in circles at the ankles. Try picking up a pencil or marble with toes.
- Walk barefoot on uneven surfaces, thick grass, or sandy beach.
- Walk daily and properly. Keep toes pointed ahead and lift rather than push the foot, letting it come down flat on the ground, placing little weight on the heel.
- Massage the feet to rest them after a tiring day.
- Lie down with feet higher than head for approximately one-half hour daily.

- Avoid wearing poorly fitted shoes or shoes with high heels and pointed toes.

Teach that the callus or other foot problems should be treated by a podiatrist. If the person scrapes or cuts a callus, there is risk of infection.

Sleep

Most middle-aged adults sleep without difficulty; seven to eight hours of sleep constitute a normal pattern. Refer to Chapter 12 for more information on normal sleep patterns. Insomnia may be a sign of a more serious underlying medical condition, for example, cardiac or thyroid disease or depression. Some medications interfere with sleep, such as some antidepressants, antihypertensives, thyroid medication, and corticosteroids. See the box entitled "Sleep Hygiene Recommendations" to promote better sleep.[170]

Sleep Hygiene Recommendations

- Establish pre-sleep routines, e.g., a warm bath or reading.
- Maintain a regular time for sleep and awakening. Use the bed only for sleeping.
- Go to bed when feeling sleepy, or do something boring to become drowsy.
- Get regular exercise, but avoid the hours just before bedtime.
- Avoid caffeine (coffee, tea, cola, and chocolate) within six hours of bedtime.
- Avoid alcohol within several hours of bedtime.
- Avoid daytime naps.
- Avoid sleep medications, if possible, since they interfere with deep sleep and have a detrimental effect if taken for too long.

Parasomnias *are conditions in which sleep is disrupted by inappropriate activation, either in the brain centres that control body movements or in the autonomic nervous system that governs physiological and emotional functions.* Some are characteristic of non-REM (NREM) sleep and occur in the first third of the night. Others are typical of REM sleep and occur in the last two-thirds of the night.[171] Hobsen and Silvestri describe various disorders and treatment.[172] However, one kind of sleep disturbance—sleep apnea—in middle age is being studied to a greater extent.

Sleep apnea, *more than five episodes of cessation of airflow for at least ten seconds each hour of sleep,* is a problem that is being increasingly recognized. This syndrome is found primarily in men over 50 and postmenopausal women, especially in people who are obese and have short, thick necks. Approximately 35% to 40% of elders have sleep apnea. Often it is first detected because the person snores loudly or dozes during the daytime. Sleep apnea can be life-threatening. There are three types:[173,174]

- *Obstructive.* Respiratory effort continues despite pharyngeal obstruction to airflow.

- *Central.* There is no respiratory effort with airflow.
- *Mixed.* Episodes of no respiratory effort initially are followed by respiratory effort and then airflow.

The person may have the symptoms or manifestations listed in Table 13-5.[175,176] A sleep diary can be kept, on which treatment and teaching can be based (see Table 13-5).

TABLE 13-5
Sleep Apnea

Pathophysiology

- Airway collapses or is restricted during sleep
- Continued effort to breathe, respiratory difficulty
- Hypoxia caused by intervals of not breathing
- Sleep disturbed

Manifestations

- Excessive daytime sleepiness
- Frequent nocturnal awakening
- Chronic heavy, loud snoring
- Severe morning headaches, sleepiness
- Unrefreshing daytime sleep
- Irritability and personality changes
- Poor concentration, impaired memory
- Hypertension
- Cardiac arrhythmias
- Depression
- Impotence, sexual dysfunction
- Right-sided heart failure

Differential Diagnosis: Narcolepsy

- Manifestations of unexpected falling asleep, sudden loss of muscle tone, REM sleep disturbed, temporary paralysis of muscles when falling asleep or awakening, hallucinations

Client Care

- Maintain sleep diary, including hours in bed, hours slept, and sleep quality
- Avoid daytime napping
- Schedule rest time before bedtime
- Establish regular bed and wakeup times
- Avoid caffeine, nicotine, alcohol, and stimulants such as decongestants
- Avoid pharmacotherapy
- If no improvement, schedule sleep-laboratory referral for evaluation

Treatment

- Weight loss of 10% of body weight
- Dental appliance worn during sleep
- Ventilation therapy such as continuous positive-airway pressure (CPAP)
- Surgery, if severe case

CRITICAL THINKING

What would be your response to a middle-aged adult who is planning to take herbal remedies to enhance sleep?

Health Promotion and Health Protection

Immunizations

All Canadian adults require maintenance of immunity to tetanus and diphtheria preferably with combined (Td) toxoids. All adults should receive adequate doses of all routinely recommended vaccines; and other vaccinations should be given from selected circumstances when appropriate. Particular emphasis should be placed on improving appropriate utilization of influenza, pneumococcal, and hepatitis B vaccines.[177]

CRITICAL THINKING

What are some methods of identification for the use of vaccines for adults in community centres?

Injury and Accidents

The gradually changing physical characteristics and preoccupation with responsibilities may contribute to the middle-aged person's having accidents. Accidents are the fourth leading cause of death in middle age.

Fractures and dislocations are the leading cause of injuries for both sexes, with more men affected than women, probably because of occupational differences. Because of the middle-aged adult's changing physical abilities, motor vehicle accidents are the most common cause of accidental deaths in the later years, especially for men. Occupation-related accidents rank second, and falls in the home rank third as causes of death. However, women suffer less than one-third as frequently as men from fatal falls during the middle years.[178,179]

The middle-aged adult is a person at work in an industry, office, school, home, or out-of-doors. Accidents that disable persons for one week or more sharply increase after age 45.[180] Because of their interest in accident protection legislation, industries and other occupational settings are increasingly health and safety conscious. Efforts must continue in this direction.

You can teach about safety as it relates to remodelling a home, maintaining a yard, or establishing a work centre. Handrails for stairways; a handgrip at the bathtub; conveniently located electric outlets; indirect, no-glare, and thorough lighting; and tools, equipment, and home or yard machines kept in proper working condition all provide ways to avoid an accident, especially in later middle age. Sensible middle-aged people plan for the gradual failing of their physical abilities by making the home as safe, convenient, and comfortable as possible as they rethink homemaking functions for the coming decades. Further, you can be instrumental in initiating or strengthening a safety program in an occupational or school setting.

CRITICAL THINKING

You have been asked to develop an exercise program for middle-aged adults in a community centre. How would you begin?

Illness Prevention

Middle age is not automatically a period of physical or psychological hazard or disease. No single disease or mental condition necessarily is related to the passage of time, although the middle-aged person should be carefully assessed for signs of illness. Major health problems of this era are cardiovascular disease, cancer, pulmonary disease, diabetes, obesity, alcoholism, anxiety, depression, and glaucoma.[181–183]

You can help the person maintain energy and improve health by teaching the information presented in this section and the chapter. The person can learn moderate eating, drinking, or smoking habits and to use only medically prescribed drugs. Many *measures promote health:*

1. Regular physical examinations
2. Pursuit of leisure activity
3. Use of relaxation techniques
4. Working through the emotional and family concerns related to middle age
5. Affirming the worth of self as a middle-aged person
6. Preparing for the later years
7. Confronting developmental tasks

The person also needs to prepare for possible accidents or illness.

Teach that the mounting statistical, experimental, and autopsy findings point to cigarette smoking as a causative factor in breast and lung cancer, cardiovascular disease, chronic obstructive pulmonary disease, and peptic ulcer. For the person who feels trapped, depressed, frustrated, or isolated, easily accessible escapes are alcoholism, drugs, and excess food intake. Assist the person in finding other ways to cope with stressors.

The medicine cabinet may look like a pharmaceutical display if the self-absorbed person retreats into hypochondriasis. Old injuries may become bothersome, and new injuries do not heal as quickly. Illness or accident proneness can also be a means of resolving serious difficulties or of escaping responsibilities. If understanding and help from others is negligible or nonexistent and the possibility of recouping losses or rearranging one's life seems unlikely, the brief care and attention given during illness or after injury may not offer sufficient gratification. Suicidal thoughts and attempted or actual suicide is a call for help or an escape from problems. The prop of ill health should not be removed without study and caution, for removing one syndrome may only result in discharge of emotional tension through another physical or emotional syndrome. Thus nursing intervention and medical treatment must be directed toward both physical and emotional factors.

Because nursing care is holistic, you can meet emotional and spiritual needs of the person while giving physical care and doing health teaching related to common health problems discussed in the following pages.

Common Health Problems: Prevention and Treatment

A variety of health problems may occur, although many middle-aged adults remain healthy. Table 13-6 lists a summary of diseases that are frequently experienced, and texts provide for more information on the diseases summarized in the table.

TABLE 13-6
Common Health Problems in Middle Age

Problem	Definition	Symptom/Signs	Prevention/Treatment
Sinusitis, nonbacterial and bacterial	Inflammation of mucous membrane lining parnasal sinuses; may be caused by bacteria, viruses, irritants, or allergies	Normal sinus drainage prohibited Usually clear drainage in nonbacterial type Purulent drainage in bacterial type, with fever (headache and tenderness of frontal and maxillary sinus to palpation frequent with bacterial involvement)	Oral antihistamine and decongestant for nonbacterial type Addition of antibiotic for bacterial type
Hiatal hernia with esophagitis	Herniation of stomach through diaphragm with reflux of acid into esophagus	Substernal pain, usually worse when bending over or lying down Sometimes nausea and vomiting	Maintenance of ideal weight Avoidance of tight clothing Eat frequently in small amounts Elevation of head of bed
Duodenal peptic ulcer disease	Ulceration of duodenal mucosa	Pain in the epigastrum or right upper quadrant usually 1–2 hours after meals	Antacids or prescription drugs (e.g., cimetidine [Tagamet] or omeprazole [Prilosec]) Small frequent meals Avoidance of caffeine, alcohol, and spices
Angina pectoris	Imbalance between oxygen needed by myocardium and oxygen supplied	Pain in substernal region but sometimes in neck, back, and arms	Workup to determine accurate diagnosis Nitroglycerine
Secondary hypertension	High blood pressure based on specific cause	Blood pressure >150/100 More common in men, but after 55 years, women likely to be affected	Following treatment plan based on cause of high blood pressure Reduction of sodium and cholesterol in diet Reduction of weight as needed Relaxation techniques
Hyperthyroidism (Grave's disease)	Too much secretion of thyroid hormone	Can mimic heart problems with accelerated or irregular heartbeat Feeling of agitation	Antithyroid medications or radioactive iodine therapy
Hyperuricemia, or gout	High uric acid level, causing acute inflammatory arthritis (can also be chronic)	Usually red, hot tender joint; often in great toe but can be in other joints	Specific drugs Rest Elevation of joint(s) Cold compresses
Diabetes mellitus (type II)	Glucose intolerance corrected by means other than insulin	High blood sugar Thirsty Weight loss Frequent urination	Diet Exercise Oral medication

(continued)

TABLE 13-6 *(continued)*
Common Health Problems in Middle Age

Problem	Definition	Symptom/Signs	Prevention/Treatment
Prostatitis, acute	Acute infection of prostate gland; often caused by *Escherichia coli*	Low back and perineal pain referred sometimes to inguinal region and testes Extremely tender prostate	Sitz baths Appropriate antibiotics
Prostatitis, chronic	Prolonged inflammation of prostate	Only slightly tender and enlarged prostate	Prostatic massage Sitz baths Increased sexual activity
Lubosacral strain, mild	Strain and inflammation of ligaments and musculature in Lubosacral region	Muscle spasm over region but no radiation No flank pain No pain on straight leg raising	Cold packs Muscle relaxant Analgesic Bed rest Chiropractic treatment Education in bending and lifting techniques Use of firm mattress
Foot callus	Thickness of the outer layers of the skin on the sole of the foot	Pain when congestion and swelling press nerve endings, and underlying bursa	Avoid shoes that put excess pressure and friction on the sole of the foot

Common health problems in middle age, in addition to those listed on Table 13-6, are atherosclerosis, coronary artery disease, asthma, impaired vision and hearing, AIDS, obesity (gaining 10 kg in adulthood increases risk by 60%), arthritis, osteoporosis, and various kinds of cancer.

Cancer

In men the primary sites for cancer are the prostate, lung, colon, rectum, and bladder. In women, the common sites are lung, breast, colon, rectum, and cervix.[184–188]

The primary site for cancer in women is the breast followed by the lung cancer.[189] The greatest risk is for women after age 50. Exposure of the breast tissue to estrogen increases cancer risk because of cell proliferation. Thus, early menarche, late menopause, and long-term use of oral contraceptives increase risk. Adipose tissue stores estrogen, thus, obesity is a risk factor. Other *gynecologic cancers* also affect the middle-aged woman:[190–192]

1. *Cervical.* Highly curable if diagnosed and treated early. A history of human papillomas virus (HPV) infection, a prevalent sexually transmitted disease, carries an 80% risk of cervical cancer. Other risk factors include first intercourse before age 18, multiple sexual partners, large number of children, and history of smoking. In Canada, the mortality and morbidity rates have fallen significantly since screening began.[193]

2. *Endometrial.* Risk factors include irregular menses (especially postmenopausal), estrogen therapy without added progestin, polycystic ovary disease, diabetes, and hypertension.

3. *Ovarian.* Higher mortality because of lack of early symptoms. Risk factors include presence of the BRCA-1 gene mutation; history of breast, colon, or endometrial cancer; and having ovulated for more than 40 years. Epithelial ovarian cancer remains the most common cause of death from tumours of the pelvis and ranks fifth among causes of death from cancer overall in Canada.[194]

The Nurse's Health Study, which obtained information from 115 000 women over a 20-year period, has looked at a wide-ranging assortment of risk factors. Their findings indicate that one in eight women will develop breast cancer and one in two will develop cardiovascular disease eventually. Annual mammography screening has been found to reduce cancer deaths by one-third in women aged 50 to 60; mammography should not be eliminated on the basis of cost.[195,196]

In Canada, the third highest primary site for cancer is the colon.[197] Colorectal cancer, the second greatest cause of death in the U.S., affects men and women about equally, and increases steadily after age 50. A variety of screening tests can detect the precancerous polyps. Surgical removal in the early stages is curative.

Regular screening for colorectal cancer should begin at age 50. The prognosis for colorectal cancer is good if diagnosed and treated in the precancerous or early stages.[198]

The rate of death from prostate cancer has recently declined in many areas of the world. Over the past 15 years, prostate-specific antigen (PSA) screening has increased in popularity, which has resulted in increases in the incidence of prostate cancer.[199] Over the same period, there have been changes in the management of the disease. Pickles states that all men older than 45 with at least a ten-year life expectancy should be informed of the potential benefits and drawbacks of PSA screening so they can make an informed decision about whether or not to have the test.[200]

CRITICAL THINKING

What are some drawbacks of PSA testing for middle-aged men?

Cardiovascular Disease
Cardiovascular disease is the underlying cause of death in 33% of Canadians.[201] Males are more likely to die from ischemic heart disease and acute myocardial infarction, while women die from congestive heart failure and cerebrovascular disease.[202] Risk factors are increasing despite knowledge that many of these hazards are preventable. Approximately 80% have at least one risk factor (smoking, physical inactivity, overweight, hypertension, or diabetes), while 10% have three or more.[203]

According to Tanuseputro and his colleagues, even though a high prevalence of potentially modifiable cardiovascular factors and a large variation exists between subgroups in the Canadian population, the burden of cardiovascular disease could be reduced through risk factor modification.[204]

CRITICAL THINKING

How can you encourage men to become more physically active?

Respiratory Conditions
Acute, as well as chronic, pulmonary diseases are a frequent cause for days absent from work. Generally middle-aged women have more disability days from work because of respiratory and other acute disorders; men have more disability days from injuries.[205,206]

Hypothyroidism
Hypothyroidism can cause weight loss, heat intolerance, insomnia, and restlessness or irritability. All individuals over 50, especially women, should have an annual thyroid test, even if there are no apparent symptoms. Either hyperthyroid or hypothyroid disease is easily treated with drugs.[207–209]

Chronic Illness
The middle-ager may experience chronic illness in self or a family member. A number of references give information about reactions to as well as coping with chronic illness in this era.[210,211]

Chronic illness of any kind represents multiple losses: threatened self-concept and low self-esteem; unpredictability, fear of the future, and feelings of loss of support; abandonment by family, friends, and health care workers; and reduced function and spontaneity.[212] Chronic sorrow is experienced with chronic illness.[213]

Help the person to:
1. Work through feelings and practical problems.
2. Formulate new meanings and understandings.
3. Discover personal strengths and new support systems.
4. Deepen a sense of hope and faith and a personal belief system.

5. Develop a sense of humour and broaden perspective as the illness is acknowledged.
6. Make choices; take control where it is possible.
7. Share insights and solutions with others in similar situation.
8. Learn how to manage the situation.

Sometimes the chronic disease osteoporosis is not prevented in the woman. The article by Dowd and Cavalieri gives practical suggestions to help the person stay as comfortable, safe, and healthy as possible.[214]

In Canada and abroad, researchers have identified the high national costs of diabetes.[215] Jacobs and his colleagues obtained data from the Manitoba Medicare database and the Manitoba Diabetes database. They concluded that the prevalence and utilization were considerably higher for the Aboriginal population.[216]

CRITICAL THINKING

What are some ways that our society could combat the escalating incidence of diabetes?

Sexual Dysfunction
Erectile dysfunction or **impotence**, an *inability to achieve or maintain an erection sufficient for satisfactory performance,* may occur as early as 40 or 45 years (5% of men) and increases in incidence through middle age and after (15% to 25% of men over age 65). The male may experience loss of psychological arousal, less frequent erections, slower orgasms, and longer recovery between ejaculations.[217]

There are various causative factors:[218–220]
1. Late-onset diabetes, probably because of autonomic neuropathy involving the sacral parasympathetic fibres that supply the penis
2. Vascular disease, hypertension, or impaired circulation, because a high blood flow is necessary to distend vascular spaces of erectile tissue (i.e., occlusion of pudendal arteries)
3. High blood cholesterol
4. Obesity
5. Endocrine problems or adrenalectomy, reducing libido
6. Depression
7. Neurological disorders, neuropathy
8. Kidney failure
9. After myocardial infarction if activity is limited
10. Prostatectomy

Contributing factors include:[221]
1. Alcohol intake or alcoholism
2. Medications, such as some antihypertensives and some antidepressants
3. Smoking
4. Poor sexual techniques, fear of failing in sexual performance
5. Unhappy or unsatisfying relationship
6. Fatigue, mental or physical
7. Anxiety, stress response, boredom

Treatment consists of adjusting lifestyle and medications; injections of prostaglandin E$_1$ (a substance found in semen), a wraparound vacuum constrictive device, or penile implant surgery. The prescription medication sidenafil citrate (Viagra) can help some men achieve erections in response to sexual stimulation. The medication should not be used by men who are taking nitrates to reduce angina pain or for other reasons. Various side effects may occur.[222]

The middle-aged person may subtly, hesitantly, or openly discuss problems of sexual function with you. Listen carefully. Let the person know that such problems are not unusual. You may not know the answers, but your listening can help the person make a decision. Decisions involve the person seeking medical care or counselling. The person must realize the need to change behaviour. You can assist in attitude and value clarification about sexuality and sexual behaviour. Refer the person or couple to a counsellor who can help with physical and emotional problems. Sometimes a change in medication dosage or modification in treatment regimen can reduce sexual dysfunction.

Mind–Body Connections

Research shows the connection between mind and body. Some personality traits carry more risk than others for heart attack and stroke. Type A traits, such as aggressiveness, competitiveness, and anger, top the list.[223,224]

One study of anger levels in 1623 heart-attack patients found the risk for heart attack was 2.3 times greater during the two hours following an anger episode. Another study of 2074 middle-aged men in Finland found that strokes were twice as common in those with high anger scores. A study of 541 premenopausal women found that high anger increased the likelihood of plaque formation in the carotid arteries of middle-aged women.[225] Other studies also link anger, hostility, resentment, depression, and heart disease.[226,227]

Teach individuals about the mind–body connection, constructive coping skills, and anger management.[228] For example, low-dose aspirin therapy, along with sound diet and exercise can protect the heart.[229] Diet and not smoking can reduce cancer risk.[230] Taking control over cognitive distortion and developing positive thinking strategies are equally powerful in improving the immune system and self-esteem[231,232] (see Chapter 5). Establishing close friendships and leisure activities also promotes positive physiological as well as emotional effects[233,234] (see Chapter 11).

PSYCHOSOCIAL CONCEPTS

The following information is relevant to understand, assess, and intervene with the middle-ager. Health promotion strategies, physical as well as psychosocial, to aid mental and emotional functioning may be used.

Factors that Influence Research Findings on Cognitive Ability

Because most studies on adult cognition have been cross-sectional, caution is necessary in interpreting the results, as many factors are influential. For the middle-aged person especially, the *following can negatively influence test scores*:

1. Amount of education
2. Experiential differences
3. Fixed attitudes
4. Number of years since formal schooling was completed
5. General health status

The gradual neuron loss that occurs over the lifetime does not affect cognitive function. Because most intelligence tests are developed for children and adolescents, the kind of test given can influence the scores. The middle-aged adult scores relatively high on tests that require general information or vocabulary abilities. At age 60 intelligence quotient (IQ) test results are equal to or better than those of young adults. Only arithmetic reasoning shows a plateau through the adult years. Speed requirements of the test may mitigate against the IQ test scores; adults show a peak in speed of performance in the 20s and a gradual decrease in overall speed of performance through the years. Adults usually value accuracy and thoroughness more than speed.[235–237] In fact, IQ tests may be irrelevant. What should be tested is how people identify problems and use reason and intuition to solve problems.[238]

In various studies, physically fit and active men were found to have a higher IQ score than men who engaged in little physical activity.[239,240]

In the past decade more middle-aged women have returned to university for baccalaureate, graduate, doctoral, and postdoctoral degrees. They have shown themselves as capable as men scholastically and in applying intellectual ability in the workplace.

CRITICAL THINKING

What motivates women to achieve academic success in our society?

Cognitive Development

Cognitive processes in adulthood include reaction time, perception, memory, learning and problem solving, and creativity. These are performed through characteristics of both concrete and formal operations, depending on the situation.[241]

Reaction time or speed of performance is individual and generally stays the same or diminishes during late middle age. The speed of response is important primarily in test situations, because much of the problem solving necessary in adulthood requires deliberation and accuracy rather than speed. Reaction time is related to complexity of the task, the habitual pattern of response to stimuli, and familiarity with the task. Time for new learning increases with age, but adults in their 40s and 50s have the same ability to learn as they did in their 20s and 30s.[242–244]

Memory is maintained through young and middle adulthood; no major age differences are evident. Some quantitative changes may occur. For example, a person in early adulthood who could recite a ten-digit span of numbers as a series of discrete units may only be able to recite eight grouped or categorized digits in late middle age. The ability to categorize or group information, to sharpen observational skills and give more attention to the phenomenon, to relate meaning to that to be remembered, and to use interactive imagery—imagining events in a story form with self in the interaction—are all ways to strengthen memory and aid learning.[245–248] The middle-aged adult memorizes less readily material that is not well organized and seems to retain less from oral presentation of information than younger students.[249]

There are different types of memory. *Sensory memory,* information stored in a sense organ, is transitory, a few seconds. *Short-term memory* may be based on recall for days or weeks. *Long-term memory* may last a lifetime. Memory is not reliable in the adult years or at any age. Most people forget or ignore episodes that do not fit the self-image or that are considered unimportant. People who think they remember an event from childhood or a number of years previously may be making up plausible scenarios, fantasies, or confabulations based on earlier reports or stories. The middle-aged adult who continues to use memory will retain a keen memory.[250-252]

Learning occurs in adults of all ages. The highly intelligent person becomes even more learned. The capacity for intellectual growth is unimpaired and is enhanced by interest, motivation, flexibility, a sense of humour, confidence, and maturity attained through experience. Learning means more; it is not just learning for learning's sake. Knowledge is applied; motivation to learn is high for personal reasons. Reluctance to learn occurs if the new material does not appear relevant or does not serve the person as well as current information.[253-257]

Problem-solving abilities remain throughout adulthood. There are no significant differences between 20-, 40-,

EVIDENCE-BASED PRACTICE

Learning to Live with Early Dementia

Much of the literature on early dementia is focused on caregiver perspectives, while little is known about the perspectives of persons with early-stage dementia such as what it is like to live with this syndrome. This study was conducted to explore the process of learning to live with early-stage dementia. Interviews were conducted with six early-stage participants (three men and three women) ranging in age from 61 to 79 years. A preliminary theoretical framework was developed from the data, which outlines a five-stage process of learning to live with dementia that begins with various *antecedents* and proceeds through the stages of *anticipation, appearance, assimilation,* and *acceptance.* This process evolved as participants' awareness of themselves and their outer world changed. Ultimately, the findings of this study have several implications for clinicians working with persons in early-stage dementia.

The term *dementia* refers to a clinical syndrome comprising a wide range of neurological diseases that typically occur with increasing age and are distinguished by progressive memory loss, impaired judgement, and decreased capacity for abstract reasoning. The most common cause of dementia is Alzheimer's disease.

Each participant was interviewed twice. Once transcripts from the first interviews were coded and analyzed, a preliminary theory comprising six categories was identified. A second interview was conducted with each participant for the purpose of verifying and clarifying emerging theory. During the second interview (one to three months later), the interview process evolved and became more unstructured and open-ended as clarification was sought on issues that emerged in the previous interview.

Practice Implications

1. Nurse-clinicians and researchers should be cognizant of the emotional strain endured by dementia sufferers and seek to minimize any further emotional distress that may result from the interview process during a nursing assessment or research study. One means of minimizing distress may be to conduct assessments or interviews in the dementia sufferer's home.

2. Denial has been identified as a common coping method used among individuals with early memory loss. In this

study, however, evidence of denial did not surface. On the contrary, participants demonstrated a striking openness and willingness to talk about their memory impairment and its effects on their lives. Intellectualizing the disease (e.g., by educating oneself about it) was another conscious means used by participants to assimilate it into their lives.

3. One of the factors participants saw as instrumental in the assimilation process was connecting with and learning from other dementia sufferers in support groups. The participants in this study who attended a support group identified (many) benefits. These findings clearly indicate that more support groups should be established for persons with early-stage dementia. Research into the design, function, and efficiency of such groups, once established, could serve to ensure maximum benefit for participants and to secure funding to staff them with educated personnel such as nurses.

4. Supportive family and friends played a key role in enabling participants to come to terms with their memory loss. Based on this finding, nurses can play a role in educating family members and others in the importance of learning to understand and support persons in early stages of the disease.

5. The clinical approach of health care professionals who work with people with early-stage dementia is important. One participant, for example, explained that the insensitivity of her physician in blurting out to her the news that she had Alzheimer's disease had discouraged her from asking the physician questions about the diagnosis. These findings suggest that nurse clinicians and researchers must become aware of the impact of their verbal and nonverbal communication on early-stage sufferers. Adopt an individualized, unhurried approach in working with early-stage sufferers, and demonstrate the recognition of and respect for the unique difficulties and concerns of these persons.

6. As persons are being diagnosed earlier in the disease process, it is becoming increasingly important to identify the coping methods that early-stage sufferers employ and (determine) whether they facilitate or hinder adaptation to early dementia.

Source: Werezak, L., and N. Stewart, Learning to Live with Early Dementia, Canadian Journal of Nursing Research, 34, no. 1 (2002), 67–85. Used with permission.

and 60-year-olds in learning a task. Generally, better-educated people perform better than less educated people in any age group. When there is no time limitation, there are no task differences in complex task solutions because young and middle-aged adults use different strategies. Young adults, knowing they can function quickly, may be more likely to use less efficient reasoning strategies, such as trial and error. In late middle age, because people know they are becoming slower, they tend to think a problem through first so they can solve it in fewer tries. Thus, they appear to be slower in grasping and solving a problem. But the wider life experiences prompt recognition of more variables in a situation and thus enhance problem solving.[258–262]

The middle-aged adult is able to do all the cognitive strategies of **Piaget's stage of formal operations** described in Chapters 11 and 12. Sometimes the practicality of a situation will call forth use of concrete operations; because not all problems in life can be solved by abstract reasoning, the middle-aged adult does both operations realistically in problem solving. He or she also uses the fifth stage of cognitive development, problem finding, described in Chapter 11. Societal, occupational, and general life experiences are crucial to cognitive operations of the middle-aged person. Thus, perceptions about the same situation, problem, or task can vary considerably in a group of middle-aged adults.[263]

Cognitive characteristics that are developed in the young adult are used throughout middle age as well. Various patterns mark the development of **intellectual skills.** The mature adult can symbolize experience and behaves in a way that shows organization, integration, stability, and unity in the cognitive process. Representing experience symbolically as hunches, words, thoughts, or other symbols is part of becoming mature. The person can reflect on past and current experience and can imagine, anticipate, plan, and hope. The person develops an inner private world that gives him or her resources for happiness and potential for anxiety. The person can recall past defeats and triumphs and monitor ongoing thoughts for consistency and logic. When the person solves a problem, he or she can explain how it was solved. Because the mature adult is more imaginatively productive, he or she is capable of producing more images, thoughts, and combinations of ideas, is able to use reflection to gain perspectives about life, and is aware of personal beliefs, values, motives, and powers. The mature person is increasingly interested in other persons and warm, enduring relationships and is adaptable, independent, self-driven, conscientious, enthusiastic, and purposeful. The person can reflect about personal relationships, the ups and downs or contradictions in relationships, and their sources of strain and satisfaction and concomitantly understand why other persons feel and act as they do.[264–267] These characteristics of cognition are part of *contextual intelligence* and *social* or *post normal intelligence*[268] (see Chapter 12).

Riegel proposed that adult thought is characterized by **dialectical thinking,** *a seeking of intellectual stimulation and even crisis; welcoming of contradictions and opposing viewpoints, creating a new order and discovering what is missing.* Adults struggle cognitively with morality, ethics, philosophy, religion, and politics; yet, they do not necessarily need to resolve the contradictions they face. Dialectical thought increases with age.[269]

Kramer proposed that another characteristic of adult thought is to *integrate, synthesize, and form metasystems.* The person does not look for one correct answer but looks at any experience from multiple perspectives. Thus, knowledge is ever-changing.[270]

Buhler[271] implies cognitive development as she describes the *maintenance* and *change* tendencies in life. *Maintenance,* through the restitution of deficiencies (need satisfaction) and upholding of the system's internal order, is necessary for cognitive function to occur. *Change,* involving self-limited adaptation and creative expansion, is part of the cognitive development of the adult. Maintenance and change occur with different emphases in various life stages. The child develops self-limiting adaptation as he or she learns; the adolescent and adult move into creative expansion; after middle age, the person assesses the past and self and wants to restore inner order, and in old age, the person either continues to follow previous adaptive and creative drives or regresses to need-satisfying tendencies.

The intellectually curious have an increased need and ability to spin new syntheses and theories, to make meaningful that which seems meaningless, to coordinate hypothesis formation and testing, to be systematic at problem solving, to seek environmental diversity, and to become more subtle, differentiated, integrated, and complex. The mature person has a progressive integration; that is, he or she is continually open, flexible, curious, and actively engaged. If cognitive efficiency becomes disrupted, a mature person is able to recover from such disorganization more quickly than an immature person, even though the two do not differ in intelligence. The person can analyze and judge information, even that which is personally relevant, in terms of demands of the information itself without being influenced by either personal desires or persuasive opinions of others. Thought becomes objective and judgment independent.[272–274]

Neugarten, in her studies, found that the person changes both cognitively and emotionally over time as the result of accumulated experience. The person abstracts from experiences and creates more encompassing and more refined categories for interpreting events. The middle-aged person differs cognitively from the young adult in that he or she was born in a different historical era and thereby has different formative experiences. The middle-aged adult thus has a greater apperceptive mass or store of past experience by which to evaluate events or make decisions. Through the adult years, perspectives and insights broaden and deepen, and attitudes and behaviours change.[275–279]

Although *Gould*[280–283] focuses more on personality than cognitive development, he described adulthood as a time of thoughtful confrontation with the self—letting go of the idealized image, the desire to be perfect, and acknowledging the realistic image of self and personal feelings. The adult continues to gain new beliefs about self and the world. Conflicts between past and present beliefs are resolved.

Assist the middle-aged adult (and others) in understanding the cognitive changes and strengths of cognitive ability. Reinforce a positive self-image related to cognitive abilities.

CRITICAL THINKING

What are some ways that our society might foster the learning of adult citizens?

Creativity

Dennis[284] found an age pattern for creative output. He found that scientists show a peak activity in early and middle adulthood. Unique, original, and inventive productions are more often created in the 20s, 30s, and 40s than later in life. The more a creative act depends on accumulated experience, the more likely it is to occur in middle age or later life. People are less productive in total creative output in their 20s than in their 30s and 40s. Poets, novelists, and scholars gain in productivity in middle and old age, and, although quality may decrease, quality increases as a greater proportion of contextual, intuitive, and social intelligence is used.[285-288] Some creative works cannot be produced without the benefit of years of experience and living, absorbing the wisdom of the culture, and the resultant development of new insights.

Creativity is seen not only in famous people or young people. The average middle-aged adult may have many responsibilities and stresses; however, typically he or she approaches a situation, task, or learning experience in a creative way.

You can encourage the middle-aged adult to pursue creative ideas and activities and to approach roles, responsibilities, and tasks in a creative way. Help the middle-aged adult overcome any self-consciousness about the unique cognitive response to a situation.

Continued Learning

With increasing emphasis on continued learning, the middle-aged person is frequently enrolled in refresher courses, continuing education courses, or workshops related to occupation or profession. He or she takes college credit and noncredit courses to deal with specific problems; learn specific content; learn for fun; find an academic program that is necessary for changing a profession or occupation; gain more personal satisfaction; relieve boredom, loneliness, or an unhappy situation; or broaden the mind and learn for the sake of learning. Rapid technologic changes in business or the professions cause obsolescence of knowledge and skills, which also forces middle-aged persons to continue to learn.

When you are teaching, use *methods that capitalize on the learning strengths of mature adults, including:*

1. Active discussion and role-play
2. De-emphasis on memorization
3. Presentation of large amounts of new information
4. Suggestions to develop cognitive strategies that will help him or her synthesize, analyze, integrate, interpret, and apply knowledge
5. Validating with the middle-aged adult and others that he or she can learn, because myths to the contrary are prevalent
6. Providing a conducive environment, one that considers sensory changes
7. Consideration of the sensory changes discussed previously

Work and Leisure Activities

Work

Work will be viewed differently by different middle-agers. Consider that the older middle-aged person grew up under the influence of the Depression and with the Protestant ethic. Both stressed the economic and moral importance of work. Thus, work became respected and sought. Being without a job or idle was a harbinger of problems and meant being lazy and worthless. How has this middle-aged adult adjusted to mechanization, waning of the work ethic, the demise of a full day's work for a full day's pay? For the young middle-ager, what was a promising career or lifetime employment may have ended in being laid off permanently by the company, forced early retirement, or forced job hunting. Finding work could be difficult.[289-293] If the person is unemployed and job hunting, see the box entitled "Suggestions for Someone Who Is Unemployed"[294] or you may want to explore career options described in the box entitled "Career Track Options in Late Middle Age."

CRITICAL THINKING

What are some strategies you might use with a middle-aged adult who is Asian and unemployed?

Suggestions for Someone Who Is Unemployed

- Offer hope and encouragement, but guard against sounding "spiritually superior." This is a dark valley, emotionally, economically, philosophically, and spiritually.
- Remind the person that unemployment is a reflection of current economic conditions, not of personal worth.
- Seek opportunities to affirm the person's talents and positive attributes.
- Help him or her consider all the options, including launching a business from home, changing careers, and working part-time.
- Allow the person to express feelings, but do not encourage self-pity. Your time with the person should leave him or her feeling uplifted and hopeful. Pray with the person if he or she desires.
- Offer to hold him or her accountable to a specific job-hunting schedule. It is often hard to stay motivated and organized without a friendly nudge.
- Talk about subjects other than unemployment.
- Encourage the person/family to relax and have fun. If you are a friend, invite them to your home or give them a gift certificate for dinner and a movie.
- If the person is a friend or relative, provide practical, but discreet, help, including food, clothing, and finances.

The person may be fortunate enough to be in a business or profession in which he or she works successfully for self or is allowed freedom within a specialized area of work. As many as 20% may be self-employed. He or she will experience the dignity of being productive and will enjoy increasing self-esteem, autonomy, and sense of achievement; however, most middle-aged adults are employed in a system in which the value is on production, not the person. Often, in contrast to union-set rules, whereby no more than a specified amount can be done within a specified time, ever-greater output is demanded on the job.

Career Track Options in Late Middle Age

Coast into Retirement

- Do the job but no more; collect the paycheque; enjoy the final years.

Go for Last Promotion

- Campaign to obtain final reward for all that was contributed to receive public acknowledgment of the importance of work done.

Try for Great Achievement

- Work to outdo the present record and others' records so that others will see you saved the best for last.

Survive Difficult Period

- Recognize the company's difficult period; learn to survive and even prosper in the challenging time.

Retire Early

- Take the attractive package being offered by the company so that the years of later maturity can be enjoyed.

Start Your Own Business

- If tired of working for others, go into business for self (e.g., consulting in work arena, turning hobby into business).

There are several categories of workers that are different from the past. They have been described as follows:

1. *Free agents.* They seek and find professional and financial independence in a variety of entrepreneurial occupations. Many work alone, out of a home office, and are involved in community services as well as business ventures. They know how to market talents to the highest and most interesting bidder.

2. *Nomads.* They have no real loyalty to the job or the boss as they move from one geographic area and job to another. They spot the next trend, find a job at a company, and are ready to move with it. In their job-hopping and hunting, they develop great contacts and a variety of skills. They take advantage of job opportunities as they arise.

3. *Globalists.* They travel from time zone to time zone around the world as they work in a borderless economy with their laptop computer. They constantly network, scout out opportunities, and improvise as necessary.

4. *Niche-finders.* They spot new markets emerging from recent social and economic trends and build, market, and manage a company to capitalize in it. They are the leaders in the new industry.

5. *Retreads.* They relish learning and stay abreast of technological change. Because of their maturity and experience, they'll never be without a job. Self-improvement, helping peers adapt, and reminding younger workers that computer skills are only one facet of the job guarantee that they will never become obsolete.

6. *Corporate leaders.* New-age bosses redesign jobs to incorporate new skills and ventures. They give workers freedom to manoeuvre as needed to hang on to valuable employees. They expand responsibilities for self and others as they dream up new projects.

But whatever the category, for employed North Americans, the biggest chunk of time goes to working for a living. The time spent at the full-time job has increased over the past two decades. There is a decline in leisure. Many feel that they are overworked and have insufficient time for family. For some, the ideal playground is the workplace. All sorts of workers carry cell phones or pagers; business-related calls come in constantly. It can be difficult in some jobs to keep up with voice mail and e-mail, let alone the necessary reading. The "baby boomers" declared their contempt for "the man in the grey flannel suit": the company-oriented worker. However, they have done more than any other generation to erase the line between work and private life in many professions, managerial jobs, or careers. Work is considered the way of such fulfillment. Work has forced the middle-ager to develop and expand skills beyond what was considered possible to accomplish.[295]

CRITICAL THINKING

What would life be like in today's society for a middle-aged person without technology?

Many middle-aged women work outside of the home; thus, they are especially in the middle in terms of the demands of various roles on their time and energy. The middle-aged woman is wife, mother, homemaker, grandmother, worker, and organization member. The women who are caregivers also have child care responsibility; some may have quit their jobs or have work conflicts. The middle-aged woman is often in the middle in terms of two competing values: (1) traditional care of elders is a family responsibility and (2) women should be free to work outside the home if they wish. Each family member feels the repercussions as the balance of roles and responsibilities changes. Most middle-aged women are working today for a variety of reasons:[296]

- Inflation and the rising cost of living
- Changes in attitudes about sex-appropriate roles as a result of the woman's movement
- The rising divorce rate that forces the woman to become economically independent
- Fewer children in the home
- Use of labour-saving devices for the home that results in free time
- Increasing educational levels that stimulate career interests or the desire to remain in the profession
- Expectancy of a higher standard of living
- Assistance with costs of sending children to university

Determine the degree of work stability, extent to which work is satisfying, and emotional factors that have operated in the person's concept of work and in the self-concept. Assess how well the middle-aged person can function as a mentally and physically healthy person. As a professional person, you will have to resolve conflicts related to your work role. Hence, you are in a position to assist the middle-aged person in talking about and resolving feelings and values related to work and other activity.

Because the demands on middle-aged adults are often overwhelming—work, home, family, church, and social and civic organizations—teach steps for effective *time management* (see the box entitled "Guidelines for Time Management").

Retirement comes for others after a layoff, and no job is found for years. Some, because of financial need, will work as long as possible. But retirement will have to come eventually (see the box entitled "Suggestions for Planning for Early Retirement"). Explore with the person various options to prepare for retirement—at age 55, 62, 65, 70, or 75.[297] Help the person to examine risks or the worst possible scenario if an option is chosen. Examine what it will take in effort and ability to make the option happen, strategies to fall back on if the option is not successful, the support system (financial, emotional, and social) to ensure success, and personal willingness both to take the risks and to enjoy the benefits. A part of planning for retirement is to study the financial plans that go with each option to ensure, to the extent possible, financial security in old age.[298–303]

Guidelines for Time Management

- Establish priorities; maintain a log if necessary. *Write goals.*
- *Do it now.* Do not procrastinate with small tasks; schedule large projects.
- Recognize *unpleasant tasks; work on them first.*
- *Clear the decks and desks.* Eliminate clutter; organize the workplace for efficiency.
- *Stick to the job.* Avoid distractions.
- *Do one thing at a time.* Finish one major task before beginning another; however, *there are times you can do two things at once*, e.g., planning while waiting in line.
- *Plan ahead.* Assemble what is needed for a task before initiating it; set aside relaxation time.
- *Consider limitations—your own,* equipment not available for a project, and other responsibilities that will interfere.
- *Learn to say "no" and suggest someone else* who would be able to handle the situation. Delegate low-priority jobs to others.
- *Anticipate delays* that are inevitable in every task; plan for interruptions and unforeseen events.
- *Plan on alternative way* to do the job; have backup activity if a selected task cannot be done as scheduled.
- *Use odd times.* Shop when stores are not crowded; carry a notebook to jot ideas while you wait.

Suggestions for Planning for Early Retirement

- Start planning early. Most successful early retirees have long-range plans in place before they reach 40.
- Stay with a good employer. Unless you are sure you can strike it rich on your own, work for secure companies with generous pension plans. Avoid excessive job hopping so you can accrue substantial pension benefits.
- Make use of employer-sponsored investment programs. Place a percentage of your paycheque into tax-deferred plans. Participate to the maximum.
- Save and invest wisely in other plans—bonds, stocks, property, other annuities, and RRSPs. You cannot count on Old Age Pension or a company pension. You may have to live off savings. You will need between 60% and 80% of preretirement income.
- Plan for unexpected medical expenses.
- Scale back your lifestyle. There are many ways to do this. You might buy a smaller house, forego extravagant vacations, or send your kids to local colleges instead of Ivy League schools.
- Explore career directions you can pursue later in life. You may want to work a few months a year or hours a week. Some individuals have turned a hobby into a way to make money.

CRITICAL THINKING

What other strategies can you use to manage time effectively?

Retirement

Some people in this era *retire* early by plan. The life decade of the 50s is a point of transition in development of consciousness about retirement. Middle-aged persons *least likely to anticipate retirement* include those who:

- Work in a company that is prospering
- Have unfinished agendas at work
- Have high job satisfaction
- Perceive retirement as unfeasible because they have not done advance financial (or emotional) planning
- Retain their health

Leadership Role

The middle-aged adult's cognitive stage is in favour of his or her being a formally designated or an informal leader, if other factors are favourable. (Usually middle-aged leaders have developed necessary qualities from childhood on, but occasionally a person does not believe that he or she has this ability until there is a measure of success in the life work.)

The *leader* usually has the *following characteristics*:[304,305]

- Adequate socioeconomic resources
- Higher level of education or success than majority of group to be led
- Realistic self-concept
- Realistic goals and ability to encourage others toward those goals

- High frustration tolerance
- Ability to express negative thoughts tactfully
- Ability to accept success or failure gracefully
- Ability to delegate authority
- Understanding of group needs
- Flexibility in meeting group needs

The middle-aged person may demonstrate this leadership ability on the job or in community or church organizations. Women who are most successful in leadership careers are those who have little conflict in the multiple roles of career woman, mother, and wife. Their husbands' support and encouragement are major assets, but women are also becoming more assertive on their own behalf about their roles outside the home.

You can encourage or reaffirm the middle-aged person in the leadership role. You may also assist him or her in working through feelings or conflicts related to the work setting or the job itself.

Leisure

The middle-aged person, taught little about how to enjoy free time, may now be faced with increasing amounts of leisure because of advances in technology, earlier retirement, and increased longevity. The average middle-aged adult who has moved up the pay scale and whose children may be grown will have more money and more time to take trips or try new hobbies. Yet *various factors hinder use of these new opportunities:*[306,307]

- Value of work learned in younger years
- Cultural emphasis on intellectual pursuits so that play is considered childish and a poor use of time and talents
- Conditioning to at least appear busy
- Fears of regression and not wanting to return to work
- Lack of previous opportunity to learn creative pursuits or hobbies
- Hesitation to try something new because of fear of failure

Help the person avoid feelings of alienation that result from inability to use leisure time. Use the suggestions in the box entitled "Teaching Use of Leisure in the Daily Schedule" with your middle-aged clients.

CRITICAL THINKING

What are some other strategies you might use to teach a client and his or her family about the effective use of leisure time?

CRITICAL THINKING

What are some leisure activities you may pursue for yourself?

Emotional Development

The middle years, the climacteric, are a period of self-assessment, and greater introspection—a transitional period. In middle age (and beyond) the person perceives life as time left to live rather than time since birth. Time is seen as finite; death is a possibility. Middle-aged adults clock themselves by their positions in different life contexts—changes in body, family, career—rather than by chronologic age. Time is seen in two ways: (1) time to finish what the person wants to do and (2) how much meaning

Teaching Use of Leisure in the Daily Schedule

- Emphasize that both play and recreation are essential to a healthy life.
- Stress the indispensability of leisure as a part of many activities, whether work or creative endeavours. Leisure is both a state of mind and use of time away from work. Have the person analyze leisure activities, whether they bring pleasure, work off frustration, make up deficits in life, or create a sense of pressure or competition.
- Help the person recognize the interplay of physical and intellectual endeavours and their contribution to mental health.
- Differentiate compulsive, competitive, and aggressive work and play from healthy, natural work and play. Intrinsic in play are spontaneity, flexibility, creativity, zest, and joy.
- Recognize the person's creative efforts to encourage further involvement in leisure activities.
- Educate the person about the importance of preparing for retirement.
- Inform the person of places, courses, or workshops at which he or she can learn new creative skills and use of talents.
- Encourage the person to enjoy change, to participate in organizations, and to initiate stimulating contacts with others.
- Encourage the person to stop the activity when it no longer meets personal needs.

and pleasure can be obtained in the time that is left. The person makes the often-agonizing reappraisal of how achievements measure up against goals and of the entire system of values. He or she realizes that the choices of the past have limited present choices. He or she can no longer dream of infinite possibilities. The person is forced to acknowledge that he or she has worked up to or is short of personal capabilities. Goals may or may not have been reached; aspirations may have to be modified. The possibility for advancement becomes more remote. The person will have to go on with ever-brighter, ever-younger men and women crowding into the competitive economic, political, and social arena.

Developmental Crisis

According to Erikson,[308] the psychosexual crisis of middle age is generativity versus self-absorption and stagnation. **Generativity** is a *concern about providing for others that is equal to the concern of providing for the self.* If other developmental stages were managed successfully, the person has a sense of parenthood and creativity; of being vital in establishing and guiding the next generation, the arts, or a profession; of feeling needed and being important to the welfare of humankind. The person can assume the responsibility of parenthood. As a husband or wife, each can see the strengths and weaknesses of the other and combine their energies toward common goals.

A biological parent does not necessarily get to the psychosocial stage of generativity, and the unmarried person or the person without children can be very generative.

The middle-aged person who is generative takes on the major work of providing for others, directly or indirectly. There is a sense of enterprise, productivity, mastery, charity, altruism, and perseverance. The greatest bulk of social problems and needs fall on this person who can handle the responsibilities because of personal strengths, vigour, and experience. There is a strong feeling of care and concern for that which has been produced by love, necessity, or accident. He or she can collaborate with others to do the necessary work. Ideas about personal needs and goals converge with an understanding of the social community, and the ideas guide actions taken on behalf of future generations.

The generative middle-aged adult may be a mentor to a young adult. A **mentor** is an *experienced adult, with experience, wisdom, patience, and understanding, who befriends, guides, and counsels a less experienced and younger adult in the work world or in a social or an educational situation.*

Mentoring differs from coaching. The mentor has the following roles:

- Advisor
- Guide
- Sponsor
- Tutor
- Advocate
- Coach
- Role model
- Protector
- Friend

Mentoring involves developing a long-term relationship with many roles. Coaching is performance-oriented. The mentor is usually approximately ten years older, is confident, warm, and flexible, enjoys sharing knowledge and skills, is trustworthy, and promotes psychosocial development and success of the younger person. The mentor is found in business, management, nursing, or other careers or professions, sponsoring the younger person as an associate, creating a social heir, teaching him or her as much as possible for promotion into a position, or recommending the one being mentored for advancement. Several authors present more information on mentoring.[309–311]

CRITICAL THINKING

What is your conceptual understanding of the process of mentoring?

The middle-aged person's adaptive mechanism and superego are strong but not rigid. There is an expansion of interests and investment in responsibilities. Youth and young adults usually are self-centred. With approaching middle age and the image of one's finite existence faintly in view, the person consciously reappraises and uses self. With introspection, the self seems less important, and the words *service, love of others,* and *compassion* gain new meaning. These concepts motivate action. In church work, social work, community fund drives, cultural or artistic efforts, a profession, or political work, the person is active and often the leader. The person's goal is to leave the world a better place in which to live. A critical problem, however, is coming to terms with accomplishments and accepting responsibility that comes with achievement. In addition, he or she must come to terms with violations of the moral codes of society (e.g., tax loopholes used by some adults) and, with superego and ego in balance, develop a constructive philosophy and an honest method of operation.

Some middle-aged adults believe the most important work of the person begins after parenthood ceases and is cognitive and emotional in nature: preserving culture, maintaining the annals of history, keeping alive human judgment, maintaining human skills, preserving and skillfully contriving the instruments of civilization, and teaching all this to oncoming generations. Although young and middle-aged adults are involved in such functions, these qualities of the human mind are best manifested in the late middle years or thereafter.

The generative person feels a sense of comfort or ease in lifestyle. There is realistic gratification from a job well done and from what has been given to others. He or she accepts self and the body, realizing that although acceptance of self is originally based on acceptance from others, unless he or she accepts self, he or she cannot really expect acceptance from others.

The mature middle-aged person has tested ways of doing things. He or she can draw on much experience; thus, he or she may have deep sincerity, mature judgment, and a sense of empathy. He or she has a sense of values or a philosophy underlying the life, giving a sense of stability and causing him or her to be reflective and cautious. The person recognizes that one of the most generative things he or she can give to society is the life led and the way he or she lives it. Consider the following statement by a 50-year-old man:

> *Those were full years—raising the kids with all its joy and frustration. I'm glad they're on their own now. This is a new stage of life. I can go fishing; Mary can go out to lunch. We have more time together for fun, and now we have more time for working at the election polls and in volunteer activities.*

CRITICAL THINKING

What do you believe is the main message of this 50-year-old man?

The middle years can be wise and felicitous, or they can be foolish and frantic, fraught with doubts and despair.

If the developmental task of generativity is not achieved, a sense of **stagnation,** or **self-absorption,** enshrouds the person. Thus, *he or she regresses to adolescent, or younger, behaviour, characterized by physical and psychological invalidism.* This person hates the aging body and feels neither secure nor adept at handling self physically or interpersonally. He or she has little to offer even if so inclined. He or she operates on a slim margin and soon burns out (see the box entitled "Consequences of Self-Absorption"). Consider the following statement by a 50-year-old woman:

> *I spent all those years raising the kids and doing housework while Bob moved up the professional ladder. We talked less and less about each other, only about the kids or his job. Now the kids are gone. I should be happy, but I'm lost. I can't carry on a decent conversation with Bob. I don't have any training for a job. And I look terrible! I sit around and eat too much. I wear high collars to hide my wrinkled neck, and no cosmetics will hide the dark circles under my eyes.*

Consequences of Self-Absorption

- Denial of signs of normal aging
- Unhappiness with advancing age, desire to stay young, fear of growing old
- Regression to inappropriate youthfulness in dress or behaviour, rebelliousness, foolish behaviour
- Preoccupation with self, self-indulgence
- Physical, emotional, social, and interpersonal insecurity
- Attempts to prove youthfulness with infidelity to spouse
- Resignation, passivity, noninvolvement with societal or life issues
- Isolation or withdrawal from others
- Despair about signs of aging (considers self old, life is over)
- Either overcompliance or excessive rigidity in behaviour
- Intolerance, cynicism, ruthless attitude
- Lack of stamina, chronic health problems that are not coped with
- Chronic defeatism, depression

Immature adults have impaired and less socially organized intellectual skills and value systems; their intellectual skills are fused by personal emotions and are coordinated in strange and unrealistic ways. The immature person seeks private self-absorption and vicarious immersion in subjective problems of others. Yet the characteristics of the self-absorbed person are health-endeavouring attempts and reparative efforts to cope or adapt. They may or may not work well, depending on the intensity of personality characteristics and the social and physical environment.

Maturity

Because **maturity,** *being fully developed as a person,* is not a quality of life reached at any one age or for all time, the characteristics described as generativity are general guidelines.

Realize that if the person is doing what is appropriate for age, situation, and culture, he or she is acting maturely for the age. As the person grows older, the ideal level of maturity and autonomy may recede further into the future and never be fully achieved. Maturity is the achievement of efficiently organized psychic growth predicated on integration of experiences of solving environmentally stimulated conflicts. The external environment is a potent force on the person; conflicts are primarily socially incurred. The psychosocial organization in maturity shows a cultural direction. As one ages, the psychic interests broaden and are less selfish. Part of maturity is staying power, the power to see it through, which is different from starting power. Seeing it through is to use faith and persistence, to continue even against great odds.

Characteristics of staying power include:

1. Integrity of consciousness and personhood
2. Remaining loyal to values, faith, philosophy, beliefs

3. Holding to a cause greater than self
4. Giving up something worthwhile rather than worrying about present risks

In adulthood there is no one set of appropriate personality characteristics. You will work with many personality types as you promote health. The great person for the time is one who stands firm in the face of opposition at a crucial moment in history. The great person is intolerant of the evils he or she is trying to combat. Each of us leads a particular life at a particular time, place, and circumstance and with a particular personal history. Success in leading that life depends on a *pattern* of qualities appropriate to that life.

The mature person is reflective, restructures or processes information in the light of experience, and uses knowledge and expertise in a directed way to achieve desired ends. No one will reach the highest ideal of self-actualization described by Maslow (Chapter 5), yet each can reach his or her own ideal and peak of well-being and functioning relatively free of anxieties, cognitive distortions, and rigid habits and with a sense of the individuality and uniqueness of the self and others.

The following *characteristics of positive mental health and maturity* were described by Jahoda:[312]

- Accepting personal strengths and limits, having a firm sense of identity, and living with the past without guilt
- Striving for self-actualization and living up to the highest potential
- Developing a philosophy of life and code of ethics, an ability to resist stress and tolerate anxiety, and the equilibrium of intrapsychic forces
- Having a sense of autonomy, independence, and ability for self-direction
- Having an adequate perception of reality and of factors affecting reality, having a social sensitivity, and treating others as worthy of concern
- Mastering the environment: working, playing, solving problems, and adapting to the requirements of life
- Valuing human relationships and feeling responsible to others

Other authors have also identified criteria for emotional maturity (see the box entitled "Criteria of Emotional Maturity").[313-316]

CRITICAL THINKING

What is your understanding of emotional intelligence?

Personality Development

Emotional or personality development has also been described by the stage theorists Jung[317,318] and Sheehy.[319]

Jung divided personality development to correspond to the first and second halves of the life cycle. In the first half, until the age of 35 or 40, the person is in a period of expansion. Maturational forces direct the growth of the ego (the conscious or awareness of self and the external world); capacities

Criteria of Emotional Maturity

- Ability to deal constructively with reality
- Capacity to adapt to change
- Relative freedom from symptoms that are produced by tensions and anxieties
- Capacity to find more satisfaction in giving than receiving
- Capacity to relate to other people in a consistent manner with mutual satisfaction and helpfulness
- Capacity to sublimate, to direct one's instinctive hostile energy into creative and constructive outlets
- Capacity to love
- Ability to use intuition, a natural mental ability associated with experience to comprehend life-events and formulate answers

unfold for dealing with the external world. The person learns to get along with others and tries to win as many of society's rewards as possible. A career and family are established. To achieve it is usually necessary for men to overdevelop the masculinity and for women to overemphasize their feminine traits and skills. The young person dedicates self to mastery of the outer world. Being preoccupied with self-doubt, fantasy, and the inner nature is not advantageous to the young adult, for the task is to meet the demands of society confidently and assertively.[320,321]

Jung believed that, during the 40s, the personality begins to undergo a transformation. Earlier goals and ambitions have lost their meaning. The person may feel stagnant, incomplete, depressed, as if something crucial is missing, even if the person has been quite successful, because success has often been achieved at the cost of personality development. The person begins to become introspective, to turn inward, and to examine the meaning of life. Separating self from ordinary conformity to the goals and values of mass society and achieving a measure of psychic balance are accomplished through individuation—finding one's individual way.[322,323]

Jung recognized that, although middle-aged persons begin to turn inward, they still have much energy and resources for the generativity described by Erikson and for making personal changes. The person may begin new or long-forgotten projects and interests or even change careers. Men and women begin giving expression to their opposite sexual drives. Men become less aggressively ambitious and more concerned with interpersonal relationships. They begin to realize that achievement counts for less and friendship for more. Women tend to become more aggressive and independent. Such changes can create midlife marital problems. Although ongoing development may create tension and difficulties, Jung believed that the greatest failures come when adults cling to the goals and values of the first half of life, holding on to the glories and beauty of youth.[324,325]

Levinson[326] describes midlife stages of development (see Tables 12-5 and 13-7).

As you work with the middle-aged person, use the concept of generativity versus self-absorption in assessment of the client's developmental level, and promote achievement of this developmental task through your listening, support, encouragement of activities, teaching, and counselling. The generative person or mentor needs to hear that what he or she is doing is indeed a worthwhile contribution. Your own generativity can be a positive model for others. Your reinforcement of another's strengths facilitates further emotional development and maturity. The self-absorbed person should be referred to a long-term counsellor.

TABLE 13-7 Levinson's Theory of Mid-Adulthood	
Age Range	Life Structure
40–65	Re-evaluate match between self-concept and achievements; are senior members in community; assume responsibility for next generation.
45–50	Enter middle adulthood bridge between past and future.
50–55	Age 50 transition; take stock of self in relation to family and occupation.
55–60	Culminate life plans and structure for middle age; new level of stability; may be peak of career.
60–65	Late adult transition; prepare for aging.
65 and beyond	Late adulthood.

Source: Adapted from Levinson, D., A Conception of Adult Development, American Psychologist, 41 (1986), 3–13; Levinson, D., A Theory of Life Structure Development in Adulthood, in K.N. Alexander and E.J. Langer, eds., Higher Stages of Human Development, New York: Oxford University Press, 1990, 35–54.

CRITICAL THINKING

What strategies could you develop to help the middle-aged person who is self-absorbed?

Body Image Development

The gradually occurring physical changes described earlier confront the person and are mirrored in others. The climacteric causes realignment of attitudes about the self that cut into the personality and its definition. Other life stresses cause the person to view self and the body differently. The person not only realizes he or she is looking older but subjectively feels older as well. Work can bring a sense of stress if he or she feels less stamina and vigour to cope with the task at hand. Illness or death of loved ones creates a concern about personal health, sometimes to excess, and thoughts about one's own death are more frequent. The person begins to believe that he or she is coming out second-best to youth, for the previous self-image of the youthful, strong, and healthy body with boundless energy becomes inadequate. Depression, irritability, and anxiety about femininity and masculinity result. In North America, more than in European or Asian cultures, youth and vigour are highly valued, a carryover from frontier days.[327] The person's previous personality largely influences the intensity of these feelings and the symptoms associated with body image changes. Difficulties are also caused by fear of the effects of the climacteric, folklore about sexuality, attitudes toward womanhood, social and advertising pressures in our culture, and emphasis on obsolescence.

Whether a man or a woman, the person who lacks self-confidence and who cannot accept the changing body has a compulsion to try cosmetics, clothes, hairstyles, and the other trappings of youth in the hope that the physical attributes of youth will be attained. The person tries to regain a youthful figure and face, perhaps through surgery; tints the hair to cover signs of grey; and turns to hormone creams to restore the skin. These people are clients at times. There is nothing wrong with dressing attractively or changing the colour of one's hair. Most people gradually adjust to their slowly changing body and accept the changes as part of maturity. The mature person realizes it is impossible to return to youth. To imitate youth denies the mature person's own past and experience. The excitement of the middle years lies in using adeptly the experience, insights, values, and realism acquired earlier. The person does not need to downgrade or agree continually with everything that young people say and do. The middle-aged person feels good about self. Healthy signs are that he or she prefers this age and has no desire to relive the youthful years.

You can promote integration of a positive body image through your communication skills and teaching. Reaffirm the strengths of being middle-aged to the client, using information presented in this chapter and emphasizing the specific strengths of the person.

Adaptive Mechanisms

The adult may use any of the adaptive mechanisms described in previous chapters. **Adult socialization** is defined as the *processes through which an adult learns to perform the roles and behaviours expected of self and by others and to remain adaptive in a variety of situations.* The middle-aged adult is expected and normally considers self to be adaptive. The emphasis is on active, reciprocal participation of the person; little preparation is directed to anticipating, accepting, or coping with failure. The ability to shift emotional investments from one activity to another, to remain open-minded, and to use past experience as a guide rather than as the rule is closely related to adaptive ability.

The adult, having been rewarded for certain behaviours over the years, has established a wide variety of role-related behaviours, problem-solving techniques, adaptations to stress, and methods for making role transitions; they may not be adaptive to current demands or crises or to increasing role diffusion. There is a continuous need for socialization in adulthood, for a future orientation, for anticipating events, and for learning to respond to new demands. Ongoing learning of adult roles occurs through observation, imitation, or identification with another, trial-and-error behaviour, the media, books, or formal education.

Coping or adaptive mechanisms or ego defences used in response to the emotional stress of the middle years depend on the person's capacity to adapt and satisfy personal needs, sense of identity, nature of interaction with others, sense of usefulness, and interest in the outside world.

The middle-aged adult must be able to channel emotional drives without losing initiative and vigour. During middle age the person is especially vulnerable to a number of disrupting events: physiologic changes and illness in self and loved ones, family stresses, changes in job or role demands or responsibilities, conflict between family generations, and societal changes. The person should be able to cope with ordinary personal upheavals and the frustrations and disappointments in life with only temporary disequilibrium. He or she should be able to participate enthusiastically in adult work and play and to experience adequate sexual satisfaction in a stable relationship. The person should be able to express a reasonable amount of aggression, anger, joy, and affection without undue effort, unnecessary guilt, or lack of adequate control. Further, the middle-aged adult is a role model of maturity for the young adult.

The person can retain a sense of balance by recognizing that each age has its unique joys and charms, and the entire life span is valued as equally precious. He or she can appreciate what is past, anticipate the future, and maintain a sense of permanence or stability. The person can adapt successfully to the stresses of middle age by achieving the developmental crisis.

You can help the middle-aged adult prevent or overcome maladaptive mechanisms. As you extend empathy and reinforce a sense of emotional maturity and health, the person may feel more able to cope with life stressors and perceived failures. If you feel unable to listen to or work with the problems of someone who may be twice your age, refer the person to a counsellor.

CRITICAL THINKING

What are some other ways that you can help a middle-aged adult from another culture to overcome maladaptive mechanisms?

Midlife Crisis

Middle age can be seen as a transition or a crisis. The **midlife crisis** is *a major and revolutionary turning point in one's life, involving changes in commitments to career or spouse and children and accompanied by significant and ongoing emotional turmoil for both the individual and others.* The term **midlife transition** has a different meaning; it includes *aspects of crisis, process, change, and alternating periods of stability and transition.*[328–333]

For some, midlife is one of the better periods of life: it is a *transition* from youth to later maturity; life expectancy is longer; psychologically and physically, midlife is healthier than ever in history; and parental responsibilities are decreasing. Most people are in their late 40s or early 50s when the last child leaves home, leaving a couple of decades for the spouses to be together without the obligations of childrearing. The couple realizes that the myth of decreasing sexual powers is not true. Women in midlife may begin or continue their education or a career. Men see midlife as a time of continuing achievement. Experience, assurance, substance, skill, success, and good judgment more than compensate for the disappearance of youthful looks and physical abilities.

Levinson[334,335] also found in his study of men that the period of midlife transition is around ages 40 to 45. For a few, the sense of change even in relation to body changes was slight, not particularly painful, and a manageable transition. For approximately 80% of the men, however, the early 40s evoked tumultuous struggles within the self and with the external world. This period involved for many a profound reappraisal, false starts, emotional turmoil, and despair. At least one-third of North American males between the ages of 40 and 60 will experience some aspect of midlife crisis.

If the person has not resolved the identity crisis of adolescence and achieved mature intimacy in young adulthood, if the person fears the passage of time, physical changes, aging,

---

CASE SITUATION
Midlife Crisis

Louise, a 48-year-old architect, had an uneasy feeling about her relationship with her husband Charles, age 49 and a teacher. The feeling had been there for some time, and she had tried a time or two to talk about it but had been rebuffed by Charles.

Louise believed that she and Charles were slowly drifting apart, each into his or her own profession. Yet the pronouncement by Charles seemed so sudden. As she joined him in the family room after dinner, he quietly looked at her and said, "I have something to tell you. I'm leaving. There's nothing here for me anymore. I'm almost 50. I've got to get on with things."

Louise was overcome with shock, grief, guilt, disbelief, helplessness, and worry. They had been married for 22 years. She had often thought about all they could do together when they retired. Because they were childless, they would be free to travel. She panicked as she thought of life and aging without him. For days she slept and ate little but managed to go to work.

In the following months Louise and Charles met to talk several times. She wanted them to see a marriage counsellor and work out their differences. As Charles continued to move his clothes, belongings, and favourite items from the home, he revealed that he would be living with another woman, a colleague from his work, and they would marry as soon as both divorces were finalized.

The divorce proceedings took more than a year. During that time Louise sought counselling for herself. Gradually she revealed her situation to her family, other relatives, and friends. She often blamed herself for Charles's leaving and talked frequently of what a wonderful person he was. She maintained a hectic pace, caring for the home and yard and handling the responsibilities of her job; however, in the months after the initial separation, Louise also re-established a daily exercise routine, which she had interrupted after Charles left home. She contacted a number of friends she had seen only occasionally in the past few years and began to attend the church of her childhood faith. She was pulling herself together—physically, emotionally, mentally, socially, and spiritually.

After the divorce was finalized, Louise continued to blame herself for several years. She worked hard, achieving recognition at the architectural firm where she was employed. She also maintained her home and neighbourhood ties and became active in her church.

After ten years Charles, who is remarried, still visits Louise occasionally and calls every few weeks. Louise has resolved the events of Charles's midlife crisis but has avoided opportunities to date or remarry. She believes the struggles and crises of the past decade, including various illnesses and the death of her parents, have prepared her for adaptation to her eventual retirement, aging, and dying. She still believes that she and Charles could re-establish a marriage and that it would be more love-filled and happy. Yet she remains fully committed to caring for a number of older friends; to the responsibilities of her profession, home, and organizational and church membership; and to continuing to deepen her spiritual and emotional maturity.

1. In your assessment you note that Louise has avoided opportunities to enlarge her social network on an intimate level. How can you assist Louise to work through her grief?

2. Discuss the psychosocial implications of Louise's belief system.

3. List, with your rationale for each, several health promotion strategies you would employ with Louise.

and mortality, *if the person cannot handle the meaning of life's routines and changes, midlife is seen as a crisis.*

Family experiences are undoubtedly integral to the direction of the midlife crisis. The midlife transition for men, often the husbands of menopausal women, brings new stresses. This period is often accompanied by sexual problems, sometimes leading to affairs, marital disruption, and the abandonment of the wife. Adolescent children may be sexually and aggressively provocative, challenging, or disappointing. Children leaving home for school or marriage change the family balance. Having no children can be a keen disappointment when the man realizes he has no heirs. Some women view their children's leaving home and marrying as an extension or expansion of parenting to include the wider interests and loci of their children. Far-flung needs of family members and expanded interests and activities lead to a different kind of parenting. Some women are restored to themselves and to their own development. Restored to themselves does not mean alone; women depend much more on their relationships for their development—not only for their emotional comfort and security but also to express the acting-on-the-world component of their aggression. The potential for autonomy, changes in relationships, and the development of their occupational skills, contacts, and self-image may start after childbearing is completed. The woman's newfound autonomy, role changes, and increased interaction with or demands on the husband may be very threatening to the man.

It is healthier in the long range for the person to acknowledge the disruptive feelings and the diffusion of identity and to work through them rather than to deny them, and to seek a healthy and constructive outlet for these feelings.

You can be instrumental in assisting the person in working through this crisis. You will use principles of communication and crisis intervention (see Chapter 5). Refer the person to a counsellor who can work with the individual and family. *The following guidelines may help the person who feels he or she is in midlife crisis. Share and use them as you work with others,* or use them in your own life.

- Do not be scared by the midlife crisis. Physical and psychological changes are normal throughout life; see them as opportunities for maturing.
- Face your feelings and your goals realistically. If you feel confused, see a counsellor who can help you sort through your feelings and goals.
- See your age as a positive asset. Acknowledge your strengths and the benefits of middle age. Take steps to adjust to your liabilities or to correct them if you can. If a change in hairstyle or clothes makes you feel better, make that change.
- Reconcile yourself to the fact that some or many of your hopes and dreams may never be realized and may not be attainable. Remain open to the opportunities that are available; they may exceed your dreams.
- If the job is not satisfying, consider another job or another field after appraising yourself realistically; or be willing to relinquish some responsibility at work.
- If you dread retirement, plan for it financially, along with leisure and other activities.

- If job pressures are great, seek outlets through recreational activities or other diversions, become involved in community service, and renew spiritual study and religious affiliations.
- Renew old friendships; initiate new ones. Invest in others and, in the process, enhance personal self-esteem and emotional well-being.
- Try to be flexible and open-minded rather than dogmatic or inflexible in meeting and solving the problems you face.
- If you are concerned about sexual potency, realize that the problem is typically transient. The more you worry, the worse it gets. Talk about your sexual feelings and concerns with your spouse. The love and concern you have for each other can frequently overcome any impotency. It is important for the woman to perceive sexuality apart from childbearing and menstruation and for the man to perceive sexuality apart from having children and love affairs. If you are so inclined, together read how-to sex manuals. Seek a marriage counsellor if together you cannot work out problems of sexual dysfunction.
- Share your feelings, concerns, frustrations, and problems with your spouse or confidante so that she or he can understand the changes you are experiencing. Keeping feelings to oneself can increase alienation and the difficulty of repairing the relationship.
- Examine your attitudes as a parent; strike a balance between care and protection of offspring. Realize their normal need for independence.
- Realize that frequently the middle-aged woman is becoming more assertive just when the middle-aged man is becoming more passive. Recognizing this as normal and talking about these changes can help the spouses better understand each other's needs and aspirations.
- Get a physical examination to ensure that physical symptoms are not indicators of physical illness. Do not think that vitamins or health foods alone will cause you to feel differently.
- Seek counselling for psychological symptoms. The counsellor may be a nurse, religious leader, mental health therapist, social worker, marriage counsellor, psychologist, or psychiatrist.

Give some specific suggestions to the spouse of the man in midlife crisis:

- Recognize and acknowledge changes in him, but do not make value judgments. Do not say, "You look awful dressed in that. Who do you think you are, a young swinger?" Say instead, "I notice you're no longer wearing your regular suits and ties. Why is that?"
- Make it easier for him to talk about his feelings and fears by listening to verbal and nonverbal messages. Avoid telling him how he should feel, dress, or behave.
- Try not to make him feel guilty by hurling your fears or anger at him. His guilt about your fears will only cause him to withdraw and refuse to discuss his problems with you.
- Emphasize to him that he does not have to leave to find what he is looking for. Try to find new joint interests,

friends, or hobbies. Be willing to see a marriage counsellor with him.

■ Focus on changing yourself. Become more alive by taking care of your appearance, keeping informed, and broadening your interests.

■ Avoid threatening his self-concept by appearing too competent in managing all areas of life while he neglects his usual family and home roles. Encourage him to maintain roles. Be prepared to pick up loose ends, however.

■ Try to re-establish the intimacy and closeness that you once shared. Be willing to compromise and change your own attitudes and behaviour.

■ Try to maintain spontaneity in your sexual life. Allow a sense of adventure to rekindle the relationship. If you can re-establish an active and satisfying sexual life at this point, you can both be certain that it will continue for many more years.

■ If he is coping with a midlife crisis symptom, focus on his strengths. But do not hand out empty praise. Instead find a real reason to praise him.

■ Do not adopt a motherly role toward him. Whereas sympathy and compassion are constructive, constant mothering and giving advice tend to diminish his sexual interest and ability to relate as your husband.

■ Do not feel guilty when your husband develops any of the midlife crisis symptoms. It is not your fault. If handled with honesty and intelligence, the midlife crisis in men can be a positive turning point in a marriage, eventually creating a more constructive, satisfying, loving relationship.

Assist individuals considering midlife career or work changes to assess their current job skills and applicability of them to new careers, explore alternatives within their current job position and external counselling services, and examine personal values.

Benefits from the midlife crisis include personality growth and deepening maturity because of personal introspection and desire to change behaviour to feel better and improve one's life. The concern about mortality can motivate the person to take better care of health and to take time to pursue new interests or reinitiate old relationships. The person can experience an invigorating rebirth, generating new energies and new commitments.

Moral-Spiritual Development

The middle-aged person continues to integrate new concepts from widened sources into a religious philosophy if he or she has gained the spiritual maturity described in Chapter 12. He or she becomes less dogmatic in his or her beliefs. Faith and trust in God or another source of spiritual strength are increased. Religion offers comfort and happiness. The person is able to deal effectively with the religious aspects of upcoming surgery and its possible effects, illness, death of parents, or unexpected tragedy.

The middle-aged person may have become alienated from organized religion in early adulthood or may have drifted away from religious practices and spiritual study because of familial, occupational, and social role responsibilities. As the person becomes more introspective, studies self and life from new perspectives, ponders the meaning of life, and faces crises, he or she is likely to return to study of religious literature, practices of former years, and organized religious groups for strength, comfort, forgiveness, and joy. Spiritual beliefs and religion take on added importance. The middle-aged adult who becomes revived spiritually is likely to remain devout and active in his or her faith throughout life. If the person does not deepen spiritual insights, a sense of meaninglessness and despair is likely in old age.

Moral development is advanced whenever the person has an experience of sustained responsibility for the welfare of others. Middle age, if it is lived generatively, provides such an experience. Although the cognitive awareness of higher principles of living develops in adolescence, consistent commitment to their ethical applications develops in adulthood after the person has had time and opportunity to meet personal needs and to establish self in the family and community. Further, the level of cognitive development sets the upper limits for moral potential. If the adult remains in the state of concrete operations, he or she is unlikely to move beyond the conventional level of moral development (law-and-order reasoning), because the postconventional level requires a deep and broad understanding of events and a critical reasoning ability.[336]

Although Kohlberg's work[337] on moral development was done on men, women generally come out at stage 3 of the conventional level (see Table 5-9 on pages 222–223), which emphasizes an interpersonal definition of morality rather than a societal definition of morality or an orientation to law and order. Perhaps the stage of moral development often seen in women, with concern for the well-being of others and a willingness to sacrifice self for others' well-being, is an aspect of stage 5 of the postconventional level.

Gilligan,[338,339] whose research centred on moral development in women, found that women define morality in terms of selfishness versus responsibility. Women subjects with high morality scores emphasized the importance of being responsible in behaviour and of exercising care with and avoiding hurt to others. Men think more in terms of general justice and fairness; women think in terms of the needs of specific individuals. Gilligan's view of moral development is outlined in Table 13-8 according to three levels and the transition points from level I to level II and from level II to level III.

Developmental Tasks

Each period of life differs from the others, offering new experiences and opportunities and new tasks to surmount. The developmental tasks of middle age have a biological basis in the gradual aging of the physical body, a cultural basis in social pressures and expectations, and an emotional origin in the individual lifestyle and self-concept that the mature adult has developed.

The following developmental tasks should be accomplished by middle-aged people. Through your care, counsel, and teaching, you can assist your clients to be aware of and to achieve these tasks.

■ Maintain or establish healthful life patterns.

■ Discover and develop new satisfactions as a mate, give support to mate, enjoy joint activities, and develop a sense of unity and abiding intimacy.

TABLE 13–8
Moral Development in Women

Level	Characteristics
I. Orientation of individual survival	Concentrates on what is practical and best for self
Transition 1: from selfishness to responsibility	Realizes connection to others; thinks of responsible choice in terms of another as well as self
II. Goodness as self-sacrifice	Sacrifices personal wishes and needs to fulfill others' wants and to have others think well of her; feels responsible for others' actions; holds others responsible for her choices, dependent position; indirect efforts to control others often turn into manipulation through use of guilt
Transition 2: from goodness to truth	Makes decisions on personal intentions and consequences of actions rather than on how she thinks others will react; takes into account needs of self and others; wants to be good to others but also honest by being responsible to self
III. Morality of nonviolence	Establishes moral equality between self and others; assumes responsibility for choice in moral dilemmas; follows injunction to hurt no one, including self, in all situations

Source: Gilligan, C., In a Different Voice: Women's Conceptions of Self and of Mortality, Harvard Educational Review, *47, no. 4 (1977), 481–517.*

- Help growing and grown children to become happy and responsible adults and relinquish the central position in their affections, free the self from emotional dependence on children, take pride in their accomplishments, stand by to assist as needed, and accept their friends and mates.
- Create a pleasant, comfortable home, appropriate to values, interests, time, energy, and resources; give, receive, and exchange hospitality; and take pride in accomplishments of self and spouse.
- Find pleasure in generativity and recognition in work if employed; gain knowledge, proficiency, and wisdom; be able to lead or follow; balance work with other roles; and prepare for eventual retirement.
- Reverse roles with aging parents and parents-in-law, assist them as needed without domineering, and act as a buffer between demands of aging parents and needs of young adults; prepare emotionally for the eventual death of parents unless they are already deceased.
- Maintain a standard of living related to values, needs, and financial resources.
- Achieve mature social and civic responsibility; be informed as a citizen; give time, energy, and resources to causes beyond self and home. Work cooperatively with others in the common responsibilities of citizenship; encourage others in their citizenship; stand for democratic practices and the welfare of the group as a whole in issues when vested interests may be at stake.
- Develop or maintain an active organizational membership, deriving from it pleasure and a sense of belonging;

refuse conflicting or too burdensome invitations with poise; work through intra-organizational tensions, power systems, and personality problems by becoming a mature statesperson in a diplomatic role, leading when necessary.
- Accept and adjust to the physical changes of middle age, maintain healthful ways of living, attend to personal grooming, and relish maturity.
- Make an art of friendship; cherish old friends and choose new; enjoy an active social life with friends, including friends of both sexes and of various ages; accept at least a few friends into close sharing of feelings to help avoid self-absorption.
- Use leisure time creatively and with satisfaction, without yielding too much to social pressures and styles; learn to do some things well enough to become known for them among family, friends, and associates; enjoy use of talents; share some leisure time activities with a mate or others and balance leisure activities with active and passive, collective and solitary, service-motivated and self-indulgent pursuits.
- Acknowledge and confront the psychological sense that the time left for cognitive, creative, emotional, social, and spiritual fulfillment is shorter and that fulfillment may never come.
- Continue to formulate a philosophy of life and religious or philosophic affiliation, discovering new depths and meanings in God or a creator that include but also go beyond the fellowship of a particular religious denomination; gain satisfaction from altruistic activities or the concerns of a

particular denomination; invest self in significant causes and movements; and recognize the finiteness of life.

■ Prepare for retirement with financial arrangements and development of hobbies and leisure activities, and rework philosophy and values.

The single or widowed middle-aged person will have basically the same developmental tasks but must find a sense of intimate sharing with friends or relatives (also see the box entitled "Key Interpersonal Relationships for Never-Married Women").

Key Interpersonal Relationships for Never-Married Woman

Blood ties:	Nieces, nephews, siblings, aging parents. Often the woman gives assistance, which involves sacrifice.
Constricted ties:	Affiliation with a nonkin family; establishment of a quasi-parental tie with a younger person who is like a son or daughter; or a long-term relationship with a same-generation companion. These relationships are voluntary and positive, but there is no assurance of care from these individuals.
Quasi-parental relations:	Acting like a parent to younger nonrelatives. There is no biogenetic tie but the relationship is modelled on parent–child tie.
Companionate:	A marriage-like interdependency in which there is much involvement over time and a sense of obligation to care for each other.
Friendship:	A close relationship that endures and provides security. Depending on the duration and closeness, the friend may provide help in time of need.

Peck[340] sees the issues, conflicts, or tasks the person must work through in middle age as encompassing four aspects:

1. *Valuing wisdom gained from living and experience versus valuing physical powers and youth.* The person needs to accept his or her age, that youth cannot be regained, and that although physical strength and power may diminish, wisdom may accomplish more than physical strength anyway.

2. *Socializing versus sexualizing in human relationships.* The middle-aged adult, although still active sexually, now sees

and relates to people as humans rather than just on the basis of men or women. The person relates to others without the sexual self-consciousness of adolescence or young adulthood and sees the intrinsic dignity and worth of all people as social and spiritual beings.

3. *Emotional flexibility versus emotional impoverishment.* The middle-aged adult, although often accused of being rigid and unable to change, remains accepting of and empathic to others, open to people of different backgrounds, and open to changing personal behaviour. The person becomes emotionally impoverished only if he or she withdraws from others, avoids learning from experience, refuses to change, or demonstrates the self-absorption described by Erikson.[341]

4. *Mental flexibility versus mental rigidity.* The middle-aged adult, although accused of being closed to new ideas and excessively cautious, remains open to learning and flexible in problem-solving strategies. The person becomes mentally rigid if he or she avoids new experiences or learning opportunities or denies social, educational, or technologic changes.

HEALTH CARE AND NURSING APPLICATIONS

Your role in caring for the middle-aged person and family has been described throughout the chapter. Assessment, using knowledge presented in this chapter, is the basis for formulating *nursing diagnoses.* Nursing diagnoses that may be applicable to the middle-aged adult are listed in the box entitled "Selected Nursing Diagnoses Related to Middle Age." Interventions may involve the health promotion or direct care measures described throughout the chapter to assist the person and family in meeting physical, emotional, cognitive, spiritual, and social needs. Stolte states that middle adulthood is generally productive with much energy placed on career development, family responsibilities, and community concerns.[342] Nurses often have contact with middle-aged adults either in hospitals or community settings. A wellness diagnosis would be helpful to enhance the person's life.

TRANSITION TO LATER MATURITY

The middle-aged adult has developed a sense of the life cycle; through introspection, he or she has gained a heightened sensitivity to the personal position within a complex social environment. Life is no longer seen as an infinite stretch of time into the future. The person anticipates and accepts the inevitable sequence of events that occur as the human matures, ages, and dies. The middle-aged adult realizes that the course of his or her life will be similar to the lives of others. Sex differences between men and women diminish in reality and perception. Turning points affect all and are inescapable. Personal mortality, achievements, and failures and personal strengths and limits must be faced if the person is to be prepared emotionally and developmentally for later maturity and the personal aging process. The person realizes that the direction in life has been set by decisions

Selected Nursing Diagnoses Related to Middle Age

Pattern 1: Exchanging

- Altered Nutrition: Less than Body Requirements
- Altered Nutrition: Risk for More than Body Requirements
- Risk for Infection
- Risk for Injury
- Risk for Trauma
- Impaired Skin Integrity
- Altered Dentition
- Energy Field Disturbance

Pattern 2: Communicating

- Impaired Verbal Communication

Pattern 3: Relating

- Impaired Social Interaction
- Social Isolation
- Altered Role Performance
- Risk for Altered Parenting
- Sexual Dysfunction
- Altered Family Processes
- Caregiver Role Strain
- Parental Role Conflict
- Altered Sexuality Patterns

Pattern 4: Valuing

- Spiritual Distress

Pattern 5: Choosing

- Ineffective Individual Coping
- Impaired Adjustment
- Defensive Coping
- Ineffective Denial
- Ineffective Family Coping: Disabling
- Ineffective Family Coping: Compromised
- Altered Nutrition: More than Body Requirements
- Family Coping: Potential for Growth
- Decisional Conflict
- Health-Seeking Behaviours

Pattern 6: Moving

- Impaired Physical Mobility
- Activity Intolerance
- Fatigue
- Risk for Activity Intolerance
- Sleep Pattern Disturbance
- Diversional Activity Deficit
- Impaired Home Maintenance Management
- Altered Health Maintenance

Pattern 7: Perceiving

- Body Image Disturbance
- Self-Esteem Disturbance
- Chronic Low Self-Esteem
- Situational Low Self-Esteem
- Sensory/Perceptual Alterations
- Hopelessness
- Powerlessness

Pattern 8: Knowing

- Knowledge Deficit

Pattern 9: Feeling

- Pain
- Chronic Pain
- Dysfunctional Grieving
- Anticipatory Grieving
- Risk for Violence: Directed at Others
- Risk for Self-Mutilation
- Post-Trauma Syndrome
- Anxiety
- Fear

Other NANDA nursing diagnoses are applicable to the ill middle-aged adult.

Source: North American Nursing Diagnosis Association, NANDA Nursing Diagnoses: Definitions & Classification 1999–2000. *St. Louis: North American Nursing Diagnosis Association, 1999.*

NARRATIVE VIGNETTE

Wellness Diagnosis: Caretaker's Role

Mrs. L, age 60, has breast cancer, which has metastasized to the bone and brain. Her husband, age 75, is somewhat fragile; and her 40-year-old daughter resides, with her family, about one hour away from their home. During your visit to Mr. and Mrs. L's home, you note that Mrs. L appears calm and comfortable, and she informs you that the medication is effectively controlling her pain. You observe that Mr. L is sitting at her bedside, holding his wife's hand. In a soft and loving tone of voice, Mr. L informs his wife not to worry and that "everything's going to be OK," adding that their daughter and family will be in later for a visit.

1. Develop a wellness diagnosis for this family.
2. List several interventions, with rationales for your diagnosis.

related to occupation, marriage, family life, and having or not having children. Although occupation and lifestyle can be changed, at least to some extent, the results of other earlier decisions cannot be changed. The consequences must be faced and resolved. The middle-aged person realizes he or she may not achieve all dreams, but remaining open to opportunities along the way may enable the person to achieve accomplishments never fantasized that are equally meaningful.

The person in late midlife realizes that life's developmental markers and crises call forth changes in self-concept and sense of identity, necessitate incorporation of new social roles and behaviours, and precipitate new adaptations. But they do not destroy the sense of continuity within the person from youth to old age. This adaptability and a sense of continuity are essential for the achievement of ego integrity in the last years of life.

INTERESTING WEBSITES

CANADIAN CAREGIVER COALITION

http://www.ccc-ccan.ca

This organization's mission is to join with caregivers, service providers, and other stakeholders to identify and respond to the needs of caregivers in Canada.

A FRIEND INDEED: MENOPAUSE & MIDLIFE NEWSLETTER

http://www.afriendindeed.ca/canada.htm

This publication provides understandable and reliable information about midlife and the menopausal transition, independent of any vested interests. It is published six times yearly and distributed to thousands of women across North America.

HEART AND STROKE MENOPAUSE CHECKLIST

http://ww1.heartandstroke.ca/Page.asp?PageID=1562&ArticleID=1397&Src+&From+SubCategory

This checklist can be filled in online, printed out, and brought on medical visits. Women and their doctors can go through the checklist and talk about a number of options.

WEIGHT WATCHERS CANADA

http://www.weightwatchers.ca/about/his/index.aspx

For over 40 years Weight Watchers has helped millions of people lose weight. The Weight Watchers plan was developed by respected health officials, but Weight Watchers is not a medical organization and cannot give medical advice.

SUMMARY

1. The middle years are filled with challenge, pleasures, and demands.
2. The middle-ager is in the "sandwich generation," caring for children and grandchildren, and aging parents and other relatives.

3. This is the prime of life, although some physical changes occur that require adaptation.
4. The middle-ager continues to learn and, in turn, is a mentor and leader in the community.
5. This is a time of generativity, of wanting to leave the world a better place.
6. The middle-ager relies on experience, resolves value conflicts, and initiates action that is relevant to the situation.
7. For some, middle age is a time of struggle, crisis, loss, or illness.
8. The box entitled "Considerations for the Middle-Aged Client in Health Care" summarizes what you should consider in assessment and intervention with the middle-aged client and family.
9. Health promotion behaviours are important for present and future well-being.

Considerations for the Middle-Aged Client in Health Care

1. Family and cultural history
2. Personal history
3. Pre-existing illness
4. Risk factors for disease in family (e.g., cardiovascular disease, cancer, osteoporosis, developmental disability, mental illness)
5. Psychosocial evaluation (age-related stresses, distress with partner, midlife crisis issues)
6. Caregiver responsibilities
7. Knowledge of normal changes in middle age and coping strategies—adaptive capacity
8. Nutrition history—weekly diet intake
9. Complete physical examination
10. For women:
    a. Menstrual history (age onset, pattern, current pattern)
    b. History of estrogen administration
    c. Reproductive history (number of pregnancies, at what age, miscarriages or abortions)
    d. Perimenstrual history (beginning of menopausal symptoms, response, whether menopause has occurred)
    e. Interest in or current administration of hormone replacement therapy; any side effects
11. Other members of household (review 1–9)

ENDNOTES

1. Gormly, A., *Lifespan Human Development* (6th ed.). Fort Worth: Harcourt Brace College Publishers, 1997.
2. Papalia, D., and S. Olds, *Human Development* (3rd ed.). Boston: McGraw Hill, 1998.
3. Sheehy, G., *The Silent Passage: Menopause.* New York: Random House, 1992.
4. Sheehy, G., *Passages for Men.* New York: Random House, 1998.
5. Santrock, J., *Life Span Development* (6th ed.). Chicago: Brown & Benchmark, 1997.
6. *Ibid.*
7. *Ibid.*
8. Gormly, *op. cit.*
9. Papalia and Olds, *op. cit.*
10. Santrock, *op. cit.*

11. Hoff, L., *People in Crisis: Understanding and Helping* (4th ed.). Redwood City, CA: Addison-Wesley, 1995.

12. Santrock, *op. cit.*

13. Papalia and Olds, *op. cit.*

14. Seifert, K., R. Hoffnung, and M. Hoffnung, *Lifespan Development.* Boston: Houghton Mifflin, 1997.

15. Sigelman, C., *Life-Span Human Development* (3rd ed.). Pacific Grove, CA: Brooks/Cole, 1998.

16. Papalia and Olds, *op. cit.*

17. Santrock, *op. cit.*

18. Sigelman, *op. cit.*

19. Martin-Matthew, A., Aging and Families: Ties over Time and Across Generations, in N. Mandell and A. Duffy, eds., *Canadian Families: Diversity, Conflict, and Change* (3rd ed., pp. 311–331). Toronto, Thomson, Nelson, 2005.

20. McPherson, B.D., *Aging as a Social Process* (3rd ed.). Toronto: Harcourt Brace, 1998.

21. Martin-Matthew, *op. cit.*

22. Boyd, M., and M. Nihart, *Psychiatric Nursing: Contemporary Practice.* Philadelphia: Lippincott, 1998.

23. Burgess, A., *Psychiatric Nursing: Promoting Mental Health.* Stamford, CT: Appleton & Lange, 1997.

24. Hoff, *op. cit.*

25. Bee, H., D. Boyd, and P. Johnson. *Lifespan Development* (Canadian ed.). Toronto: Pearson Education Canada, 2003.

26. Chappell, N., E. Gee, L. McDonald, and M. Stone, *Aging in Contemporary Canada.* Toronto: Pearson Education Canada, 2003.

27. *Ibid.*

28. Mitchell, B.A., and E.M. Gee, Young Adults Returning Home: Implications for Social Policy, in B. Galaway and J. Hudson, eds., *Youth in Transition to Adulthood: Research and Policy Implications* (pp. 61–65). Toronto, Thomson Educational Publishing, 1996.

29. Mitchell and Gee, *op. cit.*

30. Gormly, *op. cit.*

31. Sheehy, G., *Passages for Men.*

32. Santrock, *op. cit.*

33. Sinnot, J., The Developmental Approach: Postformal Thought as Adaptive Intelligence, in F. Blanchard-Fields and T.M. Hess, eds., *Perspectives on Cognitive Change in Adulthood and Aging* (pp. 358–386). New York: McGraw-Hill, 1996.

34. Gormly, *op. cit.*

35. Santrock, *op. cit.*

36. Gormly, *op. cit.*

37. Papalia and Olds, *op. cit.*

38. Santrock, *op. cit.*

39. Seifert et al., *op. cit.*

40. Gormly, *op. cit.*

41. Papalia and Olds, *op. cit.*

42. Sheehy, G., *Passages for Men.*

43. Sigelman, *op. cit.*

44. Statistics Canada, *Population by Marital Status and Sex*, Website: http://www.statcan.ca/english/Pgdb/Famil01.htm, October 2004.

45. Papalia and Olds, *op. cit.*

46. Hoff, *op. cit.*

47. Lund, D.C., and M.S. Caserta, Older Men Coping with Widowhood, *Geriatrics & Aging*, 7, no. 6 (2004), 29–33.

48. Caserta, M.S., D.A. Lund, and S.J. Rice, Pathfinders: A Self-Care and Health Education Program for Older Widows and Widowers, *Gerontologist*, 39 (1999), 615–620.

49. *Ibid.*

50. Chappell et al., *op. cit.*

51. Rosenthal, C.J., M.A. Martin, and S.H. Matthews, Caught in the Middle? Occupancy in Multiple Roles and Help to Parents in a National Probability Sample of Canadian Adults, *Journal of Gerontology*, 51B (1996), S274–S283.

52. *Ibid.*

53. Chappell et al., *op. cit.*

54. Martin-Matthew, *op. cit.*

55. Clemens-Stone, S., D.G. Eigsti, and S. McGuire, *Comprehensive Community Health Nursing: Family, Aggregate, and Community Practice* (4th ed.). St. Louis: C.V. Mosby, 1995.

56. Gormly, *op. cit.*

57. Papalia and Olds, *op. cit.*

58. Sigelman, *op. cit.*

59. Statistics Canada, *Caring for an Aging Society*, Website: http://www.statcan.ca/english/freepub/89-582-XIE/, March 2004.

60. *Ibid.*

61. *Ibid.*

62. Ward-Griffin, C., and V. W. Marshall, Reconceptualizing the Relationship between "Public" and "Private" Eldercare, *Journal of Aging Studies*, 17 (2003), 189–208.

63. Brody, E.M., S.J. Litvin, C. Hoffman, and M.H. Kleban, Marital Status of Caregiving Daughters and Co-residence with Dependent Parents, *The Gerontologist*, 35, no. 1 (1995), 75–84.

64. Fink, S.V., The Influence of Family Resources and Family Demands on the Strains and Well-being of Caregiving Families, *Nursing Research*, 44, no. 3 (1995), 139–146.

65. Franks, M.M., and M.A.P. Stephens, Social Support in the Context of Caregiving: Husband's Provision of Support to Wives Involved in Parent Care, *Journal of Gerontology*, 51B, no. 1 (1996), P43–P52.

66. Fredman, L., M. P. Daly, and A. M. Lazur, Burden among White and Black Caregivers to Elderly Adults, *Journal of Gerontology*, 50B, no. 2 (1995), S110–S118.

67. Gormly, *op. cit.*

68. Mathews, S. H., Gender and the Division of Filial Responsibility between Lone Sisters and Their Brothers, *Journal of Gerontology*, 50B, no. 5 (1995), S312–S320.

69. Sheehy, G., *Passages for Men.*

70. Picot, S.J., Rewards, Costs, and Coping of African American Caregivers, *Nursing Research*, 44, no. 3 (1995), 147–152.

71. Pohl, J.M., C. Boyd, J. Liang, and C.W. Given, Analysis of the Impact of Mother-Daughter Relationships on the Commitment to Caregiving, *Nursing Research*, 44, no. 2 (1995), 68–75.

72. Sigelman, *op. cit.*

73. Young, R.F., and E. Kahana, The Context of Caregiving and Well-being Outcomes Among African and Caucasian Americans, *The Gerontologist*, 35, no. 2 (1995), 225–232.

74. Brody et al., *op. cit.*

75. Fink, *op. cit.*

76. Gormly, *op. cit.*

77. Mathews, *op. cit.*

78. Mui, A.C., Caring for Frail Elderly Parents: A Comparison of Adult Sons and Daughters, *The Gerontologist*, 35, no. 1 (1995), 86–93.

79. Papalia and Olds, *op. cit.*

80. Pohl et al., *op. cit.*

81. Sigelman, *op. cit.*

82. Fast, J.E., and N.C. Keating, *Informal Caregivers in Canada: A Snapshot.* Ottawa: Health Canada, 2001.

83. Taylor, S., and M.H. Kopot, The Breakfast Club: Providing Support for Male Caregivers of Persons with Alzheimer Disease or Related Dementia, *Geriatrics Today: Journal of the Canadian Geriatric Society*, 4, no. 3 (2001), 136–140.

84. *Ibid.*

85. Fink, *op. cit.*

86. Gormly, *op. cit.*

87. Papalia and Olds, *op. cit.*

88. Sigelman, *op. cit.*

89. Zarit, S.H., P.A. Todd, and J.M. Zarit, Subjective Burden of Husbands and Wives as Caregivers: A Longitudinal Study, *The Gerontologist*, 26 (1986), 260–266.

90. Perry, J., Wives Giving Care to Husbands with Alzheimer's Disease: A Process of Interpretive Caring, *Research in Nursing & Health,* 25 (2002), 307–316.

91. Bar-David, G., Three Phase Development of Caring Capacity in Primary Caregivers for Relatives with Alzheimer Disease, *Journal of Aging Studies,* 13, no. 2 (1999), 177–197.

92. *Ibid.*

93. Eakes, G., M. Burke, and M. Hainsworth, Middle-Range Theory of Chronic Sorrow, *IMAGE: Journal of Nursing Scholarship,* 30, no. 2 (1998), 179–184.

94. Martin-Matthew, *op. cit.*

95. *Ibid.*

96. Andrews, M., and J. Boyle, *Transcultural Concepts in Nursing Care* (3rd ed.). Philadelphia: Lippincott, 1999.

97. Bee, H., *Lifespan Development* (2nd ed.). New York: Longman, 1998.

98. Gormly, *op. cit.*

99. Papalia and Olds, *op. cit.*

100. Santrock, *op. cit.*

101. Seifert et al., *op. cit.*

102. Putting Polish on the Golden Years, *Postgrad: St. Louis University School of Medicine,* 17, no. 1 (1995), 8–12.

103. Santrock, *op. cit.*

104. Wasaha, S., What Every Woman Should Know About Menopause, *American Journal of Nursing,* 96, no. 1 (1996), 24–32.

105. Putting Polish on the Golden Years.

106. Santrock, *op. cit.*

107. Wasaha, *op. cit.*

108. Lock, M., Menopause in Cultural Context, *Experimental Gerontology,* 29 (1997), 307–317.

109. Santrock, *op. cit.*

110. *Ibid.*

111. Sheehy, G., *Passages for Men.*

112. Lock, *op. cit.*

113. Santrock, *op. cit.*

114. Lock, *op. cit.*

115. *Ibid.*

116. Sheehy, G., *Passages for Men.*

117. *Ibid.*

118. Boyd and Nihart, *op. cit.*

119. Guyton, A., *Textbook of Medical Physiology* (9th ed.). Philadelphia: W.B. Saunders, 1995.

120. *Ibid.*

121. Wasaha, *op. cit.*

122. Hoff, *op. cit.*

123. Bee, *op. cit.*

124. Doreso-Worters, P., and D. Siegal, Managing Menopause, *Modern Maturity,* May–June (1995), 40–42, 76

125. Gormly, *op. cit.*

126. Guyton, *op. cit.*

127. Papalia and Olds, *op. cit.*

128. Putting Polish on the Golden Years.

129. Santrock, *op. cit.*

130. Seifert et al., *op. cit.*

131. Wasaha, *op. cit.*

132. Whipple, B., Common Questions About Osteoporosis and Menopause, *American Journal of Nursing,* 95, no. 1 (1995), 69–70.

133. Health Canada, *It's Your Health, Benefits and Risks of Hormone Replacement Therapy (Estrogen with or without Progestin),* Website: http://www.hc-sc.gc.ca/english/iyh/medical/estrogen.html, July 2004.

134. *Ibid.*

135. *Ibid.*

136. Blake, J.M., J.A. Collins, R.L. Reid, D.M. Fedorkow, and A.B. Lalonde, The SOGC Statement on the WHI Report on Estrogen and Progestin Use in Postmenopausal Women, *Journal of Obstetrics and Gynaecology Canada,* 24, no. 10 (2002), 783–787.

137. *Ibid.*

138. *Ibid.*

139. *Ibid.*

140. *Ibid.*

141. Lemay, A., The Relevance of the Women's Health Initiative Results on Combined Hormone Replacement Therapy in Clinical Practice, *Journal of Obstetrics and Gynaecology Canada,* 24, no. 9 (2002), 711–715.

142. Humphries, K., and S. Gill, Risks and Benefits of Hormone Replacement Therapy: The Evidence Speaks, *Canadian Medical Association Journal,* 168, no. 8 (2003), 1001–1010.

143. Lock, *op. cit.*

144. Papalia and Olds, *op. cit.*

145. Lock, *op. cit.*

146. Papalia and Olds, *op. cit.*

147. The Phytoestrogen Question, *The New England Journal of Medicine Health News,* 3, no. 15, (1999), 1, 4.

148. (21c)

149. Calgary Health Region, *Grace Women's Health Centre, Nutrition and Bone Health,* Website: http://www.crha-health.ab.ca/clin/women/Nutrition_bone.htm, July 2004.

150. *Ibid.*

151. Health Canada, Office of Nutrition Policy and Promotion, Website: http://www.hc-sc.gc.ca/hpfb-dgpsa/onpp-bppn/weight_book_04_e.html, July 2004.

152. *Ibid.*

153. Duyff, R., *The American Dietetic Association's Complete Food and Nutrition Guide.* Minneapolis, MN: Chronimed Publishing, 1998.

154. Low Fat Mind Games, *Tufts University Diet and Nutrition Letter,* 13, no. 9 (1995), 1.

155. Williams, S., *Nutrition and Diet Therapy* (10th ed.). St. Louis: C.V. Mosby, 1995.

156. Doreso-Worters and Siegal, *op. cit.*

157. Williams, *op. cit.*

158. Duyff, *op. cit.*

159. Wasaha, *op. cit.*

160. Williams, *op. cit.*

161. Edelman, C., and C. Mandel, *Health Promotion Throughout the Lifespan* (4th ed.). St. Louis: C.V. Mosby, 1998.

162. Fenstermacher, K., and B. Hudson, *Practice Guidelines for Family Nurse Practitioners.* Philadelphia: Saunders, 1997.

163. Guyton, *op. cit.*

164. Nelson, M., *Strong Women Stay Slim.* New York: Bantam Books, 1998.

165. Tierney, L., S. McPhee, and M. Papadakis, *Current Medical Diagnosis and*

166. Back Protection for Daily Sitters, *Staying Well Newsletter,* May–June (1991), 1–2.

167. Edelman, and Mandel, *op. cit.*

168. Getting Relief: Your Aching Feet, *Harvard Health Letter,* 24, no. 5 (1999), 1–3.

169. *Ibid.*

170. Trouble Sleeping? *Mount Sinai School of Medicine Focus on Healthy Aging,* 2, no. 2 (1999), 2.

171. Hobson, J., and L. Silvestri, Parasomnias, *The Harvard Mental Health Letter,* 15, no. 8 (1999), 3–5.

172. *Ibid.*

173. *Ibid.*

174. Sleep Apnea: No Rest for the Weary Without Proper Diagnosis, *Harvard Health Letter,* 23, no. 1 (1997), 4–5.

175. 62

176. Sleep Apnea: No Rest for the Weary Without Proper Diagnosis.

177. Health Canada, *Canadian Immunization Guide* (6th ed.). Ottawa: Minister of Public Works and Government Services Canada, 2002.

178. Bee, *op. cit.*
179. Edelman and Mandel, *op. cit.*
180. Health Risks, *Women's Health Advocate Newsletter,* 2, no. 11, (January 1996), 2–3.
181. Bee, *op. cit.*
182. Fenstermacher and Hudson, *op. cit.*
183. Tierney et al., *op. cit.*
184. Health Risks.
185. Hoole, A., G. Pickard, R. Ouimete, J. Lohr, and W. Powell, *Patient Care Guidelines for Nurse Practitioners* (5th ed.). Philadelphia: J. B. Lippincott, 1999.
186. Risk: What It Means to You, *Harvard Women's Health Watch,* 3, no. 3 (1995), 3–4.
187. Tierney et al., *op. cit.*
188. Health Canada, *Population and Public Health Branch, Centre for Chronic Prevention and Control Cervical Cancer,* Website: http://www.hs-sc.gc.ca/pphb-dgspsp/ccdpc-cpcmc/cc-ccu/facts_e.html, July 2004.
189. Cole, David E. C., New genetic Technologies: Clinical Application and Ethical Issues in Familial Ovarian Cancer, *Clinical and Investigative Medicine,* 27, no. 1 (2004), 16–18.
190. Fenstermacher and Hudson, *op. cit.*
191. Spencer-Cisek, P., Overview of Cancer Prevention, Screening, and Detection, *Nurse Practitioner Forum,* 9, no. 3 (1998), 134–146.
192. Tierney et al., *op. cit.*
193. Health Canada, Population and Public Health Branch, Centre for Chronic Prevention and Control Cervical Cancer.
194. Cole, *op. cit.*
195. Risk: What It Means to You.
196. Routine Mammograms Found to be Cost-effective for Women Age 40–49, says UC—Davis Study, *The Nation's Health,* 25, no. 10 (1995), 12.
197. Statistics Canada, Canadian Statistics, *New Cancer Cases by Primary site of Cancer, by Sex,* Website: http://www.statcan.ca/english/Pgdb/hlth61.html, July 2004.
198. Tierney et al., *op. cit.*
199. Coldman, A.J., N. Phillips, and T.A. Pickles, Trends in Prostate Cancer Incidence and Mortality: An Analysis of Mortality Change by Screening Intensity, *Canadian Medical Association Journal,* 168, no. 1 (2003), 31–35.
200. Pickles, T., Current Status of PSA Screening, *Canadian Family Physician,* 50, no. 1 (2004), 57–63.
201. Svendsen, A., The Current Status of Cardiovascular Disease in Canada—A Call to Action, *Canadian Journal of Cardiovascular Nursing,* 14, no. 1 (2004), 5–7.
202. *Ibid.*
203. *Ibid.*
204. Tanuseputro, P., D.G. Manuel, M. Leung, K. Nguyen, and H. Johansen, Risk Factors for Cardiovascular Disease in Canada, *Canadian Journal of Cardiology,* 19, no. 11 (2003), 1249–1259.
205. Health Risks.
206. Tierney et al., *op. cit.*
207. Fenstermacher and Hudson, *op. cit.*
208. Thyroid Testing for Women Over 50, *Mount Sinai School of Medicine Focus on Healthy Aging,* 2, no. 2 (1999), 2.
209. Tierney et al., *op. cit.*
210. Cancer and The Mind, *The Harvard Mental Health Letter,* 14, no. 9 (1998), 1–5.
211. Schaefer, K., Women Living in Paradox: Loss and Discovery in Chronic Illness, *Holistic Nursing Practice,* 9, no. 3 (1995), 63–74.
212. *Ibid.*
213. Eakes et al., *op. cit.*
214. Dowd, R., and J. Cavalieri, Help Your Patient Live with Osteoporosis, *American Journal of Nursing,* 99, no. 4 (1999), 56–60.
215. Jacobs, P., J.F. Blanchard, R.C. James, and N. Depen, Excess Costs of Diabetes in the Aboriginal Population of Manitoba, Canada, *Canadian Journal of Public Health,* 91, no. 4 (2000), 298–301.
216. Dowd and Cavalieri, *op. cit.*
217. Papalia and Olds, *op. cit.*
218. Guyton, *op. cit.*
219. Fink, *op. cit.*
220. Tierney et al., *op. cit.*
221. Boyd and Nihart, *op. cit.*
222. *Ibid.*
223. Hearts and Mind: Part I, *Harvard Mental Health Letter,* 14, no. 1 (1997), 1–4.
224. Taking Anger to Heart, *Johns Hopkins Medical Newsletter: Health after 50,* 11, no. 5 (1999), 1–3.
225. *Ibid.*
226. Hearts and Mind: Part I.
227. The Broken Heart: An Overlooked Risk Factor for Heart Disease? *Women's Health Advocate Newsletter,* 4, no. 10 (1997), 7.
228. Taking Anger to Heart.
229. Tierney et al., *op. cit.*
230. *Ibid.*
231. Boyd and Nihart, *op. cit.*
232. Burgess, *op. cit.*
233. Gormly, *op. cit.*
234. Seifert et al., *op. cit.*
235. Gormly, *op. cit.*
236. Papalia and Olds, *op. cit.*
237. Sigelman, *op. cit.*
238. Gormly, *op. cit.*
239. *Ibid.*
240. Papalia and Olds, *op. cit.*
241. Wadsworth, B., *Piaget's Theory of Cognitive and Affective Development: Foundations of Constructivism* (5th ed.). New York: Longman, 1996.
242. Gormly, *op. cit.*
243. Papalia and Olds, *op. cit.*
244. Seifert et al., *op. cit.*
245. Gormly, *op. cit.*
246. Papalia and Olds, *op. cit.*
247. Santrock, *op. cit.*
248. Seifert et al., *op. cit.*
249. Santrock, *op. cit.*
250. Gormly, *op. cit.*
251. Papalia and Olds, *op. cit.*
252. Sigelman, *op. cit.*
253. Gormly, *op. cit.*
254. Papalia and Olds, *op. cit.*
255. Santrock, *op. cit.*
256. Seifert et al., *op. cit.*
257. Wadsworth, *op. cit.*
258. Gormly, *op. cit.*
259. Papalia and Olds, *op. cit.*
260. Santrock, *op. cit.*
261. Seifert et al., *op. cit.*
262. Wadsworth, *op. cit.*
263. *Ibid.*
264. Gormly, *op. cit.*
265. Papalia and Olds, *op. cit.*
266. Santrock, *op. cit.*
267. Seifert et al., *op. cit.*
268. Gormly, *op. cit.*
269. *Ibid.*
270. *Ibid.*
271. Buhler, C., The Developmental Structure of Goal Setting in Group and Individual Studies, in C. Buhler and F. Massarik, eds., *The Course of Human Life.* New York: Springer, 1968.
272. Gormly, *op. cit.*

273. Papalia and Olds, *op. cit.*
274. Seifert et al., *op. cit.*
275. Neugarten, B., The Awareness of Middle Age, in R. Owen, ed., *Middle Age.* London: British Broadcasting Corporation, 1967.
276. Neugarten, B., Women's Attitudes Toward Menopause, in B. Neugarten, ed., *Middle Age and Aging.* Chicago: University of Chicago Press, 1968.
277. Neugarten, B., Dynamics of the Transition of Mid-Age to Old Age, *Journal of Geriatric Psychiatry,* 4 (1970), 71–87.
278. Neugarten, B., Adaptation and the Life Cycle, *The Counseling Psychologist,* 6, no. 1 (1976), 16–20.
279. Neugarten, B., and J. Moore, The Changing Age-Status System, in B. Neugarten, ed., *Middle Age and Aging.* Chicago: University of Chicago Press, 1968.
280. Gould, R., Adult Life Stages: Growth Toward Self-tolerance, *Psychology Today,* 8, no. 7 (February 1975), 74–78.
281. Gould, R., *Transformations: Growth and Change in Adult Life.* New York: Simon & Schuster, 1978.
282. Gould, R., Transformation in Mid-life, *New York University Education Quarterly,* 10, no. 2 (1979), 2–9.
283. Gould, R., Old Wine in New Bottles: A Feminist Perspective on Gilligan's Theory, *Social Work,* September–October (1988), 411–415.
284. Dennis, W., Creative Production Between the Ages of 20 and 80, *Journal of Gerontology,* 21, no. 1 (1966), 8.
285. Bee, *op. cit.*
286. Gormly, *op. cit.*
287. Newman, B., and P. Newman, *Development Through Life: A Psychosocial Approach* (7th ed.). Belmont, CA: Brooks/Cole, 1999.
288. Papalia and Olds, *op. cit.*
289. Bee, *op. cit.*
290. Gormly, *op. cit.*
291. Newman and Newman, *op. cit.*
292. Papalia and Olds, *op. cit.*
293. Seifert et al., *op. cit.*
294. Parton, D., Out of Work: One Family's Journey, *Focus on the Family,* January (1994), 2–4.
295. Hunter, M., Work, Work, *Modern Maturity,* May–June (1999), 36–49.
296. Papalia and Olds, *op. cit.*
297. Boyd and Nihart, *op. cit.*
298. Bee, *op. cit.*
299. Early Retirement: A Disappearing American Dream, *Capper's,* March 14 (1995), 18.
300. Gormly, *op. cit.*
301. Hardy, M., and J. Quadnagno, Satisfaction with Early Retirement: Makeup Choices in the Auto Industry, *Journal of Gerontology: Social Sciences,* 50B, no. 4 (1995), S217–S228.
302. Newman and Newman, *op. cit.*
303. Papalia and Olds, *op. cit.*
304. Bee, *op. cit.*
305. Gormly, *op. cit.*
306. *Ibid.*
307. Seifert et al., *op. cit.*
308. Erikson E., *Childhood and Society* (2nd ed.). New York: W.W. Norton, 1963.
309. Gormly, *op. cit.*
310. Newman and Newman, *op. cit.*
311. Vance C., and Olson, R. *The Mentoring Connection in Nursing.* New York: Springhill, 1998.
312. Jahoda, M., *Current Concepts of Positive Mental Health.* New York: Basic Books, 1958.
313. Bee, *op. cit.*
314. Newman and Newman, *op. cit.*
315. Papalia and Olds, *op. cit.*
316. Seifert et al., *op. cit.*
317. Jung, C., *Modern Man in Search of a Soul.* New York: Harcourt, Brace & World, 1955.
318. Kelleher, K., The Afternoon of Life: Jung's View of the Tasks of the Second Half of Life, *Perspectives in Psychiatric Care,* 28, no. 2 (1992), 25–28.
319. Sheehy, G., *Passages for Men.*
320. Jung, *op. cit.*
321. Kelleher, *op. cit.*
322. Jung, *op. cit.*
323. Kelleher, *op. cit.*
324. Jung, *op. cit.*
325. Kelleher, *op. cit.*
326. Sheehy, G., *Passages for Men.*
327. Body Image: The Last Frontier of Women's Rights, *Women's Health Advocate Newsletter,* 4, no. 10 (1997), 4–6.
328. Bee, *op. cit.*
329. Gormly, *op. cit.*
330. Newman and Newman, *op. cit.*
331. Papalia and Olds, *op. cit.*
332. Sheehy, G., *Passages for Men.*
333. Sigelman, *op. cit.*
334. Levinson, D., A Conception of Adult Development, *American Psychologist,* 41 (1986), 3–13.
335. Levinson, D., A Theory of Life Structure Development in Adulthood, in K.N. Alexander and E.J. Langer, eds., *Higher Stages of Human Development,* New York: Oxford University Press, 1990, 35–54.
336. Kohlberg, L., *Recent Research in Moral Development.* New York: Holt, Rinehart & Winston, 1977.
337. *Ibid.*
338. Gilligan, C., In a Different Voice: Women's Conceptions of Self and of Mortality, *Harvard Educational Review,* 47, no. 4 (1977), 481–517.
339. Gilligan, C., N. Lyons, and T. Hammer, eds., *Making Connections.* Cambridge, MA: Harvard University Press, 1990.
340. Peck, R.C., Psychological Developments in the Second Half of Life, in B. Neugarten, ed., *Middle Age and Aging.* Chicago: University of Chicago Press, 1968.
341. Erikson E., *Childhood and Society* (2nd ed.). New York: W.W. Norton, 1963.
342. Stolte, K.M., *Wellness: Nursing Diagnosis for Health Promotion,* Philadelphia: Lippincott, 1996.

Chapter 14

ASSESSMENT AND HEALTH PROMOTION FOR THE PERSON IN LATER ADULTHOOD

Old age, to the unlearned, is winter: to the learned, it is harvest time.

Yiddish Proverb

OBJECTIVES

STUDY OF THIS CHAPTER WILL ENABLE YOU TO:

1. Define terms and theories of aging related to understanding of the person in later maturity.

2. Explore personal and societal attitudes about growing old and your role in promoting positive attitudes in the community.

3. Compare and contrast relationships in the late years with those of other developmental eras, including with spouse, offspring, grandchildren, other family members, friends, pets, and other networks.

4. Compare and contrast the status of either singlehood or widow(er)hood in later adulthood to that status in early and middle adulthood.

5. Describe signs of and factors contributing to elder abuse and contrast with child and spouse abuse.

6. Examine physiologic adaptive mechanisms of aging and influences on sexuality, related health problems, and assessment and intervention to promote and maintain health, comfort, and safety.

7. Discuss the cognitive, emotional, body-image, and spiritual development and characteristics of the aged person, their interrelationship, and your role in promoting health and a positive self-concept.

8. Compare and contrast the adaptive mechanisms used by the person in this period with those used in other periods of life.

9. Describe the developmental crisis of later maturity, the relationship to previous developmental crises, and your role in helping the person meet this crisis.

10. List the developmental tasks for this era, and describe how to facilitate their accomplishment.

11. Identify changing home, family, social, and work or leisure situations of this person and your responsibility in helping the person face retirement, loss of loved ones, and changes in roles and living arrangements. Discuss selection of an adequate personal care home or residence for seniors.

12. Describe major federal, provincial/territorial, and local programs to assist the elderly financially, socially, and in health care, and describe your professional and personal responsibility in this regard.

13. Define remotivation and reminiscence; discuss the value, purpose, and use of these and other group processes with the elderly.

14. Summarize the needs of the elderly, standards of nursing care to assist in meeting those needs, and future trends in care of the person in later maturity.

15. Assess and work effectively with a person in later adulthood, using the information presented in this chapter and showing empathy and genuine interest.

I really don't like being labelled a golden-ager. I acknowledge my age and my limits, but I certainly didn't turn incompetent at 65.

When does later adulthood begin? Historically, it was designation of an eligible age for receipt of Old Age Pension benefits that established age 65 as the beginning age for this period in the life cycle. In reality, the age span for this period is continually changing. Images once associated with later maturity are no longer clear. The chronologic age of 65 no longer determines or predicts behaviours, life events, health status, work status, family status, interests, preoccupations, or needs. Individuals undergo aging at different rates, and their view of the aging process is influenced by many factors—culture, generation, and occupation. Some individuals, especially members of ethnic minorities and lower socioeconomic levels, view the onset of old age as taking place earlier than age 65.[1,2] Younger generations may misperceive how the old view themselves.

The rapid increase of the number of older adults between the years 2000 and 2030 reflects the aging of the "baby boom" generation.[3] As mothers of the post–World War II baby boom reach old age, the current trend of elderly women living alone will increase, according to a study in 21 European and North American countries. Four-generation families will be the norm (Figure 14–1), and five-generation families will be increasing in number.

Recently, the elderly population has been growing faster among non-whites than Caucasians. By 2025, 15% of the elderly population is projected to be non-white, in contrast to 10% in 1980. This continued aging trend in the population requires changes in all aspects of our social structure—employment, housing, education, leisure activities, transportation, industrial development, and health care.

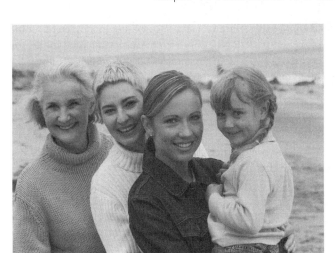

FIGURE 14–1

Four-generation families, once unusual, will become the norm as the population ages.

DEFINITIONS

Because the terms describing this age group are not clearly defined by the general public or health care professionals, it is important to clarify some of the terms used in this chapter.[4–9]

Aging, which *begins at conception and ends at death, is a process of growing older, regardless of chronologic age.*

Biological age is the *person's present position with respect to the potential life span, which may be younger or older than chronologic age,* and encompasses measures of functional capacities of vital organ systems.

Social age, which *results from the person's life course through various social institutions,* refers to *roles and habits of the person with respect to other members of society.* Social age may be age-appropriate or older or younger than that of most people in the social group. Social age includes such aspects as the person's type of dress, language usage, and social deference to people in leadership positions.

Psychological age refers to *behavioural capacity of the person to adapt to changing environmental demands and includes capacities of memory, learning, intelligence, skills, feelings, and motivation for exercising behavioural control or self-regulation.*

Cognitive age includes the *age the person feels and looks to self, plus the fit of behaviour and interests to his or her chronologic age.* The person says, "I do most things as if I were _____ years old."

Senescence is the *mental and physical decline associated with the aging process.* The term describes a group of effects that lead to a decrease in efficient function.

Later maturity is the *last major segment of the life span; this stage begins at the age of 65 or 70.* The World Health Organization (WHO) divides this segment of life into the elderly (65–75), the old (76–90), and the very old (over 90). Some authors divide this group into **young-old,** *ages 65 to 74, or 65 or 70 to 80;* **mid-old,** *75 to 84;* and **old-old,** *80 or 85 and older.* The term **frail-old** is sometimes used instead of **old-old** or **very old.**

Developmental tasks and cultural age timetables for life eras and family transitions exist for all stages of life, but they are not the same for everyone or all cultures. These tasks and timetables influence the life course but are likely to be flexible in the minds of individuals, especially older individuals. However, there are age "norms" in key areas of life, which have been addressed in previous chapters and in this chapter as well.[10]

Senility is a *wastebasket term still used to denote physical and mental deterioration often associated with old age. It is used when other options have not been carefully considered.* The correct term would be related to a specific disease, such as senile dementia, Alzheimer's type.[11] Yet what looks like senility or Alzheimer's disease may be the result of drug reactions; malnutrition; dehydration; delirium; hypothyroidism; microstrokes and hypertension; toxicity in the system; disorders resulting from lack of communication and experiencing sensory deprivation for physical reasons or because of institutionalization; or the expectations of caregivers.[12,13]

CRITICAL THINKING

What are the stages of decline due to Alzheimer's disease?

Gerontology is the *scientific study of the individual in later maturity and the aging process from physiologic, pathologic, psychological, sociologic, and economic points of view.*

Geriatrics is a *medical specialty concerned with the physiologic and pathologic changes of the individual in later maturity and includes study and treatment of the health problems of this age group.*

Later maturity is divided into three sequential segments. The first segment may be regarded as a *sociopolitical or cultural-organizational perspective.* Offspring are in a creative period, and the mature adult is in the ruling, protective stance as he or she assumes parental hierarchical leadership over the family of families. The older person becomes concerned with the creation, ordering, and maintenance of a larger society. The second segment is characterized by a *reaffirmation of social, moral, and ethical standards* necessary for establishment of pacific relationships among the oncoming generations as they are involved in rendering decisions, planning, erecting social guideposts, and selecting subordinate leaders. The judgmental functions of the mind are most highly developed at this time, created out of actual and vicarious experience with conflict situations and from cultural learning and values. The last segment of psychic maturity involves *retrospective examination,* the need to correlate the present with the past to determine the true nature of accomplishments, errors, and rediscoveries. Cultural vision is at its broadest possible development, embracing one nearly complete life cycle and its interrelatedness with a multitude of other life cycles. The person compares and contrasts his or her values with cultural values and, through reasoning and intuition, evaluates meaning and purpose and has an increased interest in the history of human development.

SOCIETAL PERSPECTIVES ON AGING

I may be old and wrinkled on the outside but I'm young and vulnerable on the inside.

Ageism refers to *any attitude, action, or institutional structure that discriminates against individuals on the basis of their age or that infers that elderly people are inferior to those who are younger.*

Your attitude, teaching, and advocacy can diminish ageism, stereotypes, and myths. Your teaching and practice must also consider cultural differences among the elderly. Ageist attitudes toward older adults are not new in North America. Generally, older women are judged more harshly than older men. Children appear most positive in their perception of elderly persons.[14–17] Elsner and colleagues give an account of when health care providers were unethical and demonstrated ageism.[18]

In North America, old age frequently is characterized as a time of dependence and disease. Negative presentation of older adults, especially women, in movies, books, and magazines, in jokes, and on television contributes to negative beliefs and attitudes.[19,20] Society's fear of the changes associated with aging such as grey hair, hearing loss, wrinkles, loss of muscle tone, slowness, and approaching death also contributes to negative attitudes. However, Kaufert and Lock examined visual images of menopausal women portrayed in pharmaceutical ads. They found a shift from a negative image in the 1970s, to a positive image in the 1990s. The new ads showed women with healthy teeth, hair, and skin.[21]

Numerous unproven *myths* and age-related *stereotypes* pervade our culture. One study revealed that of three age groups, young, middle-aged, and elderly adults, the elderly reported more stereotypes than did either of the other age groups. Interestingly, the young adults reported the fewest stereotypes.[22] These myths and stereotypes obscure the truth and may prevent us from achieving our own potential as we grow older. Society stereotypes the older adult as being asexual, unemployable, unintelligent, and socially incompetent. Some of these myths and the contrasting realities are listed in the box entitled "Myths and Misconceptions and Their Realities for the Elderly Person."[23–27]

CRITICAL THINKING

What are some other prevalent myths in our society? What fact goes furthest to dispel such myths?

Many of the myths and stereotypes associated with aging are culturally determined. The older adult in North America lives in a culture oriented to youth, productivity, and rapid pace. Because of this orientation, older people may feel that they are not respected, valued, or needed.

There is no one criterion for successful aging. A study by Roos and Havens[45] of more than 3500 people in Manitoba, from 1971 to 1983, found few consistent predictors of successful aging. As more people live longer, are healthy, and are aging successfully, attitudes are becoming more positive. The elderly are more and more perceived as powerful, admired, healthy, active, sexy, and affluent.[46–49]

Culture, ethnicity, and socioeconomic level influence the role of the older adult in family relationships and determine health practices. Differences exist among cultural populations in how they esteem and care for the elderly, how the elderly stay involved in family matters, and the types of health care services used.[50–58] Differences also exist among urban and rural families of the elderly.[59,60] Many older adults continue to follow health practices that are linked to their cultural heritage. Respect must be shown for these cultural aspects of aging and cultural influences on health practices and healing methods.[61–66]

Myths and Misconceptions and Their Realities for the Elderly Person

Myth 1: Age 65 Is a Good Marker for Old Age.

Fact: Factors other than chronologic age cause the person to be old. Many people are more youthful than their parents were at age 65. With increased longevity, perhaps 70 or 75 should be the chronologic marker.[28]

Myth 2: Most Old People Are in Bed or in Institutions and Are Ill Physically and Mentally.

Fact: Approximately 5% are institutionalized; 95% are living in the community. Although 67% of older persons outside institutions have one or more chronic conditions, 14% do not. Chronic conditions range from mild and correctable to more severe. Approximately 81% of the aged living in the community has no mobility limitations, 8% have trouble getting around; 6% need the help of another person; and 5% are homebound. The average number of restricted activity days is only twice that for young adults. Some report no physical illness, and some with physical disease processes do not consider themselves ill.[29]

Myth 3: All Old People Are Alike.

Fact: Each older adult is unique and *quite diverse*. This segment of the life span covers more years than any other segment—sometimes more than 35 years. The older people are, the more varied are their physical capabilities, personal style, economic status, and lifestyle preferences. From birth, physical and mental elaboration continues through life to make people more and more unlike one another.[30,31]

Myth 4: The Next Generation of Older Adults Will Be the Same as This Generation.

Fact: The next generation will be better educated, healthier, more mobile, more youthful in appearance, more accustomed to lifestyle change and technology, and more outspoken. The world

Myths and Misconceptions and Their Realities for the Elderly Person (continued)

is changing so quickly that each successive generation is vastly *different* from the ones that came before.[32]

Myth 5: Old Age Brings Mental Deterioration.

Fact: Approximately 5% of older adults show serious mental impairment, and only 10% demonstrate even mild to moderate memory loss. Many professionals work past 65 to 70 years.[33]

Myth 6: Old People Cannot Learn and Are Less Intelligent.

Fact: Older adults *can* and *do* learn; however, they may need a longer period in which to respond to questions and stimuli. When learning problems occur, they are usually associated with a disease process. Intelligent people remain so.[34]

Myth 7: Most Older Adults Are Incompetent.

Fact: Older people may have a slower reaction time and take longer to do psychomotor tasks; however, they have more consistent output, less job turnover, greater job satisfaction, fewer accidents, and less absenteeism.[35]

Myth 8: Most Older Adults Are Unhappy and Dissatisfied with Life.

Fact: How happy or sad the person feels reflects basic temperament throughout life, the adaptation to past and current life events, and social support. Positive social ties and realistic expectations buffer psychological distress. Older people tend to be satisfied with their lives as middle-aged people, even when they have lower incomes and poorer health.[36]

Myth 9: The Elderly Are Self-Pitying, Apathetic, Irritable, and Hard to Live With.

Fact: Research shows that mood is related to the present situation and past personality. The older person is as likely as a younger one to have an interesting and pleasant personality.[37,38]

Myth 10: The Elderly Are Inactive and Unproductive.

Fact: Many young children have working grandparents. Thirty-six percent of men over 65 years are employed in some type of job. Older women often do their housework into their 80s or 90s.

Older workers have a job attendance record that is 20% better than that of young workers, and they also sustain fewer job-related injuries.[39]

Myth 11: The Elderly Do Not Desire and Do Not Participate in Sexual Activity.

Fact: Recent research refutes this assertion. Sexual activity may decline because of lack of a partner or misinformation about sexuality in late life. The person who has been sexually active all along is able to continue sexual activity, and sexual activity involves more than intercourse between the partners.[40]

Myth 12: The Elderly Are Isolated, Abandoned, and Lonely, and They Are Unlikely to Participate in Activities.

Fact: Many elderly prefer to live in a separate household. Many elderly live with someone and do not feel lonely. Approximately 10% of people over 65 years never married and have adjusted to living alone. Elderly people who do not have children often have siblings or friends with whom they live. Other elderly live in institutions or residences for the aged where they make friends. The percentage of purposefully abandoned elderly is small; often the person who is a loner in old age has always been alone.[41,42]

Myth 13: Retirement Is Disliked by All Old People and Causes Illness and Less Life Satisfaction.

Fact: Although this may be true for some people, many older people look forward to retirement and are retiring before 65 so that they can continue other pursuits. Most are not sick from idleness and a sense of worthlessness. More than three-fourths of them have satisfying lives.[43]

Myth 14: Special Health Services for the Aged Are Useless Because the Aged Cannot Benefit Anyway.

Fact: At age 65 the average person can look forward to 15 more years of life. The elderly have fewer acute illnesses and accidental injuries, and these conditions are correctable, although older people take longer to recover than younger people do. Common chronic conditions are cardiovascular disease, cancer, arthritis, diabetes, sensory impairments, and depression, which can be treated so that the person can achieve maximum potential and comfort.[44]

CRITICAL THINKING

What changes have you noticed that occur in people in later life?

THEORIES OF AGING

There is no single model of longevity. Centenarians reach that milestone because of a unique mix of environmental, behavioural, and genetic factors. Risks for heart disease,

cancer, and stroke can be reduced by eating a healthful diet, exercising, and avoiding carcinogens, such as cigarettes, sunburn, and radon, especially for people under 75 years of age.[67–73]

Genetic processes that lengthen life include the following:[74]

1. A rare gene that causes people to produce extraordinary amounts of beneficial high-density lipoprotein (HDL), which guards against atherosclerosis.

2. A gene, Apo A01 Melano, that quickly clears cholesterol from the bloodstream.

3. Apolipoprotein E (Apo E2, Apo E3, Apo E4), which has been linked to cardiovascular and Alzheimer's disease. Two copies of Apo E4 increase risk for atherosclerosis and late onset of Alzheimer's disease. Two copies of Apo E2 lengthen life.

4. Werner's gene produces helicase, a special enzyme that is involved in repairing DNA. Lack of the enzyme causes premature aging and death before 50.

The oldest-old are probably endowed with genes that protect them against common diseases and with traits that keep their cells in good working order longer than expected. Gender differences emerge among super-survivors. Women outnumber men at age 95, but men fare better in terms of mental function and physical health. Men with dementia die before 90; women with the same amount of impairment live longer.[75]

Five personality traits affect longevity: sociability, self-esteem and confidence, conscientiousness, social dependability, cheerfulness and optimism, and energy levels.[76]

In a study of 1500 people who were followed, beginning in 1921, from age 11 every five to ten years, 60% of the original sample is still alive in their late 80s. The risk of dying before age 70 was higher for people who had been optimistic, cheerful, and good-humoured children. The likelihood of dying before 70 was lowest for those who had been cautious and conscientious as children. Conscientious people may have better and less risky health habits.[77]

In a four-year study of 1300 men and women over 71 years of age, those that scored highest for depression were about 50% more likely than the others to undergo a drop in physical ability. Decreased capability was seen even when the depressed

14–1 BONUS SECTION IN CD-ROM

Research Abstract: Robust Aging among the Young-Old, Old-Old, and Oldest-Old

The purpose of the study was to examine relationships between four predictors for robust aging: productive involvement, affective status, cognitive status, and functional status.

people had started the study with physical function nearly intact. Apparently, depressed people are less likely to exercise and seek medical care, which may be factors. Psychological distress also causes neural, hormonal, and immunologic alterations that depress the body's stamina or ability to fight illness. The physical decline reinforces depression.[78]

Knowledge of these theories can be useful as you help the elder and the family to understand the aging process.

CRITICAL THINKING

What is the most outstanding contribution to the aging process made by the study of genetics?

Biological Theories

Biological theories can be categorized as nongenetic cellular, physiologic, and genetic. See Table 14-1 for definitions or explanations and limitations related to the theories.[79–85]

TABLE 14-1 Theories of Physical Aging		
Theory	Definition/Explanation	Applications/Limitations
Nongenetic Cellular Theories		
Wear and Tear Theory	Body systems wear out because of accumulation of stress of life and effects of metabolism. Most general and obvious explanation of aging compares body to a machine.	Little scientific evidence. Theory does not consider self-repair mechanisms of body or differences of life span within the human species.
Cross-linkage or Faulty DNA Repair Theory	Bonds or cross-linkages develop between molecules or peptides: these bonds change the molecules' properties physically and chemically. Thus collagen in intracellular or extracellular material is chemically altered and function affected. When collagen is cross-linked with other molecules, changes range from wrinkling, to atherosclerosis, to inelasticity of tissue. When cross-linkages occur with DNA molecules that carry genetic program, DNA is damaged and repairs slowly; mutation or death of cell occurs.	A viable theory.

(continued)

TABLE 14-1 *(continued)*
Theories of Physical Aging

Theory	Definition/Explanation	Applications/Limitations
Accumulation of Waste or of Senescent Cells Theory	Substances, such as metabolic waste materials and lipofuscins, which interfere with cellular metabolism and cause cell death, accumulate in cells. Examples of accumulation of metabolic waste are cataracts of the eye, cholesterol in the arteries, and bone brittleness. Cells that cannot divide any more accumulate in older people.	These substances may be a result rather than cause of senescence.
Accumulation of Errors Theory	As cells die, they must synthesize new proteins to make new cells; sometimes an error occurs. When enough errors occur, organ failure results.	Little scientific evidence.
Free Radical (or Oxidative Damage) Theory	Oxygen-free radicals (charged or unstable molecules) or chemicals that contain oxygen in a highly activated state and react with other molecules during normal metabolism cause damage to cells and aging. Exposure to radiation and certain enzymes may interfere with life activities.	Oxidation, as explained by theory, implicated in atherosclerosis, cancer, neurologic disease, and reduced immune function.
Deprivation Theory	Aging is caused by deprivation of essential nutrients and oxygen to cells.	Little scientific evidence. It is likely that deprivation is the result of aging.
Physiologic Theories		
Biological Clock or Aging by Program Theory	Each organism contains genes or evolutionary processes that govern or control speed at which metabolic processes are performed. These genes or processes act as a genetic clock dictating occurrence of aging and dying. Cells are genetically programmed to reproduce only a certain amount of time; human limit may be 100 to 120 years. Hypothalamus may be the timer that keeps track of age of cells and determines how long they will keep reproducing.	Humans may be able to outlive inner governing processes because of medical technology and improvements in lifestyle. Cells in nervous system and muscles do not reproduce themselves; all other cells do, at least to some extent.
	Reproduced older cells do not appear to pass on information accurately through the DNA, which weakens functioning ability of older cells.	Cells are more likely to reproduce imperfectly as they get older.
Neuroendocrine Theory	Hormonal changes produce free radicals, cross-linkages, and autoimmunity.	Free radicals may be a special form of cross-linkage; may cause free radicals.
Immune (or Mounting Mutations) Theory	Ability of immune system to deal with foreign organisms or processes diminishes with age. Greatest decline is observed in thymus-derived immunity (T-cell production reduced). Production of antibodies declines after adolescence. **Autoimmune responses** may occur, *whereby normal cells are engulfed and digested*, making person more vulnerable to disease.	A viable theory. Autoimmunity may result from production of new antigens caused by (1) mutations that cause formation of altered RNA or DNA; or (2) the new antigens may have been hidden in the body earlier in life and are not recognized by body in late life. Implications for cancer.
Genetic Gene Theory	Aging is programmed; *the program exists in certain harmful genes. Genes that direct many cellular activities in early life may become altered in later years, which alters function* and may be responsible for functional decline and structural changes associated with aging.	Genetic basis exists for longevity, although environmental factors such as vaccines, nutrition, pollutants, safety factors, and medical care and technology can alter life span.

Psychosocial Theories

Just as one biological theory does not adequately address biological aging, one single psychosocial theory of aging is not adequate to explain psychological or social aging. The **Continuity Theory** proposes that *an individual's patterns of behaviour are the result of a lifetime of experiences, and aging is the continuation of these lifelong adjustments or personality patterns.* Personality traits remain stable, and early personality function is a guide for the retirement years.[86–89] Continuity Theory, as first proposed by Brim and Kagan, assumes neither a necessary reduction in activity levels (Disengagement Theory) nor the necessity of maintaining high activity levels (Activity Theory). They associated successful aging with the ability of the person to maintain patterns of behaviour that existed before old age. Continuity in behavioural patterns and lifestyle exists over time, regardless of the actual level of activity present. Each of us has a powerful drive to maintain the sense of identity or continuity that allays fears of changing too fast or being changed against one's will by external forces. There is a simultaneous drive to develop and mature further, which fosters continuing change in at least small ways. Adult development is not in the genes but in the intricacies of life experiences. Two psychological mechanisms, selective perception and situational reinforcement, are used to maintain a sense of continuity. **Selective perception** means that *experiences are reacted to on the basis of their relative congruence with currently held values, beliefs, and attitudes.* Noncongruent ideas are screened out of awareness, ignored, or not attended to. **Situational reinforcement** means that the *behaviours used are those that are rewarded. Previously established behaviour patterns tend to have a long history of reinforcement.* Continuity Theory may explain why, when one spouse was relocated to a long-term institution, the other spouse did not appear to perceive the marriage much differently than before the move.[90]

Developmental Theories

Several developmental theories have addressed psychosocial aging. **Erikson's Epigenetic Theory**[91] suggests that *successful personality development in later life depends on the ability to resolve the psychosocial crisis known as integrity versus despair.* Erikson's theory is psychodynamic and is part of a life cycle approach that emphasizes that the developmental tasks of each stage must be met before the person can work through the next tasks. The theory is discussed in detail later in this chapter.

Peck's Theory[92] hypothesizes that *there are three psychological developmental tasks of old age: ego differentiation versus work-role preoccupation, body transcendence versus body preoccupation, and ego transcendence versus ego preoccupation* (see Chapter 13). Reed[93] also identified these tasks. These issues are an extension and further development of Erikson's stage, with emphasis on change and growth in later life. Havighurst[94] presents several major developmental tasks that must be mastered or achieved to meet the developmental needs of later maturity (see the section entitled "Developmental Tasks" later in this chapter). He uses an eclectic approach that combines previously developed concepts into one theory. According to

all developmental theories, the older adult's behaviour and response depend on how earlier developmental crises were handled.

Levinson theorizes that late adulthood is characterized by a *transition period which occurs between 60 and 65 years of age; the person does not become suddenly old, but physical and mental changes increase awareness of aging and mortality.*[95]

Sociologic Theories

Disengagement Theory suggests that individuals in a society undergo a self-disengagement process during the middle and later years of life. This process is characterized by a reduction in general energy levels, reduction in societal involvement, and increased preoccupation with one's own needs and desires. Studies do not support the Disengagement Theory.

CRITICAL THINKING

Which of the following theories would researchers use to direct their research in gerontology?

Cross-cultural studies show **disengagement** is not inevitable, and it is generally not applicable to family relationships. Sill's research[96] reveals that awareness of **finitude,** *estimate of time remaining before death,* and physical incapacity were more important than age in predicting level of activity. The person who perceives self as near death begins to constrict life space; psychological preparation for death may lead to disengagement. The person may consciously or unconsciously be aware of **terminal drop,** *the period preceding the person's death from a few weeks up to two years,* which may account for some intellectual decline, changed verbal abilities, withdrawal from the world, and mood changes, as well as onset of physical illness.[97]

Activity Theory implies that the older adult has essentially the same psychological and social needs as do middle-aged people. According to this theory, the older adult must compensate for the loss of roles experienced in later maturity. The older adult does not disengage but needs to maintain a moderately active lifestyle. In reality, the response to aging by older adults is a combination of the two theories.[98–102]

In her study of women in their 70s, 80s, and 90s, Sheehy found that many are, indeed, very actively pursing a second adulthood.[103] They have remained active, creative, involved in various organizations; they may be returning to college or acting as consultants. They are full of zest and have a passion and purpose in life. They may concentrate on a few priorities intensely or volunteer in a number of projects. They demonstrate wisdom, discussed by Erikson,[104] and ego and spiritual transcendence rather than self-preoccupation, as discussed by Peck.[105]

CRITICAL THINKING

What do you aspire to be like when you are elderly? Describe your profile.

Mead first articulated the **Symbolic Interaction Theory** in 1934, from which many of our present theories have grown. This theory holds that *the person develops socially according to the* *continuous bombardment of self-reflections perceived from others.* The aged in our culture are generally seen as having little social validity, and if this attitude is perceived consistently, it can become a self-fulfilling prophecy. People may expect to become inept and forgetful. Social and cultural expectations may strongly colour self-view and consequent behaviour. Symbolic Interaction Theory attempts to consider the interrelationships of several dimensions of the aging process, including:[106]

- Sociocultural dimensions that set the limits on available alternatives for the person.
- Contextual dimensions within which the individual's life course develops (e.g., includes biological change, past experiences).
- Personal evaluation of life experience, health status, and the future foci of energy and roles.

Biological changes, psychological changes, societal circumstances, and past and present experiences all are considered as relevant for explaining the aging process.[107]

Brown developed the **Urban Ecologic Model of Aging,** which is based on *person-environment interaction and the fact that human behaviour and subjective well-being are reflected in the social interaction that occurs between the individual and the environment.* Individual adaptive behaviour and subjective well-being are balanced when demands of the environment do not exceed level of ability to manage the demands. The older person is more vulnerable than the younger counterpart, especially if the person is impoverished, experiences environmental stress or social problems, or has multiple problems or needs. The greater the individual vulnerability, the greater the environmental impact on the person.[108]

Brown expanded the model to include (1) consideration of the suprapersonal environment and characteristics of the neighbourhood, (2) personal characteristics of residents in the locale, (3) perceptions of the surrounding environment, (4) effects of media reports on the person's perception, (5) factual data about the surrounding environment, and (6) residential satisfaction and subjective well-being. The elder's personal experience or perception may differ from the factual reports of the neighbourhood or environment, especially in urban, inner-city, or poverty-stricken areas.[109]

CRITICAL THINKING

Does research support Brown's Urban Ecological Theory?

FAMILY DEVELOPMENT AND RELATIONSHIPS

The changing demographic profile of developed countries has been associated with an increased number of four- and five-generation families. In such families it is common to have two generations at or near old age, with the oldest person frequently over 75 years. The "generation in the middle" may extend into retirement years in many families. Thus the "young-old," facing the potential of diminished personal resources, may be the group increasingly called on to give additional support to aged kin—the old-old and very or frail-old.

Relationship with Spouse

In later life, responsibilities of parenthood and employment diminish with few formal responsibilities to take their place. There is usually a corresponding decline in social contacts and activities. The factors that affect the social life of the elderly are found in personal social skills and in resources available in the private life. Marital status remains a major organizing force for personal life. With children gone and without daily contact with co-workers provided by employment, the elderly lose the basis for social integration. Declining health, limited income, and fewer daily responsibilities may create greater needs for social support. Thus, having a spouse provides the possibility for increased companionship. Having a spouse also increases longevity, especially for older males.

Interestingly, spouses may not increase in their support of each other into late life, perhaps because of increased **interiority** *(introspection)* with aging. Time may erode bases of respect, affection, and compatibility. Sometimes marriages have not been filled with mutual emotional or social support in earlier years, so there is no foundation for increasing mutual emotional support. Women are often the sole support for men. Older women tend to feel the husband is not supportive emotionally or in health care; however, women tend to rely on a more extensive network of family and friends for support.

The greater the number of adult children living nearby, the more likely the elderly mother is to have a weekly conversation or visit with at least one child. Women with two or more children are more likely than women with only one child to see the children as a source of potential help. Interestingly, adult children with siblings are more likely to report a higher-quality relationship with the mother than are adults who are only children.[110–112]

For the woman continually to have a spouse in the house or with her, wanting to share in her activities can be distressing, even though it has been anticipated. The loss of privacy and solitude, doing tasks in her own way and at her own pace, loss of independence, and loss of contact with friends may all be issues. The increased accommodation to meeting husband's needs, however, is offset by increased opportunities for nurturing and being nurtured and for sharing mutual interests.[113–115]

Your listening and teaching may assist the elderly person in making the necessary adjustments to the spouse.

CRITICAL THINKING

How do intimate partnerships contribute to happiness in later adulthood?

Relationships with Offspring and Other Family Members

Historical trends toward smaller families, longer life spans, increasing employment of women, and increasingly high mobility of both young and old have important implications for children being a primary resource in old age.

The number of children influences the recency with which older parents have seen their child, the amount of assistance older parents receive, and factors influencing older parents' interaction with children. Parents with one child report fewer visits and less help received, especially if the only child is an employed daughter. Older parents expect children, especially the daughter(s), to assume an appreciable level of responsibility in meeting important health, economic, and emotional needs, regardless of how many offspring there are to share in the assistance. Geographic proximity is a stable predictor of older parent–child interaction, more than offspring gender or health status of the parent. Daughters who are primarily blue-collar workers provide more assistance to older parents and have more association with parents than corresponding sons. Parents receive more help from offspring as income for the offspring increases.[116–120]

Older parents receive and perceive their children's help in several ways. Younger parents receive more help with automobile maintenance and help in the form of gifts. Older parents receive help with shopping and transportation. Parents who most strongly valued family are most desirous of and satisfied with family support. Parents may tend to expect less help from children when they live at a distance or when they work outside the home. Further, they appreciate most the help that keeps them self-reliant or autonomous, maintains social integration, maximizes choice and expressive interactions, and forestalls reliance on more extensive services. Parents with a greater degree of ill health express less satisfaction with children's help, possibly because it symbolizes dependency and loss of social integration.[121–123]

Some elderly people have a limited number of family members; some couples have no children. The childless couple will probably have adapted to childlessness psychologically; however, they are especially vulnerable at crisis points such as episodes of poor health and death of spouse or housing companion. If those persons or couples cannot drive or have no transportation, they will have a greater need for help, although they may hesitate to ask for help.

Your teaching and referrals may enable the elderly person with few relatives or resources to manage more effectively.

CRITICAL THINKING

To what extent do you believe that the number of male caregivers will increase in the future?

Grandparenthood and Great-Grandparenthood

Grandparenthood has multiple meanings for the person, depending in part on age at the initial time of grandparenthood, and the number and accomplishments of the grandchildren are probably a source of status.[124–129] The stage of grandparenthood may come to middle-aged persons, depending on age of their own childbearing and age of their children's childbearing. The relatively young grandparent may either like and accept or resist the role and may not like the connection of age and being a grandparent. Relative youth of grandparents contributes to the complex patterns of help and relationships

between the generations. Traditionally, the central figure, especially in the poor black family, has been the mother or grandmother, who has been responsible for maintenance of family stability and a source of socialization.[130,131] The increasing divorce rate also adds to the complexity of grandparent relationships. The child may have eight sets of grandparents. The grandparents may be the main caretakers for the children, or there may be a part-time commitment, sharing child care with their adult children. Likewise, grandchildren have a special tie to grandparents.[132] Research indicates that even when there was divorce in the family, adult children from divorced families continued their relationships with grandparents.[133]

Grandparents increasingly are the main caretakers of children, often in the custodial role, although legal custody is unlikely even if the children have a permanent home. Sometimes the grandparents serve as babysitter or a daycare service. When mothers also live in the home, the grandmother's being the main caregiver may have a negative impact on both the mother's and grandmother's parenting.[134–140] Grandparents are often happy with their role in that they can enjoy the young person and enter into a playful, informal, companionable and confiding relationship (Figure 14–2). The grandchild is seen as a source of leisure activity, someone for whom to purchase items that are also enjoyable to the grandparent. The number of **great-grandparents** and **great-great-grandparents** is increasing as more people live longer.

Great-grandparents may be as active in the grandparenting role as they were as grandparents; but advanced age, geographic distance, and cohabitation, divorce, and remarriage of family members tend to limit their participation.[141,142] Great-grandparents want to influence the younger generation with their wisdom, remain connected, share values and family stories, and give meaning to their transcendence.[143]

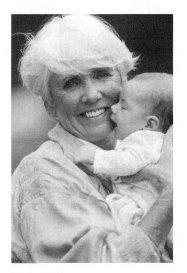

FIGURE 14–2

Grandparents often look forward to their role.

Source: Sherwen, L.N., M.A. Scoovena, and C.T. Weingarten, Nursing Care of the Childbearing Family. Stamford, CT: Appleton & Lange, 1991, p. 764.

CRITICAL THINKING

What are some tips for grandparents when they are caring for preschool grandchildren?

Social Relationships

Social networks of family, friends, and neighbours provide instrumental and expressive support. They contribute to well-being of the senior by promoting socialization and companionship, elevating morale and life satisfaction, buffering the effects of stressful events, providing a confidant, and facilitating coping skills and mastery. For example, social supports buffer the effects of stressful life events and represent more than the quantity or proximity of social ties but also the extent to which social ties fulfill needs of the senior. Also, the components of informal support networks—spouses, children, close relatives, distant kin (cousins, aunts, uncles, nieces, nephews), co-workers, close friends, neighbours, members of volunteer community support services, and acquaintances—have a variety of functions and vary in importance to the senior. Some members of the community act as lay gatekeepers. Mail carriers, veterinarians, utility workers, the sheriff's department, and farm, implement, and grain dealers provide informal social support and help look out for the rural elders.[144] Instrumental help is given in the form of advice, information, financial aid, and assistance with tasks. Socioemotional aid is given in the form of affection, sympathy, understanding, acceptance, esteem, and referral to services.[145–149] Planning for contact between the generations (e.g., with preschoolers or adolescents) also contributes to meaningful social interactions for both generations.[150,151]

Formal health-related support services include government and private agencies that provide a service. Examples include home maintenance services, chore services, home-delivered groceries or meals, pharmacies that deliver drugs or medical supplies, assistance of home health aides, home visits by professional therapists or nurses, and case management services. Formal support services that are available to elderly adults but that do not always come to the home include medical and social services, daycare, respite care, and the church.[152]

Frequency of use of social networks is not related to physical health. As income decreases, visiting with neighbours declines, but visits to close friends or relatives increase, as does the tendency to talk to family members about feelings and to talk to friends about events. The elderly rate helpfulness of children and other family members as important. Lower income increases the senior's reliance on friends and relatives and the value placed on their help. Higher income may provide resources that facilitate social visiting and a broader network of relationships. A higher frequency of social contacts and greater intensity of kin and friend relationships have been found for women in comparison to men. Apparently intimacy or close friendship ties and having a confidant are less important to the male.[153,154]

Supportive ties become smaller and more unstable in old age; and social support may provide burdens for those who provide support to the senior. Burdens and costs may result in being less willing or able to help, physical or psychological distancing, increasing the social isolation of the dependent senior, or becoming enmeshed in the caregiver role to the exclusion of other relationships or roles. Informal networks ideally are integrated with formal support services.[155–157]

A system of informal assistance through family, friends, and neighbours is the major source of help for the elderly. Among and for seniors, there are three types of neighbourhood exchange types:

1. High helpers, who exhibit a more formal quasi-professional style of helping without reciprocation.
2. Mutual helpers, who show an interdependent style of give and take.
3. Neighbourhood isolates, whose social ties and help sources are primarily outside the neighbourhood.

High helpers with neighbours are those who also do volunteer work or are active in self-help groups. Mutual helpers have more neighbourhood contact and are generally quite outgoing. Isolates have little contact with others and view themselves as quiet people. They may be in poor health and in need of help themselves.[158–160]

Many of the events of later life are exit events, involving continuous threat, stress, and loss such as widow(er)hood, chronic or poor health, retirement, change in residence, and lower income. Socialization contributes to well-being by lending continuity and structure to the transitions encountered by people.

Often you will be able to assist the elderly in asking for and accepting help from others, or in becoming familiar with community resources.

Caregiver Role

The role of the middle-aged offspring in caring for the elderly parent has been described in Chapter 13. Refer to Chapter 13 and the references in the endnotes of that chapter and this chapter for more information on the caregiver role.[161–170] Even as elders are being cared for, they are also a source of support—emotionally, socially, and financially (by providing living arrangement)—for the adult child.

The caregiver in an elderly couple is most frequently the wife, as women live longer than men and are usually younger than their spouses. If the woman is impaired, the husband is often the caregiver. The spouse is the primary source of help for married elderly with impaired capacity, and adult daughters are the major helpers when a spouse is not present or not able to sufficiently help. In some cultures, the grandchild or great-grandchild may be the major caregiver, especially if they were raised by the now-frail great-grandparent. This is discussed in Burton's research.[171] The probability of relying on friends is highest among impaired elderly who are unmarried and have few family members within an hour's travel. The more frail the person, the more likely a family member will be the primary caregiver rather than formal systems or nonrelated people.[172,173] The majority of noninstitutionalized elderly are self-sufficient.

When the spouse cannot manage care for the elderly parent, children try to assist. Sons tend to become caregivers only in the absence of an available female sibling and are more likely to rely on their own spouses for support and help. Sons tend to provide less direct care assistance and to be less involved; hence, they do not feel as stressed by the caregiving experience.

The elderly person who cares for a disabled or ill spouse is a hidden victim, at risk for physical and emotional stresses of caregiving superimposed on stresses of the aging process. He or she is likely to experience a barrage of feelings and role overload, including being head of the household. The woman, or man, as the spouse who is the caregiver, may also be chronically ill or disabled. Thus, the family caregiver for the noninstitutionalized elder is in need of help from supportive services.[174–176] These services for the spouse could include a wives' support group sponsored by a senior centre; home health care; adult daycare; foster home placement; extended respite care; homemaker, visitor, or respite services and individual counselling. Sometimes the elder is the caregiver for an adult child with developmental disability, mental retardation, or mental illness. The gratification, frustration, and stress are related to the adult child's diagnosis, size of the women's support system, the family's social climate, and adult child's participation in out-of-home programs.

Be aware of feelings of the middle-aged or elderly caregiver and the family; needs and feelings of the elderly person; issues and conflicts for the family; and ways to help families manage the caregiving experience. Education and support group programs appear to hold great promise as a means for assisting family caregivers of older relatives. You will have an important role in implementing both of those interventions. A number of strategies can be helpful to the caregiver both in preventing decline in the caregiver and in administering care to the elder.[177–181] Various *programs can be effective for reducing stress for caregivers of elderly family members who are emotionally or physically disabled:*

- Support groups, especially for caregivers of patients with Alzheimer's or other dementias, which offer practical solutions to problems as well as emotional support
- Respite care programs based at the person's home or in agencies, to care for the ill person when the caregiver needs time off (a day, weekend, or week)
- Education about stress management techniques that enhance abilities to care for the self as well as the family member
- Telephone crisis counselling to elders and their caregivers and use of telecommunication services may be increasingly available.[182]

Widow(er)hood

Because widow(er)hood may occur before late life, the feelings, problems, and issues pertinent to the widow(er) have been discussed in Chapter 13. Refer to Chapter 13 and the references in the endnotes for this chapter for additional insights. Bereavement does not permanently affect health status for most seniors, although the grief reaction may induce physiologic symptoms initially. Stress appears to increase as the death approaches, and then health status may deteriorate. Regardless of the predeath mourning done by the survivor, the elderly widow(er) has great increase in psychological distress.[183–187]

Widow(er)hood disrupts couple-based relationships and obligations to a spouse and introduces emotional and material burdens on those relationships that outlive the marriage. Widow(er)hood, especially after a period of caregiving, may also introduce both a measure of freedom to make new contacts and a stimulus to do so. The widowed person may have greater intimacy with friends than those who are married, for married people interact more with their spouses.[188–192]

The elderly widowed are not more isolated than elderly married, and elderly women have some advantage over elderly men in their ability to develop or maintain social relationships. Patterns of social relationships established among the married apparently provide the parameters within which social relationships continue among the widowed. Both married and widowed women are more likely to talk to close friends and relatives and to talk to family about worries and to children about crises than are married or widowed men. Loss of spouse allows for expansion or addition of new roles; frequency of contact increases with widow(er)hood. Widow(er)hood results in greater involvement with informal social relationships than marriage.

The widow who lives alone in her own home may be in need of a great deal of help. Neighbours often provide this help, especially if children reside out of town. The childless widow, however, may not receive any more help from neighbours than widows with children, despite greater needs. Perhaps adult children are able to elicit neighbour assistance; such requests for extra help are not forthcoming if there are no children.

Your teaching, emotional support, referral to services, and encouragement to continue as active a life as possible are important to the widow or widower as she or he adjusts to losses and new roles.

Divorce and the Elderly

Be prepared to give emotional support or crisis intervention to the older person who is encountering divorce or who is reworking the conflicts, dilemmas, and losses of having experienced divorce.

An increased number of seniors will fall in the ever-divorced and currently divorced categories because those entering old age in the future will be more accepting of divorce as a solution to an unpleasant marriage. Further, in the future more elderly women will have economic independence because of their years in the workforce, and this may encourage higher divorce rates.[193–196] Novak and Campbell state that little research exists on divorced older people.[197] However, there appears to be an increasing number of divorces in older people.[198]

Being divorced in old age, or in any age, may negatively affect a person's economic position and may increase demands for social welfare support. Typically divorce is associated with deterioration in the standard of living for women, although it has little effect for men. Further, family and kinship relationships are affected by divorce. The children or other relatives who would provide physical help and psychosocial support may not be available to one of the parents in his or her old age.

Remarriage also establishes a new set of nuclear family relationships. To assure economic safety, some elders establish a **prenuptial** or **antenuptial agreement.** *This contract is made before marriage to settle, in advance, respective property and financial rights of each party and the children of each person in the event of divorce or death.* In formulating a contract, the man and woman should each retain their own lawyers, fully disclose all assets, and finalize the pact well before the wedding. For some people, the prenuptial contract, with all the legal work involved, becomes a reality check. The couple may decide not to marry, realizing that the relationship will not really meet each person's needs. Some elders choose to forego a contract and formal marriage but do reside together for companionship.[199] The experience of being divorced can help the senior cope with bereavement. The person knows survival is possible after a marital relationship ends.[200–203]

CRITICAL THINKING

Undertake a content analysis of several academic journals focusing on prenuptial agreements between elderly couples. What trends do you observe?

Singlehood

A small percentage of the elderly population remains single and never marries. They have no spouse or children. They may or may not have living family members. They may or may not live alone. Never-married elders do not constitute a single "social type"; their situations are more complex. Like other elders, they are affected by social opportunities and restraints and the cultural values and changes that impinge on their life situations. Some older people are homosexual. Some live in locations in which women outnumber men, causing an imbalance in mate selection. Others may have chosen the single lifestyle as a means to some end, such as a career. Some have had family responsibilities that precluded marriage or were otherwise unable to break out of their families of orientation. Others have been lifelong isolates and have had poor health or a stigmatized social identity. Possibly the factors for singlehood have been multiple.

Well-being in old age can be at least partly explained by a supportive relationship with the parent in early life. Elders who had a supportive relationship are more likely to be adaptive and cope with adversity effectively in old age.[204–207] As practitioners, we should be sensitive to these differences and to their effects on the lives and identities of never-married elders.

There are prior relationships for never-married older women that help reduce social isolation and loneliness and increase life satisfaction and social support (see Chapter 4 and Chapter 12).

Issues of attachment may be different for the widowed and the never married, but this does not mean that there are no loss issues, although it is clear that there are some never-married elders who do not develop such attachments. There are a range of attachments and bereavement experiences for the never married in late life, not just an absence of personal loss issues. Having lived independently all during adult life, the person may have developed effective adaptive mechanisms and a supportive social network. The single person may be no lonelier than the married person. He or she does not experience the desolation of widow(er)hood or divorce.[208]

Few studies have been done on *health status* of the single senior. They generally conclude that the well-being of single people is equivalent to that of married persons, whereas widowed, divorced, and separated persons have lower well-being. A decline in functional capacity greatly increases the likelihood that the unmarried older person will move in with others or become institutionalized.

Psychological integrity and social independence are features of the single personality. The single person views *fluidity and variety in social relationships,* rather than the exclusivity of marriage, as an advantage in promoting opportunities for personal growth while still protecting autonomy. Lifestyle is geared to preserving personal independence and the development of self, with privacy, self-expression through work, freedom of movement, and preoccupation with expanding experiences, philosophic insights, and imaginative conceptions of life as goals for the person. Single women are happier and better adjusted than single men; marital roles may be less beneficial and more stressful for women than for men. Although single women are happier than single men, they are nevertheless less happy than married women.

Friends are important. Friendship is a process that occurs throughout life. Older adults rarely terminate friendships, though they may fade away because of lifestyle changes, geographic moves, or illness. Friends can also act as family and promote healing—emotionally, physically, and socially. Positive social interaction lowers the stress hormone levels, helps preserve cognitive functions, and prevents depression. Sharing ideas, talking, and listening are the main value of friendships. Men talk more about topics, such as past careers, politics, and sports. Women talk more about relationships and feelings.[209]

Be alert to special emotional and social needs of the single elderly, to their reticence at times to ask for help, and to the need for information about community resources. You may become a significant confidant.

CRITICAL THINKING

Compare and contrast health promotion strategies required by the single elderly person and the married elderly couple.

Elders and Pets

Pets are great companions for older people. Pets are therapeutic in the home and in the centre or institution for the elderly. They offer companionship and unconditional love, they soothe and lift the spirits, and a specially trained dog can offer assistance and security (e.g., as a brace for the neurologically impaired). Dogs can pull wheelchairs and even help load them into cars. Pets have a beneficial effect on physical health: they lower stress response and lower blood pressure. Touches from the pet and stroking the pet provide physiologic release; and they tend to lower anxiety. Pets can promote verbal communication skills; birds can even "talk" back. Although animals and birds do carry disease, healthy pets can be obtained from well-run shelters and shops or the Humane Society. Canine Companions for Independence is an organization that supplies highly trained service dogs for helping people who use wheelchairs or are hearing impaired or deaf, and social companions for people with disabilities. Pets are chosen for temperament, not breed. There is no charge for the dog. The person or family may need help in keeping the pet immunized, cleaned, and given the care that prevents unnecessary decline in the pet's health. Today, volunteers regularly take their animals to visit residents in hospitals, personal care homes, and other institutions across Canada. Katz states that pet facilitated therapy (PFT), which has emerged during the past few decades, is refreshingly simple, low-tech, and effective.[210]

Explore accessible pet services. Mobile veterinarians, grooming vans, and other services are available in some areas.[211] You can be instrumental in promoting pet therapy.[212]

The death of a pet can precipitate a deep grief, and mourning will result because of the loss. Crisis counselling, giving the person a helping hand and shoulder to cry on, may help the person work through the pet's death or work through feelings related to having to put the pet to sleep. Be aware that the senior who wants euthanasia for an apparently healthy pet may be contemplating suicide or suicide may follow the death of a pet. Death of a pet can be the last straw in a series of stresses and losses.

Elder Abuse and Neglect

The abuse and neglect of older adults is not a new problem.[213] The 65-and-older age group comprises one of the fastest-growing segments of the Canadian population. According to Hawranik and McKean, this changing profile has heightened concern about the possible increase in the incidence of abuse and neglect among seniors.[214] Most Canadian research on elder abuse has used convenience samples, at times with low response rates; consequently, generalizations from these results are uncertain.[215]

CRITICAL THINKING

What are your attitudes and beliefs about elder abuse?

Usually the abuser is a relative (spouse more often than offspring) residing with the victim. However, abusers need not be blood relatives, or even family members. The abuse and neglect of older persons can occur either in the home or in community programs such as recreation centres and adult day programs.[216] Refer to the box entitled "Types and Manifestations of Elder Abuse" for further description.[217–221]

Hypotheses about the causes of elder abuse are listed in the box entitled "Causes of Elder Maltreatment, Abuse, or Neglect."[222]

Ways to prevent or reduce abuse are listed in the box entitled "Tips for the Older Person for Preventing or Reducing Abuse."

Types and Manifestations of Elder Abuse

Physical Abuse

- Neglect of physical care (food, eyeglasses, hearing aid, or information withheld)
- Slap, bruise, push
- Beating
- Burns, broken bones
- Brandishing a knife, cutting, stabbing
- Restraint (chain to toilet or tie to bed), resulting in skin breakdown or decubitus ulcers, as well as fractures
- Sexual molestation, rape

Psychological Abuse

- Verbal abuse (curse, scream, insult, demean, treat like a child)
- Verbal threats, name calling
- Decision making, voting denied
- Exclusion from family activities, isolation
- Placement in nursing home without consent or knowledge

Financial Abuse

- Confiscation of pension or other income cheques
- Person forced to sign over property or assets
- Other financial exploitation
- Theft of property and personal items for sale
- Takeover of trust, guardianship
- Exploitation of resources for profit

Social Abuse

- Forced isolation from family, friends
- Constant switching of doctors
- Refusal of home health care or other community resources (daycare, home health aide, Meals-on-Wheels)
- Inability to accept help or acknowledge difficulty with care
- Geographic isolation, e.g., rural, inner-city ghetto
- Caregiver or client minimize injuries or situation

Causes of Elder Maltreatment, Abuse, or Neglect

- Elder becomes more dependent or disabled.
- Elder is cognitively impaired or has Alzheimer's disease.
- Family is under economic stress.
- Caregiver is exhausted or loses control; unable to cope.
- Adult offspring is unemployed, lives in parent's home, and expects to be cared for.
- Adult offspring is mentally ill or alcohol- or drug-addicted.
- Family interaction pattern of screaming, hitting, and violence has existed through lifetime of marriage or childrearing.
- Retirement and lack of role clarity for both spouses result in much frustration in retired man.
- Man who was abusive to co-workers now abuses most available person, the wife.
- Woman is financially dependent on spouse.
- Elder is abandoned or seldom visited by children.
- Victim is unwilling or unable to report the problem.

Tips for the Older Person for Preventing or Reducing Abuse

- Remain sociable and stay active in the community; enlarge your circle of friends; join a community group.
- Plan for possible disability by completing an advance medical directive and arranging for power-of-attorney.
- Familiarize yourself with community resources that help older people remain as independent as possible.
- Do not share a household with anyone who has a history of violent behaviour or substance abuse.
- Do not move in with a child or relative if your relationship is troubled.
- Avoid taking into your home new or unknown people in a live-in arrangement.
- Ask for help when you need it from a lawyer, physician, or trusted family member.
- Check the *Directory of Services and Programs Addressing the Needs of Older Adult Victims of Violence in Canada*.[223] For example, residents in Nova Scotia may call the Health and Community Service Office, the Public Health Nurse, or the RCMP.

Signs and symptoms of the abused or neglected elder include the following:

- Bruises, fractures, malnourished status
- Undue confusion not attributable to physiologic consequences of aging
- Conflicting explanation about the senior's condition
- Unusual fear exhibited by the senior in a presumed safe environment, in the home, or in the presence of the caregiver
- A report of the daily routine that has considerable gaps in the sequence
- Apparent impaired functioning or abnormal behaviour in the caregiver
- Indifference or hostility displayed by caregiver in response to questions

During assessment of potential abuse or neglect, do not let stereotypes about the elder or caregiver(s), an emphasis on family privacy, or denial prevent you from identifying the problem. Avoid a censuring tone of voice or judgmental expression or stance. Show a willingness to listen to the caregiver's perspective. Solicit the caregiver's early memories of relationships with the senior to learn of long-term conflicts. Most abused seniors are reluctant and ashamed to report abuse or neglect because of (1) fear of retaliation, (2) exposure of offspring to community censure or legal punishment, and (3) fear of potential removal from their home.

Three questions help detect partner violence. These questions are applicable to spouse abuse at any age:

1. Have you been hit, kicked, punched, or otherwise hurt by someone within the past year? If so, when?
2. Do you feel safe in your current relationship?
3. Is there a partner from a previous relationship who is making you feel unsafe now?

From the answers given, ask related questions in order to gain full information. Be gentle and give the person time to give what may be painful answers.

CRITICAL THINKING

What nursing interventions can be developed in working with the abused elderly?

In Canada, it is the older adult's right to make his or her decisions. It is critical to note that if the older adult who is being abused is considered mentally competent, then he or she is supported in the decision to report or not to report. Some service providers believe that criminal prosecution is of little assistance to the older victim because the focus is on punishing the offender rather than helping the victim.[224] However, anyone (victim, family member or friend, a witness to the abuse, or a service provider) can report a suspected occurrence to the police. Reports can be made anonymously if desired. In provinces and territories with mandatory reporting legislation, service providers who know of, or suspect, abuse are required to report the incident to the authorities.[225] Victim assistance programs can be most helpful in supporting older adults and their families as they proceed through the criminal justice system. Examples of victim assistance programs can include law information lines, seniors' advocacy centres, and legal aid services. In Manitoba, for example, there is a Senior Abuse Line, which is a confidential information service aimed at providing seniors, family members, professionals, and others with a one-stop information resource on elder abuse.[226] Other provinces and territories have similar sources of assistance.

CONTROVERSY DEBATE

Elder Abuse

Robert and Sarah Hughes have been married to each other for almost 50 years. Robert ran his own gasoline and automobile service station with two or three auto mechanics. Five years ago he sold the business and seemed to become a changed person since he stopped spending long hours each day at work. Sarah had been a cashier in a large local grocery store. Robert insisted she stop work when he sold the business—so they could "do things together." Reluctantly she gave up her job when she was 68 years old. Because of Sarah's memory loss in recent years, Robert has allowed home-care workers into the home to help her with eating and to perform personal care. The workers report that Robert yells at Sarah when she forgets things. They have even seen him attempting to force feed her when she could not finish eating her entire meal. He sometimes swears at her and calls her names. Recently, they have seen bruises on Sarah's arms and welts on her legs. You are the home-care coordinator to whom the home-care workers report.

1. What intervention options are open to you to address the elder abuse that seems clearly evident here?

2. What is the role of the home-care nurse in introducing and implementing interventions?

3. What barriers should you expect to encounter when the interventions are applied?

4. How will you address these barriers?

PHYSIOLOGIC CONCEPTS

Use this information to assess, teach, and implement health promotion measures.

Physical Characteristics

When we are born, regardless of our genetic background or external influences, we all have one thing in common—the element of aging. From the day of birth, we begin the aging process in our unique way. There is much diversity in the aging process.

The rapidity and manifestations of aging in each individual depend on heredity, past illnesses, lifestyle, patterns of eating and exercise, presence of chronic illnesses, and level of lifetime stress. Some generalized physiologic changes do occur, however; they include a decrease in rate of cell mitosis, a deterioration of specialized nondividing cells, an increased rigidity and loss of elasticity in connective tissue, and a loss of reserve functional capacity.[227–229]

Certain *other characteristics* have been observed *about aging*:[230–234]

- Time of onset, type, and degree of aging differ between men and women and are more distinctive between the sexes in middle life than in the later years.
- Senescent alterations in one organ or in the whole organism can be either premature or delayed in relation to the body's total chronology.
- The progression of aging in cellular tissues is asymmetric: the characteristics of old age may be displayed prominently in one system (brain, bone, cardiovascular apparatus, lungs) and be less obvious elsewhere (liver, pancreas, gastrointestinal tract, muscles).
- Certain pathology is a manifestation of aging.
- **Organ reserve,** *the extra capacity of the organs that is drawn on in times of stress or illness,* lessens with age. (In young adulthood, the body can put forth four to ten times its usual effort when stressed.)
- A direct relationship exists between the sum of common aging traits and the length of survival.

General Appearance

The general appearance of the older adult is determined in part by the changes that occur in the skin, face, hair, and posture. Old women have significantly more body fat, greater truncal skin-folds, and greater circumferences than old men and young adult women and less fat-free body mass than young adult women.[235]

Skin. The overall appearance of the skin changes dramatically (Table 14-2).[236,237]

Head. Even the appearance of the face changes as the nose and ears tend to become longer and broader and the chin-line alters. Wrinkles on the face are pronounced because of the repeated stress produced by the activity of facial muscles. The predominant mood expressed by the facial muscles of the individual becomes permanently etched on the face in the form of wrinkles (smile or frown lines) above the eyebrows, around lips, over cheeks, and around the outer edges of the eye orbit. Shortening of the platysma muscle produces neck wrinkles.[238–240]

Grey hair is the universal phenomenon associated with aging, but it is not a reliable indicator of age, as some individuals begin greying as early as their teen years. The hair gradually greys; the exact shade of grey depends on the original hair colour. Eventually all the pigmented hair is replaced by nonpigmented hair; gradually the overall hair colour turns pure white. Both males and females are affected. The loss of hair occurs on the scalp, in the pubic and axillary areas, and on the extremities. In older adults there is also increased growth of facial hair due to the change in the androgen-estrogen ratio.[241–243]

Posture. The posture of the older adult is one of general flexion. The head is tilted forward; hips and knees are slightly flexed. Muscles in the torso are held rigidly. The older adult stands with the feet apart to provide a wide base of support. He or she takes shorter steps, which may produce a shuffling gait. A shift in the centre of gravity occurs as well, which affects movement and balance.[244–246]

Neurologic System

Nervous System Changes. With aging there are major changes in the nervous system that occur normally and alter

TABLE 14-2
Alterations in Integumentary System Related to Aging

Tissue/Organ	Alteration and Rationale	Implications for Health Promotion
Epidermis	Skin manufactures less collagen, elastin, and other proteins. Cellular division decreases; thus, skin cells are replaced more slowly. (Skin cells live an average of 46 days in 70-year-old, compared with 100 days in 30-year-old.)	Wounds heal more slowly. Maintain nutrition and hygiene.
	Elastin fibres are more brittle. Loss of collagen fibres causes decreased turgor and loss of elasticity, wrinkles, and creases.	Use emollients and lotion to maintain moisture on skin. Avoid hot water baths, excessive soap. Rinse skin well; pat dry.

(continued)

TABLE 14-2 *(continued)*
Alterations in Integumentary System Related to Aging

Tissue/Organ	Alteration and Rationale	Implications for Health Promotion
	Permeability increases and cells are thinner. Ability to retain fluids decreases, causes skin to become drier, less flexible. Fair-skinned persons lose pink tones, become paler. **Lentigo senilis,** *irregular areas of dark pigmentation on dorsum of hands, arms, and face* and uneven pigmentation occur. Capillaries and small arteries on exposed skin surface become dilated. Decreased response to pain sensation and temperature changes may cause accidents or burns.	Some medications make skin more fragile and susceptible to bruising: aspirin, prednisone, steroid topical creams. Cosmetics may be used. Protect from direct sun. Use sunscreen, protective factor of 15 or higher, with UVA and UVB protection. Assist person in accepting appearance changes. Teach safety factors. Care with heating pads or hot water bottles and ice packs.
Subcutaneous tissue (hypodermic)	Loss of fat cells, especially in face and limbs, causes sagging and wrinkles. Lack of tissue over bony prominences contributes to decubitus ulcers. Lower cutaneous blood flow and loss of fat contribute to decreased insulation and susceptibility to chilling.	Assist adjustment to appearance and changes. Protect bony prominences from pressure, abrasions, injury, and decubitus ulcers. Provide adequate clothing and heat control for comfort.
Dermis	Decreased fat, water, and matrix content cause translucent appearance of skin. Larger and coarser collagen fibres decrease flexibility of collagen, reduce elasticity, and cause sags and wrinkles. Decreased number of fibroblasts and fibres cause thinning tissue.	Emollients, lotions, and cosmetics may be used. Assist person in accepting appearance changes. Avoid bumps, scrapes, and lacerations of skin. Wear protective clothing.
Hair	Reduced melanin production causes greying. Thinning, stiffness, and loss of lustre are due to change in germ centre that produces hair follicles. Baldness is genetic. In women increased facial hair on upper lip and chin result from diminished estrogen.	Use hair colouring or cosmetic techniques if desired. Assist person in integrating appearance changes into body image.
Sebaceous oil glands	Decreased lubrication with oil causes skin to be drier, rougher, and scaly.	Use emollients/lotions. Avoid hot water, use minimal soap, rinse well. Pat dry. Use room humidifiers.
Sweat glands	Reduced number interferes with ability to sweat freely and regulate body temperature.	Prevent heat stroke. Drink adequate water. Dress in garments that allow heat transmission from body. Use fan or air conditioner as needed in hot weather.
Nails	Growth is slower. Increased calcium deposition causes ridges and thickening.	Encourage visit to podiatrist for care of toenails and cosmetologist for care of fingernails.

the individual's sensory response:[247–254]

- Loss of nerve cells
- Decrease in neurotransmitters
- Slower nerve impulse transmission
- Decrease in nerve conduction velocity
- Decline in electric activity
- Increase in sensory threshold
- Decline in integration of sensory and motor function

All of these neurologic changes create problems for the older adult. For example, by age 70, upper body stiffness, slower voluntary movement, slower decision making, visual changes, and slowed startle response are seen. Because of these particular neurologic changes, older adults do not respond as quickly to changes in their external environment. This slower response affects many facets of their life (e.g., there is greater risk to overall safety, and drivers over 65 years of age are involved in a higher percentage of automobile accidents per kilometre driven than are drivers aged 25 to 54 years). The older adult's increase in sensory threshold affects pain and tactile perception and response to stimuli, resulting in increased susceptibility to burns or other injuries.[255–259]

Brain. By age 90 the brain's weight has decreased 10% from its maximum and reduction in size is not uniform throughout the brain. This weight loss is accompanied by a reduction of cells in the cerebral cortex and a decrease in the number of functioning neurons in the grey matter, rather than in the brain stem. The white matter is not significantly different than in young people. The void left by these anatomic changes is filled by expanding ventricular volumes in the form of cerebrospinal fluid.[260]

The amount of space between the skull and brain tissue doubles from ages 20 to 70. Reduced cerebral blood flow and oxygenation of the brain and reduced glucose metabolism may alter thought processes and perceptual function. Altered brain waves and sleep patterns, including reduced REM (dream) sleep, contribute to nighttime wakefulness. (Measures to reduce insomnia are discussed in Chapter 12.) Increased activity of monoamine oxidase enzymes may contribute to depression.[261–263] The anatomic and physiologic changes in the brain of the older adult are not always directly related to performance abilities. Declining human performance in advanced age may be due to deficits in systems peripheral to the central nervous system and/or to other behavioural factors.[264–268]

Vestibular and Kinesthetic Response. The response to vestibular and kinesthetic stimuli decreases with age. The vestibular division of the vestibulocochlear nerve is associated with balance and equilibrium. With aging there is a decrease in the number of nerve fibres, thus affecting balance and equilibrium. Reduction in the number of sensory cells in the utricle, saccule, and semicircular ducts further affects balance. These reductions may begin as early as 50 years of age but are especially noticeable after 70. Vestibular sense receptors are located in muscles and tendons; these receptors relay information about joint motion and body position in space to the central nervous system. Loss of neurons in the cerebellum that receive the sensory information also contributes to diminished balance.[269–273] (See Table 14-3.)

TABLE 14-3
Health Promotion Implications for Other Neurologic Changes

Change	Health Promotion Implication
Vestibular and kinesthetic	Teach safety factors, such as ways to maintain balance and safe walking. Canes, walking sticks, or walkers can be helpful. Make home fall-proof. Wear flat, rubber-soled, properly fitting shoes.
Tactile	Use firm but gentle pressure on hand, arm, or shoulder to indicate your presence or soothe with touch. Teach safety factors: 1. Walk more slowly to allow feet to fully touch surface and to be cognizant of foot placement, e.g., on stairs, uneven surfaces, or outdoors. 2. Monitor use of hot water bottles, heating pads, or ice bags to avoid burns or frostbite. 3. Teach ways to avoid bumps or abrasions. Bed-ridden or chair-bound person *must* have position changed frequently to prevent decubitus ulcer.
Taste and smell	Teach need for more seasoning, preferably spices and herbs rather than sugar or salt, to better enjoy food and discriminate tastes. Encourage adequate nutrition. Teach safety factors related to reduced smell, e.g., how to monitor for burning food or gas leaks.

Vision. Visual changes occur. Loss of vision is gradual; fewer than 1% have extremely severe visual impairment. The number of fibres composing the optic fibre decreases over time. Lacrimal glands produce fewer tears, causing the cornea to become dry and irritated. The lens thickens and yellows; objects take on a yellowish hue; and the cells within the lens lose water and shrink. The diameter of the pupil decreases and the pupil is less able to accommodate to light changes. The lack of pupillary response, increased lens opacity, and irregular corneal surface, which causes light to scatter, together result in intolerance to glare and difficulty in adjusting from brightly to dimly lit areas, or vice versa. Visual contrast sensitivity for size and light decreases. These changes interfere with the ability to transmit and refract light. Because of loss of elasticity in the lens and slower response in accommodation, **presbyopia,** *inability to change lens shape for near vision,* is present in most adults after age 45 or 50. Even with corrective lenses, the individual may need longer to focus on near objects.[274–279]

Colour vision is also altered after age 60, because of retinal changes (rods and cones), loss of sensitivity of photoreceptors, and slower transmission of visual impulses to the nervous system. The reception of short wavelengths (blue) is affected first, followed by middle-wavelength hues (green, greenish yellow), and, last, by the long wavelengths (red). Thus, for the older adult, colours such as green, blue, and violet are more difficult to see than are red, orange, and yellow. Pastels fade so that they are indistinguishable from each other; monotones, whites, and dark colours are also difficult to see. Brighter colours compensate for decline in colour discrimination and yellowing and opacity of the lens.[280–284]

Cataract development and glaucoma frequently occur in this age group. With **cataracts** the *lens becomes opaque,* accompanied by diminished vision and increased sensitivity to glare. **Glaucoma** is caused by damage to the optic nerve from increased intraocular pressure. These conditions and the other visual changes such as **arcus senilis,** the *accumulation of lipids on the cornea,* can be assessed during periodic eye examinations. The elder with lens-opacifying disease has increased risk for macular degeneration, regardless of age, sex, or systolic blood pressure.[285–289]

Age-related macular degeneration (AMD), a common, often slow-to-be-detected, eye disease in elders, *occurs when the macula, the most light-sensitive portion of the retina, begins to deteriorate.* An intact macula is necessary for good central vision and to see fine details. One-fourth of elders over 65 and one-third over 80 experience some AMD. Teach that prevention may involve an adequate diet of antioxident vitamins or carotenoids (pigments found in yellow, orange, red, and dark green fruits and vegetables). In addition, smoking should be avoided and eyes protected from bright sunlight by wearing polarized sunglasses and a wide-brimmed hat.[290,291]

See Table 14-4 for health promotion implications related to visual changes, as well as the box entitled "Guidelines for Helping the Blind Person."[292–296]

CRITICAL THINKING

What are the resources in your community to assist the blind older adult?

Hearing. With age, the pinna (external ear) becomes longer, wider, and less flexible; this change does not appear to affect hearing. As cerumen production diminishes and the wax becomes drier, however, blockage of the ear canal can occur. The presence of dried, packed wax can interfere with sound transmission. Any auditory changes that occurred in middle age continue through later life. Men are twice as likely as women to have hearing loss. The tympanic membrane becomes thinner and less resilient and may show some sclerotic changes. In some older adults calcification of the ossicles occurs. There are also changes in the organ of Corti, loss of nerve cells in the eighth cranial nerve, and an increased rate of time for passage of impulses in the auditory nerve. Because of the changes to the inner ear and cochlea, a hearing aid (many are small) or corrective surgery may partially improve hearing; however, a hearing aid magnifies all sounds. If there is sensorineural deafness,

---

Guidelines for Helping the Blind Person

- Talk to the blind person in a normal tone of voice. The fact that he or she cannot see is no indication that hearing is impaired.
- Be natural when talking with a blind person.
- Accept the normal things that a blind person might do such as consulting the watch for the correct time, dialling a telephone, or writing his or her name in longhand without calling attention to them.
- When you offer assistance to a blind person, do so directly. Ask, "May I be of help?" Speak in a normal, friendly tone.
- In guiding a blind person, permit him or her to take your arm. Never grab the blind person's arm, for he or she cannot anticipate your movements.
- In walking with a blind person, proceed at a normal pace. You may hesitate slightly before stepping up or down.
- Be explicit in giving verbal directions to a blind person.
- There is no need to avoid the use of the word *see* when talking with a blind person.
- When assisting a blind person to a chair, simply place his or her hand on the back or arm of the chair. This is enough to give location.
- When leaving the blind person abruptly after conversing with him or her in a crowd or where there is a noise that may obstruct hearing, quietly advise that you are leaving so that he she will not be embarrassed by talking when no one is listening.
- Never leave a blind person in an open area. Instead, lead him or her to the side of a room, to a chair, or some landmark from which he or she can obtain direction.
- A half-open door is one of the most dangerous obstacles that blind people encounter.
- When serving food to a blind person who is eating without a sighted companion, offer to read the menu, including the price of each item. As you place each item on the table, call attention to food placement by using the numbers of an imaginary clock. ("The green beans are at 2 o'clock.") If he or she wants you to cut up the food, he or she will tell you.
- Be sure to tell a blind person who the other guests are so that he or she may know of their presence.

---

damage to the auditory nerve or the hearing centre of the brain from bacterial or viral infections, head injuries, or prolonged exposure to loud noise, a hearing aid will not improve hearing.[297–299]

Of all individuals over 65, 13% suffer severe **presbycusis,** *progressive loss of hearing and sound discrimination.* The consonants, especially *s, sh, ch, th, dg, z,* and *f,* and high-frequency sounds produce problems for the individual with presbycusis. The ability to locate the direction from which sound is coming diminishes, and older people have difficulty hearing individuals who speak rapidly or in high tones.[300–303] For some helpful suggestions, see the box entitled "Guidelines for Communicating with the Hearing-Impaired Person."[304–307]

TABLE 14-4
Neurologic Changes in the Eye—Implications for Health Promotion

Change	Health Promotion Measure
Dry cornea	Use artificial tears if needed.
	Wear glasses to protect eyes from dust, flying debris.
Lens changes Presbyopia Spatial-depth vision changes	Wear corrective glasses or contact lenses. Use hard lens to magnify print for reading. Obtain books and periodicals in large print or tape-recorded materials. Teach safety considerations; take time to focus for vision. Teach safety factors related to doorways, space, and objects. It is important for institutions to place colour guards on stair steps; to clearly mark doorways; to avoid having carpet, furniture, walls, and drapes all of same or similar colour; walls, floor, doors, door frames, and furniture should be clearly delineated.
Pupillary and lens changes Decreased tolerance to glare or light changes	Wear tinted glass or brimmed hat to reduce glare or bright light. Turn on light in dark room before entering. Stand in doorway or at stairwell briefly to adjust to light changes from either bright light or dark. Teach need for more *indirect* but adequate illumination to perceive stimuli, do visual work. Avoid white or glossy surfaces. It is important for institutions to cover windows and avoid shiny wax on floor. Avoid glare on floor in bedroom, dining areas, lounges, or hallways. Teach safety considerations, especially with driving in bright sunlight or at night. Use nightlight to allow low-lighted visibility.
Retinal changes Colour-vision altered	Teach implications for personal grooming and dress, enjoyment of colours in nature, interior decoration, and design of living environment. Brighter colours are enjoyed. Teach family implications for selecting greeting cards and gifts. Adapt to yellow vision; teach implications for selecting clothing, cosmetics, or interior decor. It is important for institutions to use colours in interior decor that can readily be seen and enjoyed and not misinterpreted by elderly. Use sharp contrasting colours on doors, strips of contrasting colour on bottom of wall, and coloured or white strip at edge of each step to assist in distinguishing colours, space, and specific areas. Teach safety considerations to avoid misinterpretation of colour or not seeing objects that are pale or light colours.

CRITICAL THINKING

Why do some seniors reject hearing aids?

Tactile Acuity. There is a decreased number of nerve cells innervating the skin and thus a decreased response or sensitivity to touch. Even the soles of the feet have fewer sensory receptors and less responsivity. Two-point threshold is one of the oldest measures of spatial acuity of the skin. Age-related deterioration of tactile acuity, like visual and hearing changes, begins in late middle age. Acuity of touch, however, varies with different body regions; the fingertip has more acuity than the forearm for texture and temperature in old age. Acuity is also related to space between stimuli; for example, the fingertip may be sensitive to a single nodule but not as sensitive to the dots of Braille, to the glucose testing monitor used by the diabetic, or to other tactile aids used by the sensory handicapped.[308–311] See Table 14-3 on page 664 for health promotion implications related to tactile changes.

Taste and Smell. With aging, there is a general decrease in taste perception because of a decline in the actual number of taste buds (about half as many as in young adulthood, but women have more than men.) Diminished taste perception is linked to the changes in the processing of taste sensations in the central nervous system. Taste perception may also be affected by the diminished salivation that occurs in older persons. Usually older adults experience an increased preference for more sugar, salt, spices, and highly seasoned foods.

The sense of smell begins to decline in most people by middle age and continues a gradual decline into old age because the number and sensitivity of receptors decrease, especially after

Guidelines for Communicating with the Hearing-Impaired Person

- When you meet a person who seems inattentive or slow to understand you, consider the possibility that hearing, rather than manners or intellect, may be at fault. Some hard-of-hearing persons refuse to wear a hearing aid. Others wear aids so inconspicuous or clearly camouflaged that you may not spot them at first glance. Others cannot be helped by a hearing aid.

- Remember the hard-of-hearing may depend to a considerable extent on reading your lips. They do this even though they may be wearing a hearing aid, for no hearing aid can completely restore hearing. You can help by trying *always to speak in a good light* and by facing the person and the light as you speak.

- When in a group that includes a hard-of-hearing person, try to carry on your conversation with others in such a way that he or she can watch your lips. Never take advantage of the disability by carrying on a private conversation in his or her presence in low tones that cannot be heard.

- Speak distinctly but naturally. Shouting does not clarify speech sounds, and mouthing or exaggerating your words or speaking at a snail's pace makes you harder to understand. On the other hand, try not to speak too rapidly.

- Do not start to speak to a hard-of-hearing person abruptly. Attract his or her attention first by facing the person and looking straight into the eyes. If necessary, touch the hand or shoulder lightly. Help him or her grasp what you are talking about right away by starting with a key word or phrase, for example, "Let's plan our weekend now," "Speaking of teenagers...." *If he or she does not understand you, do not repeat the same words.* Substitute synonyms: "It's time to make plans for Saturday," and so on.

- If the person to whom you are speaking has one "good" ear, always stand or sit on that side when you address him or her. Do not be afraid to ask a person with an obvious hearing loss whether he or she has a good ear and, if so, which one it is. The person will be grateful that you care enough to find out.

- Facial expressions are important clues to meaning. Remember that an affectionate or amused tone of voice may be lost on a hard-of-hearing person.

- In conversation with a person who is especially hard-of-hearing, do not be afraid occasionally to jot down key words on paper. If he or she is really having difficulty in understanding you, the person will be grateful for the courtesy.

- Many hard-of-hearing persons, especially teenagers who hate to be different, are unduly sensitive about their disability and will pretend to understand you even when they do not. When you detect this situation, tactfully repeat your meaning in different words until it gets across.

- Teach the family to avoid use of candles. Electric light will give the person a better chance to join the conversation because he or she can see the lips during conversation. Similarly, in choosing a restaurant or nightclub, remember that *dim lighting may make lip-reading difficult.*

- Teach family members that they do not have to exclude the hard-of-hearing person from all forms of entertainment involving speech or music. Concerts and operas may present problems, but movies, plays, ballets, and dances are often just as enjoyable to people with a hearing loss as to those with normal hearing. (Even profoundly deaf persons can usually feel rhythm, and many are good and eager dancers.) For children, magic shows, pantomimes, and the circus are good choices.

- When sending a telegram to someone who does not hear well, instruct the telegraph company to deliver your message, not telephone it.

- The speech of a person who has been hard-of-hearing for years may be difficult to understand since natural pitch and inflection are the result of imitating the speech of others. To catch such a person's meaning more easily, watch the face while he or she talks.

- Do not say such things as "Why don't you get a hearing aid?" or "Why don't you see a specialist?" to a person who is hard-of-hearing. Chances are he or she has already explored these possibilities, and there is no need to emphasize the disability.

- *Use common sense* and tact in determining which of these suggestions apply to the particular hard-of-hearing person you meet. Some persons with only a slight loss might feel embarrassed by any special attention you pay them. Others whose loss is greater will be profoundly grateful for it.

age 80. It is believed that the sense of smell decreases because the olfactory nerves have fewer cells. This diminished sense of smell combined with the decline in taste sensation may account for the loss of appetite experienced by many older adults. The inability to smell also presents hazards for the individual, as he or she cannot quickly detect leaking gas, spoiled food, smoke, or burning food.[312–315]

See Table 14-3 on page 664 for health promotion implications related to changes in taste and smell.[316–318]

Cardiovascular System

Although the cardiovascular system undergoes considerable changes with aging (Table 14-5), in the absence of heart disease it is usually able to maintain the daily cardiac and circulatory functions of the older adult. However, the cardiovascular system may not be able to meet the needs of the body when a disease process is present or when there are excess demands caused by stress or excessive exercise. Obesity, physical inactivity, and abdominal fat distribution also reduce physiologic function. See Table 14-5 for cardiovascular changes and implications for health promotion.[319–328]

Respiratory System

Changes produced by aging affect both internal and external respiration; the older adult has difficulty taking oxygen from the atmosphere and delivering it to internal organs and tissues. See Table 14-6 for physiological changes and implications for health promotion.[329–333] Be prepared to do the Heimlich manoeuvre if the person chokes because of a weaker gag reflex or musculature (Figure 14–3).

TABLE 14-5
Cardiovascular Changes with Aging and Health Promotion Implications

Organ/Tissue	Change and Rationale	Implication for Health Promotion
Heart Internal	At age 70, cardiac output at rest is 70% of that at age 30.	Medication may be needed to maintain adequate function. Exercise routine should be maintained.
	Number and size of cardiac muscle cells decrease, causing loss of cardiac muscle strength, reduction in stroke volume, and less efficient pumping and cardiac output.	Assess for myocardial damage, muscle damage, and congestive heart failure.
	Thickening of collagen in heart valves reduces efficiency of closure because of rigidity. Calcification of valves increases.	Assess for aortic and mitral murmurs, valve stenosis or insufficiency, and endocarditis.
	Thickness of left ventricle wall increases; left ventricle is unable to pump volume of blood in cardiac cycle. Blood flow is maintained to brain and coronary arteries to greater extent than other body parts.	Cognitive, visceral, and muscular functions may not be adequately maintained with less cardiac output and inadequate blood supply.
	Pacemaker cells in sinoatrial node and atrioventricular nodes are replaced by fibrous and connective tissue, causing delay in nerve transmission and more time to complete the cardiac cycle.	Assess for ectopic activity, arrhythmias, and conduction defects.
External	Increased amount and stiffening of collagen surrounding heart, causing inelasticity. Increased fat deposits on surface of heart, reducing oxygen supply to body.	Maintain fluid balance and adequate aeration; avoid standing too long or constipation to reduce strain on heart. Straining to defecate strains right side of heart as blood suddenly pours through vena cava after pressure is decreased.
Blood vessels	Reduced elastin content and increased collagenous connective tissue in arterial walls reduce elasticity of walls of peripheral vessels, aorta, and other arteries.	Assess for increased systolic and diastolic blood pressure, abdominal pulsation, bruits, and aneurysms.
		Orthostatic hypotension may occur; blood pressure falls sharply on standing. Instruct person to rise to sitting position from lying position and stand slowly to allow for adjustment.
	Atherosclerosis, *increased accumulation and calcification in arterial walls,* makes smaller lumen diameter; vessel walls harder, thicker, and resistant to blood flow; and less rebound to vessel after being stretched. Blood flow is reduced to vital organs; cerebrovascular accidents (strokes) and multifarct dementia may occur.	Low-cholesterol diet should begin in early life, as these changes may occur in early life. Lifestyle: exercise, weight loss, no smoking, low-salt diet (under 3 g/day) can reduce blood pressure by 10/mm/Hg. Moderately elevated blood pressure may have protective effect on brain. Assess for hypertension and other circulatory problems.
	Walls of veins are thicker due to increased connective tissue and calcium deposits, decreasing elasticity.	Wear support hose to reduce varicose veins, beginning in early life. Sit with feet and lower legs elevated to enhance blood return to heart.
	Valves in large veins may become incompetent; varicose veins are common.	Avoid prolonged standing.

Musculoskeletal System

The major age-related change in the skeletal system is the loss of calcium from bone. Bone loss is accelerated with the loss of gonadal function at menopause. Therefore, bone loss is greater in females than in males and in older than younger females. Some studies have shown that by age 70 a woman's skeletal frame may have lost 30% or more of its calcium. With this change in bone composition comes a gradual decrease in height, on the average of 1.2 cm for each 20 years of life in both men and women and all races. Decreased synthesis of bone and increased decalcification, or osteoporosis in vertebrae, cause collapse, and loss of collagen and atrophy in intervertebral disks cause the spinal column to compress and posture to become curved or stooped and shorter. In addition to the decrease in height, bone strength is progressively lost because of loss of bone mineral content. Osteoporosis (which is discussed later) is seen as the extreme version of the universal process of adult bone loss.[334–340]

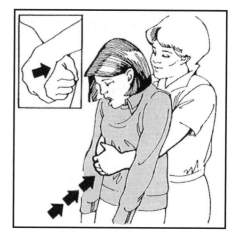

FIGURE 14–3

Heimlich manoeuvre.

Source: Berger, K.J., and M.B. Williams, Fundamentals of Nursing: Collaborating for Optimal Health. *Norwalk, CT: Appleton & Lange, 1992, p. 317.*

TABLE 14–6
Respiratory System Changes and Health Promotion Implications

Organ	Change and Rationale	Implication for Health Promotion
Nose	Reduced number and activity of cilia cause reduced bronchoelimination.	Less effective clearing of respiratory tract predisposes to infections. Avoid smoke-filled environment. Wear mask if air pollution exists. Avoid allergens. Maintain health status and avoid crowds in winter to prevent respiratory infections and pneumonia.
Throat	Cough reflex decreased. Sensitivity to stimuli decreased.	Teach safety factors, especially when eating (cut food into small portions, chew well, eat slowly).
Trachea	Flexibility is decreased; size of structure is increased.	
Rib cage and respiratory muscles	Calcification of chest wall causes rib cage to be less mobile. Decreased strength of intercostal and other respiratory muscles and diaphragm impairs breathing. Osteoporosis of ribs and vertebrae weakens chest wall and respiratory function. Calcification of vertebral cartilage and kyphosis stiffen chest wall and impair respiratory movements.	Maintain exercise, deep breathing, and erect posture to enhance respiratory muscle function. Avoid pressure to ribs to prevent rib fracture (e.g., leaning chest on edge of bath tub).
Lungs	Capacity to inhale, hold, and exhale breath decreases with age. Vital capacity at 85 is 50%–65% of capacity at 30. Elastin and collagen changes cause loss of elasticity of lung tissue; lungs remain hyperinflated even on exhalation, and proportion of dead space increases. Decreased elasticity and increased size of alveoli. Increased diffusion and surface area across alveolar-capillary membrane.	Encourage deep breathing, full exhalation, and erect posture throughout life. Maintain exercise to enhance lung function. Activity should be adjusted to respiratory efficiency and ventilation-perfusion ratio.

Decreased sensorimotor functions affect postural stability. Increased body sway is associated with reduced visual acuity, tactile sensitivity, vibration sense, joint position sense, ankle dorsiflexion strength, quadriceps muscle strength, and increased reaction time. Peripheral sensation ability is also a factor in sway and maintenance of postural stability.[341]

Maintaining upright posture and balance is a complex task. As postural control mechanisms deteriorate with disease and age, the person is more susceptible to falls. Standing on one leg and tandem walking become more difficult. The centre of pressure tends not to approach the edges of the base of support as closely as in younger years. One way to determine stability is to measure **functional reach**, *the maximum distance one can reach beyond arm's length while maintaining a fixed base of support in standing position.* Height and age affect reach, but the general ability to reach and the length of reach are related to ability to maintain stability when walking.[342]

The older adult experiences a gradual loss of muscular strength and endurance. Muscle cells atrophy, and lean muscle mass is lost. Studies have shown a 30% loss in muscle fibre between ages 30 and 80. In addition, as the elastic fibres in the muscle tissues decrease, the muscles become less flexible, and stiffness is noted more frequently.[343–346]

Changes in body weight also occur in the older adult. These changes follow definite patterns. Men usually exhibit an increase in weight until their middle 50s and then gradually lose weight. Women continue to gain weight until their 60s before beginning a gradual reduction in weight. The most significant weight loss occurs near 70 years of age and is probably due to decreased number of body cells, changes in cell composition, and decreased amounts of body tissue. See Table 14-7 for health promotion implications related to aging changes in the musculoskeletal system.[347–350]

Urinary System

As with the other body systems, major changes in structure and function of the urinary system are associated with aging. The kidneys, bladder, and ureters are all affected by the aging process.
Kidney. The aging kidney suffers a decrease in renal function as one ages. There is a loss of nephrons, the size of the kidney diminishes, and there is a loss of glomeruli—as much as 30% to 40% by age 70. Vascular changes affect the blood flow. Narrowing of blood vessels and vasoconstriction often due to arteriosclerosis and hypertension produce a decreased total renal blood flow. This is more significant than renal tissue loss[351–353] and causes reduced glomerular filtration rate and tubular function. See Table 14-7 for health promotion implications.[354–356]
Bladder. The bladder of an elderly person has a diminished capacity—less than 50% that of the young adult—because of atrophy, decreased size and elasticity, and reduced tone.[357] Coupled with a delayed desire to void, the elderly often have problems with frequent urination and a severe urgency to void. Aged women are especially prone to incontinence as the pelvic muscles become more flaccid. The pelvic diaphragm is the muscle mass that helps maintain bladder tone and proper closure of the bladder outlet. Weakening of the pelvic diaphragm leads to stress incontinence. More than 20% of

admissions to geriatric facilities are due to the inability to deal with incontinence.[358]

The same factors involved in the problem, reduced urinary capacity resulting in frequency and retention of residual urine, often lead to chronic cystitis, skin irritation, frequent need for antibiotics, and withdrawal from society.[359] Urinary tract infections (UTIs) are three times more prevalent in patients who are bowel incontinent. In a study done in a U.S. Veteran Affairs Medical Center, *Escherichia coli* was the main organism found in the urine cultures of patients with bowel incontinence. Nurses need to be aware of this when assisting the patient who may suffer from repeated UTIs.[360] It may not stem from frank bowel incontinence but there may be sufficient staining to provide contamination, and therefore more frequent hygiene may be advisable. Measures to combat urinary incontinence include regulation of fluid intake, pelvic muscle exercises (Kegel exercises) a regular pattern of voiding, and the use of drugs that block the hyperactivity of voiding. Teach the woman to control pelvic muscles and do the *Kegel exercise* as follows:

1. Tighten the muscles at least five times each day to help strengthen the pelvic floor muscles.
2. Don't tighten other muscles such as your hips or legs, during the pelvic floor exercises.
3. Sit, lie down, or stand during practice.
4. Practise this important exercise without anyone knowing.

Nurses can help immeasurably by establishing routines for toileting and reinforcing the patient with a positive attitude, helping to foster self-esteem and independence.

CRITICAL THINKING

Look at media advertisements for products used for incontinence. What type of message is sent to the older adult?

Hypertrophy of the prostate in the older man is very common and can begin as early as age 40. Irregular changes in the smooth muscle fibres and the prostate tissue occur with age. The problem consists of frequency, especially at night, difficulty starting the stream, dribbling, and retention with overflow. Cancer of the prostate is the most prevalent malignancy in men. Therefore, regular physical examinations should be encouraged to screen out the possibility of a malignancy. Some men are concerned about their sexual potency if surgery is to be performed.[361] Care should be taken to explain that although external ejaculation will be absent, erection and orgasm are likely to be unaffected.

See Table 14-7 for health promotion implications.[362–364]

Gastrointestinal System

Changes occur throughout the gastrointestinal system.
Mouth. The oral mucosa atrophies; the connective tissue becomes less elastic; vascular tissue becomes calcified and fibrotic; and nerve cells diminish in number. Tooth decay, loss of teeth, degeneration of the jawbone, progressive gum recession, and increased resorption of the dental arch interfere with the older adult's ability to chew food. Saliva flow decreases and becomes more alkaline as the salivary glands secrete less ptyalin and amylase. Thirst sensation decreases. All of these

TABLE 14-7	
Aging Changes and Health Promotion Implications	
System/Organ	**Implications for Health Promotion**
Musculoskeletal	Maintain calcium intake, normal nutrition, and exercise to slow degradation of bone or osteoporosis, to overcome stiffness, and to maintain strength, endurance, and joint mobility.
	Teach safety measures related to less coordination and strength, postural and structural changes, and slower reaction time to avoid falls and fractures.
	Teach ways to arrange the home environment and needed supplies to avoid excessive reach or climbing.
	Use devices to extend arm reach to obtain objects or supplies.
Renal	
Kidney	Avoid polypharmacy or *excessive medication intake.*
	Assess for drug side effects and toxicity because kidneys are major route of excretion.
	Assess for renal insufficiency if person is dehydrated, hypotensive, feverish, or using diuretics.
Bladder	Maintain adequate fluid intake and frequent toileting.
	Avoid diuretic use in afternoon or before long travel.
	Pads may be worn in underpants or lined pants can be worn as precaution.
	Assess for urinary tract infections.
	Explore self-esteem issues related to incontinence.
	Engage in bladder retraining.
Gastrointestinal	
Mouth	Encourage drinking 8 glasses of water daily to avoid dry mouth and dehydration.
	Maintain dental hygiene and care to prevent periodontal disease and loss of teeth.
	Teach new brushing techniques, daily flossing, and use of toothpaste with fluoride additive.
	Teach safety factors related to prevention of choking and use of Heimlich manoeuvre if needed.
Stomach	Encourage adequate nutritional intake, adjusting food texture and taste, as necessary, and with vitamin-mineral supplements if necessary.
	Promote nutrition through programs like senior nutrition sites or Meals on Wheels, as needed.
Liver/gallbladder	Encourage adequate protein intake to overcome hepatic synthesis.
	Avoid high-fat foods.
	Avoid polypharmacy because of reduced metabolism and excretion.
Bowel	Encourage bulk, vegetables, fruits, and cereals; especially water; exercise; and regular toileting patterns to prevent constipation.
	Avoid daily laxatives if at all possible, but if self-administered for years, it will need to be continued. Mild stool softener is preferred.
Immune	Maintain nutrition, hygiene, and health status to overcome delayed immune response and trend to infections.
	Observe for masked signs of inflammation or infection; e.g., temperature or white blood cell count may not be as elevated as in middle age.
	Teach safety measures and stress management strategies to overcome delayed or inadequate body response to stress.
	Treat symptomatically for comfort if autoimmune processes occur.

changes alter the digestive process at the onset.[365–368] See Table 14-7 for health promotion implications.[369,370]

Gastrointestinal Tract. Because of decreased stimuli from the autonomic nervous system, peristalsis is slowed the entire length of the gastrointestinal tract. Emptying of the esophagus and stomach is delayed. The gastric mucosa shrinks, causing decreased secretion of pepsinogen and hydrochloric acid, which delays digestion. Digestion is decreased further by the reduction in secretion of hydrochloric acid and pancreatic enzymes. Bile tends to be thicker, and the gallbladder empties more slowly. Hepatic synthesis is reduced. These changes result in a decreased absorption of nutrients and drugs by gastrointestinal

tract. In addition, some older adults do not have enough intrinsic factor and develop pernicious anemia.[371–374]

Elimination of waste products is of equal importance to gastrointestinal function in the aged. The changes in the cell, and therefore in tissue structure, and the loss of muscle tone may decrease intestinal mobility. Elimination depends on fluid intake, muscle tone, regularity of habits, culture, state of health, and adequate nutrition—all of which interrelate. Alterations in many of these areas occur with aging. Poor nutrition and lack of exercise add to the problem.

In the majority of persons over age 65, there is some degree of immobility, either physical, social, or environmental.

Physical changes in the tissues combine with this immobility to produce constipation or fecal impaction in circumstances that might not so affect a younger person.

See Table 14-7 for health promotion implications.[375,376]

Endocrine System

During aging, the ability of endocrine glands to synthesize hormones appears to remain within normal limits, although one study revealed significantly lower total body potassium and total body water levels in older than younger females. The number or sensitivity of hormonal receptors, however, may decrease. This means that, even though blood levels remain adequate, there is a lack of response to some hormones; this is especially true of the hormones produced by the adrenal and thyroid glands. Failure to respond to these hormones decreases the individual's ability to respond to stress.[377–379]

Beta cell activity of the pancreas appears altered with age, although the extent varies among people. Decreased insulin response causes hyperglycaemia. Aging is associated with elevated glucose levels after ingestion of glucose under the standard conditions of oral glucose tolerance testing. After ingestion of more physiologically mixed meals, a mild degree of postprandial hyperglycemia and hyperinsulinemia can still be demonstrated in the elderly compared with young adults. Postprandial elevations in glucose and insulin levels, however, are much lower after mixed meals compared with that observed during the standard glucose tolerance test. Increased circulating glucose and insulin levels are accompanied by a detectable elevation in hemoglobin A_{1c} concentration. These modest abnormalities, sustained over many years, may contribute to the development of atherosclerosis or other manifestations of aging.[380,381]

The chemical composition of fluids surrounding body cells must be closely regulated, and when analysis of blood shows alterations in blood volume, acidity, osmotic-pressure, or protein and sugar content, older adults require a longer time to recover internal chemical equilibrium. Insulin, secreted by cells in the pancreas, normally accelerates the removal of sugar from the blood. In older adults given intravenous insulin with extra glucose, the glucose is removed from the bloodstream at a slower rate than in younger people because of poorer hormone production. Stress intensifies glucose intolerance. Elderly persons undergoing the stress of surgery, illness, injury, or emotional stress may manifest diabetic symptoms; the elevated blood and urinary glucose levels usually return to normal when the stressor subsides.[382–384]

There is decreased metabolic clearance rate and plasma concentration of aldosterone. An increased response by antidiuretic hormone to hyperosomolarity contributes to hyponatremia.[385]

Growth hormone, estrogen, and testosterone blood levels do decrease in later maturity. Because of the decrease in estrogen levels after menopause, the breasts of the female have more connective tissue and fat and less glandular tissue. The breast tissues lose elasticity and begin to sag. The lack of estrogen causes the uterus and fallopian tubes to decrease in size. The fallopian tubes also become less motile. The decline of testosterone secretion is not abrupt like that of estrogen. Therefore

the changes are less obvious; however, the gradual decline of hormone does increase the incidence of benign prostatic hypertrophy in the older man and affects physical reserves, as testosterone has a nitrogen-conserving effect.[386]

CRITICAL THINKING

What services are available for the community-living diabetic elderly person?

Immune System

During the aging process, the thymus gland starts to involute and degenerate; the total number of circulating lymphocytes decreases by approximately 15%, and antibody–antigen reactions decline. In addition, lymphoid tissue decreases, and a general decline occurs in immune responses, including both cell-mediated and humoral immunity.[387–390] The immune system becomes less efficient with aging because of reduced production and function of T and B cells. The reduced T cells may be a factor in increased malignancy rates. Autoimmune responses may increase, causing diseases such as rheumatoid arthritis and other collagen diseases.[391] See Table 14-7 for health promotion implications.[392,393]

Hematopoietic System

There are minor changes in the blood components of the older adult; hemoglobin level, red blood cell count, and circulatory blood volume are not significantly changed. Most of the changes that occur are related to specific pathologic conditions instead of normal aging.[394]

Reproductive System and Changes that Influence Sexual Function

Although men and women experience some common changes as a result of aging, they are considered separately because of certain particular physiologic changes relating to sexual response and vigour.

Male Changes. The production of testosterone continues throughout the man's lifetime, and this hormone is available longer and at a higher level than its counterpart, estrogen, in the woman. As the concentration of the male hormone diminishes, the testes become smaller and softer; the testicular tubes thicken and begin to degenerate; and sperm production decreases or is inhibited. In addition, the prostate gland enlarges, contractions weaken, force of ejaculation decreases, and volume and viscosity of seminal fluid are reduced.[395–398]

In 1970, Masters and Johnson found that as a sexual partner, the older man experiences reduction in the frequency of intercourse, the intensity of sensation, the speed of attaining erection, and the force of ejaculation. *Excitement phase* builds more slowly, and erection takes longer to attain; with diminished vasoconstriction of the scrotum, there is less elevation of the testes. The *plateau phase* preceding orgasm lasts longer, with less muscle tension. There is a reduced or absent secretory activity by Cowper's gland before ejaculation. The *orgasmic phase* is of shorter duration, and the expulsion of the seminal fluid is usually completed with one or two contractions as compared with four or more in the young male. In the *resolution stage,* loss of erection may take seconds as compared with the young man's minutes or hours. **Refractory time,** *time needed for another erection,* is extended from several to 24 hours. A number of diseases and some medications can cause impotence.[399,400]

Female Changes. In the older adult woman there is a decline in the blood level of estrogen because of reduced ovarian function after menopause. This reduction in hormone causes the vaginal wall to shrink and thin and the vaginal and cervical secretions to diminish and become more acid. These changes may produce pruritis as well as dyspareunia (pain on intercourse), which can restrict sexual activity. In addition, the size of the clitoris is slightly smaller, and lubrication from the Bartholin glands decreases. With the loss of subcutaneous body fat, the vulva and external genitalia shrink.[401–404]

Female sexual performance in later maturity reveals no reduction in sexual desire or excitability with advancing age. Regular sexual stimulation and activity seem to overcome the effects of estrogen starvation. Studies reveal an increase in masturbation for relief of sexual tension in postmenopausal women into their sixth and seventh decades and for men over age 65. There may be an increased level of sexual desire among women after hysterectomies, indicating that there is no connection between fertility and libido.[405–407]

Neural and hormonal changes can combine to affect her sexual activity. In the *excitement phase* of coitus, vaginal lubrication is reduced and takes longer to appear. There is less flattening and separation of the labia major and decreased vasocongestion of the labia minora. Atrophy or thinning of vaginal walls causes the vagina to be less elastic (less depth and breadth). Muscle tension is reduced. During the *plateau phase,* there is less vasocongestion and less secretion from the Bartholin glands. All of these changes make penetration more difficult and less comfortable. During the *orgasmic phase,* there are fewer contractions of the uterus and vagina. During the *resolution phase,* the vasocongestion of the clitoris and orgasmic platform quickly subsides. Burning and frequency of urination may follow intercourse as the atrophic bladder and urethra are not adequately protected. Thus, the sex act may become less satisfying and even painful.[408,409]

See Chapter 13 for a discussion of hormonal replacement therapy.

Sexuality. It is well known that stress, hormonal activity, general health, and aging can each be assessed according to measurable standards. The data are sufficient to infer that psychological influences can be exerted to produce physiologic change in young and old alike. Because of the relationships between the mind and body and the interdependence of all body systems, societal attitudes regarding the characteristics and needs of older citizens are crucial to their quality of life.

There is no doubt that normal aging of the reproductive system decreases efficiency and lengthens time for response for both men and women, but unlike other organ systems that perform more specific functions, the reproductive system extends far beyond procreation. It is deeply tied to the need for interpersonal communication, and it involves that warmth and comfort found only in body contact. When one is old, the yearning for intimacy, security, and belonging becomes intensified as other privations are felt keenly: loss of friends,

job status, active participation in parenting or career, and decision making.

The older person is a sexual person. Research about sexuality in people between the ages of 60 and 91 years indicates that:[410,411]

- Ninety-seven percent like sexual activity.
- Seventy-five percent think intercourse feels as good now, or better, than it did when they were young.
- Seventy-two percent are satisfied by their sexual experiences.
- Ninety percent think sexual activity is good for their health.
- Women are more satisfied with activities such as sitting close to someone and talking and saying and hearing endearments, if sexual intercourse is not a choice.
- Men are more satisfied with reading or watching erotic materials and caressing another person's body if sexual intercourse is not a choice.

The person's sense of self-worth and the partner's physical health status are positively related to the continuance of sexual intercourse.[412–414]

Nutritional Needs

Nutrition is the fundamental element of healthy human development and an essential contributor to the overall health of older adults. Energy needs are believed to decline with age because of decreased basal metabolism hormonal functions, reduction in lean body mass, and a more sedentary lifestyle.[415] However, sufficient energy intakes (at least 1500 calories or 6.3 MJ) distributed among appropriate food choices are essential for adequate nutrient intakes.[416] Although the protein needs of seniors are still subject to controversy, it has been suggested that their protein requirements exceed those of younger adults (1.0 to 1.25 g/kg versus 0.8 g/kg of body weight, respectively).[417]

Appetite in older adults is strongly influenced by medication and the presence of a physical or psychological disease such as chronic disease and depression. Psychological sensory functions such as taste and smell could also be factors affecting appetite. Daily energy intake is determined by the level of physical activities.[418] Functional limitations in food intake–related activities, such as shopping and cooking, negatively affect energy and nutrient intake.[419]

Special problems exist in the nutrition of older people. Factors that affect nutrition and their clinical manifestations are described in Table 14-7 (page 671) and Table 14-8.[420–425]

Utilize the *Canada Food Guide to Healthy Living* to assist the older adults to plan meals for themselves.[426]

CRITICAL THINKING

Outline a general teaching plan you would use to instruct an older adult about dietary needs.

Sufficient water or other fluid intake is essential. Fluid intake is often reduced in seniors for several reasons:

- The aging process reduces the thirst sensation.

TABLE 14-8
Factors that May Affect Nutrition in Later Maturity

Factor and Process	Effect	Clinical Manifestation
Ingestion		
Loss of teeth; poor dentures; atrophy of jaws	Improper mastication; deletion of important foods from diet	Irritable bowel syndrome; constipation; malnutrition
Dietary habits	Overeating; eccentric diets	Obesity; malnutrition
Psychological losses and changes; changes in social environment; lack of socialization	Poor appetite	Anorexia; weight loss
Reduced income; difficulty with food preparation and ingestion	Excessive ingestion of carbohydrates	Obesity; malnutrition
Decreased fluid intake	Dry feces	Impacted stools
Digestion and Absorption		
Decreased secretion of hydrochloric acid and digestive enzymes	Interference with digestion	Dietary deficiencies
Hepatic and biliary insufficiency	Poor absorption of fats	Fat-soluble vitamin deficiency; flatulence
Atrophy of intestinal mucosa and musculature	Poor absorption; slower movement of food through intestine	Vitamin and mineral deficiencies; constipation
Decreased secretion of intestinal mucus	Decreased lubrication of intestine	Constipation
Metabolism		
Impaired glucose metabolism and use	Diabetic-like response to glucose	Hyperglycemia; hypoglycemia
Decrease in renal function	Inability to excrete excess alkali	Alkalosis
Impaired response to salt restriction	Salt depletion	Low-salt syndrome
Decline in basal metabolic rate	Lower caloric requirements but same amount of food eaten	Obesity
Changes in iron and calcium (phosphorus, magnesium) metabolism	Iron deficiency; increased requirements for calcium	Anemia; demineralization of bone; osteoporosis
Changes in vitamin metabolism	Deficiency in vitamins K and C, especially	Peripheral neuropathy, sensorimotor changes; easy bruising and bleeding tendencies

- The senior who has incontinence problems limits fluid intake to reduce output.
- Fewer meals are eaten; opportunity for fluid intake is less apparent.
- The senior who takes a diuretic often wrongly assumes fluid intake should be reduced.

At least six or seven glasses (8 ounces or 250 mL) of water should be ingested daily to (1) soften stools; (2) maintain kidney function; (3) aid expectoration; (4) moisturize dry skin; and (5) aid absorption of medications, bulk laxatives, and high-fibre foods.

You can help make mealtime pleasant for the older person:

- Encourage the person to prepare menus that are economical and easy to shop for, prepare, and consume.
- Encourage the person to do meal preparation to the extent possible.
- The environment should be a comfortable temperature and well lighted so that food can be seen.
- Place food where the person can smell, see, and reach it.
- If needed, open cartons and food packets of various sorts and help season the food.
- Keep the tray attractive, neat, and uncluttered to ensure an appetizing appearance.
- Use foods that can be easily chewed and digested.
- Ensure that dentures and eyeglasses are clean and in place on the person at mealtime, instead of in the drawer or on the bedside table.
- Oral hygiene is important and contributes to greater enjoyment of food. Mouth care also promotes healthy tissues in the mouth, thereby keeping the beginning of the alimentary canal intact and functional.
- Do not give medications with meals if avoidable, especially if the medication has an unpleasant taste.
- Offer foods when the person is hungry rather than only at set meal or snack times.
- If necessary, use adaptive feeding devices to help the person feed self.

Keller and McKenzie conducted a Canadian study to measure nutritional risk in a sample of vulnerable community-living seniors, and to determine patterns of nutritional risk in these seniors.[427] The majority of the sample was female and the average age was 79 years. Common nutritional risk factors were weight change, restricting food, low fruit and vegetable intake, difficulty with chewing, cooking, or shopping, and poor appetite. The principal components analysis identified four independent components within the *Seniors in the Community: Risk Evaluation for Eating and Nutrition* questionnaire. These components were low food intake, poor appetite, physical and external challenges, and instrumental activity challenges. The pattern of nutritional risks identified in this vulnerable population may help providers identify useful strategies for deleting risks.[428]

Rest and Sleep

Rest is important. Though older adults may not sleep as many hours as they once did, frequent rest periods and sensible pacing of activities provide the added energy for a full and active life. Rest may consist of listening to soft music, reading, thinking of happy experiences, napping, or merely lying with eyes closed. Some older adults have several 15- to 60-minute naps during the daylight hours.

With so much diversity among the individuals in this age group, it is difficult to state how many hours of *sleep* are recommended. Older adults in reasonably good health probably do not require any more sleep than was required during their middle adulthood.

Aging affects the process of sleep in three areas: length of sleep, distribution of sleep during the 24-hour day, and sleep stage patterns. The older adult requires a somewhat longer period to fall asleep, and sleep is lighter, with more frequent awakenings. The total amount of daily sleep declines as the spontaneous interruption of sleep increases. The older adult may actually spend more time in bed but sleep less, waking with the feeling of inadequate sleep. The time spent in stage IV, the deepest sleep period, and REM sleep decreases. This also contributes to feelings of fatigue.[429–434]

Sleep apnea, described in Chapter 12, occurs in many elderly adults. Persons with sleep apnea are more sleepy during the day than nonapneic individuals; apnea during sleep has a detrimental effect on the well-being of elderly adults, even if oxygen desaturation is mild or moderate. Greater levels of depression and cognitive impairment are seen in sleep apneic elders.[435]

Insomnia is a common problem in the older adult. Many factors contribute to this. Determine the person's usual sleeping patterns, the amount and type of daily activity, and the existence of disturbing environmental conditions. Assess the presence of pain, fear, anxiety, lack of exercise or depression.

CRITICAL THINKING

What are a few health promotion strategies you can suggest to an older adult to combat insomnia?

Exercise and Activity

According to a substantial body of scientific evidence, regular physical activity can bring significant health benefits to people of all ages and abilities.[436] According to *Canada's Physical Activity Guide to Healthy Active Living for Older Adults*, 60% of older adults are not sufficiently active to achieve optimal full health benefits.[437] The guide serves as a roadmap to promote physical activity in an aging society.[438] Being active is very safe for most people. The guide recommends for an older adult to begin exercise slowly and build up slowly, listening to the body. It advocates a period of 30 to 60 minutes of moderate physical activity most days.[439] One can even exercise 10 minutes at a time, adding up the time to the 30 to 60 minutes.

See Table 14-9 for physical, psychological, and social benefits of exercise.[440–447]

TABLE 14-9 Benefits of Regular Exercise
Physical
■ Helps slow aging process, regardless of age
■ Maintains good health and energy
■ Improves general strength and body agility and balance
■ Improves respiration and circulation
■ Promotes muscle mass, strength, and endurance
■ Protects against ligament injuries
■ Promotes bone mass formation; slows loss of bone tissue
■ Induces better sleep patterns
■ Normalizes blood cholesterol and triglyceride levels
■ Controls blood glucose levels
■ Normalizes blood pressure
■ Improves appetite, digestive processes, and bowel function
■ Promotes weight control (moderate exercise burns 240–420 calories/hour)
■ Reduces risk of heart disease
Psychological
■ Reduces age-related decline in brain's oxidative capacity and improves memory and information processing
■ Promotes faster reaction time
■ Contributes to improved mood and morale
■ Improves cognitive test scores
■ Enhances self-confidence
■ Maintains interest in life and alertness
■ Contributes to sense of control
■ Prevents depression
Social
■ Promotes socialization when exercise is included in group activity
■ Maintains independence

One group of active people is farmers, and farmers age 65 or older generally enjoy better health then city or small-town dwellers of the same age. They have fewer medical conditions and excel at performing tasks. Farmers may be healthier because of their lifestyle, and 70% are married. If you are looking for a 75-year-old who still works, that person is more likely to farm than do anything else; 61% of farmers say they do not expect to stop working.[448]

Even if the individual has a decreased exercise tolerance, with supervision a plan can be developed to help him or her achieve higher levels of physical fitness. It is, however, important that the older adult not start a walking exercise program without consulting the physician, who would be aware of any needed limitations.

Table 14–10 lists consequences of not having sufficient exercise.[449–452]

For the individual who is not especially interested in planned exercise programs, you can suggest bowling, golf, swimming, dancing, games such as shuffleboard and horse-shoes, and home and garden chores. All of these activities can improve the well-being of the older adult (Figure 14–4). Also, see the box entitled "Guidelines for Walking Exercise."[453–458]

An exercise program regularly followed may bring a dimension of dynamic fitness to life that helps him or her move vigorously and live energetically as long as possible. Histories of vigorous persons in their 80s and 90s and even over age 100 show that the majority have been physically and mentally active throughout their earlier lives.[459] Movement therapy programs such as tai chi and other movement patterns contribute to improved morale, self-esteem, and attitudes toward aging.[460]

Carter and his research group from the University of British Columbia Bone Health Research Group found that women aged 65 to 75 who had been diagnosed with osteoporosis and who participated in an exercise program experienced improvements in dynamic balance and strength. Both are important determinants of risk for falls, especially in this sample of older women.[461]

CRITICAL THINKING

What information would you include in a health education plan on osteoporosis?

TABLE 14-10
Consequences of Not Exercising and Being Sedentary

- Decline in all body systems
- General weakness
- Lower energy level
- Stooped posture
- Muscle tissue replaced by adipose tissue
- Atrophy of tissues and functions
- Higher blood cholesterol and triglyceride levels
- Greater risk for heart disease
- Weight gain
- Lower self-concept, self-esteem
- Depressive mood

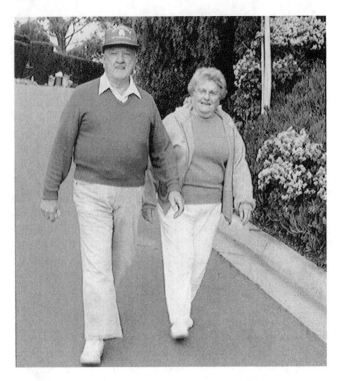

FIGURE 14–4

Older adults can maintain health and prevent illness by participating in regular exercise.

Source: Berger, K.J., and M.B. Williams, Fundamentals of Nursing: Collaborating for Optimal Health. *Stamford, CT: Appleton & Lange, 1992, p. 1317.*

Guidelines for Walking Exercise

1. No single program will work for all elders. Determine first the meaning and perceived value of exercise among sedentary elders before developing the following plan.
2. Begin, if previously sedentary, by walking slightly above a stroll for 15 to 30 minutes.
3. Aim to walk a mile in about 15 to 20 minutes. Then build to 2 miles in 30 minutes.
4. A "training heart rate" is 60% to 90% of your fastest pulse rate per minute.
   - Subtract age from 220.
   - Multiply the result by 0.6 and 0.9 to get the bottom and top of target zone for aerobic training.
5. Walk 3 to 5 times a week, with a heart rate in the target zone for 15 to 60 minutes.
6. Develop a strategy to ensure a commitment to walking.
7. Wear shoes with a firm heel cup for stability, a rocker sole for smooth heel-to-toe motion, and plenty of toe room for push-off. Wear loose, comfortable clothing.
8. Maintain erect posture; lean forward from the ankles, not the waist. Keep head level and chin up.
9. Keep elbows bent at a 90° angle and swing arms at the shoulder. The hand should end its forward swing at breastbone height. On the backswing, the upper arm should be parallel to the ground.
10. Stretch before and during the walk and keep a long, smooth stride during the walk.

Devices to Assist Mobility

When we see persons using canes, walkers, wheelchairs or electric scooters, we tend to think of them as not being an active part of the community. Actually, various assistive devices, when used correctly, can be a means of promoting mobility and independence. Often, the person who refuses to use a cane or walker develops a shuffling gait, characterized by short steps, and over time leg muscles become flaccid, the back may weaken, and posture suffers.

Electric scooters are another means of providing mobility for some people. They encourage more participation in social activities, the ability to get around in a retirement complex or a nearby store. They can be transported by car to outside events as well: going to the zoo, the shopping mall, or concerts where handicapped access is provided. The theory held by some that an electric cart keeps people from walking is not a valid one. If the client is able to walk at all, he or she should be given an appropriate walking and exercise program by the physician or therapist. Combining the use of cane, walker, and electric cart with an exercise program is the ideal arrangement.

In Canada, the guide *Go for It: A Guide to Choosing and Using Assistive Devices* was developed to assist seniors, veterans, and individuals with disabilities and their caregivers with issues before starting the process of obtaining an assistive device. The guide covers comprehensive information about available assistive devices, and includes contact information.[462]

CRITICAL THINKING

Describe your plans for a fall-prevention program for the older adult.

Health Promotion and Health Protection

Male and female differences in longevity result from hormones, genetic makeup, natural immunity, and lifestyle behaviour. Because of the immunity effects of estrogen, women, statistically, develop heart disease ten years later than men. In the past, lifestyle choices of women also gave them a biological advantage—less drinking of alcoholic beverages, less cigarette smoking, more attention to personal health care, and less exposure to risks at work and play. As women are changing their lifestyles, however, the gap between the sexes in health status and longevity is narrowing.[463]

Today's elders, overall, are healthier, better educated, more politically astute, more mobile and youthful in appearance, and more accustomed to changing lifestyles than their counterparts of yesteryear. In a study of people ages 57 to 83, age was not related to differences in healthy behaviours. Many reported no digestive or sleep difficulties. All were active, kept in touch with family and friends, were confident that the environment was safe, and managed stress well. All but one attributed their health, quality of life, and zest to remaining active, eating healthily, exercise, pacing self, doing preferred activities, and reading the Bible or feeding the mind.[464]

CASE SITUATION

Mrs. B, an 85-year-old resident of a life-care facility, is an example of someone who uses mechanical means to help maintain her participation in the life around her, to do volunteer work, enhance her ability to walk long distances, and to promote a normal posture while walking.

Mrs. B has had both knees replaced as a result of arthritis. She has osteoarthritis of the spine and rheumatoid arthritis in both hands. She uses a cane for short distances, such as from car to church, shops, or private homes. However, her greatest help is that afforded by one of the newly designed four-wheel walkers. It has rack- and pinion-steering, 12 cm wheels with hand brakes, a seat to sit on when tired or waiting in line, and a basket for purse or packages. This type of walker is the first to have handles that are adjustable to allow the person to stand upright, supporting the back in a normal posture. Thus, she can stride forward without having to lift or turn the walker, because of the ease of steering.

Mrs. B finds that she uses her walker most of the time, thereby being able to maintain a normal gait and an erect posture and therefore uses the electric cart less often. She is able to use the shopping carts in supermarkets as she would a walker, and because her walker can be folded, it can go with her on more extensive shopping trips by car or bus. Her electric cart takes her to the swimming pool six days a week, where she does water aerobics. Her exercise program, combined with the use of assistive devices, has given Mrs. B a more enriched life in her elder years.

1. What are the specific benefits to a client like Mrs. B of the type of exercise she does?
2. What safety concerns should you be aware of regarding walkers?
3. What other health promotion strategies do you need to consider for clients like Mrs. B?

Five conditions shorten life expectancy: coronary artery disease, stroke, cancer, diabetes, and confusion. Arthritis decreases functional ability. Decreasing the prevalence of arthritis would reduce functional limitation. Advances against common nonfatal disabling conditions would be more effective than advances against fatal conditions in reducing the anticipated increase in the functionally limited older population anticipated in the 21st century.[465]

Menec, Chipperfield, and Perry conducted a four-year study of 1406 older adults, ages 65 to 74, 75 to 84, and over 85, who lived in rural and urban communities (not in institutions). It was found that persons who had high perceptions of self-control and used active coping strategies had better perception of their health.[466] Self-perception of health is an important indicator of mortality. Older adults who rated their health as "bad or poor" and "fair" were more than twice as likely to die in three to five years as those who rated their health positively. Older adults who experienced some functional impairment were three times more likely to die than those who were unimpaired. Being hospitalized during the year doubles the risk of dying. More research is needed on factors that contribute to health as we age.[467]

Overall, about 25% of today's elders want to live to be 100 years old. Most would prefer to live to be 90 to 91. The main criteria for deserving longevity is to be able to care for self, to be able to do what fulfills contentment, and to be without intense pain.[468–470]

The focus of health care for individuals in this period of life should be on the *prevention of disease and the promotion of health.* Although numerous body changes occur with aging, many older adults live active, productive lives. Thorough assessment is essential. Several references are useful.[471–477]

Immunizations

All Canadian adults require maintenance of immunity to tetanus and diphtheria, preferably with combined (Td) toxoid.[478] Those 65 years of age and over should receive influenza vaccine every year and, on a one-time basis, a dose of pneumococcal vaccine. Special recall strategies may be necessary to ensure high coverage, particularly for those who are at a greatest risk of influenza-related complications. Such older adults would include those with chronic cardiopulmonary disease.[479]

Safety Promotion and Accident Prevention

Older people have a disproportionate share of accidents that cause body injury or death. This is especially true for accidents that occur in the home. Many of these accidents are directly related to physiologic changes that result from normal aging.

Teach that falls in the elderly may occur for a number of reasons:

- Improper use of or incorrectly fitted assistive devices
- Lower-extremity disability
- Decrease in functional base of support
- Vision and hearing impairment
- Arrhythmias, cardiovascular disease, strokes
- Kinesthetic changes, changes in postural reflexes, sway
- Vertigo and syncopal (fainting) episodes
- Peripheral neuropathy
- Inadequate swing foot clearance, tripping
- Depression, inattention
- Excess ingestion of alcohol
- Use of certain medications, such as diuretics, sedatives, antibiotics, antidepressants, antipsychotics
- Excess cigarette smoking or osteoporosis, which reduces bone mineral density and can cause fractures resulting in falls

Teach the following safety measures to be used by the elderly to avoid injury to the skin or other injury:[480,481]

- Place padding on hard edges of wheelchairs and over rough or sharp corners or surfaces of furniture, tables, or countertops.
- Pad the wooden or metal arms of chairs used by elders.
- Wear gloves to wash dishes or work in the garden to protect hands.
- Wear long sleeves to protect arms.
- Wear long pants to protect the legs.
- Work and walk more slowly to avoid collisions with objects or falls.
- Wear flat, rubber-soled, well-fitted shoes; avoid walking in socks, stockings, or loose slippers. Grip handrails (and place feet on the diagonal if a long foot) when going up and down steps; put nonskid treads on stairs.
- Use nonslip mats; remove throw rugs; tack rugs to floor if not wall-to-wall.
- Use seat and grab bars in bathtub or shower.
- Maintain exercise to improve gait and mobility; tai chi and yoga also steady movements and improve posture and balance.
- Make sure house is well lit and lights are easy to reach; motion sensitive lights are useful.
- Remove or repair unstable furniture.
- Have vision and hearing checked annually.
- Review with physician any medications that could increase risk of falling.

Older adults are also particularly vulnerable to fraudulent sales pitches and seemingly honest requests for help by strangers. Use the box entitled "Safety in the Home: Do Not Be a Victim of the Con Game" to teach elders to avoid fraud, scams, or unethical or illegal schemes. Encourage them to report such incidents promptly.[482,483]

CRITICAL THINKING

Use the Internet to find more information about safety in the home.

Visual Changes. Changes in visual acuity produce numerous hazards for the older adult. The older adult's problems with colour interpretation, light intensity, and depth perception should be considered in the home and institutional environment. Use Table 14-4 on page 666 for suggestions on how to assist the elder in maintaining vision comfort and safety. Other suggestions follow.

Teach that the environment should be kept free of hazards—no articles on the floor, no furniture with sharp edges, no scatter rugs. The baseboards should be painted a darker colour than the walls. Signs should be prepared with dark backgrounds and light lettering. Blues and greens on signs should be avoided. Numbers on doors, elevators, and telephones should be large enough for the older adult to see. Encourage use of a magnifying glass for close vision work, a small flashlight to illuminate dim areas, and having properly fitted and cared for eyeglasses. Teach proper care of contact lenses.

Teach that television should be viewed with normal room illumination and at a distance, at least 1.8 metres from the screen. Some persons with impaired vision may have to sit closer. Glasses correcting distance vision should be worn while watching television, and the set should be adjusted as clearly as possible.

Some signs and symptoms indicate the need for appropriate referral to an ophthalmologist:

- Pain in and around eyes
- Headaches, especially at night or early morning
- Mucous discharge from eyes

Safety in the Home: Do Not Be a Victim of the Con Game

- **Carpet cleaner:** Ad offers very low price to clean carpeting in one or more rooms of your house. Workers flood room, ruin carpet and scheme to charge more than quoted to replace damaged material, which may not be replaced.
- **City inspector:** "Inspector" knocks at the door to check plumbing, furnace, heater, wiring, trees, or whatever. Once inside, he or she may rob you or insist something needs repair and charge excessively for the job.
- **Home repair:** "Contractor" offers to repair or remodel your home, exterminate pests, or check for radon or offers work with leftover materials from another job in area. The person will find "work" that is unnecessary, resulting in unnecessary expense.
- **Product demonstration:** Agent offers to describe only (not sell) new product if you will sign paper "for my boss" proving he or she did it. Once inside the house, anything can happen.
- **Contest winner:** You are told you have won vacation, auto, or other prize but must send $5 for postage or registration or call 800 number for details. Cost for anything will exceed worth.
- **Lottery:** Person offers to sell you winning lottery ticket he or she cannot cash because "I'm an illegal immigrant," or "I'm behind in my child-support payments." Or "law firm" says anonymous donor has bequeathed a winning lottery ticket to you, but first you must send $20 for a computer search to verify your identity.
- **Lend sale:** You are promised cheap land or complete retirement and recreational facilities in sunny gorgeous site. The land may not exist, even if you paid for it.
- **Credit or phone card:** Person asks for your credit or phone card number to send you a product, check unauthorized charges, verify insurance, and so on. They can then use your number to charge items.

- **Governmental service:** Official-sounding firm offers governmental service that is "required" (e.g., plastic-coated identification cards), "critically needed" (e.g., to help keep agency solvent), or useful (e.g., earnings form). The money sent obtains no service.
- **Mail-order health care or laboratory tests:** You are promised medical care by mail or laboratory screening for AIDS, cholesterol, cancer, hair loss, and so on. The results are likely to be phoney if received at all for the money you sent.
- **Medical products:** You buy health, beauty care, or "cure" product by mail, or you are sent newspaper clipping extolling magic diet with note scribbled across it, "It works—try it!" signed "J." Avoid such products.
- **Obituary:** You are recently widowed; COD box arrives for product "your husband (or wife) ordered." Return unless actually ordered.
- **Pigeon drop:** Person offers to share "found" money with you if you will put some of your own money with it "to show good faith."
- **Need help:** Man says his wife is sick, his car has been impounded, he has run out of gas, or some such tale; he needs just $10 or $20, promises to pay it back, and shows extensive identification.
- **Unknown callers:** Woman with child knocks on door and asks for some favour requiring entrance.
- **Travel club:** Firm offers bargain airfare or hotel package in glamorous foreign locale. You may never get anything that was promised.

Source: Modified from Marklein, M., Con Games Proliferate: New Threats Haunt City Folks, AARP Bulletin, 32, no. 2 (1991), 1, 16–17.

- Obvious inflammation or irritation of the eyes and surrounding tissue
- Avoidance of activities requiring sight
- Glasses not being worn, missing, or not fitting properly
- Change of previous visual habits (requiring different light or reading distance)

When you are caring for a blind person, follow the guidelines presented in the box entitled "Guidelines for Helping the Blind Person" on page 665. Teach other health care providers and family members these guidelines also.

Hearing Impairment. Changes in hearing acuity may predispose the person to accident risks. Many elderly persons have been diagnosed as being mentally ill, whereas in reality they were suffering from a gradual loss of hearing. If one is unable to hear clearly, it is easy to imagine one is being talked about or ignored. This leads to depression, and then behaviour often is categorized as irrational, suspicious, or hostile. This produces isolation and further frustrations, and the vicious cycle that ensues may in the end cause real paranoia to develop.

Refer to the suggestions on effective communication with the hearing-impaired person given in the box entitled "Guidelines for Communicating with the Hearing-Impaired Person" on page 667. Encourage the hearing-impaired person to consult with a physician about use of a hearing aid rather than going to a nonqualified practitioner.

Tactile Changes. Changes in *temperature regulation* and the inability to feel pain also produce **safety problems.** Utilize Table 14-3 on page 664 for teaching and implementing health promotion.

The elderly usually *feel cold* more easily and may require more covering when in bed; a room temperature somewhat higher than usual may be desirable.

Assess for *hypothermia risk or presence,* as follows:

- Medications to treat anxiety or depression, hypothyroidism, vascular disease, alcoholism, and immobility reduce the body's response to cold.
- Living alone or anything that increases nighttime accidents can increase risk, as do poverty and poor housing.

■ The elder may insist he or she is comfortable in a cool environment; the person is unaware of the temperature of surroundings.

■ The person is not thinking clearly or acting as usual.

■ Low body temperature, irregular or slow pulse, slurred speech, shallow respirations, hypotension, drowsiness, lack of coordination, and sluggishness may be present, singly or in combination.

■ Coma may occur and is probable when the body temperature is 32.2°C (90°F) or less.

Severe hypothermia can cause complications of kidney, liver, or pancreatic disorders, ventricular fibrillation, and death. Recovery depends on severity and length of exposure, previous health, and the rewarming treatment.[484,485]

Teach the elderly person the following measures to prevent hypothermia in cold weather:[486,487]

1. Stay indoors as much as possible, especially on windy, wet, and cold days.
2. Wear layered clothing, and cover the head when outdoors.
3. Eat high-energy foods such as some fats and easily digested carbohydrates and protein daily.
4. Keep at least one room warm at 20°C (70°F) or above.
5. Use extra blankets, caps, socks, and layered clothing in bed.
6. Have contact with someone daily.
7. Avoid drinking alcoholic beverages.

Hyperthermia must also be prevented. Assess for the three types of heat-related illnesses that may affect any age, especially the older adult. The older adult is especially vulnerable if he or she has circulatory impairment or is taking psychotropic or beta-blocker medications, which interfere with heat regulation.[488]

Teach the elder and family members about differences between each type of hyperthermia and general causes:

1. **Heat cramps.** *Mild disorder that involves large skeletal muscles,* caused by sudden sodium depletion.[489]
2. **Heat exhaustion.** *More serious, not life-threatening, but a precursor to heat stroke.* This occurs if the person has inadequate fluid or sodium intake. Signs and symptoms are diaphoresis, thirst, fatigue, headache, elevated body temperature, flushed skin, nausea, vomiting, possible diarrhea.[490]
3. **Heat stroke. Classic:** *Occurs during extremely hot weather, during a "heat wave" when the elder is in a closed apartment with no cooling system or outdoors in the heat.* **Exertional:** *Occurs during strenuous physical exertion (or for the elder with even moderate activity) when temperature and humidity are high.* Increased sweating depletes sodium, but high humidity interferes with ability of the body to lower its core temperature. Several physiological mechanisms operate to maintain normal body temperature; thyroid function decreases and aldosterone and the antidiuretic hormone (ADH) production increases to conserve body water and sodium. If these mechanisms are overwhelmed, peripheral vasoconstriction conserves central circulatory volume, but the core body temperature

rises dramatically. *Signs and symptoms* include:[491]

a. Fever
b. Headache
c. Vertigo
d. Faintness
e. Confusion
f. Hyperpnea
g. Abdominal distress

At the higher body temperature, skin is hot and dry; respirations are weak, and tachycardia, agitation, delirium, hallucinations, and convulsions may occur.[492]

Complications, especially for heat stroke, include:[493]

1. Cerebral edema, brain damage
2. Pulmonary edema
3. Liver necrosis
4. Acute renal failure
5. Myocardial necrosis or infarction
6. Gastrointestinal bleeding or ulceration

Prompt recognition and treatment of heat-related illness is essential to prevent organ damage or death. *Teach prevention,* including staying in a cool environment, increasing fluid intake, wearing a sunblock outdoors, loose, light clothing, and sponging off or taking cooling showers. *Treatment* includes removing the person to a cool place, applying cool clothes, loosening clothing, and giving fluids. Emergency department care may be necessary, to assess for and prevent complications when body temperature continues to rise.[494]

Pain perception and reaction may be decreased with age. Because pain is an important warning device serving the safety of the organism, use caution when applying hot packs or other hot or cold applications. The elderly person may be burned or suffer frostbite before being aware of any discomfort. More accurate assessment of physical signs and symptoms may be necessary to alleviate conditions underlying complaints of pain such as abdominal discomfort and chest pain, which may be more serious than the older person's perception indicates.

Dulling of *tactile sensation* occurs because of a decrease in the number of areas of the body responding to all stimuli and in the number and sensitivity of sensory receptors.[495] Use the following information in your care. *Teach* the elder and family about these changes and their implications. There may be clumsiness or difficulty in identifying objects by touch. The person may not respond to light touch but needs to be touched. Because fewer tactile cues are received from the bottom of the feet, the person may get confused about position and location. These factors, combined with sensitivity to glare, poorer peripheral vision, and a constricted visual field, may result in disorientation, especially at night when there is little or no light in the room.[496] Because the aged person takes longer to recover visual sensitivity when moving from a light to a dark area, night lights and a safe and familiar arrangement of furniture are essential. Sensory alterations may require modification of the home environment and extra orientation to new surroundings. Simple explanations of routines, location of the bathroom, and the way the signal cord works in the hospital are just a few examples of information the older client needs. Objects in a familiar environment should not be moved. Use touch, if acceptable to the person. Increased hairbrushing or combing, back rubs, hugs, and touch of shoulders, arms, or hands increase tactile sensation.

Understand that some of the changed behaviour, discussed later under the heading "Psychological Concepts," is directly related to physical changes in nerve and sensory tissue and influences nursing practice, whether you are giving physical care, establishing a relationship, providing a safe environment, or planning recreational needs. Research indicates that hand, foot, and eye preference becomes more right-sided and ear preference becomes more left-sided with advancing age. Adapt nursing care measures to accommodate these changes. The whole area of client teaching is also affected, because you must understand the altered responses and the changing needs of the elderly before beginning their health education.

CRITICAL THINKING

Outline the content of your health promotion program on hypothermia and hyperthermia.

Special Considerations in the Physical Examination of Older Patients

The *health history* of the elder should include:[497]

1. Current problems
2. Complete history of past medical problems
3. Smoking, alcohol, and drug history
4. Medication list
5. Psychosocial history and mental status
6. Nutritional patterns
7. Review of body systems focusing on functional abilities
8. Exercise patterns
9. History of immunizations
10. Support systems
11. Caregiver roles, caregiver stress, possible neglect or abuse
12. Advance directives

Physical examination should include:[498]

1. Vital signs and weight
2. Mobility screening
3. Hypertension and vascular disease screening
4. Cancer screening
5. Hearing and vision screening
6. Breast examination: mammography for women up to age 75 (and perhaps to age 85)
7. Papanicolaou smear, if inadequately screened at younger age or if history of abnormalities

In carrying out any particular physical assessment in the older adult, the nurse may need to modify some procedures to glean the most information. Even helping the patient undress gives the nurse opportunity to observe the patient's ability to perform the task and to note anything unusual, for example, condition of clothing, personal hygiene, or clothing that may be inappropriate for the season or temperature (e.g., thermal underwear in August).

CRITICAL THINKING

Describe the questions you would ask and the observations you would make to assess the skin, exercise patterns, and medication list of an 85-year-old person.

Orthostatic vital signs are valuable in the elderly, as heart rate response to postural change may alter decisions regarding hypertension or hypotension.

Attention must be given to avoid discomfort, maintain the patient's dignity, and distinguish signs of disease from changes typical of normal aging.

Another important observation is the palpation of temporal arteries. Checking for tenderness or thickening may raise the possibility of temporal arteritis, especially in a patient with jaw pain, temporal headaches, earache, or unexplained fever.

The following are specific ways to *increase patient comfort:*

- Warm the examining room sufficiently
- Use chairs that are high enough to make rising easy.
- Provide a footstool for getting on and off the table.
- Place a pillow under the head and perhaps under the knees, as many elders feel a strain on the back when lying supine.
- Place grab bars near the scale.
- Minimize positional changes during the examination.

Other important areas of exploration in the elderly are hearing acuity; condition of dentures; suspicious lesions under the tongue; jugular venous pulse; carotid arteries for bruits; and breast examination, including the skin under pendulous breasts.

Suspected urinary incontinence can be tested by having the patient hold a small pad over the urethral area and coughing three times in a standing position. Cystocele, rectocele, or uterine prolapse should be ruled out, and in the man, a digital rectal examination should be done to check the prostate.

Examination of the elder patient's feet is most important; also, have the patient sit up and hang the feet down to check the venous flow. Are the patient's shoes appropriate for good balance and prevention of falls? The patient's gait can offer significant clues, for example, the Parkinsonian gait shown by short, shuffling steps, short or absent arm swing, and a stooped trunk.

Common Health Problems: Prevention and Treatment

The health problems of the older adult may be associated with the aging process, a disease state, or both. Yet more than 90% of elders need no help with activities of daily living. Consider all of the aspects of aging before deciding on a course of action. Refer to a medical-surgical nursing text for in-depth information on health problems. Other references will also be useful.[499–503]

Table 14-11 summarizes common neurologic and respiratory diseases: blood dyscrasias; genitourinary, skeletal, and cardiovascular diseases; and tuberculosis. Sexual function diseases and substance abuse are also presented in overview.[504–508] Use the information in assessment, teaching, health promotion, and illness prevention.

TABLE 14-11
Common Health Problems in Later Maturity

Problem	Definition	Symptom/Signs	Prevention/Treatment
Neurologic diseases			
Herpes zoster (shingles)	Caused by same virus that causes chicken-pox	Unilateral vesicular eruption that follows dermatomes of affected nerve root	Analgesics; cool soaks; acyclovir (Zovirax)
	Involves dorsal root ganglia	Severe pain; rash that progresses from macules to crusting pustules	Investigation of underlying immunologic problems
Parkinson's disease	Slowly progressive degenerative disorder of nervous system	Resting tremor; masklike face; shuffling gait, forward flexion; muscle weakness; rigidity	Symptomatic, medicine to correct depleted dopamine and rid excessive acetylcholine
Alzheimer's disease	Presenile dementia or neural atrophy	Cognitive, physical, and emotional deterioration	Treatment extremely varied, depending on areas affected
			Much support and understanding needed from families and caretakers; in turn, families and caretakers need support
Respiratory diseases			
Chronic obstructive pulmonary disease	Consists of three components: bronchitis, bronchoconstriction, and emphysema	Three components: (1) bronchitis—excessive mucus and sputum production with inflammation of the bronchi; (2) bronchoconstriction—narrowing airways; (3) emphysema—irreversible destruction of distal air space	Smoking cessation; increased fluids; yearly influenza vaccine; one-time pneumonia; vaccine; bronchodilator; expectorants as necessary; avoidance of sedatives and cold, wet weather, postural drainage; antibiotics if infection
		Shortness of breath, sputum production, wheezing, tachypnea, hyperinflation	General attention to proper nutrition, rest, and hygiene
Blood dyscrasias			
Pernicious anemia	Progressive megaloblastic microcytic anemia that results from lack of intrinsic factor essential for absorption or vitamin B_{12}	Weakness, numbness, tingling of extremities; fever, pallor; anorexia, weight loss	Vitamin B_{12} injections; folic acid and iron medications
Secondary anemia	Reduced hemoglobin level, hematocrit, and red blood cells counts, resulting from nutritional deficiency, blood loss, and primary problem	Fatigue, shortness of breath, light-headedness, skin pallor; sometimes arrhythmia	Iron preparation or perhaps blood transfusion; maintenance or stable activities of daily living; attention to primary issue

(continued)

TABLE 14–11 *(continued)*
Common Health Problems in Later Maturity

Problem	Definition	Symptom/Signs	Prevention/Treatment
Chronic lymph-ocytic leukemia	Neoplasm of blood-forming tissue	Characterized by small, long-lived lymphocytes, chiefly B cells in bone marrow, blood, liver, and lymphoid tissue	Complexity of disease dictates seeking medical-surgical text or physician
Hodgkin's disease	Malignant disorder	Characterized by painless progressive enlargement of lymphoid tissue	Complexity of disease necessitates seeking medical-surgical text or physician
Genitourinary diseases			
Benign prostatic hypertrophy (BPH)	Overall enlargement of prostate gland via enlargement of fibrous and muscular tissue	Difficulty in stopping and starting urinary flow; voiding frequent small amounts Diffuse enlargement of prostate; landmarks preserved	Medication such as Hytrin; possible surgical inter-vention; rule out cancer
Skeletal diseases			
Osteoporosis	Absence of normal quantity of bone Predisposes to fracture	Loss of normal cortical thickness; increased porosity in cortical bone; thinning, fragmentation, and loss of trabeculae in can-cellous bone	Prevention: diet in earlier years containing adequate calcium, vitamin D, phosphorus, protein, and fluoride
Osteoarthritis	Degeneration of articular cartilage and hypertrophy of bone	Pain and stiffness, mainly in weight-bearing joints and dorsal interphalangeal joints of fingers	Exercise to improved stiffness; rest to help pain; heat, antiphyretic, adequate nutrition, physical therapy, Fosamat or other stabilizer
Cardiovascular diseases			
Congestive heart failure	Cardiac function altered so that there is not enough cardiac output to meet demands of tissue meta-bolism; consequently sodium and body water are retained	Arteriosclerotic heart disease and hypertension precursors; depressed breathing (unless sitting or standing); ankle swelling; frequent nighttime voiding; weight gain; distended neck veins; rales in lungs; heart with "gallop rhythm"	Low-sodium diet; correct high blood pressure with angiotensin-converting enzyme (ACE) inhibitors, nitrates, and other vasodila-tors, chemical trials being done with calcium channel blockers, prostacycline analogues, and oral inotropes; rate and rhythm regulated with digitalis preparation; urinary output increased with diuretics

(continued)

TABLE 14–11 *(continued)*
Common Health Problems in Later Maturity

Problem	Definition	Symptom/Signs	Prevention/Treatment
Chronic occlusive arterial disease of the extremities	Because of partial or complete occlusion of one or more peripheral blood vessels, decreased blood flow to one or more extremities	Diabetes often a precursor; cramping pain in the muscles during exercise that is relieved by rest; sometimes nighttime cramping; extremity may feel cool; pulses may be decreased; skin may lose hair and appear shiny	Evaluate for revascularization; practise good skin care; avoid excess heat or cold; avoid tobacco and caffeine; drugs not effective
Stasis ulcer of the lower extremity	Chronic ulcerative skin lesion caused by venous stasis and consequent poor circulation	Peripheral pulses intact; **pitting edema** *(induration remains after pushing in skin and tissue with a finger)* or **brawny edema** *(thickened and hardened skin)* around ulcer site	Rest and elevation of involved leg; once or twice daily cleaning with povidone iodine (Betadine) or hydrogen peroxide solution; occasionally application of moist heat or Unna boot; watch for widening of lesion and cellulitis
Infectious diseases			
Tuberculosis (not yet common, but re-emerging)	Infectious disease transmitted by airborne route and caused by *Mycobacterium tuberculosis;* infection refers to successful colonization in a host; active disease indicates pathogenic process	Chronic flulike cough, decreased appetite, weakness, weight loss, continued slightly elevated temperature, night sweats, dyspnea on exertion, pain with respiratory movements if pleura involved, rales over apex of lung, hoarseness if larynx involved, dysphagia if pharynx involved	TB skin testing, x-ray if indicated, sputum testing, multiple-drug therapies (isoniazid, rifampin, pyrazinamide, and ethambutol or streptomycin); appropriate infection control techniques for both patient and those in contact with patient

Heart disease is the number one killer for men and women; however, men and women differ in the classic warning symptoms. Men are likely to experience angina, *a severe squeezing pain that radiates to the neck, upper abdomen, or left arm and occurs during stress or exertion.* Women are more likely to experience shortness of breath or profound fatigue that occurs in activities they previously found easy to do. Or they may have nausea, heartburn, or indigestion unrelated to anything recently eaten.[509–511]

Stroke (cardiovascular accident) is the third most common cause of death. Excessive adiposity in adults aged 65 to 74 seems to influence risk of stroke in conjunction with hypertension, diabetes, and other cardiovascular disease risk factors; therefore, control of weight and fat consumption remains an important concern as people age.[512–514]

Cancer is the second leading cause of death; pneumonia, influenza, and chronic obstructive lung disease rank fourth and fifth as causes of death.[515] Other prevalent disorders are arthritis, diabetes, hypertension, and osteoporosis.[516] Elderly men are more likely to commit suicide than any other age group in North America, and Caucasians, in contrast to other racial groups, are the most likely to use firearms for suicide.[517]

CRITICAL THINKING

Describe your suicide assessment plan.

Diseases that Affect Sexual Function

Health problems associated with the *sexual changes* of aging are of concern to the older adult. Certain diseases in the elderly female have been linked to estrogen deficiency. There is a statistical rise in atherosclerosis attacking the coronary arteries in aged females (and in younger women who have had ovaries removed); women treated with estrogen therapy have had fewer myocardial infarctions. Although there is no clear-cut case for a cause-and-effect relationship, the female hormones apparently are crucial to the enzymatic system in the metabolism of fats and proteins.

Factors that contribute to *sexual dysfunction* are essentially the same as those that affect performance at any age: disease or mutilating surgery of the genitourinary tract, diverse systemic diseases, and emotional disturbance coupled with societal attitudes. Treatment of the aged for a physical complaint often contributes to widespread use of drugs. Tranquilizers can give way to excessive use of alcohol or marijuana. They weaken erection, reduce desire, and delay ejaculation. Many of the metabolic disorders are overlooked and go untreated; anemia, diabetes, malnutrition, and fatigue may negatively affect the quality of life and cause impotence. Obesity may impose a hazard for cardiac and vascular integrity and at best is damaging to a healthy self-image.

Many older persons are under the false impression that any sexual activity will increase the danger of illness or even death because of stress on heart or blood pressure. In truth, oxygen consumption, heart rate, and blood pressure increase only moderately during intercourse and may actually afford a distinct therapeutic and preventive measure. In persons with arthritis, for example, the increase in adrenal corticosteroids during sexual activity relieves some of the symptoms. The present-day practice of prescribing exercise for cardiac patients attests that sexual intercourse need not be considered dangerous for anyone able to walk around a room.

Radical surgery or dysfunction of the genitourinary tract produces the most devastating effects on sexual capacity and libido. Extensive resectioning due to malignancy may make intercourse difficult if not impossible. Although a decline in desire and capacity for climax may follow hysterectomies, they are by no means inevitable. The loss of childbearing ability and the lack of an ejaculation are for some women and men psychologically traumatic, and these clients may need some support and guidance in adjusting to change.

Nursing care involves a re-examination of one's own bias about sex and sexuality in the aged.

Human sexuality covers a wide spectrum, and the pattern for each individual is a product of prenatal development and postnatal learning experiences coupled with one's inherent sense of personal identity within a sex classification. This basic pattern is not altered simply by age. It continues to mediate one's capacity for involvement in all life activities.

CRITICAL THINKING

Discuss the attitudes of society, older adults, and health professionals that can interfere with healthy sexual function in older adults.

Nursing and health care planning for the elderly can be effective. Realizing the need for sexual expression in some form or other, nurses can be open and nonjudgmental when clients display a desire for warmth, close contact, and companionship. Touch is particularly important to the older person who has been bereft of family ties, perhaps for many years. Some people require more relief from sexual tension than others. If incidents arise that seem unduly unorthodox, such as open masturbation or unusual behaviour with the opposite sex, the nurse can be a support person if there is a sincere desire for counselling. The nurse in a sensitive way should focus on the person and not on any specific act.

Exploring alternate lifestyles with persons who are single, alone, and old may be a way for the nurse to assist. Teaching

that includes information about therapy available, such as estrogen replacement, when there are emotional or physiologic problems associated with the climacteric can help the elderly woman to choose treatment. A thorough knowledge of anatomy and physiology of normal aging is essential for the nurse who cares for the elderly. Only then can information be accurate and teaching effective. The nurse may want to involve the older adult's spouse or partner during the assessment.[518]

Intervention can include the following:

- Becoming better educated about sexuality
- Increasing self-awareness
- Discussing sexuality openly with peers, staff, and students
- Attempting to manipulate the environment of the aged client to provide a healthier milieu in which relationships can be a source of comfort
- Evaluating own behaviour in terms of intimacy, touch, friendships, and interest in the aged
- Above all, accepting the challenge ourselves to live fully and to assist the aged in our care to do the same

Pharmacokinetics and Aging Changes

Changes in brain structure and function in the aging process may potentiate the effects of alcohol and other psychoactive drugs. Total body water content decreases by 10% to 20% from ages 20 to 80, and extracellular fluid volume decreases by 35% to 40%. An increase of 18% to 36% in total body fat occurs in men and an increase of 33% to 45% occurs in women from 20 to 80 years. Alcohol, which distributes in body water, has a smaller water distribution volume in the elderly, resulting in higher blood alcohol levels. Medications that are fat soluble have a large distribution volume, lower serum levels for a single dose, longer elimination times, and, thereby, greater cumulative and toxic effects. Albumin is the major drug-binding protein; a decrease in albumin level may result in higher levels of free medication, less therapeutic effect, and increased drug-drug interactions. Aging affects both the liver and kidneys, reducing the rate of medication elimination and increasing the side effects or toxicity. Blood flow and oxidative enzyme levels decrease with age, which affects disposition of medications and contributes to less therapeutic effects.[519,520]

Magnesium toxicity may occur in older people who regularly ingest large doses of magnesium-containing antacids for indigestion and constipation. Symptoms include muscle weakness and incoordination, drowsiness, and confusion; coma occurs in severe cases.[521]

CRITICAL THINKING

Review a few scholarly journals that provide information on magnesium toxicity.

Table 14-12 lists magnesium-containing drugs that are often used by the elderly.[522] Many medications are affected in action by the foods eaten. Table 14-13 presents medication-food interactions that may occur.[523–525]

You need to be observant about medications ingested by the elderly and to educate about potential and unexpected adverse affects, related to physiologic changes and lifestyle.

TABLE 14-12
Magnesium-Containing Medications

Antacids

Gaviscon
Maalox Heartburn Relief
Mylanta
Di-Gel
Mylagen II
Milk of Magnesia
Simaal Gel
Mag-Ox-400
Uro-Mag
Riopan

Laxatives

Citrate of magnesia
Epsom salts
Milk of Magnesia

Analgesics

Backache caplets
Doan's Arthritis Pain Formula
Bufferin
Bayer Select Backache Pain Formula

CRITICAL THINKING

What tips about taking medications would you give a group of older adults?

Polypharmacy and Adverse Drug Reactions

In Canada, Gill, Misiaszed, and Brymer conducted a study to determine the prevalence and predictors of potentially inappropriate prescribing of medications in long-term settings. They found that a total of 69 potential inappropriate prescriptions were found in 65 of 355 long-term care patients.[526] The most common types of potentially inappropriate prescriptions were anticholinergic drugs to manage antipsychotic cases (17 cases), tricyclic antidepressants with active metabolites (916 cases), and long-acting benzodiazepines (14 cases). The researchers concluded that potentially inappropriate prescribing in the long-term care setting is common and can be improved by providing a follow-up letter that suggests improving the alternatives.[527]

Health Canada developed a kit called "Medication Matters: How You Can Help Seniors Use Medications Safely." It was designed to help health professionals give older adults information they need to use medication safely.[528]

Teach elders and family members the following:

1. To learn as much as possible about the medication being taken and the disease process.
2. How to keep track of medications, prescribed and over-the-counter, as well as vitamin-mineral supplements and herbs, the doses, times consumed, and any reactions that are unusual.
3. To inform each of the physicians about all of the prescribed and over-the-counter medications that are taken daily.
4. To follow the directions for taking the medications, such as drinking a tall glass of water to reduce side effects.
5. Consult a physician or pharmacist about any questions or symptoms. Report problems promptly.

CRITICAL THINKING

You are asked to give a 30-minute presentation on "Medications and the Older Adult" to a local senior citizen group. What educational materials would you use?

Substance Abuse

There has been considerable publicity about the recommendation of a glass of wine with dinner to lower risk of heart disease. Less has been written about the pitfalls of excessive consumption of alcohol. A safe amount of alcohol is far less than most people think, especially for older adults and women, who are especially vulnerable to intoxication and drug interactions. Whatever the age or gender; experts do *not* recommend starting to drink, because of alcohol's potential for harm and addiction. There are safer ways to protect the heart.[529] Further, certain medical conditions require alcohol abstinence: hypertension, cardiac arrhythmias, ulcers, liver disease, and dementia. Alcoholism is the second major cause of preventable death in the U.S. (second only to cigarette smoking).[530,531]

Older adults are especially vulnerable to effects of alcohol because of their unique physiology. Aging increases alcohol sensitivity in elders because their tissues hold less water than that of younger persons. Thus, alcohol has greater potential for intoxication, drug interactions (elders typically take two to seven, or more, medications), and side effects.[532]

Women are more sensitive to alcohol than men because they produce less of the enzyme that breaks down alcohol. The average woman achieves a higher alcohol blood level and becomes more intoxicated after drinking half of the amount of alcohol consumed by the average man. Small body size increases alcohol potency because there is less body water to dilute the alcohol, especially in elders, who are more likely to be dehydrated.[533]

Many elderly people are alcoholics, and an increasing number are abusing not only prescription drugs, but also heroin, LSD, marijuana, and cocaine. Contrary to popular opinion, they can be successfully treated.

There are two types of elderly alcoholics: those who began alcohol abuse in their youth (approximately two-thirds of elderly persons who are alcoholics) and those whose minimum drinking habits increased in old age as a reaction to and way to cope with various problems and losses. Widowers constitute the largest proportion of late-onset elderly alcoholics.[534]

Because alcohol is a central nervous system depressant, there are some adverse effects of alcohol abuse. With low

TABLE 14-13
Common Medication–Nutrient Interactions in the Elderly

Drug	Interaction
Methyldopa	Should be taken at times of day when high-protein foods are not being consumed, since absorption is competitive between this drug and amino acids in foods.
Antihypertensive drugs	May influence potassium and magnesium status.
Antibiotics	Influence intestinal absorption.
Aspirin	Can increase gastric acidity and cause anorexia. May require increased need for folic acid and vitamin C. May cause GI bleeding and subsequent iron deficiency.
Laxatives	Can cause gas, cramps, and anorexia. Can affect vitamin D absorption and in turn worsen calcium balance. Mineral oil can interfere with the absorption of vitamins A, D, E, and K.
Tetracycline	Calcium in dairy products makes the drug less effective.
Anticoagulants	Can be adversely affected when liver, green leafy vegetables, and other foods high in vitamin K are eaten in excess.
Monoamine oxidase inhibitors	Foods high in tyramine such as aged cheese, Chianti wine, pickled herring, salami, pepperoni, yogurt, sour cream, raisins, meat prepared with tenderizers, and chicken livers can increase blood pressure and may cause severe headaches, brain hemorrhage, and even death. Cola beverages, coffee, and chocolate should be taken in moderation.
Alcohol	Certain drugs may increase intoxication. Consumed with depressants, alcohol can compound the depressant effect; can cause anticonvulsants and anticoagulants to be metabolized more quickly, causing exaggerated responses; can raise blood sugar levels and interfere with medication prescribed for diabetes; can increase blood pressure when take with MAO inhibitors; can reduce blood pressure when take with diuretics; with antibiotics, it can cause cramps, nausea, and vomiting. Alcohol may destroy the coating of time-release capsules, causing more rapid absorption of a drug. Can increase requirements for nutrients, such as folic acid, thiamine, vitamin B_6, zinc, and magnesium.
Diuretics	Can promote loss of potassium, can increase calcium excretion.
Antacids	Some contain aluminium hydroxide, which can contribute to phosphate deficiency. As a result, blood phosphate may be high but only at the expense of phosphorus released from the bone.

blood levels, the person may feel relaxed and comfortable; depression is an adverse effect. With increased blood levels, the person may feel a sense of stimulation, but in reality the brain centres lose ability to check belligerent or antisocial behaviour. Alcohol also interacts with various drugs, through either potentiation of or interference with medication action, as shown in Table 14-14. (Alcohol interacts adversely with at least 50% of the commonly used over-the-counter drugs.) Other effects such as loss of coordination, slower reflex reaction time, and slower mental response cause the person to be accident prone, which may in turn cause injury, fractures, or death. Excess alcohol intake and, as a result, poor dietary intake, malabsorption, and progressive liver damage cause hypomagnesemia and hypocalcemia, resulting in osteoporosis and avitaminosis. Various deficiency states result. Esophagitis, erosive gastritis and ulcer formation, pancreatitis, and liver cirrhosis are serious diseases that may hasten death. Cancer of the mouth, pharynx, and esophagus is more common in the alcoholic. Finally, excessive alcohol intake may cause pneumonia, respiratory failure, or cardiac failure and death.[535,536]

Your acceptance of, listening to, and assessment of the elderly person in various health care settings can be critical for diagnosis and treatment. You are a liaison between the client and other professionals and can facilitate treatment of the alcoholism and prevention or treatment of various complications. Further, your counselling, education, and support of the family and client can foster their acceptance of the diagnosis and pursuit of treatment.

CRITICAL THINKING

Outline a plan for teaching older adults about substance abuse.

TABLE 14–14
Alcohol Interactions with Medications

Medication Taken with Alcohol	Effect on Person
Antidiabetic agents	Increased hypoglycemia; increased effects of alcohol
Anticoagulants	Increased effect; possible hemorrhage
Barbiturates	
Tranquilizers	
Narcotics	Increased central nervous system depression, oversedation
Antidepressants	
Antihistamines	
Anaesthetics	
Antibiotics	Inhibition of antimicrobial action

PSYCHOLOGICAL CONCEPTS

The psychological and socioeconomic concepts about aging are significant for all who work with the aged, and you will find older people concerned and needing to talk about the many changes to which they must adjust. Knowledge of the crises in this life stage is necessary if you are to aid clients and families in the attainment of developmental tasks, in meeting the crises, and in the early or appropriate treatment of these crises.

Cognitive Development

One universal truth that concerns the process of aging is that its onset, rate, and pattern are singularly unique for each person. Within the individual, the cognitive functions do not change or decline at the same pace. Some will not decrease at all; for example, memorization of facts may be difficult but wisdom will be evident. This is especially true of psychological and mental changes, which generally have a later and more gradual onset than physical aging. Unless the person develops Alzheimer's or another dementia or a vascular disease, age alone does not ruin memory. The person continues to encode general features of experience but may leave out details. Too little sleep (or too many sleeping pills), too much alcohol, or a dysfunctional thyroid gland and depression disrupts formation of new memories.[537,538]

Many factors must be considered when assessing the intellectual functioning of older people:

- Overall health status, as physical health can affect the level of psychological distress, life satisfaction, and cognitive ability (that is, anemia, lung disease, poor circulation, blood pressure or blood sugar changes, hypothyroidism, and fluid or nutritional imbalance can profoundly affect mental status).
- Medications (prescribed and over-the-counter) that are being taken (some drugs slow or interfere with cognitive processes because of toxicity related to slower elimination from the body; drug overdose or **polypharmacy,** *taking excess and unneeded combinations of drugs, may cause drug interactions, toxicity, confusion, or depression,* and must be avoided with careful monitoring and adjustments).
- Sensory impairments (vision, hearing) that interfere with integration of sensory input into proper perception, consequent learning, and appropriate behaviours
- Sociocultural influences
- Motivation
- Interest
- Educational level
- Time since school learning
- Isolation from others
- Deliberate caution
- Using more time to do something, which others may interpret as not knowing
- Adaptive mechanism of conserving time and emotional energy rather than showing assertion

The initial level of ability is important: a bright, 20-year-old will be a bright 70-year-old. Overall, mental ability increases with age.[539–542]

The elder demonstrates **crystallized intelligence,** *knowledge and cognitive ability maintained over the lifetime, dependent on sociocultural influences, life experiences, and broad education, which involve the ability to perceive relationships, engage in formal operations, and understand the intellectual and cultural heritage.* Crystallized intelligence is measured by facility with numbers, verbal comprehension, general information, and integrative and interpretive ability. It is influenced by the amount the person has learned, the diversity and complexity of the environment, the person's openness to new information, and the extent of formal learning opportunities. Self-directed learning opportunities and educational opportunities to gain additional information increase crystallized intelligence after 60 years of age.[543]

A decline occurs in many people after the late 70s. The loss of biological potential is offset by acquired wisdom, experience, and knowledge. In contrast, **fluid intelligence,** *independent of instruction, social or environmental influences, or acculturation and dependent on genetic endowment, is less apparent. It consists of ability to perceive complex relationships, use of short-term or rote memory, creation of concepts, and abstract reasoning.* Fluid intelligence is measured by ability to do tasks of memory span, inductive reasoning, and figural relations. There is, however, no uniform pattern of age-related changes for all intellectual abilities, nor is there a consistent decline in all elders.[544]

Intellectual plasticity refers to the fact that the *person's performance or ability can vary a great deal, depending on social, environmental, and physical conditions;* for example, time to do a task, anxiety about evaluation, attention to or motivation for task, amount of environmental stimulation, or cognitive training or education.[545]

The *senior performs certain cognitive tasks more slowly for several reasons:*

- Decreased visual and auditory acuity
- Slower motor response to sensory stimulation
- Loss of recent memory
- Divided attention
- Greater amount of prior accumulated knowledge and learning that must be scanned and appropriately placed mentally
- Perceived meaninglessness of task
- Changed motivation

He or she may be less interested in competing in timed intellectual tests. Reaction time is also slower when the person suffers significant environmental or social losses, is unable to engage in social contact, and is unable to plan daily routines. The person who is ill often endures environmental and social losses by virtue of being in the client role. Thus, he or she may respond more slowly to your questions or requests.[546–550]

Studies indicate that elderly adults are equivalent to young adults in cue use, encoding, specificity, decision-making speed, design recognition, and spatial memory or awareness of location, especially when distinctive cues are available. Other studies indicate that cognitive performances of young and old adults are comparable when the task is divided or attention has not been interrupted, on assessing contents and products of memory and on recall and recognition of factual information.[551–558]

Older women excel over men in verbal ability and speed of reaction. Older people are able to tolerate very extensive degenerative changes in the central nervous system without serious alteration of behaviour if their social environments are sufficiently supportive. If their environment was restricted in early life, however, learning is inhibited in later life. *Mental functions, especially vocabulary and other verbal abilities, do not deteriorate appreciably until six to 12 months before death.*[559–561]

Table 14-15 summarizes types of cognitive functions, characteristics of the elderly, and health promotion implications.[562–569]

TABLE 14-15
Cognitive Development in Person

Characteristic	Change during Aging	Implication for Health Care
Sensory memory		
	Large amount of information enters nervous system through the senses; selective attention occurs. Some information is sent to short-term memory for further processing; some is lost because nervous system cannot process. First step of memory process involves recall that lasts a few minutes.	Avoid sensory overload. Assist hearing, visual, and tactile functions. Recognize that person may be inattentive to your teaching or to their symptoms or situation. Use variety of teaching methods, include visual aids. Teach importance of health maintenance, as healthy elders maintain general intellectual function.
Short-term memory		
	Brain holds information for immediate use: conceptualization, rehearsal, memorization, association with long-term memory. Deals with current activities or recent past of minutes to hours. Remains consistent with earlier abilities. Older person can repeat string of digits as well as younger person unless asked to repeat them backward; information about digits fades in about a minute unless person rehearses it. Overall mental status is poorly correlated with short-term memory. Recall is better for logically grouped, chunked, or sequenced information.	Give attention for memory abilities. Teach importance of continuing to use memory, memory retrieval tricks, or cues. Teach person to use variety of associative and memory strategies to enhance recall. Teach relaxation methods to reduce anxiety about memory and enhance attention, rehearsal, motivation, and general function. Teach cognitive tricks or use of lists or ways to organize information to improve memory or remember essential information. Teach person to overcome interferences. Let person set own pace to enhance learning and memory.

(continued)

TABLE 14-15 *(continued)*
Cognitive Development in Person

Characteristic	Change during Aging	Implication for Health Care
Long-term memory		
	Use of information acquired, transferred for storage, and stored over years. Unlimited, permanent storehouse of memories, which may not have to pass through short-term memory. Involves images (mental pictures) and verbalization. Three encoding systems are used: visual-spatial, verbal sequential, and abstraction.	Give attention for memory abilities. Recognize that dysfunctions in short- and long-term memories occur independently. Encourage person to use memories and associations in tasks.
Declarative (episodic)		
	Conscious memory of specific persons, places, events, or facts that is acquired quickly, but may not be accurately or easily recalled. Requires intact hippocampus. Older person stores long-term memories, but does not retrieve as quickly as younger person unless he or she uses memory tricks.	Give person adequate time for recall. Encourage use of memory tricks and associations.
Recognition		
	Involves selecting correct response from incoming information rather than recall or retrieval. Ability is retained with age for words, background, familiar objects.	Give support and recognition for ability to recognize and use information.
Implicit (reflexive)		
	Unconscious learning of information or skill through experience or practice (e.g., playing piano, riding bicycle). Requires intact cerebellum. Ideas, concepts, or ability to perform readily remembered. Does not weaken with age in absence of pathology, as person can demonstrate if not discuss.	Use practice in learning new skills for self-care. Reinforce use of habits. Encourage reminiscence or life review. Use habits and well-practised skills when possible in teaching or assisting them. Encourage continued practice of implicitly learned tasks or information.
Reaction time (RT)		
	Speed of response slows during life, and is more obvious after age 60 because of central nervous system changes; shorter duration of alpha rhythm in brain wave (RT fastest between ages 20 and 30). RT remains faster in males than females. Reaction time remains accurate even if slower in both sexes in older adult.	If the person is hurried, response quality and quantity will be reduced. Allow person to proceed at own pace in learning, making decisions, or doing tasks. Do not consider slower response the same as confusion or dementia.

(continued)

TABLE 14-15 *(continued)*
Cognitive Development in Person

Characteristic	Change during Aging	Implication for Health Care
Attentional selectivity		
	Gradual reduced ability in focusing on a specific idea or event, especially as the information processing demands of the task increase. As capable as younger people in correcting unanticipated errors.	Call attention to specific tasks or ideas that the person must focus on when teaching or counselling. Recognize and reinforce capabilities.
Problem solving		
	Skills increase steadily into old age; performance unrelated to IQ test scores or formal education. Person adopts simpler judgmental strategies and relies on pre-existing knowledge more so than young adult. In low-memory–demand tasks, elder is more efficient than young adult. Is better at complex judgmental strategies than young adult.	Teach importance of continuing cognitive function. Engage person in goal setting and problem solving.
Dialectical thinking		
	Older people better able to see all sides of a situation and come to conclusion that integrates different viewpoints and contradictory ideas when given time and when experience rather than memory is required. Is better at solving conditional-probability problems than young adult. Is better at telling integrated story than young adult.	Listen to what may appear to be rambling or loose associations as ideas are likely to be related and pertinent.
Social awareness		
	Increased knowledge and empathy related to culture, living, value systems, or application of ethical and moral principles. Social responsibility traits remain stable or increase in older adult.	Recognize and reinforce capabilities. Use older people as consultants and teachers of the culture.
Higher mental functions: calculations, abstract reasoning		
	Involves integrity of several cognitive functions and exercising values and judgment in decision making and problem solving, logical thinking, future planning, comparison and evaluation of alternatives in context of reality and social responsibility, considering consequences of action. These functions are vulnerable to neurologic pathology; loss of abstraction ability may be first sign of disease or dementia.	Encourage person to remain active in situations or roles that require use of cognitive abilities, e.g., volunteer, mentor, teaching aide, organizational committees, political activities.

(continued)

TABLE 14–15 *(continued)*
Cognitive Development in Person

Characteristic	Change during Aging	Implication for Health Care
Creativity		
	Productivity continues into old age. Aesthetic sense and appreciation of beauty continue to develop.	Provide pleasing environment and opportunities for creativity. Teach family and elder that intellectual and creative mastery of the world exists in many forms and manifests itself daily.
General knowledge		
	Maintains or improves into old age, especially in vocabulary, verbal abilities, and verbal comprehension. General task-specific skills remain equal to those of young adult.	Encourage person to remain active in family and community; participation is a predictor of ability. Reinforce knowledge and wisdom and combat ageism. Teach health promotion as physical health can affect mental function.
Academic performance		
	Elderly students in college perform as well as younger students, tend to have fewer problems, and are able to use new technology and equipment.	Encourage elder to participate in classes, continue learning in credit or non-credit courses or in elder hostel.
Spatial discrimination		
	High-level cortical function related to (1) visual and kinesthetic senses; (2) frontal lobe (motor skill) and parietal lobe (association) functions; (3) ability to produce accurate representations of the way in which objects or parts of objects relate to each other in space; (4) interpretation of directions and top/bottom and visual and spatial cues. Loss of impairment occurs independent of altered sensory function, language dysfunction, or position sense. Older adult tends to need more time and be less accurate in case of maps or finding directions.	Teach spatial cues. Recognize impact on rehabilitation. Test for constructional ability (copy geometric figure or draw face of clock) and general orientation to determine early brain dysfunction. Observe for unilateral neglect of body, inattention to objects or people in left half of sensory field. Assist with and teach family about self-care and safety implications.
Wisdom		
	Superior knowledge and judgment with extraordinary scope, depth, and balance applicable to specific situations and the general life condition. Increases because of empathy and understanding developed over the years. Depends on cognitive and personality factors as well as virtue (character).	Acknowledge the elder's wisdom, creative ability, and productivity. Encourage family to use elder as confidant and consultant.

Cognition and intellectual development are part of maturity. It is in the last half of life that the person best draws on cumulative experiences to establish social, moral, and ethical standards; render decisions; assist in planning; erect social guideposts; and establish pacific relationships between oncoming generations. The judgmental functions of the mind are most highly developed after midlife.[570–575]

Creativity is evident in the later years. The following are important to remember as you teach, assist, and advocate for the elderly:[576]

- People are not identical to others in creative output at any age. Expected age decrement in creativity varies across disciplines; in some there is scarcely a decline at all.
- Creative output of the person in her or his 60s or 70s will most often exceed that produced in the 20s as long as the person is healthy.
- Creative output changes in relation to role changes in career or profession rather than in relation to age.
- The person with a late start in career or profession usually reaches a later peak and higher output in the last years.
- Reduced creative output does not mean corresponding loss of intellectual or motivational capabilities.
- Factors such as health and reduced vigour may interfere with creative output but can be overcome with individual motivation and assistance to the person.
- Creativity can resurge in life's last years.

In your care of the older person and in teaching about cognitive characteristics of later maturity, recognize that the normal aging brain, free of disease, may function as effectively and efficiently as the normal young adult brain except for speed and recent memory. Significant cognitive impairment is related to disease, not normal aging.

Everyone experiences mild forgetfulness as they age. However, **mild cognitive impairment (MCI),** *persistent memory problems in which important information is forgotten regularly,* may be a forerunner of late-life memory disorders or Alzheimer's dementia (AD). The person with MCI has normal abstract language ability but may ask the same question over and over and have difficulty remembering details. In contrast, the person with AD has additional symptoms, including confusion, attention deficit, language impairment, disorientation, and difficulty performing once-familiar tasks.[577]

More research is being done on the association between MCI and AD. The elder can be taught to remember essential information (utilize suggestions in the box entitled "Effective Memory Strategies").

CRITICAL THINKING

You have been asked to present an in-service program on medications used to treat dementia and the management of dementia-related behaviours. What information would you present?

Use the following *suggestions when you teach:*

- Always approach the teaching situation in a way that enhances the person's self-concept and self-confidence.

Effective Memory Strategies

Selective Encoding (getting information into memory)

- Actively and creatively try to find meaning in facts
- Underline selectively; outline
- Distinguish between important and nonimportant points and facts
- Summarize main points
- Reconstruct facts; test self

Elaboration

- Use imagery, visualization of content
- Use metaphor
- Use analogy
- Paraphrase in own words
- Encode more than one strategy

Organization

- Understand how information is organized
- Choose appropriate and effective retrieval cues
- Be aware that related items may cue memory
- Reorganize information so new material better relates to previous knowledge

External Representation

- Take notes; outline
- Make charts, diagrams, tables, or graphs
- Make a conceptual map

Monitoring

- Test self
- Check where errors are made; correct errors

- Keep in mind and assess the elder's experiences, current knowledge, needs, interests, questions, health status, and developmental level as you plan and implement teaching.
- Minimize distracting noise; select a comfortable setting.
- Tell the person that you are planning a teaching session, state the general topic, and emphasize importance. Get the person's attention and increase anticipation.
- Arrange for the person to be near the teacher, teaching aids, or demonstration.
- Consider the aged person's difficulty with fine movement and failing vision when you are using visual aids.
- Provide adequate lighting without glare; do not have the person face outdoor or indirect light.
- Use sharp colours with a natural background and large print to offset visual difficulties.
- Explain procedures and directions with the person's possible hearing loss and slowed responses in mind.
- Use a low-pitched, clear speaking voice; face the person so he or she can lip read if necessary.

- Teach slowly and patiently, with sessions not too long or widely spaced and with repetition and reinforcement.
- Mentally "walk through" or imagine a task through verbal explanation before it is to be done to enhance recall.
- Material should be short, concise, and concrete; present material in a logical sequence; summarize often.
- Break complex tasks or content into smaller and simpler units; focus on a single topic to promote concentration.
- Match your vocabulary to the learner's ability and define terms clearly and as frequently as needed.
- Give the aged person time to perceive and respond to stimuli, to learn, to move, to act.
- Help the person make associations between prior and new information and emphasize abilities that remain constant to enhance recall and application.
- Have the person actively use several sensory modalities to make motions and repeat the content aloud verbally while seeing or hearing it.
- Plan extra sessions for feedback and return demonstrations and extra time for these sessions.
- Whenever possible, include a significant other in the teaching session to ensure further interpretation and support in using the information.

Two forms of recall serve as therapeutic interventions: reminiscence and life review.[578–583] Reminiscence and life review differ but share some characteristics: (1) both use memory and recall for enjoyment or to cope with difficulties and look at accomplishments, (2) both can be structured or free-flowing; (3) both are integrative and can involve happy or sad feelings; (4) both serve a therapeutic function; and (5) both are implemented primarily with elderly but can be used with middle-agers or young adults, especially in terminal illness.

Reminiscence involves *informal sharing of bits and pieces of the past that surface to the consciousness and involves the feeling related to the memories. Thus, this memory process includes affective and cognitive functions.* It is an oral history.

Goals for use of reminiscence include the following:

- Provide pleasure and comfort (but sad and angry feelings and memories also come forth)
- Improve self-confidence, self-esteem, and mood
- Improve communication skills and cognitive function; stay oriented
- Increase socialization, decrease isolation
- Improve alertness, connectedness with others
- Increase deeper friendships; put relationships in order
- Promote role of confidant
- Promote ego integrity and satisfaction with life; find meaning in life cycle
- Provide strength to face new life challenges
- Obtain data
- Facilitate grieving for losses

During reminiscence therapy, your role is to:

- Encourage informal, spontaneous discussion
- Be supportive, provide positive atmosphere
- Avoid probing or pushing for insight

- Allow repetition in the person's discussion
- Encourage the person to integrate the happy and sad memories
- Allow the person to evaluate implications or prior outcomes as memories are recalled, if desired
- Validate and support the meaningful contributions and activities of past life
- Use themes or props, if desired, to stimulate discussion, especially in a group
- Avoid focusing on issues or judgment of memories

Reminiscence may be done with individuals, with family and clients, or with a group of clients. You have a role in all of these.

CRITICAL THINKING

You are asked to give an in-service talk on "Reminiscence Therapy" to a group of nurses in a personal care home. What are your goals?

Life review involves *deliberately recalling memories about life events; it is the life history or story in a structured autobiographical way. It is a guided or directed cognitive process, used with a goal in mind.* It may include reminiscence and affective functions.

Goals for use of life review include the following:

- Increase self-esteem
- Increase life satisfaction, or well-being
- Increase sense of wisdom, validate wisdom
- Increase sense of peace about life
- Decrease depression
- Integrate painful memories, crises, unmet needs, unfulfilled aspirations
- Promote ego integrity, resolve self-despair
- Work through prior crises, events, traumas, relationships

During life review therapy, your role is to:

- Accept the story and accompanying photographs or memorabilia but encourage a life span approach
- Convey empathy for experiences and feelings (happy and sad)
- Validate and support values being expressed
- Allow repetition to promote necessary catharsis
- Discuss issues that arise so they can be resolved
- Reframe events if the person cannot do so
- Encourage the person to evaluate prior responses, achievements, or ways of handling a situation
- Allow the focus to remain on the person's own self
- Validate that which has been meaningful in life to the person
- Recognize that the person may not ever really resolve or accept the multiple losses that have occurred (sadness may remain)

These measures, combined as necessary, allow for comprehension and appropriate response and compensate for decline in perception, memory, and slower formation of associations and concepts.

Emotional Development

The older person experiences emotions at least as intensely as young adults.[584] Emotional responses become less unidimensional with age; for example, love may be less euphoric and become more bittersweet the second or third time around. Positive emotions acquire negative loading over time, and vice versa. Identical events may elicit different emotions over time, and events that elicited emotional response earlier may no longer do so. Multiple roles in old age are linked to greater psychological well-being and flexibility in emotional responses overall.[585–589]

Erikson,[590] describing the eight stages of man, states: the developmental or psychosexual task of the mature years is ego integrity versus despair. A complex set of factors combines to make the attainment of this task difficult for the elderly person.

Ego integrity is the *coming together of all previous phases of the life cycle*.[591] Having accomplished the earlier tasks, the person accepts life as his or her own and as the only life for the self. He or she would wish for none other and would defend the meaning and the dignity of the lifestyle. The person has further refined the characteristics of maturity described for the middle-aged adult, achieving both wisdom and an enriched perspective about life and people (see the box entitled "Wisdom: Expert Knowledge"). Even if earlier development tasks have not been completed, the aged person may overcome these handicaps by associating with younger persons and helping others resolve their own conflicts. Historical situation, family environment, marital status, and individual development all influence the integrity achievement.[592,593]

Use the consultative role to enhance ego integrity. Ask the person's counsel about various situations that relate to him or her personally or to ideas about politics, religion, or activities current in the residence or institution. Although you will not burden the person with your personal problems, the senior will be happy to be consulted about various affairs, even if his or her advice is not always taken. Acting as a consultant enhances ego integrity. Having the person reminisce also promotes ego integrity, and reintegration and recasting of life events put traumatic events into perspective.

The person who has achieved ego integrity remains creative. Decrement in achievement is rarely so substantial that the person becomes devoid of creativity at life's end. Even an octogenarian can expect to produce many notable contributions to any creative activity, as has been witnessed with artists, composers, and politicians. Creativity in the late years depends on initial creative potential, but creativity may lie dormant during the demanding young adult years. The older adult has many of the necessary qualities for creativity: time, accumulated experience, knowledge, skills, and wisdom. Often the changes mandated by retirement and late life trigger new creative levels, including those in ordinary people.

CRITICAL THINKING

In what ways can you promote creative expression?

Without a sense of ego integrity, the person feels a sense of **despair** and **self-disgust**. *Life has been too short and futile. The person wants another chance to redo life.* Refer to the box entitled "Consequences of Self-Despair or Self-Disgust" for a list of feelings and behaviours that are part of self-despair.[594,595] Feelings of despair and disgust about self are compounded by the relationship losses suffered and the consequent loneliness and hopelessness that may occur. Having no confidant or companion and physical health status are both related to the emotional status.[596–598] Suicidal thoughts or attempts may result; this is a growing problem.[599]

Nursing care for the person in despair involves use of therapeutic communication and counselling principles, use of touch and relaxation techniques, and being a confidant so that the person can work through feelings from the past and present ones of sadness and loneliness. **The maintenance phase of the nurse–client relationship** is important, as the person needs time to resolve old conflicts and learn new patterns of thinking and relating. The person can move to a sense of ego integrity with the ongoing relating of at least one caring person—a person who listens; meets physical needs when the person cannot; nurtures and encourages emotionally; brings in spiritual insights; validates the senior's realistic concerns, fears, or points of anguish; and listens to the review of life, patching together life's experiences.

Wisdom: Expert Knowledge

Knowledge that is both factual and strategic in the fundamental aspects of life.
Knowledge that considers the context of life and social changes.
Knowledge that considers relativism of values and life goals.
Knowledge that considers uncertainties of life.
Knowledge that reflects good judgment in important but uncertain matters of life.

Consequences of Self-Despair or Self-Disgust

- Discuss unresolved conflicts related to people or life situations
- Wishes to relive life, redo life course; fears death
- Suspicious or hypercritical of others; angry toward others, especially significant others
- Has a sense of overwhelming guilt, shame, self-doubt, self-disgust, inadequacy
- Disengages from others; withdraws from people or life's interests
- Feels worthless, a burden
- Demonstrates decreasing cognitive competence
- Discusses lack of accomplishments in life or unfinished endeavours
- Is lonely, has had few relationships
- Describes desire for relationships, a confidant, companion
- Feels hopeless, helpless, sad, depressed
- Has suicidal thoughts or behaviour

Personality Development and Characteristics

Encourage the uniqueness of the individual. Realize and explain to others that the earlier personality traits are maintained.[600,601]

No specific personality changes occur as a result of aging: values, life orientation, and personality traits remain consistent from at least middle age onward. *The older person becomes more of what he or she was.* The older person continues to develop emotionally and in personality but adds on characteristics instead of making drastic changes.[602–606] If he or she were physically active and flexible in personality and participated in social activities in the young years, these characteristics will continue appropriate to physical status and life situation. If the person was hard to live with when younger, he or she will be harder to live with in old age.

CRITICAL THINKING

What communication skills can a nurse use with an older adult who is rigid in his or her ways?

Personality and Lifestyle

Personality problems in old age are related to problems in early life. Even when the younger years are too narrowly lived or painfully overburdened, the later years may offer new opportunities. Different ways of living can be developed as the social environment changes and as the person also changes. Later maturity can provide a second and better chance at life.[607]

A study found that older adults tend to cling or become more committed to highly valued roles when they encounter stress in the role or in life in general. If the person gains a strong sense of self-esteem from the role (e.g. caregiving, community volunteer), it is less likely to be devalued, regardless of how high the associated stress. However, there may be a time that the person gives up the role in a sense of relief if stress is ongoing and deleterious to well-being. Further, the context of the role situation must be considered when determining how the senior values the role (e.g., great-grandparenthood or grandparenthood).[608]

CRITICAL THINKING

What approach would you use to identify spiritual health?

Young-Old Personality

In the *young-old* person (ages 65 to 75 or 80 and sometimes beyond), the personality is frequently flexible, shows characteristics commonly defined as mature, and is less vulnerable to the harsh reality of aging.[609] The person manifests self-respect without conceit; tolerates personal weakness while using strengths to the fullest; and regulates, diverts, or sublimates basic drives and impulses instead of trying to suppress them. He or she is guided by principles but is not a slave to dogma; maintains a steady purpose without pursuing the impossible goal; respects others, even when not agreeing with their behaviour; and directs energies and creativity to master the environment and overcome the vicissitudes of life.[610–613]

Motivations change; the senior wants different things from life than he or she did earlier. Concerns about appearance, standards of living, and family change. Stronger incentives, support, and encouragement are needed to do what used to be eagerly anticipated. He or she avoids risks or new challenges and is increasingly introspective and introverted.

Yet generosity is a common trait of the elderly; the person gives of self fully and shares willingly with people who are loved and who seem genuinely interested in him or her.

The elderly person hopes to remain independent and useful as long as possible, to find contentment, and to die without being a burden to others. Increasingly, dependency may undermine self-esteem, especially if the person values independence.

Personality characteristics differ for men and women, especially in relation to assertiveness. The man becomes more dependent, passive, and submissive and more tolerant of his emerging nurturant and affiliative impulses. The woman becomes more dominant and assertive and less guilty about aggressive and egocentric impulses. Perhaps the reversal in overt behaviour is caused by hormonal changes. Perhaps the man can be more open to his long-unfulfilled emotional needs when he is no longer in the role of chief provider and no longer has to compete in the work world. Perhaps the woman reciprocates in an effort to gratify needs for achievement and worth; she expresses more completely the previously hidden conflicts, abilities, or characteristics.[614]

Old-Old Personality

Old-old age (age 80 or 85 years and beyond) is a time for meditation and contemplation, not camaraderie.[615,616] Camaraderie is for young people who have energy and similarities in background, development, and interest. Old-old people may be friendly and pleasant, but they are also egocentric. Egocentricity is a physiologic necessity, a protective mechanism for survival, not selfishness. Old-old people are even more unique in the life pattern than young-old people because they have lived longer. Further, they have less energy to deal with challenging situations, and relating to a group of oldsters can be challenging.[617] There is increased interiority in the personality.[618]

The person in later maturity, especially in old-old age, may be called childish. Only the very simple, those who have not grappled with the complexities of life, or the very ill and regressed will be infantile.

The old-old have greater need than ever to hold onto others. They are often perceived as clingy, sticky, demanding, loquacious, and repetitious. This often causes the younger person to want to be rid of the senior, which causes a vicious circle of increased demand and increased rejection.

Preoccupation with the body is a frequent topic of conversation, and other elderly people respond in kind. The behaviour is analogous to the collective monologue and parallel play of young children. The talk about the body satisfies narcissistic needs, and it is an attempt magically to relieve anxiety about what is happening. This pattern alienates the young and the young old, and they tend to avoid or stop conversing with the aged.

Old-old persons intensely appreciate the richness of the moment, the joys or the sorrows. They realize the transience of life, and they are more likely to start each day with a feeling of expectancy, not neutrality or boredom. Their future is today. As a result, they become more tolerant of others' foibles, more thrilled over minor events, and more aware of their own needs, even if they cannot meet them.

CRITICAL THINKING

What is your definition of an old-old personality?

Irritating behaviour of the old-old person is frequently related to the frustration of being dependent on others or helpless and the fear that accompanies dependency and helplessness. The tangible issue at hand—coffee too hot or too cold, visitors too early, too late or not at all, or the fast pace of others—is often not really what is irritating, although the person attaches complaints to something that others can identify. The irritability is with the self, loss of control, lost powers, and present state of being.

Perhaps the *most frequent error in assessing* the elderly is the diagnosis of senility. Conditions labelled as such may actually be the result of physiologic imbalances, depression, inadequacy feelings, or unmet affectional and dependency needs. Psychological problems in the elderly are often manifested in disorientation, poor judgment, perceptual motor inaccuracy, intellectual dysfunction, and incontinence. These problems are frequently not chronic and may respond well to supportive therapy. Just as few young adults reach complete maturity, few older persons attain an ideal state of personality integration in keeping with their developmental stage.

Carry out principles of care previously described to meet emotional and personality needs of the elderly.

CRITICAL THINKING

What cultural differences would you expect in the emotionality of the older adult?

Adaptive Mechanisms

Nursing and all health care professionals need a strong commitment to assist the elderly in maintaining adaptive mechanism appropriate to this period of life, although each person will accomplish them in his or her unique way, pertinent to life experiences and cultural background.

Persons in their older years are capable of changes in behaviour but find changing difficult. As new crises develop from social, economic, or family restructuring, new types of ego defences may be needed. At the same time, the need to change may interfere with developing a sense of ego integrity.

Changing adaptive mechanisms must be developed for successful emotional transition in these later years. They help the person maintain a sense of self-worth and control over external forces, which in turn promotes a higher level of function.[619] Peck[620] lists three developmental tasks related to adaptation, and they serve to show not only the tasks involved but also the mechanisms undergoing change as the older personality strives to become integrated.

Ego differentiation *versus work-role preoccupation is involved in the adaptation to retirement, and its success depends on the ability to see self as worthwhile not just because of a job but because of the basic person he or she is.* **Body transcendence** *versus body preoccupation requires that happiness and comfort as concepts be redefined to overcome the changes in body structure and function* and, consequently, in body image and the decline of physical strength. The third task is **ego transcendence** *versus ego preoccupation, the task of accepting inevitable death.* Mechanisms for adapting to the task of facing death are those that protect against loss of inner contentment and help to develop a constructive impact on surrounding persons.[621]

Certain adaptive or defensive mechanisms are used frequently by the aged. **Regression,** *returning to earlier behaviour patterns,* should not be considered negative unless it is massive and the person is incapable of self-care. A certain amount of regression is mandatory to survival as the person adapts to decreasing strength, changing body functions and roles, and often increasing frustration. Regression is an adaptive mechanism used by the older adult who is dying, and it is manifested differently than in younger years. The regression is a complex of behaviours not associated solely with a return to former levels of adaptation.

To integrate into self-concept and handle the anxiety created by a complex of losses, changes, and adaptation related to aging and dying, the older person behaves in a way that may be confused with dementia or drug reactions. Careful assessment is needed, using history of the person's normal patterns and history of illness.

CRITICAL THINKING

How can you encourage the older adult to use adaptive mechanisms to enhance his or her health?

The dying elderly person may express regression in any or all of the following behaviours:[622–625]

- Massive denial and projection
- Misuse of words, confusion about familiar concepts, fragmentation of speech, misinterpretation
- Preoccupation with minutiae, impaired ability to deal with simple abstractions
- Awkward childlike thinking

The dying elderly person will invest little emotionally into goal setting and care planning. Any goal must be short term. Caregivers, including family, must provide physical and emotional support, recognizing the dying person's need to disengage from self-care and significant others. During the care process you must support the family caregivers and encourage them to talk about perceptions and feelings and to explain behavioural changes and needs of the dying person.

Other commonly used adaptive mechanisms are described in Table 14-16.[626] McCrae[627,628] found in a study that controlled for types of stress that older persons did not consistently differ from younger ones in using 26 of 28 coping mechanisms, including rational action, expression of feelings, and seeking help. Middle-aged and older persons were less likely than younger ones to use immature and ineffective mechanisms

TABLE 14-16
Adaptive Mechanisms Used by the Older Adult

Mechanism	Description
Emotional Isolation	*By repressing the emotion associated with a situation or idea while intellectually describing it,* the person can cope with very threatening situations and ideas such as personal and another's disease, aging, and death and can begin to resolve the associated fears. Thus, aged persons can appear relatively calm in the face of crisis.
Compartmentalization	*Narrowing of awareness and focusing on one thing at a time* so that the aged seem rigid, repetitive, and resistive.
Denial	*Blocking a thought or the inability to accept the situation* is used selectively when the person is under great stress and aids in maintaining a higher level of personality integration.
Rationalization	*Giving a logical sounding excuse for a situation* is often used to minimize weakness, symptoms, and various difficulties or to build self-esteem.
Somatization	*Complaints about physical symptoms and preoccupation with the body* may become an outlet for free-floating anxiety. The person can cope with vague insecurities and rapid life changes by having a tangible physical problem to deal with, especially because others seem more interested and concerned about disease symptoms than feelings about self.
Counterphobia	*Excessive behaviour in an area of life to counter or negate fears about that area of life* is observed in the person who persists at activities such as callisthenics or youthful grooming or fashion to retain a youthful appearance.
Rigidity	*Resisting change or not being involved in decision making* is a common defence to help the person feel in control of self and life. A stubborn self-assertiveness is compensatory behaviour for the person who has been insecure, rigid, and irritable.
Sublimation	*Channelling aggressive impulses into sociably acceptable activity* can be an effective defence to meet old age as a challenge and maintain vigour and creativity. Often the elderly desire to live vicariously through the younger generation, and they become involved with the young through mutual activities and listening or observing their activities.
Displacement	*Expressing frustration or anger onto another person or object that is not the source of the feelings* provides a safe release and disguises the real source of anxiety. The elder may blame another for his or her deficiencies, bang furniture, throw objects, or unjustly criticize family or health care workers.
Projection	*Attributing personal feelings or characteristics, usually negative, to another* allays anxiety, releases unpleasant feelings, or elevates self-esteem and self-concept. Projection is done unconsciously, usually to those closest to the person; a milieu free of counteraggression helps the person feel secure.

of hostile responses and escapist fantasy. Health threats in all ages elicit wishful thinking, faith, and fatalism. Using **insight** (*intellectual understanding*) and reminiscence is also adaptive.[629] Resilience is also a part of adaptation. *Characteristics of the successfully adjusted older woman* include the following:[630]

- **Equanimity:** *balanced perspective of one's life and experiences*
- **Perseverance:** *persistence despite adversity or discouragement*
- **Self-reliance:** *belief in oneself and one's abilities*
- **Meaningfulness:** *realization that life has purpose and the value of one's contribution*
- **Existential aloneness:** *realization that each person's path is unique and some experiences must be faced alone*

The following are *components of an adaptive old age*:[631,632]

- High mental status

- Absence of organic brain damage or disease
- High morale
- Counterphobic rather than passive-dependent behaviour
- Denial of aging
- Vitality, interest, and enjoyment
- Adequate income
- Relatively good health
- Personal adaptability
- Available family
- Psychosocial stimulation
- Maintenance of meaningful goals
- Acceptance of death
- Sense of legacy

CRITICAL THINKING

What may be other adaptive mechanisms of the older adult that you see in the community?

Hoarding may be an adaptive behaviour, although it is usually regarded as a disagreeable, messy, and unsafe characteristic of the elderly or a sign of illness or dementia (it may be maladaptive behaviour signalling illness at any age). The elderly may hoard and collect various or specific items for various *reasons*:[633]

■ It may be a lifelong habit; in the younger years the person was considered a "pack rat," or someone who always had what was needed in an emergency, or "someone who had everything handy." The behaviour, if part of the person's self-concept and previously rewarded, is likely to continue to be valued and practised.

■ It may be the mark of a creative, intelligent person, an artist, or former teacher who keeps supplies that can be used in the vocation or hobby.

■ The articles that are saved, potentially useful or likely to be used, represent security, especially if the person (a) lived through the Great Depression and World War II and remembers severe scarcity or poverty, and will not waste; (b) was an immigrant or displaced person from another country; or (c) buys food or supplies in large quantities to save money, even if not used.

■ The articles may be symbolic of a happier past or represent a future.

■ The gathered objects may represent a sense of control.

■ The articles may compensate for loneliness and recent losses or be a way to keep in touch with family or friends now dead or relocated.

■ Collecting, observing, handling, and sorting objects may be a pleasant diversion, especially for the old who are less socially active.

■ Articles may be kept close at hand rather than stored in cabinets or closets to save energy in retrieving them when needed.

■ When cognitive impairment occurs, the person may be unable to discriminate between needed and unneeded objects and thereby keep everything.

Table 14-17 lists interventions that can be used by you, family, or friends, if the hoarding poses a problem.

The box entitled "Characteristics of Successful Aging" summarizes a holistic perspective about successful aging.[634–639] Holistic care will contribute to these characteristics.

Acute illness at any age influences behaviour, affective responses, and cognitive function. These aspects of the person are also affected by chronic illness, but their effects and adaptive mechanisms used are less well known.

Your approach during care can either increase or decrease *motivation to participate in treatment or rehabilitation* even when the person already feels self-motivated. *Helpful approaches* include the following:

■ Set a definite goal with the client.

■ Reinforce and support the basic drives or character/personality structure of the client. Do not label the preoccupation

---

TABLE 14–17
Interventions for Hoarding Behaviour

1. Discuss the situation with the person. Let the person show you collections and tell the stories; learn the meaning of behaviour.

2. Offer to assist with cleanup, filing, or discarding if the person wishes and lacks energy or motivation. Never throw away objects without consent of the person unless dementia is present.

3. Set limits firmly if the hoarding is hazardous; e.g., help the person clean out the refrigerator with spoiled or inedible food, straighten up a room, and make a clear walkway to avoid falls.

4. Do not argue or nag about insignificant articles or out-of-the-way collections.

5. Discuss the need to discard some of the accumulation but tell the person he or she can decide what to discard, store, give to family or friends, and keep.

6. Reward behaviours that reduce hoarding.

7. Arrange for the person to engage in outside activities, groups, and relationships. Keep the person busy with interesting activities.

8. Evaluate the person's need for possible relocation to the home of a family member or to an assisted living retirement centre for close supervision and assistance.

9. Refer the person, after consultation with family, guardian, or health care team, to a treatment facility if the behaviour is indicative of depression, obsessive–compulsive disorder, paranoia, or dementia.

10. Assist family and friends, if necessary, in determining whether a legal guardian should be appointed.

---

with achieving or the persistence in practice as obsession or compulsion. Realize that the former "toughness" or "survival traits" of the person are now an asset, not to be diminished by your traditional approach.

■ Convey caring, be kind, share "power" or control with the client rather than trying to be the boss. In turn, the client will feel, and be, more "cooperative."

■ Encourage or reinforce with attention to the attempts as well as achievements.

■ Use humour gently and appropriately to release tension or encourage. Do not use sarcastic humour.

■ Convey a positive attitude that the person can achieve the goal, at least to the extent possible. Avoid negative comments, an attitude that "puts down" the client, or nonverbal behaviour that conveys you do not perceive capability.

■ Avoid a power struggle, insistence on the client doing an activity your way, or domination of the client. Let the person go at his or her own pace and in a way that is safe but will still achieve results.

Characteristics of Successful Aging

High Degree of Life Satisfaction

- Feels life has been rewarding; has met goals
- Has few regrets
- Has positive attitude about past and future
- Feels life is stimulating, interesting; sets new goal
- Is able to relax; has good health habits

Harmonious Integration of Personality

- Has developed ego strength, unity, and maturity over the years
- Demonstrates self-actualization, satisfaction, individuation, authenticity
- Makes use of potentials and capabilities throughout life
- Has an accurate self-concept and body image
- Has meaningful value system, and spiritual fulfillment

Maintenance of Meaningful Social System

- Keeps involved with caring network of family and friends
- Maintains interest in life through social attachments
- Feels affection for and from others and sense of belonging

Personal Control over Life

- Feels independent and autonomous
- Makes own decisions, in charge of self to extent possible
- Maintains sense of dignity, self-worth, positive self-concept

Establishment of Financial Security

- Has made careful and effective financial plans
- Uses community resources to extent necessary

CRITICAL THINKING

What does successful aging mean to you?

Body Image Development

Physical changes discussed earlier have both private and public components and combine to change the appearance and function of the older individual and thereby influence the self-image. Both young and older adults revealed no differences in private body consciousness;[640] however, as the person ages, loss of muscle strength and tone is reflected in a decline in the ability to perform tasks requiring strength. The old-old or frail person sees self as weakened and less worthwhile as a producer of work either in actual tasks for survival or in the use of energy for recreational activities.

The loss of skin tone, although not serious in itself, causes the aged in a society devoted to youth and beauty to feel stigmatized. Changing body contours accentuate sagging breasts, bulging abdomen, and the dowager's hump caused by osteoporosis. These changes all produce a marked negative effect. This stigma can also affect the sexual response of the older person because of perceived rejection by a partner.

Loss of sensory acuity causes alienation from the environment. Full sensory status cannot be regained once it is lost through aging. Although eyeglasses and better illumination are of great help in fading vision, the elderly recognize their inability to read fine print and to do handwork requiring good vision for small objects. The danger of injury caused by failure to see obstacles in their paths because of cataracts, glaucoma, or senile macular degeneration makes the elderly even more insecure about the relationship of their body to their environment. They often seek medical help too late because they do not understand the implications of the diagnosis or the chances for successful correction.

Hearing loss, the result of degeneration of the central and peripheral auditory mechanism and increased rigidity of the basilar membrane, is likely to cause even more negative personality changes in the older person than loss of sight. Behaviour such as suspiciousness, irritability, and impatience, and paranoid tendencies may develop simply because hearing is impaired. Again the person may fear to admit the problem or to seek treatment, especially if he or she is unaware of the possibilities of help, through either hearing aids or corrective surgery.

Often the elderly view the hearing aid as another threat to body image. Eyeglasses are worn by all age groups and hence are more socially acceptable, but a hearing aid is conceived as overt evidence of advanced age. Adjustment to the hearing aid may be difficult for many people, and if motivation is also low, the idea may be rejected.

Be especially alert as you assess visual and auditory needs of the elderly. One of the modern medical miracles is lens implant surgery for those with cataracts. Seeing the senior before and after surgery allows you to share the joy of blindness-to-sight and to do necessary teaching. Surgery and discharge are usually the same day.

Hearing needs may not be met as easily, but astute observation can change the situation quickly. There are a number of specific ways to modify the environment for persons with sensory impairments.

Encourage the senior to talk about feelings related to the changing body appearance, structure, and function. Provide a mirror so that he or she can look at self to integrate the overt changes into his or her mental image. Photographs can also be useful in reintegrating a changing appearance. Help the senior to stay well groomed and attractively dressed, and compliment efforts in that direction. Touch and tactile sensations are important measures to help the person continue to define body boundaries and integrate structural changes.

CRITICAL THINKING

What nursing responsibilities would you implement with an older adult who has a hearing impairment?

Moral–Spiritual Development

The elderly person with a mature religious outlook and philosophy still strives to incorporate broadened views of theology and religious action into the thinking. Self-transcendence is related to lower loneliness scores and to mental and spiritual health.[641] Because the elderly person is a good listener, he or she is usually liked and respected by all ages. Although not adopting inappropriate aspects of a younger lifestyle, he or she can contemplate the fresh religious and philosophic views of adolescent thinking, thus trying to understand ideas previously missed or interpreted differently. Similarly, others listen to him or her. The elderly person feels a sense of worth while giving experienced views. He or she is concerned about moral dilemmas and conflict and offers suggestions on ways to handle them. Basically he or she is satisfied with living personal beliefs, which can serve as a great comfort when he or she becomes temporarily despondent over life changes or changes in the family's life, or when confronting the idea of personal death.

Spiritual beliefs enable the older person to cope with painful or unexpected events and to be more productive and adaptive in a threatening environment. The spirit can be considered the primary locus of healing, since it is the basic characteristic of humanness. Spiritual health is necessary for physical, emotional, and mental well-being, satisfaction with life, happiness, and a sense of energy. Isaia, Parker, and Murrow, in their study of 37 people in a senior centre, found that these elders, regardless of age, perceived themselves to be highly spiritual. Women had higher scores for spirituality and well-being than did men.[642]

A study of life satisfaction in 166 black seniors ranging in age from 65 to 88 years (87 males and 79 females) revealed that men and women differed. High life satisfaction in women and men was related to church participation, religious faith, and family role involvements (often associated with the religious roles). High life satisfaction in men was also related to income and education levels.[643]

Life experience that is meaningful has a spiritual quality. *Four themes give life meaning and promote spiritual well-being:*[644]

1. Concern for the welfare of others
2. Opportunity to be helpful or useful as needed
3. Becoming involved in activity that is useful to someone else
4. Maintaining positive feelings about self and others

Religious belief and participation are important for most elders, regardless of ethnicity; however, different ethnic groups vary in how they participate, and they differ in the role religion plays in providing a resource for coping with adversities of aging. Nonorganizational religious participation includes reading religious materials, watching or listening to religious programs, prayer, and requests for prayer. Demographics, religious denomination, and health disability factors influence participation in these and organizational activities.

Elderly persons who have not matured religiously or philosophically may sense a spiritual impoverishment and despair as the drive for professional and economic success wanes. These persons need help to arrive at an adequate spiritual philosophy and to find some appropriate religious or altruistic activities that will help them gain feelings of acceptance, self-esteem, and worth.

CRITICAL THINKING

What coping mechanism would you like to develop to prepare yourself for older adulthood?

Nursing Care to Meet Spiritual Needs

Care of clients' spiritual needs is an essential part of holistic care. This includes talking with the elderly, listening to statements that indicate religious beliefs or spiritual needs, and reading scriptures or praying with the person when indicated or requested. Giving spiritual care to the elderly person may involve providing prompt physical care to prevent angry outbursts and accepting apologies as the person seeks forgiveness for a fiery temper or sharp tongue. Quoting or reading favourite scripture verses, saying a prayer, providing religious music, or joining with the person in a religious song may calm inner storms. Acknowledging realistic losses and feeling with those who weep can provide a positive focus and hope. Helping the aged person remain an active participant in church, religious programs, or Bible study in the nursing home can maintain his or her self-esteem and sense of usefulness. Finally, in dying and near death, the religious person may want to practise beloved rituals and say, or have quoted, familiar religious or scriptural verses.

Developmental Tasks

The following developmental tasks are to be achieved by the aging couple as a family and by the aging person living alone. You can assist the elderly person to meet these tasks:[645–647]

- Recognize the aging process, define instrumental limitations, and adjust to societal views of aging.
- Adjust to decreasing physical strength and health changes.
- Decide where and how to live out the remaining years; redefine physical and social life space.
- Continue a supportive, close, warm relationship with the spouse or significant other, including a satisfying sexual relationship.
- Find a satisfactory home or living arrangement and establish a safe, comfortable household routine to fit health and economic status.
- Adjust living standards to retirement income and reduced purchasing power; supplement retirement income if possible with remunerative activity.
- Maintain culturally assigned functions and tasks.
- Maintain maximum level of health; care for self physically and emotionally by getting regular health examinations and needed medical or dental care, eating an adequate diet, and maintaining personal hygiene.
- Maintain contact with children, grandchildren, and other living relatives, finding emotional satisfaction with them.
- Establish explicit affiliation with members of own age group.
- Maintain interest in people outside the family and in social, civic, and political responsibility.
- Pursue alternate sources of need satisfaction and new interests and maintain former activities to gain status, recognition, and a feeling of being needed.

CASE SITUATION
Later Maturity

Mrs. Bertini, 78 years old, has been a widow for 20 years. She and her husband had no children, but two nieces and a nephew who live in another city visit occasionally. Mrs. Bertini has coped with arthritis for many years and, with the help of a home health agency and friends, has been able to remain in her home after suffering a broken hip. She has taken medication for cardiac disease and hypertension since experiencing a mild heart attack ten years ago.

Despite increasing physical disability, Mrs. Bertini has maintained close ties with three female friends, two of whom had worked with her in a hat factory when they were young. These friends and their husbands were also friends of her husband. The four couples often played cards and attended social functions together.

Mrs. Bertini has begun to find it increasingly difficult to do her housework and shopping. Although the neighbourhood pharmacy still delivers medication, the family-owned grocery on the block where she has lived for 20 years recently closed, and she cannot manage the four-block walk to the bus stop. She has admitted to her friends that she needs assistance, but on her limited income of a small pension from her husband and the minimum amount from the Old Age Security pension, she cannot afford to hire help.

Although Mrs. Bertini has occasionally considered entering a nursing home, the decision is forced when her landlord announces a rent increase of $90 monthly. With great reluctance, she asks her closest friends to take her to several nursing homes in her area of the city. As a devout Catholic, her decision is immediate; she feels most comfortable with the home operated by Little Sisters of the Poor. It is accredited, looks homey, and is clean. The sisters and other workers are friendly and kind. Her friends help her sell her furniture and move to the nursing home. She takes her television and stand, her favourite chair and footstool, and her most treasured mementos and clothes with her.

The first few days in the nursing home are eventful as Mrs. Bertini meets new people and attends the planned activities. Then she begins to feel confined by having only a small room. She misses her independence and occasionally feels lonely. In her own home she used to sleep until 9 a.m., but now if she wants breakfast, she must be in the dining room no later than 8 a.m. Although mobility is painful, slow, and possible only with aid of a walker, Mrs. Bertini makes a point to attend the activities given in the home and accepts invitations from her friends to go out to eat at favourite restaurants. She looks forward to the letters, gifts, and holiday visits from her nieces and nephews and writes short notes to keep in touch with them. She also attends chapel services weekly. She tells her visitors that she is not afraid of death; her only wish is that she does not suffer long.

1. Suppose that one of Mrs. Bertini's friends had contacted you, a health care professional, at the time when her rent increase had just been announced. The friend asked for your assistance for Mrs. Bertini. What steps would you have taken?

2. What municipal and provincial agencies are available for you to call upon for help and direction for Mrs. Bertini should this situation have presented itself to you in the area where you now live?

3. If you were a health care professional working in the Little Sisters of the Poor home on Mrs. Bertini's ward, how would you deal with her thoughts about death and suffering?

- Find meaning in life after retirement and in facing inevitable illness and death of oneself, spouse, and other loved ones.
- Work out values, life goals, and a significant philosophy of life, finding a comfort in a philosophy or religion.
- Reassess criteria for self-evaluation.
- Adjust to the death of spouse and other loved ones.

McCoy[648] describes similar developmental tasks for this era:

- Disengage from paid work.
- Reassess finances.
- Be concerned with personal health care.
- Search for new achievement outlets.
- Manage leisure time.
- Adjust to more constant marriage companion.
- Search for meaning of life.
- Adjust to single state.
- Solve problems.

- Manage stress accompanying change.
- Be reconciled to death.

Brown[649] refers to different developmental tasks for young-old and old-old persons because the changing life situations necessitate different attitudes, efforts, and behaviours. The tasks are listed as follows for each age group.

Young-Old

- Prepare for and adjust to retirement from active involvement in the work arena with its subsequent role change (especially for men).
- Anticipate and adjust to lower and fixed income after retirement.
- Establish satisfactory physical living arrangements as a result of role changes.
- Adjust to new relationships with one's adult children and their offspring.

- Learn or continue to develop leisure time activities to help in realignment of role losses.
- Anticipate and adjust to slower physical and intellectual responses in the activities of daily living.
- Deal with the death of parents, spouses, and friends.

Frail-Old or Old-Old

- Learn to combine new dependency needs with the continuing need for independence.
- Adapt to living alone in continued independence.
- Learn to accept and adjust to possible institutional living (nursing and/or proprietary homes).
- Establish an affiliation with one's age group.
- Learn to adjust to heightened vulnerability to physical and emotional stress.
- Adjust to loss of physical strength, illness, and approach of one's death.
- Adjust to losses of spouse, home, and friends.

SOCIOECONOMIC CONCEPTS

Retirement

Age, sex, health status, family background, ethnicity, type of job or profession, lifetime work experience, and economic incentives all influence when the person voluntarily or involuntarily ceases the career or job. These variables all influence the retirement experience.[650–652] By 2030, there will be more grandparents than grandchildren. However, many of the "Baby Boomers" say they will continue to work part-time rather than retire completely.[653] As corporations reduce their workforce numbers, the older worker is most likely to be released because of salary and pension costs, despite job discrimination legislation. Yet keeping the older worker may be less costly because of retraining costs and lower turnover and absenteeism. He or she is loyal and committed to the company, is flexible about accepting new assignments, and often is a better salesperson. Many people are living longer but are working shorter careers; yet the proportion of young to old people is diminishing. As the 21st century progresses, it is likely that more older people will be needed in the workplace to relieve the labour shortage.[654–659]

Retirement affects all the other positions the person has held and the relationships with others. Retirement is a demotion in the work system. It will, for many people, mean a reduction in income, or the person may seek a new job, either part- or full-time, for financial reasons but also for emotional and socialization reasons. Inability to keep up with the former activities of an organization or group may result, and a change in status may require a changing social life.[660,661] See the box entitled "Phases of Retirement" for more understanding of the experience.[662,663]

In Canada, it appears that the median age of retirement has fallen from age 62 to 61.[664] Depending upon the educational attainment and gender, the average retirement age of a

---

Phases of Retirement

Pre-Retirement

Remote

Adult works intensely and enjoys fruits of labour, job or professional status, financial security, and competence. Little thought or preparation for retirement.

Near Retirement

Adult begins thinking about and planning time for end of job, structured work, or professional position. Duties and obligations are gradually given up. Active planning for retirement.

Retirement

Leaving paid employment, its structure, and its stresses.

Post-Retirement

Honeymoon

Adult is enthusiastic and feels euphoric about change immediately following retirement. Feels enthusiasm and excitement of self-initiated activities. Feels frustrated, angry, and anxious about the future, if forced to retire because of company policy, health, or some other life situation.

Disenchantment

Retiree's plans are beyond financial means, health status interferes, or plans are not as satisfying as anticipated. Feels disappointed, let down, depressed, cynical, or angry.

Reorientation

Retiree comes to grips with reality of retirement, reorients self to the future, and re-evaluates goals and strategies for their potential for achievement.

Stability

Retiree determines and implements long-term choices or goals. This stage may occur after the honeymoon; some people do not experience disenchantment and reorientation. Achieves long-term goals with contentment.

Terminal

The person becomes ill, disabled, or is facing death. Retirement, and the associated lifestyle, has lost its significance or meaning. Or the person may be dissatisfied with retirement goals, activities and leisure and re-enters employment, usually part-time. Becomes a worker again, sometimes in a field unrelated to earlier career(s).

---

person may be as low as 57, or as high as 65. Self-employed individuals continued to retire at approximately age 65. There is evidence to suggest that in the future there may be pressure on people of both genders to delay retirement. The smaller "baby bust" generation will be the source of labour within the economy, and production in the economy may slow due to the decreased labour force, resulting in price inflation.[665] This may force some potential retirees to postpone retirement, since the value of their assets will have decreased.[666]

In Canada more women than men retire.[667] Tompa states that a number of personal conditions lead people to choose retirement, including health, unemployment, a spouse's decision to retire, and attitudes toward work.[668]

Health professionals who work with the elderly need to be sensitive to their wishes regarding retirement and to reinforce their plans and dreams for retirement.

CRITICAL THINKING

How old do you expect to be when you retire?

Retirement as an experience and the tasks achieved differ among Canada, the United States, and other countries.[669]

Retirement Planning

You are often with persons nearing retirement and may be asked directly or through nonverbal cues and disguised statements to help them sort out their feelings as they face retirement. Planning will help in the transition from worker to retiree. Although some persons who disliked their jobs, have an adequate income, and participate in a variety of activities eagerly look forward to a pleasurable retirement, many seniors would prefer and are able to work past age 65.[670–672]

Despite much work in recent years at both the national and local levels to develop comprehensive programs for elders, few business organizations have recognized the many ways in which they might assist the potential retiree. Private organizations with large numbers of employees are, for the most part, the only ones having effective retirement preplanning programs. The retiree may be faced with these questions:

1. Can I face loss of job satisfaction?
2. Will I feel the separation from people close to me at work?
3. If I need continued employment on a part-time basis to supplement pension payments, will the old organization provide it, or must I adjust to a new job?
4. Shall I remain in my present home or seek a different one because of easier maintenance or reduced cost of upkeep?
5. Might a different climate be better and, if so, will I miss my relatives and neighbours?

Whatever the elderly person's need, your role will be supportive. Advocate retirement planning. Recommend agencies that may be useful in making plans, and provide current information.

CRITICAL THINKING

What coping mechanisms would you like to develop to prepare yourself for retirement?

Use of Leisure

The constructive use of free time is often a problem of aging. What a person does when he or she no longer works is related to past lifestyle, continuous core activities, accumulated experiences, and the way in which he or she perceives and reacts to the environment.

Leisure time, *having opportunity to pursue activities of interest without a sense of obligation, demand, or urgency,* is an important aspect of life satisfaction, expression of self, and emotional and social development. Leisure activity is chosen for its own sake and for the meaning it gives to life, but it involves both physical or mental activity and participation. It is a way to cope with change. Adults value most the leisure activity that involves interaction with others or a pet, promotes development, or is expressive and maintains contact with the broader community. Most people have a core of activities that they enjoy. Reading and viewing television are popular pastimes; interestingly, television preferences are similar for older and younger adults, but reading preferences vary strongly with age and sex.

A Canadian study found that physically active leisure contributes directly to higher levels of physical health and well-being and lower levels of ill-health among Canadians.[673]

The *elder can contribute in many ways to the community and society after his or her retirement:*

- Through volunteer or part-time work with hospital, community agency, or social, welfare, or conservation organization of choice
- Through a friendly visitor program to other old or home-bound people
- Through a telephone reassurance program (calling the same person at the same time each day to determine the status)
- Through foster grandparent programs in nurseries, with failure-to-thrive children, and in preschool or daycare settings, homes for abused or orphaned children, or juvenile detention centres
- To homes for battered women or children, providing mothering or fathering skills
- To shelters for the homeless, and providing counselling
- To churches and church-related organizations in many capacities
- To Habitat for Humanity, an organization that builds or remodels homes for poor people in various rural and urban areas
- As a volunteer for a crisis hotline (e.g., suicide, drug use, child care, prayer line)
- Through collaboration with police, clergy, or community leaders, working to create drug-free and gun-free neighbourhoods and schools

The box entitled "Questions to Consider before Volunteering" lists questions to consider before assuming the volunteer role or questions the senior should ask key people in an agency that is being considered for a volunteer role. Explore these questions with the person.

14-2 BONUS SECTION IN CD-ROM

Research Abstract: Giving Up the Car: Older Women's Losses and Experiences

This section reveals the emotional experiences of older adults when they have to give up driving an automobile.

Questions to Consider before Volunteering

- Do you have the time to give?
- Do you make punctuality a habit?
- Do you take responsibility seriously?
- Can you give reasonable advance notice if you must cancel plans or appointments?
- Do you consistently follow through on projects?
- Do you work well with others?
- Do you adhere to an organization's policies and procedures?
- Do you accomplish tasks that have been assigned?
- Would you receive orientation or training that you want or need?
- Do you understand and agree with the details of the position and the demands it will place on you?
- Would you have enough responsibility or authority to challenge you if you desired the challenge?
- Is the organization respected in your community?
- Does the organization respect its volunteers' time?
- Are the current volunteers dedicated to the organization or cause?
- Would you be able to use your experience or educational background?

As population shifts occur and society becomes more technologically complex, causing earlier retirement for some workers, the definition of productivity must be changed from that which involves exchange of money. Toffler has coined the word **"prosumers,"** *people who produce goods and services for their families and friends but not for monetary gain.*[674] Family roles are also likely to change, with an older family adopting or nurturing a younger family, giving assistance with child care or other tasks. The elderly will be needed as caregivers across family lines as home care becomes an important aspect of the health care system, and the caregiving role can give added meaning to life.

CRITICAL THINKING

What are some of the Canadian research findings on retirement?

14–3 BONUS SECTION IN CD-ROM

Federal Planning for the Aged in the United States

In this section the reader will gain information about the arrangements made by the U.S. government for the aged in the United States.

Federal Planning for the Aged in Canada

The 2004 Liberal Task Report states that all Canadians have a right to receive equal and accessible universal health care, be it at home or within a public institution. It recommends that the federal, provincial, and territorial governments collaborate to develop a set of national home care objectives.[675] Many other recommendations were also developed to present a unique perspective on the experience of aging.

With respect to health status, the *2001 Report Card on Seniors in Canada* identified three areas needing improvement: injury prevention, promotion of physical activity, and suicide prevention—especially for men.[676] The updated information from the *2003 Report Card on Seniors* indicated that fewer unintentional injuries occurred in 1999–2000. Seniors aged 65 to 74 showed an improvement in their physical activity levels, and suicide among senior men aged 85 and older decreased slightly between 1997 and 1998. Seniors' life expectancy is increasing, yet more seniors than any other age group have become ill or died because of new infectious diseases. The National Advisory Council on Aging (NACA) will expect the Minister of Health to pay particular attention to the needs of older Canadians in developing the Pan-Canadian Healthy Living Strategy to emerging infectious diseases.[677] The NACA was created on May 1, 1980, to assist and advise the Minister of Health on all matters related to the aging of the Canadian population and the quality of life of older adults.[678]

Old Age Security/Guaranteed Income Supplement

In Canada the foundation of the governmental system is to assure income for the elderly. It is provided by the Old Age Security (OAS) pension, the Guaranteed Income Supplement (GIS), and the Spouse's Allowance (SPA), as well as several provincial and territorial programs that augment the federal benefits.[679]

Canada Pension Plan

The Canada Pension Plan (CPP) is a contributory, earnings-related social insurance program that applies throughout Canada except in the province of Quebec. In 1997, following a year of public comment, substantial reforms were implemented to the CPP. From 5.8% in 1997, the contribution rate is scheduled to rise to 9.9% in 2003 and beyond.[680] The Quebec Pension Plan (QPP) covers workers in Quebec. Like the CPP, the QPP is compulsory and covers almost all workers.[681] Almost all of today's seniors receive income from the CPP or QPP.

Community Planning

Planning and policy and program development must not be bound by ageism and myths about people in later maturity. More and more people who are very old are taking care of themselves in their own home and should be allowed to remain independent to the extent possible. Elsner et al. gives vivid accounts of ethical and policy considerations—and abuses—by health care providers when they did not assess accurately or when they intervened inappropriately.[682]

As people become older, infirm, and less mobile, a battery of community services is needed, not only to provide social activities and a reason to remain interested in life, but also to enable them to live independently. Most older adults require health care that is specific to their aging-related and disease-related needs, including their need to be cared for in a holistic way with diverse experiences, perspectives, and resourcefulness.[683]

CRITICAL THINKING

What will the future of health care be like for the older adult?

Community Services

Discuss available and needed services with the elder and family. Refer as appropriate. Advocate for needed services. Supportive services may include the following:

- Referral services
- Visiting and telephone-reassurance programs, sometimes offered through churches or private organizations
- Services that provide shopping aides
- Portable meals, sometimes from an agency called Meals on Wheels, for those who cannot shop for or prepare their own food
- Transportation and handy-person services, including home upkeep
- Daycare or foster home placement for the elderly (patterned after services for young children but modified for older adults)
- Recreation facilities geared to the older person
- Senior citizen centres that provide recreation and a place for the lonely to belong
- Respite services so that the family can get relief from care-giving while the elderly person receives needed care

All of these services can be used to promote health, prevent dysfunction, enhance a sense of independence, and aid family caregivers. *Adult daycare services* allow the person to remain at home and avoid institutionalization; the elder has daytime supervision and care, and the family member can continue employment (Figure 14–5). Help clients use the box entitled "Criteria for Selecting Personal Daycare." *Home care* prevents lengthy hospitalization, assists families and the elder with the tasks of care, and permits respite for the family. You may be giving care in either setting.

Another helpful community service for elders is the senior centre. Senior centres are found in almost all communities and are based in a variety of settings. Some are operating in buildings built for this purpose, but most are housed in facilities originally planned for other purposes: church halls, community buildings, old schools, mobile home park clubhouses, and the like. A small staff is maintained, and most of the help with programs, maintenance, and materials comes from volunteers among the older persons who attend the centre. Programs include activities such as crafts, social events from cards to dancing, exercise classes, and a full meal served at noon most weekdays. Other services may be daily telephone calls to homebound elderly, information and referral services, home-delivered meals, minor profit-making endeavours, and discount programs in cooperation with local merchants.

Group work among the aged has been done with much success in a number of communities and in a variety of settings.

Criteria for Selecting Personal Daycare

- Is agency accredited?
- Is the agency designed in space, furniture, decor and colour, equipment, and safety features for the elderly, including frail but ambulatory elderly and the cognitively impaired?
- What meals are served? Are special diets served? Ask the attendees about food.
- Are nurses and social workers employed? Physical therapists? Occupational therapists? Are attendants certified? Professionals should be available to the extent that the agency enrolls elders with physical or cognitive problems.
- Is transportation provided? Some agencies have van service to pick up and deliver the senior home—within a certain radius and at certain hours—for a nominal fee.
- How do staff members handle medical or psychiatric emergencies? What is the policy if the elder becomes ill during the day?
- What is the schedule for the day? Are a variety of activities available? Are trips taken to the community? Are there activities of interest to and for participation by individuals and groups?
- What is the cost per day? Are there extra fees for activities? For clients with special physical or cognitive problems?
- How do staff members interact with clients and families?
- How do the clients interact? Do they appear to be satisfied with the care? Talk with them.

Some of this work has been initiated in centres operated for the elderly and has been used not only to encourage the individual to participate in a group activity, but also to carry out health teaching. Many types of groups can be developed for the elderly.[684,685]

As a citizen of the community, you can be active in initiating and supporting local programs. See Elsner et al. for information about ethical and policy considerations for promoting health in centenarians.[686]

Extended-Care Facility

The concept of long-term care for the elderly has broadened to be less custodial, more homelike, more holistic, and community focused. The names for the institutions vary: extended-care facility or campus or senior health care centre. The term *nursing home* is used less frequently. The facility must be approved for skilled nursing, although it may have both skilled and intermediate care levels for residents.

The extended-care facility may serve as a transitional stop between hospital and home (generally for those over 65); in some cases, however, the stay is permanent.

The goals of the modern-day facility are to provide supervision by a physician, 24-hour nursing services, hospital affiliation, written client care policies, and specialized services in dietary, restorative, pharmaceutical, diagnostic, and social services. Unfortunately, these are sometimes hollow goals, even though the physical plant is new, licensing is current, and government funds are being used. Often the homes are

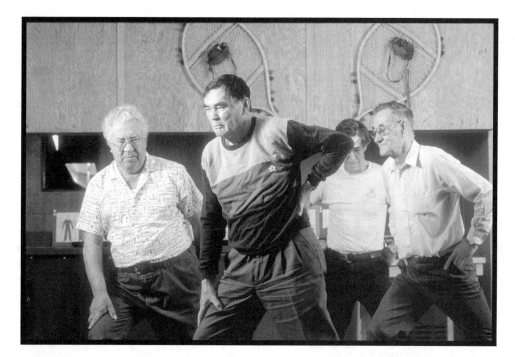

FIGURE 14–5

Adult daycare centres offer meals, nutritional counselling, mental health services, exercise classes, physical therapy, and social activities to elders.

Source: Berger, K.J., and M.B. Williams, Fundamentals of Nursing: Collaborating for Optimal Health. *Stamford, CT: Appleton and Lange, 1992, p. 1717.*

operated for profit by those outside the nursing or medical profession. The residents are not always physically or mentally able to protest if care is poor, and often families of the residents do not monitor the care. Exposure of blatant neglect in some of the facilities has awakened public and government consciousness; perhaps this exposure will correct the most glaring problems and alert other facilities to their obligation to follow prescribed goals. If standards are met, the nursing home provides an excellent and needed service to society because the elderly must be discharged from expensive acute care hospital beds as soon as possible. Prolonged hospitalization can foster confusion, helplessness, and the hazards of immobility. Further, some elderly persons cannot care for themselves. There are ways to individualize care, give holistic care, and prevent neglect or abuse of residents in long-term care settings.[687,688]

Selecting a Care Facility. When you help the family or senior select a nursing home, the following questions should be asked:

- What type of home is it, and what is its licensure status?
- What are the total costs, and what is included for the money?
- Is the physical plant adequate, clean, and pleasant? How much space and furniture are allowed for each person?
- What safety features are evident? Are fire drills held?
- What types of care are offered (both acute and chronic)?
- What is the staff-to-resident ratio? What are the qualifications of the staff? What are staff attitudes toward the elderly?

- What are the physician services? Is a complete physical examination given periodically?
- What therapies are available?
- Are pharmacy services available?
- Are meals nutritionally sound and the food tasty?
- Is food refrigerated, prepared, distributed, and served under sanitary conditions? Is eating supervised or assisted?
- Are visitors welcomed warmly?
- Are residents aware of their Bill of Rights? (For example, see the box entitled "Bill of Rights for Residents of Extended-Care Facilities."[689])
- Do residents appear content and appropriately occupied? (Observe on successive days and at different hours.) Are they treated with dignity and warmth by staff? Is privacy afforded during personal care?
- Has the local Better Business Bureau received any complaints about this facility?
- Does the administrator have a current licence?
- Is the home certified to participate in government or other programs that provide financial assistance when needed?
- Is an ombudsman available to investigate complaints of residents or family?

Bill of Rights for Residents of Extended-Care Facilities

The Bill of Rights is available for the people who live in Ontario long-term care facilities.

Assisted Living

Assisted living is a *residential and social-model* that is an *alternative to the medical model of institutionalization.* The living arrangement is for people who are frail or have physical limitations that necessitate help with care beyond the home health care model. The elder who lives alone, needs help with care, is lonely and feels isolated, may choose this option. Assisted living is staffed with a registered nurse (RN) and other levels of care providers.

The services typically offered in a nursing home are offered in a residential setting, at a lower cost. A comprehensive social, functional, and Medicare assessment is obtained. The RN starts the flow of resources, delegating care to professionals from various disciplines. The resident is to have independence, individuality, choice, privacy, dignity, and greater control over life than would be possible in long-term care. There is not the confinement to one room. There is a choice about activities. Transportation to outside events and shopping is available. This setting, just like the long-term care setting, also requires an ombudsman or consumer protection advocate to assure the original intent is maintained.[690,691]

Life Lease

Life lease is a unique housing option for mature adults and seniors. A life lease project provides an opportunity to purchase an interest in the project and to "share" in any appreciated value of the building and property.[692]

Translocation

The elderly person who is moved to a nursing home or long-term care facility (often rest-of-the-lifetime care facility) or who is moved from one room to another within the same facility undergoes a crisis called **translocation syndrome**, *physical and emotional deterioration as a result of changes or movement.* A move may be made because of changes in health, in staffing, or in the residents or because families desire it. Such a move may be life threatening, however.

People at greater risk are those who are depressed, highly anxious, severely ill, intermittently confused, or over 85 years of age. People who need structure, who cannot stand changes, or who deny problems or feelings are also more likely to experience difficulty.

Reducing relocation's impact begins with enlisting the resident's understanding of the need for the move and participation. The person should be prepared for the move. When he or she can make decisions about the move and predict what will happen, the person maintains a sense of control, which diminishes the move's impact. Moving to a similar environment also reduces the problems. The ability to express fears, concerns, and anger helps. If the person to be moved to an institution is relatively young, has good morale, and has an opportunity to select and then feel satisfied with the new surroundings, the translocation syndrome may be minimum.

One way to reduce the crisis of admission to a nursing home or long-term care centre or to reduce translocation shock is to have preschool or school children visit in the home. Both generations benefit from the exchange of affection. The youngsters bring stimulation to the elderly generation; the older generation can demonstrate stability, wisdom, and coping with adversities, and the qualities of ego integrity.

Taking one's frail loved one to a nursing home is not easy at that point in life when he or she can no longer care for self and home, at that point when the person has lost about everything that was precious and gave life meaning. Many family members have given poignant accounts of the pain for the elder and for the family and how the elder works to retain personal integrity and dignity despite the emotional assault.

Remotivation

Remotivation is one form of group therapy that can be conducted in a hospital, extended-care facility, elder daycare, or senior centre for disengaged or regressed elderly. The goal of this therapy is to remotivate the unwounded areas in the personality of the older adult. It can be used by the average employee—nurse or ancillary—who is closest to the client or

---

NARRATIVE VIGNETTE
New Horizons

Mr. and Mrs S are now 75 and 73 years old, respectively, and they have moved to an assisted-living facility where you are the nurse. Their health conditions have not changed significantly in the last two years, except that Mrs. S. now has more difficulty walking because of her arthritis. Mr. and Mrs. S recently moved to the facility because they needed help with transportation, and wanted to live in a place where they had fewer responsibilities and more time to enjoy life. Mrs. S has become tearful and says she has been disappointed in their move from their own home. She says, "Now we have the time to enjoy our life together, but we seem to be in each other's way all the time. When we lived in our own home, we were so busy with yard and housekeeping and all

the daily chores, we never had time to think about what we enjoy together. Now I don't have to cook meals and worry about getting to the grocery store, but we aren't enjoying the time we have together."

1. How do you respond to Mrs. S. when she shares this concern with you?

2. What activities will you suggest for her?

3. What are the strengths of this family?

4. What health promotion strategies can you develop based on those strengths?

5. Is there a problem here that needs your help, or will it just "go away"?

resident. It is designed to stimulate self-respect, self-reliance, and self-esteem in the older person who has become disengaged.[693–695] It encourages the person to focus attention on the simple, objective aspects of everyday life.

The method consists of a series of meetings, usually of about 12 clients, led by a person who has been trained in the technique. The sessions last about an hour. The leader guides the group through five steps:[696–698]

1. Creating a climate of acceptance by greeting each person by name, making them welcome, and making remarks that encourage replies, such as comments on the weather or a familiar incident.

2. Creating a bridge to the world by relating a current event or referring to a topic of general interest. (Each client is encouraged to comment.)

3. Sharing the world we live in, expanding step 2 through the use of appropriate visual aids.

4. Appreciating the work of the world through discussion of jobs, how goods are produced, how jobs are done, or the type of work the clients have done in the past.

5. Creating a climate of acceptance by showing pleasure in their attendance and speaking of plans for the next meeting.

Remotivation increases communication and strengthens contact with everyday features of the world for the person who may still have areas of intact personality. You may use remotivation technique as an adjunct to other interventions.

Group Action among Older Citizens

Interest in civic, social, political, and economic issues is shown in various action groups that have been organized among older citizens through community projects.

Older persons can help isolated elderly persons in their community. A survey of community services can determine which services are most and least used, which are inadequate, what changes are needed, and what sort of problems the elderly in the area have to face. In one community a one-to-one visiting service was needed; it brought joy and met needs of the isolated elderly. It also provided the elderly visitors with a sense of independence, social acceptability, recognition, status, and a sense of meaning in their lives at a time when losses of one sort or another had left them vulnerable.

Action groups have been formed in many major cities in recent years. Their members are elderly persons who are concerned about the needs of their peers and who believe that group action is effective in bringing about legislative change, especially in the area of financial assistance to meet rising costs. Many of these groups have exerted a considerable influence on federal and local planning. Such issues as tax relief, transportation, health care, and nutrition are of vital interest to many concerned elderly citizens who still feel responsible for themselves and their community.

You may have the opportunity to work with action groups in either an advisory, consultative, or direct participation role.

Retirement Communities

Retirement brings many changes, which are discussed by several authors.[699–710] Along with our increased life span and the development of social planning for retirement has come the emergence of a distinct social phenomenon: the retirement apartment complex community.

Apartment complexes are financed privately, by religious organizations, or by the government. The senior must be able to maintain self, although visiting nurse services are acceptable. These complexes may include a central dining room, a nurse and doctor on call, planned social events, transportation services, and religious services. Essentially all living needs are within easy access. Additionally, the seniors have the company of each other if they so desire.

In many cities, hotels have been converted to residence facilities for the elderly. Reminiscent of old-style rooming houses, they provide more supervision and services, such as meals, laundry facilities, and shopping. In most of these residences each person is responsible for his or her own room, laundry, and breakfast.

Many couples opt for continuous care facilities. One- or two-bedroom apartments or cottages are available for a one-time endowment and a monthly fee for two persons. Services include one meal a day, maid service, all utilities including local telephone bill, full maintenance, a full recreational and social program, and many extras. The residents have at their disposal a fully equipped health centre with 24-hour nursing care service as long as needed in the intermediate or long-term care sections of the nursing home facility.

In many regions of the United States, especially in Florida, the desert Southwest, and California, planned communities have been built that are specifically designed for and restricted to those persons over 55. Some are carefully planned miniature cities of low cost with simply designed homes built around clubhouse activities, golf courses, and swimming and therapy pools. Activities such as bingo games, dance instruction, foreign-language study, crafts, and bridge lessons are offered. Other communities are mobile home parks in which often elaborate coaches cost as much as and are set up as permanent homes.

One sociologic aspect of these communities bearing such names as Sun City, Leisure World, and Carefree Village is the lifestyle adopted by the residents as they try to establish a secure base in a new life that is often far removed from family, former friends, and familiar patterns of living. They show concern for the safety, health, and well-being of each other by watching to see that lights are on at accustomed hours in each other's homes, signifying all is well. Celebration of birthdays with special parties and remembrances, entertaining for visiting friends and relatives of one's neighbours, visiting the sick members, and providing food and transportation to the hospital for the spouse of a sick resident all become part of the new life. The residents participate in activities that either are completely new or have not been indulged in for many years, such as golf, bicycle riding, hiking, and dancing. Even clothes become brighter for both sexes, and the popularity of casual dress provides for the members of the snowbird set—those who have moved to a warm climate—a new freedom and a chance to try bright colours and styles they may not have worn in a former setting.

This phenomenon gives you insight into the needs for security, a sense of maximum personal effectiveness and belonging, and a feeling of self-actualization, especially when old patterns are put aside either by choice or because of circumstances mediated by health or socioeconomic conditions. Further, the older adult needs a suitable place to live, supportive relationships a sense of community, financial security, and a sense of setting and achieving goals.

Discuss the information in the box entitled "Guidelines for Selecting a Retirement Community" with elders and their families.

Effect of the Able Elderly

The emergence of a population group identified as the well elderly is the result of social and demographic progress in the industrial world. More people are living longer, and poverty, frailty, and dependence are not the common characteristics of most of these older people. In the future there will be more healthy elderly who are better educated and physically and emotionally capable. Our society can already use the elderly population's capabilities; in the future we shall have a rich human resource in larger numbers.

The elderly often give financial support and other kinds of assistance to their younger family members; most old people are not a drain on the family. An aging society offers expanding opportunities for family life. Four types of new potentials are present because of recent demographic change: (1) increased complexity of social networks, (2) increased duration of relationships, (3) prolonged opportunities to accumulate experience, and (4) new chances to complete or change role assignments.

The elder's accumulated shared experience builds family bonds but also helps others deal with a changing historical context. As the elder leaves certain roles behind, he or she can pick up new ones—whether as a grandparent; in a second career; as an activist in the political, social, or community arena; as a decision maker; as an advocate for ethical and moral actions; or as a participant in policy making or creative pursuits in the arts. Well elderly are and will be making contributions to society; it is important to perceive the well older person as a contributing resource.

Outlook for the Future

The current generation of older persons is where we shall all be one day; therefore, planning for them is planning for all of us. Areas such as health care delivery, distribution of income over a long life span, sustaining adequate social involvement, coping with organizational systems, and use of leisure are all problems of now and the future. Intervention that seems costly now may be, in the long run, the most economical in terms of tax dollars.

In the face of increasing shortages that raise the cost of living and the change in age and sex distribution by that time, future planning for the elderly will include employment and the attendant problems usually associated with younger persons. Our society will need the experience and wisdom of the senior generation. If persons are employed as late as age 75, health maintenance programs, industrial planning, and awareness of safety needs are a few of the necessary considerations.

For the older, less active persons of the future, Burnside[711] suggests intervening in loneliness through listening, exploring what may be significant to the seniors, and helping them to compensate in some way for personal losses. In addition, she suggests that nurses record the experiences of the elderly for posterity. Day schools for the elderly might encourage research projects, family therapy, and the study of successful aging.

Thus you, the professional of the future, will be challenged to be the innovator. You will be called on to devise and use new treatment methods so that the elderly will function more effectively in society. It is your goal to help them:

1. Use the potential they have developed throughout life.
2. Pass through the years of late maturity with ego intact and satisfying memories.
3. Leave something of their philosophy for posterity.

HEALTH CARE AND NURSING APPLICATIONS

Assessment and Nursing Diagnoses

Your role in caring for the elderly person or couple has been described throughout the chapter. Assessment, using knowledge presented about normal aging changes versus pathology in the elderly, provides the basis for *nursing diagnoses*. Use the box entitled "Selected Nursing Diagnoses Related to Persons in Later Adulthood."

Guidelines for Selecting a Retirement Community

- Check climate and cultural and recreational facilities in relation to your preferences and lifestyle.
- Visit the facility; talk with residents; eat a meal. Is it an active, lively community?
- Call regulators, Chamber of Commerce, and Better Business Bureau to check track record of the developer or owner(s).
- Ask what insurance or bonding instruments will protect you in case the facility experiences financial difficulty. Get copies.
- Review all documents you are asked to sign and seek competent legal advice before signing.
- Ask about lease termination policies. How much notice must the owner give? What are the refund policies?
- Get terms of the deposit in writing. If it is refundable, how and at what percentage? Will interest be applied; if so, at what rate?
- Determine if monthly fees are tied to an index. If so, which one? Ask for a history of increases to date, and check the index at a library.
- If it is a lifetime or continuing care community, are nursing home costs prepaid? If not, what are the additional costs?
- Ask about restrictions and policies about visitors (overnight, for how long), parking a recreational vehicle, parking more than one car, and use of facilities by visitors.
- Take your time to decide. Visit different facilities.

Selected Nursing Diagnoses Related to Persons in Later Adulthood

Pattern 1: Exchanging

Altered Nutrition: More than Body Requirements
Altered Nutrition: Less than Body Requirements
Hypothermia
Hyperthermia
Risk for Constipation
Stress Incontinence
Risk for Fluid Volume Imbalance
Risk for Injury
Risk for Trauma
Risk for Disuse Syndrome
Impaired Skin-Integrity
Altered Dentition
Energy Field Disturbance

Pattern 2: Communicating

Impaired Verbal Communication

Pattern 3: Relating

Impaired Social Interaction
Social Isolation
Risk for Loneliness
Altered Role Performance
Sexual Dysfunction
Altered Family Processes
Caregiver Role Strain
Altered Sexuality Patterns

Pattern 4: Valuing

Spiritual Distress
Potential for Enhanced Spiritual Well-Being

Pattern 5: Choosing

Ineffective Individual Coping
Impaired Adjustment
Defensive Coping
Ineffective Denial
Ineffective Family Coping: Disabling
Ineffective Family Coping: Compromised
Family Coping: Potential for Growth
Potential for Enhanced Community Coping

Decisional Conflict
Health-Seeking Behaviours

Pattern 6: Moving

Impaired Physical Mobility
Fatigue
Risk for Activity Intolerance
Sleep Pattern Disturbance
Diversional Activity Deficit
Impaired Home Maintenance Management
Altered Health Maintenance
Bathing/Hygiene Self-Care Deficit
Dressing/Grooming Self-Care Deficit
Toileting Self-Care Deficit
Relocation Stress Syndrome

Pattern 7: Perceiving

Body Image Disturbance
Self-Esteem Disturbance
Chronic Low Self-Esteem
Situational Low Self-Esteem
Sensory/Perceptual Alterations
Unilateral Neglect
Hopelessness
Powerlessness

Pattern 8: Knowing

Knowledge Deficit
Acute Confusion
Altered Thought Processes
Impaired Memory

Pattern 9: Feeling

Pain
Chronic Pain
Dysfunctional Grieving
Anticipatory Grieving
Risk for Violence: Self-Directed
Post-Trauma Syndrome
Anxiety
Death Anxiety
Fear

Other of the NANDA diagnoses related to physiologic phenomena are applicable to the ill individual in this group.

Source: North American Nursing Diagnosis Association, NANDA Nursing Diagnoses: Definitions & Classification 1999–2000. *Philadelphia: North American Nursing Diagnosis Association, 1999.*

CRITICAL THINKING

Design several wellness diagnoses for the older adult and his or her family.

Interventions

Interventions may involve direct care, use of verbal and non-verbal skills, availability of self and therapeutic relationship, support, counselling, education, spiritual care, use of remotivation techniques, or referral as you assist the person in later maturity to meet physical, emotional, cognitive, spiritual, or social needs.

You represent a whole cluster of psychological potentials for the elderly person; you become the supportive figure, interpreter of the unknown, symbol of the people close to him or her, and possessor of important secrets or privileged information. You become guide and companion. All this occurs if an empathic regard for the elderly person is reflected in your attitude and actions, even though your initial image of him or her may have been that of punitive parent. Of prime importance is your willingness to listen, explain, orient, reassure, and comfort the elderly person. Your role is crucial, for you are the one who is most likely to maintain personal contact with the client either in an institutional setting or in a community agency.

Involve the person's family if possible. The interest of a family member does much to increase motivation on the part of the elderly. Determine family attitudes and evaluate relationships during teaching-learning or visiting sessions at which the family is present. This procedure helps the family members alter their attitudes to a more realistic acceptance of their relative's health needs. Social support of family and friends is critical for maintaining lifestyle behaviours, emotional and physical health, and coping skills, including for the frail elderly.[712–715]

The *cognitive and emotional needs of the elderly person can be met in many ways:*

1. Ensure an adequate environmental conditions to overcome sensory impairment.
2. Use clear communication, including explanations of procedures and the necessity for them.
3. Use demonstration and written instructions along with the verbal message, divided into small units, for teaching skills related to self-care.
4. Combine explanations with practice sessions.
5. Organize information so that content is logically grouped and sequential, when a larger amount of data is given.
6. Indicate how and when the essential information is relevant to the person's needs, interests, and life experience. He or she is likely to recall this information when necessary.
7. Plan for a new task to overlap with the execution of a previous one and allow the older person to work slowly and with care.
8. Simulate the real situation as much as possible so that essential steps of the task can be clearly perceived and the teaching can be adapted to the individual's pattern and ability.
9. Allow the person ample time to respond to a task.
10. Convey an understanding attitude to prevent discouragement and depression.

As in all communication, false assurance can only inhibit the person's ability to develop a trusting attitude and suggest paternalism. The display of genuine interest and a receptive attitude will show the older person that he or she is not alone and will help immeasurably in allaying fear. Candour helps decrease anxiety, and the person's fear of death, the dark, or the unknown may be overcome to a great degree through your presence.

Encourage the senior to *reminisce and do life review,* through discussion or use of photographs, music, or literature. Ask questions about his or her early years, work experience, family, special events, travel, hobbies, and treasured objects. Listen as the person shares life philosophy and gives counsel.

Loneliness is an outgrowth of age-related losses and psychological changes in the elderly. It implies a need to assess carefully situations to determine the signs as described in the following case study:

> An elderly man living alone made no complaint of loneliness, but the astute community health nurse found his home in deplorable untidiness and unsafe clutter, his diet extremely limited, and his personal hygiene poor. After a homemaker was sent in to help him clean the house, sit with him during meals, and provide a chance for a trusting relationship with another person, he became receptive to suggestions for modifying his living habits and eventually began to visit a senior-citizen group regularly and to make new friends. He came to realize that adaptation to isolation had been unsafe. Interest and patience showed by others restored the feeling of being a valued and accepted human being again.

The authors know of other individuals who would not modify living habits but chose to remain (from a health care viewpoint) in unsafe and unsanitary conditions. Yet instead of giving the person up as a "hopeless case," the nurses continued to foster a relationship of trust, listened to reasons for remaining in the present situation, and helped the person live out the remaining life on his or her own terms.

Help the elderly person to remain in contact with the environment by providing devices such as clocks, watches, and calendars and letting him or her be the one who winds the clock and turns the calendar page each day. If a hearing aid is worn, check its effectiveness. Sudden moves, even within the same institution, increase mortality rates and psychological and physical deterioration. The person should be permitted to remain in familiar territory and with the desired clutter. If a move is essential, he or she should have some choice in the decision, an opportunity to keep valued possessions, and time to adjust to the idea. The person needs to have a personal lounging chair or specific place

EVIDENCE-BASED PRACTICE

Positive Aspects of Caregiving: Rounding Out the Caregiving Experience

The negative consequences of caregiving have been clearly documented and include caregiver depression, poor perceived health, and increased risk of mortality. Recent research has tried to further elaborate the meaning of caregiving by examining not only the negative consequences of caregiving but also those seen as positive by the caregivers themselves. Four reasons have been emphasized for exploring these positive psychological factors: (1) caregivers want to talk about them, (2) clinicians will be assisted in knowing what works most effectively, (3) knowing these will be an important determinant of quality care provided to older adults, and (4) the need to enhance the theory in this area. The "satisfactions of caregiving" have been conceptualized into three dimensions: (1) satisfactions derived mainly from the interpersonal dynamic between carer and cared-for persons, (2) satisfactions derived mainly from the intrapersonal or intrapsychic orientation of the carer, and (3) satisfactions deriving mainly from a desire to promote a positive or avoid a negative outcome for the recipient. The study focused on 289 caregivers who were caring for someone residing in the community.

Results

The majority of caregivers were women (68.5%). Spouses comprised 34.3% of the sample. The mean age of the recipients was 84.4 years with a range of 71 to 100. The caregivers' ages ranged from 29 to 96, with a mean age of 64 years. Almost half (49.1%) were offspring of the care recipient, and 46.4% lived with the recipient.

Two hundred and eleven (73%) of the caregivers said they could find one positive aspect of caregiving, and an additional 6.9% could identify more than one. In terms of specific positive aspects of caregiving, 65 (22.5%) mentioned companionship; 63 (21.8%) fulfilling/rewarding; 37 (12.8%)

enjoyment; 30 (10.4%) duty/obligations; 21 (7.3%) provide quality of life; 17 (5.9%) meaningful/important; 16 (5.5%) love people; 1 (0.3%) likes making decisions, and 3 (1%) other. On a seven-point scale rating overall feelings of caring, 88 (30.4%) gave the happiest rating and 210 (72.7%) rated within the top three ratings.

Practice Implications

1. Because positive feelings about caretaking were significantly related to the negative consequences of caregiving (caregiver depression, burden, and self-assessed health), clinicians should be asking about positive aspects of caring if they want to understand the caregiver experience and assist caregivers.

2. Satisfactions can be used as a quality control measure or indicator to determine if services are meeting carer needs.

3. When carers feel that only they can provide the appropriate care or that companionship is very important to them, they may refuse to allow others to assist with care. Therefore asking more specifically about satisfactions of caring may help to identify carers who will be more difficult to link to services and may be helpful in clarifying which services will be most acceptable to caregivers.

4. Satisfactions of caring might be helpful as a "risk" indicator. Caregivers who cannot identify any positive aspects of caring may be at a particular risk for depression and poor health outcomes. They also may be more at risk of institutionalizing their care recipient earlier than others.

5. Clinicians should consider incorporating the feelings about caring measure used in this study as a quick screen in their caregiver assessments. By doing so they are more likely to improve their understanding of the caregiving experience and target interventions more appropriately.

Source: Cohen, C.A., A. Colantonio, and L. Vernich, Positive Aspects of Caregiving: Rounding Out the Caregiver Experience, International Journal of Geriatric Psychiatry, 17, (2002), 184–188. Reproduced by permission of John Wiley & Sons Limited.

---

in the dining room. Room furniture should be arranged for physical safety and emotional security. Privacy must be respected.

Darkness is a cause of confusion. Night-lights should be left on and call bell, tissues, and water placed within easy reach. In the hospital room contact should be available to the client through frequent, quietly made rounds at night. Sometimes a client remains oriented more easily if the room door is open so that he or she can see the nurses' station and be reassured of not being alone.

The *use of touch* is very beneficial, for the older person has little physical contact with others. The need for contact comfort is great in the human organism, and you can satisfy

this need to a degree, provided you remember that touch is a language and has a special power. In giving medications, physical care, and treatments, touching is a crucial encounter. Often the person will pay close attention to instructions and cooperate more in his or her care when you use touch on the hand or shoulder while speaking. The success of this aid depends on what your hands are saying.

To the elderly, all things connected with *food service* have psychological implications. Food represents life; it nurtures. Mealtime is thought of as a time of fellowship with others and a sharing of pleasure, and this attitude should be retained as much as possible for older people. Making the food more attractive, talking with the person, comforting and touching, cajoling if need be, may help, especially if food is being refused. Appetizers and special drinks have been successfully used as an aid to therapy.

During any crisis in which the organism is under stress, there are several alternatives: exhaustion, recuperation through the help of others, or despondency and dependency. You and the elder may *work toward resolution of the crisis.* Share the following suggestions with the person:

- Acknowledge the sadness, anger, guilt, and other feelings that are a part of the loss. It is not a sign of weakness to have those feelings.
- Allow self to express the feelings; cry alone or talk and cry with someone who is understanding. If you have always been stoic, it is all right to show feelings. Others may feel more comfortable with you.
- Indulge self constructively. Feelings of fatigue, confusion, and even depression occur with grief. Pay attention to basic needs of nutrition, sleep, and exercise. Do something pleasurable for yourself. Resist artificial consolers such as alcohol, sleeping pills, other drugs, and cigarettes.
- Ask for support and accept it. Determine wishes, needs, and wants. It is all right to ask for help. You have done your share of nurturing; now is your time to allow others to help you.
- Say "No" to major stressors. Take your time in making major decisions. Do not undertake too many life-changing events at once.
- Move beyond regret—the "if only" or "I should have." Do what is needed in the situation. Learn from mistakes. Forgive self and others.
- Affirm your power to heal the wounds. Life will not be the same after a loss; however, life can go on. Talk to others. Call forth inner reserves and spiritual strength. Imagine the person is present. State aloud or in a letter or tape to the person that which was left unsaid.
- Focus memory on the valued or favourite times, the happy scenes, and the pleasant instead of the disease, death, or the traumatic.

The fine line between independence and dependence is difficult to maintain with clients of any age, but especially in the elderly because of society's view of them. Expectations of those around us generally foster behaviour to match. Conflict between independent and dependent feelings can be avoided, usually first by assuming a firm control based on professional competence and then later by relaxing and allowing the client to emancipate self.

Working with the elderly person is very rewarding if you are able to suspend youth-directed attitudes and not measure the person against standards that are inappropriate and perhaps too demanding. As with other age groups and in all our relationships, acceptance of the other person as he or she is, not as you wish him or her to be, is extremely important.

INTERESTING WEBSITES

HEALTH CANADA'S PHYSICAL ACTIVITY UNIT FOR OLDER ADULTS

http://www.hc-sc.gc.ca/hppb/paguide/older
This guide serves as a roadmap for older adults—explaining why physical activity is important, offering tips and easy ways to increase their physical activity, and stating how much is needed to maintain good health and improved quality of living later in life.

NATIONAL CLEARINGHOUSE ON FAMILY VIOLENCE PUBLICATION: ABUSE AND NEGLECT OF OLDER ADULTS

http://www.hc-sc.gc.ca/hppb/familyviolence/html/agenegl_e.html
This fact sheet provides information on abuse and neglect of older adults living in the community. The information will be of greatest interest to professionals and community service providers.

SENIORS CANADA ONLINE

http://www.seniors.gc.ca/scolPortSearchScreen.jsp?lang=en
This is Canada's trusted source of seniors-related information on the Internet. Seniors Canada Online provides single-window access to Web-based information and services that are relevant to seniors, their families, caregivers, and supporting service organizations.

NATIONAL FRAMEWORK ON AGING

http://www.phac-aspc.gc.ca/seniors-aines/nfa-cnv/index_e.htm
The National Framework on Aging is a conceptual tool useful in guiding current and future policy and program development. Designed to address the priorities of seniors and to assist policymakers in reviewing proposed policy changes, the NFA reflects the changing demographic reality of a maturing Canadian society.

SUMMARY

1. Later adulthood spans many years; thus, the era is divided into young-old, mid-old, and old-old (or frail-old). Certainly the person at age 90 or 100 is different from the 70-year-old.
2. No theory of aging fully explains older adulthood.
3. Numerous changes occur over the life span; yet the person maintains many characteristics and abilities typical of the younger years.
4. Generally, the older person is more adaptive and able than is expressed in attitudes of ageism and stereotypes.
5. There are more well elders and more older adults living longer.

Considerations for the Elderly Client in Health Care

- Personal history
- Family ties; family history; widow(er)
- Cultural history
- Current responsibilities with a spouse or other family members
- Impact of physiologic changes on functional status and activities of daily living
- Behaviours or appearance that indicate person is being abused or neglected
- Implementation of safety measures, immunizations, and health practices
- Pre-existing illness
- Risk factors, past or current measures used to reduce or prevent them
- Current illness
- Behaviours that indicate age-appropriate cognitive status; ability to manage own affairs
- Behaviours that indicate age-appropriate emotional status, including ego integrity instead of self-despair, and moral-spiritual development
- Behaviours that indicate that retirement and losses that occur in late life have been grieved and integrated into the self-concept and life patterns
- Satisfactory living arrangements
- Involvement in the community to the extent possible
- Behavioural patterns that indicate adult has achieved development tasks

6. Older adults will continue to contribute to society and their contributions will be needed.
7. Well elders will have an increasing influence on their communities and local, provincial, and national legislation.
8. Because of the increasing number of older adults, a wider variety of resources will be needed and implemented.
9. Some changes may be the result of disease, rather than the aging process, and should be prevented or treated.
10. The box entitled "Considerations for the Elderly Client in Health Care" summarizes what you should consider in assessment and health promotion of the elderly.

ENDNOTES

1. Andrews, M., and J. Boyle, *Transcultural Concepts in Nursing Care* (3rd ed.). Philadelphia: Lippincott, 1999.
2. Bee, H., *Lifespan Development* (2nd ed.). New York: Longman, 1998.
3. *Ibid.*
4. *Ibid.*
5. Ebersole, P., and P. Hess, *Toward Health Aging: Human Needs and Nursing*
6. Gormly, A., *Lifespan Human Development* (6th ed.). Fort Worth, TX: Harcourt Brace College Publishers, 1997.
7. Papalia, D., and S. Olds, *Human Development* (3rd ed.). Boston: McGraw Hill, 1998.
8. Seifert, K., R. Hoffnung, and M. Hoffnung, *Lifespan Development.* Boston: Houghton Mifflin, 1997.
9. Sigelman, C., *Life-Span Human Development* (3rd ed.). Pacific Grove, CA: Brooks/Cole, 1998.
10. Settersen, R., and Hagestad, G., What's the Latest? Cultural Age Deadlines for Family Transitions, *The Gerontologist,* 36, no. 2 (1996), 178–188.
11. American Psychiatric Association, *Diagnostic and Statistical Manual of Mental Disorders* (4th ed.). Washington, DC: American Psychiatric Association, 1994.
12. *Ibid.*
13. Ebersole and Hess, *op. cit.*
14. Bee, *op. cit.*
15. Lookinland, S., and K. Anson, Perpetuation of Ageism Attitudes Among Present and Future Health Care Personnel: Implications for Elder Care, *Journal of Advanced Nursing,* 21, no. 1 (1995), 47–56.
16. Rohan, E., B. Berkman, S. Walker, and W. Holmes, The Geriatric Oncology Patient: Ageism in Social Work Practice, *Journal of Gerontology: Social Work,* 23, no. 1/2 (1994), 201–221.
17. Seifert et al., *op. cit.*
18. Elsner, R., M. Quinn, S. Fanning, S. Cueldner, and L. Poon, Ethical and Policy Considerations for Centenarians: The Oldest Old, *IMAGE: Journal of Nursing Scholarship,* 31, no. 3 (1999), 263–267.
19. Bee, *op. cit.*
20. Seifert et al., *op. cit.*
21. Kaufert, P. A., and M. Lock, 1997. Medicalization of women's third age, *Journal of Psychosomatic Obstetrics and Gynaecology,* 18, 81–86.
22. Hummert, M., T. Garstka, J. Shaner, and S. Strahm, Stereotypes of the Elderly Held by Young, Middle-aged, and Elderly Adults, *Journal of Gerontology: Psychological Sciences,* 49 (1994), P240–P249
23. Ebersole and Hess, *op. cit.*
24. Gormly, *op. cit.*
25. Papalia and Olds, *op. cit.*
26. Seifert et al., *op. cit.*
27. Sigelman, *op. cit.*
28. Ebersole and Hess, *op. cit.*
29. *Ibid.*
30. Edelman, C., and C. Mandle, *Health Promotion Throughout the Lifespan* (3rd ed.). St. Louis: C. V. Mosby, 1994.
31. Emerg, C., F. Huppert, and R. Schein, Relationships among Age, Exercise, Health, and Cognitive Function in a British Sample, *The Gerontologist,* 35 (1995), 378–384.
32. Ebersole and Hess, *op. cit.*
33. *Ibid.*
34. *Ibid.*
35. *Ibid.*
36. *Ibid.*
37. *Ibid.*
38. Newman, B., and P. Newman, *Development Through Life: A Psychosocial Approach* (7th ed.). Belmont, CA: Brooks/Cole, 1999.
39. *Ibid.*
40. *Ibid.*
41. Ebersole and Hess, *op. cit.*
42. Edelman and Mandle, *op. cit.*
43. Ebersole and Hess, *op. cit.*
44. *Ibid.*
45. Roos, N., and B. Havens, Predictors of Successful Aging: A 12 Year Study of Manitoba Elderly, *American Journal of Public Health,* 81, no. 1 (1991), 63–68.
46. Becker, G., The Oldest Old: Autonomy in the Face of Frailty, *Journal of Aging Studies,* 8 (1994), 59–76.
47. Bowling, A., and E. Grundy, Activities of Daily Living: Changes in Functional Ability in Three Samples of Elderly and Very Elderly People, *Age and Aging,* 26 (1997), 107–114.
48. Laws, G., Understanding Ageism: Lessons From Feminism and Postmodernism, *The Gerontologist,* 35 (1995), 112–118.

49. Papalia and Olds, *op. cit.*
50. Beattie, E., Long-Term Care for the Elderly in Australia, *IMAGE: Journal of Nursing Scholarship,* 31, no. 2 (1999), 134–135.
51. de Barros, A., Long-Term Care for Elders in Brazil, *IMAGE: Journal of Nursing Scholarship,* 31, no. 2 (1999), 135–136.
52. Dickerson, A., and A. Fisher, Culture Relevant Functional Performance Assessment of the Hispanic Elderly, *Occupational Therapy Journal of Research,* 15, no. 1 (1995), 50–68.
53. Manion, P., J. Specht, L. Sitler, et al., Family Involvement in Care Intervention: Comparison of Effects for Caucasian and African-American Family Caregivers, *District Three Profile: Missouri Nurse Association,* 42, no. 1 (1998), 3.
54. Pascucci, M.A., and G.L. Loving, Ingredients of an Old and Healthy Life: A Centenarian Perspective, *Journal of Holistic Nursing,* 15, (1997), 199–213.
55. Rowe, J.W., R.L., Kahn, Successful Aging. *The Gerontologist,* 37 (1997), 433–440.
56. Ruffing-Rahal, M., Individuation and Varieties of Well-Being Experience among Older Women. *Advances in Nursing Science,* 20 (1998), 13–20.
57. Tashiro, J., Long-Term Care for the Elderly in Japan, *IMAGE: Journal of Nursing Scholarship,* 31, no. 2 (1999), 133–134.
58. Uyer, G., Long-Term Care for the Elderly in Turkey, *IMAGE: Journal of Nursing Scholarship,* 31, no. 3 (1999), 136–137.
59. Andrews and Boyle, *op. cit.*
60. Browne, C., and A. Broderick, Asian and Pacific Island Elders: Issues for Social Work Practice and Education, *Social Work,* 39 (1994), 252–259.
61. Barusch, A.S., Self-Concepts of Low-Income Older Women: Not Old or Poor, but Fortunate and Blessed, *International Journal of Aging and Human Development,* 44 (1997), 269–282.
62. Barusch, *op. cit.*
63. Fenstermacher, K., and B. Hudson, *Practice Guidelines for Family Nurse Practitioners.* Philadelphia: Saunders, 1997.
64. Heidrich, S.M., Older Women's Lives through Time, *Advances in Nursing Science,* 20 (1998), 65–75.
65. Manion et al., *op. cit.*
66. Sigelman, *op. cit.*
67. Bee, *op. cit.*
68. Gormly, *op. cit.*
69. Longevity: Biology Isn't Destiny: But It's Part of It, *Harvard Health Letter,* 22, no. 6 (1997), 1–3.
70. Newman, B., and P. Newman, *Development Through Life: A Psychosocial Approach* (7th ed.). Belmont, CA: Brooks/Cole, 1999.
71. Papalia and Olds, *op. cit.*
72. Seifert et al., *op. cit.*
73. Sigelman, *op. cit.*
74. Longevity: Biology Isn't Destiny: But It's Part of It.
75. *Ibid.*
76. *Ibid.*
77. *Ibid.*
78. Depression Leads to Physical Decline in Older Men and Women, *Tufts University Health and Nutrition Letter,* 16, no. 7 (1998), 7.
79. Bee, *op. cit.*
80. Edelman and Mandle, *op. cit.*
81. Gormly, *op. cit.*
82. Longevity: Biology Isn't Destiny: But It's Part of It.
83. Papalia and Olds, *op. cit.*
84. Seifert et al., *op. cit.*
85. Sigelman, *op. cit.*
86. Ebersole and Hess, *op. cit.*
87. Gormly, *op. cit.*
88. Papalia and Olds, *op. cit.*
89. Sigelman, *op. cit.*
90. Gladstone, J., The Marital Perceptions of Elderly Persons Living in or Having a Spouse Living in a Long-term Care Institution in Canada, *The Gerontologist,* 35 (1995), 52–59.
91. Erikson, E. *Adulthood.* New York: W. W. Norton, 1978.
92. Peck, R. C., Psychological Development in the Second Half of Life, in B. Neugarten, ed., *Middle Age and Aging.* Chicago: University of Chicago Press, 1968.
93. Reed, P., Self-transcendence and Mental Health in Oldest-old Adults, *Nursing Research,* 40, no. 1 (1991), 5–11.
94. Havighurst, R., *Developmental Tasks and Education* (3rd ed.). New York: David McKay, 1972.
95. Levinson, D., A Theory of Life Structure Development in Adulthood, in K.N. Alexander and E.J. Langer, eds., *Higher Stages of Human Development.* New York: Oxford University Press, 1990, 35–54.
96. Sill, J., Disengagement Reconsidered: Awareness of Finitude, *The Gerontologist,* 20, no. 4 (1980), 457–462.
97. White, N., and W. Cunningham, Is Terminal Drop Pervasive or Specific? *Journal of Gerontology,* 43, no. 6 (1988), 141–144.
98. Bee, *op. cit.*
99. Gormly, *op. cit.*
100. Papalia and Olds, *op. cit.*
101. Seifert et al., *op. cit.*
102. Sigelman, *op. cit.*
103. Sheehy, G., *New Passages.* New York: Random House, 1995.
104. Erikson, *Adulthood.*
105. Peck, *op. cit.*
106. Mead, G., Mind, Self, and Society, in A. Strauss, ed., *George Herbert Mead: On Social Psychology.* Chicago: University of Chicago Press, 1964.
107. *Ibid.*
108. Brown, V., The Effects of Poverty Environments on Elders' Subjective Well-being. A Conceptual Model, *The Gerontologist,* 35 (1995), 541–548.
109. *Ibid.*
110. Anderson, L., and N. Stevens, Associations with Parents and Well-being in Old Age, *Journal of Gerontology: Psychological Sciences,* 48 (1993), P109–P118.
111. Papalia and Olds, *op. cit.*
112. Sigelman, *op. cit.*
113. Gormly, *op. cit.*
114. Pina, D., and V. Bengston, Division of Household Labour and the Well-being of Retirement-aged Wives, *The Gerontologist,* 35 (1995), 308–317.
115. Seifert et al., *op. cit.*
116. Ebersole and Hess, *op. cit.*
117. Gormly, *op. cit.*
118. Papalia and Olds, *op. cit.*
119. Seifert et al., *op. cit.*
120. Sigelman, *op. cit.*
121. Bee, *op. cit.*
122. Newman and Newman, *op. cit.*
123. Papalia and Olds, *op. cit.*
124. Bee, *op. cit.*
125. Gardner, J., et al., Grandparents' Beliefs Regarding Their Role and Relationship with Special Needs Grandchildren, *Education and Treatment of Children,* 17, no. 2 (1994), 185–196.
126. Edelman and Mandle, *op. cit.*
127. Papalia and Olds, *op. cit.*
128. Seifert et al., *op. cit.*
129. Sigelman, *op. cit.*
130. Callandro, G., and C. Hughes, The Experience of Being a Grandmother Who Is the Primary Caregiver for Her HIV-Positive Grandchild, *Nursing Research,* 47, no. 2 (1998), 107–113.
131. Menec, V., Chipperfield, and R. Perry, Self Perceptions of Health: A Prospective Analysis of Mortality, Control, and Health, *Journal of Gerontology: Psychological Sciences,* 54B, no. 2 (1999), 85–93.

132. Solomon, J., and J. Marx, "To Grandmother's House We Go": Health and School Adjustment of Children Raised Solely by Grandparents, *The Gerontologist,* 35, no. 3 (1995), 386–394.

133. Cooney, T., and L. Smith, Young Adults' Relations with Grandparents Following Recent Parental Divorce, *Journal of Gerontology: Social Sciences,* 51B, no. 2 (1996), S91–S95.

134. Bee, *op. cit.*

135. Gardner et al., *op. cit.*

136. Papalia and Olds, *op. cit.*

137. Newman and Newman, *op. cit.*

138. Papalia and Olds, *op. cit.*

139. Seifert et al., *op. cit.*

140. Solomon and Marx, *op. cit.*

141. Don't Fall For a Telephone Line, *Modern Maturity,* 40, no. 3 (1997), 83.

142. Reese, C., and R. Murray, Transcendence: The Meaning of Great-Grandmothering, *Archives of Psychiatric Nursing,* 10, no. 4 (1996), 245–251.

143. *Ibid.*

144. Collins, C.E., F.R. Butler, S.H. Gueldner, and M.H. Palmer, Models for Community-Based Long-Term Care for the Elderly in a Changing Health System. *Nursing Outlook,* 45 (1997), 59–63.

145. Bee, *op. cit.*

146. Newman and Newman, *op. cit.*

147. Papalia and Olds, *op. cit.*

148. Seifert et al., *op. cit.*

149. Thompson, E., A. Futterman, D. Gallagher-Thompson, J. Rose, and S. Lovett, Social Support and Caregiving Burden in Family Caregivers of Frail Elders, *Journal of Gerontology: Social Sciences,* 48, no. 5 (1995), S245–S254.

150. Bee, *op. cit.*

151. Papalia and Olds, *op. cit.*

152. Jackson, S.A., and M.B. Mittelmark, Unmet Needs for Formal Home and Community Services Among African-American and White Older Adults: The Forsyth County Aging Study. *The Journal of Applied Gerontology,* 16 (1997), 298–316.

153. Bee, *op. cit.*

154. Papalia and Olds, *op. cit.*

155. Bee, *op. cit.*

156. Papalia and Olds, *op. cit.*

157. Seifert et al., *op. cit.*

158. Bee, *op. cit.*

159. Papalia and Olds, *op. cit.*

160. Seifert et al., *op. cit.*

161. Bee, *op. cit.*

162. Boland, D., and S. Sims, Family Care Giving: Care at Home as a Solitary Journey, *IMAGE: Journal of Nursing Scholarship,* 28 (1996), 55–58.

163. Chang, B., Cognitive-Behavioral Interventions with Homebound Caregivers of Persons with Dementia, *Nursing Research,* 48, no. 3 (1999), 173–182.

164. Papalia and Olds, *op. cit.*

165. Picot, S., J. Zauszniewski, S. Debanne, and E. Holston, Mood and Blood Pressure Responses in Black Female Caregivers and Non-caregivers, *Nursing Research,* 48, no. 3 (1999), 150–161.

166. Roberts, J., et al., Problem-Solving Counseling for Caregivers of the Cognitively Impaired: Effective for Whom? *Nursing Research,* 48, no. 3 (1999), 162–172.

167. Seifert et al., *op. cit.*

168. Kart, S., E.K. Metress, and S. Metress, *Human Aging and Chronic Disease.* Boston/London: Jones & Bartlett, 1992.

169. Szabo, V., and V. Shang, Experiencing Control in Caregiving, *IMAGE: Journal of Nursing Scholarship,* 31, no. 1 (1999), 71–75.

170. Thompson et al., *op. cit.*

171. Burton, L., Age Norms, the Timing of Family Role Transitions, and Intergenerational Caregiving Among Aging African-American Women, *The Gerontologist,* 36, no. 2 (1996), 199–208.

172. Boland and Sims, *op. cit.*

173. Seifert et al., *op. cit.*

174. Chang, *op. cit.*

175. Roberts et al., *op. cit.*

176. Szabo and Shang, *op. cit.*

177. Chang, *op. cit.*

178. Ebersole and Hess, *op. cit.*

179. Roberts et al., *op. cit.*

180. Kart et al., *op. cit.*

181. Szabo and Shang, *op. cit.*

182. Boyd, M., and M. Nihart, *Psychiatric Nursing: Contemporary Practice.* Philadelphia: Lippincott, 1998.

183. Bee, *op. cit.*

184. Boland and Sims, *op. cit.*

185. Newman and Newman, *op. cit.*

186. Papalia and Olds, *op. cit.*

187. Seifert et al., *op. cit.*

188. Bee, *op. cit.*

189. Gormly, *op. cit.*

190. Newman and Newman, *op. cit.*

191. Papalia and Olds, *op. cit.*

192. Seifert et al., *op. cit.*

193. Bee, *op. cit.*

194. Gormly, *op. cit.*

195. Papalia and Olds, *op. cit.*

196. Sigelman, *op. cit.*

197. Novak, Mark, and Lori Campbell. *Aging and Society: A Canadian Perspective, Fourth Edition,* Scarborough: Nelson Thomson Learning, 2001.

198. Moire, E., M.W. Rosenberg, and D. McGuiness, *Growing Old in Canada: Demographic and Geographic Perspectives,* Toronto: ITP Nelson and Statistics Canada, 1997.

199. Couture, D., For Better, For Worse, *Modern Maturity,* July–August (1998), 64–65.

200. Bee, *op. cit.*

201. Gormly, *op. cit.*

202. Papalia and Olds, *op. cit.*

203. Seifert et al., *op. cit.*

204. Gardner et al., *op. cit.*

205. Gormly, *op. cit.*

206. Seifert et al., *op. cit.*

207. Sigelman, *op. cit.*

208. Seifert et al., *op. cit.*

209. The Johns Hopkins Prescription for Longevity, *The Johns Hopkins Medical Letter Health After 50,* 10, no. 10 (1998), 4–6.

210. Canoe.ca, Wired and Retired: Pet Therapy, 2004. [Database online] [cited 21 July, 2004] Available @ www.canoe.ca/Lifewise FamilyRetired00/0704_retired.html

211. Bassett B., All Creatures Great and Small, *Arthritis Today,* March–April (1995), 28–34.

212. *Ibid.*

213. Health Canada, Community Awareness and Response: Abuse and Neglect of Older Adults, 2001. [Database online] Ottawa [cited 20 October, 2004] Available @ www.hcsc.gc.ca/hppb/familyviolence/pdfs/agecommuni_e.pdf

214. Hawranik, Pamela, and Elizabeth McKean. *The Abuse of Older Adults: Issues and Prevention Strategies.* In Within our Reach: Preventing Abuse across the Lifespan, 90, 91. (Christine Ateah and Janet Mirwaldt, Editors, Winnipeg: Fernwood Publishing, 2004.

215. Novak, Mark, and Lori Campbell. *Aging and Society: A Canadian Perspective, Fourth Edition,* Scarborough: Nelson Thomson Learning, 2001.

216. Health Canada, Community Awareness and Response: Abuse and Neglect of Older Adults, 2001. [Database online] Ottawa [cited 20 October, 2004] Available @ www.hcsc.gc.ca/hppb/familyviolence/pdfs/agecommuni_e.pdf

217. Bee, *op. cit.*

218. Edelman and Mandle, *op. cit.*
219. Gormly, *op. cit.*
220. Papalia and Olds, *op. cit.*
221. Seifert et al., *op. cit.*
222. Bee, *op. cit.*
223. Government of Canada, Directory of Services and Programs Addressing the Needs of Older Adult Victims of Violence in Canada, Ottawa: Minister of Health, 2002. Cat No. H72-21/170–2002 [Database online] Ottawa [cited 20 October, 2004] Available @ www.hcsc.gc.ca/hppb/familyviolence/pdfs/2002-olderadultvictims.pdf
224. Health Canada, Community Awareness and Response: Abuse and Neglect of Older Adults, 2001. [Database online] Ottawa [cited 20 October, 2004] Available @ www.hcsc.gc.ca/hppb/familyviolence/pdfs/agecommuni_e.pdf
225. *Ibid.*
226. Manitoba Government, Manitoba Seniors' Guide, 2004/2005. Winnipeg: Minister Responsible for Seniors, 2004.
227. Ebersole and Hess, *op. cit.*
228. Gormly, *op. cit.*
229. Sigelman, *op. cit.*
230. Ebersole and Hess, *op. cit.*
231. Gormly, *op. cit.*
232. Papalia and Olds, *op. cit.*
233. Seifert et al., *op. cit.*
234. Sigelman, *op. cit.*
235. Guyton, A., *Textbook of Medical Physiology* (9th ed.). Philadelphia: W. B. Saunders, 1995.
236. Ebersole and Hess, *op. cit.*
237. Gormly, *op. cit.*
238. Ebersole and Hess, *op. cit.*
239. Gormly, *op. cit.*
240. Hampton, *op. cit.*
241. Ebersole and Hess, *op. cit.*
242. Gormly, *op. cit.*
243. Hampton, *op. cit.*
244. Ebersole and Hess, *op. cit.*
245. Hampton, *op. cit.*
246. Papalia and Olds, *op. cit.*
247. Burke, J., and G. Kamen, Changes in Spinal Reflexes Preceding a Voluntary Movement in Young and Old Adults, *Journal of Gerontology: Medical Sciences,* 51A, no. 1 (1996), M17–M22.
248. Ebersole and Hess, *op. cit.*
249. Edelman and Mandle, *op. cit.*
250. Gormly, *op. cit.*
251. Hampton, *op. cit.*
252. Papalia and Olds, *op. cit.*
253. Seifert et al., *op. cit.*
254. Sigelman, *op. cit.*
255. Ebersole and Hess, *op. cit.*
256. Edelman and Mandle, *op. cit.*
257. Gormly, *op. cit.*
258. Papalia and Olds, *op. cit.*
259. Seifert et al., *op. cit.*
260. Guyton, *op. cit.*
261. Boyd and Nihart, *op. cit.*
262. Edelman and Mandle, *op. cit.*
263. Guyton, *op. cit.*
264. Bee, *op. cit.*
265. Ebersole and Hess, *op. cit.*
266. Gormly, *op. cit.*
267. Hampton, *op. cit.*
268. Papalia and Olds, *op. cit.*
269. Bee, *op. cit.*
270. Gormly, *op. cit.*
271. Guyton, *op. cit.*
272. Hampton, *op. cit.*
273. Papalia and Olds, *op. cit.*
274. Bee, *op. cit.*
275. Burnside, I., ed., *Nursing and the Aged* (3rd ed.). New York: McGraw-Hill, 1988.
276. Ebersole and Hess, *op. cit.*
277. Gormly, *op. cit.*
278. Papalia and Olds, *op. cit.*
279. Seifert et al., *op. cit.*
280. Burnside, *Nursing and the Aged.*
281. Gormly, *op. cit.*
282. Guyton, *op. cit.*
283. Hampton, *op. cit.*
284. Papalia and Olds, *op. cit.*
285. Bee, *op. cit.*
286. Gormly, *op. cit.*
287. Hampton, *op. cit.*
288. Kelly, J., Visual Impairment Among Older People, *British Journal of Nursing,* 2, no. 2 (1993), 110, 112–113, 115–116.
289. Papalia and Olds, *op. cit.*
290. Macular Degeneration: Researchers Get Sights on Vision Disease, *Harvard Health Letter,* 23, no. 10 (1998), 3–4.
291. New Ways to Protect Your Vision, *The Johns Hopkins Medical Letter Health After 50,* 10, no. 3 (1998), 3.
292. Burnside, *Nursing and the Aged.*
293. Ebersole and Hess, *op. cit.*
294. Edelman and Mandle, *op. cit.*
295. Jacobson, W.H., *The Art and Science of Teaching Orientation and Mobility to Persons with Visual Impairments.* New York: American Foundation for the Blind, 1993.
296. Norris, R., Commonsense Tips for Working With Blind Patients, *American Journal of Nursing,* 89, no. 3 (1989), 360–361.
297. Burnside, *Nursing and the Aged.*
298. Edelman and Mandle, *op. cit.*
299. Gormly, *op. cit.*
300. Ebersole and Hess, *op. cit.*
301. Edelman and Mandle, *op. cit.*
302. Gormly, *op. cit.*
303. Hampton, *op. cit.*
304. Burnside, *Nursing and the Aged.*
305. Ebersole and Hess, *op. cit.*
306. Gormly, *op. cit.*
307. Kaakinen, J., Living with Silence, *The Gerontologist,* 32 (1992), 258–264.
308. Burnside, *Nursing and the Aged.*
309. Ebersole and Hess, *op. cit.*
310. Gormly, *op. cit.*
311. Guyton, *op. cit.*
312. Burnside, *Nursing and the Aged.*
313. Ebersole and Hess, *op. cit.*
314. Hampton, *op. cit.*
315. Making Sense of Taste and Smell, *Tufts University Diet and Nutrition Letter,* 13, no. 9 (1995), 3–6.
316. Burnside, *Nursing and the Aged.*
317. Ebersole and Hess, *op. cit.*
318. Making Sense of Taste and Smell.
319. Bee, *op. cit.*
320. Burnside, *Nursing and the Aged.*
321. Ebersole and Hess, *op. cit.*
322. Edelman and Mandle, *op. cit.*
323. Gormly, *op. cit.*
324. Guyton, *op. cit.*
325. Hampton, *op. cit.*

326. Papalia and Olds, *op. cit.*
327. Seifert et al., *op. cit.*
328. Sigelman, *op. cit.*
329. Burnside, *Nursing and the Aged.*
330. Ebersole and Hess, *op. cit.*
331. Edelman and Mandle, *op. cit.*
332. Guyton, *op. cit.*
333. Hampton, *op. cit.*
334. Bee, *op. cit.*
335. Gormly, *op. cit.*
336. Guyton, *op. cit.*
337. Hampton, *op. cit.*
338. Papalia and Olds, *op. cit.*
339. Seifert et al., *op. cit.*
340. Sigelman, *op. cit.*
341. Guyton, *op. cit.*
342. Duncan, P., et al., Functional Reach: A New Clinical Measure of Balance, *Journal of Gerontology: Medical Sciences,* 45, no. 6 (1990), M192–M197.
343. Gormly, *op. cit.*
344. Guyton, *op. cit.*
345. Hampton, *op. cit.*
346. Papalia and Olds, *op. cit.*
347. Burnside, *Nursing and the Aged.*
348. Ebersole and Hess, *op. cit.*
349. Edelman and Mandle, *op. cit.*
350. Hampton, *op. cit.*
351. Guyton, *op. cit.*
352. Hollenberg, N.K., and T.J. Moore, Age and the Renal Blood Supply: Renal Vascular Responses to Angiotensin Converting Enzyme Inhibition in Healthy Humans, *Journal of the American Geriatrics Society,* 42, no. 8 (August 1994), P805–P808.
353. Papalia and Olds, *op. cit.*
354. Burnside, *Nursing and the Aged.*
355. Ebersole and Hess, *op. cit.*
356. Edelman and Mandle, *op. cit.*
357. Guyton, *op. cit.*
358. Ebersole and Hess, *op. cit.*
359. Burnside, *Nursing and the Aged.*
360. Lara, L. L., P. R. Troop, and M. Beadleson-Baird, The Risk of Urinary Infection in Bowel Incontinent Men, *Journal of Gerontological Nursing,* 16, no. 5 (1990), P24–P26.
361. Kart et al., *op. cit.*
362. Burnside, *Nursing and the Aged.*
363. Ebersole and Hess, *op. cit.*
364. Edelman and Mandle, *op. cit.*
365. Gormly, *op. cit.*
366. Guyton, *op. cit.*
367. Hampton, *op. cit.*
368. Papalia and Olds, *op. cit.*
369. Burnside, *Nursing and the Aged.*
370. Ebersole and Hess, *op. cit.*
371. Gormly, *op. cit.*
372. Guyton, *op. cit.*
373. Hampton, *op. cit.*
374. Papalia and Olds, *op. cit.*
375. Burnside, *Nursing and the Aged.*
376. Ebersole and Hess, *op. cit.*
377. Gormly, *op. cit.*
378. Guyton, *op. cit.*
379. Papalia and Olds, *op. cit.*
380. Guyton, *op. cit.*
381. Hampton, *op. cit.*
382. Burnside, *Nursing and the Aged.*
383. Ebersole and Hess, *op. cit.*
384. Hoole, J., C. Pickard, R. Ouimette, J. Lohr, and W. Powell, *Patient Care Guidelines for Nurse Practitioners* (5th ed.). Philadelphia: J.B. Lippincott, 1999.
385. Guyton, *op. cit.*
386. Hampton, *op. cit.*
387. Gormly, *op. cit.*
388. Guyton, *op. cit.*
389. Hampton, *op. cit.*
390. Papalia and Olds, *op. cit.*
391. Guyton, *op. cit.*
392. Burnside, *Nursing and the Aged.*
393. Ebersole and Hess, *op. cit.*
394. Hampton, *op. cit.*
395. Gormly, *op. cit.*
396. Guyton, *op. cit.*
397. Hampton, *op. cit.*
398. Sigelman, *op. cit.*
399. Gormly, *op. cit.*
400. Masters, W., V. Johnson, and R. Kolodny, *Masters and Johnson on Sex and Human Loving.* Boston: Little, Brown, 1988.
401. Gormly, *op. cit.*
402. Guyton, *op. cit.*
403. Hampton, *op. cit.*
404. Masters et al., *op. cit.*
405. Burnside, *Nursing and the Aged.*
406. Ebersole and Hess, *op. cit.*
407. Gormly, *op. cit.*
408. *Ibid.*
409. Masters et al., *op. cit.*
410. Gormly, *op. cit.*
411. Papalia and Olds, *op. cit.*
412. Burnside, *Nursing and the Aged.*
413. Ebersole and Hess, *op. cit.*
414. Edelman and Mandle, *op. cit.*
415. Health Canada. *Healthy Aging: Nutrition and Healthy Aging,* Ottawa: Minister of Public Works and Government Services Canada, 2002. Cat. No. H39-612/2002-3E
416. *Ibid.*
417. *Ibid.*
418. *Ibid.*
419. *Ibid.*
420. Burnside, *Nursing and the Aged.*
421. Duyff, R., *The American Dietetic Association's Complete Food & Nutrition Guide.* Minneapolis: Chronimed Publishing, 1998.
422. Ebersole and Hess, *op. cit.*
423. Guyton, *op. cit.*
424. Morrison, S., Feeding the Elderly Population, *Nursing Clinics of North America,* 32, no. 4 (1997), 791–801.
425. Williams, S., *Nutrition and Diet Therapy* (10th ed.). St Louis: C. V. Mosby, 1995.
426. Health Canada. *Food Guide Facts: Background for Educators and Communicators,* Ottawa: Minister of Supply and Services Canada, 1992. Cat No. H39-253/11-1992E
427. Keller, Heather H., and Jacquelyn D. McKenzie, 2003. Nutritional risk in vulnerable community-living seniors, *Canadian Journal of Dietetic Practice and Research,* 64, no. 4, 195–201.
428. *Ibid.*
429. American Nurses Association, *Integrating an Understanding of Sleep Knowledge Into Your Practice.* Washington, DC: Author, 1995.
430. Dowling, G., Sleep Problems in Older Adults, *The American Nurse,* April–May (1995), 24–25.
431. Gormly, *op. cit.*
432. Guyton, *op. cit.*

433. Papalia and Olds, *op. cit.*
434. Werner, K., D. Christoph, J. Born, and H. Fehm, Changes in Cortisol and Growth Hormone Secretion During Nocturnal Sleep in the Course of Aging, *Journal of Gerontology: Medical Sciences,* 51A, no. 1 (1996), M3–M9.
435. American Nurses Association, *Integrating an Understanding of Sleep Knowledge Into Your Practice.*
436. Health Canada. *Healthy Aging: Physical Activity and Older Adults,* Ottawa: Minister of Public Works and Government Services Canada, 2003. Cat. No. H39-612/2002-4E
437. *Ibid.*
438. Health Canada. Physical Activity Unit–Physical Activity Guide for Older Adults, 2003. [Database online] Ottawa [cited 10 September, 2004] Available @ www.hcsc.gc.ca/hppb/paguide/older/index.htm
439. Health Canada. Physical Activity Unit–Physical Activity Guide for Older Adults, 2003. [Database online] Ottawa [cited 10 September, 2004] Available @ www.hcsc.gc.ca/hppb/paguide/older/index.htm
440. A Little Activity Yields Big Returns, *The Johns Hopkins Medical Letter Health After 50,* 9, no. 10 (1997), 2–3.
441. Blumenthal, J., et al., Long-term Effects of Exercise on Psychological Functioning in Older Men and Women, *Journal of Gerontology: Psychological Sciences,* 46, no. 6 (1991), P352–P361.
442. Burnside, *Nursing and the Aged.*
443. Ebersole and Hess, *op. cit.*
444. Edelman and Mandle, *op. cit.*
445. Gormly, *op. cit.*
446. Papalia and Olds, *op. cit.*
447. The Johns Hopkins Prescription for Longevity.
448. Center for Aging Studies, *Rural Elderly* (Online), available: iml.umkc.edu/casww (1999).
449. Clark, C., Wellness Self-Care by Healthy Older Adults, *IMAGE: Journal of Nursing Scholarship,* 30, 4 (1998), 351–355.
450. Edelman and Mandle, *op. cit.*
451. Gormly, *op. cit.*
452. Papalia and Olds, *op. cit.*
453. A Little Activity Yields Big Returns.
454. Clark, D., Age, Socioeconomic Status, and Exercise Self-Efficacy, *The Gerontologist,* 36, no. 2 (1996), 157–164.
455. Edelman and Mandle, *op. cit.*
456. Gleich, G., Health Maintenance and Prevention in the Elderly, *Primary Care,* 22, no. 4 (1995), 697–711.
457. Strategies for Preventing Falls, *Mount Sinai School of Medicine Focus on Healthy Aging,* 2, no. 1 (1998), 3.
458. Wolinski, F., T. Stamp, and D. Clark, Antecedents and Consequences of Physical Activity and Exercise Among Older Adults, *The Gerontologist,* 35, no. 4 (1995), 451–462.
459. Burnside, *Nursing and the Aged.*
460. Tse, S. and D. Bailey, T'ai Chi and Postural Control in the Well Elderly, *The American Journal of Occupational Therapy,* 46, no. 4 (1992), 295–299.
461. Carter, Nick D., Karim M. Khan, Heather A. McKay, Moira A. Petit, Constance Waterman, Ari Heinonen, Patti A. Janssen, et al. 2002. Community-based exercise program reduces risk factors for falls in 65- to 75-year-old women with osteoporosis: Randomized controlled trial, *Canadian Medical Association Journal,* 167, no. 9, 997–1004.
462. Government of Canada. *Go for it! A guide to choosing and using assistance devices,* Ottawa: Minister of Public Works and Government Services Canada, 2002. Cat. No. H39-631/2002E
463. Edelman and Mandle, *op. cit.*
464. Clark, Wellness Self-Care by Healthy Older Adults.
465. Boult, C., M. Altmann, D. Gilbertson, C. Yu, and R. Kane, Decreasing Disability in the 21st Century: The Future Effects of Controlling Six Fatal and Nonfatal Conditions, *American Journal of Public Health,* 86, no. 10 (1996), 1388–1393.
466. Menec, V., Chipperfield, and R. Perry, Self Perceptions of Health: A Prospective Analysis of Mortality, Control, and Health, *Journal of Gerontology: Psychological Sciences,* 54B, no. 2 (1999), 85–93.
467. *Ibid.*
468. Bee, *op. cit.*
469. Papalia and Olds, *op. cit.*
470. Seligson, S., Anti-Aging Comes of Age, *Health,* April (1998), 63–81.
471. Bee, *op. cit.*
472. Burnside, *Nursing and the Aged.*
473. Ebersole and Hess, *op. cit.*
474. Fenstermacher, K., and B. Hudson, *Practice Guidelines for Family Nurse Practitioners.* Philadelphia: Saunders, 1997.
475. Hoole et al., *op. cit.*
476. Papalia and Olds, *op. cit.*
477. Sigelman, *op. cit.*
478. Health Canada. *Canadian Immunization Guide,* Ottawa: Her Majesty the Queen in Right of Canada, 2002. Cat. No. H498/2002E
479. *Ibid.*
480. Aging Skin, *Harvard Women's Health Watch,* 11, no. 10 (1995), 4–5.
481. Aging Skin: Handle With Care, *Harvard Health Letter,* 20, no. 10 (1995), 6–7.
482. Don't Fall For a Telephone Line, *Modern Maturity,* 40, no. 3 (1997), 83.
483. Marklein, M., Con Games Proliferate: New Threats Haunt City Folk, *AARP Bulletin,* 32, no. 2 (1991), 1, 16–17.
484. Burnside, *Nursing and the Aged.*
485. Ebersole and Hess, *op. cit.*
486. Burnside, *Nursing and the Aged.*
487. Ebersole and Hess, *op. cit.*
488. Batscha, C., Heat Stroke: Keeping Your Clients Cool in the Summer, *Journal of Psychosocial Nursing,* 35, no. 7 (1997), 12–17.
489. *Ibid.*
490. *Ibid.*
491. *Ibid.*
492. *Ibid.*
493. *Ibid.*
494. *Ibid.*
495. Hampton, *op. cit.*
496. Burnside, I. *Working with Older Adults: Group Process and Techniques.* New York: Jones, 1994.
497. Gleich, *op. cit.*
498. *Ibid.*
499. Burnside, *Nursing and the Aged.*
500. Ebersole and Hess, *op. cit.*
501. Fenstermacher and Hudson, *op cit.*
502. Hoole et al., *op. cit.*
503. Tierney, L., S. McPhee, and M. Papadakis, *Current Medical Diagnosis and Treatment, 1999* (38th ed.). Stamford, CT: Appleton-Lange, 1999.
504. Burnside, *Nursing and the Aged.*
505. Ebersole and Hess, *op. cit.*
506. Fenstermacher and Hudson, *op cit.*
507. Hoole et al., *op. cit.*
508. Tierney et al., *op. cit.*
509. For Women Sick at Heart, *Tufts University Diet and Nutrition Letter,* 13, no. 9 (1995), 2.
510. Health Risks: Perception and Reality, *Harvard Women's Health Watch,* 1, no. 10 (1994), 1.
511. Tierney et al., *op. cit.*
512. Fenstermacher and Hudson, *op cit.*
513. Hoole et al., *op. cit.*
514. Tierney et al., *op. cit.*
515. Health Risks: Perception and Reality.
516. Tierney et al., *op. cit.*

517. Boyd, and Nihart, *op. cit.*
518. Pangman, Verna C., and Marilyn Seguire, 2000. Sexuality and the chronically ill older adult: A social justice issue, *Sexuality and Disability*, 18, no. 1, 49–59.
519. Boyd and Nihart, *op. cit.*
520. Guyton, *op. cit.*
521. Avoiding Magnesium Overdose, *Tufts University Diet and Nutrition Letter*, 13, no. 9 (1995), 7.
522. *Ibid.*
523. Boyd and Nihart, *op. cit.*
524. Duyff, *op. cit.*
525. Williams, *op. cit.*
526. Gill, Sudeep S., Brian C. Misiaszek, and Chris Brymer, 2001. Improving prescribing in the elderly: A study in the long term care setting, *Canadian Journal of Clinical Pharmacology*, 8, no. 2, 78–83.
527. *Ibid.*
528. Health Canada. *How You Can Help Seniors Use Medication Safely*, Ottawa: Div. of Aging and Seniors, nd. Kit.
529. When Alcohol and Aging Don't Mix, *The Johns Hopkins Medical Letter Health After 50*, 10, no. 12 (1999), 4–5.
530. The Johns Hopkins Prescription for Longevity.
531. When Alcohol and Aging Don't Mix.
532. *Ibid.*
533. *Ibid.*
534. Ebersole and Hess, *op. cit.*
535. Boyd and Nihart, *op. cit.*
536. When Alcohol and Aging Don't Mix.
537. Boyd and Nihart, *op. cit.*
538. Papalia and Olds, *op. cit.*
539. Bee, *op. cit.*
540. Emerg et al., *op. cit.*
541. Gormly, *op. cit.*
542. Papalia and Olds, *op. cit.*
543. Schaie, K., and S. Willis, Adult Personality and Psychomotor Performance: Cross-sectional and Longitudinal Analysis, *Journal of Gerontology: Psychological Sciences*, 46, no. 6 (1991), P275–P284.
544. *Ibid.*
545. Gormly, *op. cit.*
546. Bee, *op. cit.*
547. Burnside, *Nursing and the Aged.*
548. Gormly, *op. cit.*
549. Papalia and Olds, *op. cit.*
550. Schaie and Willis, *op. cit.*
551. Bee, *op. cit.*
552. Burnside, *Nursing and the Aged.*
553. Edelman and Mandle, *op. cit.*
554. Gormly, *op. cit.*
555. Newman and Newman, *op. cit.*
556. Papalia and Olds, *op. cit.*
557. Seifert et al., *op. cit.*
558. Sigelman, *op. cit.*
559. Bee, *op. cit.*
560. Gormly, *op. cit.*
561. Papalia and Olds, *op. cit.*
562. Bee, *op. cit.*
563. Burnside, *Nursing and the Aged.*
564. Edelman and Mandle, *op. cit.*
565. Gormly, *op. cit.*
566. Newman and Newman, *op. cit.*
567. Papalia and Olds, *op. cit.*
568. Seifert et al., *op. cit.*
569. Sigelman, *op. cit.*
570. Bee, *op. cit.*
571. Erikson, *Adulthood.*
572. Gormly, *op. cit.*

573. Lidz, T., *The Person: His and Her Development Throughout the Life Cycle* (2nd ed.). New York: Basic Books, 1983.
574. Papalia and Olds, *op. cit.*
575. Sigelman, *op. cit.*
576. Duncan, *op cit.*
577. A New Slant on Memory Loss, *The Johns Hopkins Medical Letter Health After 50*, 11, no. 9 (1999), 1–2.
578. Bee, *op. cit.*
579. Burnside, *Nursing and the Aged.*
580. Erikson, *Adulthood.*
581. Newman and Newman, *op. cit.*
582. Papalia and Olds, *op. cit.*
583. Seifert et al., *op. cit.*
584. Sheehy, *op. cit.*
585. Bee, *op. cit.*
586. Gormly, *op. cit.*
587. Papalia and Olds, *op. cit.*
588. Seifert et al., *op. cit.*
589. Sigelman, *op. cit.*
590. Erikson, E., *Childhood and Society* (2nd ed.). New York: W. W. Norton, 1963.
591. *Ibid.*
592. Erikson, *Adulthood.*
593. Lidz, *op. cit.*
594. Erikson, *Adulthood.*
595. Erikson, *Childhood and Society.*
596. Bowling, A., and P. Browne, Social Networks, Health and Emotional Well-being Among the Oldest-Old in London, *Journal of Gerontology: Social Sciences*, 46, no. 1 (1991), S20–S32.
597. Erikson, *Adulthood.*
598. Erikson, *Childhood and Society.*
599. Boyd and Nihart, *op. cit.*
600. Kolanowski, A., and A. Whall, Life-Span Perspective of Personality of Dementia, *IMAGE: Journal of Nursing Scholarship*, 28, no. 4 (1996), 315–320.
601. Light, J., J. Grigsby, and M. Bligh, Aging and Heterogeneity: Genetics, Social Structure, and Personality, *The Gerontologist*, 36, no. 2 (1996), 147–156.
602. Jung C., Psychological Types, in G. Adler et al., eds., *Collected Works of Carl G. Jung*, Vol. 6. Princeton, NJ: Princeton University Press, 1971.
603. Maas, H., and J. Kuypers, *From Thirty to Seventy.* San Francisco: Jossey-Bass, 1974.
604. Neugarten, B., Grow Old Along With Me! The Best is Yet to Be, *Psychology Today*, 5, no. 7 (1971), 45ff.
605. Neugarten, B., Adult Personality: A Developmental View, in Charles, D., and W. Looft, eds., *Readings in Psychological Development Through Life*. New York: Holt, Rinehart & Winston, 1973, pp. 356–366.
606. Schaie and Willis, *op. cit.*
607. Erikson, *Adulthood.*
608. Krause, N., Stress and the Devaluation of Highly Salient Roles in Late Life, *Journal of Gerontology: Social Sciences*, 54B, no. 2 (1999), S99–S108.
609. Lidz, *op. cit.*
610. Buhler, C., The Developmental Structure of Goal Setting in Group and Individual Studies, in C. Buhler and F. Massarik, eds., *The Course of Human Life*. New York: Spring, 1968.
611. Erikson, *Adulthood.*
612. Erikson, *Childhood and Society.*
613. Lidz, *op. cit.*
614. Neugarten, B., The Future and the Young-Old, *The Gerontologist*, 15, Part 2 (1975), 4–9.
615. Buhler, *op. cit.*
616. Lidz, *op. cit.*
617. Buhler, *op. cit.*

618. Neugarten, B., Adaptation and the Life Cycle, *Counseling Psychologist,* 6, no. 1 (1976), 16–20.
619. Lidz, *op. cit.*
620. Peck, *op. cit.*
621. *Ibid.*
622. Burnside, *Nursing and the Aged.*
623. Ebersole and Hess, *op. cit.*
624. Lidz, *op. cit.*
625. Sigelman, *op. cit.*
626. Lidz, *op. cit.*
627. McCrae, R., Age Differences in the Use of Coping Mechanisms, *Journal of Gerontology,* 37 (1982), 454–460.
628. McCrae, R., and P. Costa, Age, Personality, and Spontaneous Self-concept, *Journal of Gerontology: Social Sciences,* 43, no. 6 (1988), S177–S185.
629. Lidz, *op. cit.*
630. Peck, *op. cit.*
631. Ebersole and Hess, *op. cit.*
632. Erikson, *Adulthood.*
633. Hogstel, M., Understanding Hoarding Behavior, *American Journal of Nursing,* 93, no. 7 (1993), 42–45.
634. Bee, *op. cit.*
635. Gormly, *op. cit.*
636. Newman and Newman, *op. cit.*
637. Papalia and Olds, *op. cit.*
638. Roos and Havens, *op. cit.*
639. Seifert et al., *op. cit.*
640. Roos and Havens, *op. cit.*
641. Reed, P., Self-transcendence and Mental Health in Oldest-old Adults, *Nursing Research,* 40, no. 1 (1991), 5–11.
642. Isaia, D., V. Parker, and E. Murrow, Spiritual Well-Being Among Older Adults, *Journal of Gerontological Nursing,* 25, no. 8 (1999), 16–21.
643. Andrews and Boyle, *op. cit.*
644. Lidz, *op. cit.*
645. Duvall, E., and B. Miller, *Marriage and Family Development* (6th ed.). Philadelphia: J.B. Lippincott, 1984.
646. Erikson, *Adulthood.*
647. Hattendorf, J., and T. Tollerud, Domestic Violence: Counseling Strategies That Minimize the Impact of Secondary Victimization, *Perspectives in Psychiatric Care,* 33, no. 1 (1997), 14–23.
648. McCoy, V., Adult Life Cycle Tasks/Adult Continuing Education Program Response, *Lifelong Learning in the Adult Years,* October (1977), 16.
649. Brown, M., *Readings in Gerontology.* St. Louis: C. V. Mosby, 1978.
650. Andrews and Boyle, *op. cit.*
651. Calasanti, T., Theorizing About Gender and Aging: Beginning with the Voices of Women, *The Gerontologist,* 32 (1992), 280–281.
652. Calasanti, T., Gender and Life Satisfaction in Retirement: An Assessment of the Male Model, *Journal of Gerontology: Social Sciences,* 51B, no. 1 (1996), S18–S29.
653. Bee, *op. cit.*
654. *Ibid.*
655. Gormly, *op. cit.*
656. Newman and Newman, *op. cit.*
657. Papalia and Olds, *op. cit.*
658. Seifert et al., *op. cit.*
659. Sigelman, *op. cit.*
660. Bosse, R., et al., How Stressful is Retirement? Findings From the Normative Aging Study, *Journal of Gerontology: Psychological Sciences,* 46, no. 1 (1991), P9–P14.
661. Papalia and Olds, *op. cit.*
662. Atchley, R., *The Social Forces in Later Life* (3rd ed.). Belmont, CA: Wadsworth, 1977.
663. Gormly, *op. cit.*
664. Rathje, Kelly. 2003. Retirement trends in Canada, The Expert Witness Newsletter, 8 no. 1, 26–32.
665. *Ibid.*
666. *Ibid.*
667. Novak, Mark, and Lori Campbell. *Aging and Society: A Canadian Perspective,* Fourth Edition, Scarborough; Nelson Thomson Learning, 2001.
668. Tompa, E. 1999. Transitions to retirement: Determinants of age of social security take up, *Social and Economic Dimensions of an Aging Society Research Program* (SEDAP) Research Paper no. 6, Hamilton, ON: McMaster University
669. Andrews and Boyle, *op. cit.*
670. Papalia and Olds, *op. cit.*
671. Seifert et al., *op. cit.*
672. Sigelman, *op. cit.*
673. Iwasaki, Yoshi, Jiri Zuzanck, and Roger C. Mandell, 2001. The effects of physically active leisure on stress-health relationships, *Canadian Journal of Public Health,* 92, no. 3, 214–218.
674. Parker, M., M. Thorslund, and O. Lundberg, Physical Function and Social Class Among Swedish Oldest-Old, *Journal of Gerontology: Social Sciences,* 48 (1994), S196–S201.
675. Government of Canada. Liberal Task Force Report, February, 2004, Ottawa: Liberal Task Force on Seniors, 2004.
676. Government of Canada, Interim Report Card: Seniors in Canada, 2003. National Advisory Council on Aging. [Database online] Ottawa [cited 21 October, 2004] Available @ www.phac-aspc.gc.ca/seniorsaines/naca/report_card2003/pdf/interim%20card%202003_e.pdf
677. *Ibid.*
678. Health Canada, Division of Aging and Seniors National Advisory Council on Aging, 2003 [Database online] Ottawa [cited 6 October, 2004] Available @ www.hc-sc.gc.ca/seniors_aines/index_pages/naca_e.htm
679. Government Retirement Benefits in Canada, 1998. [Database online] Calgory [cited 28 July, 2004] Available @ www.ucalgary.ca/MG/inrm/finplan/retire/cdn_gov.htm
680. *Ibid.*
681. *Ibid.*
682. Elsner, R., M. Quinn, S. Fanning, S. Cueldner, and L. Poon, Ethical and Policy Considerations for Centenarians: The Oldest Old, *IMAGE: Journal of Nursing Scholarship,* 31, no. 3 (1999), 263–267.
683. King, T. 2004. Status and standards of care for older adults, *Canadian Nurse,* 100, no. 5, 23–26.
684. Boyd and Nihart, *op. cit.*
685. Burnside, I. *Working with Older Adults: Group Process and Techniques.*
686. Elsner et al., *op. cit.*
687. Burnside, *Nursing and the Aged.*
688. Edelman and Mandle, *op. cit.*
689. Community Legal Education Ontario (CLEO). *Every Resident: Bill of Rights for People who Live in Ontario Long Term Care Facilities,* Advocacy Centre for the Elderly (ACE) and CLEO, 2004.
690. Papalia and Olds, *op. cit.*
691. Seifert et al., *op. cit.*
692. Life Lease Associates of Canada, What is Life Lease [Database online] Toronto [cited 15 October, 2004] Available @ www.life-lease.com/whatis.htm
693. Burnside, *Nursing and the Aged.*
694. Ebersole and Hess, *op. cit.*
695. Tolbert, B.M., Reality Orientation and Remotivation in a Long-term Care Facility, *Nursing and Health Care,* 5, no. 1 (1984), 40–44.
696. Burnside, *Nursing and the Aged.*
697. Ebersole and Hess, *op. cit.*
698. Tolbert, *op. cit.*
699. Bailey, L., and R. Hanssen, Psychological Obstacles to Job or Career Change in Late Life, *Journal of Gerontology: Psychological Sciences,* 50B (1995), P280–P288.

700. Bee, *op. cit.*
701. Burnside, *Nursing and the Aged.*
702. Calasanti, Gender and Life Satisfaction in Retirement: An Assessment of the Male Model.
703. Gormly, *op. cit.*
704. Hayward, M., S. Friedman, and H. Chen, Race Inequities in Men's Retirement, *Journal of Gerontology: Social Sciences,* 51B, no. 1 (1996), S1–S10.
705. Newman and Newman, *op. cit.*
706. Papalia and Olds, *op. cit.*
707. Pienta, A., J. Burr, and J. Mutchler, Women's Labor Force Participation in Later Life: The Effects of Early Work and Family Experiences, *The Journal of Gerontology,* 49 (1994), S231–S238.
708. Seifert et al., *op. cit.*
709. Sigelman, *op. cit.*
710. Szinovacs, M., and C. Washo, Gender Differences in Exposure to Life Events and Adaptation to Retirement, *Journal of Gerontology: Social Sciences,* 47 (1992), S191–S196.
711. Burnside, *Nursing and the Aged.*
712. *Ibid.*
713. Ebersole and Hess, *op. cit.*
714. Edelman and Mandle, *op. cit.*
715. Schank, M., and M. Lough, Profiles of Frail Elderly Women, Maintaining Independence, *Journal of Advanced Nursing,* 15, no. 6 (1990), 674–682.

Chapter 15

DEATH, THE LAST DEVELOPMENTAL STAGE

Death is universal, but there is no universal meaning to death. Meaning comes from a merging of philosophical, spiritual, emotional, sociocultural, historical, and geographical factors.

Ruth Beckmann Murray

OBJECTIVES

STUDY OF THIS CHAPTER WILL ENABLE YOU TO:

1. Explore personal reactions and ethical issues associated with active and passive euthanasia and the right-to-die movement versus extraordinary measures to prolong life.

2. Compare and contrast the concept of death held by each of: the child, the adolescent, and the adult.

3. Examine personal feelings about death and the dying person.

4. Discuss the stages of awareness and related behaviour as the person adapts to the crisis of approaching death.

5. Describe the sequence of reactions when the person and family are aware of terminal illness.

6. Dialogue with another about how to plan for eventual death.

7. Determine response options to the wishes and needs of a dying client and family members.

8. Plan and administer care to a client, based on a firm professional understanding of his or her awareness of eventual death. The administration of care should include consideration of behavioural and emotional reactions, and physical needs.

9. Intervene appropriately and in a professional manner, to meet the needs of the family members of the dying person.

10. Compare and contrast home or hospice care with hospital or nursing home care.

11. Evaluate the effectiveness of care given.

ISSUES RELATED TO DYING AND DEATH

Definitions of Death

Death has been avoided in name and understanding. There is no harm in saying "he passed" instead of "he died." There is harm in suddenly facing a client's death without sufficient emotional preparation.

The aged differ from persons in other life areas in that their concept of future is realistically limited. The younger person may not live many years into the future but generally thinks of many years of life ahead. The older person knows that, despite medical and technical advances, life is limited.

Death is the last developmental stage. It is more than simply an end process; it can be viewed as a goal and as fulfillment. If the person has spent his or her years unfettered by fear, if he or she has lived richly and productively, and if he or she has achieved the developmental task of ego integrity, he or she can accept the realization that the self will cease to be and that dying has an onset long before the actual death. Research on near-death experiences also conveys that death is another stage.[1,2,3,4,5]

If death is considered the last developmental phase, it is worth the kind of preparation that goes into any developmental phase, perhaps physically, and certainly emotionally, socially, philosophically, or spiritually.

CRITICAL THINKING

How do you personally view death?

Most people want to die at home surrounded by their loved ones. However, Canadian research indicates that in some provinces, up to 90% die in hospital.[6] Wilson and her researchers conducted an interdisciplinary historical investigation of twentieth century influences on location of death in Canada.[7] The findings revealed two key influences on location of death: (1) health care and health-system developments that have amalgamated health care in hospitals, while at the same time increasing and sustaining public expectancies about curative, or least beneficial hospital care. The increase in hospital death rate throughout much of the twentieth century may be considered largely due to the shift in illness care from home to the hospital; (2) The other key influence on the location of death was the decreased availability of home-based formal and informal caregivers available to the dying member. Regarding caregivers, Stajduhar examined the social context of home-based palliative caregiving. The results indicated a need for interventions to improve support for caregivers at home, and to examine how assumptions influence, and at times, drive, the provision of home health care.[8] In fact, a need exists to examine more closely the type and intensity of services required to give care to clients and their families in the final stage of a terminal illness.[9]

Calls to enhance home care services for the dying have been voiced across Canada. As palliative care continues to expand, it is evident that a shift from hospital care to community and home-based care is evident.[10] Many terminally ill clients would like to die at home for reasons that would benefit both them and their families. For example, one benefit that clients may experience within their home is a sense of security and freedom of control. Benefits experienced by the family while caring for their loved one may be feelings of satisfaction and gratitude.

Because of technologic advances, the determination of **death** is *changing from the traditional concept that death occurs when the heart stops beating.* In the U.S., the *Uniform Determination of Death Act* (UDDA), or similar legislation, is recognized in all 50 states. The Act defines death as *irreversible cessation of circulatory and respiratory functions, or irreversible cessation of all functions of the brain, including the brain stem.* Death based on neurological criteria is true death.[11]

Medically accepted standards for *brain death* include the following neurological criteria:[12]

- Underlying cause of condition or brain injury must be known and diagnosed as irreversible.
- Declaration of death can be made only if patient is not suffering from hypothermia (32.2°C) or receiving central nervous system depressants, either of which may present the appearance of brain death.
- Person must manifest cerebral unresponsiveness and no reflexes.
- Apnea testing must not produce spontaneous respiration.

Institutions may also have other criteria for their policies and procedures for pronouncing brain death. Most institutions require an electroencephalogram (EEG) to confirm absence of brain activity. Some require a cerebral radionuclide scan or four-vessel arteriogram to verify absence of blood flow.

Shemie, Doig, and Belitsky claim that in Canada, brain death is legally defined as "according to accepted medical practice," and that procedures associated with neurological death are determined individually by each hospital setting.[13] The Canadian Neurocritical Care Group recently published Guidelines for the Diagnosis of Brain Death. These guidelines closely resemble the American Academy of Neurology Guidelines.[14] In fact, the guidelines established by the Canadian Congress Committee on Brain Death in 1988, as well as the guidelines developed by the Canadian Neurocritical Care Group in 1999, began to clarify a set criteria; but the work has not led to any standardization of diagnostic criteria or uniform practice.[15,16] It is interesting to note that, according to Wijdicks, national and international variability and inconsistency exists in the "accepted medical practices" for determining neurological death.

Brain death is differentiated from **coma,** a *persistent vegetative state* in which the person, not assistive devices, maintains basic vital homeostatic functions and therefore is not dead, even though he or she is not responding verbally or nonverbally. In brain death, the appearance of life continues when the ventilator is used to deliver enough oxygen to keep the heart beating and the skin warm. The ventilation is maintained until there is a decision about tissue or organ donation. If there is no organ procurement, the ventilator is discontinued.

The Canadian Association of Critical Care Nurses (CACCN) firmly attests to the fact that critical care nurses play a significant role in how decision-making processes regarding the withholding, or withdrawing, of life support occur for the critically ill.[17] The position of the CACCN statement is based on the following beliefs and principles:

- Patients have a right to autonomy in decision-making regarding their own health care
- Patients' health decisions must be made on an individual basis
- Health care professionals should behave in ways that best benefit the patient
- Life support refers to the provision of taking into account any or all of the following: assisted ventilation, inotropic support, and all or any of the mechanisms utilized to maintain and/or support the life of the patient who is deteriorating. The removal of fluids and/or nutrition may be examined and discussed on an individual basis.

The CACCN believes that all health care institutions and provincial associations have a responsibility in managing and directing the process of withdrawing or withholding life support treatments.

To address the ethical issues affecting the practice of registered nurses, the Canadian Nurses Association (CNA), in collaboration with other national health related organizations, has prepared a Joint Statement on Resuscitative Interventions. The Canadian Bar Association also played a part in the development of this Joint Statement. The statement includes the following: guiding principles for health care facilities when developing cardiopulmonary-resuscitation (CPR) policy, CPR as a treatment option, competence, the treatment decision, and its communication, implementation and review, palliative care, and other treatment.[18] Finally, the Canadian Nurses Association Code of Ethics for Registered Nurses (2002) provides an ethical framework for the practice of nursing.[19] It reflects changes in Canadian social values and conditions that not only affect the health care delivery system, but create challenges and opportunities for nurses in their practice setting. Nurses must discover and honour an individual's wish regarding the manner in which they want to live the remainder of their life. In fact, decisions about life-sustaining treatments are guided by such considerations. Nurses must advocate for health and well-being as well as social conditions that allow individuals to live and to die with dignity. Nurses must also intervene if other individuals fail to respect the dignity of persons in care.

CRITICAL THINKING

Review the CNA Code of Ethics (2002). What does fair treatment of individuals and groups mean to you?

The family, more than anyone else, must live with the memories of their loved ones and the events surrounding death. It is a violation of the family's dignity to rush death. Even though a less-involved person might say, "Why don't they turn the machines off!" this person should be ignored until all those closely involved with the client can say with acceptance and assurance, "Now is the time." Increasingly, the *person* is saying that he or she has a right to decide how long machines should maintain personal life or that of a loved one. Family, health care providers, ethical committee, and hospital legal counsel may all be involved in discussions about when to end life. The nurse may advocate for the patient when he or she cannot speak for self.

Organ and Tissue Donation

Although organ transplantation is growing in Canada, shortages of needed organs still exist.[20] Molzahn, Starzomski, and McCormick claim that over a five-year period from 1996 to 2000, the waiting list grew by 62%, while the available transplants increased 22%. By the end of 2001, almost 4000 Canadians were waiting for organ transplants—a 15.6% increase in three years.[21] CNA Fact Sheet on Organ Donation and Tissue Transplantation claims that heading the list of single organ transplants in Canada are kidneys (62%), followed by livers (22%), and hearts (10%). Eighty-six percent of transplant recipients are between 18 and 64 years of age; and men make up the majority (64%) of those requiring transplants, particularly heart transplants.[22] All provinces and territories have enacted legislation, which is remarkably uniform across Canada, dealing with organ donation before and after the death of the donor.[23]

The reasons for the shortage of organs are varied, numerous, and complex. Some of the reasons include: (a) fewer accidental deaths due to the enhancement of safety on the road; (b) society's perception regarding organ donation; (c) individuals' or families' reluctance to approve organ donations and signing cards, that is many individuals have fears and misconceptions about organ donations. Other reasons include professional attitudes and knowledge regarding, first, the acceptability of organ donation, and, second, the issue of identifying potential organ donors. It is interesting to note that a review of all deaths in 2000 in Quebec was undertaken by the College des Medecins du Quebec.[24] They found that of all patients who appeared brain dead on the basis of the chart review, 23% had not been identified as potential organ donors at the time. In addition, for patients with a diagnosis of brain death, 24% of the families were not consulted for consent to donation. Finally, the values and beliefs of the families regarding organ transplantation and the ethnocultural considerations in Canada provide a list of "reasons" which can interfere with

organ donation. Bowman and Richard claim that the effects of culture on attitudes toward organ donation may be overlooked by examining more pragmatic explanations for organ transplants, by discussing the organization of medical care, or the relationship between the health care system and the public. As a result, we may significantly underestimate the effect of culture on Canadian attitudes toward organ donation.[25] For example, the practices of autopsy and organ removal are both in opposition of the belief system of the First Nations people in Canada.[26]

CRITICAL THINKING

What other cultural groups might not support organ donation?

The Canadian Nurses Association states that nurses can support organ donation and tissue transplantation in the following ways:

- Collaborate with and support other members of the transplant team, taking into account the client/family during the donation, retrieval, and transplantation phases;
- Acknowledge, differentiate, and comprehend the roles of members of the health care team, volunteer agencies, and organ procurement service;
- Encourage and support health care facilities to provide support programs for clients, family members, and health care providers in transplantation service;
- Know about agency policies and procedures regarding organ and tissue transplantation. Formulate interdisciplinary policies and procedures to direct the team in the transplantation process;
- Be aware of policies related to legal and ethical issues, such as consent and confidentiality;
- Comprehend the cost-benefit aspects of organ and tissue transplantation.

Many ethical issues exist around the matter of organ donation and tissue transplantation. In recent years, xenotransplantation (the adoption of animal organs for transplantation into human beings) has received renewed attention in the medical field as well as in the media. At the same time, scientists are exploring cloning as a means of producing organs for transplants. Emerging ethical issues surrounding new discoveries are complex. It is critical that the nursing profession participate in future developments.

CRITICAL THINKING

What are your thoughts and feelings regarding organ donation and tissue transplantation?

Stem cell research holds great potential to treat human disease and prevent suffering. A stem cell can be thought of as a blank cell that has yet to become specialized. Scientists are fascinated by the ability of stem cells to become any type of cell. At present, Canada has no laws to govern stem cell research, nor are there any guidelines for researchers, research ethics boards, or funding agencies governing how stem cells may be derived and used.[27] The organization of Canadian

Institutes of Health Research has introduced Human Pluripotent Stem Cell Research: Guidelines for CIHR Funded Research. This introduction of the guidelines results from the recognition of an urgent need for specific guidelines—guidelines that allow for response to a growing, evolving science and shifting public opinion, as well as to ensure ethical and scientific oversight. With the introduction of these guidelines, Canadian researchers will be able to move forward and remain at the forefront of their field, while conducting their research according to ethical standards.

On the other hand, regarding human cloning, there have been consistent calls in Canada, since the 1993 Report of the Royal Commission on New Reproductive Technologies, to ban human reproductive cloning.[28] Recognizing the health and safety concerns, as well as opposition from the public sector in relation to human cloning, the Assisted Human Reproduction (AHR) legislation prohibits human cloning for any purpose (i.e., whether for reproductive, therapeutic, or research purposes). Penalties for contravening the prohibition are severe—a maximum fine of $500 000, ten years in prison, or both.

CONTROVERSY DEBATE

Howard is a 14-year-old boy who has been diagnosed with leukemia. He wants to donate his corneas for transplant if he should die. His parents strongly disapprove of his wish and believe it is wrong for him to do so. They have said that they will not co-sign a donor card for him. Howard has asked you to be his advocate in this matter.

1. As a health professional how will you support Howard?

2. How will you counsel this family? What is your rationale?

Euthanasia

Euthanasia is legally defined as the *act or practice of painlessly putting to death persons suffering from incurable or distressing diseases.* Commonly referred to as "mercy killing," it is seen as a means to finalize the suffering and pain of patients who otherwise would experience an undignified and distressed death.

Although maintaining life beyond all reason is an ethical dilemma for the nurse, an equally taxing ethical dilemma occurs when the doctor deliberately hastens the client's death by increasing the dose of a narcotic analgesic such as morphine to the point of lethality. Responsible, moral caregivers promote quality of life and right to die with dignity. If each human life is seen as of infinite value, it will be worth the efforts to ease pain and help the person find meaning in the current situation.

Euthanasia is illegal throughout the world. In the Netherlands, immunity is granted to the physician who follows specific guidelines.[29,30,31] In Canada, attempts to make euthanasia legal have so far failed to win support. Most

nurses do not support active euthanasia; support for it is based on patient autonomy, informed consent, and suffering. Religious beliefs may be the most accurate predictor of the person's stance on euthanasia. Many nurses who are opposed to active euthanasia operate on the basis of sanctity of life, traditional rules, and laws prohibiting the taking of life. They are worried about the double effect of giving medication for pain that may also shorten life and their own professional integrity and responsibility. Nurses who support active euthanasia define professional integrity and responsibility as being an advocate for patients who make a decision to end his or her life. If they see that death is eminent, they believe that euthanasia makes the process more compassionate. Most Western countries consider **active euthanasia,** *deliberately hastening death,* as first-degree murder. On the other hand, court decisions have been inconsistent about **passive euthanasia,** *omission of care or inaction to prolong life.* The recent court case involving Robert Latimer, a Saskatchewan farmer, who was convicted for the second degree murder of his severely disabled daughter, has received much publicity. After his conviction following a second trial ordered by the Supreme Court of Canada, Latimer was sentenced to time served plus two years in jail. Some may claim that Latimer's sentence highlighted a turning point in the law's attitude toward euthanasia. However, Latimer's sentence was overturned on appeal by the Crown to the Saskatchewan Court of Appeal, which substituted the minimum ten-year sentence mandated by the *Criminal Code of Canada.* The case is on further appeal to the Supreme Court of Canada. Another case in Nova Scotia involved Dr. Nancy Morrison, who was charged with the murder of a terminally ill cancer patient. At the preliminary hearing, charges were dropped against Dr. Morrison owing to insufficient evidence that she had committed any fault to hasten the patient's death. Although she enjoyed much public support for her cause, Dr. Morrison accepted a reprimand from her provincial College of Physicians and Surgeons.

Euthanasia is based on two fundamental legal premises: the right to privacy and the right to refuse treatment when informed. The competent client may decline treatment for religious reasons, fear of pain or suffering, exhaustion of finances, and unlikelihood of recovery. The incompetent client is not allowed the right to refuse in similar situations for fear of an irrational choice. Medical practice defers to wishes of the family. Nurses and other health care workers must explore their personal beliefs and stance in active euthanasia, passive euthanasia, and physician-assisted death; their professional obligations to patients who request these; and ethical principles that balance the conflicting moral claims.[32,33,34,35]

In any discussion of euthanasia, it becomes important to recognize the problems surrounding the concept. It is of equal importance to note the difference between the act of intentionally ending a life, and that of withdrawing treatment that is no longer appropriate.[36] As a society, we are obligated to think carefully about all aspects of the matter. Ultimately, health professionals are expected to make sure people can live well until they die. When the time of death approaches, the health professional's main responsibility is to determine how the patient can achieve a good death. This is a critical discussion, and we are all involved.

Leininger[37] believes quality of life is culturally defined and patterned, and issues related to life, death, health, and well-being must be studied from a transcultural rather than individual perspective.

Right-to-Die Movement, the Compassionate Health Network, and Advance Directives

An increasingly publicized facet with moral and ethical aspects is the right-to-die movement, which began in England, Holland, and the Scandinavian countries, and which has gained momentum in the United States. Originally the Right-to-Die Society and the movement insisted that people should have the last word about their own lives, either to maintain or to discontinue treatment when ill or dying. In 1991, the Right to Die (Society) of Canada was developed for the purpose of allowing Canadians a practical means of changing the law to permit choice-in-dying. In 1998, the Society restructured to become an "umbrella organization" known as the Right to Die Network Canada. The network's basic field of operation is in Ottawa to work with federal politicians to change certain laws.[38] It has a 24-hour toll-free line with a bilingual operator.

It is noteworthy to mention that the Compassionate Health Network (CHN) was founded in 1991 by President Cheryl M. Eckstein, who is an anti-euthanasia activist. The organization's work includes providing material on euthanasia, assisted suicide, suicide, and palliative care to health professionals, government officials, students, disability rights advocates, lawyers, and the public at large on a national and international basis (www.chni-nternational.com/cheryl_e_dossier.htm).[39]

Advance Directives

Advance directives are written instructions provided by patients to identify their future health care preferences for the event they become incompetent to make such decisions.[40] All provinces, except New Brunswick, have legislation that recognizes the directives expressed in living wills. Living wills have several formats depending upon the province or territory in which you reside.[41]

The Canadian Nurses Association states that there are two major groups/forms: (a) instructional—commonly referred to as the living will. A living will allows individuals to identify life-sustaining treatments they would like, or not like, in given situations, (b) the proxy directive—a document which allows individuals to specify who is to make health care decisions in the event that they become incompetent.[42] Proxy is a legal term used to designate a substitute decision-maker. Such a designation is frequently referred to as a power of attorney for personal care. A wide selection of Power of Attorney Forms is available on the internet. Advance directives must be signed by the person and one witness, who is neither the proxy nor the proxy's spouse. The health professionals involved with counselling and implementation of

advance directives need to be aware of the current legislation in their own province or territory.[43] It is noteworthy that another, commonly used, advance directive is the University of Toronto's Centre for Bioethics Living Will. It has been translated into several different languages and has been adapted for people with HIV/AIDS and cancer.

Even though advance directives are promoted widely in our society, health professionals should be aware of a few of their advantages and limitations. One of the primary advantages of advance directives is to support individuals in making decisions on their own behalf, promoting the principle of self-determination. They provide directives in advance for the fair treatment of individuals, who are incompetent by providing a mechanism whereby prior wishes regarding life-sustaining treatment can be communicated. Advance directives decrease the dilemmas faced by families and loved ones of an individual in a life-threatening situation. One of the main arguments against advance directives is that the written documentation may be somewhat vague, as well as challenging to apply, in a specific clinical situation. They may also lead to inappropriate treatment decisions if situations arise that an individual could not foresee or consider at the time of writing the directive. Patients may change their mind regarding the type of treatment they wish to receive, but inadvertently forget to change their advance directives. Other advantages and limitations do exist.

The role of the nurse is important in advance directives. The Canadian Association of Critical Care Nurses (CACCN) states that the nurse should have adequate knowledge to provide patients and family members with information about the goals, advantages, and limitations of advance directives. Values taken from The CNA Code of Ethics for Registered Nurses (2002) are important to end-of-life decision making and advance directives. These values include health and well being, choice, and dignity. Further, the CNA argues that the first step in supporting clients who are considering end-of-life decisions must be for nurses to reflect on their values and beliefs associated with these issues, and to become comfortable with those values and beliefs. Another important end-of-life step is for the nurse to enter into dialogues with clients to assist them to clarify their beliefs, values, and awareness of themselves in the context of their current situation. It becomes imperative that: (1) individuals make their own decisions autonomously about advance directives, and (2) they are not coerced by any family member or health professional. The nurse's role is to ensure the effective communication to other members of the health care team regarding the client's treatment wishes as written in the advance directive.[44]

In summary, the nursing profession as a whole views and supports advance directives as an effective tool that enhances the quality of nursing care being delivered. However, the nurse must be mindful of the legal and ethical implications of advance directives.[45]

CRITICAL THINKING

What is the importance of cultural values regarding advance directives?

Assisted Suicide

In Canada, the assisted suicide debate received considerable attention during the early part of the 1990s. Keatings and Smith define assisted suicide as an act whereby an individual, who is lacking the means of completing the act of taking one's own life requires the assistance of another to complete the act. Under Section 241 of the *Criminal Code*, it is an offence to counsel, aide, or support anyone to commit suicide.[46] The CNA Code of Ethics for Registered Nurses does not address the issue of assisted suicide. Meanwhile, the much publicized case of Sue Rodriguez in British Columbia has made it clear that it is the responsibility of every nurse to become prepared for the moral challenges involved in the debate over assisted suicide.[47,48]

Assisted suicide is defined by the American Nurses Association (ANA) *as making a means of suicide available to the patient with the knowledge of the person's intended use of the equipment, medication, object, or weapon.* It differs from euthanasia, where the professional directly ends the patient's life. The ANA has issued a statement against assisted suicide or acting deliberately to terminate a patient's life; in most states in the U.S., such action is illegal. The nurse's role is to assist the person, to comfort, and to be present and available as a support.[49,50] Kirk explains how Oregon's *Death with Dignity Act*, enacted in 1998, affects nursing practice with terminally ill adults, and Murphy[51] also discusses the role of the nurse in assisted suicide.

Certain measures, when covered by a physician's order, are not considered assisted suicide or euthanasia:

- Giving a patient who is hypotensive enough morphine to control his or her pain (here the principle of double effect applies, in which an action intended to reduce pain and suffering is permissible even if it may have the unintended effect of death).
- Giving a dyspneic patient enough morphine to control his or her pain symptoms (again, double effect applies).
- Sedating a symptomatic or distressed patient at his or her request (the principle of autonomy applies).
- Withholding or withdrawing nutrition or hydration at the request of a patient (autonomy applies).

Withholding food and water or discontinuing a feeding tube and intravenous fluids to the chronically or terminally ill, or those in a persistent vegetative state, is a form of passive euthanasia, and may become assisted suicide; it is of growing ethical concern for nurses. The nurse is taught to be an advocate for the client—a very special responsibility. Although it is difficult, it enables one to provide a committed kind of caring related to the client's needs and rights.

Ferdinand discusses *guidelines to help you determine reasons for a patient's desire to die and how to respond without compromising professional principles*:

- Talk with the patient about suicidal statements.
- Assess emotional as well as physical pain and work to reduce both through a variety of pain management methods.
- Allow the patient to express fears about "losing his (or her) mind" as a result of the disease or aging process and how this can be prevented, prepared for, or coped with in late stages of AIDS, brain cancer, or liver or kidney disease.
- Assess and treat underlying depression, which is likely to remove the desire to die.
- Explore losses with the patient and how to cope with or overcome these, and enhance the person's autonomy and control to the extent possible.
- Discuss the patient's idea of death with him or her. Encourage the person to make plans via advance directives or options of hospice care.
- Encourage the patient to discuss faith, hope, and meaning of life. Refer to pastoral care.
- Listen nonjudgmentally, with compassion and concern.
- Encourage the person to do what he or she can for themself and to ask others for help when necessary.
- When thoughts of suicide persist, the principle of confidentiality does not prevent you from sharing the patient's disclosure with the physician and health care team, or from facilitating discussion between the patient and family.

As people live longer, they fear there may be a longer period of frailty, disability, depression, and social disconnectedness. Some will choose death rather than survive with pain, isolation, tubes, and machines. In spite of available access to palliative care and symptom management, there is an increasing movement for the person who is mentally alert, but in great pain or disability, to make a life termination decision.[52] The nursing profession and all health care providers have a great deal at stake. It is important that nurses be aware of their own beliefs and personal feelings regarding assisted suicide while recognizing the acceptable ethical and legal implications within the scope of their practice.

CRITICAL THINKING

Reflect for a moment and determine what your opinion of assisted suicide really is.

Physician-assisted suicide (PAS) is the *prescription of medication or counselling of an ill patient so that he or she may use a drug overdose to end his or her own life.* Dr. Jack Kevorkian, well-known for PAS, has attended numerous deaths by suicide. He is responsible for developing the "suicide machine" to inject lethal drugs into those seeking his help in dying. Boehnlein, a physician, discusses ethical, social, and economic opposition to PAS. He maintains that it is not a compassionate act and that dignified death does not come from inappropriate use of medical technology and expertise.[53]

This issue encompasses the autonomy and individual rights of the patient, the nurse's or physician's role, and society's stake. Each perspective is a complicated issue. We need to establish safeguards so that the true wishes of the patient can be expressed and legally accounted for. Many people know they can write living will directives but do not do so.

Our society shows that we still hope for the quick fix with technology, but the aging population reminds us otherwise. We are faced with the Oregon *Death with Dignity Act* of 1994. We are looking at the Netherlands' experience, referred to as the

Issues in Death and Dying

Mrs. Morton is a 94-year-old widow who has resided in the same farmhouse since her marriage in the early 1920s. She has a 45-year history of cardiac disease. She now has a pacemaker and takes medication for her heart daily. She has had a bilateral modified mastectomy but has had no further recurrence of cancer. Several times she has been hospitalized, and during the last two hospitalizations, she required resuscitation after suffering cardiac arrest.

Mrs. Morton is a very determined, devout, Christian woman, and each time she has been gravely ill, she has proclaimed her faith and has been discharged to her home. She firmly refused admittance to a senior residence centre after the last hospitalization, insisting that if she had a visiting nurse and continued help from her grandson, she could live alone in her farm home. Her grandson, who has shopped for her for the last ten years, agreed to do more tasks as necessary. Reluctantly, her physician agreed and ordered home health aide and nurse services. Because of her grave condition and inability to walk, except for a few steps, the physician also made occasional home visits.

In the nine months since her discharge, Mrs. Morton has regained her strength and her circulation has improved. She now walks in her home with a walker and cooks meals for herself and her grandson. She does receive help with bathing and vacuuming. Thus she contributes to the employment of several people. Recently her divorced granddaughter, Jean, and two great-grandchildren have come to live with her because Jean is on welfare and cannot pay rent and other expenses.

Mrs. Morton acknowledges that having three more people in her home is stressful but says she believes she must help them. She has loaned or given considerable money from her farm income and Old Age Pension cheque to all three of her grandchildren and several of her great-grandchildren. Thus she contributes to the economic support of three, and sometimes more, people. She doubts that anyone will ever repay her.

Because Mrs. Morton is very alert, friendly, and indeed very wise, she is a joy to visit. When her many friends come to visit, she shares a piece of cake she has baked and chats about local news. She reminisces some, but not excessively. She seldom complains, even briefly. Although her physical condition is marginal, her mental health is excellent. Possibly because of those healthy components, her physical condition has improved. Mrs. Morton is very much alive and looking forward to her 95th birthday.

QUESTIONS

1. As a health professional, what steps would you take to assist Mrs. Morton to prepare an advance directive?
2. List two advantages and one limitation of advance directives.
3. What would you say and do to prepare Jean and her children for Mrs. Morton's eventual death?

"slippery slope" where, in 1990, there were 8100 intentional opiate overdoses, 1000 lethal injections *without request,* and physician-assisted suicides of which only 41% met regulatory requirements. A study conducted by Wilson and his researchers regarding attitudes of terminally ill patients toward euthanasia and physician-assisted suicide revealed that many patients with advanced cancer favour policies that would allow them access to both euthanasia and physician-related suicide in the event that pain and physical symptoms became intolerable. However, the results also indicated that, for patients who would actually make the requests for a physician-assisted suicide, the psychological considerations may be at least as prominent as the physical symptoms.[54]

It is important for nurses to struggle with the values and issues of death—accidental death, long-term dying, active or passive euthanasia, and right-to-die choices—and consequently the issues and values of life. You will often be asked about your thoughts and beliefs; it is impossible to be value-free, but you can be non-judgmental and accepting of another's values. How you proceed with nursing care of the chronically ill or dying person will be influenced by your beliefs. Do not force your beliefs and values on another, but often the client will appreciate your open sharing of values and beliefs. Such sharing may even give him or her energy to continue to live with quality of life against overwhelming odds. *Certainly do all possible so that the person does not face dying and death alone.*

DEVELOPMENTAL CONCEPTS OF DEATH

As you work with people of all ages, well and ill, you will need to understand how people perceive death. A review is given here of how the child, adolescent, and adult perceives death. The concept of death is understood differently by persons in the different life eras because of general maturity, experience, ability to form ideas, and understanding of cause and effect. Culture, the religious beliefs, and the historical era also influence the concept of death, of how to grieve, and customs for handling the dead person and the mourners.

Children's Concepts of Death

Nagy[55] found three stages in the child's concept of death: (1) death is reversible, until age 5 years; (2) death is personified, ages 5 to 9; and (3) death is final and inevitable, after age 9 or 10.

The *child younger than age 5* sees death as reversible, a temporary departure like sleep or a trip, being less alive or a decrease in life functions, very still, or unable to move. Children think grown people will not die—nothing can happen to them. There is much curiosity about what happens to the person after death. The child connects death with external events, what is eaten, cemeteries, and absence. He or she thinks dead persons are still capable of growth, that they can breathe and eat and feel, and that they know what is happening on earth. Death is disturbing because it separates people from each other and because life in the grave seems dull and unpleasant.

Fear of death in the child of this age may be related to parental expression of anger; presence of intrafamily stress such as arguing and fighting; physical restraints, especially during illness; or punishment for misdeeds. At times, the child feels anger toward the parents because of their restrictions, and wishes they would go away or be dead. Guilt feelings arising from these thoughts may add to the fear of death. De Arteaga[56] discusses how to help a young child deal with death, answer questions, and grieve.

The *child from ages 5 to 9* accepts the existence of death as final and not like life. Around age 7 (at the Concrete Operations stage), he or she thinks of death as final, irreversible, and universal. Death is perceived as a person such as an angel, a frightening clown, or a monster who carries off people, usually bad people, in the night. Personal death can be avoided; he or she will not die if he or she runs faster than death, locks the door, or tricks death, unless there is bad luck. The biological changes that result in death are not understood. Parental disciplining techniques inadvertently add to this belief if they threaten that bad things will happen to the child. Traumatic situations also can arouse fear of death.

The *child, after age 9 or 10,* realizes that death is inevitable, final, happens according to certain laws, and will one day happen to him or her. If he or she is terminally ill, the child may acknowledge approaching death before the parents do. Death is the end of life, like the withering of flowers or falling of leaves, and results from internal processes. Death, for many children, is associated with being enclosed in a coffin without air, or being slowly eaten by bugs. Unless the notion of cremation is taught the child tends to think of death as a slowly rotting process. The child may express thoughts about an afterlife, depending on ideas expressed by parents and other adults and their religious philosophy.[57,58]

Death is an abstract concept, and Nagy's stages offer a guide; however, not all children's thinking about death fits into those stages. Children (and adults) may have a concept of death that contains ideas from all three stages. The ability to think abstractly is acquired slowly and to varying degrees by different people. Usually the child is unable to understand death until he or she is preadolescent or in the chum stage, for until then he or she has not learned to care for someone else as much as for themself.

The child's ideas and anxiety about separation and death and the ability to handle loss are influenced by many factors:

1. Experiences with rejecting or punitive parents
2. Strong sibling rivalry
3. Domestic or social violence
4. Loss, illness, or death in the family
5. Reaction and teaching of adults to separation or death
6. Ability to conceptualize and assimilate the experience

Children who live in a war-torn area have a more complete concept of death than do children who grew up in a peaceful environment. Terrorist attacks, acts of war, and sudden violent attacks are upsetting for children, even if they only view them on television or, conversely, observe the impact on the adults they care about. One of the most important things that parents or significant caregivers can do is to reassure children that they are safe and that they will be protected from danger.[59]

The child may think of the parent's death as deliberate abandonment for which he or she is responsible and expect death to get him or her next. The child may fear death is catching and for that reason avoid a friend whose parent has just died. If the child perceives death as sleep, he or she may fear sleep to the point of being unable to go to bed at night or even to nap. He or she may blame the surviving parent for the other parent's death, a feeling that is compounded when the surviving parent is so absorbed in personal grief that little attention is given to the child. The child may use magical thinking, believing that wishing to have the parent return will bring the parent back.

The child's fascination with and fear of death may be expressed through the games he or she plays or concern about sick pets or a dead person. Short-lived pets such as fish or gerbils help the child deal with death. Parents should handle these concerns and the related questions in a relaxed, loving manner.[60]

Self-Knowledge of Death

Can the sick child realize his or her own approaching death? Often children know more about death than adults may realize, especially chronically or terminally ill children. Children are harmed by what they do not know, by what they are not told, and by their misconceptions.

Often children acknowledge their lack of future and may say, "I'm not going anywhere." They may request an early celebration of a birthday or holiday. Parents should monitor the child's television viewing carefully, for programs often give an unrealistic impression of death, for example, cartoons and movies that show that death is reversible (or that there is survival or no harmful effects after obviously lethal injuries). Other researchers are finding similar results about children and the subject of death.[61] Although it is not easy for adults to talk with children about death, see the book *Talking About Death: A Dialogue Between Parent and Child* by Grollman.

Children's Attendance at Funerals

There are age-based guidelines for a child's involvement in a funeral. Children from 2 to 3 can view the body or be given a brief explanation, depending on their level of understanding and relationship to the deceased. But 3- to 6-year-olds benefit from a short private funeral home visit or the service itself. Seven- to 9-year-old children should attend the funeral unless they resist. Eleven- and 12-year-olds should be included in making the arrangements and the funeral service itself. In the teen years, friends of the adolescent should be encouraged to share the grief, and all should be treated as adults (see the box, entitled "Dos and Don'ts for Discussing Death with Children").

CRITICAL THINKING

What important losses did you experience in your own childhood? How did you cope with them?

Adolescents' Concepts of Death

Adolescents ponder the meaning of life. They are concerned about their bodies and a personal future. They are relatively realistic in thinking, but because of dependency–independency conflicts with parents and efforts to establish individuality, there is a low tolerance for accepting death. The healthy young person perceives self as invincible and may engage in risky behaviour. He or she seldom thinks about death, particularly as something that will happen to themselves, despite the fact that media reports of school violence have probably influenced his or her thoughts. He or she fears a lingering death and usually views death in religious or philosophic terms. He or she believes death means lack of fulfillment; there is too much to lose with death.[62,63,64]

Because of inexperience in coping with crisis and the viewpoints of death, and wanting to appear in control, the adolescent may not cry at the death of a loved one or parent. Instead he or she may continue to play games, listen to records, engage in antisocial behaviour, withdraw into seclusion or vigorous study, or go about usual activities. If the young person cannot talk, such activities provide a catharsis. Mastery of feelings sometimes comes through a detailed account of the parent's death to a peer or by displacing grief feelings onto a pet. Also, the adolescent may fantasize the dead parent as perfect or feel much the way a child would about loss of a parent. Often the adolescent's behaviour hides the fact that he or she is in mourning but carries on an internal dialogue with the dead person for weeks or months. *Be attuned to the thoughts and feelings of the adolescent who has faced death of a loved one so that you can be approachable and helpful.* One study found that the father had a more accurate view of the adolescent child's grief than did the mother.

Adolescents are more interested in world events than are children. Adolescents may be affected strongly by stressful events such as terrorist attacks, acts of war, and other violent events such as the disasters of floods and blizzards. Even though most adolescents can cope with stressful events, parents and significant caregivers can help by being present to them, listening, and supporting them as necessary.[65]

Adults' Concepts of Death

The adult's attitudes toward and concepts about dying and death are influenced by cultural and religious backgrounds. A number of references provide information.[66,67,68,69,70] The adult's reactions to death are also influenced by the experience of death of loved ones, or of others and whether the death event is sudden or has been anticipated. Fear of death is often more related to the process of dying than to the fact of death—to mutilation, deformity, isolation, pain, loss of

Dos and Don'ts for Discussing Death with Children

Do

- Ask the child what he or she is feeling. Bring up the subject of death naturally in the context of a dead pet, a book character, television show, movie, or news item.
- Help the child have a funeral for a dead pet.
- Help the child realize he or she is not responsible for the death.
- Tell the child what has happened on his or her level (but not in morbid detail).
- Explain the funeral service briefly beforehand; attendance depends on the child's age and wishes.
- Answer questions honestly, with responses geared to the child's age.
- Remember that expressions of pain, anger, loneliness, or aloneness do not constitute symptoms of an illness, but are part of a natural process of grieving.
- Help the child realize that the adults are also grieving and feeling upset, anger, despair, and guilt.

Don't

- Admonish the child not to cry; it is a universal way to show grief and anxiety.
- Tell a mystical story about the loss of the person; it could cause confusion and anxiety.
- Give long, exclusively detailed explanations beyond the level of understanding.
- Associate death with sleep, which could result in chronic sleep disturbances.
- Force the child to attend funerals or ignore signs of grieving in the child.

control over body functions and one's life, fear of the unknown, and permanent collapse and disintegration. Premonitions about coming death, sometimes correct, may occur.

Anticipation of Death

There are four responses to viewing death: positivist, negativist, activist, and passivist. Fear or anxiety about death is less in the person who believes that most of the valued goals have been attained. This person is likely to reflect positively on present activities and death as an aspect of the future and is referred to as a *positivist*. If the person believes that the time left is short, fears loss of ego integration, wishes that he or she could relive part of life, and fears death, the person is referred to as a *negativist*. A person may perceive death as diminishing the opportunity for continued fulfillment of goals. The achieved goals do not offset the fear of death. Death as a foreclosing of ambition is more distasteful than the prospect of loss of life. A person with such an attitude is referred to as an *activist*. Finally, the person may not view death with concern or fear, but as a respite from disappointments of life because attempts to attain life goals may have been so overshadowed by failure. Death may be accepted as a positive adjustment to life. Such a person is referred to as a ***passivist***.

Women are more likely to integrate the anticipation and actual experience of widowhood than are men, and greater stability of friendships through the life cycle eases adaptation to the loss of a spouse. The widow is likely to seek intimacy with same-sex friends, who replace family ties in late life.[71]

The importance of will-to-live, or lack of it, has been recognized by nurses and others for many years. The person may not be terminally ill yet, but because of the loss of a loved one, loss of feelings of self-worth and usefulness, boredom, or disillusionment with life, they may lose the will to live and rapidly decline and die. Often there are few or no causes for death apparent on autopsy.

Meaning of Death

To the adult facing death because of illness, particularly the elderly, death may have many meanings. Death may convey some positive meanings: a teacher of transcendental truths not comprehended during life; an adventure; a friend who brings an end to pain and suffering; or an escape from an unbearable situation into a new life without the present difficulties. Highly creative artists and scientists who believe they have successfully contributed their talents to society, and people with a strong belief system may have little fear of death. The great destroyer who is to be fought, punishment and separation, and a means of vengeance to force others to give more affection than they were willing to give in the past, are examples of negative meanings.[72]

The person who is dying may have suicidal thoughts or attempt suicide. Suicide is a rebellion against death, a way to cheat death's control over him or her. The elderly may be more likely to commit suicide to avoid pain, loneliness, and helplessness, or if the spouse has died.

The time comes in an illness or in later life when both the person and the survivors-to-be believe death would be better than continuing to suffer. The client has the conviction that death is inevitable and desirable and works through feelings until finally he or she has little or no anxiety, depression, or conflicts about dying. The body becomes a burden and death holds a promise. There is little incentive to live.

CRITICAL THINKING

What sorts of death-related losses do you think are most frequently experienced among middle-aged adults?

Near-Death Experience

A phenomenon that has gained public interest through Moody's publication *Life After Life*[73] is the **near-death experience (NDE)** of *"coming back to life" after just being declared clinically dead or near dead.* The stories (those told to Moody and those heard before and since) have a sameness, although details and interpretation depend on the personality and

beliefs of the person.[74] Atwater, who has distinguished herself as one of the best researchers in the field of near-death experiences, argues that health care providers are at a loss in how to recognize it if one of their patients had a near-death experience. This particular inability also holds true for the general public.[75]

There is additional publicity about men and women of a wide range of age, education, background, religious and nonreligious belief, and temperament who came close to death or had a near-death experience or who had an **out-of-body experience (OBE)**, *a feeling that one's consciousness or centre of awareness is at a different location than one's body,* often reported in relation to being resuscitated.

The person may have difficulty describing the feelings; as there has been more researched and written, individuals are more willing to share what several decades ago was not talked about readily. People who have experienced a positive near-death experience speak of a spiritual encounter that parallels the writings in the Bible in relation to the afterlife, a paradise, heaven, and express a stronger spiritual faith and no fear of death. They report a feeling of bliss about a life to come and new meaning in this life. Some people have had a negative, unpleasant, or fear-producing near-death experience; they remain afraid to die unless they turn their life around spiritually.[76]

Nearing-Death Awareness

Nearing-death awareness (NDA) differs from near-death experiences. It is an *extraordinary awareness of how death will unfold and what the person will need to die well.* This awareness is often communicated symbolically or in obscure messages by people who are dying slowly. Typically the person describes seeing or being visited by a dead loved one or a spiritual figure, and may be heard talking with this visitor (these are not pathologic hallucinations). The person may talk of getting in line for a journey (departure from this life) while lying in the hospital bed (the person is not confused). Family may think the person is losing his or her mind; reassure them by explaining the nearing-death awareness phenomenon and the need to stay with and talk to the person, and listen and learn. The person may speak of a reunion or a wonderful place, describe heaven or Jesus, talk about having a dream, or talk about a certain day being sad (and die on that day). The person may call to someone, seeking reconciliation and forgiveness. A spiritual care provider should be called.[77,78]

Keep in mind that dying patients in any setting—intensive care unit, emergency department, home, or hospice—may express nearing-death awareness. Talk to co-workers about this phenomenon, and make sure to chart patients' comments and behaviour suggesting it. If we listen with care to our dying patients, we may be able to comprehend their special awareness and help loved ones to share in it—to receive the parting gifts the dying want to give. We too may benefit. We have much to learn about dying. Our patients are the best possible teachers.

CRITICAL THINKING

What is your assessment of what near-death experiences can tell us about life after death?

BEHAVIOUR AND FEELINGS OF THE PERSON FACING DEATH

When death comes accidentally and swiftly, there is no time to prepare for death. However, death is a normal, expected event to the old, and most old people anticipate death with equanimity and without fear. The crisis is not death but where and how the person will die. Studies show that old persons living in their own homes or having adjusted to living in an institution do not fear death. Those who are close to death and are on a waiting list for admission to an institution score the highest for fear of death. The prospect of dying in conformal, unexpected circumstances creates the crisis.[79,80] Widowhood is more expected as the person ages.

Awareness of Dying

When the person approaches death gradually by virtue of many years lived or from a terminal illness, he or she will go through a predictable sequence of feelings and behaviour.

Glaser and Strauss[81,82,83] describe the stages of awareness that the terminally ill or dying person may experience depending on the behaviour of the health team and family, which, in turn, influences interaction with others.

Closed awareness *occurs when the person is dying but has neither been informed nor made the discovery.* He or she may not be knowledgeable about the signs of terminal illness, and the health team and family may not want the person to know for fear that "he will go to pieces." Maintaining closed awareness is less likely to occur if the dying person is at home.

The client and family have no opportunity to review their lives, plan realistically for the family's future, and close life with the proper rituals. Even legal and business transactions of the client may suffer as he or she tries to carry on life as usual, starts unrealistic plans, and works less feverishly on unfinished business than he or she would if the prognosis were known.

Despite the intentions and efforts of the health team and family, however, the client may become increasingly aware. He or she has a lot of time to observe the surroundings, even when very ill. He or she has time to think about the nonverbal cues and indirect comments from the staff, the inconsistent answers, the new and perplexing symptoms that do not get better despite reassurance that they will improve. At times, others may relax their guard when they think he or she does not understand and say something about the prognosis that is understood.

Suspicious awareness *develops for the reasons previously described. The person may or may not voice suspicions to others, and they are likely to deny his or her verbal suspicions.*

The client watches more closely for signs to confirm suspicions. The changing physical status; the nonverbal and verbal communications of others, with their hidden meanings; the silence; the intensity of or challenges in care; and the briskness of conversation usually will inadvertently tell or imply what he or she suspects.

Mutual pretence *occurs when staff and family become aware that the client knows he or she is dying, but all continue to pretend otherwise.* There is no conversation about impending death unless the client initiates it, although on occasion staff members may purposely drop cues because they believe the client has a right to know.

There has been a movement toward no pretence, where there is frank discussion between patient and health care providers. The talks may indicate the family is reluctant to let go or is letting go prematurely. The patient and family are helped to resolve the mutual pretence.

Open awareness *exists when the person and family are fully aware of the terminal condition, although neither may realize the nearness nor all the complications of the condition and the mode of death.*

With the certainty of death established, the person may plan to end life in accord with personal ideas about proper dying, finish important work, and make appropriate plans for and farewells with the family. He or she and the family can talk frankly, make plans, share grief, and support each other. The anguish is not reduced but it can be faced together.

The health team in the hospital has ideas, although not always verbalized, about how the person ought to die, morally and stylistically. The wishes of the client and the family should always have priority, particularly when they ask that no heroic measures be taken to prolong life. Extra privileges, special requests, or the client's discharge to the family can be granted. Most people wish to die without pain, with dignity, in privacy, and with loved ones nearby. Often dying in the hospital precludes both privacy and dignity, and the health team should continuously work to provide these rights. Cultural and religious beliefs, as well as rituals following a death, must be respected by all health professionals. Wright, Watson, and Bell, in their book *Beliefs: The Heart of Healing in Families and Illness*, outline clearly in table form, the death and dying issues related to religious beliefs.

Sequence of Reactions to Approaching Death

When the person becomes aware of the diagnosis and prognosis, whether he or she is told directly or learns by advancing through the stages of awareness discussed previously, he or she and the family usually go through a predictable sequence of reactions described by Kübler-Ross.

In your practice, assessment and intervention must be individualized. Do not assume that everyone is experiencing each stage as the research results describe.

Denial and Isolation
Denial and **isolation** are the *initial and natural reactions when the person learns of terminal illness:* "It can't be true. I don't believe it's me." The person may go through a number of rituals to support this denial, even to the point of finding another

doctor. He or she needs time to mobilize resources. Denial serves as a necessary buffer against overwhelming anxiety.

The person is denying when he or she talks about the future; avoids talking about the illness or the death of self or others; or persistently pursues cheery topics. Recognize the client's need; respond to this behaviour, and let him or her set the pace in conversation. Later the person will gradually consider the possibility of the prognosis; anxiety will lessen; and the need to deny will diminish.

Psychological isolation occurs when the *client talks about the illness, death, or mortality intellectually but without emotion as if these topics were not relevant.* Initially the idea of death is recognized, although the feeling is repressed. Gradually, feelings about death will be less isolated, and the client will begin to face death but still maintain hope.

If the client continues to deny for a prolonged time despite advancing symptoms, he or she will need much warmth, compassion, and support as death comes closer. Your contacts with the client may consist of sitting in silence, using touch communication, giving meticulous physical care, conveying acceptance and security, and looking in on him or her frequently. If denial is extensive, he or she cannot grieve or face the inevitable separation. Yet Kübler-Ross found that few persons maintain denial to the end of life.

Anger

The second reaction, **anger,** *occurs with acknowledgment of the reality of the prognosis.* It is necessary for an eventual acceptance of approaching death. As denial and isolation decrease, anger, envy, and resentment of the living are felt. Often, direct expression of anger is unacceptable, so this stage is difficult for the client and others. Anger is displaced onto things or people: "The doctor is no good," "The food is no good," "The hospital is no good," "The nurses are neglectful," and "People don't care." The family also bears the brunt of the anger.

Anger results when the person realizes life will be interrupted before he or she finishes everything planned. Everything reminds the person of life while he or she is dying, and he or she feels soon-to-be-forgotten. He or she may make angry demands, frequently ring the bell, manipulate and control others, and generally make the self heard. He or she is convincing self and others that he or she is not yet dead and forgotten.

Do not take the anger personally. The dying person whose life will soon end needs empathy. The person who is respected, understood, and given time and attention will soon lower the angry voice and decrease demands. The person will realize he or she is considered a valuable person who will be cared for and yet allowed to function at maximum potential as long as possible. Your calm approach will lower anxiety and defensive anger.

Bargaining

The third reaction, **bargaining,** occurs when *the person tries to enter into some kind of agreement that may postpone death.* He or she may try to be on the best behaviour. He or she knows the bargaining procedure and hopes to be granted the special wish—an extension of life, preferably without pain. Although

the person will initially ask for no more than one deadline or postponement of death, he or she will continue the good behaviour and will promise to devote life to some special cause if he or she lives.

Bargaining may be life promoting. As the person continues to hope for life, to express faith in God's willingness to let him or her live, and to engage actively in positive, health-promoting practices, the body's physical defences may be enhanced by mental or emotional processes yet unknown. This process may account for those not-so-uncommon cases in which the person has a prolonged, unexpected remission during a malignant disease process. Hope, which is involved in bargaining and which you can support, gives each person a chance for more effective treatment and care as new discoveries are made.

Depression

Depression is the fourth reaction and occurs when *the person gets weaker, needs increasing treatment, and worries about mounting medical costs and even necessities.* Role reversal and related problems add to the strain. Depression about past losses and the present condition; feelings of shame about the illness, sometimes interpreted as punishment for past deeds; and hopelessness enshroud the person and extend to the loved ones.

Depression is normal. The family and staff need to encourage the person by giving realistic praise and recognition, letting him or her express feelings of guilt, work through earlier losses, finish mourning, and build self-esteem. You will need to give more physical and emotional help as the person grows weaker. He or she should stay involved with the family as long as possible.

Preparatory Depression

Preparatory depression is the next stage and differs from the previous depression. Now *the person realizes the inevitability of death and comes to desire the release from suffering that death can bring.* He or she wishes to be a burden no more and recognizes that there is no hope of getting well. The person needs a time of preparatory grief to get ready for the final separation of impending loss: not only are loved ones going to lose him or her, but the person is losing all significant objects and relationships. The person reviews the meaning of life and searches for ways to share insights with the people most significant to him or her, sometimes including the staff. Often the fear that he or she cannot share aspects of life or valued material objects with people of his or her own choosing will cause greater concern than the diagnosis of a terminal illness or the knowledge of certain death. As a person thinks of what life has meant to them he or she begins to get ready to release life. Such a release, however, does not come without feelings of grief. Often he or she will talk repetitiously to find a meaning in life.

The family and health team can either inhibit the person during this stage or promote emotional comfort and serene acceptance of death. The first reaction to depressed, grieving behaviour and life review is to cheer him or her. This meets your needs but not those of the client. When the person is preparing for the impending loss of all love objects and relationships, behaviour should be accepted and not changed.

Acceptance of the final separation in life will not be reached unless he or she is allowed to express a life review and sorrow. There may be no need for words if rapport, trust, and a working nurse–client relationship have been previously established. A touch of the hand and a warm accepting silence are therapeutic. Too much interference with words, sensory stimuli, or burdensome visitors hinders rather than helps emotional preparation for death. If the person is ready to release life and die and others expect him or her to want to continue to live and be concerned about things, the person's own depression, grief, and turmoil are increased. He or she wishes quietly and gradually to disengage self from life and all that represents life. He or she may request few or no visitors and modifications in the routines of care and repeatedly request no heroic measures to prolong life.

Honour the client's requests but at the same time promote optimum physical and emotional comfort and well-being. Explain the feelings and needs of the client to the family and other members of the health team so that they can better understand his or her behaviour. The family should know that this depression is beneficial if the client is to die peacefully and that it is unrelated to their past or present behaviour.

Acceptance

The final reaction, **acceptance** or a *kind of resolution,* comes if the person is given enough time, does not have a sudden, unexpected death, and is given some help in working through the previous reactions. He or she will no longer be angry or depressed about the fate and will no longer be envious or resentful of the living. He or she will have mourned the loss of many people and things and will contemplate the end with a certain degree of quiet expectation. Now the ultimate of ego integrity, described by Erikson,[85] becomes evident. Acceptance is difficult and takes time. It depends in part on the client's awareness of the prognosis of illness so that he or she can plan ahead—religiously, philosophically, financially, socially, and emotionally. This last stage is almost devoid of feeling.

Priorities change; family and close friends become more important. Gradually the person is able to plan for the not-too-far future. Money is less important. Negative friends are avoided. The person must adjust to fatigue, changes in body function or structure, effects of chemotherapy or radiation, the continuing treatment appointments, and loss of control.

The healthy aged person will also go through some aspects of the reactions discussed previously, for as the person grows old, he or she contemplates more frequently personal mortality and begins to work through feelings about it.

Whereas Kübler-Ross looks at the dying *person* with the family implied, Giacquinta[86] looks at the *family* with the dying person implied. Table 15-1 outlines the four main stages and the 10 phases the family will experience from the time of diagnosis through the post death period.

Both the Kübler-Ross and the Giacquinta models are helpful. They are built on observations of hundreds of dying persons and families, but you must not stereotype responses into these stages. Sometimes the person or family will not go through every one of these stages, and the stages will not always follow in this sequence. The person or family may remain in a certain stage or revert to earlier stages. Feelings related to several of the researched stages may exist.

Do not convey that the client or family should be in a certain stage or reacting a certain way. Avoid social and religious clichés. Rather, be a caring, concerned, available person, willing to do nondramatic, simple, but helpful tasks such as bringing the family member something to drink, watering the flowers sent by a friend, and offering to call a significant person. Equally important will be doing physical care procedures in a thorough but efficient manner so that visiting family members can spend as much time with their dying loved one as possible. Listen to feelings when the person wants to talk but do not probe.

CRITICAL THINKING

Think about a loved one in your family who was gravely ill or dying. How did you respond initially to the seriousness of the situation?

Anniversary Reaction and Emotionally Invested Deadlines

Anniversary reaction *refers to feelings of grief and sadness or a reliving of the mourning process about a year after the death of the loved one.* Or the *grief and mourning response, including physical symptoms, may be more intense at the person's birth date or at one of several of the major holidays* throughout the year.

Predilection to Death and Postponement of Death

The phenomenon of **predilection to death** is seen in *people who, although lacking any signs of emotional conflict, suicidal tendencies, severe depression, or panic, correctly anticipate their own deaths.* These persons are firmly convinced of their impending death yet feel no depression or anxiety toward it, regarding it as completely appropriate. Such clients are resigned to death; to fight against it is unthinkable, for death is a release from the burden of their life or body. Research shows that death comes to the predilection clients just as they have anticipated it would, although medically their condition does not warrant such a quick demise or, in some cases, any death at all.[87]

Postponement *refers to the person making an overt (conscious or spoken) or covert (unconscious) decision about the choice of date or event for time of death. Death seems inevitable but the person holds onto life unexpectedly.* Typically, the choice may be associated with waiting for return of a loved one or an emotionally invested date for the person. Some people die just before entry into a nursing home from their residence or the hospital.[88]

TABLE 15-1
Family's Response to Dying and Death

Four Main Stages	Family Experiences	Nurse Can Foster
Living with Terminal Illness		
Person learns diagnosis, tries to carry on as usual, and undergoes treatment	*Impact:* emotional shock, despair, disorganized behaviour	
	Functional disruption: much time spent at hospital (if traditional surgery or treatment chosen), ignoring of home tasks and emotional needs, weakening of family structure, emotional isolation	Hope as different treatment methods are used, communication, seeking helpful resources, family cohesiveness
	Search for meaning: questioning why this happened; casting blame on various persons, deity, institutions, habits; realization that "Someday I will die too"	Security
	Informing others (family and friends): ascent from isolation, with moral and practical support, or feeling of rejection: others do not understand, do not care, or are afraid; possible need to retreat again into emotional isolation	Courage, reliable help, understanding of why some people cannot help
	Engaging emotions: beginning grieving, fearing loss of emotional control, assumption of roles once carried by dying person	Problem solving; idea that life will change but will be ongoing
Living–Dying Interval		
Person ceases to perform family roles, is cared for, either at home or in hospital; person needs to come to terms with accomplishments and failures and to find renewed meaning in life	*Reorganization:* firmer division of family tasks	Cooperation instead of competition; analysis to see if new role distribution is workable
	Framing memories: reviewing life of dying person—what he or she has meant and accomplished, new sense of family history, relinquishment of dependency on dying member	Focus on life review rather than only on what person is now
Bereavement		
Death occurs	*Separation:* absorption in loneliness of separation as person becomes unconscious	Intimacy among family members; release of grief as normal
	Mourning: guilt, "Could I have done more?"	
Reestablishment		
	Expansion of the social network: overcoming feelings of alienation and guilt	Looking back with acceptance and forward to new growth and socialization with a reunited, normally functioning family

---

NARRATIVE VIGNETTE

You are the only health care professional—an occupational nurse, in a gold mine in a small rural community. You have been on the job for three months. One of your family members has become gravely ill. You need to stay with your loved one for a few weeks until your sister comes from New Brunswick to stay with your relative. You have heard about Compassionate Care Benefits.

1. How do you apply for this benefit in your province/territory?
2. What assistance can you expect to receive?

Some individuals, despite impending death, maintain hope and endurance and apparently refuse to die and live beyond the time of expected death. A person can program, through unconscious or conscious will onset of illness, recovery from severe illness, or time of death. A strong will to live is often associated with the person's being interested, involved, or active in life or having a loved one, spouse, or dependant whom he or she desires to be with or for whom he or she feels' responsible. For some, the death month is related to the birth month in that some people postpone death to witness their birthdays or another important holiday. The person with excessive fear of death may be unable to die until able to express and work through conscious fears or phobias.

"Scared to Death" (Death by Autosuggestion)

Unlike the predilection client, who, convinced of impending death, anticipates it, the **scared-to-death individual** does not see death as appropriate.[89,90,91] He or she *believes self the victim of a curse, hex, or prediction and therefore cannot be saved by anyone or by any means.* **Psychic death** is said to occur when *a person is convinced of and accurately predicts his or her own death when no medical cause for death exists.* **Auto-suggestion** is the most accurate description for the cause of psychic death; it implies that the *person responded in such a way as to convince self of imminent death.* A synonym for autosuggestion might be "self-hypnosis."

Planning for Death

While the person is still healthy and capable of making the many decisions in relation to death, he or she can do much to relieve worries and take the burden of those decisions off others. You are in a position to provide professional information to others. In working with the family, you may wish to inform them that the Government of Canada announced, in 2003, a new type of Employment Insurance Benefit called the Compassionate Care Benefit. This benefit allows a person to temporarily leave their place of employment to care for a dying family member—and receive support from the Federal Government Employment Insurance Program.[92]

Representatives from some nursing and funeral homes and cemeteries are educating people to keep a folder, revised periodically, of all information that will be used by those

making arrangements at the time of death. Such a folder might include names of advisors such as attorney, banker, life insurance broker, and accountant. Personal and vital information should be included such as birth certificate, marriage licence, military discharge papers, and copies of wills, including willing of body parts to various organizations. Financial records (or a copy of those held in a safety deposit box), estimated assets and liabilities, and insurance and social insurance information should be there. Personal requests and wishes, listing who gets what, should be written along with funeral arrangements and cemetery deeds.

These are intellectual preparations. They cannot ease the sense of loss in the living, but they can foster peace of mind, realizing that the deceased's wishes were carried out.

CRITICAL THINKING

With which aspects of emotional preparation might you be able to assist family members as the death of a loved one nears?

HEALTH CARE AND NURSING APPLICATIONS

Death is an intensely poignant event, one that causes deep anguish, but one you may frequently encounter in client care.

Self-Assessment

Personal assessment, being aware of and coping with your personal feelings about death, is essential to assess accurately or intervene helpfully with the client, family, or other health care providers. How do you protect yourself from anxiety and despair resulting from repeated exposure to personal sufferings? The defences of isolation, denial, and "professional" behaviour are common in an attempt to cope with feelings of helplessness, guilt, frustration, and ambivalence about the client's not getting well or the secret wish for the client to die. It takes courage and maturity to undergo the experience of death with clients and families and yet remain an open, compassionate human being. You are a product of the culture, just as the client and the family are, and hence will experience many of the same kinds of reactions. Religious, philosophic, educational, and family experiences and general maturity also affect your ability to cope with feelings related to death.

The dying client may seek an identification and partnership with someone, and often this person is the nurse. If you

15-1 BONUS SECTION IN CD-ROM

Coping with Mom's Cancer Diagnosis

In this first-person account we are able to live one person's experience of caring for their dying mother.

are the nurse, think of this as a positive experience, where it may be a privilege to share with someone the last hours or days of their life.

Dying in the hospital has become so organized, and care so fragmented, that you are not necessarily vulnerable to personal involvement in the client's death. However, you are more likely to be personally affected by and feel a sense of loss from the client's death if an attachment has been formed to the client and family because of prolonged hospitalization, hospice care, and if the death is unexpected. Also, if you perform nursing measures you believe might have contributed to the client's death, if you have worked hard to save a life, or if the client's social or personal characteristics are similar to your own, you will feel the loss.

Glaser and Strauss describe how health care workers judge a client's value according to social status and respond accordingly. The client's death is considered less a social loss (and is therefore less mourned by the nursing staff) if he or she is elderly, comatose, or confused, of a lower socioeconomic class or a minority group, poorly educated, not famous, unattractive, or is considered "responsible" for having the disease. The dying client in these categories is likely to receive less care or only routine care. The client with high social value, whose death is mourned and who receives optimum care by the nursing staff is the person who is young, alert, or likable, has prominent family status, has a high-status occupation or profession, is from the middle or upper socioeconomic class, or is considered talented or pretty.

If the client's death is very painful or disfiguring, you may avoid the client because of feelings of guilt or helplessness. In addition, you may be aware of the callous attitudes of health team members or of the decision of the family and doctor about prolonging life with heroic measures or not prolonging life. These situations can provoke intense negative reactions if you disapprove of the approaches of other members of the health team.

You must attempt to deal with the various pitfalls of working with the dying. These include:

1. Withdrawal from the client
2. Isolation of emotions
3. Failure to perceive own feelings or feelings of client and family
4. Displacing own feelings onto other team members
5. "Burning out" from intense emotional involvement
6. Fearing illness and death

Support for Nurses

A support system should be available. Specific times should be set aside for staff members to share emotional needs related to a specific dying client or to learn specifics of the dying process. Often nurses can help each other, but there should also be a specialist with whom to confer: a master's educated nurse with additional psychiatric consultation liaison skill, a religious leader, a nun, a psychologist, or a psychiatrist. The specialist should also be available for spontaneous sessions.

The administration may also encourage and sponsor the nurses in taking courses other than in nursing (sociology, philosophy, religion) to gain different perspectives. Health care professionals should join professional organizations in which they can share problems or solutions and gain support. Staff may change departments either temporarily or permanently to feel the accomplishment of working with those who recover. Two primary care nurses (if that is the system) can work together so that they can share emotions and support each other.

If you work with cancer clients exclusively, you may also need special assistance. Optimism and logical thinking must be encouraged in the client and maintained in your self. You may hear many opinions about helpful treatment, both inside and outside the medical establishment; and you may see that some of the established treatments have unpleasant side effects. The question arises: Why must the client endure so much?

If you can think of death as the last stage of life and as fulfillment, you can mature and learn from the client as he or she comes to terms with personal illness. The meaning of death can serve as an important organizing principle in determining how the person conducts his or her life, and it is as significant for you as for the client. With time and experience, you will view the role of comforter as being as important as that of promoting care. Then the client who is dying will be less of a personal threat.

Some *guidelines for the nurse working with dying clients* are presented:

- Individual staff members should be encouraged to gain personal insight and acknowledge their own limits. Extra support or time off may be necessary when staff members are under a high degree of stress. The needs of clients deserve priority, however; if certain staff members constantly require considerable support, they may be encouraged to seek employment elsewhere.
- A healthy balance must be maintained between work and an outside life. This type of work demands considerable personal involvement. There must be times when each member of staff is left totally off call so they might pursue personally affirming activities.
- The individual must be careful when the "need to be needed" becomes too great and he or she attempts to be everything to everyone. This work is probably best accomplished by a team.
- The individual must maintain a support system at work and outside the work setting. Hospice units must make provision for ongoing staff support through the use of visitation, psychiatric consultants for the staff, or weekly

staff support meetings. In addition, individuals should be encouraged to seek relationships outside the work setting for additional support.

■ For those working in isolation, it may be wise to consider ongoing sessions with an outside consultant and therapist who can offer guidance and provide support.

Dean claims that humour can function as a coping mechanism to deal with the potential vulnerability that accompanies constant exposure to loss and death.[93] At times, of course, humour may be considered inappropriate in a hospice/palliative care setting. Experienced health professionals will recognize, however, the importance of sensitivity and intuition, as indicators of when, and how, humour may be introduced.

CRITICAL THINKING

What guidelines for the use of humour by a nurse do you think are important?

Assessment of Client and Family

Assessment of the client and family is done according to the standard methods of assessment. The total person (physical, intellectual, emotional, social, and spiritual needs and status) must be assessed to plan effective care. Learn what the client and family know about the client's condition and what the doctor has told them, to plan for a consistent approach.

Recognize also that people differ in the way they express feelings about dying and death. Mourning may be private or public. Listen to the topics of conversation the person discusses, observe for rituals in behaviour, and learn of typical behaviour in health from him or her or the family to get clues to what is important. The routines that are important in life may become more important now, and they may assist in preparation for death. Observe family members for pathologic responses—physical or emotional—as grief after loss from death increases the risk of mortality for the survivor, especially for the male spouse or relative who is in late middle age or older.

Nursing Diagnoses

The box entitled, "Nursing Diagnoses Related to the Dying Person," is a list of diagnoses that may be pertinent to the dying person and are related to assessment and need for holistic care. Stepnick and Perry relate the phase of resolving death according to the Kübler-Ross format to what could be nursing diagnoses. They list four stages of spiritual development (chaotic, formal, skeptic, and mystic) and nursing strategies to assist the client at each stage of spiritual development as the client approaches death.

Intervention with the Family

The family will be comforted as they see *compassionate care being given to their loved one.* Your attitude is important, for both family members and clients are very perceptive about your real feelings, whether you are interested and available,

giving false reassurance, or just going about a job. Family members often judge your personal relationship with the loved one as more important than your technical skill. In order to give sensitive, quality care, note the cultural differences and structure of each family. For example, the structure of the First Nation families is not based on the nuclear family, but upon the extended family. It is very common to find multigenerational households in First Nation communities. As a result, when a health crisis arises within the family, it is not unusual for a large extended family to gather around. This gathering demonstrates respect for the ill or dying individual and indicates support for those family members most affected by the crisis.[94]

Try to *help the relatives compensate for their feelings of helplessness, frustration, or guilt.* Their assisting the client with feeding or grooming or other time-consuming but nontechnical aspects of care can be helpful to them, the client, and the nursing staff. The family may be acting toward or caring for the client in a way that seems strange or even nontherapeutic to the nursing staff. Yet these measures or the approach may seem fine to the client because of the family pattern or ritual. It is not for you to judge or interfere unless what the family is doing is unsafe for the client's welfare or is clearly annoying to the client. In turn, recognize when family members are fatigued or anxious and relieve them of responsibility at that point. Encourage the family to take time to rest and to meet needs adequately. A lounge or other place where the family can alternately rest and yet be near the client is helpful.

Show acceptance of grief. By helping the family members express their grief and by giving support to them, you are helping them, in turn, to support the client.

Prepare the family for sudden, worsening changes in the client's condition or appearance to avoid shock and feelings of being overwhelmed.

The crisis of death of the loved one may result in a life *crisis for the surviving family members.* The problems with changes in daily routines of living, living arrangements, leisure-time activities, role reversal and assuming additional responsibilities, communicating with other family members, or meeting financial obligations can seem overwhelming. The failure of relatives and friends to help or the insistence by relatives and friends on giving help that is not needed is equally problematic. Advice from others may add to rather than decrease the burdens. The fatigue that a long illness causes in a family member may remain for some time after the loved one's death and may interfere with adaptive capacities. You can help by being a listener, exploring with the family ways in which to cope with their problems, and making referrals or encouraging them to seek other persons or agencies for help. Often your willingness to accept and share their feelings of loss and other concerns can be enough to help the family mobilize their strengths and energies to cope with remaining problems. It is important to be sensitive to their cultural beliefs and practices around death.

The most heartbreaking time for the family may be the time *when the client is disengaging from life* and from them. The *family will need help to understand this process* and recognize it as normal behaviour. The dying person has found peace. His or her circle of interests has narrowed, and he or she wishes to be

Nursing Diagnoses Related to the Dying Person

Pattern 1: Exchanging

Altered Nutrition: Less than Body Requirements
Risk for Infection
Ineffective Thermoregulation
Constipation
Diarrhea
Bowel Incontinence
Altered Urinary Elimination
Altered Tissue Perfusion (specify type)
Risk for Injury
Impaired Tissue Integrity
Impaired Skin Integrity
Energy Field Disturbance

Pattern 2: Communicating

Impaired Verbal Communication

Pattern 3: Relating

Impaired Social Interaction
Social Isolation
Altered Role Performance
Altered Family Processes
Caregiver Role Strain
Altered Sexuality Patterns

Pattern 4: Valuing

Spiritual Distress

Pattern 5: Choosing

Ineffective Individual Coping
Impaired Adjustment
Defensive Coping
Ineffective Denial
Ineffective Family Coping: Disabling
Ineffective Family Coping: Compromised
Family Coping: Potential for Growth
Decisional Conflict
Health-Seeking Behaviours

Pattern 6: Moving

Impaired Physical Mobility
Activity Intolerance
Fatigue
Risk for Activity Intolerance
Sleep Pattern Disturbance
Diversional Activity Deficit
Impaired Home Maintenance Management
Altered Health Maintenance
Feeding Self-Care Deficit
Impaired Swallowing
Bathing/Hygiene Self-Care Deficit
Dressing/Grooming Self-Care Deficit
Toileting Self-Care Deficit

Pattern 7: Perceiving

Body Image Disturbance
Self-Esteem Disturbance
Sensory/Perceptual Alterations
Hopelessness
Powerlessness

Pattern 8: Knowing

Knowledge Deficit
Acute Confusion
Altered Thought Processes

Pattern 9: Feeling

Pain
Chronic Pain
Anticipatory Grieving
Anxiety
Fear

Other NANDA diagnoses are applicable to the dying person.

Source: North American Nursing Diagnosis Association, NANDA Nursing Diagnoses: Definitions & Classification 1999-2000. Philadelphia: North American Nursing Diagnosis Association, 1999.

left alone and not disturbed by any news of the outside world. Behaviour with others may be so withdrawn that he or she seems unreachable and uncooperative. He or she prefers short visits and is not likely to be in a talkative mood. The television set remains off. Communication is primarily nonverbal. This behaviour can cause the family to feel rejected, unloved, and guilty about not doing enough for the client. They should understand that the client can no longer hold onto former relationships as he or she accepts the inevitability of death. The family needs help in realizing that their silent presence can be a very real comfort and shows that he or she is loved and not forgotten. Concurrently, the family can learn that dying is not a horrible thing to be avoided.

This may be the time when family insist on additional life-sustaining or heroic measures, although they will only prolong suffering. The nurse can listen to their desire to prolong life, explain the needs and what is happening to the patient, act as a mediator when various family members make contradictory statements, calm angry tempers, and start a rational discussion about what's best for the patient. Having a meeting that includes family, nurse, pastoral care, the physician, members of an ethics committee, and other health care workers or significant others is useful. Keeping lines of communication open and maintaining a bond with the family, being non-judgmental, and encouraging family contact with the patient are essential and challenging, even difficult at times.[95,96]

EVIDENCE-BASED PRACTICE

Factors which Influence Coping: Home-based Family Caregiving of Persons with Advanced Cancer

In a qualitative study, 15 family caregivers were interviewed following the death of their particular family member, for whom they had provided care. Coping emerged as a category needing further analysis. Factors were identified which either facilitated or interfered with caregiving coping. The caregivers in the study ranged in age from 37 to 81 years. Of the 11 women in the study, six were wives; three were daughters, one a daughter-in-law, and one a sister. Of the four men, three were husbands and one a son. The length of time in the primary caregiving role ranged from one to 11 months. The first of two interviews occurred from one to 12 months following the death of the family member.

Results

A. Three main categories that *facilitated* their coping included: the characteristics of the caregivers themselves, the contributions made by the dying person, and supportive networks, both formal and informal, available to the caregivers.

B. Interfering factors, evident to a lesser extent in the data, related to their experiences with the informal and formal systems. For example, caregivers identified the less than adequate coordination and scheduling of health services coming into the home.

Practice Implications

1. Clinicians are challenged to recognize the centrality of the reciprocal caring partnership between caregivers and the dying person.
2. Service providers, external to the intimate duality, must seek to support both of its members in order to facilitate the coping capacity and emotional tenacity of both.
3. The dying person must be recognized as not just the passive recipient of care, but an active and participating member in the caregiving process.
4. Clinicians must recognize the emotional intensity of home-based palliative caregiving and be sensitive to the tremendous responsibility carried by family caregivers. They must work with family caregivers, the dying persons, and with each other as true and equal partners in the caregiving process.
5. Clinicians must be available to families for support and guidance through the maze of caregiving.
6. Clinicians must recognize the effect their attitudes and values have on the care they deliver.
7. Health care providers must continually engage in anticipatory guidance, interpretation, and monitoring of the inevitable decline and dying process of the ill person with caregivers so that they can feel secure and supported in their emotionally exhausting work.

Source: Strang, Vicki R., and Priscilla M. Koop, Factors which Influence Coping: Home-based Family Caregiving of Persons with Advanced Cancer, Journal of Palliative Care, 19, no. 2 (2003), 107–114. Used with permission.

News of impending or actual death is best communicated to a family unit or group rather than to a lone individual to allow the people involved to give mutual support to each other. This should be done in privacy so they can express grief without the restraints imposed by public observation. Stay and comfort the person facing death, at least until a religious leader or other close friends can come.

Requests by an individual or family to see the dead person should *not* be denied on the grounds that it would be too upsetting. The person who needs a leave taking to realize the reality of the situation will ask for it; those for whom it would be overwhelming will not request it.

Sometimes the survivor of an accident may ask about people who were with him or her at the time of the accident. The health team should confer on when and how to answer these questions; *well-timed honesty is the healthiest approach;* otherwise the person cannot adapt to the reality of the accidental death. The person's initial response of shock, denial, and tears or later grief will neither surprise nor upset the medical team who understand the normal steps in resolving crisis and loss. Cutting off the person's questions or keeping him or her sedated may protect the staff, but it does not help the survivor.

The parents who grieve for their dying or fatally injured child must be respected, be given the opportunity to minister to the child when indicated, and be relieved of responsibilities at times. Encourage the parents to share feelings, and work to complement, not compete with, the parents in caring for the child. Also, remember that grandparents, siblings, peers, and sometimes the babysitter will need understanding in their grieving. The timing and type of support given after accidental death of a child are important. Nelson and Wiener et al. give some practical suggestions for care of the parents.

Accident, suicide, and homicide are the leading causes of death before age 40. Thus, survivors often include children and adolescents. The grief and mourning that surrounds each of these death events differ from an anticipated death. The suddenness of each causes shock, confusion, helplessness, emptiness, and intense sadness. With suicide comes guilt and shame, a sense of being responsible, as well as anger at the person who committed suicide. With homicide come the feelings of intense anger, rage, revenge, with the sadness intensified by the imagery related to brutality and what the person suffered in the last moments alive. With each of these types of death, the family longs to undo certain acts and to be able to say goodbye in a loving way. Long-term therapy is often needed.

CRITICAL THINKING

What role (if any) do you believe serious accidents play in one's encounters with death?

Other Grief Responses

As you care for the family of the dying person, or interact with the family after death, you may perceive that they are not grieving in what you consider the usual or normal way. You may assess their grief and mourning, both in anticipation of and at the time of death as absent or delayed, as complicated, pathologic, neurotic, and dysfunctional, or as a clinical depression.[97]

Delayed grief response may be identified when *there is no anticipatory grieving or no expression of grief at death.* Later, there may be manifestations of not having grieved the loss:

- Continuing to act as if the person still lives, or looking for them
- Various physical symptoms, such as insomnia, loss of appetite and weight, pain, and actual malfunction of the body
- Expressions of frustration or anger that is out of context or excessive, or personality changes
- Complaints of excessive stress at work or home
- Increased smoking and use of alcohol or other drugs
- Difficulty in interpersonal and family relationships
- Nightmares, illusions of seeing the person and then realizing the person was someone else, or hallucinations of the person
- Statements about "shutting down at the time of death"

Complicated grief response may occur *when the person is experiencing unresolved grief associated with the past.* It is manifested in several ways:

- Multiple physical complaints, often with no significant findings or physical examination (Often the symptoms mimic those of the deceased.)
- Suicidal ideas or attempts, wanting to join the dead person
- Intense grief when speaking of the deceased, or inappropriate, angry affect, or the mechanism of emotional isolation, e.g., smiling while talking about the dead person
- Withdrawal from others, failure to participate in the usual family or social activities, radical life changes
- Inability to talk about the deceased without intense grief expressions
- Intense grief reactions triggered by minor events
- Repeated verbalization of themes of loss
- Extreme sadness at certain times of the year, e.g., anniversary dates or special holidays

Through counselling, the person may remember past losses or rejections and grieve these as well as the current loss.

Dysfunctional grief response may occur when (1) *the person had a very dependent or ambivalent relationship with the deceased;* (2) *the circumstances surrounding death were uncertain, sudden, or overwhelming,* such as homicide, *or complicated with assault,* such as rape or violent attack; *or* (3) *a loss that is socially unspeakable or socially negated,* such as capital punishment or death or murder of someone who had been a gang member or molester of children or had a criminal history. If there has been a history of mental illness or suicide, or if the person has minimal support systems, another loss will be more difficult to handle.[98,99,100,101]

Pathologic grief response is an *intensification of grief to the point that the person is overwhelmed, demonstrates prolonged maladaptive behaviour, manifests excessive symptoms and extensive interruptions in healing,* and does not progress to integration of the loss, finding meaning in the loss, and resolution of the mourning process.

Intervention for the Dying Person

Care of the dying client falls primarily on the nurse. You have sustained contact with the client and understand dying and the many needs of the dying person. You know the value of compassionate service of mind and hands. You can protect the vulnerable person and understand some of the distress felt by client and family. You have an opportunity to help the client bring life to a satisfactory close, truly to live until he or she dies, and to promote comfort. The client needs your unqualified interest and response to help decrease loneliness and make the pain and physical care or treatment bearable.

To assist you and other health care professionals, a publication referred to as *A Guide to the End of Life Care for Seniors* has been developed to present a manual of national guidelines. This Guide is intended to support end of life care for seniors in Canada. In addition, this Guide provides health care information for other groups, such as family caregivers and social service providers. Ethical issues concerning end of life and how to deliver end-of-life care are provided. Spirituality and cultural issues are presented with significant focus on the diverse needs of Canada's Aboriginal peoples.

While providing care to *the dying person* you will experience many frustrations. There is the challenge of talking with or listening to the client. Will he or she talk about death? Pain may be constant and difficult to relieve, causing you to feel incompetent. He or she may be demanding, nonconforming to the client role, or disfigured and offensive to touch or smell. The family may visit so often and long that they interfere with necessary care of the client. Accusations from the client or family about neglect may occur or be feared. It is no wonder that despite good intentions, religious convictions, and educational programs, you may avoid the dying client and family. They are left to face the crisis of death alone. As you rework personal feelings about crisis, dying, and death and become more comfortable with personal negative feelings and emotional upset, you will be able to serve more spontaneously and openly in situations previously avoided. You will be able to admit, without guilt feelings, personal limits in providing care, to use other helpers, and yet to do as much as possible for the client and family without showing shock or repugnance about the client's condition.

Physical care of the dying person includes providing for nutrition, hygiene, rest, elimination, relief of pain or other symptoms; care of the mouth, nose, eyes, skin, and peripheral circulation; positioning; and environmental considerations. Hospital personnel should not focus exclusively on the client's complaints of pain or other physical symptoms or need to avoid the subject of death. Complaints may be a camouflage for anxiety, depression, or other feelings and covertly indicate a desire to talk with someone about the feelings. Analgesics and comfort measures to promote rest can be used along with crisis therapy. Spend sufficient time with the client to establish a relationship that is supportive. Provide continuity of care. Try to exchange information realistically within the whole medical team, including client and family, to reduce uncertainty and feelings of neglect. Clients can withstand much pain and distress as long as they feel wanted or believe their life has meaning.

Thorough, meticulous physical care is essential to promote physical well-being but also to help *prevent emotional distress*. During the prolonged and close contact physical care provides, you can listen, counsel, and teach, using principles of effective communication. But let the client sleep often, without sedation if possible. The many physical measures to promote comfort and optimum well-being can be found in texts describing physical care skills. *Nursing care is not less important because the person is dying.*

Avoid too strict a routine in care. Let the client make some decisions about what he or she is going to do as long as safe limits are set. Modify care procedures as necessary for comfort. Through consistent, comprehensive care you tell the client you are available and will do everything possible for continued well-being.

During care, conversation should be directed to the client. Explain nursing procedures, even though the client is comatose, as hearing is the last sense lost. Response to questions should be simple, encouraging, but as honest as possible. Offer the person opportunities to talk about self and feelings through open-ended questions. When the client indicates a desire to talk about death, listen. There is no reason to expound your philosophy, beliefs, or opinions. Focus your conversation on the present and the client. Help the client maintain the role that is important to him or her. Convey that what he or she says has meaning for you. You can learn by listening to the wisdom shared by the client. Recognize when the client is unable to express feelings verbally, and help him or her to reduce tension and depression through other means—physical activity, crying, or sublimate activities.

If the client has an intense desire to live and is denying or fearful of death, be accepting but help him or her maintain a sense of balance. Do not rob the person of hope or force him or her to talk about death. Follow the conversational lead; if the topics are concerned with life, respond accordingly.

Encourage communication among the doctor, client, and family. Encourage the client to ask questions and state needs and feelings instead of doing it for him or her, but be an advocate if the person cannot speak for self.

Explore with family members the ways they can communicate with and support the client. Explain to the family that because the comatose client can probably understand what is being said, they should talk in ways that promote security and

should avoid whispering, which can increase the person's fears and suspicions.

Psychological care includes showing genuine concern, acceptance, understanding, and promoting a sense of trust, dignity, or realistic body image and self-concept. Being an attentive listener and providing for privacy, optimum sensory stimulation, independence, and participation in self-care and decision making are helpful. You will nonverbally provide a feeling of security and trust by looking in frequently on the client and using touch communication.

Spiritual needs of the dying person, regardless of the spiritual beliefs, can be categorized as follows:[102]

- Search for meaning and purpose in life and in suffering, including to integrate dying with personal goals and values, to make dying and death less fearful, to affirm the value of life, and to cope with the frustration caused by anticipated death.

- Sense of forgiveness in the face of guilt about unfulfilled expectations for self, accepting nonfulfillment or incompleteness and making the most of remaining life, acts of omission or acts of commission toward others, resolving human differences.

- Need for love through others' words and acts of kindness and silent, compassionate presence. If family and friends are not present, the nurse may be the primary source of love.

- Need for hope, which connotes the possibility of future good. Concrete hope consists of objects of hope within the person's experience such as freedom from pain or other symptoms or ability to perform certain tasks or to travel. Abstract hope or transcendent hope is characterized by distant and abstract goals and incorporates philosophic or religious meanings. Hope may be expressed as belief about afterlife, reunion with deceased loved ones, and union with God, a superior alternative to present existence. If there is no belief in the afterlife, hope may be expressed as belief about transfer of physical energy from the deceased body, belief about contributing to another's life through an organ donation, or belief in leaving a legacy in his or her children or community or organizational contributions.

You may assist with meeting the person's spiritual needs if requested and if you feel comfortable in doing so. Certainly you should know whom to contact if you feel inadequate. The religious advisor is a member of the health team. If the client has no religious affiliation and indicates no desire for one, avoid proselytizing.

Consider the social needs of the client until he or she is comatose or wishes to be left alone. Visitors, family, or friends can contribute significantly to the client's welfare when visiting hours are flexible. If possible, help the client dress appropriately and groom to receive visitors, go out of the room to a lounge, meet and socialize with other clients, or eat in a client's dining room or the unit.

Community health nurses have found two distinct attitudes in families of dying clients. The first attitude is, "If he is going to die soon, let's get him to the hospital!" For these families the thought of watching the actual death is abhorrent.

They feel personally unable to handle the situation and feel comforted by the thought of their loved one dying in a place where qualified professionals can manage all the details. If possible, these families should have their wishes met.

The second attitude is, "I want her to die at home. This is the place she loved. I can do everything that the hospital personnel can do." This attitude can be supported by the visiting nurse. The visiting nurse can usually coordinate community resources so that a home health aide, homemaker services, proper drug and nutrition supplies, and necessary equipment can be available in the home. Even the comatose client who requires a hospital bed, tube feedings, catheter change and irrigation, daily bed bath, feces removal, and frequent turning can be cared for in the home if the health team, family, and friends will share efforts. The families who desire this approach and who are helped to carry out their wishes seem to derive great satisfaction from giving this care.

Clients and family members often select the *home as the place of care in the terminal stages of disease and as the place to die.* Being with family and friends and living in their own home are often high priorities for clients. Home represents their life's work and helps to maintain a sense of dignity, identity, and control over dying. They realize at home they would not have to battle extraordinary measures. The family wants the client at home because it is his or her wish and because they believe they would desire to be at home if they were dying. Clients and families who choose the hospital as the place of death believe clients would receive better care there. Clients do not want to burden families. Families are concerned about their loved one's comfort.[103,104]

CRITICAL THINKING

Suppose someone in your family has died. What activities or rituals would you like to have carried out at the funeral or memorial service?

Findings from a research study, conducted by Dr. Harvey Max Chochinov, who is the Head of the Psychosocial Oncology Department at Cancer Care Manitoba, and a member of the Department of Psychiatry, University of Manitoba, resulted in a dignity-conserving care model complete with practical tools for palliative care providers.[105] Dr. Chochinov explains that dignity has a unique meaning for each patient and their family; and it must be discovered by health care providers in order for them to be able to provide comprehensive, empathetic care.

Hospice and Palliative Care

The first hospice palliative care programs in Canada were developed in the 1970s to respond to the needs of the dying. Initially, these programs were largely grass roots initiatives that evolved gradually into a single movement that aims to relieve suffering and to advance the quality of life for those who are living with, or dying from, an illness.[106] In a consensus-building process led by the Standards Committee of the Canadian Hospice Palliative Care Association, caregivers,

organizations, and consumers joined to share their experiences and to formulate a clear vision for hospice palliative care that everyone could use. This resulted in a national model for hospice and palliative care based on nationally accepted principles and norms of practice. All are encouraged to use the model to guide activities related to it. The new Model to Guide Hospice Palliative Care is now available free online (http://www.chpca.net).

The Canadian Hospice Palliative Care Association consensus building process (2001) regarding standards (norms) of practice has directed the development of hospice palliative care nursing standards. The purpose of those nursing standards is fourfold:

- To establish knowledge for the nursing care of individuals and families with advanced illness
- To support an ongoing development of hospice palliative care nursing
- To promote hospice palliative care nursing as a speciality
- To serve as a base for the development of certification in hospice palliative care nursing.[107]

The focus of the hospice palliative care nurse is to bring comprehensive, coordinated, and compassionate care to all individuals and families living with advanced illness.

In Canada, the Quality End-of-Life Care Coalition (QELCC) was formed in 2000 with a group of 24 national stakeholders who met in Toronto, Ontario. At that time the Blueprint for Action (2000) was created. The Coalition developed an action plan for 2002–2004 and its primary mandate is to act as an advocate for quality end-of-life care for all Canadians.[108]

Evaluation

Throughout intervention with the dying client or his or her family you must continually consider whether your intervention is appropriate and effective, based on their needs rather than yours. Observation alone of their condition or behaviour will not provide adequate evaluation. Ask yourself and others how you could be more effective, whether a certain measure was comforting and skilfully administered, and how the client and family perceived your approach and attitude. Assigning a person unknown to the client and family to ask these questions will help obtain an objective evaluation. Because of your involvement, you may be told only what people think you want to hear. If you and the client have established open, honest communication that encompasses various aspects of dying and if the client's condition warrants it, perhaps you will be able to interview the dying to get evaluation answers. You might ask if and how each member of the health team has added physically, intellectually, emotionally, practically, and spiritually to the person's care. You may also ask how each member of the health team has hindered in these areas.

Through careful and objective evaluation you can learn how to be more skilful at intervention in similar situations in the future.

INTERESTING WEBSITES

CANADIAN HOSPICE PALLIATIVE CARE ASSOCIATION

http://www.acsp.net

The Canadian Hospice Palliative Care Association (CHPCA) is the national association which provides leadership in hospice palliative care in Canada. CHPCA offers leadership in the pursuit of excellence in care for persons approaching death so that the burdens of suffering, loneliness, and grief are lessened

CANADIAN VIRTUAL HOSPICE

http://www.virtualhospice.ca

The Canadian Virtual Hospice (CVH) will facilitate equitable distribution of mutual support, the exchange of information, easier and more efficient communication and collaboration between and amongst health care professionals, palliative care researchers, the terminally ill and their families. To create a sense of community amongst key stakeholder groups across Canada, the CVH will create a community of mutual support, accessible through internet technology. Another primary goal of this project is to enable caregivers to conduct interactive consultations with professionals having expertise in palliative care, via a Web-based forum, the "Canadian Virtual Hospice." The website does not offer direct medical advice or clinical care but offers information and resources that may help people better understand the physical, emotional, and spiritual aspects of their experiences.

WORLD HEALTH ORGANIZATION (WHO)

http://www.who.int/about/en

The World Health Organization, the United Nations specialized agency for health, was established on April 7, 1948. WHO's objective, as set out in its Constitution, is the attainment by all peoples of the highest possible level of health. Health is defined in WHO's Constitution as a state of complete physical, mental, and social well-being and not merely the absence of disease or infirmity. WHO is governed by 192 Member States through the World Health Assembly. The Health Assembly is composed of representatives from WHO's Member States. The main tasks of the World Health Assembly are to approve the WHO program and the budget for the following biennium, and to decide major policy questions.

LIVING WILLS REGISTRY CANADA

http://www.sentex.net/~lwr

The Living Wills Registry Canada is unique to this country. The Registry was established by Dr. David Williams, a Stratford family physician, and his wife Maureen in 1992. The Registry's mandate is to assist people in directing their own medical treatment in the event of incapacitating illnesses or injuries. The website contains information about living wills, the organization, ordering a living will, and links.

SUMMARY

The concept of and reaction to dying and death depend on the person's cultural background and developmental level, the kind of death, the extent of support from significant others, and the quality of care given by nurses and other health care providers. Nurses and other health care workers must work through their own feelings as they face ethical and moral dilemmas related to use of technology and either prolonging or shortening life deliberately. There is much to learn from people who have a nearing-of-death awareness, a near-death experience, premonitions about death, or other kinds of dying experiences. The dying process and the afterlife are indeed the last stage of development.

REFERENCES

1. Callahan, M., Back from Beyond, *American Journal of Nursing,* 94, no. 3 (1994), 20–23.
2. Gormly, A., *Lifespan Human Development* (6th ed.). Fort Worth: Harcourt Brace College Publishers, 1997.
3. Newman, B., and P. Newman, *Development Through Life: A Psychosocial Approach* (7th ed.). Belmont, CA: Brooks/Cole, 1999.
4. Schoenbeck S., Exploring the Mystery of Near-death Experiences, *American Journal of Nursing,* 93, no. 5 (1993), 43–46.
5. Schoenbeck S., Exploring the Mystery of Near-death Experiences, *American Journal of Nursing,* 93, no. 5 (1993), 43–46.
6. Manitoba Centre for Health Policy Report, On Death and Dying in Manitoba, 2004. [Database online] Winnipeg [cited 21 April 2004] Available on World Wide Web @ http://www.umanitoba.ca/centres/mchp/reports/reports_04/end.htm
7. Wilson, Donna M., Susan L. Smith, Marjorie C. Anderson, Herbert C. Northcott, Robin L. Fainsinger, Michael J. Stingl, and Corrine D. Truman, Twentieth-century social and health care influences on location of death in Canada, *Canadian Journal of Nursing Research,* 34, no. 3 (2002), 141–161.
8. Stajduhar, Kelli I., Examining the perspectives of family members involved in the delivery of palliative care at home, *Journal of Palliative Care,* 19, no. 1 (2003), 27–35.
9. Dudgeon, Deborah J., and Linda Kristjanson, Home versus hospital death: Assessment of preferences and clinical challenges, *Canadian Medical Association Journal,* 152, no. 3 (1995), 337–340.
10. Critchley, P., A. R. Jada, A. Taniguchi, A. Woods, R. Stevens, L. Reyno, and T. J. Whelan, Are some palliative care delivery systems more effective and efficient than others? A systematic review of comparative studies, *Journal of Palliative Care,* 15, no. 4 (1999), 40–47.
11. Chalalewski, F., and M. Norris, The Gift of Life: Talking to Families About Organ and Tissue Donation, *American Journal of Nursing,* 94, no. 6 (1994), 28–33.
12. Tierney, L., S. McPhee, and M. Papadakis, *Current Medical Diagnosis & Treatment, 1999* (38th ed.). Stamford, CT: Appleton & Lange, 1999.
13. Schemie, Sam D., Christopher Doig, and Philip Belitsky, Advancing toward a modern death: The path from severe brain injury to neurological determination of death, *Canadian Medical Association Journal,* 168, no. 8 (2003), 993–997.
14. Wijdicks, Eelco F. M. Brain death worldwide, *Neurology,* 58, no. 1 (2002), 20–25.
15. Canadian Congress Committee on Brain Death, Death and brain death: A new formulation for Canadian medicine. *Canadian Medical Association Journal,* 138, no. 5 (1988), 405–406.
16. Canadian Neurological Care Group. Guidelines for the diagnosis of brain death, *Canadian Journal of Neurological Science,* 26, no. 1 (1999), 64–66.

17. Canadian Association of Critical Care Nurses (CACCN), 2001. Withholding and withdrawing of life support. [Database online] Ottawa [cited 21 April 2004] Available on World Wide Web @ http://www.caccn.ca/life_support.htm

18. Canadian Nurses Association Policy Statement, Joint Statement on Resuscitative Interventions, 1995. [Database online] Ottawa [cited 16 May 2004] Availanle at www.cna-nurses.ca. Site Navigation: Position/Policy Statements, Ethics, PS21.

19. Canadian Nurses Association, Code of Ethics for Registered Nurses, 2003. Ottawa: CNA. ISBN 1-55119-890-8.

20. Shemie, Sam D., Christopher Doig, Graeme Rocker, and Philip Belitsky, How to improve organ donation rates, *Canadian Medical Association Journal*, 170, no. 3 (2004), 318–320.

21. Molzahn, A. E., R. Starzomski, and J. McCormick, The supply of organs for transplantation: Issues and challenges. *Nephrology Nursing Journal*, 30, no. 1 (2003), 17–26.

22. Canadian Nurses Association, Fact Sheet, 2000, Organ Donation and Tissue Transplantation. [Database online] Ottawa [cited 16 May 2004] Available at www.cna-nurses.ca. Site Navigation: CNA Publications, CNA Fact Sheets, Title, FS-16.

23. Keatings, Margaret, and O'Neil B. Smith, *Ethical & Legal Issues in Canadian Nursing, Second Edition*. Toronto: W. B. Saunders Canada, 2000.

24. Transplant Committee Report, Potential Donors in Quebec Hospitals Year 2000, 2003. [Database online] Montreal [cited 16 May 2004] Available at www.cmq.org/uploadedfiles/transplantationEng.pdf

25. Bowman, Kerry W., and Shawn A. Richardson, Cultural considerations for Canadians in the diagnosis of brain death, *Canadian Journal of Anesthesia*, 51, no. 3 (2004), 273–280.

26. Canadian Nurses Association, n.d. Everyday Ethics: Putting the code into practice, Ottawa: CNA. ISBN 1-55119-027-3.

27. Canadian Institutes of Health Research (CIHR), Human Pluripotent Stem Cell Research: Guidelines for CIHR-Funded Research, 2002. [Database online] Ottawa [cited 24 August 2004] Available at www.cihr-irsc.gc.ca/e/1487.html

28. Health Canada, Human Cloning, 2004. [Database online] Ottawa [cited 24 August 2004] Available at www.hc-sc.gc.ca/english/media/releases/2004/2004_10bk2.htm

29. Gordon, C., Euthanasia: It's No Dutch Treat, *Focus on the Family*, June (1997), 10–11.

30. Papalia, D., and S. Olds, *Human Development* (3rd ed.). Boston: McGraw Hill, 1998

31. Seifert, K., R. Hoffnung, and M. Hoffnung, *Lifespan Development*. Boston: Houghton Mifflin, 1997.

32. Aroskar, M., Legal and Ethical Concerns: Nursing and the Euthanasia Debate, *Journal of Professional Nursing*, 10, no. 1 (1994), 5.

33. Ferdinand, R., I'd Rather Die Than Live This Way, *American Journal of Nursing*, 95, no. 12 (1995), 42–47.

34. Kirk, K., How Oregon's Death with Dignity Act Affects Practice, *American Journal of Nursing*, 98, no. 8 (1998), 54–55.

35. Miles, A., Am I Going to Die? *American Journal of Nursing*, 94, no. 7 (1994), 20.

36. St Joseph's Healthcare, Euthanasia—The Right to Die, n.d., [Database online] Hamilton [cited 17 May 2004] Available at www.stjosham.on.ca. Site Navigation: St. Joseph's Healthcare Home Page, Consumer Health Information Centre, Health Extension, Health Extension Topics, Index-E, #1809 Euthanasia—The Right to Die.

37. Leininger, M., Quality of Life From a Transcultural Nursing Perspective, *Nursing Science Quarterly*, 7, no. 1 (1994), 22–28.

38. Right to Die Society of Canada (RTDSC), n.d. The Right to Die Network of Canada. [Database online] Victoria [cited 17 May 2004] Available at www.rights.org/RTDSC.html

39. Compassionate Healthcare Network, n.d. [Database online] Surrey, B.C. [cited 17 May 2004] Available at www.chninternational.com

40. Canadian Association of Critical Care Nurses, Advance Directives, 1999. [Database online] London, ON [cited 11 May 2004] Available at www.caccn.ca/advance_directives.htm

41. Bee, Helen, Denise Boyd, and Paul Johnson. *Lifespan Development, Canadian Edition, Study Edition.* Toronto: Pearson Education Canada, Inc., 2005.

42. Canadian Nurses Association, Policy Regulations and Research Division, 1998. Advance Directives: The Nurse's Role. *Ethics in Practice*, May. ISSN 1480-9990.

43. University of Toronto Joint Centre for Bioethics, Living Will. [Database online] Toronto [cited 17 May 2004] Available at www.utoronto.ca/jcb

44. Molly, D. William, and Virginia Mepham. *Let Me Decide.* Toronto: Penguin Books Canada, 1996.

45. Molinski, Bonnie, "Advance Directives: What are the Ethical and Legal Implications for Nursing," St. Francis Xavier University, Canada. Distance Nursing Paper. www.stfx.ca/distancenursing/paper_BM.html

46. Galbraith, Kim M., and Keith Dobson, The role of the psychologist in determining competence for assisted suicide/euthanasia in the terminally ill. *Canadian Psychology*, 41, no. 3 (2000), 174–183.

47. Van Weel, Heleen, Euthanasia: Mercy, morals and medicine. *Canadian Nurse*, 91, no. 8 (1995), 35–40.

48. Shapiro, Carla, Ruth Dean, and Marilyn Seguire, Assisted suicide: A challenge for today's nurses. *Canadian Nurse*, 98, no. 1 (2002), 24–26.

49. Kowalski, S., Assisted Suicide: Where Do Nurses Draw the Line? *Nursing and Health Care*, 14, no. 4 (1993), 70–76.

50. Professor at School of Law Issues Warnings about Cybermedicine, *Saint Louis University Grand Connections*, 6, no. 3 (1999), 3.

51. Murphy, P., Nursing's Role in the Assisted Suicide Debate, *American Journal of Nursing*, 97, no. 6 (1997), 80.

52. Malcolm, A., The Right to Die, *New Choices*, July/August (1991), 68–70.

53. Boehnlein, J., The Case Against Physician-Assisted Suicide, *Community Mental Health Journal*, 35, no. 1 (1999), 5–24.

54. Wilson, Keith G., John F. Scott, Ian D. Graham, Jean F. Kozak, Susan Chater, Raymond A. Viola, Barbara J. de Faye, Lynda A. Weaver, and Dorothyann Curran, Attitudes of terminally ill patients toward euthanasia and physician-assisted suicide. *Archives of Internal Medicine*, 160 (2000), 2454–2460.

55. Nagy, M., The Child's View of Death, in H. Fiefel, ed., *The Meaning of Death*. New York: McGraw-Hill, 1959.

56. Durham, E., and L. Weiss, How Patients Die, *American Journal of Nursing*, 97, no. 12 (1997), 41–46.

57. Grollman, E., Explaining Death to Young Children: Some Questions and Answers, in E.A. Grollman (ed.), *Bereaved Children and Teens*. Boston: Beacon Press,

58. Nelson, L., When a Child Dies, *American Journal of Nursing*, 95 no. 3 (1995). 61–64.

59. Health Canada, Helping Your Child Cope—Responding to the Stress of Terrorism and Armed Conflicts, 2002. [Database online] Ottawa [cited 16 May 2004] Available on World Wide Web @ http://www.hc-sc.gc.ca/pphb-dgspsp/publicat/oes-bsu-02/child_e.html

60. Miles, A., Anger at God after a Loved One Dies, *American Journal of Nursing*, 98, no. 3 (1998), 64–65.

61. Diaz, M., When a Baby Dies, *American Journal of Nursing*, 95, no. 11 (1995), 54–56.

62. Corr, C.A., Entering Into Adolescent Understanding of Death, in E.A. Grollman (ed.), *Bereaved Children and Teens*. Boston: Beacon Press, 1995.

63. Noppe, L., and I. Noppe, Ambiguity in Adolescent Understandings of Death, in C.A. Corr and D.E. Balk (eds.), *Handbook of Adolescent Death and Bereavement*. New York: Springer, 1996.

64. Noppe, I., and L. Noppe, Evolving Meanings of Death During Early, Middle, and Later Adolescence, *Death Studies,* 21 (1997), 253–275.

65. Health Canada, Population and Public Health Branch, Helping Your Teens Cope, Responding to Stress of Terrorism and Armed Conflicts, 2002. [Database online] Ottawa [cited 16 May 2004] Available on World Wide Web @ http://www.hc-sc.gc.ca/ pphb-dgspsp/publicat/oes-bsu-02/teens_e.html

66. Kennard, M., A Visit from an Angel, *American Journal of Nursing,* 98, no. 3 (1998), 48–51.

67. Kübler-Ross, E., ed., *On Death and Dying.* New York: Collier-Macmillan, 1969.

68. Kubler-Ross, E., *Death, the Final Stage of Growth.* Englewood Cliffs, NJ: Prentice-Hall, 1975.

69. Kubler-Ross, E., ed., *Living with Dying.* New York: Macmillan, 1981

70. Stepnick, A., and T. Perry, Preventing Spiritual Distress in the Dying Client, *Journal of Psychosocial Nursing,* 30, no. 1 (1992), 17–24.

71. Stroebe, M., and W. Stroebe, The Mortality of Bereavement: A Review, in M. Stroebe, W. Stroebe, and R. Hansson (eds.), *Handbook of Bereavement: Theory, Research, and Intervention.* Cambridge: Cambridge University Press, 1993.

72. Jecker, N., and L. Schneiderman, Is Dying Young Worse Than Dying Old? *The Gerontologist,* 34, no. 1 (1994), 66–71.

73. Moody, R.A., *Life after Life.* New York: Bantam Books, 1975.

74. Eadie, B., and C. Taylor, *Embraced by the Light.* Riverside, NJ: McMillan, 1992

75. Atwater, P. M. H., 1998. In Search of a Common Criteria for Identifying Near-Death States. [Database online] Charlottesville, VA [cited 18 May 2004] Available on World Wide Web @ http://www.cinemind.com/atwater/ Site Navigation: At home-page enter title in Search Box.

76. Callahan, M., Breaking the Silence, *American Journal of Nursing,* 94, no. 1 (1994), 22–23.

77. Boltz, L., A Time to Every Purpose, *American Journal of Nursing,* 98, no. 11 (1998), 47.

78. Callahan, M., Farewell Messages, *American Journal of Nursing,* 94, no. 5 (1994), 18–19.

79. Palker, N., and B. Nettles Carlson, The Prevalence of Advance Directives: Lessons from a Nursing Home, *Nurse Practitioner,* 20, no. 2 (1995), 7–21.

80. Zerwekh, J., The Truth-tellers: How Hospice Nurses Help Patients Confront Death, *American Journal of Nursing,* 94, no. 2 (1994), 31–34.

81. Glaser, B., and A. Strauss, The Social Loss of Dying Patients, *American Journal of Nursing,* 64, no. 6 (1964), 119ff.

82. Glaser, B., and A. Strauss, *Awareness of Dying.* Chicago: Aldine, 1965.

83. Glaser, B., and A. Strauss, *Time for Dying.* Chicago: Aldine, 1968.

84. Wright, Lorraine M., Wendy L. Watson, and Janice M. Bell. *Beliefs: The Heart of Healing in Families and Illness.* New York: Basic Books, 1996.

85. Erikson, E.H., *Childhood and Society* (2nd ed.). New York: W.W. Norton, 1963.

86. Giacquinta, B., Helping Families Face the Crises of Cancer, *American Journal of Nursing,* 77, no. 10 (October 1977), 1585–1588.

87. Wiener, L., A. Alberta, M. Gibbins, and S. Hirschfeld, Visions of Those Who Left Too Soon, *American Journal of Nursing,* 96, no. 9 (1996), 57–59, 61.

88. Eaves, S., Permission to Leave, *American Journal of Nursing,* 96, no. 3 (1996), 80.

89. Gomez, E., and N. Carazos, Was Hexing the Cause of Death? *American Journal of Psychiatry,* 1, no. 1 (April 1981), 50–52.

90. Rahe, R, and M. Romo, Recent Life Changes and the Onset of Myocardial Infarction Sudden Death in Helsinki, in E. Gundason and R. Rahe, eds., *Life, Stress, and Illness.* Springfield, IL: Charles C. Thomas, 1974, pp. 105–120.

91. Richter, G., On the Phenomenon of Sudden Death in Animals and Man, *Psychosomatic Medicine,* 19 (1959), 191.

92. Canadian Hospice Palliative Care Association, A History, 2003. [Database online] Ottawa [cited 10 May 2004] Available on World Wide Web @ http://www.chpca.net/ Site navigation: From Home-page, About Us, History.

93. Dean, Ruth. *Death, Humor, and Spirituality: Strange Bedfellows?* 73,75 In Making Sense of Death (G. R. Cox, R. A. Bendiksen, and R. G. Stevenson, Editors. 2003.).

94. Health Canada. *A Guide to End-of-Life Care for Seniors.* Faculty of Medicine, University of Toronto and University of Ottawa, 2000. ISBN 0-9687122-0-7.

95. Gaguski, M., A Private Place, *American Journal of Nursing,* 99, no. 4 (1999), 18–19.

96. Miles, A., Caring for the Family Left Behind, *American Journal of Nursing,* 93, no. 12 (1993), 34–37.

97. Levin, B., Grief Counselling, *American Journal of Nursing,* 98, no. 5 (1998), 69–71.

98. Bateman, A., D. Broderick, L. Gleason, R. Kardon, C. Flaherty, and S. Anderson, Dysfunctional Grieving, *Journal of Psychosocial Nursing,* 30, no. 12 (1992), 5–9.

99. Bereavement after Homicide for a Loved One, *The Menninger Letter,* 3, no. 6 (1995), 3.

100. Brown, M., Lifting the Burden of Silence, *American Journal of Nursing,* 94, no. 9 (1994), 62–63.

101. Joffrian, L., and T. Douglas, Grief Resolution: Facilitating Self-transcendence in the Bereaved, *Journal of Psychosocial Nursing,* 32, no. 3 (1994), 13–19.

102. Conrad N., Spiritual Support for the Dying, *Nursing Clinics of North America,* 20, no. 2 (1985), 415–426.

103. Devich, L., B. Fields, and R. Carlson, Supportive Care for the Hopelessly Ill, *Nursing Outlook,* 36, no. 3 (1990), 140–142.

104. Zerwekh, J., Do Dying Patients Really Need IV Fluids? *American Journal of Nursing,* 97, no. 3 (1997), 26–30.

105. Chochinov, Harvey Max, Dignity-conserving care—A new model for palliative care. *Journal of American Medical Association,* 287, no. 17 (2002), 2253–2260.

106. Canadian Hospice Palliative Care Association, A Model to Guide Hospice Palliative Care, 2002. [Database online] Ottawa [cited 16 May 2004] Available on World Wide Web @ http://www.chpca.net Publications & Resources.

107. Canadian Palliative Care Association, Hospice Palliative Care Nursing Standards of Practice, 2001. [Database online] Ottawa [cited 19 May 2004] Available on World Wide Web @ http://www.chpca.net/home.htm Site Navigation: Interest Groups, Nurses, Nursing Standards of Practice.

108. Canadian Hospice Palliative Care Association, Quality End-of-Life Care Coalition, 2002. [Database online] Ottawa [cited 11 May 2004] Available on World Wide Web @ http://www.chpca.vet/ quality_end-of-life_care_coalition.htm

Dietary reference intakes (DRIs), 260
Dietary taboos, 13
Diethyl pyrocarbonate, 73
Diethylstilbestrol (DES), 74, 492
Differentiation, 199
Dioxin emissions, 78
Dioxin, 73, 277
Disasters, 237–238
  see also Crisis
Discipline. *See* Guidance and discipline.
Discrimination, 206
Disease
  see also specific diseases
  cardiovascular, 625
  respiratory, 625
  cultural causes of, 6
  of later adulthood, 685
  nutrition and, 544–545
  genetics of, 192, 193
  sexual function, 684–685
Disenchanted phase, 37
Disengagement or contraction stage,
  of family development, 149
Disengagement theory, 654
Dismemberment, 234
Displacement, 210, 335, 698
Disposal
  nuclear waste, 77
  toxic agents, 88
  waste, 78
Disqualifying the positive, 215
Dissociation, 210
Dissonance stage, 35
Distress, 227
Divine liturgy, 114
Divorce, 591–592
  children and, 420, 592
  in early adulthood, 601–602
  families and, 138, 145, 149, 156, 157
  in later adulthood, 658–659
  preschoolers and, 378
  in special-needs families, 142
  in various cultures, 160–161
Dizygotic twins, 190, 253
Dizziness, 64
Domestic violence, 273, 585–591
Dopamine, 195
Doping, 280
Doubt, 366, 367
Down syndrome, 257, 259, 273, 312
Dramatic play, 404
Drives, 208
Drowsiness, 64
Drug(s), 32, 318
  see also Drug abuse; Substance abuse
  effects on fetus, 263, 266–268
  fertility, 253
  reactions, in later adulthood, 686
  as teratogens, 263
Drug abuse, 110, 199
  see also Addiction; Drug(s); Substance abuse
  in adolescence, 507–509, 523
  in young adulthood, 583–584
Drug dependence, 507
Drug resistance, 74
Drug tolerance, 507
Drug toxicity, 74
Dust mites, 67
Dwarfism, 259, 385

Dyad, 149, 162, 295, 379
Dysfunctional grief response, 17
Dysmenorrhea, 537

E

E coli, 68, 71
Ear position, in neonate, 312
Early school experiences, 382
Easter, 114
Eastern Orthodox church, 114
Eating. *See* Nutritional needs.
Eating disorders, 476, 477–478, 584
Ecchymoses, 40, 353
Ecologic systems theory, 201
Ecologic theories of human
  development, 198–201
  ecologic systems theory, 201
  general systems theory, 199–201
Ecology, 198
Ectoderm, 254
Eddy, Mary Baker, 120
Education
  see also Learning; Health promotion;
    Programs
  about pollutants and toxins, 94
  about sexuality, 378–379
  child, 189
  childbirth, 180
  in behaviour theory, 201
  in comparative cultures, 20
  cultural change and, 7
  in existential and humanistic theories, 224
  health and, 35
  in infancy, 331–332
  nutrition, 546–547
  parent, 183
  poverty and, 33
  prenatal, 336
  on preventing poisonings, 359
  in psychoanalytic theories, 207
  safety, 492
  sex, 184, 458, 523, 536–537
Effective function phase, 37
Ego, 208, 214
  adolescent, 487
  functions of the adult, 555
Ego adaptive (defence) mechanisms, 210–211
Ego differentiation, 697
Ego ideal, 208
Ego integrity, 695
Ego transcendence, 697
Egocentrism, 219, 362, 398
Eida-Fita, 110
Elder abuse, 660–661
Elderly people. *See* Aging; Later adulthood.
  poverty and, 31
Elders, 10
Electra complex, 377
Electroencephalograms (EEGs), 551
Ellis, Albert, 215, 239
Embryo, teratogens and, 263
Embryonic disk, 254
Embryonic stage, 254, 255
Emerging values, 12
Emissions, 63
Emotional competency, 251
Emotional development,
  in adolescence, 483–484

  in infancy, 333
  in later adulthood, 695
  in middle-age, 617, 632–635
  in preschoolers, 406
  in school-age children, 453–455
  theories of, 560–561
  in toddlers, 366–368
  in young adults, 559
Emotional health, 582–591
Emotional intelligence, 560
Emotional isolation, 210, 698
Emotional maltreatment, 279, 301
Emotional reasoning, 215
Emotions, maternal, 272–273
Employment Equity Act, 3
Empty nest syndrome, 149, 602, 608
Encephalopathy, 392
Endocrine system, 196
  in childhood, 277
  in infancy, 316
  in later adulthood, 672
  in pregnancy, 259
  in toddlers, 372
  in young adulthood, 535
Endoderm, 254
Engagement, 146
Engrossment, 295
Enuresis, 393
Environment, 11–81, 95
  see also Ecologic theories; Pollution
  in a system, 199, 200
  patient's, 94–95
  personal lifestyle changes, 91
  professional responsibility for, 89
  teratogens in, 262, 263
  solutions for, 88, 89
  affecting disease, 193
  historical perspective on, 59–60
  human interrelationship with, 60
Environmental and mechanical hazards, 79
Environmental Protection Act, 60
Environmental Protection Agency (U.S.), 77
Epidural block, 274
Epigenetic theory of personality
  development, 213, 238, 654
Epilepsy, 435
Epinephrine, 228
Equanimity, 697
Equilibrium, 217
Equilibrium, in a system, 200
Erectile dysfunction, 625
Erikson, Erik, 213, 238, 333, 366, 554,
  635, 654
Erythema, 40
Escape behaviour, 206
Essential fatty acids, 262
Establishment stage, of family
  development, 146
Estrogen, 195, 259, 473, 535
Eternal progression, 119
Ethchlorvynol, 266
Ethnic, defined, 3
Ethnicity, defined, 3
Ethnocentrism, 37
Eucharist, 113, 114
Europe, family life in, 161
Euthanasia, 5
Evil eye, 24
Evolutionary processes, in a system, 200

attachment behaviours of, 294–300
changing role of, 159
in expectancy phase, 568
postpartum needs of, 181–182
surrogate, 178
Motivation, 217
Maslow's theory of, 225
Motor control, 217
in preschoolers, 386
in toddlers, 350
Motor vehicle crashes (VMCs), 367
Motor Vehicle Safety Act, 60
Mould, 67
Mounting mutations theory, 653
Mouth, in later adulthood, 670
Muhammad, 110
Multiculturalism, 3, 5–10, 37–38
Multiculturalism Act, 11
Multiple births, 151–153, 253, 379
Multiple intelligences, 443
Multiplication, 439
Muscular dystrophy, 257
Musculoskeletal system
in adolescence, 474
in later adulthood, 669–671
in school-age children, 424–425
in young adulthood, 534
Muslim society, 21
see also Islamic culture; Middle
Eastern culture
Mutagenic effects, 94
Mutual pretence, of death, 11
Myelinization, 350
Myopia, 359
Myths
about battered women, 588
family, 145
about menopause, 609

N

Narcotics, 510
see also Drug(s); Drug abuse
Narrative vignette, 13
Nation of Islam, 111, 115
National Aboriginal Council on HIV/AIDS
(NACHA), 35
National Ambient Air Quality Objectives
(NAAQOs), 63
National Forum on Health, 25–26
National identify, 10–11, 12
National Initiative for Telehealth Framework
of Guidelines, 50
National Institutes of Health, 193
National Pollutant Release Inventory
(NPRI), 60, 79
National Population Health Survey 1998, 25
Native American church, 120
Natural family planning, 538–539
Nature versus nurture, 189
Near poverty, 31
Near-death awareness (NDA), 11
Near-death experience (NDE), 10–11
Needs, hierarchy of, 225–226
Negative reinforcement, 203, 205
Neglect, 279, 301, 376, 413, 471–472
elder, 660–661
Neglectful parenting style, 376
Neighbourhoods, 198, 301

Neighbours-are-irrelevant model, 198
Neighbours-do-not-matter-but-
neighbourhoods-do model, 198
Neo-analytical theory, 207–214
Erickson's epigenetic, 213
Jung's, 213–214
Sullivan's interpersonal, 209–212
Neo-behaviourists, 201
Neonatal period, complications in, 267
Neonate, 292–312
see also Infancy
in Neo-Piagetian theory, 218
physical characteristics of, 303–312
sensory abilities of, 309–311
Neoplasms, 492
Nesting, 439
Net Generation, 10
Neurochemistry, 195
Neuroendocrine theory, 653
Neurological system, 195–196
in adolescents, 512
in later adulthood, 662
in young adulthood, 535
in school-age children, 424–425
Neuromuscular development, in
school-age children, 424–425
Neuromuscular maturation, 350
Neurophysiologic factors. See Neurological
system.
Neurotoxicitiy, 78
Neurotransmitters, 195
Never-married women, 641
New Age, 120
Newborn. See Neonate.
Niacin, 262
Niche-finders, 630
Nicotine, 510
see also Tobacco smoking
Nidation, 194
Nightingale, Florence, 102
Nirvana, 108
Nitrogen oxides, 62, 67
Nocturnal emissions, 473
Noise pollution, 75–76
Noise, as teratogen, 263
Nomads, 630
Nonmalfeasance, 121
Nonpoint sources, of water pollution, 68
Non-rapid eye movement (NREM)
sleep, 551–552
Nonspatial relationships, 7
Non-traditional health care. See Alternative
health care; Home remedies.
Non-verbal communication, 38
see also Body language
culture and, 6
in interviews, 166
Norepinephrine, 195, 228, 266
North America
see also Western culture
culture of, 25–26
aging in, 650
poverty in, 31–33
North American Indians, 3, 13
see also First Nations culture
Hopi, 6
Navaho, 7
nutrition and, 545
religions of, 120

North American Nursing Diagnosis
Association (NANDA), 43
Northern Contaminants Program (NCP), 74
Not-me, 368
Nuclear family, 138, 601
Nuclear waste, 77
Nursery school, 375, 382
Nursing
see also Assessment; Intervention; Nursing
diagnoses
for adolescents, 489–490, 509–523, 524
culture and, 28, 36–37
for dying patients, 13
for the elderly, 677–681
for expectant parents, 568
for infants, 336–340
for middle-aged adults, 641, 643
for pregnancy and childhood, 280–281
for preschoolers, 410–412, 413
for school-age children, 413, 460–461
for spiritual needs, 122–126, 701
for young adults, 572–641
theoretical approaches to, 238–242
for young adults, 593
Nursing diagnoses
see also Assessment; Physical examinations
for adolescents, 489–490, 491
cross-cultural, 42, 43
for environment-related illness, 89–95
for family issues, 171–174, 337
for infants, 336
for middle aged adults, 641–642
for preschoolers, 410
for school-age children, 460–461
for spiritual needs, 126
for toddlers, 371, 490
wellness, 490
for young adults, 571
Nursing homes, 706
Nutrition
see also Nutritional needs
in childhood, 276
culture and, 323, 545–546
disease and, 544–545
education, 546–547
for infants, 318–324
maternal, 259–262
medications interfering with, 687
for toddlers, 353–354, 357
for young adults, 544–545
Nutritional Labelling Regulations, 74
Nutritional needs
see also Nutrition
in adolescence, 476
in later adulthood, 673–675
in middle age, 617–618
in preschoolers, 385–387
in school-age children, 429–432

O

Obesity, 74, 191, 478–479, 534, 545
in Canada, 25
in childhood, 276
Object space, 396
Objective reality, 216
Occipital lobe, 196
Occupational hazards, 79–81, 263
Occupational Health and Safety (OHS)
Code, 77, 79

"As-Is" License Agreement And Limited Warranty

READ THIS LICENSE CAREFULLY BEFORE OPENING THIS PACKAGE. BY OPENING THIS PACKAGE, YOU ARE AGREEING TO THE TERMS AND CONDITIONS OF THIS LICENSE. IF YOU DO NOT AGREE, DO NOT OPEN THE PACKAGE. PROMPTLY RETURN THE UNOPENED PACKAGE AND ALL ACCOMPANYING ITEMS TO THE PLACE YOU OBTAINED THEM. THESE TERMS APPLY TO ALL LICENSED SOFTWARE ON THE DISK EXCEPT THAT THE TERMS FOR USE OF ANY SHAREWARE OR FREEWARE ON THE DISKETTES ARE AS SET FORTH IN THE ELECTRONIC LICENSE LOCATED ON THE DISK:

1. GRANT OF LICENSE and OWNERSHIP: The enclosed computer programs and any data ("Software") are licensed, not sold, to you by Pearson Education Canada Inc. ("We" or the "Company") in consideration of your adoption of the accompanying Company textbooks and/or other materials, and your agreement to these terms. You own only the disk(s) but we and/or our licensors own the Software itself. This license allows instructors and students enrolled in the course using the Company textbook that accompanies this Software (the "Course") to use and display the enclosed copy of the Software for academic use only, so long as you comply with the terms of this Agreement. You may make one copy for back up only. We reserve any rights not granted to you.

2. USE RESTRICTIONS: You may not sell or license copies of the Software or the Documentation to others. You may not transfer, distribute or make available the Software or the Documentation, except to instructors and students in your school who are users of the adopted Company textbook that accompanies this Software in connection with the course for which the textbook was adopted. You may not reverse engineer, disassemble, decompile, modify, adapt, translate or create derivative works based on the Software or the Documentation. You may be held legally responsible for any copying or copyright infringement that is caused by your failure to abide by the terms of these restrictions.

3. TERMINATION: This license is effective until terminated. This license will terminate automatically without notice from the Company if you fail to comply with any provisions or limitations of this license. Upon termination, you shall destroy the Documentation and all copies of the Software. All provisions of this Agreement as to limitation and disclaimer of warranties, limitation of liability, remedies or damages, and our ownership rights shall survive termination.

4. DISCLAIMER OF WARRANTY: THE COMPANY AND ITS LICENSORS MAKE NO WARRANTIES ABOUT THE SOFTWARE, WHICH IS PROVIDED "AS-IS." IF THE DISK IS DEFECTIVE IN MATERIALS OR WORKMANSHIP, YOUR ONLY REMEDY IS TO RETURN IT TO THE COMPANY WITHIN 30 DAYS FOR REPLACEMENT UNLESS THE COMPANY DETERMINES IN GOOD FAITH THAT THE DISK HAS BEEN MISUSED OR IMPROPERLY INSTALLED, REPAIRED, ALTERED OR DAMAGED. THE COMPANY DISCLAIMS ALL WARRANTIES, EXPRESS OR IMPLIED, INCLUDING WITHOUT LIMITATION, THE IMPLIED WARRANTIES OF MERCHANTABILITY AND FITNESS FOR A PARTICULAR PURPOSE. THE COMPANY DOES NOT WARRANT, GUARANTEE OR MAKE ANY REPRESENTATION REGARDING THE ACCURACY, RELIABILITY, CURRENTNESS, USE, OR RESULTS OF USE, OF THE SOFTWARE.

5. LIMITATION OF REMEDIES AND DAMAGES: IN NO EVENT, SHALL THE COMPANY OR ITS EMPLOYEES, AGENTS, LICENSORS OR CONTRACTORS BE LIABLE FOR ANY INCIDENTAL, INDIRECT, SPECIAL OR CONSEQUENTIAL DAMAGES ARISING OUT OF OR IN CONNECTION WITH THIS LICENSE OR THE SOFTWARE, INCLUDING, WITHOUT LIMITATION, LOSS OF USE, LOSS OF DATA, LOSS OF INCOME OR PROFIT, OR OTHER LOSSES SUSTAINED AS A RESULT OF INJURY TO ANY PERSON, OR LOSS OF OR DAMAGE TO PROPERTY, OR CLAIMS OF THIRD PARTIES, EVEN IF THE COMPANY OR AN AUTHORIZED REPRESENTATIVE OF THE COMPANY HAS BEEN ADVISED OF THE POSSIBILITY OF SUCH DAMAGES. SOME JURISDICTIONS DO NOT ALLOW THE LIMITATION OF DAMAGES IN CERTAIN CIRCUMSTANCES, SO THE ABOVE LIMITATIONS MAY NOT ALWAYS APPLY.

6. GENERAL: THIS AGREEMENT SHALL BE CONSTRUED AND INTERPRETED ACCORDING TO THE LAWS OF THE PROVINCE OF ONTARIO. This Agreement is the complete and exclusive statement of the agreement between you and the Company and supersedes all proposals, prior agreements, oral or written, and any other communications between you and the company or any of its representatives relating to the subject matter.

Should you have any questions concerning this agreement or if you wish to contact the Company for any reason, please contact in writing: Editorial Manager, Pearson Education Canada, 26 Prince Andrew Place, Don Mills, Ontario M3C 2T8.